PASS CCRN®!

FIFTH EDITION

Robin Donohoe Dennison, DNP, CCNS, CNE, NEA-BC
Director of Nursing Programs
University of Saint Augustine for Health Sciences
Saint Augustine, Florida

ELSEVIER

ELSEVIER

3251 Riverport Lane
St. Louis, Missouri 63043

PASS CCRN®!, FIFTH EDITION　　　　　　　　　　　ISBN: 978-0-323-59531-5
Copyright © 2019, Elsevier Inc. All rights reserved.
Previous editions copyrighted 2013, 2007, 2000 and 1996

No part of this publication may be reproduced or transmitted in any form or by any means, electronic or mechanical, including photocopying, recording, or any information storage and retrieval system, without permission in writing from the publisher. Details on how to seek permission, further information about the Publisher's permissions policies and our arrangements with organizations such as the Copyright Clearance Center and the Copyright Licensing Agency, can be found at our website: www.elsevier.com/permissions.

This book and the individual contributions contained in it are protected under copyright by the Publisher (other than as may be noted herein).

Notices

Practitioners and researchers must always rely on their own experience and knowledge in evaluating and using any information, methods, compounds or experiments described herein. Because of rapid advances in the medical sciences, in particular, independent verification of diagnoses and drug dosages should be made. To the fullest extent of the law, no responsibility is assumed by Elsevier, authors, editors or contributors for any injury and/or damage to persons or property as a matter of products liability, negligence or otherwise, or from any use or operation of any methods, products, instructions, or ideas contained in the material herein.

Library of Congress Cataloging-in-Publication Data

Dennison, Robin.
　Pass CCRN! / Robin Donohoe Dennison. – 5th ed.
　　　p. ;cm.
　Includes bibliographical references and index.
　ISBN 978-0-323-59531-5 (pbk. : alk. paper)
　I. Title.
　[DNLM: 1. Critical Care–Examination Questions. 2. Critical Care–Outlines. 3. Critical Illness–nursing–Examination Questions. 4. Critical Illness–nursing–Outlines. 5. Nursing Assessment–Examination Questions. 6. Nursing Assessment–Outlines. WY 18.2]
　　　616.028–dc23
　　　　　　　　　　　　　　　　　　　　　　　　　　　　　　2012041668

Executive Content Strategist: Lee Henderson
Content Development Specialist: Laura Bayless
Publishing Services Manager: Deepthi Unni
Senior Project Manager: Umarani Natarajan
Design Direction: Bridget Hoette

Printed in the United States of America
Last digit is the print number: 9　8　7　6　5　4　3　2　1

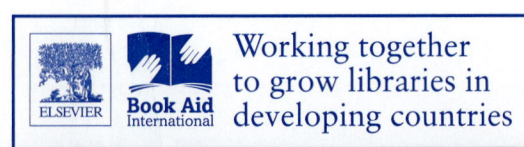

CONTRIBUTORS

Frank K. Agyapong, MS, RN, AGACNP-BC, ACCNS-AG, CEN
Clinical Nurse Specialist
Emergency Department
Brooke Army Medical Center
Fort Sam Houston, Texas

Caroline Broden, MS, RN, ACNP-BC, FNP-BC
Hospitalist
Lieutenant Colonel, U.S. Army Nurse Corps
Fort Wainwright, Arkansas

Jennifer L. Easley, MSN, RN, AGACNP-BC, CCNS-AG, CCRN
Major, U.S. Army Nurse Corps
Deputy Commander for Nursing
Fox Army Health Center
Redstone Arsenal, Alabama

K. Marie Geslak, MSN, CCNS
LTC, U.S. Army Nurse Corps
Chief, Critical Care Nursing Services
Brooke Army Medical Center
San Antonio, Texas

Jennifer D. Lorilla, MSN, RN, CCNS
Critical Care Clinical Nurse Specialist
Lieutenant Colonel, U.S. Army Nurse Corps
William Beaumont Army Medical Center
El Paso, Texas

Jana L. Nohrenberg, MSN, RN, CCNS, CCRN-K
Colonel, U.S. Army Nurse Corps
Consultant to the Army Surgeon General for
    Critical Care Nursing
Fort Hood, Texas

Lisa D. Phillips, MSN, RN, CCRN
Critical Care Nursing Services
San Antonio Military Medical Center
Fort Sam Houston, Texas

Johnnie Robbins, EJD, MSN, RN, CCNS, CCRN
Critical Care Clinical Nurse Specialist
EnRoute Care Branch Director
United States Army School of Aviation Medicine
Fort Rucker, Alabama

Traceee J. Rose, MSN, APRN, CCNS-BC, CCRN
Critical Care Clinical Nurse Specialist
Tripler Army Medical Center
Honolulu, Hawaii

Marianne Saunorus Baird, MN, RN, ACNS-BC
Corporate Director, Magnet Recognition Program
Emory Healthcare
Atlanta, Georgia

JoEllen Schimmels, DNP, PMHNP-BC
Assistant Professor
Uniformed Services University
Bethesda, Maryland

REVIEWERS

Katherine F. Alford, MSN, RN, CCRN, PCCN
Quality Management
South Texas Veterans Health Care System
San Antonio, Texas

Marianne Saunorus Baird, MN, RN, ACNS-BC
Corporate Director, Magnet Recognition Program
Emory Healthcare
Atlanta, Georgia

Marylee Bressie, DNP, RN, CCNS, CCRN-K, CEN
Core Faculty/Nurse Planner
Capella University School of Nursing and Health Sciences
Capella University
Minneapolis, Minnesota

Joyce Foresman-Capuzzi, MSN, RN-BC, CCNS, CEN, CPN, CTRN, CPEN, CCRN, TCRN, AFN-BC, SANE-A, EMT-P, FAEN
Clinical Nurse Educator
Department of Nursing
Lankenau Medical Center
Wynnewood, Pennsylvania

Linda R. Littlejohns, MSN, RN, CNRN, SCRN, FAAN
Neuroscience Clinical Nurse Consultant
San Juan Capistrano, California

Kathleen M. Stacy, PhD, RN, APRN-CNS, CCNS
Critical Care Clinical Nurse Specialist
Clinical Associate Professor
Hahn School of Nursing and Health Science
University of San Diego
San Diego, California

This fifth edition is dedicated to nurses who are serving or who have served in active duty in the branches of the Unites States military and nurses who serve our veterans. Thank you for your willingness to serve.

Preface

Welcome to *Pass CCRN®!* and congratulations—you have chosen the most up-to-date, comprehensive review of critical care nursing available on the market today. If you are a registered nurse planning to take the CCRN® examination for certified critical care practice offered by the American Association of Critical Care Nurses (AACN) Certification Corporation, this book is the tool that you need to prepare for the examination with confidence.

Information in this text is organized according to the latest CCRN® examination blueprint, which is available on the AACN website (https://www.aacn.org). This test plan, issued by the AACN Certification Corporation, identifies the content areas tested and the percentage of the examination devoted to each. Only content included in the test blueprint is covered in this book, eliminating extraneous information that can be distracting. The book also offers an array of learning activities to help you understand and retain key concepts. Also, more than 1000 additional multiple-choice questions are provided on the Evolve website so that you can practice your test-taking skills in an interactive format that simulates the examination itself.

I have written this book for nurses who are preparing to take the CCRN® examination. Teaching exam-preparation seminars for the past 30 years has helped me learn what information will best equip nurses to sit the examination and has familiarized me with the strengths and weaknesses of current exam-preparation books on the market. My goal is to provide a pertinent content review, fun but challenging learning activities, realistic practice questions, and comprehensive simulated examinations that reflect the content and complexity of the CCRN® examination.

Content Review

Pass CCRN®! uses a succinct outline format that makes the information easy to read, understand, and remember. Illustrations and tables further explicate and clarify content, highlight key concepts, and enhance written explanations. This fifth edition includes concept maps to illustrate the pathophysiology of critical care conditions to aid understanding of the linkage between pathophysiology and clinical presentation.

This edition of *Pass CCRN®!* offers significantly revised content throughout the book along with a new chapter on the integumentary and musculoskeletal systems. Critical care pharmacology is integrated throughout the book. Also, new sections have been added to remain consistent with the current blueprint.

Coverage of each body system begins with a brief review of anatomy and physiology. This refresher lays the foundation for introducing more complex topics in the areas of assessment, intervention, and evaluation. Assessment includes health history, physical examination, diagnostic studies, and system-specific assessment methods. For example, the cardiovascular chapter discusses hemodynamic monitoring and electrocardiography, the pulmonary chapter covers interpretation of arterial blood gases, and the neurologic chapter presents intracranial pressure monitoring. The format varies for the Multisystem, Professional Caring and Ethical Practice, and Behavioral and Psychosocial chapters because of the nature of the content in these chapters.

Pathologic conditions listed on the CCRN® examination blueprint are included in the content review. Each condition is first defined followed by separate sections that explore Etiology, Pathophysiology, and Clinical Presentation (including subjective, objective, and diagnostic) and concludes with Collaborative Management, which includes medical and nursing management.

Learning Activities

Sometimes we learn best when information is organized and accessed in unfamiliar ways—that's the principle at work behind the diverse learning activities in this book. Every chapter features a range of question styles, including matching, fill-in-the-blank, comparison, case studies, and crossword puzzles, to test comprehension and improve recall for readers with a variety of learning styles.

You won't be asked to complete a crossword puzzle or a matching exercise when you take the CCRN® examination, of course, but doing so helps you learn and retain an astonishing amount of information. It also makes your study sessions more enjoyable, encouraging you to stick to the timetable that you have set for yourself. I hope that working through these activities, many of which are new to this edition of the book, will be a pleasurable way to review terminology, anatomy and physiology, and pharmacology.

Practice Questions and Examinations on the Evolve Website

Another great way to study is to use the practice questions and examinations on the Evolve website. The Evolve site contains more than 1000 review questions written in a format that represents the actual CCRN® examination. The practice examinations have been thoroughly updated to reflect the percentages set forth for each content area on the most recent test blueprint and current practice.

The Evolve website offers two modes: a quiz mode, in which practice questions are arranged by body system, and a test mode that offers realistic practice CCRN® examinations. The quiz mode allows you to select topic areas in which you need additional review and create quizzes that target those areas. The test mode, on the other hand, replicates the actual CCRN® examination as closely as possible. This timed exam mode draws questions from all content areas in the number and proportion called for in the latest CCRN® examination blueprint. The program will reshuffle the questions randomly (but retaining the correct percentages in each content area) to create as many practice tests as you like. Both modes are self-scoring. Instant rationales are given to explain which answer is correct and why it is the best answer among the possible choices. Test-taking strategy tips are provided as appropriate to show you how to think through the questions if you are not sure of the content. Both of these features will boost your confidence and make you a better test taker on the important day of the CCRN® examination. Analyzing your performance on several practice exams will help you focus your final preparation on your weakest areas.

Other Helpful Features

Appendix A is a list of abbreviations and acronyms used in this book and common in critical care. Each term is spelled out in the text the first time it is used, but this appendix will help you identify abbreviations later if you don't remember them. Appendix B lists laboratory studies important in the care of critically ill adults, including the normal range of values for each. I recommend that you study this list just before taking the exam because you are expected to know common normal laboratory values. Appendix C is a list of formulae commonly used in the evaluation of critically ill patients. Appendix D contains a review of dysrhythmias, including their etiology, criteria, significance, and management.

This book is not a comprehensive critical care textbook, nor is it intended to be. Instead, I've focused selectively on the information likely to be covered on the CCRN® examination. I believe *Pass CCRN®!* is the only book you need to prepare for the examination, but if you would like an additional text to strengthen your knowledge of particular areas, I recommend *Critical Care Nursing: Diagnosis and Management*, by Linda D. Urden, Kathleen Stacy, and Mary Lough, published by Elsevier.

Critical care nursing has never been more exciting. For those of us who thrive on this challenge, keeping up with new research and clinical developments is a continual test of our mettle. CCRN® certification is a prestigious credential for those of us who specialize in critical care nursing. I am confident that if you study this book and use the Evolve website to practice your test-taking skills, you will pass the examination.

I would love to hear from you about your success with the examination, how this book helped you, and how you think it could be even more useful. E-mail me at rddennison@aol.com.

I believe that this book will be your most valuable resource in preparing for the CCRN® examination. Good luck!

Robin Donohoe Dennison, DNP, CCNS, CNE, NEA-BC

ACKNOWLEDGMENTS

I would like to acknowledge my Elsevier team for this edition. I am fortunate to have worked with Lee Henderson, Laurie Gower, Laura Bayless, and Umarani Natarajan. I have worked with most of this team for multiple books, and their support has been, once again, superb.

Most of the contributors to this edition are nurse experts on active duty in branches of our United States military. I am so thankful to have contacted Jana Nohrenberg, who assembled a team of nurse experts to review and revise chapters of this edition. Thanks to all of you for being willing to share your knowledge and expertise.

I continue to thank the previous editions clinical consultants: Karen Allard, MSN, RN, ACNS-BC, CCNS; Marylee Bressie, DNP, RN, CCRN, CCNS, CEN; Lori A. Catalano, JD, MSN, RN, CCNS, PCCN; Madelyn Danner, MS, RN, CCRN, CEN, CNE; Anita Dempsey, PhD, APRN, PMHCNS-BC; Maurice Espinoza, MSN, BSN, CNS, CCRN; Wendi Kai Fox, BSN, RN; Daniel J. Mueller, BSN, RN; Betty Nash, MSN, RN, CCRN; Jill Roberts, RN, MNSc, ACNP; Brenda Shelton, MS, RN, CCRN, AOCN; and John J. Whitcomb, PhD, RN, CCRN, FCCM.

Contents

1. The Critical Care Certification Examination, 1
2. Professional Caring and Ethical Practice, 12
3. The Cardiovascular System, 49
4. The Pulmonary System, 252
5. The Neurologic System, 378
6. The Endocrine System, 465
7. The Gastrointestinal System, 489
8. The Renal System, 564
9. The Hematologic and Immunologic Systems, 614
10. Integumentary/Musculoskeletal Systems, 666
11. Multisystem, 679
12. Behavioral/Psychosocial on the Blueprint, 721

Learning Activities Answers, 742

References and Suggested Readings, 792

Appendices

A. Common Abbreviations and Acronyms Used in Critical Care Nursing, 797
B. Normal Laboratory Values, 810
C. Formulae Significant to Critical Care Nursing, 812
D. Dysrhythmias: Etiology, Criteria, Significance, and Management, 815

Index, 833

The Critical Care Certification Examination

CHAPTER 1

Certification
Definition
1. The process by which a nongovernmental agency validates an individual nurse's qualification and knowledge for practice in a defined functional or clinical area of nursing
   a. Functional role, such as educator, executive, or advanced practice role, such as clinical nurse specialist or nurse practitioner
   b. Clinical specialty, such as critical care, progressive care, or oncology
2. This validation is based on predetermined standards of practice
   a. Determined by role delineation studies or job analyses
   b. Conducted periodically

Purposes
1. Demonstration to "patients, employers and the public that a nurse's knowledge, skills, and abilities meet rigorous national standards" (American Association of Critical-Care Nurses [AACN], 2016)
2. Protection of consumers (Kaplow, 2011)
   a. Licensure
      1) Indicates a minimum level of knowledge
      2) Granted by a governmental agency (e.g., state board of nursing)
      3) Usually renewed annually or biannually
   b. Certification
      1) Indicates an expert level of knowledge
      2) Granted by a nongovernmental agency (e.g., nursing specialty organization)
      3) Usually renewed every 3 to 5 years

Benefits of Achieving CCRN® Certification
1. For the nurse
   a. Self-satisfaction and validation of your knowledge and clinical judgment in your chosen nursing specialty
   b. Recognition and respect of others
   c. Professional challenge and motivation to update and maintain your knowledge base
   d. Career mobility: national certification is as prestigious in one state as another.
   e. Clinical advancement and promotion
      1) Most critical care unit nurse managers encourage their nursing staff to become certified, and the majority prefers to hire certified nurses over noncertified nurses when other qualifications are equal.
      2) Certification is often recommended or required for promotion up a clinical career ladder.
   f. Financial remuneration
      1) Some hospitals offer a bonus for CCRN® certification.
      2) Some hospitals offer an hourly differential for CCRN® certification.
      3) Some hospitals prefer certified nurses for clinical or administrative promotion.
      4) Most hospitals reimburse the nurse for the expense of taking the test if a passing score is attained (Teal, 2011).
   g. Certified nurses are more likely to feel empowered (Fitzpatrick, Campo, Graham, & Lavandero, 2010).
   h. Certified nurses report higher job satisfaction and autonomy (Fritter & Shimp, 2016).
   i. Continued practice in critical care: some hospitals require CCRN® certification to continue to practice in critical care settings.
2. For the institution
   a. Assurance to the general public that the nurse is competent
   b. Evidence of excellence for marketing and awards such as Magnet Recognition Program by the American Nurses Credentialing Corporation (ANCC), AACN Beacon Award for Critical Care Excellence, or Malcolm Baldrige National Quality Award
   c. Financial incentives from insurance carriers
   d. Improved retention of nurses (Fitzpatrick et al., 2010; Fritter & Shimp, 2016)
3. For patients and their families
   a. Assurance that the nurse is currently competent and knowledgeable regarding critical care nursing
   b. Improved patient safety (Kendall-Gallagher & Blegen, 2009)

c. Improved competence in detecting signs and symptoms of complications and initiating prompt intervention (Cary, 2001)
d. Reduced incidence of hospital-acquired infections (Boev, Xue, & Ingersoll, 2015)
4. Perceived barriers (Teal, 2011; Altman, 2011)
   a. Cost of the examination
   b. Fear of testing or failure
   c. Lack of institutional support
   d. Lack of rewards
   e. Lack of time for preparation and maintenance of renewal requirements
   f. Lack of experience

The Synergy Model

The Synergy Model serves as the organizing framework for the certification examinations offered by the AACN (2016a) (Fig. 1.1).

Definition of Synergy

"[A]n evolving phenomenon that occurs when individuals work together in mutually enhancing ways toward a common goal" (AACN, 2016a).

Core Concept

The needs or characteristics of patients and families influence and drive the characteristics or competencies of nurses.
1. Nursing practice should be based on the needs of the patient and family.
2. Patients with more complex needs require nurses with advanced knowledge and skills.
3. The desired result is optimal outcomes for the patient, the nurse, and the system.

Assumptions

1. Patients are biologic, psychological, social, and spiritual entities who present at particular developmental stages.
2. The patient, family, and community all contribute to providing a context for the nurse–patient relationship.
3. Patients can be described by a number of characteristics.
   a. Resiliency: the capacity to return to a restorative level of functioning using compensatory coping mechanisms; the ability to bounce back quickly after an insult
   b. Vulnerability: susceptibility to actual or potential stressors that may adversely affect patient outcomes
   c. Stability: the ability to maintain a steady-state equilibrium
   d. Complexity: the intricate entanglement of two or more systems (e.g., body, family, therapies)
   e. Resource availability: extent of resources (e.g., technical, fiscal, personal, psychological, social)
   f. Participation in care: extent to which the patient and family engage in aspects of care
   g. Participation in decision making: extent to which the patient and family engage in decision making
   h. Predictability: a summative characteristic that allows one to expect a certain trajectory of illness
4. Nurses can be described in a number of dimensions.
   a. Clinical judgment: clinical reasoning, which includes clinical decision making, critical thinking, and a global grasp of the situation, coupled with nursing skills acquired through a process of integrating formal and experiential knowledge
   b. Advocacy/moral agency: working on another's behalf and representing the concerns of the patient, family, and community; serving as a moral agent in identifying and helping to resolve ethical and clinical concerns within the clinical setting
      1) Nurses are expected to read, understand, and observe the American Nurses Association (ANA) Code of Ethics, which is available at http://nursingworld.org/MainMenuCategories/EthicsStandards/CodeofEthicsforNurses/Code-of-Ethics-For-Nurses.html (ANA, 2015).
   c. Caring practices: the constellation of nursing activities that are responsive to the uniqueness of the patient and family and that create a compassionate and

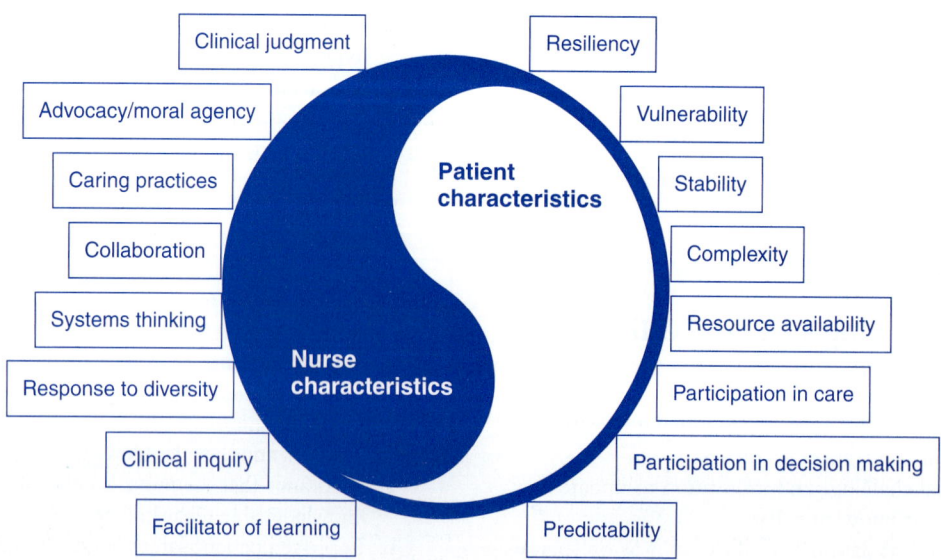

Fig. 1.1 The Synergy Model with patient and nurse characteristics.

therapeutic environment, with the aim of promoting comfort and preventing suffering
  d. Collaboration: working with others in a way that promotes and encourages each person's contributions toward achieving optimal and realistic patient goals; collaboration involves intradisciplinary and interdisciplinary work with all colleagues
  e. Systems thinking: the body of knowledge and tools that allow the nurse to appreciate the care environment from a perspective that recognizes the holistic interrelationship that exists within and across health care systems
  f. Response to diversity: the sensitivity to recognize, appreciate, and incorporate differences into the provision of care
  g. Clinical inquiry or innovator/evaluator: the ongoing process of questioning and evaluating practice, providing informed practice, and innovating through research and experiential learning
  h. Facilitator of learning as patient/family educator: the ability to facilitate patient and family learning
5. A goal of nursing is to restore a patient to an optimal level of wellness as defined by the patient.

Although this model serves as the theoretical model for the CCRN® examination, you are not tested regarding knowledge of the synergy model or terminology; rather, you are tested on application of the model.

The Adult CCRN® Examination

Basic Information about the CCRN® Examination

1. Critical care is considered to be at the most acute end of the critical care continuum; patients in critical care
   a. Are unstable and complex
   b. Require intense resources such as staffing, monitoring, and supplies
      1) Frequently require invasive hemodynamic monitoring, intravenous medication titration, and mechanical ventilation
   c. Require persistent nursing vigilance
2. The test is designed to evaluate your understanding of the common body of knowledge needed to function effectively in a critical care setting.
   a. The test consists of 150 multiple-choice questions to be completed within 3 hours; 25 of these items are not scored but are test items for the development of future exams.
   b. The questions relate to patient problems unique to critical care and to nationally recognized practice with the focus being on clinical decision making rather than memorization and recall.
3. Test plan for the CCRN® examination (Table 1.1)
   a. The test plan identifies the categories tested and the percentage of questions in each category or category group.
   b. The test plan is based on a National Practice Analysis of Critical Care Nurses conducted by the AACN in 2013 (AACN, 2015); in essence, this study identified tasks, knowledge, and experiences required of a registered nurse practicing in a critical care setting and what should be on the examination.
   c. The test plan identifies what percentage of questions is in each area as well as what disease entities are on the examination.
      1) NOTE: This book includes only content and disease entities that are on the test plan and the examination. For example, although it may be important to understand myxedema coma, it is not on the test plan, not on the examination and not in this book; focus on what is on the test plan and the examination.

Cognitive Levels of Questions

1. Questions on the examinations are distributed across these cognitive levels, but the majority of the questions are at the application and analysis levels (AACN, 2016b)
2. Summary of cognitive levels
   a. Remembering requires you to remember previously learned information.
   b. Understanding requires you to understand the information.

Table 1.1 Test Plan for the CCRN® Examination Indicating Distribution of Questions on Each System[a]

Content Areas	Approximate Percentage	Approximate Number of Questions
Clinical Judgment	80%	100
Cardiovascular	18%	22
Pulmonary	17%	21
Endocrine	20%	5
Hematology/Immunology		3
Gastrointestinal		7
Renal/Genitourinary		7
Integumentary		2
Musculoskeletal	14%	2
Neurology		10
Behavioral/Psychosocial		4
Multisystem	14%	17
Professional Caring and Ethical Practice	20%	25
Advocacy/Moral Agency		
Caring Practices		
Collaboration		
Systems Thinking		
Response to Diversity		
Clinical Inquiry		
Facilitatory of Learning		
Totals	100%[b]	125

[a]Note that this is the most recent version of the CCRN® test plan; discrete percentages are not given for some systems but rather system groups are combined for one percentage

[b]The sum of these percentages is not 100 because of rounding.

c. Applying requires you to use information.
d. Analyzing requires you to break down information into its component parts and recognize commonalities, differences, and interrelationships.
e. Evaluating requires you to judge the value of information.
f. Creating requires you to put parts of information together to form a new conclusion.

Distribution of Questions Related to the Nursing Process
All phases of nursing process are included on the examination.

Passing Score
1. The passing score for these examinations is approximately 70%.
2. About two thirds of nurses taking the CCRN® examination for the first time pass the exam; nurses retaking the test for recertification have a higher passing rate.

For more specific information about the examinations, the application and application process, and the testing process, download the CCRN® Exam Handbook at https://www.aacn.org/certification/get-certified/ccrn-adult

Plan for Passing the CCRN® Examination (Fig. 1.2)

Permission to Take the Examination
1. Requirements (AACN, 2016a)
   a. Current unrestricted RN license in the United States or in any of its territories that use the NCLEX® for RN licensure
   b. Clinical practice in critical care:
      1) Two-year option: minimum of 1750 hours in direct care of acutely or critically ill adult patients during the previous 2-year period with 875 of the hours accrued in the most recent year preceding application to take the examination (AACN, 2016a)
      2) Five-year option: minimum of 2000 hours in direct care of acutely or critically ill adult patients during the previous 5-year period with 144 of the hours accrued in the most recent year preceding application to take the examination (AACN, 2016a)
      3) These clinical practicum hours must be completed in a United States–based or Canada-based facility or in a facility determined to be comparable to U.S. standards for acute and critical care nursing practice and verifiable by an immediate supervisor (AACN, 2016a).
      4) CCRN® certification is a clinical credential, and you must maintain a clinical practice to maintain your certification.
      5) Eligible hours are those spent caring for adult patients in a critical care setting; examples include intensive (or critical) care units, cardiac care units, combined intensive care unit–coronary care units (ICU-CCUs), medical or surgical ICUs, trauma critical care units, neurologic critical care units, and critical care transport.
      6) Other settings may also be considered "critical care" depending on the characteristics of the patient population cared for in the setting; AACN can assist you in determining your eligibility to take the exam.

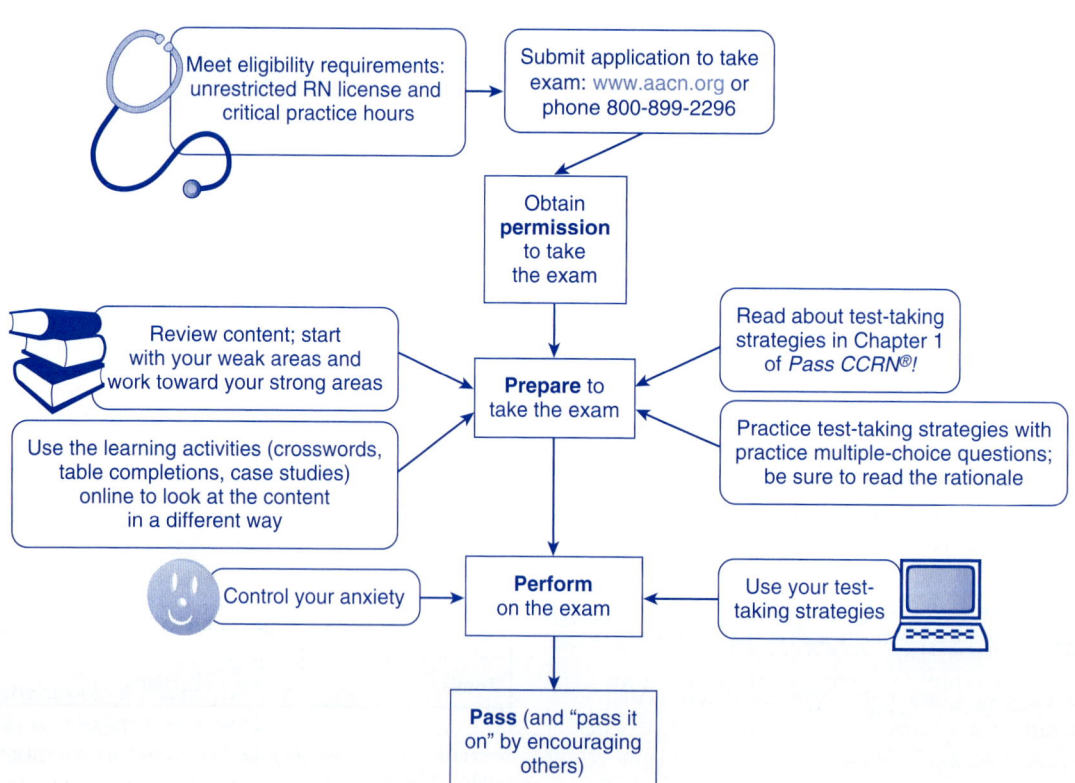

Fig. 1.2 Plan for passing the CCRN® examination.

c. BSN is not a requirement: although the ANCC requires a BSN to sit for some of its certification examinations, the AACN Certification Corporation is not a member of the ANCC and does not require a BSN to sit for the CCRN® examination.
2. To obtain an application, contact the AACN Certification Corporation.
   a. Website: https://www.aacn.org/certification/get-certified/application?code=CCRNA_IE
   b. Phone: 949-362-2050 or 800-394-5995
   c. Email: certcorp@aacn.org
3. After completion of the application process, approval to take the exam is received by mail; you must schedule testing within the next 90 days.
   a. Computer-based testing is available most weekdays year round; a pencil and paper version is available only once a year at the location of the AACN National Teaching Institute.
   b. The computerized form of the test is administered by Applied Measurement Professionals (AMP) at its testing centers nationwide.

Preparation for the Exam

1. Be positive!
   a. Avoid negative self-talk; "I'll never pass this exam" can be a self-fulfilling prophecy because you begin to believe it.
   b. Practice positive self-talk.
      1) Write down some affirmations (positive statements) related to your preparation and performance on this examination; suggested affirmations are listed in Box 1.1.
      2) Say these and other affirmations that you have written over and over again throughout your preparation time; say them like you believe them, and you will!
      3) Record your affirmations on your smartphone and play them often; play them in the car, while you walk or do dishes, or any other time when you can listen and repeat them.
2. Schedule the examination.
   a. Complete the application online.
   b. You will be sent an authorization letter indicating that you meet the requirements to take the examination, along with instructions on how to schedule the examination.
      1) Call the testing service to schedule your examination date and time; you must schedule the examination within 90 days of the date printed on your authorization letter.
      2) This flexibility in scheduling allows you to avoid scheduling conflicts between the examination and major life events such as a family wedding, graduation, or birth.
      3) Schedule the time of the examination according to when you do your best thinking or are most productive: schedule for morning if you are a lark or afternoon if you are an owl.
   c. DO SCHEDULE THE EXAM so that you have a target date; you can reschedule up to 4 business days before the scheduled test day if something comes up that interferes with your ability to complete the examination on the scheduled day.
3. Prepare for the test.
   a. Establish a realistic schedule for your preparation; 1- to 2-hour time slots are probably the most helpful.
      1) Study examination content: plan to review a system per evening, day, or weekend, depending on how much time you have left before the examination.
         a) Set priorities.
            i) Study your weak areas first.
            ii) Study the large percentage content areas even if you feel confident about them: you should feel especially confident about cardiac, pulmonary, and multisystem content because these three areas constitute 49% of the examination.
         b) Review content using this review book.
            i) Highlight areas that you do not feel confident about; you may need to refer to more comprehensive critical care texts or articles when you need additional clarification.
            ii) Complete the learning activities at the end of each chapter to consolidate your knowledge by looking at the information in another way.
         c) Practice using your test-taking skills by doing practice questions.
            i) In addition to looking at the answer, read the rationale; remember that the question may not be written exactly the same as the practice question, but the concept may be on the examination.
            ii) If you still do not understand why you missed the question, refer to the section in this book or a critical care text to understand why the correct answer is better than your answer.
            iii) In addition to looking at the answer and the rationale, read the test-taking strategy; this information will help you identify how to approach a similar question to which you do not know the answer.
            iv) Analyze why you missed a question; consider:
               (a) Did you not know the content? Study this content again.
               (b) Did you misread the question? Slow down and read the question more thoroughly.

Box 1.1 Affirmations

I understand the information important for this examination.
I am a knowledgeable critical care nurse.
I feel prepared for this exam.
I am an excellent test taker.
I will pass this exam.

- (c) Did you misread the options? Slow down and read all of the options and select the best one.
- (d) Did you miss an important element such as age, diagnosis, or parameter? Again, slow down and read the question carefully; mentally highlight the critical points in the case study that you feel are important.
- (e) Did you read into the question?
  - (i) Do not assume information that is not given; take the question at face value.
  - (ii) Do not assume that the question is intended to "trick" you; there are no "trick" questions on the practice exam questions on the website associated with this book or on the CCRN® exam.
- d) Study in a quiet place with minimal distractions.
  - i) Turn off the television, radio, and stereo; let your voice mail pick up phone calls.
  - ii) Avoid getting too comfortable; sit upright at a desk or table so that you can spread out your study materials; avoid trying to study while in bed or a recliner.
  - iii) Ensure adequate lighting.
  - iv) Reading, repeating, and writing are methods that improve remembering.
  - v) Use margins to write down memory joggers or additional thoughts.
- b. If you like study groups, organize a study group of nurses who are also preparing for the CCRN® examination.
  1) Include only members who will fulfill their obligation to participate.
  2) Establish guidelines for the group.
     a) When will you meet?
     b) What will you do at the meetings?
        i) A selected member may present essential content related to his or her specific area of interest.
        ii) Members may collect resource materials related to the specified content area and distribute them to fellow members.
        iii) Members may discuss review questions related to the specified content area.
     c) What are the group members' expectations?
- c. Create memory joggers.
  1) Almost everyone knows "On old Olympus' towering tops a fin and German viewed some hops" to remember the 12 cranial nerves; establish others that help you identify things that you have trouble remembering.
- d. Remember case study links: for example, you remember a patient with a triglyceride level over 2000 mg/dL who developed acute pancreatitis, and then ARDS helps you remember that a major risk factor for acute pancreatitis is hypertriglyceridemia and that a major complication of acute pancreatitis is ARDS.
4. Take a practice test 1 week before the examination; use this test to identify weak areas for final study time.
   a. Analyze which categories (systems) are your weakest and strongest.
   b. Analyze which cognitive level question is the most difficult for you.
   c. Analyze which component of the nursing process is most difficult for you.
5. Final preparations
   a. Don't "cram" the night before the examination; cramming usually just decreases your self-confidence and increases your anxiety.
   b. Go to bed at your usual time; if you go to bed early, you probably won't go to sleep anyway and will just worry about the test.
   c. Do not consume alcohol or other sedating drugs the night before or the day of the examination.
   d. Choose comfortable clothes that allow layering so you can remove or add clothing in response to the room temperature; wear bright colors (e.g., yellow, red, hot pink, orange) to project a more optimistic image.
   e. Take a watch, a sweater, tissue, and hard candy; don't forget your glasses if you wear them.
   f. Eat a healthy but light meal before the examination; avoid simple carbohydrates such as a doughnut or Danish pastry; rather, eat peanut butter on whole wheat toast or an egg sandwich to sustain you through the exam.
   g. Be sure to take two forms of identification with one of them being government-issued photo identification that contains a signature.
   h. Make sure that you know where the testing site is located and how long it will take to get there considering traffic at the time your test is scheduled; getting lost or just having to rush to arrive on time causes anxiety and may affect your performance.
   i. Plan to arrive 15 minutes before your scheduled appointment; if you arrive later than 15 minutes after the scheduled testing time, you may not be admitted.
   j. Take the time to visit the restroom before you check in.

Performance During the Examination

1. Control of anxiety
   a. Remember that some anxiety increases your performance; panic does not.
   b. Feeling adequately prepared decreases anxiety; take the time to prepare for this examination, including practicing your test-taking strategies.
   c. Use visualization: see yourself receiving your passing score.
   d. Use deep breathing or progressive muscle relaxation.
      1) Deep breathing is performed by putting your hand below your costal margin and breathing deeply enough to raise your hand; focus on your breathing instead of anything else.
         a) Use this method at any time during the examination when you feel frustrated or stressed.
      2) Progressive muscle relaxation is performed by contracting a group of muscles and then relaxing it: leg, leg, arm, arm, back, face.

a) Use this technique in the car before you go in to take the examination and at any time during the examination when you feel tense.
   e. Use meditation or prayer depending on your religious beliefs: these techniques are also helpful in verbalizing your goals and desires.
   f. Don't let a memory lapse or a difficult question affect your attitude or throw you into panic mode; move on to the next question to which you are likely to know the answer.
2. Instructions are given at the beginning of the examination; take the time to read the instructions carefully.
3. Test-taking skills
   a. Reading questions thoroughly
      1) Mentally highlight key points as you read the question.
         a) Age and gender of the patient
         b) Setting: prehospital, emergency, critical care, progressive care, home care
         c) Medical diagnosis and other coexisting diagnoses
         d) Time frame in relation to admission, trauma, surgery, pain, medication, visitation
      2) Look for qualifying words such as:
         a) *All, most, some, few, none*
         b) *Always, usually, frequently, seldom, never*
         c) *First, last*
         d) *Best, worst*
         e) *Most, least*
         f) *Smallest, largest*
         g) *Acute, chronic*
         h) *Partial, total*
         i) *Early, late*
         j) Answers that include global answers such as *all, always, never,* or *none* are seldom the correct answer.
      3) Pay particular attention to negative words such as *not, except, contraindicated,* and *inappropriate.*
      4) Read all the options as well as the stem.
      5) After you read the stem, answer the question without looking at the options; if your answer is there, it's probably right; however, still go ahead and read all options—there may be one better than your answer.
   b. Choosing the correct answer
      1) Make sure that you understand what the question really is; answer *the* question, not just *a* question.
      2) Always choose the best answer; even if there are two answers that you consider correct, choose the one that best answers the question being asked.
         a) If more than one option appears correct, look for the most comprehensive option.
      3) Assumptions
         a) Do not assume information that is not given; the only assumption is an ideal situation unless the question indicates otherwise.
         b) All important information is included.
            i) Do not read into the question such as "maybe she's a diabetic" or "maybe he has COPD"; if information is important to the question, it would be included
         c) Included information is probably important.
            i) Extraneous information is not usually included, so if the case study or question gives you information that you think is extraneous or superfluous, ask yourself why this information was given and how it is important to this situation.
      4) Answer questions according to national standards of care and national guidelines rather than regional, local, or specific physician's practices.
      5) Select options that are therapeutic based on evidence and show respect and acceptance for the patient and the family; eliminate options that are based on tradition rather than science and options that are inappropriate, disrespectful, or punitive.
      6) Repetition of a word or a synonym of the word in the stem and an option may help you to identify the correct answer.
      7) If the answers are numbers or number ranges, the extremes are less likely to be the correct option than the middle number or number range.
      8) This exam is computerized, and answers are random; therefore, C is no more likely to be the correct answer than A, B, or D; also, there are no patterns to the answers, so don't look for one.
   c. Answering priority questions
      1) Priority one is always whatever must be done to prevent death; always follow current ACLS guidelines.
      2) Priority two is whatever must be done to prevent disability or serious complication; consider this D for disability.
      3) Priority three is pain or discomfort; if nothing in the case study or question could cause death or disability, pain should be considered the priority.
      4) Actual problems always take precedence over potential problems; for example, actual hypoxemia takes precedence over potential oxygen toxicity.
      5) If there are two potential problems, the priority is the one that is more likely to cause death or disability.
   d. Answering questions where the answers have multiple answers (also referred to as multiple or multiples)
      1) If the option has more than one answer (such as x and y or even w, x, y, and z), both or all of the answers must be correct for the option to be correct.
      2) Elimination works well with this type of question; if there is one answer in the option that is incorrect, that option may be eliminated.
   e. Guessing
      1) Don't leave any question blank; unanswered questions are counted as incorrect, so you should never not answer a question even if you must guess.
      2) You are not penalized for guessing, but it should be used only as a last resort.
      3) First eliminate any choices that you can; it is better to guess between two choices than to guess among four.
         a) Eliminate clearly wrong answers.
         b) Eliminate any response that has no relationship to the question.

c) Eliminate similar options that say essentially the same thing because they cannot both be correct.
d) *All, always, never, none,* and *only* options are usually incorrect.
4) If you cannot even eliminate to two, then look for the option that is different from the others; for example:
a) Three antibiotics and an antifungal: choose the antifungal option.
b) Three beta-blockers and a calcium channel blocker: choose the calcium channel blocker.
c) Three very specific and one very comprehensive option: choose the comprehensive option.
5) If you are unsure of your answer and want to look at it again:
a) Go ahead and answer it with your first impression.
b) Click on "mark" at the bottom of the screen so that you can go back to it at the end of the exam.
c) At the end of the exam, the computer allows you to go back to these marked items and review them.
d) Review the question again during this review process and see if there is something in the question that changes your answer about the correct answer.
e) When you are set on the correct answer you want to submit for that question, "unmark" it and then continue to the end of the examination.
f. Changing answers
1) You may have been told to never change answers, and you should not change an answer unless you have a good reason for changing it; one good reason is that you missed a negative qualifier, such as *not, except,* or *contraindicated,* when you read it the first time.
2) If may be helpful to change answers in a different color when doing a practice test; then evaluate how many you changed from wrong to right and how many you changed from right to wrong.
a) If you change more from wrong to right, you most likely miss questions because you don't read them thoroughly, so when you realize that you misread a question, then by all means, change your answer.
b) If you change more from right to wrong, don't change your initial answer (unless you realize in this case that you had misread the question) because first impressions tend to be correct more often.
g. Answering math questions
1) Math questions are usually drug calculations, such as dopamine in micrograms per kilogram per minute, but could be other critical care calculations.
2) You are allowed to use only the computer calculator, and you are provided with scratch paper and pencil.
3) Recheck your math if you have time.

h. Maintaining concentration
1) Write down things such as formulae, normal values, and toxic levels that you are afraid that you might forget on your scratch paper before you do the first question.
2) Change your process of reading the case study, the question, and the options.
a) Read the options in reverse order from option *d* to option *a*. Use this action especially when you suspect that option *a* or *b* is the correct option.
b) Make this change every 25 to 50 questions OR
i) When you are physically tired, mentally anxious, or lose your concentration abilities
ii) When you come to the easier or the more difficult questions
3) Rephrase the question rather than rereading the same question over and over.
4) Use three slow deep breaths to regroup and get refocused at any time.
5) Sign out and go to the restroom and splash water on your face if you are losing your ability to concentrate but remember that the clock does not stop during this time.
i. Budgeting your time
1) If you are a slow test taker, you may run short on time, but more likely you will run out of mental energy because concentration for a 2- to 3-hour period is very difficult.
2) You should try to be at least halfway through the examination in 75 minutes; this halfway point will leave you some time to recheck your math and go back to the marked items.
3) One helpful technique to save time is to read the question (at end of case study) and then go back and read the case study; because we frequently read the case study, then read the question at the end of the case study, and then reread the case study, this technique saves you time by knowing what you are looking for in the case study.
4) Do not be distressed by people finishing before you; we all take examinations at different speeds, and the others may not even be taking the AACN Certification Corporation examinations because several exams are given at the same place and same time.

Pass and Pass It On

1. Test results: you will be given your test results at the completion of computerized testing and within 6 to 8 weeks by mail for pencil and paper testing.
2. If you pass
a. Use your new credential proudly.
1) You should display your credential on your hospital name badge.
2) You should proudly write it after RN when you sign your name; CCRN® is not written with periods so, for example, it is written as Your Name, RN, CCRN.
b. Pass it on by encouraging others to become certified; offer to tutor, mentor, and share study materials to assist your colleagues to become certified, too.

3. If you fail, try again!
    a. Reasons for failing the examination
        1) Knowledge deficit
            a) Prepare to take the examination even if you believe that you are an experienced critical care nurse because we all have our chosen areas of interest and our weak areas.
            b) Use this book to review the content for the examination and complete the learning activities at the end of each chapter.
            c) Take a practice examination 1 week before the examination to identify your weak areas; use your final study time focusing on those weak areas.
        2) Testing errors
            a) Practice using your test-taking skills with the questions on the Evolve Resources included with this book and pay close attention to both the rationale and the test-taking strategy included with each question.
            b) Use the learned test-taking strategies during the CCRN® examination.
        3) Test anxiety and negative thinking: believe in your ability to pass the exam and control your anxiety with any combination of prayer, meditation, deep breathing, or progressive relaxation.
    b. You will likely do better the next time because the fear of the unknown is now gone, and you know clearly what your weak areas are from the score breakdown that was given to you as you left the testing site.
        4) Prepare by focusing on your weak areas and then reapply to take the test again.

Maintaining Your CCRN® Certification

Certification as a CCRN® is for a 3-year period.

5.1 Recertification

Recertification is achieved by providing evidence of continued practice (432 hours over the 3-year period with 144 of those hours accrued in the year prior to recertification) and either retaking the examination or submitting the appropriate information about your continuing education and professional activities for review for renewal.

LEARNING ACTIVITIES

CHAPTER 1

1. What are your personal reasons for becoming CCRN® certified?
   a. _____
   b. _____
   c. _____

2. List your top five life priorities for the next year. Is CCRN® certification on this list? What is the ranking for CCRN® certification?
   1st _____
   2nd _____
   3rd _____
   4th _____
   5th _____

3. Prioritize this list from 1 (least comfortable) to 10 (most comfortable). Use this list to schedule your preparation with 1 being first and 10 being last.

Knowledge Area	Comfort Level
Cardiovascular	
Professional caring and ethical practice	
Pulmonary	
Integumentary	
Musculoskeletal	
Neurology	
Multisystem	
Gastrointestinal	
Renal	
Endocrine	
Behavioral/Psychosocial	
Hematology/Immunology	

4. Describe your plan to prepare for the CCRN® examination.
   a. Identify how many study days you have until the day that you have scheduled your examination.
   _____
   b. Decide if content review, case studies, or practice questions are the most effective method for you.
   _____
   c. Set up a schedule for your study with your weakest content areas scheduled early.
   _____

5. Explore the AACN website (www.aacn.org) focusing on the Certification tab.

6. List three new test-taking strategies that you have learned from this chapter and will use while taking the CCRN® examination.
   a. _____
   b. _____
   c. _____

Web Resources

Website Address	Resources Available
www.aacn.org	Complete test plan Application Information about the Synergy Model
http://nursingworld.org/MainMenuCategories/EthicsStandards/CodeofEthicsforNurses/Code-of-Ethics-For-Nurses.html	ANA Code of Ethics

Professional Caring and Ethical Practice

CHAPTER 2

Critical Care Nursing: General Concepts

Nursing
1. Definition: "Nursing is the protection, promotion, and optimization of health and abilities, prevention of illness and injury, alleviation of suffering through the diagnosis and treatment of human response, and advocacy in the care of individuals, families, communities, and populations" (American Nurses Association [ANA], 2017a).
2. The nursing process (ANA, 2017b)
   a. Assessment: collecting and analyzing physical, psychological, and sociocultural data about a patient
   b. Diagnosis: making a clinical judgment about the client's response to actual or potential health conditions or needs
   c. Planning: setting short- and long-term goals with the patient and developing a plan of care to achieve those goals
   d. Implementation: supervising or carrying out the actual care plan
   e. Evaluation: continuous assessment of the effectiveness of the care plan and the patient's status; the care plan is modified as needed

Critical Care Nursing
1. Acute and critical care nursing is "the specialty that manages human responses to actual or potential life-threatening problems" (American Association of Critical-Care Nurses [AACN], 2015).
   a. Standards for Acute and Critical Care Nursing Practice are available at www.aacn.org.
2. A critical care nurse is "a licensed professional nurse who is responsible for ensuring that acutely and critically ill patients and their families receive optimal care" (AACN, 2015).
3. Acute and critical care patients require "complex assessment and therapies, high-intensity interventions, and high-level, continuous nursing vigilance" to address both acute critical illness and injury as well as complex, chronic conditions. Critical care patients are "highly vulnerable, unstable, and complex" (AACN, 2015).
4. Although critical care nursing is generally delivered in specialized and designated critical care units, AACN defines the practice setting as anywhere "patients require complex assessments and interventions." The practice setting, therefore, is not tied to a specific location but by the "needs of the patient" (AACN, 2015).

The Future of Nursing
1. The Institute of Medicine (IOM) (2010) recently published a report regarding the future of nursing.
   a. Four key messages are:
      1) Nurses should practice to the full extent of their education and training.
      2) Nurses should achieve higher levels of education and training through an improved education system that promotes seamless academic progression.
      3) Nurses should be full partners with physicians and other health care professionals in redesigning health care in the United States.
      4) Effective workforce planning and policy making require better data collection and information infrastructure.
   b. Eight recommendations are:
      1) Remove scope-of-practice barriers.
      2) Expand opportunities for nurses to lead and diffuse collaborative improvement efforts.
      3) Implement nurse residency programs.
      4) Increase the proportion of nurses with a baccalaureate degree to 80% by 2020.
      5) Double the number of nurses with a doctorate by 2020.
      6) Ensure that nurses engage in lifelong learning.
      7) Prepare and enable nurses to lead change to advance health.
      8) Build an infrastructure for the collection and analysis of interprofessional health care workforce data.
2. This report resulted in the creation of the Campaign for Action (http://campaignforaction.org), which is a collaboration between the Robert Wood Johnson Foundation, the AARP Foundation, and The Center to Champion Nursing in America. The goal of this collaborative network is to work toward achieving the recommendations from the IOM report and to ensure "everyone in

America can live a healthier life, supported by a system in which nurses are essential partners in providing health care and promoting health" (Campaign for Action, 2016).

Synergy Model Nurse Competencies

1. Critical care nursing requires a dynamic relationship between the patient, family, and the nurse. Keeping the patient and family as the central focus of delivery of nursing care means that the associated nurse competencies are determined by the patient's needs (AACN, 2015).
2. The Synergy Model identifies nurse competencies (Box 2.1).

Clinical Judgment

Description

"Clinical reasoning, which includes clinical decision making, critical thinking and a global grasp of the situation, coupled with nursing skills acquired through a process of integrating education, experiential knowledge, and evidence-based guidelines" (AACN, 2016d).

Decision Making

1. Involves a number of steps by which information is assimilated, integrated, weighed, and valued to arrive at the selection of a course of action from among a number of possible alternatives
2. Steps in the decision-making process
   a. Information collection and problem identification
   b. Identification of possible solutions or actions
   c. Analysis of the possible consequences of each solution or action
   d. Selection of the best possible solution or action for implementation
   e. Implementation of the solution or action
   f. Evaluation of the results

Critical Thinking, Clinical Judgment, and Clinical Reasoning

1. Definitions
   a. Critical thinking: "a disciplined process that requires validation of data, including any assumptions that may influence your thoughts, and then careful reflection on the entire process while evaluating the effectiveness of what you have determined is the necessary action to take" (Jackson, Ignatavicius, & Case, 2006)
   b. Clinical judgment: "the development of opinions in the clinical practice setting, based on experience and knowledge, to guide the decisions you will make regarding the care of the patient" (Jackson et al., 2006)
   c. Clinical reasoning: use of "clinically specific data regarding specific populations or disease processes and making evaluations regarding their meaning" (Jackson et al., 2006)
2. The terms *critical thinking, clinical judgment,* and *clinical reasoning* are often used interchangeably. However, critical thinking and clinical reasoning are the PROCESS, and clinical judgment is the RESULT of the process (Alfaro-LeFevre, 2013) (Fig. 2.1).
3. The 4-Circle Critical Thinking Model (Alfaro-LeFevre, 2013) identifies four components to develop critical thinking and clinical judgment.
   a. Develop critical thinking characteristics of honesty, fair-mindedness, creativity, patience, and confidence.
   b. Take responsibility for professional knowledge and education and seek opportunities for learning experiences to develop theoretical and experiential knowledge.
   c. Gain interpersonal skills such as teamwork, conflict resolution, and patient and family advocacy.
   d. Practice related technical skills until they are automatic, freeing the nurse to see the bigger picture and synthesize data elements to understand the patient's response to care.
4. Development of critical thinking and clinical judgment are not solely related to the passage of time.
   a. Experience gained in the time spent providing critical care nursing and application of that experience and knowledge gained to each subsequent patient cared for drive development of these skills.
   b. The AACN describes levels of expertise as ranging from competent (level 1) to expert (level 5). Characteristics of nurses at various stages along the

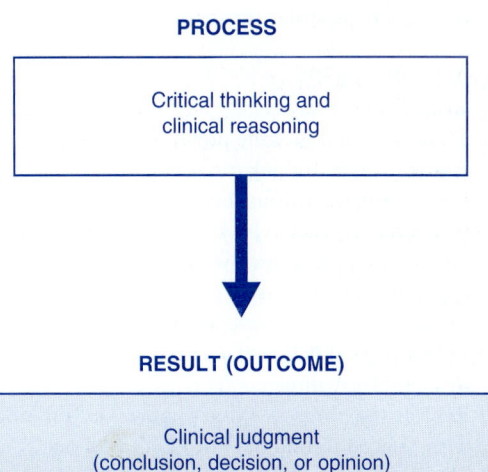

Fig. 2.1 Relationship between clinical judgment, clinical reasoning, and critical thinking. (From Alfaro-Lefevre, R. [2013]. *Critical thinking, clinical reasoning, and clinical judgment: A practical approach* [5th ed.]. St. Louis: Saunders.)

Box 2.1 Nurse Competencies According to the Synergy Model

- Clinical Judgment
- Advocacy and Moral Agency
- Caring Practices
- Collaboration
- Systems Thinking
- Response to Diversity
- Clinical Inquiry
- Facilitation of Learning

continuum of clinical judgment development can be described as follows:
- 1) Level 1: collects basic data; follows algorithms or protocols with all populations; rely upon "delegating up" to more senior nurses; focused on mastering technical skills; often includes extraneous details
- 2) Level 3: collects and interprets patient data; recognizes patterns and trends that may predict the patient response or trajectory of illness; recognizes limits and seeks assistance; able to sort out extraneous information or details
- 3) Level 5: synthesizes data points from multiple sources that may be conflicting; makes judgments based on immediate grasp of the whole picture; leverages past experiences to anticipate complications and problems; seeks multidisciplinary collaboration and consultation without feeling inferior (AACN, 2016c)

5. Ten key questions to ask to assist in determining your approach to critical thinking (Alfaro-LeFevre, 2013):
   a. What major outcomes do you and key stakeholders expect to observe in the patient after care is complete?
   b. What problems, issues, or risks must be managed to achieve the major outcomes?
   c. What are the circumstances in this particular patient situation?
   d. What knowledge and skills are required to care for this patient?
   e. How much room is there for error?
   f. How much time do you have?
   g. What human and information resources can help?
   h. Whose perspectives must be considered?
   i. What's influencing thinking?
   j. What must be done to monitor, prevent, manage, or eliminate the problems, issues, and risks identified in question 2?
6. The following strategies enhance critical thinking (Alfaro-LeFevre, 2013):
   a. Anticipate questions others might ask.
   b. Ask, "What else?"
   c. Ask, "What if?"
   d. Ask, "Why?"
   e. Think out loud or write down your thoughts.
   f. Ask an expert to think out loud.
   g. Look for flaws in your thinking.
   h. Ask someone else to look for flaws in your thinking.
   i. Paraphrase in your own words.
   j. Compare and contrast.
   k. Organize and reorganize information.
   l. Develop good habits of inquiry.
   m. Revisit information.
   n. Replace the phrases "I don't know" or "I'm not sure" with "I need to find out" or "Let's find out."
   o. Turn mistakes into learning opportunities.
7. Alfaro-LeFevre (2013) identifies 10 strategies that can be used as the nurse develops clinical judgment from clinical experiences.
   a. Keep references (e.g., texts, pocket guides, smartphone applications, personal cheat sheets) handy.
   b. Apply principles of the nursing process. This fundamental baseline of nursing practice will provide a foundation to assist in thinking through new clinical problems and make decisions based on evidence.
   c. Learn to think ahead, think in action, and think back.
   d. Follow policies, procedures, and standards of care carefully. Learn and understand the reasons behind them.
   e. Determine a system that helps you prioritize tasks or actions that must be done now and what can wait.
   f. Never perform actions if you don't know why they are indicated, the rationale, and the risks.
   g. Learn from human resources (educators, preceptors, supervisors, peers, members of the multidisciplinary care team).
   h. Seek out simulated experiences.
   i. Remember the importance of caring.
   j. When planning time for nursing care, remember to consider time for both direct and indirect care interventions.

Clinical Knowledge and Skills by System
Refer to Chapters 3 to 12.

Advocacy and Moral Agency

Description
"Working on another's behalf and representing the concerns of the patient/family and nursing staff; serving as a moral agent in identifying and helping to resolve ethical and clinical concerns within and outside the clinical setting" (AACN, 2016d).

Foundations of Ethical Nursing Practice
1. ANA Code of Ethics for Nurses (2015) (http://nursingworld.org/DocumentVault/Ethics-1/Code-of-Ethics-for-Nurses.html)
   a. Provides the foundation for ethical nursing practice
   b. Ethics are systems of valued behaviors and beliefs that govern proper conduct to ensure the protection of an individual's rights; involves judgments that help to differentiate.
   c. Values: personal beliefs about the truth and the worth of thoughts, objects, and behavior

Ethical Decision Making
1. Ethical principlism is the guiding approach to ethical decision making.
2. Four bioethical principles (Beauchamp & Childress, 2013)
   a. Respect for autonomy specifies the obligation to respect a person's right of self-determination, independence, and freedom.
      1) The nurse must be willing to respect the patient's right to make decisions about his or her own care even if the nurse does not agree with those decisions.
      2) Limitations to autonomy include the following:
         i. When the rights of one person interfere with another individual's rights, health, or well-being
         ii. When there is a high probability that a person may self-injure or injure others

b. Nonmaleficence: an individual's obligation to do no harm, intentionally or unintentionally
   1) It includes protecting mentally incompetent persons, nonresponsive persons, children, and all other person who cannot protect themselves.
   2) This principle is not absolute; an example of a conflict related to nonmaleficence is when surgical trauma causes an ultimate cure or improvement in the patient's condition.
c. Beneficence: an individual's obligation to promote good and prevent or remove harm and to promote the welfare, health, and safety of society and individuals in accordance with their beliefs, values, preferences, and life goals. Conflicts that may occur include the following decisions:
   1) What is best for another person
   2) Who should make the decision
   3) Long- or short-term benefit (a temporary harm may eventually produce a greater good)
d. Justice: a moral obligation to be fair and promote equity; ensure nondiscrimination; distribute resources in a fair and equitable manner
   1) Individuals have the right to be treated fairly and equally regardless of race, sex, marital status, medical diagnosis, social standing, economic level, or religious belief; also includes equal access to health care for all

Additional Concepts Related to Ethical Decision Making

1. Advocacy refers to respecting and supporting the basic values, rights, and beliefs of the critically ill patient.
   a. The nurse should do the following (Hayes, 2000):
      1) Respect and support the right of the patient or the patient's designated surrogate to autonomous informed decision making.
      2) Intervene when the best interest of the patient is in question.
      3) Help the patient obtain necessary care.
      4) Respect the values, beliefs, and rights of the patient.
      5) Provide education and support to help the patient or the patient's designated surrogate make decisions.
      6) Represent the patient in accordance with the patient's choices.
      7) Support the decisions of the patient or the patient's designated surrogate or transfer care to an equally qualified critical care nurse.
      8) Intercede for patients who cannot speak for themselves in situations that require immediate action.
      9) Monitor and safeguard the quality of care the patient receives.
      10) Act as liaison between the patient, the patient's family, and health care professionals.
2. Moral agency: ability to serve as a moral agent in identifying and resolving ethical and clinical concerns (Curley, 2007)
3. Accountability: answerability or responsibility
   a. Personal accountability: to oneself and the patient
   b. Public accountability: to employer, community, and society
4. Veracity: an individual's obligation to tell the truth and to not intentionally deceive or mislead the patient
   a. This principle is not absolute; an example of a conflict related to veracity is when telling the patient the truth may cause harm.
5. Paternalism: an individual's obligation to assist another person in making a decision when that person does not have sufficient data or expertise
   a. It is one of the key elements of accountability.
6. Fidelity: an individual's obligation to be faithful or loyal to agreements and responsibilities that the individual has accepted
   a. It is one of the key elements of accountability.
   b. A conflict may occur between fidelity to patients and fidelity to employer, government, and society.
7. Egoism: actions are right or wrong based on self-interest and self-preservation.
8. Social contract theory: people give up some rights to a government in exchange for social order.
9. Natural law: actions are morally or ethically right when they are in accord with human nature.
10. Confidentiality: an individual's responsibility to respect privileged information
    a. Access to patient data is limited to individuals with a "need to know."
    b. Others wishing access to patient data must have the patient's permission.
    c. Information about the patient (status or presence in the health care institution) is limited to persons whom the patient has identified.
    d. The patient has the right to access his or her medical record; if this occurs while the patient is still hospitalized, a nurse should be available to explain entries about which the patient has questions.
    e. Computerized patient records introduce new challenges to ensuring the confidentiality of patient data.
       1) Never give out your password.
       2) Never leave unattended a computer terminal where you have signed in; log off when leaving the terminal.
       3) Do not allow anyone to view the screen while you are viewing patient data.
       4) Do not view things that you don't "need to know."
11. Moral distress: when one knows the right thing to do but cannot pursue the right action; obstacles may be internal or external (Savel & Munro, 2015)
    a. Four As to rise above moral distress (Wavra, 2006)
       1) Ask: determine whether the nurse is experiencing moral distress.
          i. Expressions of anger, resentment, and frustration
          ii. Statements such as, "Why are we doing this?"
          iii. Physical symptoms such as change in weight, sleep patterns, and depression
       2) Affirm
          i. Acknowledge the distress.
          ii. Affirm professional obligations to act as described in the ANA Code of Ethics for Nurses.

3) Assess
   i. Identify sources and severity of moral distress.
   ii. Assess readiness to act by analyzing risks and benefits.
4) Act
   i. Prepare personally and professionally to act.
   ii. Take action based on self-exploration regarding obligations, responsibilities, and risks.
   iii. Anticipate setbacks and manage accordingly.
12. Moral residue: after a health care provider experiences moral distress, she or he does not necessarily immediately return to her or his normal moral baseline, this phenomenon is referred to as moral residue (Savel & Munro, 2015). Long-term consequences include:
    a. Becoming morally numb to future ethical situations
    b. Clinical burnout or leaving the profession
13. Moral courage: can be described as feeling fear but performing clinical functions anyway. Examples of strategies to overcome fear include cognitive reframing, recognizing that there is a professional obligation that outweighs the fear, developing risk tolerance (Savel & Munro, 2015).

Ethical Approaches: The Basis for Ethical Decisions

1. Deontology: actions are right or wrong based on a set of morals or rules.
   a. Emphasizes duty or obligation to another person
   b. Only acceptable ethical theory for decision making in health care
2. Teleology: actions are right or wrong based on the action's consequences and usefulness; it looks at outcome; the end justifies the means.
3. Utilitarianism: the morally right thing to do is whatever produces the greatest good for the greatest number; it is derived from teleology.

Ethical Dilemmas

Situation that requires a choice between two or more equally undesirable alternatives
1. Characteristics of an ethical dilemma (Curtin, 1982)
   a. The problem cannot be solved using only empirical data.
   b. The problem is so perplexing that it is difficult to decide what facts and data should be used to make the decision.
   c. There are far-reaching effects to the decision.
2. Conflicts related to rights of the individual: autonomy versus paternalism
   a. Informed consent
   b. Technology versus quality of life
   c. Resuscitate versus do not resuscitate (DNR)
   d. Behavior control
      1) May be misused to suppress personal freedom (e.g., use of restraints or sedating drugs)
      2) Individual's right to freedom may conflict with society's obligation to maintain social order.
3. Conflicts related to resource allocations: justice versus utilitarianism
   a. Triage decisions
   b. Quality-of-life decisions
   c. Inability to pay or lack of health insurance
   d. Organ transplantation decisions
      1) Living donors: rights of donor, recipient, families, and society
      2) Choice of one recipient over another: potential for elitism
      3) Utilization of health care resources: tremendous cost of organ transplantation
      4) Designation of death: when can an organ or organs be removed
4. Conflicts related to the role of the nurse: veracity versus fidelity
   a. Withholding therapy
   b. Right to die
      1) Positive euthanasia (also referred to as active euthanasia or mercy killing): life support systems are withdrawn or a medication, treatment, or procedure is used to cause death (e.g., assisted suicide).
      2) Negative euthanasia (also referred to as passive euthanasia): no extraordinary or heroic life-support measures are used to save a person's life (e.g., do-DNR orders).
5. Conflicts related to personal values: professional integrity versus personal ethical and moral beliefs
   a. Nurse participation in treatments or therapies against the nurse's ethical or moral beliefs (e.g., abortion)
   b. Nurse providing care for patients whose practices are against the nurse's ethical or moral beliefs (e.g., domestic violence)

Factors Affecting Ethical Issues and Decision Making

See Fig. 2.2.

Rights

1. Ethical rights (moral rights)
   a. Based on moral or ethical principle
   b. Backed by general opinion of society or culture
   c. Often privileges allotted to certain individuals or groups of individuals

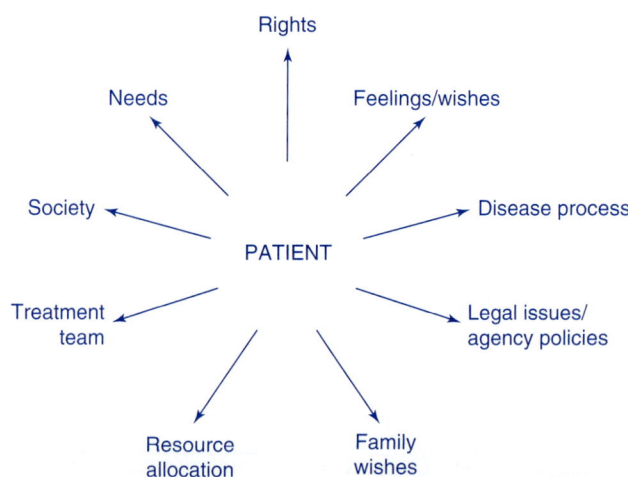

Fig. 2.2 Factors affecting ethical issues and ethical decision making in nursing. (From Kinney, M., Dunbar, S., Brooks-Brunn, J.A., Molter, N., & Vitello-Cicciu, J. [1998]. *AACN's clinical reference for critical care nursing* [4th ed.]. St Louis: Mosby.)

2. Legal rights: life, liberty, property, individual freedoms, and due process
   a. Based on a legal entitlement to some good or benefit
   b. Guaranteed by laws and, if violated, can be upheld in the legal system
3. Entitlements: statutory rights for a defined group (e.g., Medicare)
4. The American Hospital Association (AHA) Patient's Bill of Rights has been replaced by a patient information brochure titled "The Patient Care Partnership," which identifies the following expectations during a hospital stay (AHA, 2003).
   a. High-quality hospital care
   b. A clean and safe environment
   c. Involvement in your care
   d. Protection of your privacy
   e. Help with your bill and filing insurance claims

Legal Issues

1. Sources of law
   a. A constitution establishes the basis of a governing system.
   b. Statutes are laws that govern.
      1) Made, voted on, and passed by legislative bodies
      2) Nurse practice acts are statutes.
         a) Define and limit the practice of nursing
         b) May vary state to state but all must be consistent with federal provisions and statutes
   c. Administrative agencies (e.g., state boards of nursing) create rules and regulations that enforce statutory laws.
   d. Court decisions are made when the courts interpret legal issues that are in dispute.
   e. Common law consists of statements made by courts, sometimes decades in the past, when no statute exists governing the particular matter.
2. Types of court cases
   a. Criminal: charges filed by the state or federal attorney general for crimes committed against an individual or society
      1) Burden of proof is on the filing agency; the defendant is presumed innocent and must be proven guilty beyond reasonable doubt.
      2) Consequences if found guilty include imprisonment or even death.
      3) An example is a nurse who intentionally administered drugs that caused a patient's death.
   b. Civil: one individual sues another.
      1) Burden of proof to be found liable is a preponderance of the evidence.
      2) Consequences are monetary.
      3) An example would be a nurse sued for wrongful death because he or she failed to do something that would have prevented the death.
      4) Intentional torts
         a) Definition: a tort is a legal wrong committed against a person or property, independent of a contract, that renders the person who commits it liable for damages in a civil action; an intentional tort is a direct invasion of someone's legal rights.
         b) Examples include assault, battery, false imprisonment, invasion of privacy, defamation, and slander.
   c. Administrative: charges filed by a state or federal governmental agency (e.g., state board of nursing)
      1) Burden of proof to be found guilty is a preponderance of the evidence.
      2) Consequences may be monetary, disciplinary, or loss of privileges (e.g., professional license).
      3) An example is failure to obtain a new license at the predetermined time.
3. Malpractice (i.e., professional negligence)
   a. Definition: failure to do something that a reasonable and prudent professional would do or doing something that a reasonable and prudent professional would not do; an unintentional tort
      1) Reasonable and prudent: average judgment, foresight, intelligence, and skill that would be expected of a person with similar training and experience
   b. Elements that must be present for a professional to be held liable for malpractice
      1) Duty: the nurse had a duty to provide care and follow an acceptable standard of care.
      2) Breach: there was a breach of duty (i.e., the nurse failed to adhere to the standard of care).
      3) Causation: the failure to meet the standard of care must have caused injury to the patient.
      4) Damages: the patient must have suffered injuries as a result of the nurse's breach of duty.
   c. Avoidance of malpractice claims (Marquis & Huston, 2011)
      1) Practice within the scope of your state's nurse practice act.
      2) Follow your institution's policies and procedures.
      3) Model your practice after established practice standards and scientific evidence.
      4) Make patients' rights and welfare the priority.
      5) Make rational decisions based on the biological, psychological, and social sciences and be aware of laws and legal doctrines.
      6) Practice within your area of competence.
      7) Continue to update and upgrade your technical skills and seek specialty certification.
      8) Purchase professional liability insurance and know the limits of your policy.
      9) Document thoroughly in the patient's record.
         a) Document
            i) Patient status with factual observations along with time, date, and signature (may be electronic signature)
            ii) Any deviations from standard practice and reasons for such deviations
            iii) Notification of physician for changes in status and the physician's response
         b) Common problems made in documentation
            i) Omissions without explanation
            ii) Vague and ambiguous language
            iii) Unapproved abbreviations
            iv) Error correction

v) Spelling and grammar errors
vi) Illegibility
vii) Time inconsistencies (especially with electronic documentation systems)
4. Consent
   a. Blanket consent: the person gives permission for routine and customary care; this type of consent is required before admission.
   b. Informed consent: the person gives consent for a specific procedure.
      1) The physician or advanced practice registered nurse (APRN) informs the patient and ensures that he or she understands the following:
         a) Explanation of the treatment or procedure
         b) Expected results or benefits
         c) Risks involved
         d) Alternatives, including absence of treatment
         e) Name of person performing the treatment or procedure
         f) That the patient may withdraw consent at any time
      2) It is the responsibility of the person who will perform the procedure to obtain informed consent, but the nurse may witness the patient's signature on the consent form; the nurse has an ethical responsibility to notify the person who will perform the procedure if the nurse believes that the patient does not understand the procedure.
   c. Implied consent: the patient is unable to sign, but treatment is needed immediately and the treatment is in the patient's best interest.
5. Incident reports
   a. These are internal documents completed for any unusual occurrence, including errors.
   b. These reports should include facts about the incident and the care given to the patient, such as diagnostic studies, medications, and consults.
   c. Avoid statements of guilt or blame in the incident report and do not allude to the incident report in the patient's medical record.
      1) Note that there is a national trend to fully disclose all errors to the patient, and some studies have found fewer lawsuits when the patient was informed of the error.
6. Terms related to end-of-life care
   a. Advance directive: a legal document that expresses the patient's preferences related to end-of-life issues
      1) Must be developed by a competent adult (i.e., 18 years of age or older)
      2) Must be witnessed by two people
      3) May be revoked verbally, in writing, or by destruction of the document at any time
      4) Becomes effective when the person is certified to be terminally ill or have an irreversible condition with loss of decision-making capability
      5) Does not contraindicate the use of treatments for pain or suffering
   b. Living will: a directive that expresses what the patient wants done if he or she becomes terminally ill and is not able to make health care decisions
   c. Durable power of attorney for health care: a directive that designates someone to make health care decisions for the patient if the patient is unable to make the decisions

Caring Practices

Nursing activities that are responsive to the uniqueness of the patient and family and that create a compassionate and therapeutic environment with the aim of promoting comfort and preventing suffering (AACN, 2016d).

Death and Dying

1. Definition: dying is a psychophysiologic process that ultimately terminates in death for the individual and grieving for significant others.
2. Stages of death and dying (Kübler-Ross, 1969)
   a. Shock and disbelief (e.g., this is a mistake)
   b. Denial (e.g., it isn't that bad)
   c. Anger (e.g., why me?)
   d. Bargaining (e.g., if I do this. . . ., I'll survive)
   e. Depression (e.g., why bother with treatment?)
   f. Acceptance (e.g., I'm ready)
3. Interventions to assist the patient to cope with death and dying
   a. Develop a personal philosophy of death to deal effectively with dying patients and living families.
   b. Do not eliminate hope.
      1) Hope is the expectation that a desire will be fulfilled.
      2) Hope aids in the tolerance of pain and suffering throughout the dying process.
   c. Encourage the patient and family to discuss their fears and concerns; listen attentively.
   d. Provide your presence and your compassion.
   e. Provide comfort measures and analgesia.
4. Interventions to assist the family
   a. Allow the family to be with the patient.
   b. Encourage the family to participate in the care of the patient.
   c. Reassure the family of the patient's analgesia and comfort.
   d. Provide information about the patient's status frequently, especially when death is imminent.
   e. Encourage ventilation of anxiety, fears, and concerns.
   f. Ensure a private, comfortable area for the family.
   g. Refer the family to other sources of support, such as the chaplain, social worker, and support group.

Pain Management

1. Definition of pain: anything the patient says it is; it occurs whenever the patient says it does (McCaffery, 1968)
   a. Acute pain: pain that follows injury and ends when healing occurs; an example is surgical pain
   b. Chronic pain: pain that lasts longer than the normal healing period; an example is low back pain
   c. Neuropathic pain: chronic pain caused by nerve damage; an example is diabetic neuropathy
2. Assessment
   a. Self-report using validated pain assessment tools or simple questions

Table 2.1	Behavioral Pain Scale	
Item	Description	Score
Facial expression	Relaxed	1
	Partially tightened (e.g., brow lowering)	2
	Fully tightened (e.g., eyelid closing)	3
	Grimacing	4
Upper limbs	No movement	1
	Partially bent	2
	Fully bent with finger flexion	3
	Permanently retracted	4
Compliance with ventilation	Tolerating movement	1
	Coughing but tolerating	2
	Fighting ventilator	3
	Unable to control ventilation	4
Total score		3–12

From Payen, J.-F., Bru, O., Bosson, J. L., Lagrasta, A., Novel, E., Deschaux, I., et al. (2001). Assessing pain in critically ill sedated patients using a behavioral pain scale. *Crit Care Med, 29*(12), 2258–2263.

1) Pain scales
   a) Numerical (0–10) pain scale
   b) Wong-Baker FACES scale
   c) Verbal graphic rating scale
   d) Behavioral Pain Scale (Table 2.1)
   e) Critical-Care Pain Observation Tool (Table 2.2)
2) Guidelines for teaching your patient to use a pain rating scale (McCaffery, 2002)
   a) Explain the purpose of the scale.
   b) Explain the increments of the scale.
   c) Explain what is meant by "pain."
   d) Ask the patient to give an example of pain to practice using the scale.
   e) Ask the patient to practice using the scale to rate the pain.
   f) Assist the patient to set a goal for an acceptable level of pain.
   b. If unable to self-report, perform a pain assessment using a validated behavioral pain scale (i.e., Behavioral Pain Scale or the Critical-Care Pain Observation Tool) (AACN, 2013).
   c. Other cues that indicate the critical care patient may be in pain include verbal (moaning or crying), nonverbal (rubbing, splinting, guarding), or facial expressions (grimacing, frowning).
   d. It is not recommended that vital signs be used as a primary means of assessing for pain in critical care patients (AACN, 2013).
3. Pharmacologic management
   a. Pharmacologic agents
      1) Opioids (e.g., morphine, fentanyl, hydromorphone)
      2) Nonsteroidal anti-inflammatory drugs (e.g., ibuprofen, ketorolac)
      3) Local anesthetics (e.g., lidocaine, bupivacaine)
   b. Drug delivery methods used in critical care areas
      1) Analgesia
         a) Oral agents, especially sustained-release agents
         b) Intravenous
            i) Continuous infusion
            ii) Intermittent injection
            iii) Patient controlled: usually consists of a continuous infusion with patient-controlled injection for breakthrough pain
         c) Epidural
            i) Continuous infusion
            ii) Patient controlled: usually consists of a continuous infusion with patient-controlled injection for breakthrough pain
      2) Regional anesthesia
         a) Transdermal
         b) Peripheral nerve catheter: delivers local anesthetic directly to the nerve sheath
         c) Intrapleural: delivers local anesthetic directly to the parietal pleura
4. Nonpharmacologic
   a. Application of heat or cold
   b. Relaxation techniques
   c. Distraction (e.g., music, television, reading, needlepoint, coloring, drawing, writing, visitors)
   d. Other complementary therapies as described later

Complementary Therapies

Definition: "A broad set of healthcare practices, therapies, and modalities that address the whole person—body, mind, emotion, spirit, and environment" (Dossey & Keegan, 2016). These therapies are intended to cause relaxation, decrease anxiety, and augment pain management. Complementary therapies may be useful adjuncts to conventional approaches when implemented in a safe, responsible, ethical manner (Kramlich, 2016).
1. Aromatherapy using essential oils may improve physical, psychological, and spiritual health.
   a. Methods of administration include inhalation and topical application.
   b. Precautions
      1) Use with caution in patients with severe asthma or multiple allergies.
      2) Do not use near eyes.
      3) Be cautious in using them during pregnancy.
      4) Understand the properties and application considerations (e.g., dilution requirements) before using.
   c. Selected aromatherapy agents
      1) Lavender: calming, useful in insomnia, agitation, depression, stress relief
      2) Peppermint: anti-nausea (inhaled), analgesic (topical)
      3) Frankincense: relaxation, meditation, spiritual renewal
2. Progressive muscle relaxation
   a. Involves progressive tensing and relaxing of successive muscle groups, frequently accompanied by diaphragmatic breathing
   b. Decreases stress, anxiety, and agitation

Table 2.2 Critical-Care Pain Observation Tool

Indicator		Score	Operational Definition
Facial expression	Relaxed, neutral	0	No muscle tension observed
	Tense	1	Presence of frowning, brow lowering, orbit tightening and levator contraction, or any other change (e.g., opening eyes or tearing during nociceptive procedures)
	Grimacing	2	All previous facial movements plus eyelid tightly closed (the patient may present with mouth open or biting the endotracheal tube)
Body movements	Absence of movement or normal position	0	Does not move at all (doesn't necessarily mean absence of pain) or normal position (movements not aimed toward the pain site or not made for the purpose of protection)
	Protection	1	Slow, cautious movements, touching or rubbing the pain site, seeking attention through movements
	Restlessness	2	Pulling tube, attempting to sit up, moving limbs or thrashing, not following commands, striking at staff, trying to climb out of bed
Compliance with the ventilator (intubated patients)	Tolerating ventilator or movement	0	Alarms not activated, easy ventilation
	Coughing but tolerating	1	Coughing, alarms may be activated but stop spontaneously
OR	Fighting ventilator	2	Asynchrony; blocking ventilation, alarms frequently activated
Vocalization (nonintubated patient)	Talking in normal tone or no sound	0	Talking in normal tone or no sound
	Sighing, moaning	1	Sighing, moaning
	Crying out, sobbing	2	Crying out, sobbing
Muscle tension	Relaxed	0	No resistance to passive movements
Evaluation by passive flexion and extension of upper limbs when patient is at rest or evaluation when patient is being turned	Tense, rigid	1	Resistance to passive movements
	Very tense or rigid	2	Strong resistance to passive movements, incapacity to do them
Total		___/8	

From Gelinas, C., Arbour, C., Michaud, C., Vaillant, F., & Desjardins, S. (2011). Implementation of the critical-care pain observation tool on pain assessment/management nursing practices in an intensive care unit with nonverbal critically ill adults: a before and after study. *Int J Nurs Stud, 48*(12), 1495–1504. http://dx.doi.org/org/j.ijnurstu.2011.03.012

3. Biofeedback
    a. Involves use of conscious mental effort to control involuntary body functions, such as blood pressure, heart rate, and respiratory rate
    b. A biofeedback instrument is used initially to alert the patient to the cues that signal a developing symptom (e.g., tension in neck and shoulders); audible tones are given.
    c. Relaxation techniques are taught to decrease muscle tension.
    d. Decreases stress and anxiety and causes muscle relaxation
4. Meditation
    a. Mindful breathing
        1) Involves instruction, practice, and encouragement in the use of breathing techniques, such as diaphragmatic breathing or pursed-lip breathing
        2) May be used with a script "Breathing in, I am aware of breathing in. Breathing out, I am aware of breathing out. In. Out. Breathing in, I am calm. Breathing out, I smile."
        3) Decreases stress and anxiety; may improve effectiveness of ventilation, especially in dyspneic patients
    b. Guided imagery
        1) Involves focusing and directing the imagination through the use of specific words and suggestions
        2) Identify the patient's concept of a relaxing location or situation and verbally guide the patient's thoughts there
        3) Decreases stress, fear, and anxiety; enhances the immune system
    c. Prayer
        1) Involves concentrating on words or sounds to awaken a higher consciousness or become one with the patient's spiritual focus or higher being
        2) Decreases stress and anxiety; brings a state of calmness
5. Hypnosis
    1) Involves suggestion to enable a person to experience the imaginary as real, allowing deep relaxation; can be led by an assistant or self-induced
    2) Decreases stress and anxiety

6. Massage
   a. Involves a technique of controlled touch to manipulate soft tissue
   b. Effects are dependent on the type and speed of movements; the pressure exerted by the hands, fingers, or thumbs; and the area of the body being massaged.
   c. Decreases stress and anxiety, reduces muscle tension and spasm, reduces edema, causes release of endorphins to augment pain relief
   d. Aromatherapy and music may enhance the effectiveness.
7. Therapeutic (or healing) touch
   a. Involves the transfer of energy from the practitioner's hands to the patient, without actually touching, to potentiate the healing process of one who is ill or injured
   b. Consists of the following steps: centering, assessment, unruffling, modulating, and evaluation
   c. Used to help restore the balance of the energy field and to provide additional energy to be used for healing
8. Purposeful touch
   a. Involves hand holding, stroking, or patting a patient's arm, hand, or face; placing one's hand on the patient's shoulder; placing one's arm around the patient's shoulder; or hugging
   b. May also be referred to as affective touch, comforting touch, or empathetic touch
   c. Reduces stress and communicates encouragement, support, or affection
9. Music therapy
   a. Involves the use of music to soothe and relax
   b. Identify the patient's music preferences; any simple, repetitive, low-pitched music is appropriate for relaxation
   c. The most soothing music has a 3/4 beat; chants, folk songs, and lullabies are very relaxing
   d. Causes endorphin release, distraction from pain or anxiety, and relaxation; improves quality and quantity of sleep
10. Pet therapy
    a. Involves visits by the patient's own pet or by pet-visitation animals (usually dogs)
    b. Decreases stress and anxiety, may decrease heart rate and blood pressure
    c. Adhere to specific guidelines to ensure the safety and security of the patient, families, and staff
11. Humor
    a. Involves using words and images to elicit laughter
    b. Decreases stress and anxiety, enhances the patient's ability to cope and feelings of well-being, decreases tension in a difficult situation, causes endorphin release, augments the immune system, and causes muscle relaxation
    c. Requires judgment to ensure appropriateness of timing and method used to elicit laughter
       1) Start by determining the patient's receptiveness to humor and asking about what type of humor he or she appreciates
       2) Consider timing of humor, inappropriate during a crisis or when laughing would cause pain
       3) Some forms of humor are inappropriate, such as humor that demeans (i.e., racial or ethnic jokes) or sexually oriented humor (i.e., dirty jokes)
12. Acupuncture
    a. Involves the insertion of very fine needles into specific points in the body for therapeutic purposes; may also involve use of heat (moxibustion), pressure (acupressure), or electromagnetic energy to stimulate acupuncture points
    b. Causes endorphin release and decrease in pain
    c. The body of knowledge continues to grow on the efficacy of acupuncture and pain management.

Rest Requirement
1. Sleep quality is poor, and sleep deprivation is a common problem for patients in critical care unit and has been shown to increase risk of delirium (Patel, Baldwin, Bunting, & Laha, 2014).
   a. Causes (Holley, 2010; Matthews, 2011)
      1) Long periods in bed
      2) Supine position with little or no activity
      3) Little or no light variation
      4) Patient–ventilator asynchrony
      5) Pain with inadequate analgesia
      6) Dyspnea
      7) Pharmacologic agents that cause agitation or wakefulness
      8) Note that although sedatives, hypnotics, and analgesics cause the appearance of sleep, it is unclear as to whether this "sleep" has the same restorative qualities as normal physiologic sleep.
      9) Ambient noise (Tainter, 2016)
   b. In a study by Tamburri, DiBrienza, Zozula, and Redeker (2004), the mean number of care interactions per night was 42.6, and patients had 2 to 3 hours of uninterrupted sleep on only 6% of the nights observed.
   c. Recommendations to improve sleep quality in the critical care unit (Holley, 2010)
      1) Promote wakefulness during the day.
      2) Use sedatives judiciously, especially during the day.
      3) Decrease light and noise during the night.
      4) Minimize disruptions and awakenings during the night.
      5) Implementation of quiet times in which minimal interventions are performed, lights are dimmed, and rest is encouraged (Tainter, 2016).
2. Noise control
   a. Noise can produce serious physical and psychological stress and may impair the healing process; the Environmental Protection Agency (1974) recommends that daytime noise levels in a hospital not exceed 45 dB and that nighttime levels not exceed 35 dB.
      1) In 2005, the average daytime sound level was 72 dB and average nighttime sound level was 60 dB (Choiniere, 2010). Decrease volume on alarms and decrease extraneous conversation and other noise; earplugs also may be used.
      2) 11.5% of arousals from sleep and 17% of awakenings are caused by environmental noise (Freedman, Gazendam, Levan, Pack, & Schwab, 2001).

b. Recommendations to reduce noise in the critical care unit (Choiniere, 2010)
  1) Half of hospital sound peaks are directly related to human behavior with staff conversations being the most disturbing noise to patients; staff should be educated and encouraged to reduce volume of conversation and close doors during reports.
  2) Reduce volume of alarms, phones, beepers, televisions, and music.
  3) Eliminate overhead pages.
  4) Limit the number of visitors to two at a time.
  5) Note and correct noisy carts.
  6) Design units with improved sound acoustics, decentralized nurses' stations, and single-patient rooms.

The Family of the Critically Ill Adult

1. Definition: individuals who are relatives or significant others with whom the patient shares an established relationship. With regards to support, the patient defines who is considered family (Davidson et al., 2016).
2. Assessment
   a. Availability of family
   b. Structure and communication patterns within the family
     1) Role of patient within the family
     2) Primary decision maker
     3) Family spokesperson
     4) Conflicts within the family
   c. Perceptions and understanding
     1) Knowledge of patient's condition
     2) Past experience with critical care
     3) Past experience with similar health situations (e.g., myocardial infarction, cancer)
     4) Need for information about the patient
     5) Expectations of patient's outcome
   d. Coping patterns
     1) Previous responses to crises
     2) Usual coping mechanism
   e. Family resources and needs related to resources
     1) Transportation
     2) Lodging
     3) Finances
     4) Spirituality
   f. Family health maintenance needs
     1) Dietary
     2) Hygiene
     3) Rest and sleep
     4) Medications
3. Stressors
   a. Observation of a loved one in a life-threatening situation
   b. Overwhelming technology in the critical care environment
   c. Separation from the family member
   d. Financial impact
4. Most important needs of families (Leske, 1991)
   a. To have questions answered honestly
   b. To be assured the best care possible is being given to the patient
   c. To know the prognosis
   d. To feel there is hope
   e. To know specific facts about the patient's progress
   f. To be called at home about changes in the patient's condition
   g. To know how the patient is being treated medically
   h. To believe that hospital personnel care about the patient
   i. To receive information about the patient daily
   j. To have understandable explanations
   k. To know exactly what is being done for the patient
   l. To know why things were done for the patient
   m. To see the patient frequently
   n. To talk to the doctor every day
   o. To be told about transfer plans
5. Responses
   a. Fear of death, pain, and discomfort of their loved one
   b. Anxiety
   c. Financial concerns
   d. Fear of temporary or permanent changes in the roles of the patient and other family members
   e. Severe dysfunction: argumentativeness, aggression, intoxication, guilt, blame, verbal or physical abuse toward health care workers
6. Interventions
   a. Introduce yourself and ask names and relationships of family members. Identify family members by name if possible.
   b. Utilize a communication approach such as the VALUE method that is inclusive of family (Davidson et al., 2016).
     1) Value family statements.
     2) Acknowledge emotions.
     3) Listen.
     4) Understand the patient as a person.
     5) Elicit questions.
   c. Provide information about the status of the patient on request; at designated times, including during visiting hours; and at the time of any significant change in condition.
   d. Be available during family visitation to answer questions and provide explanations.
   e. Encourage family members to make notes regarding information that the physicians or nurses have given or questions that they would like to ask during the next interaction with the nurse or physician.
   f. Provide a brochure describing the unit, usual activities, visitation policies, and other useful information.
   g. Use touch therapeutically as indicated and allowed by the family members.
   h. Individualize visiting times based on the needs and response of the patient and the family.
     1) In a recent AACN practice alert, it is stated that "evidence shows that the unrestricted presence and participation of a support person (i.e., family as defined by the patient) can enhance patient and family satisfaction." and "unrestricted visitation from such a support person can improve communication, facilitate a better understanding of the patient, advance patient- and family-centered care, and enhance staff satisfaction" (AACN, 2016b).

2) Previous cited concerns about unrestricted visiting hours that have not been supported through research (AACN, 2016b).
   a) Physiologic stress for the patient
   b) Barriers to the provision of care
   c) Exhaustion of family and friends
   d) Increased risk of infection
3) Benefits of flexible visitation for the patient include the following (AACN, 2016b):
   a) Decreased anxiety
   b) Decreased confusion and agitation
   c) Reduced cardiovascular complications
   d) Decreased length of stay in the critical care unit
   e) Improved feelings of security
   f) Increased satisfaction
   g) Increased quality and safety
4) Benefits of flexible visitation for the family include the following (AACN, 2016b):
   a) Increased satisfaction
   b) Decreased anxiety
   c) Improved communication
   d) Improved understanding of the patient
   e) More opportunities for participation in care
5) Facilitate unrestricted access of the critical care patient to the chosen support person(s). Establish and implement liberal visitation policies.
i. Explain to the family if visitation is interrupted or postponed by a procedure or crisis.
j. Warn the family and explain the reason for a patient's unusual behavior (e.g., confusion).
k. Encourage family members to talk to and touch the patient, hold the patient's hand, and express their feelings.
l. Involve the family in decision making to include participation in interdisciplinary team rounds (Davidson et al., 2016).
m. Encourage family participation in care if they desire.
n. Respect the cultural beliefs and rituals of the family; accommodate these beliefs and rituals if at all possible.
o. Encourage family members to take care of their own basic needs (eating, sleeping, and attending to hygiene).
p. Provide a comfortable area for visitors, close to the unit, with bathroom facilities and a telephone; have private area available for family meetings and family–physician discussion.
q. Encourage participation in a support group if available.
r. Be empathetic; empathy is a "special emotion that comes as the result of a close identification and connection with another person" (Dracup & Bryan-Brown, 1999).

7. Family presence for invasive procedures and resuscitation interventions
   a. Policies should be developed and implemented that allow family members to have the option to be present at the bedside for procedures and resuscitation if the patient wishes (AACN, 2016a).
   b. Benefits
      1) Less anxiety about what is happening to the patient
      2) More likely to believe that everything possible was being done
      3) Greater ability to provide emotional support to the patient
      4) Studies have shown that almost all family members would be present again if a similar event were to occur, and patients reported feeling comfort and support because the family member(s) were present.
   c. Commonly stated concerns that have *not* been demonstrated in research studies on the subjects
      1) Disruption in the delivery of emergency care
      2) Adverse psychological effects to the family
   d. Role of family facilitator is recommended (Mangurten et al., 2005).
      1) Prepares the family and explains that patient care is the priority
      2) Provides the family with personal protective equipment if appropriate
      3) Escorts family members (maximum of two) to the bedside and remains with the family to provide comfort measures, facilitate seeing, touching, and talking to the patient, and provide opportunities for asking questions
      4) Escorts family members from the room if they become ill, disruptive, or overwhelmed
      5) Provides debriefing, comfort, and answers to questions after medical procedures or resuscitation

8. Guidelines for giving bad news
   a. Present information clearly; ask if there are any questions.
   b. Avoid euphemisms such as "passed" because they may be misunderstood; also avoid platitudes such as "he's better off now."
   c. Be silent if you don't know what to say; offer your presence.
   d. Offer to call the family's pastor, priest, rabbi, or other religious leader; honor the family's cultural and religious beliefs.
   e. Monitor the family for any physical complaints because stress may cause exacerbation of any preexisting condition.
   f. Provide privacy for saying goodbye and assist as the family packs the deceased's belongings; explain what to expect so they will not be surprised.
   g. If the patient is a candidate to be an organ donor, work with the organ donation coordinator to discuss donation and organ procurement with the family.

9. Guidelines for giving bad news by phone
   a. Ask for the closest family member by name.
   b. Introduce yourself: name, title, and hospital.
   c. Inform the closest family member of the incident that caused the patient to be brought to the hospital or of a change in status if the patient has been in the hospital.
   d. Ask if the family member can come to the hospital; suggest that he or she come to the hospital with another relative or friend if possible.

e. Avoid telling the family by phone that the patient has died but tell the truth if they ask; if the family lives a long distance from the hospital, they need to be informed of the death by phone, preferably by the physician, but it may be the responsibility of the nurse in some situations.
   f. If the patient is a candidate to be an organ donor, work with the organ donation coordinator to discuss donation and organ procurement with the family.

Collaboration

Description
Working with others in a way that promotes and encourages each person's contributions toward achieving optimal and realistic patient and family goals; collaboration involves intradisciplinary and interdisciplinary work with colleagues and community (AACN, 2016d).

Definitions
1. Collaboration: working together
   a. Attributes of an effective team (Yoder-Wise, 2011)
      1) Working environment: informal, comfortable, and relaxed
      2) Discussion: focused and shared by almost everyone
      3) Objectives: well understood and accepted
      4) Listening: respectful, facilitation of participation
      5) Ability to handle conflict: comfortable with disagreement, open discussion of conflicts
      6) Decision making: usually reached by consensus, general agreement necessary for action; dissenters free to voice opinions
      7) Criticism: frequent, frank, and constructive
      8) Leadership: shared; changes from time to time
      9) Assignments: clearly stated, accepted by all despite disagreements
      10) Feelings: freely expressed and open for discussion
      11) Self-regulation: frequent and ongoing, focused on solutions
   b. Basic rules to create synergy (Yoder-Wise, 2011)
      1) Establish a clear purpose
      2) Listen actively
      3) Be compassionate
      4) Tell the truth
      5) Be flexible
      6) Commit to resolution
2. Collaborative practice: when members of the medical and nursing professions, together with members of other related health care disciplines, work together to assure quality patient and family care; includes the following critical aspects
   a. Sharing in planning, decision making, problem solving, goal setting, and responsibility
   b. Communicating openly and respectfully
   c. Coordinating
   d. Cooperating
   e. Recognizing and accepting of separate and interrelated spheres of practice
3. Consultation: process of seeking, giving, and receiving help; may be formal (written) or informal (verbal)

Essential Elements of Collaboration
1. Communication
2. Trust
3. Respect
4. Understanding and acceptance of team members' roles
5. Competence
6. Shared responsibility and accountability
7. Shared goal setting
8. Flexibility
9. Administrative support

Components of Collaborative Practice
1. Unit co-directors: a physician and a nurse
2. Collaborative practice committee
3. Primary nurse and primary physician
4. Autonomy for clinical decision making
5. Integrated patient records
6. Multidisciplinary review of care

Blocks to Collaboration
1. Nurses and physicians
   a. Authoritative (sometimes aggressive) physicians
   b. Nonassertive (sometimes submissive) nurses
   c. Team members satisfied with traditional hierarchy
2. Misunderstanding or lack of understanding regarding the role and practice of professional nursing
   a. Nurses have their own license; they do not practice under the license of the physician.
   b. Physicians cannot discipline or fire nurses employed by the hospital.
   c. Nursing is not medicine; these are two separate and interrelated professions. If an umbrella term is needed, let it be *health care*, not *medicine*.
   d. Nurses have independent functions as well as dependent functions; they can perform these independent functions without a physician's prescription.
   e. Nursing research has established a unique body of scientific knowledge.
   f. Nursing practice is controlled by nurses through state nurse practice acts, not by physicians.
3. Ineffective or lack of communication between the professions
4. Lack of administrative support
5. Systems issues

Strategies for Improving Collaboration
1. Evaluate current interdisciplinary relationships in your institution and on your unit.
   a. Are team members sought out for communication about the patient?
   b. Is communication peer to peer?
   c. Is there recognition of each team member's role in enhancing patient outcomes?
   d. Are team members willing to accept responsibility and accountability for patient outcomes?
   e. What are the steps taken when conflicts arise between team members?
2. Establish a multidisciplinary critical care committee co-chaired by a nurse and a physician.
   a. Disciplines have equal representation and decision making.

b. The committee should handle issues related to practice, communication, and improving effectiveness or efficiency of clinical care.
3. Establish multidisciplinary professional activities such as the following:
    a. Rounds
    b. Patient records
    c. Orientation
    d. Education programs
    e. Quality and safety programs
    f. Task forces for problem resolution
    g. Research
4. Establish a professional nursing environment.
    a. Assurance of competency
    b. Knowledge of and ability to articulate the unique role of nursing
    c. Encouragement of professional development of nursing staff
5. Implement fundamentals of TeamSTEPPS(r) 2.0 (AHRQ, 2016).
    a. Team structure: patient is the focus; collaborative teams are developed with focus of patient needs. The team includes the patient, family, physicians, nurses, ancillary staff, and so on.
    b. Communication: effective communication is vital for patient safety. Standards of effective communication are that it is complete, clear, brief, and timely.
        1) Use tools such as SBAR to ensure effective, clear transmission of information.
        2) Call-outs are used to communicate critical information.
        3) Check-back is a form of closed-loop communication that ensures information is heard and understood by receiver.
        4) Handoff communication is essential during care transitions. Offers opportunities to ask questions, clarify, and confirm. I PASS the BATON is one tool that may be used.
        5) Leading teams: Leadership is essential for holding a system based upon teamwork together. There are usually both formal and informal leaders, but it is imperative that the leader of the team is clearly identified.
        6) Situation monitoring using the STEP mnemonic:
            Status of patient
            Team members
            Environment
            Progress toward the goal
        7) Mutual support involves team members assisting each other, providing feedback, and assuring safety of the patient through advocacy and assertive behaviors.
            i. Characteristics of effective feedback include that it is timely, respectful, specific, directed toward improvement, and it is considerate.
            ii. When patient safety is compromised (or potentially compromised), any team member can implement the two-challenge rule. Assertive statements include the CUS words (C—I am concerned; U—I am uncomfortable; S—this is a Safety issue).

Communication

1. Types of communication
    a. Spoken
    b. Nonverbal
    c. Symbolic gestures
    d. Written words
    e. Visual images
    f. Multimedia
2. Rules for good communication
    a. Be clear in your mind as to what you want to communicate.
    b. Deliver the message as succinctly as possible.
    c. Ensure that the message has been clearly and correctly understood; ask for feedback.
3. Pitfalls (Yoder-Wise, 2011)
    a. Advice giving
    b. Making others wrong
    c. Defensiveness
    d. Judging the other person
    e. Patronizing
    f. Giving false reassurance
    g. Asking "why" questions
    h. Blaming others

Conflict Resolution

1. Types of conflict (Yoder-Wise, 2011)
    a. Intrapersonal: within a person
    b. Intergroup: between two or more groups
    c. Interpersonal: between two or more people
2. The conflict process
    a. Frustration
    b. Conceptualization
    c. Action
    d. Outcomes
3. Common strategies
    a. Avoiding: parties involved in the conflict do not acknowledge it or try to resolve it.
    b. Cooperating: one party sacrifices and allows the other party to win.
    c. Smoothing: another person calms the parties involved in the conflict.
    d. Competing or coercing: one party pursues what it wants at the expense of the other party.
    e. Negotiating or compromising: each party gives up something it wants.
    f. Collaborating: all parties set aside their original goals and work together to establish a common goal.
4. Guidelines for dealing with interpersonal conflict
    a. Communicate with the angry person.
    b. Identify common goals (e.g., quality patient care).
    c. Discuss only one issue at a time; don't bring up old issues and anger.
    d. Discuss facts, not opinions, judgments, or what others are saying; don't make personal attacks.
    e. Communicate with the person involved; do not engage others in the conflict or jump to a higher organizational level.

Delegation

1. Definition: "achieving performance of care outcomes for which you are accountable and responsible by sharing activities with other individuals who have the appropriate authority to accomplish the work" (Yoder-Wise, 2011)
    a. Direct delegation: the delegation is the result of the registered nurse (RN) actively deciding what to delegate.
    b. Indirect delegation: the decision to delegate is the result of organizational protocols that designate specific tasks as appropriate for another to perform.
2. Process (ANA & National Council of State Boards of Nursing [NCSBN], 2006)
    a. Assess and plan the delegation based on the patient needs and available resources.
    b. Communicate directions to the delegate, including any unique patient requirements and characteristics as well as clear expectations regarding what to do, what to report, and when to ask for assistance.
    c. Surveillance and supervision of the delegation, including the level of supervision needed, implementation, and follow-up to problems or a changing situation
    d. Evaluation and feedback to consider the effectiveness of the delegation, including any need to adjust the plan of care
3. The five rights of delegation (ANA & NCSBN, 2006)
    a. The right task
    b. Under the right circumstances
    c. To the right person
    d. With the right directions and communication
    e. Under the right supervision and evaluation
4. Delegation to unlicensed assistive personnel (ANA, 2012)
    a. Recognize what may not be delegated.
        1) Initial and subsequent nursing assessments requiring the professional judgment of a registered nurse
        2) Determination of nursing diagnoses, care goals, care plans, and progress
        3) Interventions that require the knowledge and skill of a registered nurse
    b. Be aware of the job description, skills, and knowledge of the individual.
    c. Never delegate any task that requires the skill or knowledge of a registered nurse.

Systems Thinking

Description
The body of knowledge and tools that allow the nurse to appreciate the care environment from a perspective that recognizes the holistic interrelationship that exists within and across health care and non–health care systems (AACN, 2016d). Systems thinking is a way of "viewing the world by looking at the structures, patterns, and events of an issue rather than just the issue itself" (Hardin & Kaplow, 2017).

System
1. Definition: "A collection of interdependent elements that interact to achieve a common purpose" (Nolan, 1998)
2. Nursing is one aspect of patient care; nurses must work together with other members of the health care team and understand the organizational structure of the institution.
3. AACN (2016c) is committed to fostering work and care environments that are "safe, healing, humane, and respectful of the rights, responsibilities, needs, and contributions of all people—including patients, their families, nurses, and other healthcare professionals." The standards for establishing and sustaining health work environments are as follows:
    a. "Nurses must be as proficient in communication skills as they are in clinical skills."
    b. "Nurses must be relentless in pursuing and fostering true collaboration."
    c. "Nurses must be valued and committed partners in making policy, directing and evaluating clinical care, and leading organizational operations."
    d. "Staffing must ensure the effective match between patient needs and nurse competencies."
    e. "Nurses must be recognized and must recognize others for the value each brings to the work of the organization."
    f. "Nurse leaders must fully embrace the imperative of a healthy work environment, authentically live it, and engage others in its achievement" (AACN, 2016c).

Types of Organizational Structure
1. Bureaucracy: formal, centralized, hierarchical
    a. Rules, policies, and procedures ensure consistency and promote efficiency and productivity.
    b. Communication and decisions flow from top to bottom with limited employee autonomy.
2. Flat: less formal and hierarchical than bureaucratic organizations
    a. Fewer rules and policies than bureaucratic organizations
    b. Provides authority to make decisions at the point of interaction with the client
3. Matrix: focus on product and function
    a. Hybrid of bureaucratic and flat structures
    b. Sometimes referred to as product line management
4. Self-governance: organizational structure that allows the staff to govern themselves
    a. Sometimes referred to as *professional practice models*
    b. Authority, responsibility, and accountability belong to the nurse delivering care.
5. Shared-governance: organizational structure with governance shared by staff and management

Patient Care Delivery Systems
1. The AACN Synergy Model for Patient Care is a professional model that provides a foundation for designing patient care delivery models for health care organizations.
    a. The Synergy Model emphasizes matching patient characteristics or needs with nurse competencies.
    b. When this synergy is achieved, a healthy environment is created, patient outcomes are optimized, and staff satisfaction is achieved (Hardin & Kaplow, 2017).
2. Commonly applied patient care delivery systems (Table 2.3)

Change Process
1. Change is one constant in health care organizations.
2. Types of change
    a. Unplanned: reactive process to change that was not planned

Table 2.3 Patient Care Delivery Systems

	Functional Nursing	Team Nursing	Primary Nursing	Total Patient Care
Description	Task oriented; nurses perform tasks (e.g., charge, medicine, treatments) as assigned	Group oriented; team leader (RN) with team members deliver care to a group of patients	Patient oriented; nurse is responsible for all aspects of care for assigned patients; accountable for care delivered during entire hospitalization	As for Primary Nursing except that the nurse is accountable for care delivered during the entire shift
Advantages	• Cost effective • Each person becomes efficient at specific tasks	• Cost effective • Increased staff satisfaction	• Increased staff satisfaction, although nurses may be dissatisfied with the number of non-nursing tasks that do not require their degree of skill and knowledge • Improved quality of care • Improved continuity of care in primary nursing	
Disadvantages	• Fragmented nursing care • Diminished continuity of care • Diminished staff satisfaction	• Diminished continuity of care • Team leader must have leadership skills, especially effective delegation skills	• Efficacy questionable because an RN is very expensive and is performing tasks that do not require the skill and knowledge of an RN; use of unlicensed assistive personnel to perform non-nursing tasks increases efficacy • Restricted opportunity for evening and night shift nurses to be assigned as "primary nurse"	

    b. Planned: active process with predetermined goals; intentional, thought-out, mutual goal setting, equal power distribution; there are many models of planned change (Table 2.4)
3. The change agent: the person who works to bring about the change
    a. Key qualities of effective change agents
        1) Excellent communication skills
        2) Observational skills to monitor change
        3) Knowledge of group dynamics
        4) Perceptive nature about political issues
        5) Supportive attitude toward change participants
        6) Ability to establish trusting relationships
    b. Tips for leading change (Kotter, 1995)
        1) Involve all stakeholders in the process of planning for the change.
        2) Share the vision and create goals.
        3) Select a change model; different models work better for different change processes.
        4) Identify champions among each of the major groups of stakeholders.
        5) Identify facilitators and barriers and adjust your plan accordingly.
        6) Create a detailed plan but be flexible.

Response to Diversity

Description
The "sensitivity to recognize, appreciate, and incorporate differences into the provision of care; differences may include, but are not limited to cultural differences, spiritual beliefs, gender, race, ethnicity, lifestyle, socioeconomic status, age, and values" (AACN, 2016d)

Cultural Diversity
1. Definitions
    a. Diversity: differences that make each person unique; includes national origin, religion, age, gender, sexual orientation, race, ethnicity, education, socioeconomic status, and abilities and disabilities
    b. Culture: the learned, shared, and transmitted values, beliefs, and practices of a particular group that guide thinking, actions, behaviors, interactions with others, emotional reactions to daily living, and one's world view; subculture: a recognizable segment of a larger cultural group that shares some characteristics of the larger group but with unique features of its own
    c. Cultural sensitivity: a learned skill in which a person has an awareness of and appreciation for another's cultural uniqueness; also referred to as ethnosensitivity
    d. Cultural competence: "a set of congruent behaviors, attitudes, and policies that come together in a system, agency, or among professionals that enables effective work in cross-cultural situations" (Health Resources and Services Administration, 2016)
    e. Culturally congruent nursing care: use of cognitively based nursing techniques that incorporate an individual's cultural values, beliefs, and lifeway; these techniques facilitate, assist, support, and enable an individual toward health and well-being or to face illness or death in culturally meaningful ways
    f. Race: a group of people related by common descent of heredity who have similar physical characteristics such as skin color, facial form, and eye shape
    g. Ethnic group: subset of culture; a smaller group that identifies itself as distinct because of shared characteristics, such as culture, language, traditions, appearance, and social heritage
    h. Nationality: a people from a place with specified political and geographic boundaries
    i. Customs: patterns and practices within a cultural group that encompass collective learned behaviors (includes diet and health behaviors)
    j. Rituals: culturally prescribed codes of behavior (may guide practices and decisions including health and wellness)

Table 2.4 Selected Models for Planned Change	
Author (Year): Model	Steps in the Planned Change Process
Lewin (1951): Model of Change	• Status quo (diagnose the problem) • Unfreezing (develop the solutions) • Disequilibrium (overcome resistance) • Moving (implement change) • Refreezing (reestablish balance) • Equilibrium
Lippitt, Watson, & Westley (1958): Seven Phases of Planned Change	• Aware of the need for change • Development of a relationship between client system and change agent • Definition of the change problem • Establishment of change goals and exploration of options for achievement • Implementation of the plan for change • Acceptance and stabilization of the change • Redefinition of the relationships of the change entities
Havelock (1973): Six Phases of Planned Change	• Building a relationship • Diagnosing the problem • Acquiring relevant resources • Choosing the solution • Gaining acceptance • Stabilizing the innovation and generating self-renewal
Rogers (1995): Diffusion of Innovation Model	• Knowledge • Persuasion • Decision • Implementation • Confirmation
Prochaska (2000) and Prochaska, Prochaska, & Levesque, (2001): Transtheoretical Model	• Precontemplation: the individual is not thinking of change. • Contemplation: the individual is thinking of but not committed to change in the near future. • Preparation: the individual intends to change in the near future. • Action: the individual actively attempts to change. • Maintenance: the individual sustains the change over time.
Kotter (1995): Process for Leading Change	• Establish a sense of urgency • Form a powerful guiding coalition • Create a vision • Communicate the vision • Empower others to act on the vision • Plan for and create short-term wins • Consolidate improvements and produce still more change • Institutionalize new approaches
Berwick (2003): From Description to Prescription	• Find sound innovations • Find and support innovators • Invest in early adopters • Make early adopter activity observable • Trust and enable reinvention • Create slack for change • Lead by change

k. Values: personal standards of what is good or useful in relationship to oneself and to others

l. Norms: commonly shared customs and standards of behavior that are acceptable within a given group of people

m. Cultural paradigms: abstract explanation used by a cultural group to account for major life events

n. Enculturation: the process by which culture is transmitted from one generation to the next by means of social learning

o. Acculturation: the process by which an individual or group takes on the behaviors and practices of the dominant culture; factors that influence the degree and pace of an individual's acculturation include length of time in the new culture, age, economic and educational status, and discriminatory practices of the dominant culture

p. Ethnocentrism: the belief that one's own ethnic group, way of life, beliefs, and values are superior to those of others

q. Cultural imposition: the practice of imposing one's cultural beliefs on others with the belief that they are best or superior

r. Cultural relativism: the attitude that the differences in ways of doing things hold equal validity

s. Cultural pain: the discomfort and suffering experienced by an individual or group resulting from the insensitivity of others who have different beliefs or cultural norms

2. Significance
  a. Of the developed countries in the world, the United States has the greatest increase in population and diversity of inhabitants; immigration accounts for at least one third of the increase.
    1) The percentage of whites of European origin (the dominant culture in the United States) will continue to decline, creating a more multicultural power base.
    2) U.S. Census Bureau population projections indicate that by 2030, one in five Americans will be older than the age of 65 years; that non-Hispanic whites will no longer compose the majority of the population in 2044; and that by 2060, nearly one in five Americans will be foreign born (U.S. Census Bureau, 2014).
  b. Nurses must be aware that issues of culture, race, gender, and socioeconomics strongly influence health status and utilization of the health care system.
    1) Culturally insensitive or inappropriate care and inattention to cultural differences in care may negatively affect health outcomes.
    2) Individuals from different cultures and illegal immigrants often delay seeking medical attention because of language, cost, and cultural barriers; these delays often result in more serious conditions.
  c. Health care reform is resulting in cultural competence guidelines and enforcement by state agencies.

3. Aspects of cultural sensitivity
  a. Acknowledgment that cultural diversity exists
  b. Avoidance of stereotypes with appreciation of the uniqueness of each patient, with culture as one aspect that enhances uniqueness

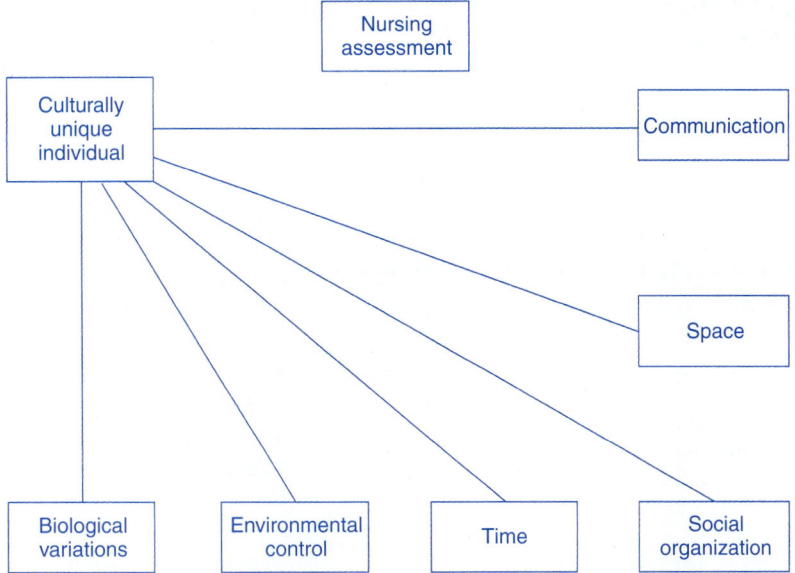

Fig. 2.3 Application of cultural phenomena to nursing care and nursing practice. (From Giger, J. [2013]. *Transcultural nursing: Assessment and intervention* [6th ed.]. St. Louis: Mosby.)

    c. Respect of the unfamiliar
    d. Appreciation that cultural values are ingrained and difficult to change
    e. Modification of care to include consistency with the patient's culture
    f. Examination of personal cultural beliefs and values
    g. Realization that the patient's health practices may be very different from yours but that each cultural group has health practices that attempt to improve health and temper illness
    h. Recognition that all people within a cultural group do not respond to illness the same; there is diversity within cultures
4. Cultural assessment
    a. Assess the degree of acculturation (e.g., how well language of the dominant culture is spoken, language spoken in the home, length of time in country, food preferences).
    b. Encourage the patient to discuss cultural beliefs and practices; definitions of health and illness and the origin of illnesses may differ within cultures.
    c. Make efforts to respect and understand different communication styles.
    d. Honor time and value orientation.
    e. Provide privacy according to individual needs; be aware that in many cultures, it is extremely important for family members to be present during assessments.
    f. Identify the decision maker within families; it may be someone other than the patient.
    g. Recognize that patients' reactions to pain are sometimes culturally driven.
    h. Be aware of biological variations among cultures, such as body structure, skin and hair color, population-specific diseases, and psychological coping characteristics.
    i. Recognize that dietary and religious practices and cultural taboos have important implications related to nursing care.
    j. Identify hobbies.
    k. Note cultural practices and modify care as necessary.
5. Cultural phenomena impacting nursing care (Fig. 2.3 and Table 2.5)
6. Cultural aspects of pain
    a. Pain is not purely a neurophysiologic response; cultural, social, and psychological denominators influence pain.
    b. Pain intensity, expression, tolerance, and expected responses from caretakers are influenced by culture.
    c. A patient's attitude and beliefs about pain are determined by culture.
    d. Each culture has its own language of distress.
        1) Facial expressions
        2) Sounds
        3) Changes in activity
        4) Words to describe feelings
    e. Nurses must always remember that regardless of the patient's cultural background, pain is what the patient says it is and it occurs when he or she says it does.
        1) All pain should be considered "real" and treated compassionately.
        2) Be aware that patients who do not verbally express the presence of pain may not be pain free.
7. Drug polymorphism
    a. Age, drug, gender, body size, and body composition affect individual responses to drugs.
    b. Factors that influence drug polymorphism vary among ethnic groups and can be categorized as environmental, genetic, and cultural; these do not include all the aspects that affect a patient's response to drugs but raise awareness regarding possible differences in response.

Table 2.5 Cultural Phenomena Affecting Nursing Care

Nations of Origin	Communication	Space	Time Orientation	Social Organization	Environmental Control	Biological Variation
Asian • China • Hawaii • Philippines • Korea • Japan • Southeast Asia (Laos, Cambodia, Vietnam)	• National language preference • Dialects, written characters • Use of silence • Nonverbal and contextual cuing	• Noncontact people	• Present	• Family: hierarchical structure, loyalty • Devotion to tradition • Many religions, including Taoism, Buddhism, Islam, and Christianity • Community social organizations	• Traditional health and illness beliefs • Use of traditional medicines • Traditional practitioners: Chinese doctors and herbalists	• Liver cancer • Stomach cancer • Coccidioidomycosis • Hypertension • Lactose intolerance
African • West Coast (as slaves) • Many African countries • West Indian Islands • Dominican Republic • Haiti • Jamaica	• National languages • Dialect: pidgin, Creole, Spanish, and French	• Close personal space	• Present over future	• Family: many female, single parent • Large, extended family networks • Strong church affiliation within community • Community social organizations	• Traditional health and illness beliefs • Folk medicine tradition • Traditional healer: root-worker	• Sickle cell anemia • Hypertension • Cancer of the esophagus • Stomach cancer • Coccidioidomycosis • Lactose intolerance
Europe • Germany • England • Italy • Ireland • Other European countries	• National languages • Many learn English immediately	• Noncontact people • Aloof • Distant • Southern countries: closer contact and touch	• Future over present	• Nuclear families • Extended families • Judeo-Christian religions • Community social organizations	• Primary reliance on modern health care system • Traditional health and illness beliefs • Some remaining folk medicine traditions	• Breast cancer • Heart disease • Diabetes mellitus • Thalassemia
Native American • 500 Native American tribes • Aleuts • Eskimos	• Tribal languages • Use of silence and body language	• Space very important and has no boundaries	• Present • Community social organizations	• Extremely family oriented • Biological and extended families • Children taught to respect traditions	• Traditional health and illness beliefs • Folk medicine tradition • Traditional healer: medicine man	• Accidents • Heart disease • Cirrhosis of the liver • Diabetes mellitus
Hispanic countries • Spain • Cuba • Mexico • Central and South America	• Spanish or Portuguese primary language	• Tactile relationships • Touch • Handshakes • Embracing • Value physical presence	• Present	• Nuclear family • Extended families • *Compadrazgo* (godparents) • Community social organizations	• Traditional health and illness beliefs • Folk medicine tradition • Traditional healers: *curandero, espiritisco, portera, senoro*	• Diabetes mellitus • Parasites • Coccidioidomycosis • Lactose intolerance

Compiled by Rachel Spector, RN, PhD, from Davidhizer, R., & Giger, J. (1999). *Transcultural nursing: Assessment and intervention* (3rd ed.). St. Louis: Mosby.

c. Drug metabolism is genetically determined.
   d. Race may affect response; also called *genetic polymorphism*
   e. Environmental factors include diet, alcohol, smoking, malnutrition, vitamin deficiencies, stress, fever, and physiologic rhythms; each of these can affect drug absorption.
   f. Cultural factors include values, beliefs, compliance, family influence, and prior drug experience; patients may be taking herbal or homeopathic remedies that can alter response to drug absorption.
   g. Nurses must become familiar with drugs that affect patients of different ethnicity.
8. Cultural behaviors relevant to nursing care (Table 2.6)
   a. Respect and embrace diversity among the patient and health care team members.
   b. Have a cultural reference available on your unit.
   c. Have a list of employees who speak another language and are willing to assist with translation and how to contact them.
9. Problems in providing culturally congruent health care; all of the following issues can lead to poor health outcomes:
   a. Stereotyping, prejudice, ignoring blind spots, and labeling
   b. Personal biases and bigotry
   c. Cultural differences, patients being labeled by nurses as "the difficult patient and/or family"
   d. Lack of interpreters and educational materials in patient's language
   e. Lack of diversity among nursing staff
   f. Lack of time (with culturally congruent care, listening to stories is important)
   g. Lack of flexibility with teaching methods

Table 2.6 Cultural Behaviors Relevant to Nursing Care

Cultural Group	Cultural Variations (Common Belief or Practice)	Nursing Implications
African Americans	• Dialect and slang terms require careful communication to prevent errors (e.g., "bad" may mean "good").	• Question the client's meaning or intent.
Mexican Americans	• Eye behavior is important. An individual who looks at and admires a child without touching the child has given the child the "evil eye."	• Always touch the child you are examining or admiring.
American Indians	• Eye contact is considered a sign of disrespect and is thus avoided.	• Recognize that the client may be attentive and interested even though eye contact is avoided.
Appalachians	• Eye contact is considered impolite or a sign of hostility. • Verbal patter may be confusing.	• Clarify statements.
American Eskimos	• Body language is important. • The individual seldom disagrees publicly with others. • Client may nod yes to be polite even if not in agreement.	• Monitor own body language closely, as well as client's, to detect meaning.
Jewish Americans	• Orthodox Jews consider excess touching, particularly from members of the opposite sex, offensive.	• Establish whether client is an Orthodox Jew and, if so, avoid excessive touch.
Chinese Americans	• Individual may nod head to indicate yes or shake head to indicate no. • Excessive eye contact indicates rudeness. • Excessive touch is offensive.	• Ask questions carefully and clarify responses. • Avoid excessive eye contact and touch.
Filipino Americans	• Offending people is to be avoided at all cost. • Nonverbal behavior is important.	• Monitor nonverbal behaviors of self and client, being sensitive to physical and emotional discomfort or concerns of the client.
Haitian Americans	• Touch is used in conversation. • Direct eye contact is used to gain attention and respect during communication.	• Use direct eye contact when communicating.
East Indian Hindu Americans	• Be aware that men may view eye contact by women as offensive. • Avoid eye contact.	• Women avoid eye contact as a sign of respect.
Vietnamese Americans	• Avoidance of eye contact is a sign of respect. • The head is considered sacred; it is not polite to pat the head. • An upturned palm is offensive in communication.	• Limit eye contact. • Touch the head only when mandated and explain clearly before proceeding to do so. • Avoid hand gesturing.

From Giger, J. (2013). *Transcultural nursing: Assessment and intervention* (6th ed.). St. Louis: Mosby.

Religious Diversity

1. Definitions
   a. Spirituality: a basic human phenomenon that helps create meaning in the world
      1) Encompasses a person's ideology, view of the world, and meaning of life
      2) Gives an individual a sense of inner peace and harmony
   b. Spiritual distress: disruption in the life principle that pervades a person's entire being and integrates and transcends one's biological and psychosocial nature
   c. Religion: a specific unified system of an expression of the belief in and reverence for a supernatural power accepted as the creator and governor of the universe
   d. Religious symbols: symbols used in the expression of faith (e.g., rosary, prayer cloth, prayer rug, medicine bundles, red ribbon, charms, "the garment")
   e. Meditation: a devotional exercise of contemplation
   f. Prayer: an intimate conversation between an individual and God or other higher being
   g. Hope: to wish for something with expectation of its fulfillment
   h. Faith: confident belief in the truth of a person, idea, or thing (e.g., God); belief not based on logical proof or material evidence
2. Significance
   a. Exclusion of the important role of spirituality for patients and families can impact on recovery and health.
   b. Care of the whole person enhances healing and health.
   c. Spiritual beliefs of providers may be an important consideration for many patients when selecting a health care provider.
3. Causes of spiritual distress
   a. Separation from religious and cultural ties
   b. Challenged belief and value systems
   c. Sense of meaninglessness or purposelessness
   d. Remoteness from God
   e. Disrupted spiritual trust
   f. Moral or ethical nature of therapy
   g. Sense of guilt and shame
   h. Intense suffering
   i. Unresolved feelings about death
   j. Anger toward God
4. Aspects of spiritual sensitivity include the following:
   a. Perform exploration of your own values and beliefs.
   b. Acknowledge that you may not agree with every aspect of the patient's spiritual beliefs and practices; be nonjudgmental and respect the patient's right to worship the Supreme Being of his or her choice.
   c. Develop good listening skills; encourage patient to discuss spiritual concerns.
   d. Know your limits; if you are uncomfortable discussing spiritual needs with a patient or praying with a patient, contact the patient's personal spiritual advisor or consult the hospital chaplain service as requested by the patient or family.
   e. Schedule physical care to allow religious rituals and practices.
   f. Respect the patient's rights and privacy.
   g. Increase your knowledge regarding different faiths. (Table 2.7 identifies selected faiths and nursing implications.)
5. Perform spiritual needs assessment.
   a. Assess the patient's spiritual or religious beliefs, values, and practices.

Table 2.7 Religious Beliefs of Selected Religions and Appropriate Nursing Interventions

Religion	Belief	Interventions
Catholicism	• God does not cause suffering but allows it for furthering human growth. • Baptism is necessary for salvation.	• Inform patient that Holy Communion is available. • Have Catholic priest or deacon available to perform Anointing of the Sick. • If patient is close to death and a Catholic religious representative is not available, any Christian may perform the baptism and then notify the priest immediately. • Make all efforts to leave religious symbols (e.g., rosary) in place.
Christian Scientist	• Sin, sickness, and death can be overcome by a full understanding of the divine principle of Jesus' teaching and healing. • Disease and illness is a delusion of the nonspiritual mind and can be overcome by prayer.	• Be aware that medical care may be refused. • May use the services of physicians for the purpose of setting bones, treatment of malignancies, and delivering babies. • Pain medications may be accepted for severe pain only. • There is no clergy or priesthood.
Hinduism	• Illness may result from misuse of the body or sins from a previous lifetime. • Meditation and prayer must be done at specific times throughout the day. • Females cannot be left in the presence of unfamiliar males.	• Plan care around religious practices. • Provide same-sex caregivers. • Provide vegetarians meals as requested. • May refuse medication by capsule because many capsules are made from beef. • Allow the family to wash the family member's body after death if desired; do not remove any sacred threads that are placed on the body.

Continued

Table 2.7	Religious Beliefs of Selected Religions and Appropriate Nursing Interventions—cont'd	
Religion	**Belief**	**Interventions**
Islam (Muslim)	• Submit to Allah's will in matters of health. • Prayer and washing required five times a day. • The left hand is considered unclean; food will not be handled with the left hand.	• Provide privacy and plan care to accommodate prayer times. • Educate regarding pain-reducing techniques. • Provide diet with dietary restrictions as requested. • Pork and some other foods are prohibited. • May refuse to take capsules because many are made from pork. • Follow patient and family wishes regarding therapies; prolonging life by life-support machinery is often seen as unacceptable. • Allow family to stay with relative during process of dying. • Allow to wash body after death. • Turn deceased person's face toward the right.
Jehovah's Witness	• Opposed to transfusions of blood obtained from a blood bank and some blood products (the source of the soul is believed to be in the blood) • Opposed to eating foods to which blood has been added • Do not celebrate national holidays (including Christmas), birthdays, or salute flags; it is believed that violators will spend an eternity in nothingness.	• Assess the patient's religious beliefs and practices before administering blood or blood products. • Most Witnesses carry cards indicating types of acceptable transfusions. • "Mature minors," according to Jehovah's Witness standards, may refuse blood transfusions. • Be aware that the patient may refuse surgical or medical interventions that will require blood transfusion. • Consider the use of volume expanders such as saline, lactated Ringer's solution, hetastarch (Hespan). • Implement blood-conservation strategies, especially in children. • Consult hematologist or medical centers familiar with bloodless medicine and surgery management, if needed. • Respect patient and family decisions to refuse blood products. • Avoid foods to which blood has been added (e.g., certain sausages, lunch meats). • Avoid attempts to involve the patient in preparations for celebrations of national holidays.
Judaism	• Sabbath begins at sundown on Friday and ends at sundown on Saturday. • There is hope for recovery until death is imminent. • May not eat nonkosher foods. • Orthodox Jews: work of any kind is prohibited on the Sabbath, including driving or using the telephone. • Orthodox Jews: prayer is required three times a day. • A person must stay with a critically ill or dying family member until death so that the soul will not feel alone.	• Provide kosher diet as requested. • Provide privacy and plan care considering prayer times. • Allow a relative to stay with the dying patient. • Notify rabbi or rebbe according to family's wishes. • Caregivers should leave the body untouched for approximately a half hour after death to allow the soul to depart. • After death, by Judaic law, the body cannot be left alone. • Autopsies generally are not allowed unless required by law. • Assist and respect practices of the Sabbath. • Do not shave body hair of Hasidic Jews. • Hasidic or Orthodox: provide same-sex caregivers.
Seventh-Day Adventist	• Sabbath is recognized as dusk on Friday to dusk on Saturday. • The body is a temple of God and should be kept healthy.	• Provide diet with dietary restrictions as requested. • The church encourages a vegetarian diet. • Be aware that the patient may avoid seafood, meat, caffeine, alcohol, drugs, and tobacco. • Protein and iodine deficiency may occur. • Be aware that the patient may refuse procedures (medical or surgical) that occur on the Sabbath.

b. Listen for verbal cues regarding spirituality (e.g., referring to God or spiritualist, talking about church, prayer, or synagogue)

c. Note the presence of religious symbols (e.g., crucifix; Star of David; Bible, Torah, Qur'an, or other spiritual books; prayer cloth) in room during interview.

d. Listen for expressions of spiritual distress (expressed hopelessness or guilt, crying, sleep disturbances, disrupted spiritual trust, loss of meaning, and purpose in life).

e. Be alert to comments related to spiritual concerns or conflicts (e.g., "Why me God?" or "I'm being punished for my sins").

Table 2.8 Characteristics of Today's Generations

Generation	Born Between	Characteristics
Silent Generation (sometimes called the Veteran Generation): ~10% of today's workforce	1925 and 1942	• Tend to be hard working, thrifty, disciplined • Value tradition • Appreciate conformity, consistency, and uniformity at work and value the system over the individual • Tend to work at large corporations that offer security and reward longevity • Prefer direct orders • Prefer assignments that are structured and task oriented
Baby Boomers: ~45% of today's workforce	1943 and 1960	• Tend to be rebellious and questioning of the status quo • Equate work with self-worth • Are driven and dedicated; willing to work overtime • May be resistant to technology • Prefer facilitation • Prefer assignments that require flexibility, independent thinking, and creativity
Generation X: ~30% of today's workforce	1961 and 1981	• Tend to be ironic, cynical, resourceful • Balance work and leisure time; less likely to work overtime • Are more independent; do not belong to any group • Are comfortable with technology • Embrace diversity • Adapt well to change • Attempt to attain several goals at once • Prefer coaching with feedback and credit for accomplishments • Prefer assignments that allow self-direction
Millennials (sometimes called Nexters or Generation Y): 15% of today's workforce	1982 and 2002	• Tend to be optimistic, assertive, self-confident, friendly • Accept authority and prefer to be led • Are cooperative team players; prefer to work in groups and teams • Have difficulty focusing on one task; prefer to multitask • Are very technology savvy • Prefer collegiality and mentoring • Prefer assignments that challenge and stretch their capabilities

    f. Determine if there are religious or spiritual practices (e.g., communion) that the patient wishes to participate in during hospitalization,

    g. Identify specific religious concerns such as dietary needs or refusal of blood.

6. Provide care that is sensitive to the patient's spiritual or religious needs.
   a. Convey a caring, nonjudgmental attitude.
   b. Inform the patient and family of the availability of spiritual or religious services (e.g., pastoral care, chapel, religious services, religious books, communion, baptism, last rites).
   c. Inform the patient and family of policies related to clergy visitation.
   d. Provide privacy and opportunities for religious practices, such as prayer and meditation.
   e. Prepare the patient for desired religious rituals.
   f. Join in prayer for reading of scripture if comfortable.
      1) If you are comfortable praying with the patient and family, the following suggestions may be helpful:
         a) Trust God or other higher being to enable you to know what to do and what to say.
         b) Really listen to the patient so that you know the patient's and family's greatest concerns.
         c) Explore the spiritual needs of the patient; ask the patient what he or she would like for God or other higher being to do.
         d) Keep prayers realistic (e.g., comfort vs miraculous healing).
         e) Be sensitive and respectful.
         f) Hold the patient's hand or stroke his or her arm, if culturally appropriate.
      2) If you are not comfortable praying with or providing other spiritual support for the patient and family, call the patient's spiritual advisor or a representative of pastoral care to pray with or comfort the patient and family.
   g. Notify the chaplain or patient's spiritual advisor of the patient's spiritual distress (with the patient's permission).
   h. Provide honest information to aid in informed decision making when spiritual beliefs and therapeutic regimens are in conflict.

7. Problems in providing spirituality-sensitive health care
   a. Avoiding or minimizing the role of spirituality in patient healing
   b. Treating religious beliefs as mental illness
   c. Failing to involve patient and family in decision making
   d. Giving information that can lead to false hope
   e. Failing to allow the patient an opportunity to work through grief

Generational Diversity

1. Each generation has a peer personality that lends itself to a collective mindset (Johnson & Romanello, 2005) (Table 2.8).

2. Avoid overgeneralizing; not everyone in each age group fits the description (or every aspect of the description) of the age group.

Barriers to Culturally Competent Healthcare (Purnell, 2014)
1. Language and health literacy
   a. Language barriers may involve both oral and written communication. May result in errors in executing the plan of care, failure to return for follow-up, or leaving against medical advice.
   b. Health literacy is the degree to which "individuals have the capacity to obtain, process, and understand basic health information and services needed to make appropriate health decisions" (HRSA, 2016).
   c. Must assess each patient for their preferred learning method and primary language and provide materials that are appropriate.
   d. Strongly recommended to not use family members as interpreters. Use language lines or staff hired specifically to provide interpreter services.
2. Availability: patients are routinely referred to emergency departments for care after their primary care provider's office is closed, leading to increased cost of care and long wait times. Patients may not have the ability to wait and may defer seeking care if not readily available.
3. Accessibility: lack of transportation to clinics, hospitals, and pharmacies may result in patients not seeking care when needed.
4. Affordability: if patients lack financial resources to obtain care, they may wait until the condition escalates in severity resulting in longer recovery time, hospitalization, and increased cost.
5. Appropriateness: it is important to have services that are congruent with the patient's cultural beliefs and physical requirements. Rural areas may lack availability of the whole spectrum of services patients may require.
6. Organizational accountability: health care providers must seek education and training opportunities about the cultures of the people that they serve. Initial and ongoing training is necessary to ensure cultural competence.
7. Adaptability: the health care system should be fluid and able to adapt to the patient's needs. For example, when a mother brings her child for routine immunizations, can she obtain a routine, screening mammogram at the same time, reducing her lost time from work and improving the overall wellness of the family?
8. Acceptability: are services available in the language preferred by the patient? It is important to match the patient's needs with the resources when possible (i.e., same gender provider is imperative in some cultures).
9. Awareness: is the population aware of the resources provided by the health care organization to the community?
10. Attitudes: health care providers need to acknowledge their own attitudes toward cultural health care practices of their population and work with the patients toward an acceptable mix of traditional practices and modern medicine.
11. Approachability: health care providers and staff must greet patients in a manner that is welcoming and culturally sensitive (i.e., avoiding eye contact in some cultures is a sign of respect).
12. Alternative practices: incorporate nonharmful alternative practices into the overall treatment plan.
13. Additional services are value-added benefits that work toward improving access to health care. For example, childcare services may be required for a parent to attend to her or his own medical needs, and if there is no access to childcare, a parent may defer seeking care.

Clinical Inquiry

Description
The ongoing process of questioning and evaluating practice, providing informed practice, and innovating through research and experiential learning (AACN, 2016d).

Evidence-Based Practice
1. Definition: the integration of the following:
   a. Best evidence
   b. Clinician expertise
   c. Patient values
   d. Circumstances
2. Five-step process for ensuring that clinical decisions are based on best evidence (Straus, Glasziou, Richardson, & Haynes, 2011)
   a. Converting information into clear questions
      1) PICOT format frequently is used (Melnyk & Fineout-Overholt, 2011)
         a) P: problem or population
         b) I: intervention
         c) C: comparison intervention
         d) O: outcome
         e) T: timing
      2) Remember: the best questions come from clinicians.
   b. Seeking evidence to answer those questions
      1) Published research reports
         a) Use search engines such as CINAHL, PubMed/MEDLINE, and Google scholar.
         b) Scour the bibliographies of the studies that you found helpful.
      2) Unpublished research reports
         a) Consult known researchers regarding the issue.
         b) Important because research studies with statistically insignificant results are frequently not published; either the researcher chooses not to publish or the report is rejected for publication (i.e., publication bias)
   c. Evaluating (critically appraising) the evidence for its validity (truthfulness) and usefulness; grading the evidence considers the following:
      1) Quality: the aggregate of quality ratings for individual studies, predicated on the extent to which bias was minimized (i.e., level of evidence)
         a) Study designs
            i) Traditional hierarchy of evidence based on study designs
               (a) Randomized controlled trials (double blinded)

Table 2.9	American Association of Critical-Care Nurses Levels of Evidence
A	Meta-analysis of multiple controlled studies or meta-analysis of qualitative studies with results that consistently support a specific action, intervention, or treatment
B	Well-designed controlled studies, both randomized and nonrandomized, with results that consistently support a specific action, intervention, or treatment
C	Qualitative studies, descriptive or correlational studies, integrative reviews, systematic reviews, or randomized controlled trials with inconsistent results
D	Peer-reviewed professional organizational standards with clinical studies to support recommendations
E	Theory-based evidence from expert opinion or multiple case reports
M	Manufacturers' recommendations only

From Armola, R., Bourgault, A. M., Halm, M. A., Board, R. M., Bucher, L., Harrington, L., Medina, J. (2009). AACN levels of evidence: What's new? *Crit Care Nurse, 29*(4), 70–73.

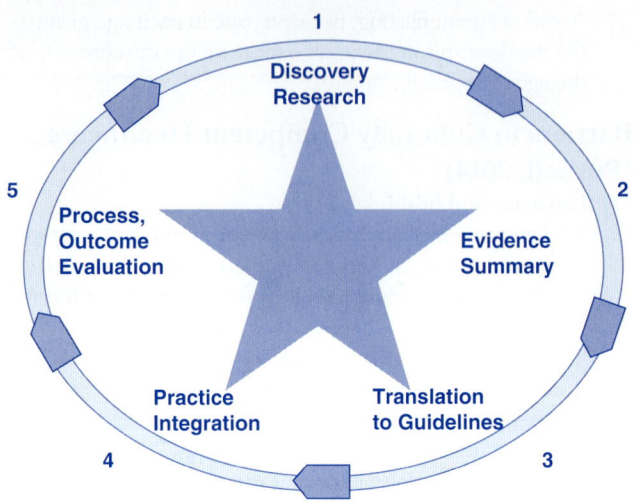

Fig. 2.4 Stevens Star Model of Evidence-Based Practice: Knowledge Transformation. (From Stevens, K. R., (2015). Stevens Star Model of EBP: Knowledge Transformation (c).)

   (b) Nonblinded randomized clinical trials
   (c) Nonrandomized clinical trials
   (d) Prospective cohort studies
   (e) Case-control studies
   (f) Case reports
   (g) Expert opinion (including consensus groups)
  ii) Randomized controlled trials are considered the "gold standard," but many nursing questions are not answered using quantitative techniques.
 b) Sample size
 c) Control of extraneous variables
2) Quantity: the magnitude of effect, numbers of studies, and sample size or power (i.e., strength of evidence)
3) Consistency: the extent to which similar findings are reported using similar and different study designs
4) Relevance: the study question's similarity to the clinical question and the extent to which the findings from the study can be applied in other clinical settings to different patients
5) Many grading scales are used to grade sources of evidence; the AACN system has recently been modified (Table 2.9).
d. Integrating findings with clinical expertise, patient values, and circumstances and, if appropriate, applying these findings
e. Evaluating performance and the outcomes of the clinical practice

The Cycle of Knowledge Transformation Using the Stevens Star Model (Stevens, 2012)

See Fig. 2.4.
1. Discovery research
 a. Primary goal of nursing research: develop a specialized, scientifically based body of nursing knowledge to facilitate improvement in patient care

 b. Definitions
  1) Scientific method: systematic approach to solving problems that controls variables and biases
  2) Basic research: research with purpose to advance knowledge; helps in understanding relationships among phenomena
  3) Applied research: research with purpose to solve a particular problem; helps in making decisions or evaluating techniques
  4) Variable: a measurable concept that varies among the subjects in a research study
   a) Independent variable: the concept that is being observed, introduced, or manipulated in a research study; may be referred to as the *treatment variable*
   b) Dependent variable: the concept that is being observed for a change after the intervention
   c) Extraneous variable: concept that is not being studied but may or may not be relevant to the results of the study; this variable can affect the dependent variable and interfere with research results
  5) Hypothesis: statement that predicts a relationship among two or more variables; may be simple, complex, directional, nondirectional, or null
 c. Research types
  1) Quantitative research: deductive process that tests hypotheses and examines cause-and-effect relationships to examine specific phenomena; emphasizes facts and data to validate or extend existing knowledge
   a) Experimental: uses randomization and a control group to test the effects of an intervention
   b) Quasi-experimental: involves manipulation of variables but lacks a comparison group or randomization
   c) Nonexperimental
    i) Descriptive: describes situations, experiences, and phenomena as they exist

ii) Ex post facto (correlational): describes relationships between variables
2) Qualitative: inductive process used to understand phenomena in a defined context; emphasizes development of new insights, theory, and knowledge
   a) Relies less on numbers and measurements and more on nursing strategies, interpersonal communication techniques, intuition, and collaboration between the nurse and patient to discover the underlying relationships
   b) Includes case studies, open-ended questions, field studies, and participant observation
d. Steps in the research process
   1) Formulate the research problem.
   2) Review the related literature.
   3) Formulate the hypothesis.
   4) Select the research design.
   5) Identify the population to be studied.
   6) Specify methods of data collection.
   7) Design the study.
   8) Conduct the study.
   9) Analyze the data.
   10) Interpret the results.
   11) Communicate the findings.
   12) Use the findings to improve patient care.
e. Ethical responsibilities related to nursing research studies
   1) Protect the rights of research participants.
   2) Ensure that the potential benefits of the study outweigh any potential risk to the participants.
   3) Submit the proposed study for review by the investigational review committee.
   4) Obtain informed consent from each participant.
f. Nursing responsibilities related to research
   1) Identify problem areas and research questions for investigation.
   2) Assist in collection of data as requested.
   3) Read and interpret reports of nursing research.
   4) Assess the quality of nursing research studies and applicability to practice.
   5) Apply research findings to change clinical practice and improve patient care.
   6) Share research findings with peers.
   7) Design and conduct nursing research.
2. Evidence summary: systematic reviews
   a. Definition: a summary of all evidence related to a specific research question using a rigorous method
      1) Quantitative systematic reviews are conducted using meta-analysis statistical techniques
      2) Qualitative systematic reviews are a descriptive summary of the review of existing studies
   b. Advantage to using systematic reviews (Stevens, 2001)
      1) Provides a usable form because the studies included in the systematic review already have been critically appraised so that high-quality studies are included; more usable for the following:
         a) For clinicians making clinical decisions
         b) For policy makers making policy decisions
         c) For administrations making economic decisions
         d) For researchers making decisions about future research designs
      2) Shortens time between research and clinical implementation
      3) Provides a distillation of large quantities of information into a manageable form with a recommendation for clinical practice
   c. Finding systematic reviews
      1) Agency for Healthcare Research and Quality: www.ahrq.gov
      2) The Cochrane Collaboration www.cochrane.org
      3) The Campbell Collaboration: www.campbellcollaboration.org
      4) The Joanna Briggs Institute: http://joannabriggs.org
3. Translation into practice recommendations: clinical practice guidelines (CPGs)
   a. Definition: a statement based on the best scientific evidence designed to assist clinical decision making about appropriate health care for specific clinical circumstances; Stevens (2012) states that CPGs "explicitly articulate the link between the recommendation and the strength of supporting evidence and/or strength of recommendation."
   b. Advantage of CPG: "can help to overcome the barriers to research use because they eliminate the need to search for journal articles, overcome nurses' limited skills in critical analysis, and minimize the impact of research jargon and unfamiliar terminology because most guidelines are published as clinical application documents" (Ciliska, Pinelli, DiCenso, & Cullum, 2001).
      1) CPG may be incorporated into standards of care, care maps, policies and procedures, and protocols.
   c. Topics of CPG
      1) A condition (e.g., myocardial infarction)
      2) A symptom (e.g., chest pain)
      3) A clinical procedure (e.g., percutaneous coronary intervention)
   d. Purposes of CPG
      1) Encourage treatment that offers individual patients maximum likelihood of benefit and minimum harm and is acceptable in terms of cost.
      2) Reduce inappropriate variations in practice.
         a) Common reasons for variations
            i) Variations in clinical decision making
            ii) Differing approaches to problem solving
            iii) Varied routines and standards
            iv) Availability of resources
            v) Lack of consensus related to appropriate treatment for given conditions
      3) Promote the delivery of evidence-based health care.
      4) Provide ready evaluation criteria by which health care professionals can be made accountable for clinical performance.
      5) Reduce the cost of health care.
   e. Finding CPG
      1) Governmental agencies
         a) National Guideline Clearinghouse: www.guidelines.gov
         b) Scottish Intercollegiate Guideline Network (SIGN): www.sign.ac.uk/guidelines/index.html

2) Select professional associations with evidence-based practice (EBP) resources
   a) Sigma Theta Tau International (STTI): www.nursingsociety.org and www.nursingknowledge.org/resources/.
   b) American Association of Critical-Care Nurses: www.aacn.org
   c) Registered Nurses' Association of Ontario: http://rnao.ca/bpg
   d) Emergency Nurses Association: www.ena.org
3) Evidence-based practice centers
   a) Joanna Briggs Institute: http://joannabriggs.org/
f. Tool for evaluation of guidelines: Appraisal of Guidelines for Research and Evaluation (AGREE) Instrument (www.agreetrust.org)
g. Toolkit for implementation of guidelines: Registered Nurses' Association of Ontario Toolkit for Implementation of CPG (http://rnao.ca/bpg/resources/toolkit-implementation-best-practice-guidelines-second-edition)
4. Integration into practice
   a. Select an EBP change model (e.g., Iowa Model of EBP to Promote Quality Care, Stetler Model of Research Utilization, Rosswurm-Larrabee Model of EBP, Johns Hopkins EBP Conceptual Model).
   b. Consider organizational barriers to EBP.
   c. Use organizational strategies to facilitate EBP.
      1) Foster an environment that values inquiry and critical thinking.
         a) Encouragement of formal education
         b) Provision of time to read research and evaluate applicability to setting
         c) Provision of access to the Internet, e-journals, library, and photocopying
         d) Provision of opportunities to attend conferences, continuing education, and in-service education, including education regarding critical appraisal of research
         e) Addition of scholarship to the nurse's role so that dissemination through local, regional, and national presentations and publication is encouraged and expected
         f) Establishment of nursing leadership to spearhead EBP activities, such as a nurse researcher, clinical nurse specialist, or nurse practitioner
         g) Encouragement of the questioning of the status quo and nursing rituals
         h) Development of collaborative teams across disciplines; "EBP is a multidisciplinary practice" (Gray, 1997)
      2) Communicate the expectation of EBP
         a) Incorporation of EBP activities in job descriptions, performance appraisals, merit raises, and career ladders promotions.
         b) Leaders asking, "Why are you doing that?" "Why are you doing that in that way?" "What is the evidence?"
         c) Requirement of evidence for practice changes and revision of policies, procedures, and protocols
      3) Increase nurse autonomy over practice.
         a) Decentralization of administration
         b) Establishment of shared governance with appropriate nursing department council and committee structures
         c) Establishment of unit-level EBP committees
      4) Eliminate the gap between research and practice (NOTE: The gap between research and practice is estimated to be approximately 10 years.)
         a) Establishment of more joint appointments between academic and practice settings
         b) Appointment of a nurse researcher on staff
         c) Use of expert consultants as necessary
         d) Provision of support for EBP committees and research activities
         e) Development of research presentations (e.g., Nursing Research Grand Rounds)
         f) Establishment of journal clubs
         g) Publication of a monthly research newsletter
      5) Use resources appropriately.
         a) Commitment of expertise, money, and time to EBP activities, including having adequate staffing
         b) Use of systematic reviews and implementation of clinical practice guidelines
5. Evaluation of the impact of EBP
   a. Formative evaluation: assessment during the change process to ensure that the change has actually occurred and preliminary effects
   b. Summative evaluation: assessment at the completion of the change process to evaluate the impact of the change; possible evaluation criteria may include the following:
      1) Patient health outcomes such as length of stay or quality of life
      2) Patient satisfaction
      3) Staff satisfaction
      4) Cost–benefit impact

Quality Management and Improvement

1. Goals
   a. Quality management (QM) emphasizes achievement of optimal patient outcomes along with the involvement of employees in the process of monitoring quality, identifying problems, and devising solutions.
   b. Quality improvement (QI) emphasizes progressive improvement through innovation.
2. Areas of focus (Yoder-Wise, 2011)
   a. Customer rather than provider
   b. Prevention rather than detection
   c. System rather than individual
3. Principles (Yoder-Wise, 2011)
   a. QM is most effective within a flat, democratic organizational structure.
   b. Managers and workers must be committed to QI.
   c. Emphasis is on improving systems and processes rather than assigning blame.
   d. Customers ultimately define quality; others involved in definition of quality include governmental agencies, accreditation agencies, and third-party payers.
   e. QI focuses on outcomes.
   f. Decisions must be based on data.

4. QI process
   a. Identify the needs.
   b. Assemble a multidisciplinary team.
   c. Collect data to measure current status.
      1) Structure evaluation: examines the components of services, such as the setting and environment, that affect quality of care
      2) Process evaluation: examines activities and behaviors of the health care provider (e.g., nurse)
      3) Outcome evaluation: measures changes in patients
         a) The "five Ds" (Elinson, 1987)
            i) Death
            ii) Disease
            iii) Disability
            iv) Discomfort
            v) Dissatisfaction
         b) Other indicators that are more positive and broader in scope (e.g., functional status, quality of life)
         c) Clinical indicators should reflect desired outcomes and represent high-quality care delivery.
   d. Establish outcomes.
      1) Comparison of observed practice with expectations
         a) Retrospective review: examination of completed health care delivery by reviewing charts, conducting conferences or interviews, and reviewing questionnaires
         b) Concurrent review: evaluation of a patient's health status (outcome audit) or management (process) while ongoing by chart reviews, interviews, and observation of the patient
      2) Benchmarks
         a) Reference points or standards against which performance or achievements can be compared
      3) Sources of standards
         a) Internal policies and procedures
         b) State nurse practice acts
         c) Accrediting bodies (e.g., The Joint Commission [TJC])
         d) Professional associations (e.g., ANA)
         e) Governmental agencies (Agency for Healthcare Research and Quality [AHRQ])
         f) Award criteria (Magnet, Beacon, & Baldwin)
         g) Other hospitals
      4) Nursing Minimum Data Set: collection of essential nursing information for comparisons across patient populations
         a) Nursing care
            i) Nursing diagnosis
            ii) Nursing intervention
            iii) Nursing outcome
            iv) Intensity of nursing care
         b) Demographics
            i) Personal identification
            ii) Date of birth
            iii) Sex
            iv) Race and ethnicity
            v) Residency
         c) Service
            i) Unique facility or service agency number
            ii) Unique health record number of the patient
            iii) Unique number of a principal registered nurse provider
            iv) Episode, admission, or encounter date
            v) Discharge or termination
            vi) Disposition of patient or client
            vii) Expected payer for most of the bill
      5) National Database of Nursing Quality Indicators (NDNQI)
         a) Developed by the ANA to promote and facilitate the standardization of information submitted by hospitals across the United States on nursing quality and patient outcomes
         b) Provides comparison data from similar hospitals and units (e.g., teaching status, number of beds, type of patient care unit)
         c) Nursing-Sensitive Indicators: indicators that capture care or its outcomes most affected by nursing care (Montalvo, 2007)
            i) Mix of RNs, LPNs, and unlicensed staff caring for patients in acute care settings
            ii) Total nursing care hours provided per patient day
            iii) Pressure ulcer rate
            iv) Patient falls
            v) Restraints
            vi) Patient satisfaction with pain management
            vii) Patient satisfaction with educational information
            viii) Patient satisfaction with overall care
            ix) Patient satisfaction with nursing care
            x) Nosocomial infection rate
            xi) Nurse staff satisfaction
            xii) Nursing turnover
   e. Select and implement a plan to reconcile discrepancies between observations and expectations.
   f. Evaluate the implementation of the plan and the achievement of outcomes.
5. Rapid cycle change for improvement
   a. The Model for Improvement (Fig. 2.5) is advocated by the Institute for Healthcare Improvement (IHI) for accelerating improvement.
   b. The model has two parts (IHI, 2011).
      1) Three fundamental questions that can be addressed in any order:
         a) What are we trying to accomplish?
         b) How will we know that the change is an improvement?
         c) What changes can we make that will result in improvement?
      2) The Plan-Do-Study-Act (PDSA) cycle to test and implement changes in real work settings
   c. Members of the improvement team should be multidisciplinary and are critical to a successful improvement effort.

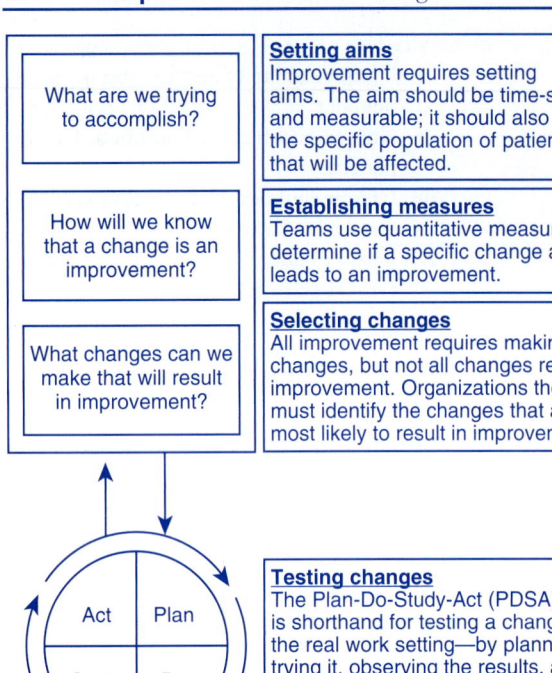

Fig. 2.5 Model for Improvement. (From Langley, G. L., Nolan, K. M., Nolan, T. W., Norman, C. L., & Provost, L. P. [1996]. *The improvement guide: A practical approach to enhancing organizational performance.* San Francisco: Jossey-Bass Publishers.)

Patient Safety

1. Recent focus on the impact of medical error on patient outcomes through several publications of the IOM (Page, 2004; Kohn, Corrigan, & Donaldson, 2000).
2. TJC has been establishing annual National Patient Safety Goals.
3. The Quality and Safety Education for Nurses (QSEN) project has established competencies for nursing and has proposed targets for knowledge, skills, and attitudes (QSEN, 2016).
    a. Categories
        1) Patient-centered care
        2) Teamwork and collaboration
        3) Evidence-based practice
        4) QI
        5) Safety
        6) Informatics
    b. Prelicensure and graduate program competencies are intended to be incorporated into curricula.
4. Medication errors
    a. Nurses are most likely to be involved in medication errors than any other form of medical errors.
    b. Prevention of medication errors (Dennison, 2005)
        1) Individual responsibility
            a) Ten rights
                i) Right patient: use two patient identifiers (i.e., not patient's room and bed number)
                ii) Right drug
                iii) Right dose
                iv) Right time
                v) Right route
                vi) Right reason
                vii) Patient's right to education
                viii) Patient's right to refuse
                ix) Patient evaluation: clarify titration parameters.
                x) Right documentation
            b) Reporting of errors and near-hits so that system analysis can occur and prevent future errors
        2) Systems thinking
            a) Nonpunitive culture
            b) Adherence to policies, procedures, and protocols
                i) Avoidance of unapproved abbreviations, and trailing zeros
                ii) Avoidance of verbal orders; if necessary, a verbal repeat should be used for confirmation
                iii) Label with drug being administered
                    (a) Bag
                    (b) Pump chamber (using channel labels on infusion pump if available)
                    (c) Tubing
            c) Use of information
                i) Patient information (e.g., laboratory values, vital signs); electronic patient record is preferred because the record is available to more than one health care professional simultaneously
                ii) Drug information: use up-to-date medication references such as Micromedex, Epocrates, and drug books that are updated annually.
            d) Use of technology
                i) Automated dispensing devices
                ii) Bar-code point of care (BPOC)
                iii) Computerized provider order entry (CPOE)
                iv) "Smart" pumps with guardrails to alert the nurse of too high or too low dose
            e) Standardization
                i) Restriction of formulary (e.g., do you really need to have three glycoprotein IIb/IIIa inhibitors, or will one or two suffice?)
                ii) Standardization of infusion concentrations (e.g., avoid double, triple, quadruple concentration)
                iii) Standardization of equipment (e.g., infusion pumps)

f) Pharmacist
   i) Review of all prescriptions
   ii) Presence on unit and on rounds
g) Medication reconciliation
h) Environment control
   i) Adequate lighting
   ii) Noise reduction
   iii) Distraction avoidance
   iv) Clean, clutter-free, organized space for preparation of medications
i) Teamwork
   i) Clarification of any unclear prescription
   ii) Use of independent double-checks of drug, dose, calculation, patient identity, infusion rate, and appropriate line for all high-alert medications (Box 2.2)
      (a) "Check this *with* me" is unacceptable because it causes confirmation error (i.e., you see what you expect to see).
      (b) Also applies to dose changes of high-alert drugs
   iii) Use of time-out if there is a question about the safety of the drug for this patient, at this time, at this dose, and by this route; never administer a drug that is unsafe
   iv) Documentation and communication of changes in patient response or adverse drug events

Peer Review

1. Component of professional autonomy and development
2. Purpose is to ensure quality and safety through maintaining standards of care.
3. Process is defined by a representative goal of nurses; it does not replace annual performance reviews by nursing leadership.
4. Six principles (Ohmart, 2013)
   a. A peer is someone of the same rank
   b. Peer review is practice focused
   c. Feedback is timely, routine, and a continuous expectation
   d. Peer review fosters a continuous learning culture of patient safety and best practice
   e. Feedback is not anonymous
   f. Feedback incorporates the nurse's developmental stage

Facilitation of Learning

Description
The ability to facilitate patient and family learning

Definitions
1. Teaching: the process of facilitating learning; an interaction designed to help a person learn to do something that he or she is currently unable to do; a two-way interaction
2. Learning: the process by which a person becomes capable of doing something he or she could not do before, including a wide range of behavior from motor skills to intellectual skills; an emotional experience which can be negative or positive, traumatic, or pleasant
3. Patient education: the process of teaching patients and their families about an illness, treatment, and other health-related matters, including how to adhere to the regimen and helping them change their behavior.

Reasons for Patient Education
1. Because the patient has a need and a right to know those things that are relevant to his or her condition, disease, or situation
2. To produce changes in knowledge, skills, attitudes, appreciation, and understanding
3. To promote and improve health
4. To encourage the patient to assume responsibility for disease management
5. To prevent illness and complications
6. To aid in coping with illness and adaptation to change
7. To promote compliance with the therapeutic regimen
8. To reduce anxiety (including family stress and anxiety)
9. To reduce the number of visits to the physician's office or emergency department and the number and length of hospitalizations
10. To comply with regulatory requirements

Box 2.2 High-Alert Medications Frequently Administered in Critical Care Areas

Adrenergic agonists (epinephrine, phenylephrine, norepinephrine)
Adrenergic antagonists (propranolol, metoprolol, labetalol)
Anesthetic agents (propofol, ketamine)
Antiarrhythmics (lidocaine, amiodarone)
Antithrombotic agents
- Anticoagulants (warfarin, low molecular weight heparin, unfractionated heparin)
- Factor Xa inhibitors (fondaparinux, apixaban, rivaroxaban)
- Direct thrombin inhibitors (argatroban, bivalirudin, dabigatran etexilate)
- Thrombolytics (alteplase, reteplase, tenecteplase)
- Glycoprotein IIb/IIIa inhibitors (eptifibatide)

Cardioplegic solutions
Chemotherapeutic agents
Dextrose, hypertonic, 20% or greater
Dialysis solutions
Epidural or intrathecal medications
Hypoglycemic agents
Inotropic medications (digoxin, milrinone)
Insulin
Liposomal forms of drugs (liposomal amphotericin B) and conventional counterparts (amphotericin B desoxycholate)
Moderate sedation agents (dexmedetomidine, midazolam)
Narcotics and opioids
Neuromuscular blocking agents (succinylcholine, rocuronium, vecuronium)
Parenteral nutrition preparations
Radiocontrast agents
Sterile water for injection, inhalation, and irrigation (excluding pour bottles) in containers of 100 ml or more
Sodium chloride for injection, hypertonic, greater than 0.9% concentration

Adapted from Institute for Safe Medication Practices. *ISMP List of high-alert medications in acute care settings*. Retrieved from http://ismp.org/Tools/institutionalhighAlert.asp

Principles of Adult Education

1. Qualities of the adult learner: a self-directed independent person who becomes ready to learn when the need to know or to perform is experienced; characteristics of the adult learner are likely to include the following:
   a. Goal oriented
   b. Less flexible
   c. Requires longer time in the performance of learning tasks
   d. Impatient in the pursuit of objectives
   e. Finds little use for isolated facts
   f. Strives for recognition and success
   g. Has multiple responsibilities, all of which draw upon his or her time
   h. Experienced in the "school of life"
   i. Requires a more constant and ideal learning environment
   j. Usually comes to the teaching program on a voluntary basis
   k. Wishes to be involved in mutual planning of learning experiences
   l. Likes to participate in diagnosing needs for learning, formulating learning objectives, and evaluating learning
   m. Expects a climate of mutual respect, trust, and collaboration that supports learning
2. Educational concepts useful with adults
   a. Pacing
      1) Allow adults to set their own pace, if possible.
      2) Tasks or methods involving significant time pressure are likely to be difficult for adults.
   b. Arousal anxiety
      1) Some degree of arousal is necessary for learning; however, older adults may become anxious in a learning situation.
      2) Allow individuals an opportunity to become familiar with a situation.
      3) Minimize the role of competition and evaluation.
   c. Fatigue
      1) Some tasks may produce considerable mental or physical fatigue, a problem likely to particularly affect older adults.
      2) Shorten the instruction sessions or provide frequent rest breaks.
   d. Difficulty: arrange materials from the simple to the complex to build the individual's confidence and skills.
   e. Errors: structure the tasks so errors are avoided and do not have to be unlearned.
   f. Practice: provide an opportunity for practice on similar but different tasks; such practice helps to develop generalizable skills.
   g. Feedback: provide information on the adequacy of previous responses.
   h. Cues
      1) Materials should be presented to compensate for the potential sensory problems of older adults.
      2) Direct attention toward the relevant aspects of the task.
      3) Reduce the level of irrelevant information to a minimum.
   i. Organization
      1) Learning and remembering often require that information be grouped or related in some way.
      2) Instruct individuals in the use of various mnemonic techniques (e.g., mental images, verbal associations) that may be used to elaborate or organize the material.
   j. Relevance and experience
      1) People learn and remember what is important to them.
      2) Attempt to make the task relevant to the individual's concerns.
      3) Performance is likely to be facilitated to the extent that the individuals are able to integrate the new information with known information.

Barriers to Teaching and Learning

1. Nurse factors: lack of time, lack of knowledge, or consideration of teaching as a lower priority than physical care
2. Physician interference (i.e., not wanting the nurse to teach the patient)
3. Patient factors
   a. Physiologic factors
      1) Instability
      2) Sedation
      3) Pain
   b. Lack of availability (e.g., procedures, physical therapy)
   c. Psychological factors (e.g., anxiety, pain)
   d. Poor language or reading skills
   e. Sensory deficits: vision, hearing
   f. Poor manual dexterity for psychomotor skills
   g. Attitudes and beliefs that conflict with teaching

Teaching and Learning Process

1. Assessment
   a. Readiness to learn
      1) Desire to know (e.g., asking questions)
      2) Absence of acute distress (e.g., pain, dyspnea)
      3) Adequate energy
   b. Sensory deficits (e.g., use of eyeglasses, hearing aid)
   c. Educational level and reading ability
   d. Learning style
      1) Environment
         a) Formal or informal
         b) Tolerance to distraction
      2) Alone or in a group
      3) Preferred learning mode
         a) Reading: print materials
         b) Seeing: pictorial materials
         c) Listening: auditory
         d) Manipulating: tactile, kinesthetic
2. Plan
   a. Identify objectives; parts of the objective should include the following:
      1) What should the learner be able to do? (behavior)
         a) Cognitive
         b) Affective
         c) Psychomotor

2) How well should the learner be able to do it? (the criteria)
3) Under what conditions should the learner be able to do it? (the condition)
b. Identify content to teach.
1) Language and terminology
2) Health care system: personnel; organization and structure; routines and procedures; norms and expectations; immediate environment
3) Basic anatomy and physiology of affected body system
4) Diagnosis, disease process
5) Therapy: treatments, medications, diet, activity, personal health habits
6) Prevention of complications
7) Skills (e.g., insulin administration, pulse taking)
8) Community resources
c. Determine methods.
1) Individual or group
a) Use individual method when you are assessing patient's knowledge, when family members or friends try to dominate teaching sessions, and when the information you'll teach provokes anxiety or is considered a topic not generally discussed in public.
b) Individual methods include programmed instruction, reading materials, audiovisual aids, and one-to-one instruction.
c) Group sessions lessen feelings of alienation and being "different"; learners learn from other learners.
d) Patient-operated groups and self-help groups offer the benefit of encouraging patients to share coping techniques and useful hints.
e) Group teaching saves time and money.
f) Family members gain support from health professionals and other patients and their families.
g) Combinations may be helpful to meet the patient's individual needs.
2) Teaching methods: the teacher of adults is a facilitator more than a teacher and uses various methods.
a) Lecture
i) May be in group session, on videotape, or on closed-circuit TV
ii) Is usually no longer than 20 minutes
iii) Includes the introduction to establish the need to know, the body to deliver content that needs to be known, and the summary to review what was covered
b) Discussion
i) Helps the patient to ask any questions about information that is in doubt
ii) Guides the nurse to assess what the patient needs to know
c) Audiovisuals
i) Includes visual and auditory stimulation to teach content
d) Printed materials
i) May be used in place of other techniques but should include a discussion with the nurses after reading for clarification of content
ii) May be used as a supplement to other methods
iii) Useful as an aid to review at a later date
iv) Should be written at no higher than sixth grade level and lower if possible (Hersh, L. et al., 2015)
v) Need to be in patient's language
e) Explanations
i) Give only as much information as requested.
ii) Ask for feedback.
f) Exploration: encourage patient to answer her or his own questions.
g) Demonstration and return demonstration
i) Used when the patient must learn a new skill
ii) Describe what you are going to do and then do it while the patient observes; then talk to patient through the process while the patient does it; finally have the patient perform the skill while the patient tells you what he or she is doing.
h) Role-playing
i) Provides practice in a safe setting
ii) Useful to see how others might respond
3. Implement
a. Assign one person to teach the patient to minimize confusion, contradiction, and incompleteness.
b. Schedule teaching sessions according to the patient's receptiveness; let the patient set the pace and choose topics of most interest first.
c. Provide ideal setting: Control the environment.
d. Know your subject area: Be competent and confident.
e. Speak the patient's language: Minimize use of medical terminology.
f. Consider your presentation style.
1) Keep the presentations of material short.
2) Place key points up front.
3) Use verbal headings.
4) Summarize at the end.
5) Obtain feedback and request questions.
g. Include "why" where appropriate.
h. Use visual aids.
i. Remember that successful learning takes time and reinforcement.
j. Provide a means for the patient to learn more, such as written information for reading and review, resource groups, and an outpatient program.
k. Coordinate education through written teaching plans, patient care conferences, and documentation.
1) Written teaching plans should include the following:
a) Objectives
b) Content
c) Teaching methods
d) Methods of evaluation

2) Documentation should include the following:
    a) Objectives
    b) Content outline
    c) Method used
    d) Evaluation of learning
        i) Objective met
        ii) Objective partially met: needs reinforcement
        iii) Objective not met: needs repeat
    e) Comments
    f) Signature
4. Evaluate learning using any of the following methods:
   a. Written tests
   b. Oral evaluation
   c. Return demonstration
   d. Analysis of physical findings (e.g., serum glucose, weight)
   e. Follow-up questionnaire

Education for Low-Literacy Individuals
1. Definition: adults with poorly developed skills in reading, writing, listening, and speaking
2. Assessing literacy level
   a. Individuals reading at a fifth-grade or higher level are considered literate; hand printing instructions and asking the patient to read them back to you is a nonthreatening way to assess reading ability.
   b. Incongruent behavior may signal a literacy problem; be alert for behavior that does not match the reported level of understanding.
   c. Low-literacy materials are preferred for low-literacy individuals.

Table 2.10 Qualities of Poor Readers and Appropriate Teaching Strategies

Qualities of Poor Readers	Teaching Strategies
Take words literally	Explain the meaning of all words
Read slowly; miss meaning	Use common words and examples
Skip over uncommon words	Use examples, review content frequently
Miss content	Describe content first, use verbal heading and visuals
Tire quickly	Use short segments

3. Teaching strategies for low-literacy patients
   a. Identify and eliminate or minimize stress, anxiety, or other distractions before teaching.
   b. Correct misconceptions that affect learning.
   c. Personalize the health message and explain the need for the information.
   d. Relate information to patient's past experiences and actively involve the patient and family in discussions.
   e. Consider the qualities of poor readers and use teaching strategies that are helpful (Table 2.10).

Learning Activities

CHAPTER 2

1. Complete the following crossword puzzle.

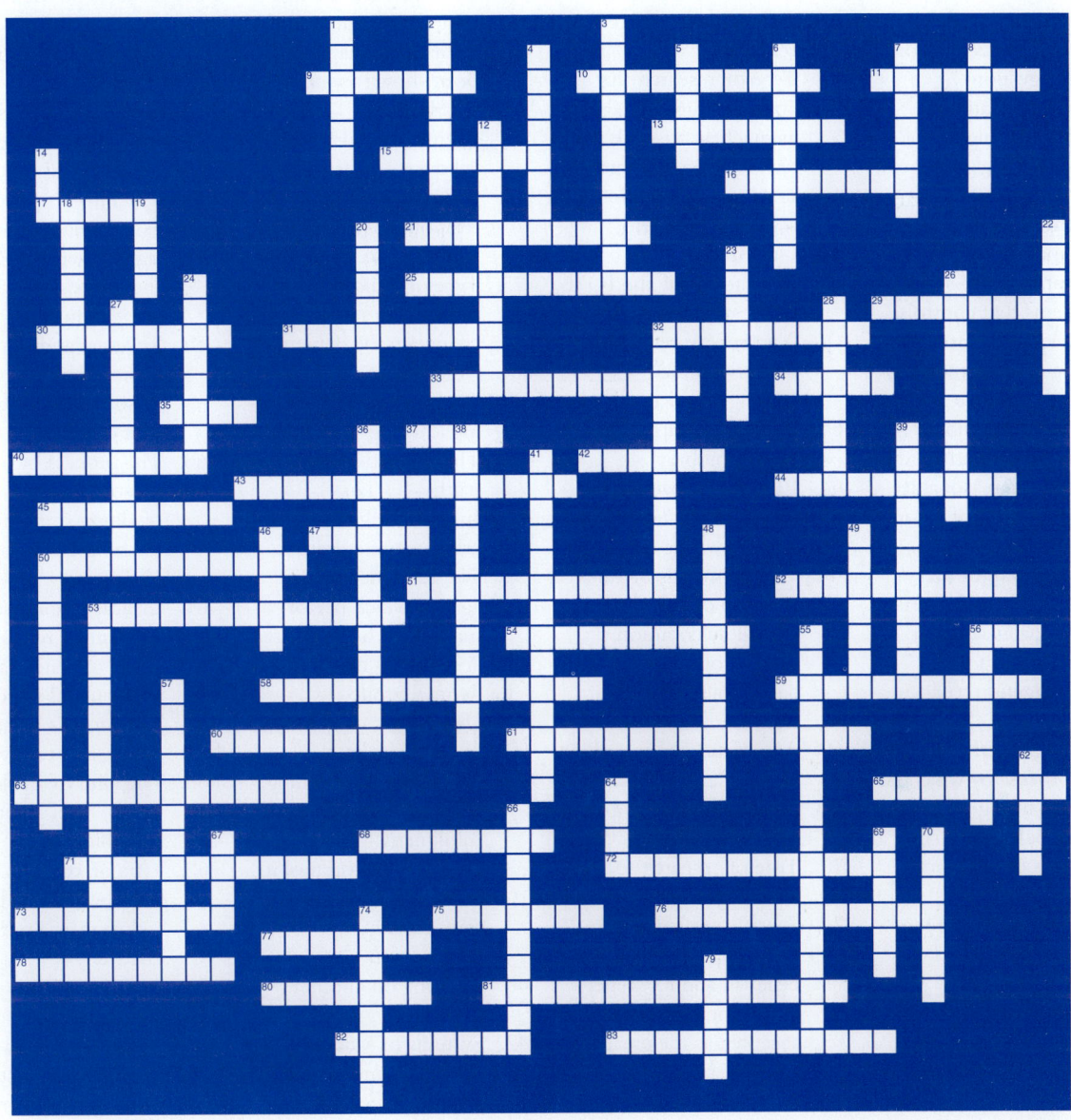

DOWN

1. Organizational structure that focuses on product and function, sometimes referred to as product line management
2. Culturally prescribed codes of behavior
3. Type of research that takes place in the individual's natural setting with emphasis on understanding human experience; results in words or phrases
4. The kind of evidence that is "best" if it is available
5. One way to eliminate the gap between research and practice is to establish _____ appointments between academic and clinical facilities
6. Ethical approach that asserts that actions are right or wrong based on consequences
7. Patterns and practices within a cultural group that encompass collective learned behaviors
8. Personal beliefs about the truth and worth of thoughts, objects, and behaviors
12. Quality _____ emphasizes innovation
14. The integration of best evidence, clinician expertise, patient values, and circumstances (abbrev)
18. This type of consent applies when the patient cannot give consent but treatment is needed immediately

45

Chapter 2 Professional Caring and Ethical Practice

19. Intentional _____ is a direct invasion of someone's legal rights
20. An intimate conversation between an individual and God or other Higher Being
22. Focusing and directing the imagination through the use of specific words and suggestions
23. The of evaluation or review that might look at a physiological parameter
24. The right to self-determination
26. This method is a systematic approach to solving problems that controls variables and biases
27. Failing to do something that a reasonable and prudent professional would do or doing something that a reasonable and prudent professional would not do
28. Type of charges that would be filed if a nurse intentionally caused a patient's death
32. The obligation to do good
36. Working together
38. The process by which an individual or group takes on the behaviors and practices of the dominant culture
39. The third point on the Stevens Star Model
41. Answerability or responsibility
46. Belief not based on logical proof or material evidence
48. Involves the use of conscious mental effort to control involuntary body functions such as blood pressure, heart rate, or respiratory rate
49. Learned, shared, and transmitted values, beliefs, and practices of a particular group that guides thinking
50. The fourth point on the Stevens Star Model
53. When one knows the right thing to do but cannot pursue the right action (2 words)
55. Quantitative research design that does not use a control group or randomization
56. This type of thinking is controlled, purposeful, and goal-directed reasoning
57. Type of research that controls study variables as much as possible and has objective and measurable data collection; results in numbers
62. One of the recommendations of the IOM publication *The Future of Nursing* is to remove the barriers on the _____ of nursing practice
64. Process for rapid cycle change (abbrev)
66. Ethical approach that asserts that actions are right or wrong based on a set of morals or rules
67. A group of people related by common descent of heredity who have similar physical characteristics
69. A collection of interdependent elements that interact to achieve a common purpose
70. Type of research to solve a particular problem
74. Specific unified system of an expression of the belief in and reverence for a supernatural power accepted as the creator and governor of the universe
79. Type of charges that could be filed if a nurse unintentionally causes a patient's death

ACROSS

9. A nurse practice act is an example of a _____
10. The "gold standard" of evidence arises from _____ controlled trials
11. The second point on the Stevens Star Model is the _____ of evidence
13. This type of report is completed for errors or other unusual occurrences
15. An ethical _____ is a situation that requires a choice between two undesirable alternatives
16. Poor sleep quality has been shown to increase the risk for _____
17. Format for posing clinical questions (abbrev)
21. Statement that predicts a relationship among two or more variables
25. Type of variable that is presumed cause of the change in the dependent variable
29. The process of facilitating learning
30. The obligation to tell the truth
31. Includes behavior, criteria, and condition
32. The reference point against which performance can be compared
33. A statutory right of a defined group
34. Using words and images to elicit laughter
35. To wish for something with the expectation of fulfillment
37. Communication tool to ensure effective, clear transmission of information
40. Working on another's behalf
42. Systems of valued behaviors and beliefs that govern proper conduct
43. The obligation to do no harm
44. Sharing nursing care activities with other individuals who have the appropriate authority to accomplish the work
45. A concept examined in a research study
47. Quality, quantity, and consistency are used to _____ the evidence
50. Assault, battery, and defamation are all examples of this type of tort
51. Insertion of needles into specific points in the body for therapeutic purposes
52. The fifth point on the Stevens Star Model, process or outcomes _____.
53. M level on the AACN Level of Evidence scale includes recommendations from _____
54. A nurse who was born in 1950 would be in this generational group
58. The ethical approach that asserts that actions are right or wrong based on the greatest good for the greatest number
59. To assist an individual to make a decision when he or she does not have the data or expertise
60. The process by which a person becomes capable of doing something he or she could not previously do
61. Critical care nurses manage human responses to actual or potential _____ problems (2 words)
63. The process of seeking, giving, and receiving help
65. The kind of evidence that is "best" if it is available
68. Type of consent that must be obtained before inclusion as a participant in a study
71. Statistical technique for conducting quantitative systematic reviews; yields a summary statistic
72. Use of scents for therapeutic purposes
73. Nursing _____ indicators are those indicators that capture care or the outcomes most affected by nursing care
75. The obligation to be fair to all people
76. Type of research that uses randomization and a control group to test the effects of an intervention
77. The nursing _____ is assess, diagnose, plan, implement, and evaluate

78. The type of variable that is the response or outcome the researcher would like to explain or predict

80. A goal for fostering EBP is to create a spirit of _____

81. The obligation to respect privileged information

82. The obligation to be faithful to agreements and responsibilities accepted

83. A basic human phenomenon that helps create meaning in the world

2. List and describe the four bioethical principles.
   a. _____
   b. _____
   c. _____
   d. _____

3. Mrs. A is admitted to the intensive care unit after a planned hysterectomy for dysfunctional bleeding related to uterine fibroids. She is 58 years old and has a supportive family made up of her husband and three adult children. Postoperatively, she has a catastrophic stroke. She did not have an advance directive in place before her surgery, and her family is now struggling with determining which treatment options are best given her very poor prognosis. Mrs. A's husband believes withdrawal of care is what his wife would have wanted, but the children disagree, and Mr. A is visibly distraught about having to be the one to make this decision.
   a. What are advance directives? Describe implications for nursing care.
   b. Which ethical principle is at the center of this dilemma?
   c. Describe the ethical concept of advocacy and discuss how the nurse could use advocacy in this scenario.

4. Match the ethical concept to the correct description.

___ 1.	Veracity	a. Responsibility to respect privileged information
___ 2.	Moral agency	b. Obligation to assist another person in making a decision when the person does not have sufficient data or expertise
___ 3.	Egoism	c. Obligation to tell the truth and not intentionally mislead or deceive
___ 4.	Paternalism	d. Obligation to be faithful or loyal
___ 5.	Fidelity	e. Ability to serve as a moral agent in identifying and resolving ethical concerns
___ 6.	Confidentiality	f. Actions are right or wrong based on self-interest and self-preservation

5. Define *moral distress* and discuss a method of assessing and responding.

6. List five complementary therapies that are helpful with patients with stress, anxiety, or pain.
   a. _____
   b. _____
   c. _____
   d. _____
   e. _____

7. List the Critical Care Pain Observation Tool (CPOT) indicators in the scoring matrix.
   a. _____
   b. _____
   c. _____
   d. _____

Chapter 2   Professional Caring and Ethical Practice

8. Describe strategies for improving collaboration within a team.
   a. _____
   b. _____
   c. _____
   d. _____
   e. _____

9. Describe teaching strategies for low-literacy patients.
   a. _____
   b. _____
   c. _____
   d. _____
   e. _____

10. List the steps in the decision-making process.
    a. _____
    b. _____
    c. _____
    d. _____
    e. _____
    f. _____

11. Which cultural groups perceive eye contact as being disrespectful or impolite?
    _____

12. Match the religious belief or nursing intervention with the religion.

____ 1.	Provide same-sex caregivers. Do not remove sacred threads from body.	a. Jehovah's Witness
____ 2.	May refuse medical care except fracture care, treatment of malignancies, delivery of babies.	b. Seventh-Day Adventist
____ 3.	Must be baptized before death to ensure salvation.	c. Islam
____ 4.	Provide kosher diet as requested. After death, body cannot be left alone.	d. Judaism
____ 5.	Sabbath is dusk on Friday to dusk on Saturday. Numerous dietary restrictions.	e. Catholicism
____ 6.	Opposed to blood transfusions	f. Hinduism
____ 7.	Turn deceased person's face toward the right; avoid pork and pork products.	g. Christian Scientist

13. Define evidence-based practice.
    _____

The Cardiovascular System

CHAPTER 3

Selected Concepts in Anatomy and Physiology

General Information About the Cardiovascular System

1. The cardiovascular system is a continuous, fluid-filled elastic circuit with a pump.
2. The cardiovascular system provides communication between all body parts through transportation of oxygen, nutrients, hormones, water, enzymes, vitamins, minerals, buffers, leukocytes, antibodies, and wastes; these functions maintain dynamic equilibrium to maintain homeostasis.
3. The cardiovascular system consists of the heart and vascular system.

The Heart

1. Bioelectrically driven, muscular, four-chamber organ that provides forward propulsion of blood into the vascular system
2. Size of a closed fist: usually approximately 9 cm wide and 12 cm long; weighs approximately 4 g/kg of ideal body weight
3. Lies in the mediastinum between the sternum (anterior) and the spine (posterior) with two thirds of the heart to the left of the midline and one third of the heart to the right of the midline (Fig. 3.1)
4. Shaped like a blunt cone
    a. Apex
        1) Inferior, anterior, and to the left
        2) Normally at fifth left intercostal space (LICS) at the midclavicular line (MCL)
        3) On the upper surface of the diaphragm
    b. Base
        1) Superior, posterior, and to the right
        2) Normally at level of second intercostal space (ICS)
5. Layers of the cardiac wall (Fig. 3.2)
    a. Pericardium: maintains the heart in a stationary position
        1) Fibrous
            a) Loose-fitting, white fibrous layer
            b) Acts as a barrier against infection and neoplastic invasion
        2) Serous
            a) Parietal layer: lines inner surface of fibrous pericardium
            b) Visceral layer: lines the surface of the heart; synonymous with epicardium
        3) Pericardial space
            a) Located between the parietal and visceral layers of the serous pericardium
            b) Contains 10 to 30 ml of lubricating fluid
                i) Protects the heart against friction and erosion
                ii) Provides a well-lubricated sac in which the heart moves during contraction
    b. Epicardium: synonymous with the visceral layer of serous pericardium
    c. Epicardial fat
        1) Thin layer of adipose tissue between the visceral pericardium and the epicardium
        2) Increased in obesity
        3) May increase risk of coronary artery disease (CAD)
    d. Myocardium
        1) Largest portion of the cardiac wall
        2) Consists of the following:
            a) Specialized conduction fibers
            b) Interlacing cardiac muscle fibers
    e. Endocardium
        1) Consists of the following:
            a) Connective tissue
            b) Elastic fibers
            c) Endothelial cells
                i) Form a smooth surface for blood contact
                ii) Deter clot formation
        2) Contiguous with the lining of the great vessels
        3) Lines the heart chambers and valves
6. Cardiac skeleton
    a. Composed of continuous dense connective tissue
    b. Located at the base of the heart and in the interventricular septum

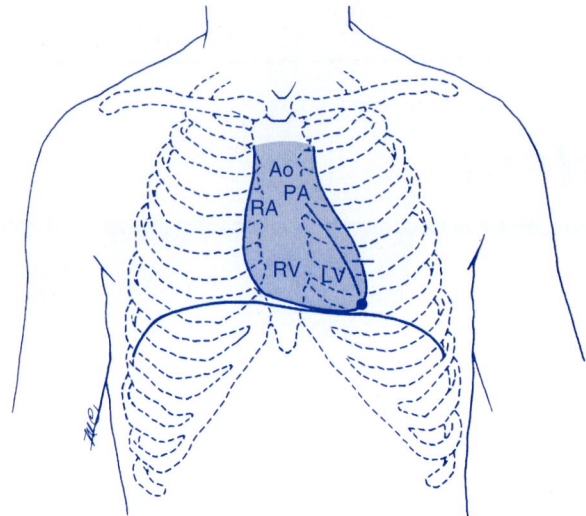

Fig. 3.1 Location and orientation of the heart chambers and great vessels within the thorax. *Ao,* Aorta; *PA,* pulmonary artery; *RA,* right atrium; *RV,* right ventricle; *LV,* left ventricle. (From Price, S., & Wilson, L. [2003]. *Pathophysiology: Clinical concepts of disease processes* [6th ed.]. St. Louis: Mosby.)

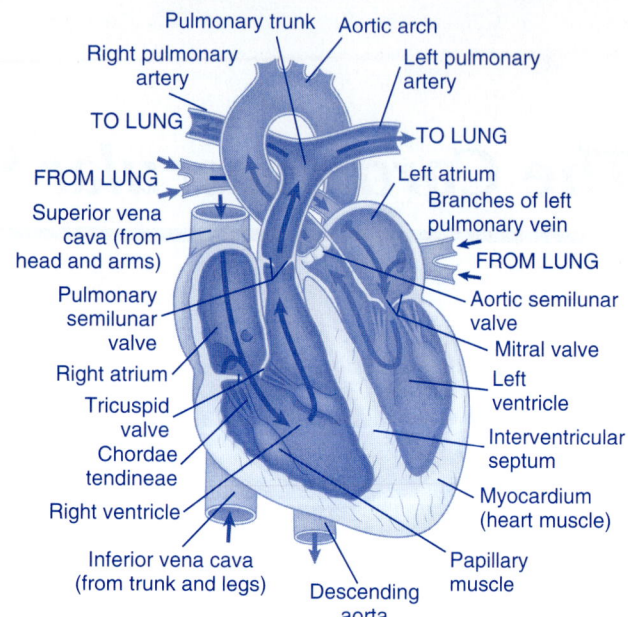

Fig. 3.3 Cardiac chambers and the structures that direct blood flow through the heart. *Arrows* indicate path of blood flow through chambers, valves, and major vessels. (From McCance, K. L., & Huether, S. E. [2014]. *Pathophysiology: The biologic basis for disease in adults and children* [7th ed.]. St. Louis: Mosby.)

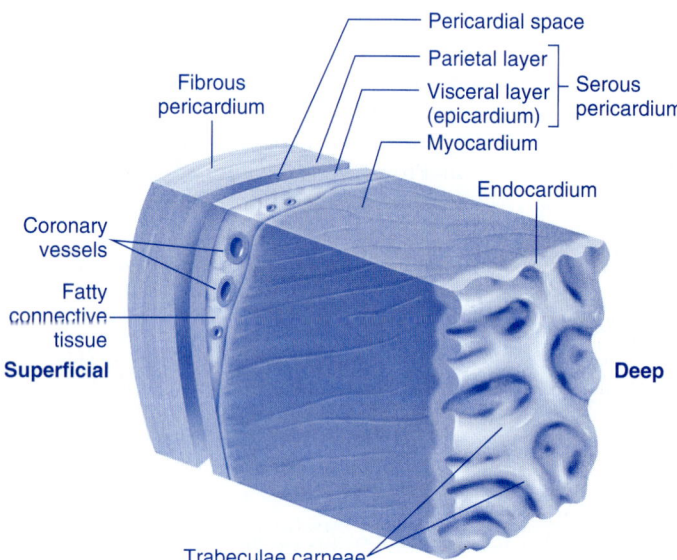

Fig. 3.2 Layers of the cardiac wall. Note the fibrous pericardium, the parietal and visceral layers of the serous pericardium, the pericardial space between the two layers of the serous pericardium, the myocardium, and the endocardium. The visceral layer of the serous pericardium is also referred to as the *epicardium.* (From Patton, K. T., & Thibodeau, G. A. [2016]. *Anatomy & physiology* [9th ed.]. St. Louis: Mosby.)

    c. Serves as the point of origin and insertion for cardiac muscle fibers
    d. Supports the heart valves; includes the four valve rings (annuli)
7. Cardiac chambers (Fig. 3.3)
    a. Atria
        1) Located posterior, superior, and to the right of the corresponding ventricles
        2) Contain the interatrial septum to divide left and right atria
        3) Contain the trabeculae to divide atria and ventricles
        4) Thin-walled, low-pressure chambers
            a) Right: 2 mm thick, 2 to 6 mm Hg pressure
            b) Left: 3 mm thick, 8 to 12 mm Hg pressure
        5) Act as reservoirs and booster pumps for the ventricles
            a) Passive ventricular filling: 70% to 75% of ventricular filling is passive as blood falls through the atrium into the ventricle
            b) Active ventricular filling: 25% to 30% of ventricular filling is active as the atrium contracts at the end of ventricular diastole
        6) Right atria
            a) Inflow tracts
                i) Superior vena cava
                ii) Inferior vena cava
                iii) Coronary sinus
                iv) Thebesian veins
            b) Outflow tract: through the tricuspid valve to right ventricle
        7) Left atria
            a) Inflow tracts: four pulmonary veins (only case of veins carrying oxygenated blood)
            b) Outflow tract: through the mitral valve to left ventricle
    b. Ventricles
        1) Located anterior, inferior, and to the left of the corresponding atria
        2) Contain the interventricular septum to divide the left and right ventricles

3) Contain the trabeculae to divide atria and ventricles
4) Act as pumps receiving blood from the atria and pumping blood into the great vessels
5) Right ventricle
   a) Thin-walled: 3 to 5 mm
   b) Low-pressure pump: 25/5 mm Hg
   c) Inflow tract
      i) Right atria via the tricuspid valve
      ii) Thebesian veins
   d) Outflow tract: pulmonary artery (only case of artery carrying deoxygenated blood)
6) Left ventricle: positioned posterior
   a) Thick-walled: 8 to 15 mm
   b) High-pressure pump: 120/5 mm Hg

c) Inflow tract
   i) Left atria via the mitral valve
   ii) Thebesian veins
d) Outflow tract: aorta

8. Cardiac valves (Fig. 3.4)
   a. Purpose: maintain unidirectional flow
      1) Permit antegrade flow; narrowing of the valvular orifice preventing normal antegrade flow is referred to as *stenosis*
      2) Prevent retrograde flow: inadequate closure of the valvular orifice allowing retrograde flow is referred to as *regurgitant, incompetent,* or *insufficient*
   b. Structure of cardiac valves (Fig. 3.5)
      1) Flexible, fibrous tissue
      2) Rings of connective tissue support the valves
   c. Atrioventricular (AV) valves: tricuspid and mitral valves
      1) Located between atria and ventricles
         a) Tricuspid valve is between right atria and right ventricle.
         b) Mitral valve is between left atria and left ventricle.
      2) Consist of annulus (fibrous supporting ring), cusps (two for mitral, three for tricuspid), and papillary muscles, which attach to valve cusps by chordae tendineae; the cusps are joined for 0.5 to 1.0 cm at the annulus (referred to as a *commissure*)
      3) Open passively during diastole
      4) Close when papillary muscles contract during systole
      5) Cause the first heart sound, S_1, when they close; two components of S_1: M_1 (mitral valve component) and T_1 (tricuspid valve component)

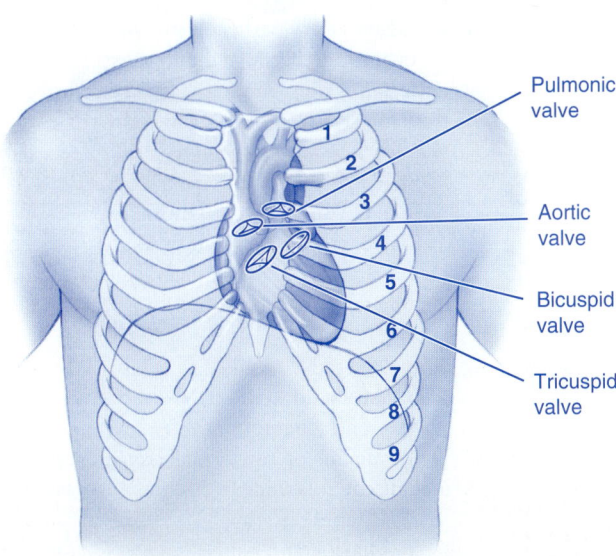

Fig. 3.4 Location of the cardiac valves. (From Herlihy, B. [2014]. *The human body in health and illness* [5th ed.]. St. Louis: Saunders.)

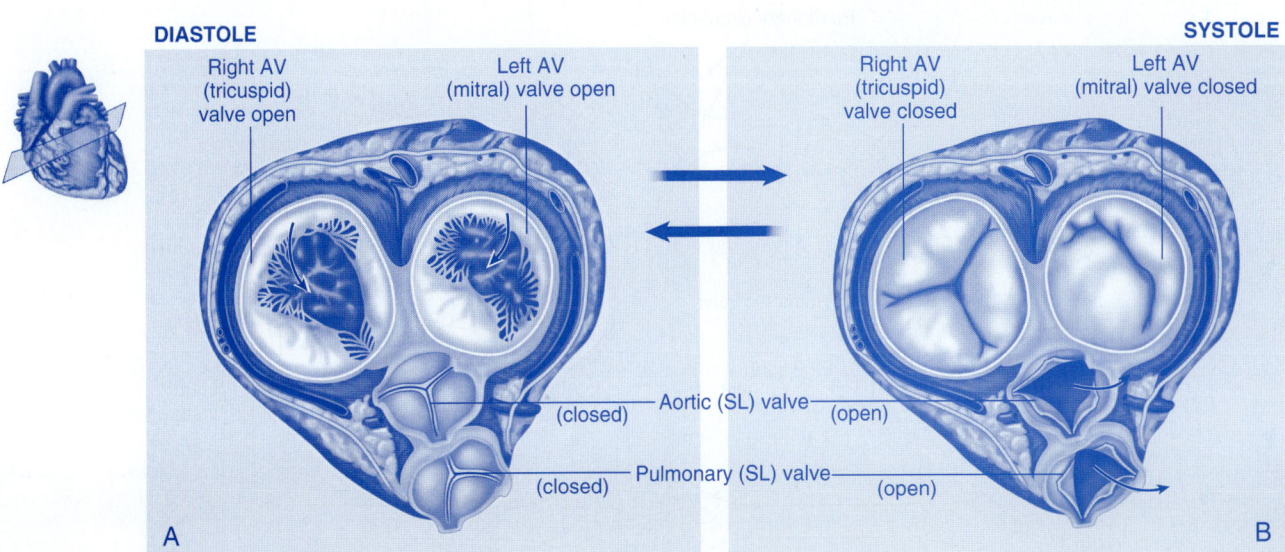

Fig. 3.5 Structure of the cardiac valves, viewed from above. **A,** Ventricular diastole when semilunar valves are closed and atrioventricular valves are open. **B,** Ventricular systole when atrioventricular valves are closed and semilunar valves are open. (From Patton, K. T., & Thibodeau, G. A. [2016] *Anatomy & physiology* [9th ed.]. St. Louis: Mosby.)

d. Semilunar valves: aortic and pulmonic valves
   1) Located between ventricles and great vessels
      a) Pulmonic valve is located between the right ventricle and the pulmonary artery.
      b) Aortic valve is located between the left ventricle and the aorta.
   2) Consist of annulus and three cusps
   3) Function by pressure gradients: pushed open with systolic and closed with diastole
   4) Cause the second heart sound, S_2, when they close; two components of S_2: A_2 (i.e., aortic valve component) and P_2 (i.e., pulmonic valve component)
9. Pathway of blood through the heart and the vascular system: venae cavae (superior and inferior) → right atrium → tricuspid valve → right ventricle → pulmonic valve → pulmonary artery → pulmonary capillary bed → pulmonary veins → left atrium → mitral valve → left ventricle → aortic valve → aorta → arteries → arterioles → capillaries → venules → veins → venae cavae (Fig. 3.6)
10. Coronary vasculature
    a. Coronary arteries are the first branch off the aorta, immediately outside the aortic valve.
    b. Coronary arteries lie on the epicardium, but branches penetrate through to the myocardium and subendocardium.
    c. The myocardium receives 5% of cardiac output (CO) and extracts 65% to 80% of oxygen in the blood even at basal rate.
       1) Blood flow through the coronary arteries is determined almost entirely by local autoregulation in response to the metabolic needs of the myocardium.
       2) Myocardial blood flow is increased by dilation of the coronary arteries.
    d. Coronary artery perfusion
       1) Effect of cardiac cycle
          a) The left ventricle is perfused primarily during diastole because of compression of musculature around intramuscular vessels during systole.
          b) The right ventricle is perfused throughout the cardiac cycle, but perfusion is greater during diastole.
       2) Effect of aortic pressure
          a) The pressure in the aorta immediately outside the aortic valve (referred to as *aortic root pressure*) is significant in coronary artery filling pressure.
          b) Coronary artery perfusion pressure (CAPP) is equal to the diastolic blood pressure (BP) minus the pulmonary artery occlusive pressure (PAOP) (previously known as *pulmonary artery wedge pressure [PAWP]* or *pulmonary capillary wedge pressure [PCWP]*); normal CAPP is 60 to 80 mm Hg.
       3) Myocardial oxygen consumption (Fig. 3.7)
          a) Determinants of myocardial oxygen demand include the following:
             i) Heart rate (HR)
             ii) Preload
             iii) Afterload
             iv) Contractility
          b) Determinants of myocardial oxygen supply include the following:
             i) Patent arteries
             ii) Diastolic pressure

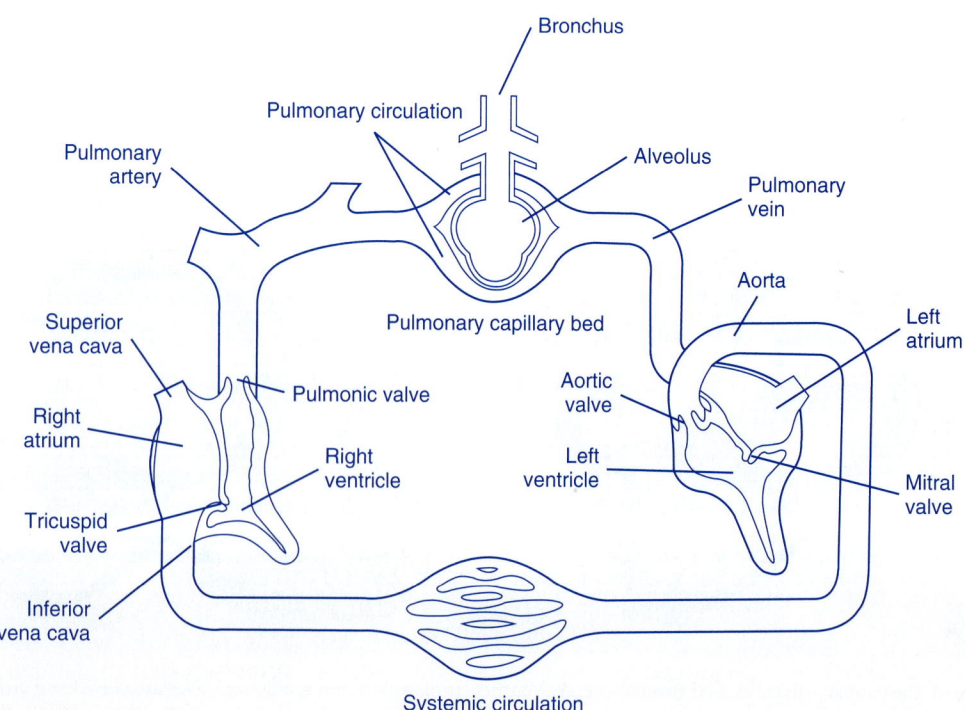

Fig. 3.6 Pathway of blood through the heart and the vascular system. (Courtesy Edwards Lifesciences, Irvine, CA.)

iii) Diastolic time
iv) Oxygen extraction
   (a) Hemoglobin (Hgb)
   (b) Arterial oxygen saturation (SaO$_2$)
c) Imbalances between supply and demand cause ischemia; prolonged imbalance causes infarction.
e. Coronary arteries and distribution (Fig. 3.8)
1) Coronary arteries are end (i.e., terminal) arteries supplying a specific area of myocardium; blockage of a coronary artery therefore results in ischemia or infarction
   a) Partial or temporary occlusion results in ischemia
   b) Complete or permanent occlusion results in infarction
2) Left coronary artery before bifurcation is referred to as the *left main coronary artery*; the left main coronary artery divides into left anterior descending (LAD) and left circumflex arteries.
   a) LAD coronary artery supplies the following:
      i) Anterior left ventricle
      ii) Anterior two thirds of the interventricular septum
      iii) Apex of left ventricle
      iv) Bundle of His and bundle branches
   b) Left circumflex coronary artery (LCA) supplies the following:
      i) Left atrium
      ii) Sinoatrial (SA) node in 45% of hearts
      iii) AV node in 10% of hearts
      iv) Marginal (or obtuse marginal) branch supplies the following:
         (a) Lateral left ventricle
         (b) Posterior left ventricle
3) Right coronary artery (RCA) supplies the following:
   a) Right atrium
   b) SA node in 55% of hearts
   c) Left posterior hemibundle (dual blood supply: LAD and RCA)
   d) AV node in 90% of hearts
   e) Marginal branch supplies:
      i) Lateral right ventricle
      ii) Inferior right ventricle
   f) In RCA-dominant hearts (approximately 80% of hearts), a branch of RCA referred to as the *posterior descending artery* supplies the following:
      i) Anterior right ventricle
      ii) Inferior wall of left ventricle
      iii) Posterior left ventricle
      iv) Posterior third of septum

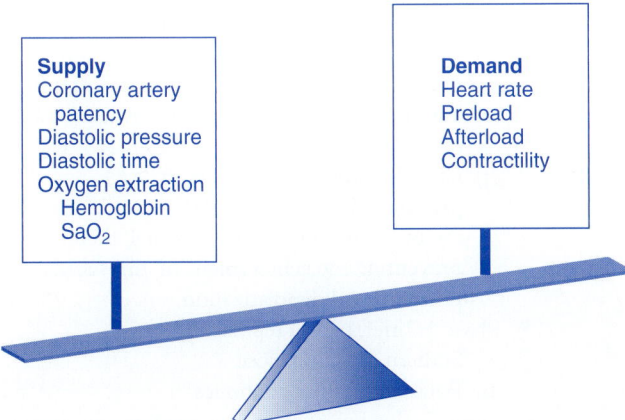

Fig. 3.7 Factors affecting myocardial oxygen supply and myocardial oxygen demand.

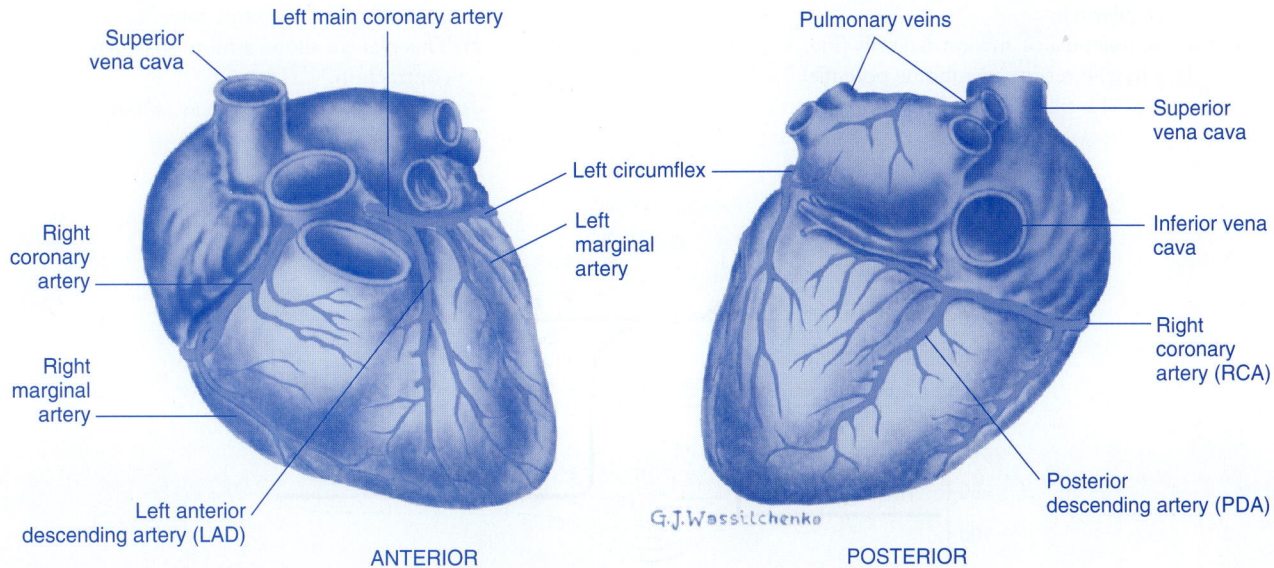

Fig. 3.8 Anterior and posterior views of the coronary artery circulation and major vessels. (From Urden, L., Stacy, K., & Lough, M. [2010]. *Critical care nursing: Diagnosis and management* [6th ed.]. St. Louis: Mosby.)

4) Collateral circulation
   a) Consists of interarterial vessels that connect, or anastomose, with each other
   b) Factors that foster development of collateral flow include: anemia, hypoxemia, and arteriosclerosis (i.e., gradual occlusion)
f. Coronary veins
   1) Most coronary veins empty into the coronary sinus, which empties into the right atrium.
   2) The thebesian veins drain some of venous blood from myocardium directly into the right atrium, right ventricle, and left ventricle rather than through the coronary sinus; this venous blood emptying directly into the left ventricle accounts for a normal physiologic shunt because it slightly decreases oxygen saturation.
g. Lymph vessels
   1) Main cardiac channel empties into the pretracheal node and then into the right lymphatic duct.
   2) Drainage system is facilitated by cardiac contraction.

11. Electrophysiology and the conduction system
    a. Types of cardiac cells
       1) Pacemaker cells
       2) Electrical conducting cells
       3) Myocardial muscle cells
    b. Properties of cardiac cells
       1) Automaticity: ability of certain cardiac cells to initiate impulses regularly and spontaneously
       2) Excitability: ability of the cardiac cells to respond to a stimulus
       3) Conductivity: ability of cardiac cells to respond to a cardiac impulse by transmitting the impulse along cell membranes
       4) Contractility: ability of the cardiac cells to respond to an impulse by muscle contraction
       5) Rhythmicity: ability of the cardiac cells to spontaneously generate an action potential at a regular rate
    c. Action potential of myocardial cells (Fig. 3.9)
       1) Phase 4: resting membrane potential
          a) This phase coincides with isoelectric line between T wave and QRS complex
          b) Electrical charge within the cell is −80 to −95 mV.
          c) Negativity is maintained by the sodium-potassium pump.
             i) An active transport system requires energy to pump sodium out of the cell and potassium into the cell.
             ii) When cellular energy (i.e., adenosine triphosphate [ATP]) supplies are low, such as during shock, this resting membrane potential cannot be maintained, and irritability occurs.
       2) Phase 0: rapid depolarization of the cell
          a) This phase coincides with QRS.
          b) It occurs when a stimulus is applied to the cell.
          c) Cell membrane permeability to sodium increases significantly so that sodium rushes into the cell (influx) and potassium begins to move out (efflux).
          d) If the stimulus is strong enough to reach a critical level known as the *threshold potential* (approximately −60 to −70 mV), then the cell responds entirely and depolarization occurs.
          e) This phase is referred to as the *sodium* (or *fast*) *channel*.
          f) Class I antidysrhythmic agents (e.g., procainamide, quinidine, lidocaine) block the influx of sodium into the cell, thereby preventing the achievement of threshold potential and depolarization.
       3) Phase 1: brief, partial repolarization
          a) Sodium channels close
          b) Potassium efflux continues
       4) Phase 2: slowing of the repolarization causing a plateau
          a) This phase coincides with ST segment.
          b) Calcium influx keeps the cell isoelectric but still depolarized as potassium efflux occurs at approximately the same rate.
          c) This plateau allows a more sustained contraction.
          d) This phase is referred to as *calcium* (or *slow*) *channel*.

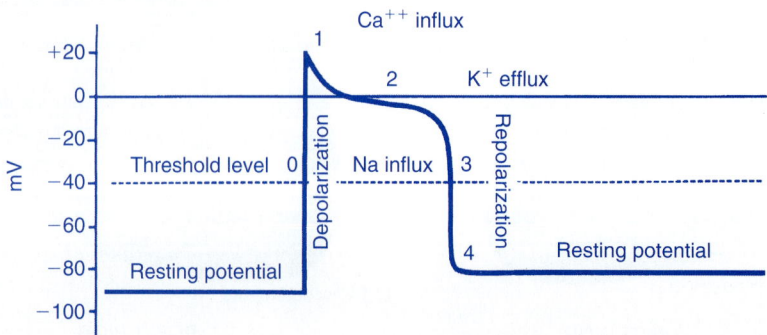

Fig. 3.9 Action potential of a nonpacemaker cell. (From Urden, L., Stacy, K., & Lough, M. [2018]. *Critical care nursing: Diagnosis and management* [8th ed.]. St. Louis: Mosby.)

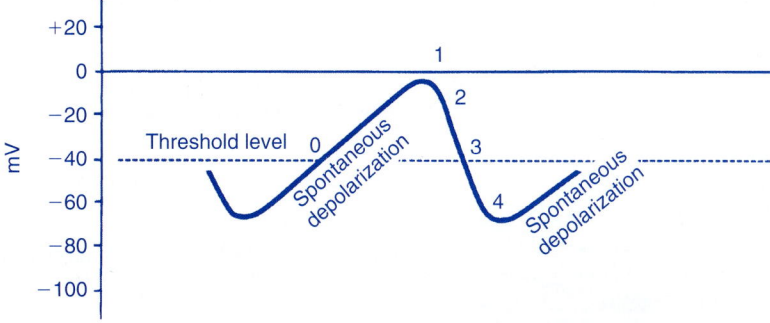

Fig. 3.10 Action potential of a pacemaker cell. (From Urden, L., Stacy, K., & Lough, M. [2018]. *Critical care nursing: Diagnosis and management* [8th ed.]. St. Louis: Mosby.)

e) Class IV antidysrhythmics (calcium channel blockers [e.g., verapamil, diltiazem]) block the movement of calcium and prolong repolarization and refractoriness.
5) Phase 3: sudden acceleration in the rate of repolarization
   a) Potassium movement accelerates during this phase; potassium efflux occurs at the beginning of phase 3 to exceed the influx of calcium and potassium influx occurs at the end of phase 3.
   b) Repolarization is completed.
   c) Class III antidysrhythmics (e.g., amiodarone, ibutilide, dofetilide) block the movement of potassium during this phase and prolong refractoriness.
6) Phase 4: resting membrane potential
d. Action potential of pacemaker cells (Fig. 3.10)
   1) Pacemaker cells have the property of automaticity.
   2) They demonstrate slow diastolic depolarization caused by a time-dependent leak of sodium into the cell.
   3) When enough sodium has entered the cell that threshold potential is reached, spontaneous depolarization occurs.
   4) Rate of diastolic depolarization determines intrinsic rate of pacemakers.
      a) SA node: 60 to 100 times per minute
      b) AV junction: 40 to 60 times per minute
      c) Purkinje fibers: 20 to 40 times per minute
e. Refractoriness (Fig. 3.11)
   1) Absolute refractory period
      a) No matter how strong the impulse is, the cell cannot be depolarized during this period.
      b) This period correlates with the period of time from phase 0 through midphase 3 on the action potential and from the QRS complex to the peak of the T wave on the electrocardiogram (ECG).
   2) Relative refractory period
      a) If the impulse is strong enough, the cell may respond but may respond abnormally (e.g., R-on-T may cause ventricular tachycardia [VT] or ventricular fibrillation [VF]).

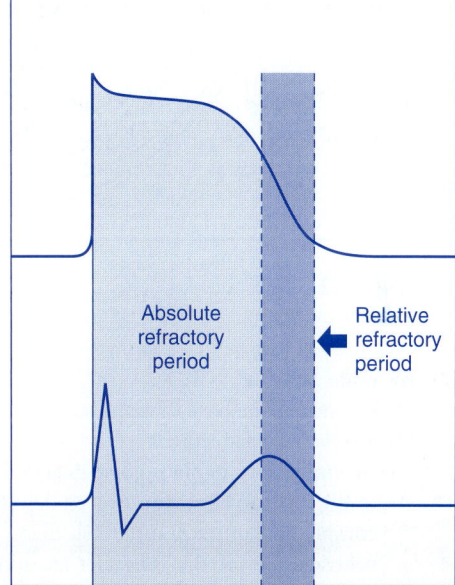

Fig. 3.11 Absolute and relative refractory periods correlated with the myocardial cell action potential and with ECG tracing. (From Urden, L., Stacy, K., & Lough, M. [2018]. *Critical care nursing: Diagnosis and management* [8th ed.]. St. Louis: Mosby.)

   b) This period correlates with late phase 3 of the action potential and the descending limb of the T wave on the ECG.
   3) Effective refractory period: the absolute refractory period plus the relative refractory period
f. Conduction system (Fig. 3.12)
   1) SA node
      a) Functions as the natural pacemaker of the heart because it has the fastest intrinsic rate (60–100 times per minute)
      b) Located in the right atrial wall near opening of superior vena cava
   2) Internodal pathways
      a) Three pathways between SA node and AV node
         i) Anterior tract (i.e., Bachmann)
         ii) Middle tract (i.e., Wenckebach)
         iii) Posterior tract (i.e., Thorel)
   3) Bachmann bundle (interatrial pathway): pathway that takes the impulse from right atrium to left atrium

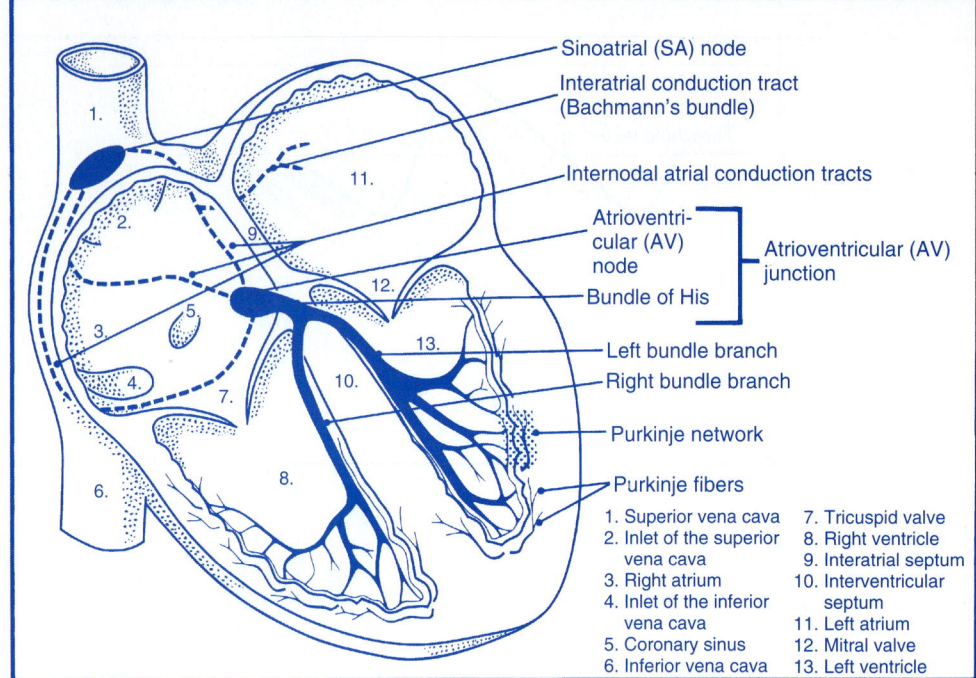

Fig. 3.12 The conduction system. (From Wesley, K. [2011]. *Huszar's basic dysrhythmias* [4th ed.]. St. Louis: Mosby.)

4) AV node
   a) Located at the base of right atrium at top of interventricular septum
   b) Accounts for the physiologic delay of 0.08 to 0.12 secs to allow the atria to depolarize completely, contract, and finish filling the ventricles before the ventricles are stimulated
   c) Contains no pacemaker cells; primary function is to slow the impulse down
5) AV junction
   a) Tissue surrounding AV node and bundle of His that contains pacemaker cells
   b) Functions as a secondary pacemaker with intrinsic rate of 40 to 60 times per minute
6) Bundle of His
   a) First portion of intraventricular conduction system
7) Bundle branches
   a) Right bundle branch (RBB) takes the impulse to the right ventricular (RV) myocardium.
   b) Left bundle branch (LBB) divides into three hemibundles.
      i) Septal hemibundle depolarizes the interventricular septum in a left-to-right direction.
      ii) Left anterior hemibundle (LAH) depolarizes the anterior and superior left ventricle.
      iii) Left posterior hemibundle (LPH) depolarizes the posterior and inferior left ventricle.
      iv) Hemiblocks
         (a) Block of the septal hemibundle does not cause a clinically identifiable situation.
         (b) The posterior hemibundle is thicker than the anterior hemibundle and has a dual blood supply so less susceptible to block than the anterior hemibundle
      c) These three major branches (i.e., RBB, LAH, LPH) are referred to as *fascicles* as in *unifascicular, bifascicular,* and *trifascicular block.*
8) Purkinje fiber system
   a) The fascicles divide into the Purkinje fibers, which continue to divide and take the impulse through the ventricular walls to terminate in the subendocardial surface of the ventricles.
   b) Acts as a final tertiary pacemaker if upper pacemakers fail at the inherent rate of 20 to 40 times per minute
9) Intercalated disks separate adjacent myocardial cells to allow rapid cell-to-cell transmission of electrical impulses and almost simultaneous activation and contraction of myocardial cells; this capability of the myocardium to respond as if it were one muscle is referred to as a *functional syncytium.*
   g. Depolarization of cardiac chambers occurs from endocardium to epicardium.
   h. Repolarization of cardiac chambers occurs from epicardium to endocardium.
12. Muscle mechanics
   a. Cardiac muscle is similar to skeletal muscle except for the following:
      1) Cardiac muscle has more mitochondria than skeletal muscle; cardiac muscle has greater ATP requirements because of the high energy requirements of the repetitive muscular action of the heart.

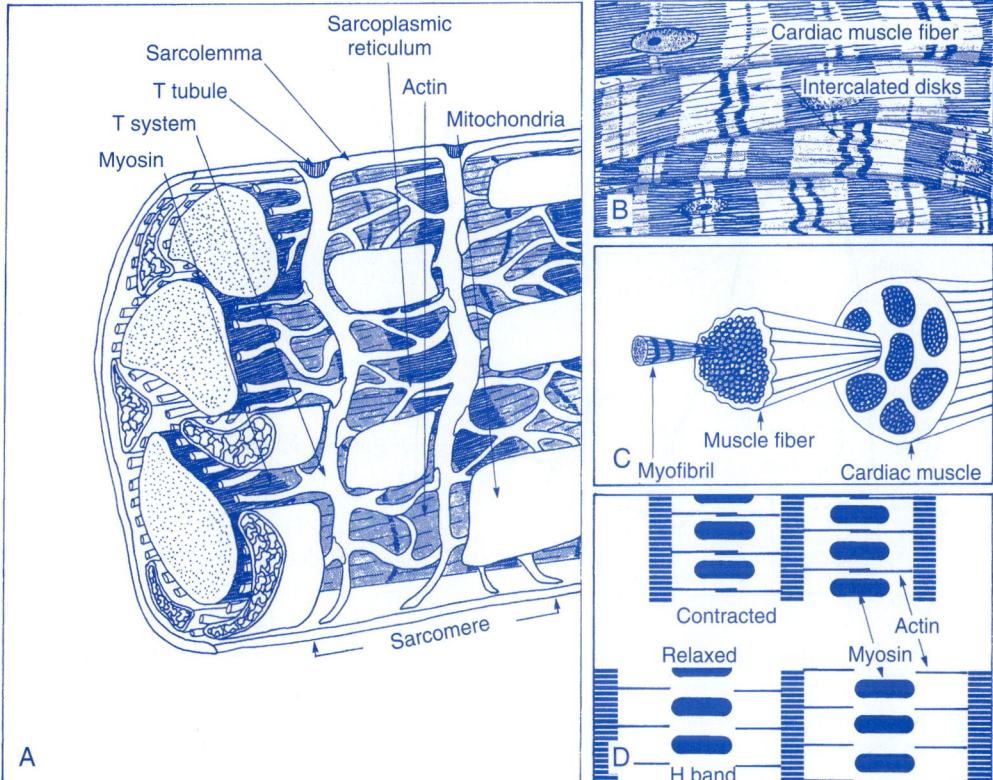

Fig. 3.13 Cardiac muscle. **A,** The ultrastructure. **B,** Intercalated disks lie between muscle cells. **C,** Myofibrils form muscle fibers, which form cardiac muscle. **D,** Actin and myosin are myofilaments, which interlace in the presence of calcium to cause muscle contraction and shortening. (From Guzzetta C. E., & Dossey, B. M. [1992]. *Cardiovascular nursing: Holistic practice.* St. Louis: Mosby.)

    2) Cardiac muscle remains contracted 150 to 300 times longer than skeletal muscle.
    3) Cardiac muscle forms a functional syncytium.
       a) Intercalated disks lie between myocardial cells; they offer low electrical impedance, allowing electrical stimuli to pass with ease from cell to cell.
       b) Stimulation of any muscle fiber results in stimulation of the entire muscle mass (all-or-none response).
       c) The heart acts as if it is one muscle (i.e., functional syncytium).
  b. Cardiac muscle ultrastructure (Fig. 3.13)
    1) A sarcomere is the basic contractile unit of the myocardium.
       a) The sarcomere measures between 1.6 to 2.2 μm; it contains a centrally placed nucleus surrounded by intracellular protein fluid called sarcoplasm, which is surrounded by a membrane called a sarcolemma.
       b) The sarcomere is composed of two sets of overlapping myofilaments, including the thick myosin myofilament and the thin actin myofilament.
       c) Troponin and tropomyosin are regulatory proteins in the sarcomere that form a troponin–tropomyosin complex to cover the myosin binding sites and inhibit cross-bridging of actin and myosin when the muscle is in a resting state.
       d) The sarcoplasmic reticulum, a continuation of the sarcolemma, penetrates the cell to form a complex tubular (T tubule) system surrounding each fibril.
       e) Calcium is stored in the sarcoplasmic reticulum and is necessary for the cross-bridging of actin and myosin.
  c. Excitation–contraction process
    1) The wave of depolarization spreads through conduction system to myocardial muscle cell.
    2) The action potential reaches the sarcoplasmic reticulum, and the T tubules transmit the action potential from sarcolemma to interior of the cell.
    3) Calcium enters the cell during phase 2 of the action potential through calcium channels in the sarcolemma and the T tubules; more calcium is released from intracellular stores in the sarcoplasmic reticulum.
    4) Calcium binds with troponin to move the troponin and tropomyosin out of the way of the myosin binding sites.
    5) Actin and myosin myofilaments interact to form crossbridges that slide these overlapping myofilaments past one another.
    6) Shortening of the sarcomere occurs.
    7) Multiple sarcomere shortening, muscle contraction, and ejection of blood from the chamber occur.

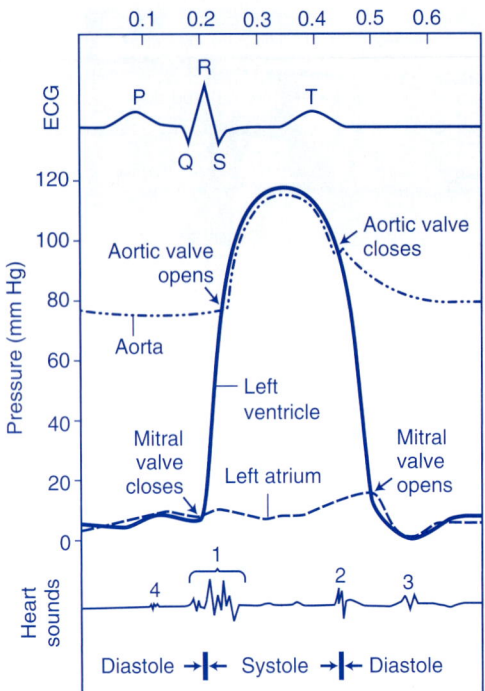

Fig. 3.14 Wigger diagram: demonstrates the cardiac cycle showing electrocardiographic events, heart sounds, and pressure curves.

8) Calcium is pumped back into the sarcoplasmic reticulum, which dissociates actin–myosin crossbridges; without the antagonist effect of calcium, troponin and tropomyosin form a troponin–tropomyosin complex, which inhibits the cross-bridging of actin and myosin.
9) Muscle relaxation occurs.

13. Cardiac cycle (Fig. 3.14)
    a. Systole: the contraction phase
        1) Isovolumetric contraction: subphase 1
            a) Contraction increases pressure in the ventricle, but there is no change in volume because the AV valves are closed, and the semilunar valves have not yet opened.
            b) Ventricular pressure must exceed the pressure in the great vessel to open the semilunar valve.
            c) This subphase accounts for two thirds of oxygen consumption of the ventricle.
            d) This subphase follows the QRS.
        2) Maximal ejection: subphase 2
            a) When the pressure in the ventricle exceeds the pressure in the great vessel, the semilunar valve opens, and blood is rapidly ejected into the great vessel.
            b) Aortic and pulmonary artery pressures (PAPs) increase rapidly, and ventricular volume decreases sharply.
            c) This subphase occurs during the ST segment.
        3) Reduced ejection (also referred to as *protodiastole*): subphase 3
            a) Blood is slowly ejected from the ventricle to the great vessel.
            b) Ventricular pressure and volume decrease.
            c) When the pressure in the great vessel is greater than the pressure in the ventricle, the semilunar valve closes, and systole ends.
            d) This subphase occurs during the T wave.
    b. Diastole: the relaxation phase
        1) Isovolumetric relaxation: subphase 1
            a) Relaxation occurs, and ventricular pressure decreases, but volume does not change because the semilunar valves have closed, and the AV valves have not yet opened.
            b) This subphase occurs after the T wave.
        2) Rapid filling: subphase 2
            a) During this subphase, the AV valves open, and blood rushes into the ventricles.
            b) Atrial and ventricular pressures decrease, and ventricular volume increases.
            c) Ventricular pressure is less than atrial pressure.
            d) This subphase occurs during the TP interval.
        3) Reduced filling (also referred to as *diastasis*): subphase 3
            a) Atrial and ventricular pressures slowly increase, and ventricular volumes increase with slow filling of ventricles.
            b) Coronary artery blood flow is optimal.
            c) This subphase occurs during the TP interval.
        4) Atrial contraction: subphase 4
            a) This subphase is also referred to as the *atrial kick*.
            b) Atrial contraction accounts for 15% to 30% of diastolic filling volume; may be up to 50% when left ventricular (LV) filling is impeded (e.g., mitral stenosis)
            c) Atrial pressure decreases, and ventricular volume and pressure increase.
            d) This subphase occurs after P wave.

14. Regulation of cardiac function
    a. Definitions
        1) CO: the amount of blood ejected by the ventricle in 1 minute
        2) Cardiac index (CI): the CO indexed for differences in body size by dividing by body surface area (BSA)
        3) Stroke volume (SV): the amount of blood ejected by the ventricle with each contraction; also defined as the difference between the end-diastolic volume and the end-systolic volume
        4) Stroke index (SI): the SV indexed for differences in body size by dividing by BSA
        5) Ejection fraction (EF): percentage of blood in the ventricle that is ejected during systole; normal is 55% to 75%
        6) Afterload: the pressure against which the ventricle must pump; the pressure required to open the semilunar valve
        7) Preload: the volume of blood in the ventricle at the end of diastole (end-diastolic pressure); determines the stretch on the myofibrils and the subsequent force of the next contraction (according to Starling law of the heart)
        8) Contractility: the force and velocity of the ejection of blood from the ventricle independent of preload and afterload

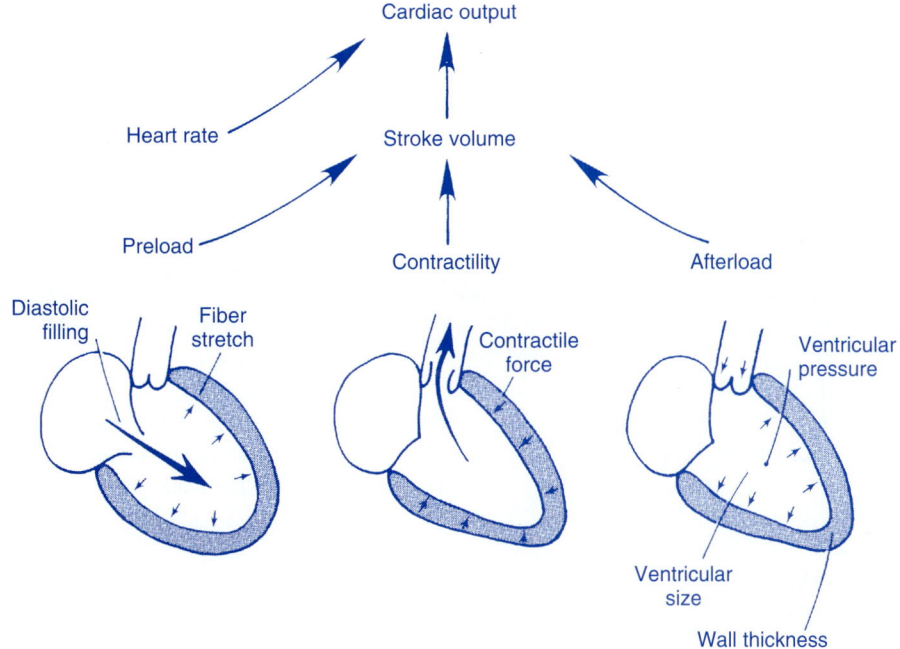

Fig. 3.15 Determinants of cardiac output. (From Price, S., & Wilson, L. [2003]. *Pathophysiology: Clinical concepts of disease processes*. [6th ed.]. St. Louis: Mosby.)

b. Intrinsic control of the heart
  1) Determinants of CO (Fig. 3.15 and Table 3.1)
    a) HR
      i) Definition: number of times per minute that the ventricles contract
      ii) Evaluation
        (a) Count the number of pulses palpable in 1 minute; the radial, brachial, femoral, or carotid pulses are most often used.
        (b) If the apical rate is auscultated with a stethoscope or the HR on ECG monitor is used to evaluate the HR, a palpable pulse with each audible heart sound or QRS must be confirmed.
      iii) Effect of HR on CO
        (a) If HR is less than 50 or greater than 150 beats/min, CO often falls, and the tendency to dysrhythmias increases.
      iv) Effect of HR on myocardial oxygen consumption
        (a) Although an increase in HR may increase CO, an increase in HR greater than 120 beats/min tends to increase myocardial oxygen demand more than the increase in coronary blood flow, potentially causing ischemia, especially in patients with CAD.
      v) Table 3.1 describes factors affecting HR.
    b) Preload
      i) Definition: the stretch on the myofibrils at the end of diastole
        (a) The degree of myofibril stretch is affected by the ventricular volume.
        (b) Although preload is a volume concept, it has traditionally been evaluated by the pressure in the ventricle at the end of diastole.
          (i) The relationship between volume and pressure is affected by the compliance of the ventricle.
          (ii) In a normally compliant ventricle, there is a linear relationship between volume and pressure.
          (iii) In a noncompliant ventricle, there is a disproportionate increase in pressure with changes in volume; this is referred to as *diastolic dysfunction*.
          (iv) Some causes of noncompliance of the ventricle include myocardial ischemia or infarction, ventricular hypertrophy, hypertrophic cardiomyopathy, restrictive pericarditis, and cardiac tamponade.
        (c) RV volumetric monitoring allows more accurate evaluation of preload through the evaluation of RV volumes rather than pressure and evaluation of RVEF.

Table 3.1 Determinants of Cardiac Output

Parameter	Conditions – Increased	Conditions – Decreased	Treatments – To increase	Treatments – To decrease

Heart rate: evaluated by palpation of pulse	• SNS stimulation (e.g., exercise, fever, infection, pain, anxiety, hypovolemia or hypervolemia, most physiologic or psychological stressors)
	• Drug effects (e.g., epinephrine, dopamine)
		• PNS (vagal) stimulation (e.g., Valsalva maneuver, coughing, suctioning, vomiting, carotid stimulation)
		• Conduction abnormalities (e.g., sinus arrest or block, second- or third-degree AV blocks) caused by ischemia, infarction, or inflammation
		• Drug effects (e.g., beta-blockers, digoxin)
			• Treatment of cause (e.g., reperfusion therapies for myocardial infarction, antiemetics for vomiting)
			• Parasympatholytic drugs (e.g., atropine)
			• Sympathomimetic drugs (e.g., epinephrine)
			• Pacemaker
				• Treatment of cause (e.g., antipyretics for fever, analgesics for pain, anxiolytics for anxiety)
				• Dependent upon rhythm:
				  • Cardiac glycosides (e.g., digoxin)
				  • Beta-blockers (e.g., propranolol, esmolol)
				  • Calcium channel blockers (e.g., verapamil, diltiazem)
				  • Other antidysrhythmic drugs dependent on rhythm
				• Vagal maneuvers
				  • Overdrive pacemaker
				  • Ablation
				  • Cardioversion or defibrillation

Preload: evaluated by PAOP (LV) and RAP (RV) or RVEDV if a right ejection fraction (REF) catheter used	• Heart failure • Hypervolemia • Bradydysrhythmias	• Hypovolemia • Excessive vasodilation (e.g., vasogenic shock) • Increased intrathoracic pressure (e.g., positive pressure mechanical ventilation) • Cardiac tamponade • Right ventricular failure or infarction (LV) • Tachydysrhythmias • Loss of atrial contraction (e.g., atrial fibrillation)	• Fluids • Isotonic crystalloids (e.g., normal [0.9%] saline, lactated Ringer solution) • Colloids (e.g., albumin, plasma protein fraction [PPF], dextran, hetastarch) • Blood and/or blood products • Adjustment of vasodilator dosage	• Diuretics (e.g., furosemide) • Venous vasodilators (e.g., nitroglycerin, morphine sulfate, nitroprusside, calcium channel blockers [e.g., nifedipine]) • ACE inhibitors (e.g., captopril, enalapril) or ARBs (e.g., losartan, valsartan) • Nesiritide
Afterload: evaluated by calculation of SVR and SVRI (LV) and PVR and PVRI (RV)	• Vasoconstriction as from SNS stimulation or vasopressors • Hypertension • Aortic stenosis • Hypercoagulability • Pulmonary hypertension (RV)	• Hypotension • Vasodilation (e.g., vasogenic shock such as septic shock, neurogenic shock, or anaphylactic shock)	• Adjustment of vasodilator dosage • Vasopressors (e.g., phenylephrine, norepinephrine, epinephrine, dopamine, vasopressin)	• Arterial vasodilators (e.g., nitroprusside, nitroglycerin greater than 1 mcg/kg/min, hydralazine, calcium channel blockers [e.g., nifedipine], alpha blockers [e.g., phentolamine, labetalol]) • ACE inhibitors (e.g., captopril, enalapril) or ARBs (e.g., losartan, valsartan), PDE inhibitors (e.g., milrinone, inamrinone) • Intraaortic balloon pump • Right ventricle specifically: oxygen, pulmonary vasodilators (e.g., aminophylline, nitric oxide, epoprostenol, bosentan)
Contractility: evaluated by calculation of stroke volume and LVSWI (LV) and RVSWI (RV)	• SNS stimulation (see heart rate for selected factors that stimulate SNS) • Sympathomimetic drugs (e.g., epinephrine)	• Myocardial ischemia or infarction • Cardiomyopathy • Hypoxemia • Acidosis • Shock (i.e., myocardial depressant factor) • Drug adverse effects (e.g., barbiturates, anesthetics, beta-blockers, calcium channel blockers, most antidysrhythmics)	• Cardiac glycosides (e.g., digoxin) • Sympathomimetics (e.g., dobutamine, dopamine at medium [~5 mcg/kg/min] dose) • PDE inhibitors (e.g., milrinone, inamrinone) • Glucagon	• Beta-blockers (e.g., propranolol, metoprolol, esmolol) • Calcium channel blockers (e.g., diltiazem, verapamil)

ACE, Angiotensin-converting enzyme; *ARB*, angiotensin receptor blocker; *LVSWI*, Left ventricular stroke work index; *PDE*, phosphodiesterase; *PVR*, pulmonary vascular resistance; *PVRI*, pulmonary vascular resistance index; *RVEDV*, right ventricular end-diastolic volume; *RVSWI*, right ventricular stroke work index; *SNS*, sympathetic nervous system; *SVR*, systemic vascular resistance; *SVRI*, systemic vascular resistance index.

Table 3.2 Clinical Indications of Hypoperfusion

Normal	Subclinical Hypoperfusion	Clinical Hypoperfusion	Shock
CI 2.5–4 l/min/m^2	CI 2.2–2.5 l/min/m^2	CI 2–2.2 l/min/m^2	CI <2 l/min/m^2
Normal	• No clinical indications of hypoperfusion, but an expert nurse may detect subtle changes in the patient • Hypoperfusion at this stage is detected by hemodynamic monitoring	• Tachycardia • Narrowed pulse pressure • Tachypnea • Cool skin • Oliguria • Diminished bowel sounds • Restlessness → confusion	• Dysrhythmias • Hypotension • Tachypnea • Cold, clammy skin • Anuria • Absent bowel sounds • Lethargy → coma

CI, Cardiac index.

ii) Evaluation
  (a) Invasive: atrial pressure correlates to end-diastolic pressure for the respective ventricle
    (i) RV preload correlates to central venous pressure (CVP) or right atrial pressure (RAP) if no tricuspid valve disease
    (ii) LV preload correlates to PAOP or left atrial pressure (LAP) if no mitral valve disease
    (iii) RV volumetric monitoring (requires right ejection fraction [REF] catheter) allows measurement of RV systolic volume, RV end-diastolic volume, and RVEF, which are more accurate reflections of preload, especially in patients with decreased ventricular compliance.
  (b) Noninvasive evaluation
    (i) RV: jugular venous distention (JVD), hepatomegaly, and peripheral edema indicate high RV preload; flat neck veins when the patient is flat, and oliguria indicate low RV preload
    (ii) LV: S$_3$, crackles, and dyspnea indicate high LV preload; clinical indications of hypoperfusion (Table 3.2) indicate low LV preload.
iii) Effect of preload on SV and CO
  (a) Starling law of the heart and the Frank-Starling mechanism: within physiologic limits, the greater the stretch on the myofibrils, the greater the force of the subsequent contraction (Fig. 3.16).
    (i) Both understretching and overstretching of the myofibrils result in a less than optimal contraction.

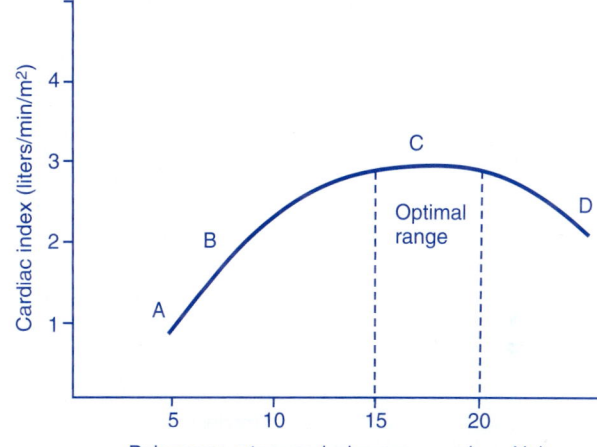

Fig. 3.16 Relationship between pulmonary artery occlusive pressure (PAOP) and cardiac index (CI). **A,** Understretched myofibrils, resulting in decreased contractility and CI. **B,** Normal stretched myofibrils, resulting in normal (but suboptimal) CI. **C,** Optimally stretched myofibrils, resulting in optimal cardiac index. **D,** Overstretched myofibrils, resulting in decreased contractility and CI.

    iv) Effect of preload on myocardial oxygen consumption: as preload increases, myocardial oxygen consumption increases.
    v) Table 3.1 describes factors affecting preload
  c) Afterload
    i) Definition: the pressure against which the ventricle must pump to open the semilunar valve; affected by vascular resistance, ventricular diameter, and the mass and viscosity of blood
    ii) Evaluation
      (a) Invasive: calculated parameter
        (i) RV afterload correlates to pulmonary vascular resistance (PVR) and pulmonary vascular resistance index (PVRI)
        (ii) LV afterload correlates to systemic vascular resistance (SVR) and systemic vascular resistance index (SVRI)

(b) Noninvasive
    (i) RV: loud P_2 and high PA diastolic pressure indicate high RV afterload; low PA diastolic pressure indicates low RV afterload.
    (ii) LV: loud A_2, cool, pale extremities, and high systemic arterial diastolic pressure indicate high LV afterload; low systemic arterial diastolic pressure indicates low LV afterload.
iii) Effect of afterload on SV and CO (Fig. 3.17)
iv) Effect of afterload on myocardial oxygen consumption: as afterload increases, myocardial oxygen consumption increases.
v) Table 3.1 describes factors affecting afterload.
d) Contractility
    i) Definition: the force and velocity of the ejection of blood from the ventricle independent of preload and afterload
    (a) Laplace law states that the amount of contractile force generated within a chamber depends on the radius of the chamber and the thickness of its walls; therefore, the smaller the radius and the thicker the wall, the greater the force of contraction.
    (b) Contractility is also significantly affected by endogenous catecholamines (e.g., epinephrine).

ii) Evaluation
    (a) Invasive: calculated parameters
        (i) RV contractility correlates to right ventricular stroke work index (RVSWI).
        (ii) LV contractility correlates to left ventricular stroke work index (LVSWI).
        (iii) EF by REF catheter
    (b) Noninvasive
        (i) Clinical indicators of hypoperfusion (Table 3.2)
        (ii) Diminished heart sounds
        (iii) EF by multiple gated acquisition (MUGA) scan or Doppler echocardiogram
    iii) Effect of contractility on SV and CO (Fig. 3.18)
    iv) Effect of contractility on myocardial oxygen consumption: as contractility increases, myocardial oxygen consumption increases.
    v) Table 3.1 describes factors affecting contractility.
c. Extrinsic control of the heart
    1) Neurologic control of the heart
        a) Autonomic nervous system
            i) Terms used to describe cardiac effects
                (a) Chronotropic: effect on HR
                (b) Inotropic: effect on contractility
                (c) Dromotropic: effect on conductivity
            ii) Sympathetic nervous system (SNS)
                (a) This branch is referred to as *fight or flight*.
                (b) SNS is innervated by physiologic or psychological stress.

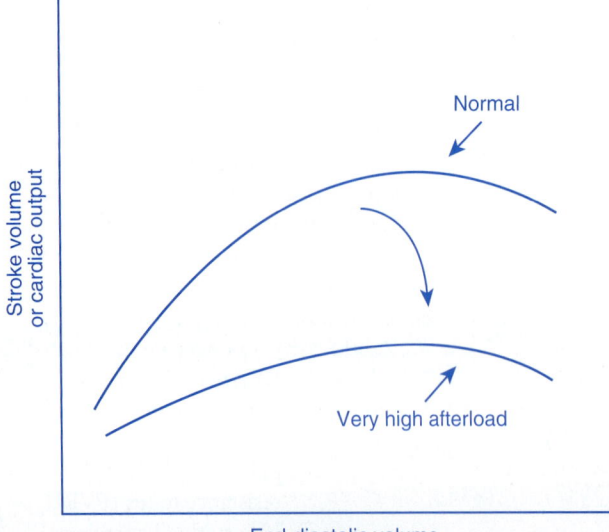

Fig. 3.17 Relationship between afterload and stroke volume. (From Hicks, G. H. [2000]. *Cardiopulmonary anatomy and physiology*. Philadelphia: Saunders.)

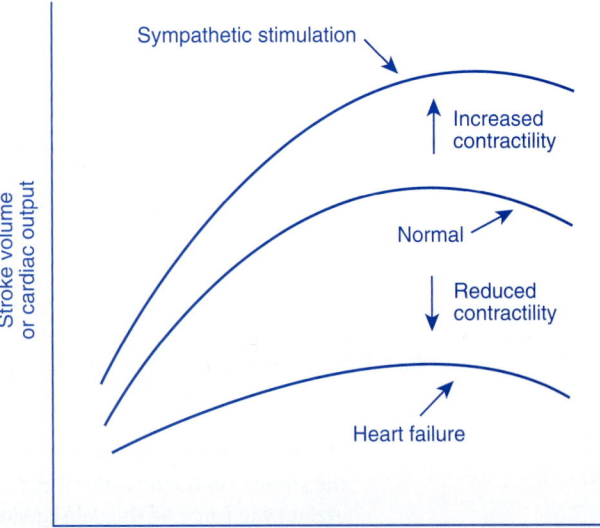

Fig. 3.18 Relationship between contractility and stroke volume. (From Hicks, G. H. [2000]. *Cardiopulmonary anatomy and physiology*. Philadelphia: Saunders.)

(c) It causes positive chronotropic, inotropic, and dromotropic effects.
(d) SNS receptors and effects are listed in Table 3.3.
(e) Sympathomimetic drugs are frequently used in critical care to augment these effects, especially after the patient's endogenous supplies are depleted; these drugs vary in their receptor stimulation and the potency of the stimulation (Table 3.4).

b) Parasympathetic (vagal) nervous system (PNS)
   i) This branch maintains steady state.
   ii) PNS causes negative chronotropic, inotropic, and dromotropic effects.
   iii) Although the cardiovascular effects of the PNS are generally undesirable in critical care, they may decrease myocardial oxygen consumption by up to 50%.
   iv) Parasympatholytic (or vagolytic) agents (e.g., atropine) block these effects.

c) Chemoreceptors
   i) Chemoreceptors are located in carotid and aortic bodies.
   ii) They are sensitive to changes in PaO_2, $PaCO_2$, and pH.
   iii) Hypoxia, hypercapnia, and acidosis cause changes in HR and ventilatory rate.

d) Baroreceptor (or aortic) reflex
   i) Baroreceptors are located in the carotid sinus and aortic arch.
   ii) They are sensitive to increased arterial pressure.
   iii) Medullary discharge causes vagal stimulation.
   iv) Vagal stimulation results in a decrease in HR and contractility, which decreases CO and arterial pressure.

e) Bainbridge reflex
   i) Baroreceptors are located in the right atrium.
   ii) They are sensitive to increased venous pressure and RAP.
   iii) Medullary discharge decreases vagal stimulation.
   iv) Decreased parasympathetic tone causes an increase in HR and CO which decreases venous pressure and RAP.

f) Respiratory reflex
   i) Inspiration decreases intrathoracic pressure, which increases venous return to the right side of the heart, which causes the Bainbridge reflex; when the increased venous return reaches the left side of the heart, LV CO increases, which increases arterial BP and decreases the HR through stimulation of baroreceptors.

Table 3.3 Sympathetic Nervous System (Adrenergic) Receptors and Effects

Receptor	Location of Receptors	Effects
Alpha$_1$	Vessels	Vasoconstriction of most vessels, especially the arterioles
Beta$_1$	Heart	Increase in heart rate (chronotropic effect), contractility (inotropic effect), and conductivity (dromotropic effect)
Beta$_2$	Bronchial and vascular smooth muscle	Bronchodilation, vasodilation
Dopaminergic	Renal and mesenteric artery bed	Dilation of renal and mesenteric arteries
Vasopressin$_1$	High concentration in vascular smooth muscle; lesser concentration in cardiac myocytes; and least concentration in the brain, renal medulla, testes, liver, cervical ganglion, and platelets	Vasoconstriction
Vasopressin$_2$	Kidneys	Antidiuresis (i.e., fluid retention)
Vasopressin$_3$	Pituitary gland	Vasoconstriction

Table 3.4 Sympathomimetic Agents and Receptor Stimulation

Drug	Alpha$_1$	Beta$_1$	Beta$_2$
Phenylephrine	++++	0	0
Norepinephrine	++++	++	0
Epinephrine	++++	++++	++
Dopamine	++ >5 mcg/kg/min; +++ >10 mcg/kg/min	++++ <10 mcg/kg/min	+
Dobutamine	+	++++	++
Isoproterenol	0	++++	++++

ii) This process is at least partly responsible for sinus dysrhythmia; an interaction between the respiratory and cardiac centers in the medulla also contributes.
  d. The endocrine function of the heart
    1) Atrial natriuretic peptide (ANP)
       a) Produced and stored by specialized atrial muscle cells
       b) Triggers for ANP release
          i) Primary cause of ANP release is increased atrial stretch.
          ii) Other causes of ANP release include acute increase in intravascular volume, exercise, and endogenous or exogenous vasopressors.
       c) Actions and effects: important regulator of blood volume and BP
          i) Inhibits sodium transport in the collecting ducts of the kidney, resulting in increased urine output
          ii) Acts as an antagonist to angiotensin II, epinephrine, and endothelin, resulting in decrease in HR and vasodilation
          iii) Diminishes the renin-angiotensin-aldosterone (RAA) system, resulting in sodium and water excretion
          iv) Decreases proliferation of cardiac fibroblasts and smooth muscle cells, resulting in the prevention of ventricular remodeling
    2) Brain natriuretic peptide (BNP)
       a) First discovered in animal brain tissue (hence the name) but is produced by ventricular muscle tissue
       b) Triggers for BNF release: increased intravascular volume
       c) Actions and effects: similar to ANP with dilation of both arteries and veins
       d) Measurement of BNP is being used both as a diagnostic study for diagnosis of heart failure (HF) as well as a therapeutic pharmacologic agent (i.e., nesiritide) for HF
    3) C-type natriuretic peptide
       a) Lowest concentration of circulating plasma natriuretic peptides; distributed predominantly in the central nervous system (CNS), kidneys, and endothelial cells
       b) Actions and effects: marked vasodilatory effects but no natriuretic effect
    4) Endothelin
       a) Potent vasoconstrictive peptides produced by endothelial cells
       b) Causes an increase in renin, aldosterone, antidiuretic hormone, and SNS effects to increase SVR

Vascular System
1. Function: supply blood, nutrients, and hormones to the tissues and remove metabolic wastes from the tissues
2. Resistance to flow

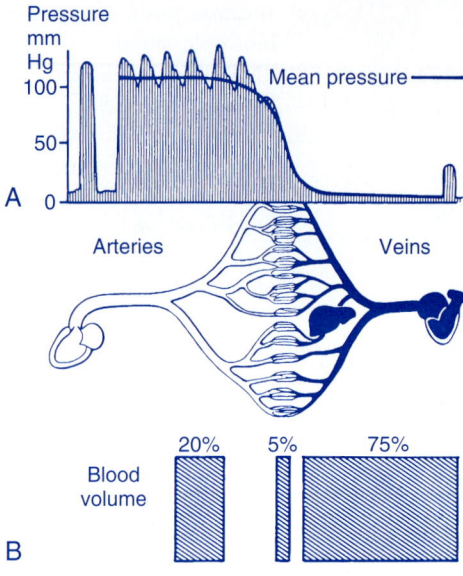

Fig. 3.19 Components of the vascular system. **A,** Mean pressure in components of vascular system. **B,** Volume in components of vascular system. (From Rushmer, R. [1976]. *Cardiovascular dynamics* [4th ed.]. Philadelphia: Saunders.)

   a. Poiseuille formula states that resistance depends on:
      1) The length of the vessel
      2) The radius of the vessel
      3) The viscosity of the blood
   b. Blood flow through the body is also influenced by neurologic stimulation affecting vascular tone and features that cause turbulence within the vascular lumen such as bifurcations or protrusions from the vessel wall into the vessel lumen (e.g., atherosclerosis).
3. Components of the vascular system (Fig. 3.19)
   a. Arteries
      1) The arteries are the delivery system that distributes and regulates the amount of oxygenated blood flow to various tissue beds.
      2) Arteries are able to stretch during systole and recoil during diastole.
      3) The arterial system is a high-pressure circuit.
      4) The layers of the arterial wall consist of the following (Fig. 3.20):
         a) Intima: thin lining of endothelium and a small amount of elastic tissue; decreases resistance to flow and minimizes the chance of platelet aggregation
         b) Media: smooth muscle and elastic tissue; changes the lumen diameter as needed
         c) Adventitia: connective tissue; strengthens and shapes the vessels
   b. Arterioles
      1) Arterioles are vital to the maintenance of BP and SVR
      2) Arterioles may lead to any of the following:
         a) Capillaries
         b) Metarterioles
         c) Precapillary sphincters which control blood flow into capillary bed

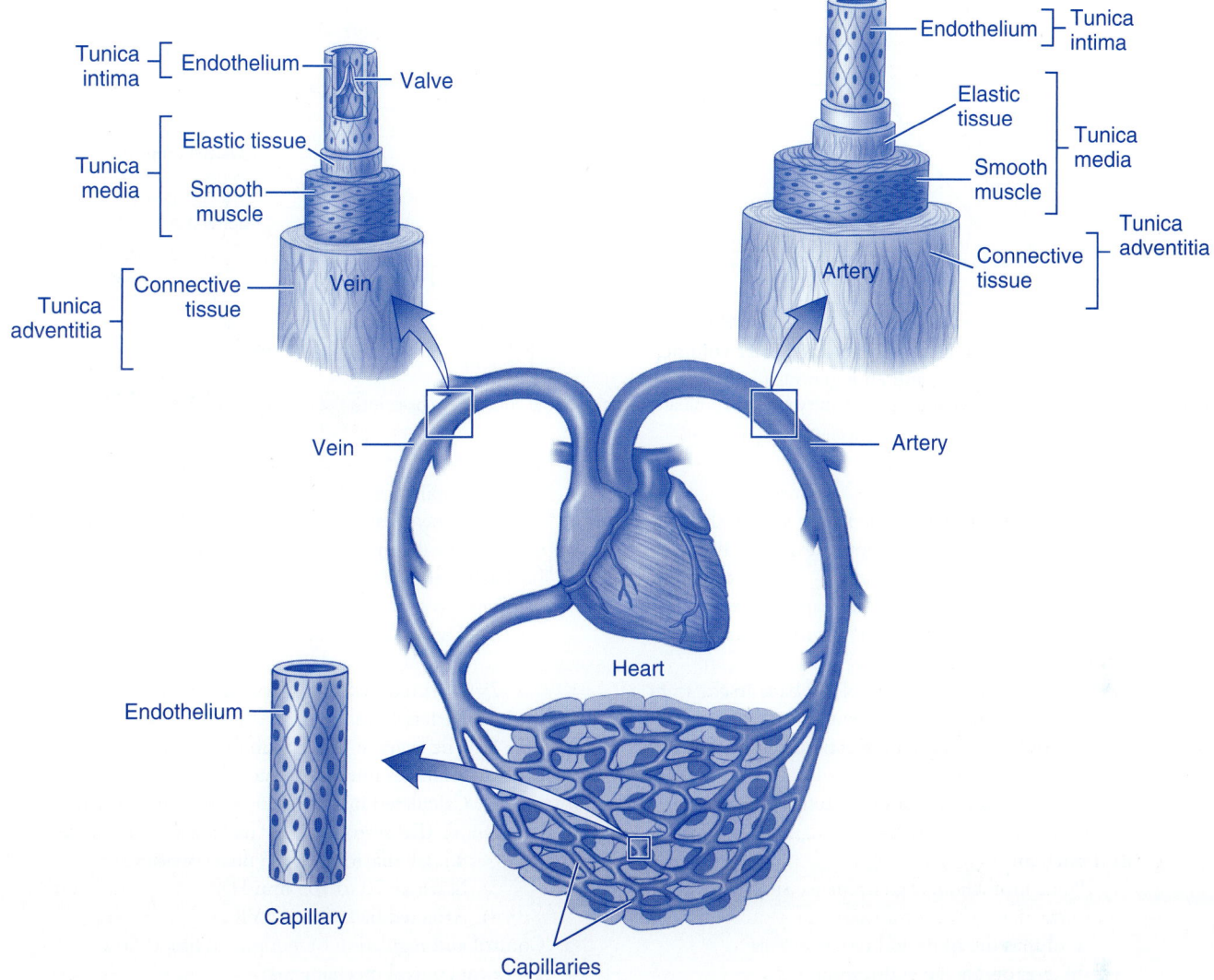

Fig. 3.20 Blood vessel wall layers. (From Herlihy, B. [2018]. *The human body in health and illness*. [6th ed.]. St. Louis: Saunders.)

c. Capillaries
   1) The capillary bed is the nutrient bed where exchange of gases, nutrients, and metabolites takes place by the process of diffusion.
   2) Capillaries contain no smooth muscle.
   3) The diameter of the capillary depends on changes in precapillary and postcapillary tone.
   4) Capillary dynamics are influenced by four pressures (Fig. 3.21).
      a) Hydrostatic pressures push.
         i) Capillary hydrostatic pressure pushes fluid out of capillary and into interstitium.
         ii) Interstitial hydrostatic pressure pushes fluid out of interstitium and into the capillary.
      b) Colloidal oncotic pressures pull.
         i) Capillary colloidal oncotic pressure pulls and holds fluid in the capillary.
         ii) Interstitial colloidal oncotic pressure pulls and holds fluid in the interstitium.
      c) Pressures pushing fluid out of the capillary dominate at the arterial end; pressures pushing fluid back into the capillary dominate at the venous end.
      d) Edema is caused by an imbalance in these pressures or an increase in capillary permeability; *third spacing* is a term used to describe fluid accumulation in any space that is not intravascular or intracellular (e.g., interstitial edema, ascites, pleural effusion, pericardial effusion, lumen of the intestine).
         i) HF: peripheral edema is caused by venous congestion and excessive hydrostatic pressure at the venous end.
         ii) Protein malnutrition or liver disease: decrease in plasma proteins decreases capillary colloidal oncotic pressure and allows excessive fluid to leak out of the capillary.

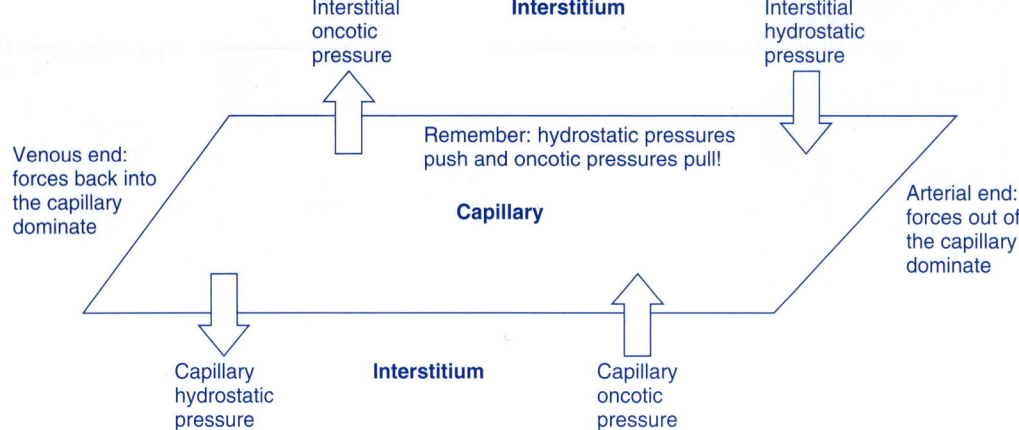

Fig. 3.21 Capillary dynamics. Forces out of the capillary dominate at the arteriole end; forces back into the capillary dominate at the venule end.

d. Veins
   1) The venous system is the return system that brings deoxygenated blood back to the heart and lungs.
   2) Veins act as a reservoir (i.e., capacitance vessels); the venous system holds 65% to 75% of total blood volume.
   3) The venous pump sends blood back to the right side of the heart; the skeletal muscles contract, compress veins, and propel blood toward the heart.
   4) Valves in the veins prevent retrograde blood flow.
e. Endothelium
   1) The endothelium is an immense single cell layer that:
      a) Lines the heart and blood vessels
      b) Surrounds the endocardium
      c) Comprises the capillary bed because capillaries are only this single endothelial layer
   2) The endothelium is instrumental in the following functions:
      a) Regulates vascular tone
      b) Prevents thrombus formation
4. BP
   a. Regulation
      1) Autonomic nervous system
      2) RAA system (Fig. 3.22)
         a) Renin secreted by the kidney in response to:
            i) Decreased BP stimulating stretch receptors in juxtaglomerular cells
            ii) SNS stimulation
            iii) Hyponatremia
         b) Renin stimulates the conversion of angiotensinogen to angiotensin I.
         c) Angiotensin I is converted to angiotensin II by angiotensin-converting enzyme (ACE) as the blood travels through the lung.
         d) Angiotensin II causes vasoconstriction and secretion of aldosterone.
         e) Vasoconstriction and sodium and water retention increases BP and decreases renin secretion.
         3) Capillary fluid shifts: especially from interstitial to intravascular
         4) Local control mechanisms
      b. Factors affecting arterial BP (Fig. 3.23)
      c. Pulse pressure (Fig. 3.24)
         1) The difference between systolic and diastolic pressures
         2) Affected by SV and arterial elastance
      d. Mean arterial pressure (MAP) (Fig. 3.24)
         1) The average pressure in the aorta and its major branches during cardiac cycle
         2) Calculated by either of the following formulae:
            a) [BP systolic + (BP diastolic × 2)] ÷ 3
            b) BP diastolic + 1/3 pulse pressure
         3) Normal: 70 to 105 mm Hg
         4) Affected by CO and SVR
5. Control and regulation of peripheral blood flow
   a. Local control mechanisms
      1) Autoregulation is the ability of the tissues to control blood flow; vasodilation is caused by hypoxia, hypercapnia, and acidosis.
      2) Precapillary sphincters, which precede every capillary bed, relax and permit more blood flow when oxygen tension falls; they constrict and restrict blood flow when oxygen tension rises.
   b. Autonomic nervous system
      1) Increased SNS stimulation: vasoconstriction
         a) Maintains arterial pressure
         b) Decreases vascular capacitance, increasing venous return to the heart and preload
      2) Decreased SNS stimulation: vasodilation
   c. Baroreceptors
      1) Increase in BP or blood volume results in the following:
         a) Decreased HR and contractility
         b) Peripheral vasodilation
         c) Decrease in SVR and BP
      2) Decrease in BP or blood volume results in the following:
         a) Increased HR and contractility
         b) Peripheral vasoconstriction
         c) Increase in SVR and BP

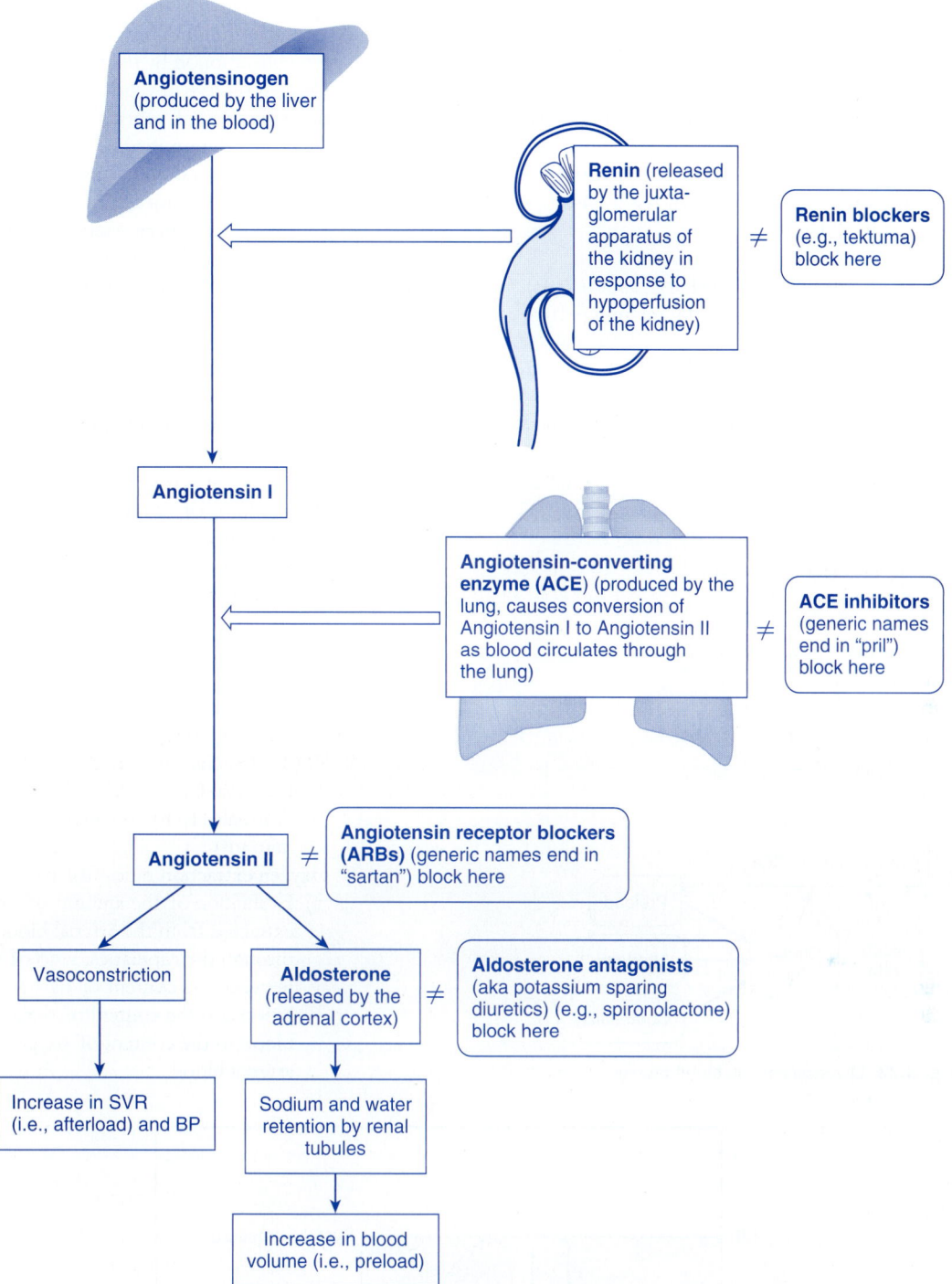

Fig. 3.22 The renin–angiotensin–aldosterone system (RAAS) and drugs that block aspects of the RAAS.

d. Vasomotor center in medulla
1) Vasoconstrictor area causes the following:
   a) Increase in HR, CO, BP
   b) Venoconstriction, which decreases vascular capacitance, thus increasing venous return to the heart, preload, and BP
2) Vasodepressor area causes the following:
   a) Decrease in HR, CO, and BP
   b) Venodilation, which increases vascular capacitance, thus decreasing venous return to the heart, preload, and BP

Oxygen Delivery to the Tissue (DO_2)/Oxygen Consumption by the Tissues (VO_2) (Fig. 3.25)

1. Parameters used to evaluate the balance between oxygen supply and oxygen consumption
   a. Oxygen delivery to the tissues (DO_2/DO_2I)
      1) DO_2 (Fig. 3.26)
         a) Product of CO and arterial oxygen content (CaO_2)
            i) CO is a product of HR and SV; SV is affected by preload, afterload, and contractility.
               (a) CI is the CO divided by the BSA.

ii) CaO_2 is a product of Hgb and arterial saturation.
  (a) CaO_2 is Hgb × SaO_2 (as a decimal) × 1.34 (the amount of oxygen that 1 g of Hgb can carry if it is 100% saturated).
  (b) CaO_2 is normally 18 to 20 ml/dl.
 b) Formula: CO × Hgb × SaO_2 × 13.4
  i) CO in l/min
  ii) Hgb in g/dl
  iii) SaO_2 as a decimal (e.g., 95% is 0.95)
 c) Normal DO_2: 900 to 1100 ml/min (~1000 ml/min)
2) DO_2I: DO_2 divided by BSA so considers body size
 a) Formula: CI × Hgb × SaO_2 × 13.4
  i) CI in l/min/m^2
  ii) Hgb in g/dl
  iii) SaO_2 as a decimal (e.g., 95% is 0.95)
 b) Normal: 550 to 650 ml/min/m^2 (~600 ml/min/m^2)
b. Oxygen consumption by the tissues (VO_2/VO_2I)
 1) Oxygen reserve in venous blood
  a) Saturation of venous blood (SvO_2)
   i) Determined by measuring the oxygen saturation in mixed venous blood in the pulmonary artery with an oximetric pulmonary artery catheter (PAC) or by blood gas analysis of a blood sample from the distal port of a PAC
   ii) Normal: 60% to 80%
  b) Venous oxygen content (CvO_2) is a product of Hgb and arterial saturation.
   i) CvO_2 is Hgb × SvO_2 (as a decimal) × 1.34 (the amount of oxygen that 1 gram of Hgb can carry if it is 100% saturated).
   ii) CaO_2 is normally 18 to 20 ml/dl.
 2) VO_2: volume of oxygen consumed by the tissues each minute
  a) Determined by comparing the oxygen content in the arterial blood with the oxygen content in the mixed venous blood (e.g., drawn from the distal tip of the PAC)
  b) Formula: CO × Hgb × 13.4 × (SaO_2 − SvO_2)
  c) Normal VO_2: 200 to 300 ml/min (~250 ml/min)
 3) VO_2I: VO_2 divided by BSA so considers body size
  a) Formula: CI × Hgb × 13.4 × (SaO_2 − SvO_2)
  b) Normal: 110 to 160 ml/min/m^2 (~150 ml/min/m^2)
 4) Oxygen extraction ratio (O_2ER)
  a) Evaluation of the amount of oxygen that is extracted from the arterial blood as it passes through the capillaries; ratio of the difference between the content of oxygen in the arterial blood and the content of oxygen in venous blood to the content of oxygen in the arterial blood

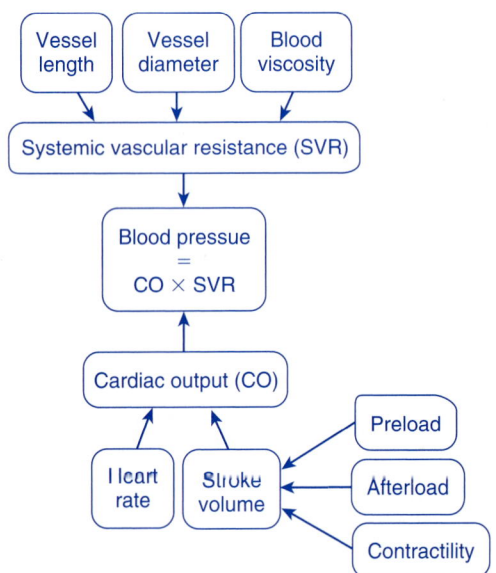

Fig. 3.23 Determinants of blood pressure.

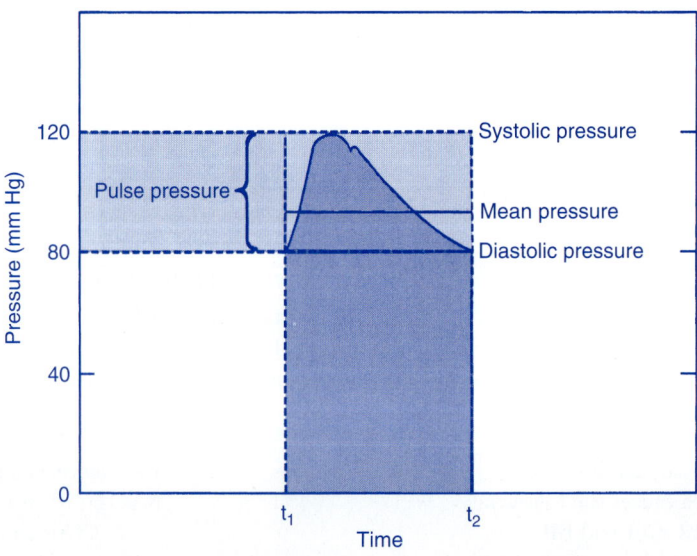

Fig. 3.24 Blood pressure, pulse pressure (difference between systolic and diastolic pressures) and mean arterial pressure (calculated or measured average pressure). (Modified from Berne, R. M., & Levy, M. N. [1997]. *Cardiovascular physiology* [7th ed.]. St. Louis: Mosby.)

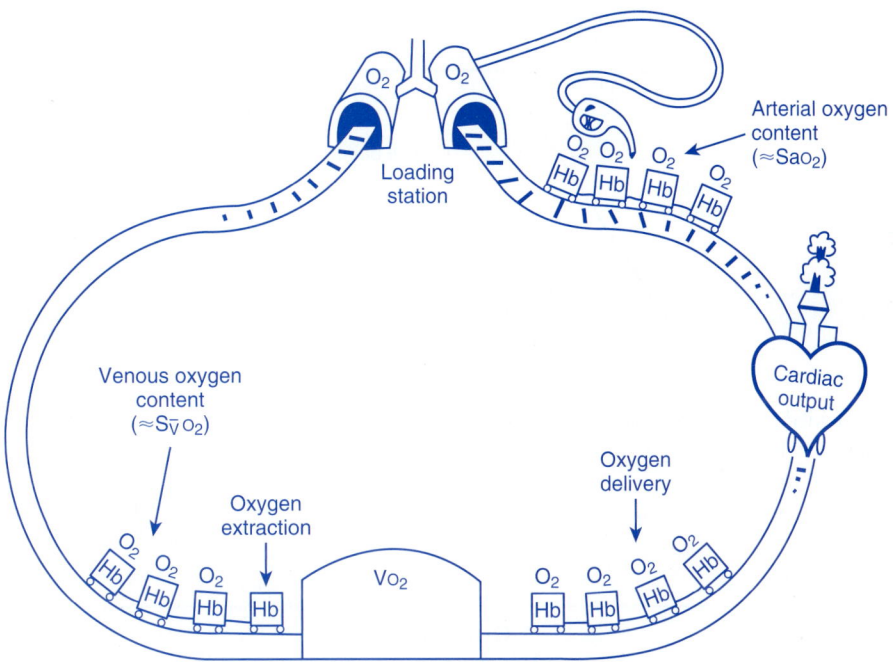

Fig. 3.25 Schematic illustrating oxygen delivery/oxygen consumption (DO_2/VO_2). (From *Understanding continuous mixed venous oxygen saturation monitoring with the Swan-Ganz TD System.* Baxter Healthcare Corporation, Edwards Critical Care.)

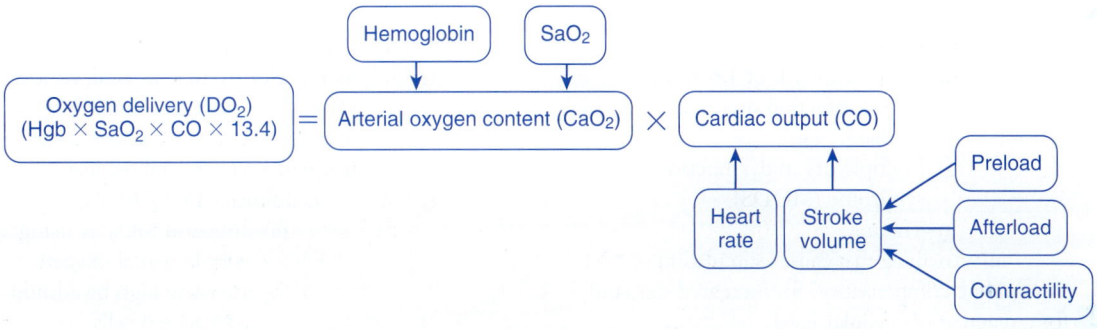

Fig. 3.26 Determinants of oxygen delivery.

  b) Formula: $(CaO_2 - CvO_2) \div CaO_2$
  c) Normal: 22% to 30% (~25%)
 5) Oxygen extraction index (O_2EI)
  a) Estimation of O_2ER calculated using only saturations
  b) Formula: $(SaO_2 - SvO_2) \div SaO_2$
  c) Normal: 20 to 27% (~25%)
c. Balance between supply and demand
 1) Key point: the tissues normally use approximately 25% of the oxygen delivered, and there is a 75% reserve.
  a) SaO_2 is normally ~100%, and SvO_2 is normally ~75%, *so the tissues used 25%, and there is a 75% reserve.*
  b) CaO_2 is normally ~20 ml/dl, and CvO_2 is normally ~15 ml/dl, *so the tissues used 25%, and there is a 75% reserve.*
  c) DO_2 is normally ~1000 ml/min, and VO_2 is normally ~250 ml/min *so the tissues used 25%, and there is a 75% reserve.*
  d) DO_2I is normally ~600 ml/min/m² and VO_2I is normally ~150 ml/min/m², *so the tissues used 25%, and there is a 75% reserve.*
 2) Oxygen reserve is reduced if DO_2 is decreased or VO_2 is increased.
  a) Factors that decrease DO_2/DO_2I
   i) Decrease in SaO_2 (e.g., acute respiratory failure, decrease in the inspired oxygen level such as smoke inhalation, decrease in barometric pressure such as high altitudes)
   ii) Decrease in Hgb (e.g., anemia, hemorrhage)
   iii) Decrease in CO (e.g., HF, hypovolemia)
  b) Factors that increase VO_2/VO_2I
   i) Patient care activities
    (a) Having a dressing change
    (b) Being bathed
    (c) Being repositioned
    (d) Having a visitor
    (e) Being suctioned
    (f) Being weighed on a sling scale
    (g) Having a physical examination
   ii) Physiologic states
    (a) Agitation
    (b) Shivering

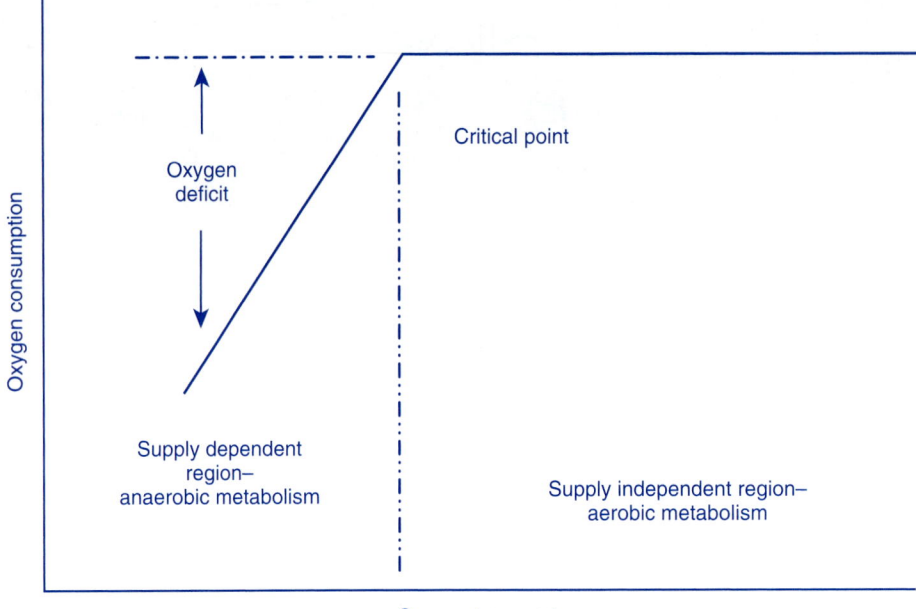

Fig. 3.27 Critical oxygen delivery point. A critical level of oxygen delivery exists whereby oxygen delivery and consumption are interdependent of each other. When this critical oxygen delivery point is exceeded, oxygen consumption becomes dependent on oxygen delivery. (From Dantzker, D. R., & Scharf, S. M. [1998]: *Cardiopulmonary critical care*. Philadelphia: Saunders.)

        (c) Fever
        (d) Increased work of breathing
        (e) Severe infection or sepsis
        (f) Burns
        (g) Multiple organ dysfunction syndrome (MODS)
        (h) Trauma
    iii) Anything that causes stimulation of SNS
  3) Physiologic compensation for increased demand for oxygen at the cellular level
    a) Increase in CO
    b) Redistribution of blood flow by recruiting underperfused capillary beds
    c) Increased oxygen extraction by the cells
  4) Critical DO_2 point (Fig. 3.27)
    a) A critical level of oxygen delivery exists where oxygen delivery and consumption are independent.
    b) When the critical oxygen delivery point is exceeded, oxygen consumption is dependent on oxygen delivery, and oxygen deficit, anaerobic metabolism, and lactic acidosis occur.
        i) If SvO_2 improves with increase in DO_2, oxygen delivery and consumption are independent.
        ii) If SvO_2 does not improve with increase in DO_2, oxygen consumption is dependent on oxygen delivery.
    c) Lactic acidosis is the result of anaerobic metabolism, and elevated serum arterial lactate level indicates a tissue oxygen deficit.
        i) Normal serum arterial lactate level is less than 1 mmol/l.
        ii) Serum lactate levels greater than 2 mmol/l are associated with increased mortality.
    d) Therapeutic efforts to decrease VO_2 and increase DO_2 may be used, although the effects of optimization of DO_2 on mortality, morbidity, length of hospital stay, and hospital costs are still unclear.
        i) Increase DO_2
            (a) Increase SaO_2 by using supplemental oxygen.
            (b) Increase Hgb by administering packed red cells.
            (c) Increase CO by using inotropic agents.
        ii) Decrease VO_2
            (a) Sedation
            (b) Muscle paralytics
            (c) Hypothermia
2. Oxygen supply and demand framework (Shackell & Gillespie, 2009) (Fig. 3.28)
  a. Used to "guide patient assessment, link patient assessment data to physiologic concepts, draw conclusions about physiologic function, and select and understand rationale for patient care interventions" (Shackell & Gillespie, 2009).
  b. Serves as knowledge map to guide thinking in identifying problems and providing care

Cardiovascular Assessment

Interview

1. Chief complaint: identifies why the patient is seeking help and the duration of the problem
2. Symptoms related to cardiac disorders
  a. Chest pain: may also be identified as indigestion; burning; discomfort; tightness; or pressure in midchest, epigastrium, or left arm. Table 3.5 describes differentiation of chest pain.

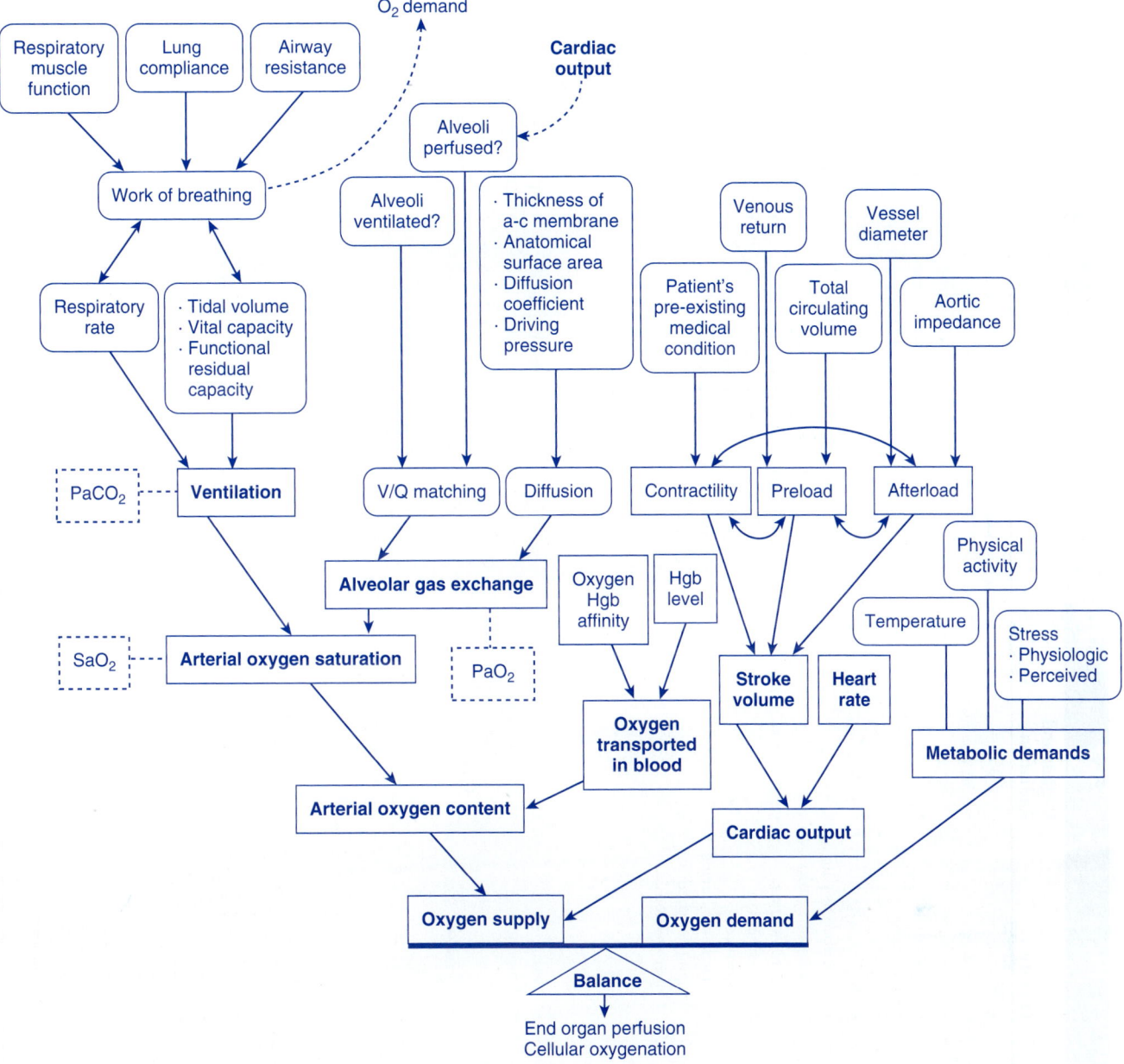

Fig. 3.28 Oxygen supply and demand framework. (From Shackell, E., & Gillespie, M. [2009]. The oxygen supply and demand framework: A tool to support integrative learning. *Dynamics*, 20[4], 15-19.)

1) PQRST format for describing complaint
    a) P
        i) Provocation: What provokes or worsens the pain?
        ii) Palliation: What relieves the pain? (Also include what was used but did not relieve pain.)
    b) Q
        i) Quality: What does the pain feel like?
    c) R
        i) Region: Where is the pain?
        ii) Radiation: If the pain radiates, to what area does the pain radiate?
    d) S
        i) Severity: How severe is the pain?
            (a) Pain scale: The most frequently used scale in adults is the 1 to 10 scale with 1 being negligible and 10 being the worst imaginable.
        e) T
            i) Timing: Is the pain intermittent or continuous? What is the relationship to other events or activities?
    b. Dyspnea
        1) Shortness of breath or "breathlessness"
        2) Exertional dyspnea
        3) Orthopnea: patient is unable to lie flat because of dyspnea
        4) Paroxysmal nocturnal dyspnea: patient awakens with a feeling of suffocation 1 to 2 hours after going to sleep; if accompanied by wheezing, may be called *cardiac asthma*
    c. Cough
        1) Quality: wet or dry
        2) Productivity: appearance of expectorant

Table 3.5 Differentiation of Chest Pain

Cause	Provocation	Palliation	Quality	Region and Radiation	Severity	Timing	Associated Signs and Symptoms
Angina pectoris	• Exercise • Exertion • Exposure to cold • Emotional stress • Eating • Smoking	• Rest • Oxygen • Nitroglycerin • Calcium channel blocker (e.g., nifedipine)	• Heaviness or pressure • Tightness • Squeezing • Dull ache • Burning • Not always described as pain but as discomfort	• Substernal • May be diffuse and vague • May radiate to arms, neck, jaw, back, upper abdomen	• Mild to severe	• Gradual or sudden onset • Duration: usually 1–4 min but may be 5–15 min	• Tachycardia, tachypnea • Dyspnea • Nausea, vomiting • Diaphoresis • Weakness • Anxiety • May have ST-T wave changes with pain
Acute myocardial infarction	• No specific precipitator • Lifestyle change and stress • Usually occurs within 3 hr of awakening	• Narcotics • Reperfusion by fibrinolytic or percutaneous coronary intervention (e.g., angioplasty, atherectomy) • No relief with rest or nitroglycerin	• As for angina • Heaviness or pressure • May show Levine sign (clenched fist over sternum)	• As for angina	• No symptoms to severe • Absence of pain is common in patients with diabetes mellitus and in older adults	• Sudden onset • Duration: longer than 30 min; usually 1–2 hr	• As for angina • Tachycardia, tachypnea • Dyspnea • Feeling of impending doom • S4 • ECG changes: T wave inversion, ST-segment elevation, eventually Q waves
Dissecting aortic aneurysm	• Peripheral vascular disease • Marfan syndrome • Aortitis • Hypertension or hypertensive crisis • Chest trauma	• Narcotics • Surgery • No relief with rest or nitroglycerin	• Tearing • Ripping	• Anterior chest • Radiation to shoulders, neck, back, abdomen	• Severe	• Sudden onset • Worse at onset • Duration: hours to days	• Tachycardia, tachypnea • Dysphagia • Confusion • Diaphoresis • Syncope • Dyspnea • Anxiety • Unilateral absence of pulse; BP differences between sides • Motor or sensory changes • Murmur of aortic regurgitation
Pericarditis	• Myocardial infarction • Cardiac surgery • Trauma • Infections • Uremia • Lupus erythematosus	• NSAIDs (e.g., ibuprofen; indomethacin) • Sitting up and leaning forward	• Sharp • Stabbing • Knifelike • Worsened by inspiration, coughing, movement, recumbent position	• Precordial • Substernal • Radiation to neck, shoulders, arms, back	• Mild to severe	• Sudden onset • Duration: days	• Tachycardia, tachypnea • Fever • Dyspnea • Pericardial friction rub • Leukocytosis • Diffuse concave ST segment

Pulmonary embolism	• Venous stasis (e.g., immobility; pelvic surgery, atrial fibrillation) • Hypercoagulability (e.g., oral contraceptives, malignancy, polycythemia) • Injury to vessel wall (e.g., IV lines, vascular surgery)	• Narcotics • High Fowler position • Splinting of chest	• Sharp • Knifelike • Shooting • Deep ache • Pressure • Worsened by deep inspiration or coughing	• Substernal or lateral chest • Radiation to shoulder or neck	• Mild to severe	• Sudden onset • Duration: minutes to hours	• Tachycardia, tachypnea • Dyspnea • Pallor or cyanosis • Cough • Anxiety, feeling of impending doom • Sinus tachycardia or atrial dysrhythmias • Accentuated P_2 • Right-sided S_4, possible right-sided S_3 • If RVF: JVD • If pulmonary infarction: pleural friction rub, hemoptysis, fever
Pneumothorax	• Congenital bleb • Emphysematous bullous • Large tidal volumes or PEEP on mechanical ventilator • Chest trauma • Exacerbated by coughing, exertion, or Valsalva maneuver	• Narcotics • Insertion of chest tube	• Tearing • Sharp • Worsened by breathing	• Lateral chest • May radiate to shoulder, back, arms	• Mild to severe	• Sudden onset • Duration: hours to days	• Tachypnea • Tachycardia • Dyspnea • Anxiety • JVD • Hyperresonance to percussion of affected side • Diminished breath sounds on affected side • Subcutaneous emphysema may be seen • Tracheal deviation may be seen, especially with tension pneumothorax
Pleuropulmonary (e.g., pleurisy)	• Respiratory infection • Aspiration	• Narcotics • Relief with sitting up	• Sharp • Worsened by coughing, inspiration, or movement	• Lateral chest • May radiate to shoulder, neck	• Moderate	• Gradual onset • Duration: days to weeks	• Tachypnea • Tachycardia • Dyspnea • Fever • Productive cough • Pleural friction rub

Continued

Table 3.5 Differentiation of Chest Pain—cont'd

Cause	Provocation	Palliation	Quality	Region and Radiation	Severity	Timing	Associated Signs and Symptoms
GI chest pain	• Cold liquids • Food intake, especially spicy foods, acidic foods or foods high in fat • Alcohol • Caffeine • Stress • Smoking • Exercise	• Sitting up • Antacids • Esophageal spasm (may be relieved by nitroglycerin)	• "Heartburn" • Dull, burning • Squeezing • Worsened by eating or supine position	• Retrosternal or lower substernal • Upper abdomen • Midline • May radiate to left arm, neck, jaw, upper abdomen, back, shoulder	• Mild to moderate	• Gradual or sudden onset • Duration: minutes to days	• Dyspnea • Diaphoresis • Anxiety • Dysphagia • Eructation • Vomiting
Musculoskeletal chest pain	• Neck or arm strain • Movement • Coughing • Deep breathing • CPR	• Rest • Heat • NSAIDs (e.g., aspirin, ibuprofen)	• Soreness • Stabbing or sticking sensation • Tenderness • Worsened with inspiration and movement	• Localized to one side of chest	• Mild to moderate	• Gradual or sudden onset • Duration: weeks	• Tachypnea • Splinting respirations • Localized tenderness over site of pain
Psychosomatic chest pain	• Stress • Fatigue	• Rest • Anxiolytics	• Dull ache • Sharp • Stabbing • Superficial	• Precordium • Localized; frequently on left side • No radiation	• Mild to moderate	• Gradual or sudden onset • Duration: minutes to days	• Hyperpnea • Dyspnea • Palpitations • Dry mouth • Dizziness • Tingling of hands, mouth • Fatigue • Frequent sighing

BP, Blood pressure; *CPR*, cardiopulmonary resuscitation: *ECG*, electrocardiogram; *GI*, gastrointestinal; *IV*, intravenous; *JVD*, jugular vein distention; *NSAID*, nonsteroidal antiinflammatory drug; *NTG*, nitroglycerin; P_2, pulmonic component of second sound; *PEEP*, positive end-expiratory pressure; *RV*, right ventricular; *RVF*, right ventricular failure; S_4, fourth heart sound;.

3) Frequency
4) Precipitating factors
5) Cardiac cough usually occurs at night and is precipitated by supine position, exertion, or by turning to one side.
6) Cough may be a side effect of ACE inhibitors or caused by HF, mitral stenosis, or pulmonary embolism (PE).
  d. Hemoptysis: may be related to pulmonary edema or PE
  e. Palpitations
1) Unpleasant awareness of the heartbeat when at rest
2) May be described as skipping, pounding, thumping sensation
3) Associated with premature beats or other dysrhythmia
4) May be accompanied by syncope or chest pain
  f. Syncope
1) Effort syncope: transient loss of consciousness that occurs shortly after heavy activity is started; may be associated with aortic or subaortic stenosis
2) Stokes-Adams attack: dramatic loss of consciousness; related to heart block or dysrhythmia
3) Pacemaker syncope: syncope caused by malfunction or failure of an artificial pacemaker
4) Hypersensitive carotid sinus syncope: syncope caused by pressure applied on a carotid sinus body of a patient with atherosclerotic and hypersensitive carotid arteries
  g. Headache: may be related to hypertension
  h. Ascites: may be related to right ventricular failure (RVF)
  i. Abdominal pain: may be related to RVF
  j. Edema or weight gain: frequently related to RVF; also described as bloated feeling, swelling, tightening of clothing, tightening of shoes, marks left from constricting garments
  k. Fatigue or weakness: may be related to RVF
  l. Nocturia: may be related to HF or diuretic use
  m. Diaphoresis: may be related to SNS stimulation or infection
  n. Unexplained joint pain: may be related to rheumatic fever
  o. Intermittent claudication: hip, thigh, or calf pain that occurs with exercise and ceases with rest; indicative of peripheral arterial disease
  p. Peripheral skin changes: a decrease in hair distribution, skin color changes, skin ulcerations that will not heal, or a thin, shiny appearance to the skin may indicate peripheral vascular disease.
  q. Calf tenderness: may be related to thrombophlebitis; may be accompanied by red, warm skin over vein
  r. Varicose veins: dilated, sometimes painful, veins
3. History of present illness: use PQRST format
  a. Provocation, palliation
  b. Quality, quantity
  c. Region, radiation
  d. Severity
  e. Timing
  f. Associated symptoms

4. Past medical history
  a. Past illnesses
1) CAD
   a) Angina
   b) Myocardial infarction (MI)
2) Cerebrovascular disease: transient ischemic attacks or stroke
3) Dysrhythmias
4) Hypertension
5) Hyperlipidemia
6) Peripheral vascular disease
7) Rheumatic fever or rheumatic heart disease
8) Murmur or known valvular heart disease
9) Pulmonary disease (e.g., asthma, chronic obstructive pulmonary disease [COPD])
10) PE
11) Connective tissue disorders
12) Endocrine disorders, especially diabetes mellitus (DM)
13) Kidney disease
14) Alcoholism
15) Anemia
16) Bleeding disorders
  b. Past chest trauma: history of recent trauma is important to differentiate MI from myocardial contusion; recent chest trauma would serve as a contraindication for fibrinolytics
  c. Past surgical procedures
1) Cardiac surgery: identify whether coronary artery bypass grafting (CABG), valve replacement, or other type of cardiac surgery
2) Percutaneous coronary intervention (PCI) procedures: angioplasty, atherectomy, stent placement, valvuloplasty
3) Pacemaker insertion
  d. Allergies and type of reaction
  e. Past diagnostic studies (e.g., stress ECG, cardiac catheterization, echocardiogram)
5. Family history
  a. CAD
  b. Cerebrovascular disease, including stroke
  c. Congenital heart defects
  d. Sudden cardiac death
  e. Peripheral vascular disease
  f. Hypertension
  g. DM
  h. Hyperlipidemia
  i. Kidney disease
  j. Bleeding disorders
6. Social history
  a. Relationship with spouse or significant other; family structure
  b. Occupation
  c. Educational level
  d. Usual activity level and ability to perform activities of daily living
  e. Stress level and usual coping mechanisms
  f. Personality type
1) Type A: sense of time urgency, hostility, aggression, ambition, competitiveness, impatience, frustration
2) Type B: none of the above qualities

- g. Recreational habits
- h. Exercise habits
- i. Dietary habits
- j. Caffeine intake
- k. Tobacco use: recorded as pack-years (number of packs per day times the number of years he or she has been smoking)
- l. Alcohol use: recorded as alcoholic beverages consumed per month, week, or day
- m. Toxin exposure
- n. Travel

7. Medication history
   a. Prescribed drug, dose, frequency, time of last dose
   b. Nonprescribed drugs
      1) Over-the-counter (OTC) drugs, including herbal supplements
      2) Substance abuse (e.g., cocaine, amphetamines)
   c. Patient's understanding of drug actions, side effects
   d. Drugs causing potential problems for patients with cardiovascular disease
      1) Sinus or cold remedies: may contain ephedrine and increase BP
      2) OTC weight reduction agents: may contain ephedrine
      3) Aspirin: prolongs blood clotting
      4) Tricyclic antidepressants (TCAs): may cause dysrhythmias (e.g., torsades de pointes)
      5) Phenytoin: may cause dysrhythmias
      6) Phenothiazines: may cause dysrhythmias, hypotension
      7) Oral contraceptives: may predispose to embolus, thrombosis
      8) Doxorubicin: may cause cardiomyopathy
      9) Lithium: may cause dysrhythmias
      10) Corticosteroids: cause sodium and fluid retention and exacerbate HF
      11) Theophylline preparations: cause tachycardia and may cause dysrhythmias
      12) Cardiac stimulants (e.g., cocaine): cause tachycardia and may cause dysrhythmias and coronary artery spasm
   e. Herbal supplements causing potential problems for patients with cardiovascular disease (Tachjian, Maria, & Jahangir, 2010)
      1) Alfalfa: may increase risk of bleeding with warfarin
      2) Black cohosh: may cause hypotension
      3) Ephedra: may increase HR and/or BP; may cause fatal interactions with many cardiac drugs
      4) Garlic: may increase risk of bleeding with anticoagulants
      5) Ginger: may potentiate warfarin
      6) Ginkgo: may increase risk of bleeding with warfarin, aspirin, or cyclooxygenase-2 (COX-2) inhibitors
      7) Ginseng: may cause hypertension
      8) Goldenseal: may potentiate warfarin; may cause hypertension, hallucinations, or delirium
      9) Grapefruit juice: increases effects of statins, calcium channel blockers
      10) Green tea: may decrease effect of warfarin
      11) Hawthorn: potentiates effects of cardiac glycosides and nitrates
      12) Kelp: increases effect of antihypertensives and anticoagulants
      13) Licorice root: may cause hypertension, hypokalemia, digoxin toxicity
      14) Oleander: may cause heart block, hyperkalemia, dysrhythmias, death
      15) St. John wort: may increase HR and/or BP; may decrease digoxin blood level

Landmarks (Fig. 3.29)

1. Anatomical
   a. Clavicle
   b. Sternum
   c. Ribs
   d. ICSs
   e. Angle of Louis
   f. Xiphoid process
   g. Costal margin
   h. Costal angle
2. Imaginary
   a. Midsternal line (MSL)
   b. Midclavicular line (MCL)
   c. Anterior axillary line (AAL)
   d. Midaxillary line (MAL)
   e. Posterior axillary line (PAL)
   f. Scapular line
   g. Midspinal line
3. Location of heart
   a. Between the sternum and spinal column
   b. Lies between second ICS and fifth ICS
   c. Apex normally at fifth LICS at MCL

Inspection and Palpation

1. Vital signs
   a. BP: sitting; lying; standing
      1) Reduction of up to 15 mm Hg in systolic and 5 mm Hg in diastolic BP when standing is normal; greater reduction indicates orthostatic changes.
         a) To assess for orthostatic changes, assist the patient to a standing position, wait 2 to 3 minutes, and then repeat measurement of BP and HR.
      2) Variation of up to 15 mm Hg between arms is normal.
      3) BP in lower extremities is expected to be 10 mm Hg higher than in upper extremities.
      4) Narrowed pulse pressure frequently indicates vasoconstriction as occurs with innervation of SNS (e.g., hypovolemic shock); widened pulse pressure frequently indicates excessive vasodilation as occurs with excessive vasodilatory mediator release (e.g., septic shock).
   b. HR
      1) Rhythm if ECG monitor available
      2) Tachycardia frequently indicates innervation of SNS.
   c. Respiratory (ventilatory) rate: tachypnea frequently indicates innervation of SNS.

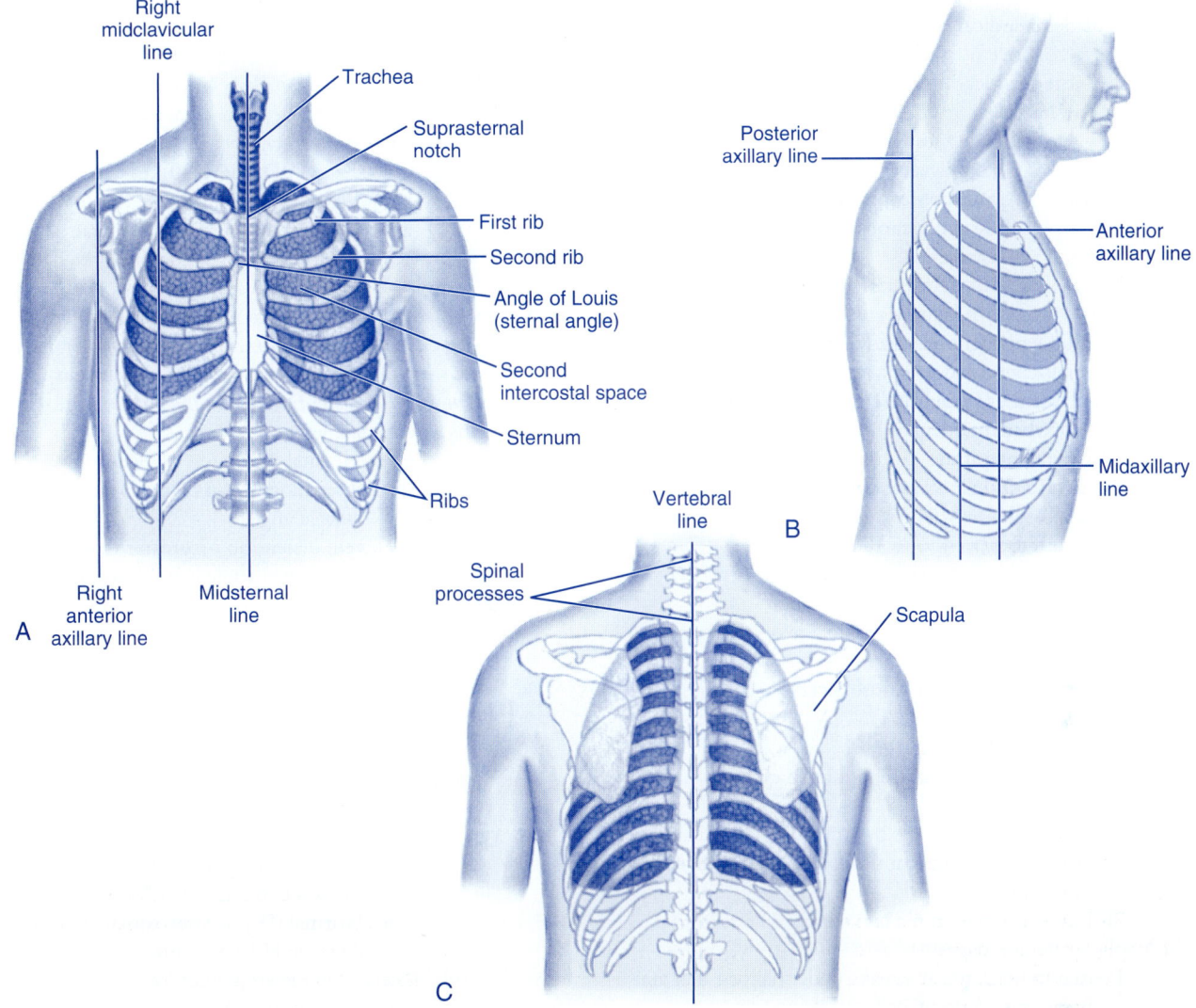

Fig. 3.29 Landmarks of the thorax. **A,** Anterior. **B,** Right lateral. **C,** Posterior. (From Urden, L., Stacy, K., & Lough, M. [2018]. *Critical care nursing: Diagnosis and management* [8th ed.]. St. Louis: Mosby.)

    d. Temperature: fever may indicate inflammatory or infectious process (e.g., MI, pericarditis, endocarditis).
    e. Height
    f. Weight: important indicator of fluid gain or loss
2. General survey
    a. Apparent health status: consistency of apparent age and chronological age
    b. Level of consciousness
    c. Gross deformity
    d. Nutritional status
    e. Stature and posture
    f. Gait
3. Skin and appendages
    a. Color
        1) Pallor: may be indication of anemia, SNS innervation, or sympathomimetic agents (e.g., phenylephrine, norepinephrine, dopamine)
        2) Cyanosis
            a) Peripheral (or cold) cyanosis is seen on fingertips, toes; associated with peripheral hypoperfusion or vasoconstriction
            b) Central (or warm) cyanosis is seen on lips, tongue, mucous membranes; associated with 5 g of deoxygenated Hgb
                i) Central cyanosis may be a late or even impossible sign of hypoxemia in severely anemic patients.
                ii) Central cyanosis may be a relatively early sign of hypoxemia in polycythemic patients; patients with chronic bronchitis are nicknamed *blue bloaters*—*blue* because of chronic hypoxemia and *bloaters* because of chronic RVF.
            c) In dark-skinned patients, cyanosis appears as an ashen color.
        3) Ruddiness: related to polycythemia or hypercapnia
    b. Moisture: diaphoresis; dryness
    c. Temperature: cold skin may be related to hypoperfusion.
    d. Turgor: decrease in skin turgor, also referred to as *tenting*, related to interstitial dehydration

e. Edema
  1) Edema indicates an increase in interstitial fluid of 30% above normal.
  2) Note the location of the edema.
     a) Facial
        i) Allergies: profound facial edema in anaphylaxis
        ii) Steroids: exogenous (e.g., prednisone) or endogenous (e.g., Cushing syndrome)
        iii) Renal disease (e.g., nephrotic syndrome)
     b) Dependent edema: RVF
     c) Generalized edema (anasarca): end-stage HF; end-stage renal failure; severe hypoproteinemia
  3) Degree of pitting
     a) Grade 1+ = 0 to ¼ inch
     b) Grade 2+ = ¼ to ½ inch
     c) Grade 3+ = ½ to 1 inch
     d) Grade 4+ = >1 inch
f. Lesions
  1) Arterial disease may cause ulcers on the toes or points of trauma.
  2) Venous disease may cause ulcers on the sides of the ankles.
4. Fingertips and nailbeds
  a. Color: bluish nailbeds with peripheral cyanosis
  b. Clubbing
     1) Loss of normal angle between base of nail and skin; clubbing present if angle is greater than 180 degrees
     2) Indicative of chronic hypoxia
  c. Splinter hemorrhages
     1) Red to black linear streaks under nailbed that run from base to tip of nail
     2) May indicate bacterial endocarditis
  d. Osler nodes:
     1) Painful red subcutaneous nodules on fingertips
     2) May indicate embolization in infective endocarditis
5. Head and neck
  a. Face
     1) Facial expression
     2) Facial flushing: episodic facial flushing may indicate pheochromocytoma
  b. Head bobbing up and down with each heartbeat
     1) Referred to as *de Musset sign*
     2) Indicates aortic aneurysm or regurgitation
  c. Eyes
     1) Xanthoma palpebrarum (also called *xanthelasma*)
        a) Benign, fatty, fibrous, yellowish plaque, nodule, or tumor on the eyelids
        b) Associated with hyperlipidemia
     2) Corneal arcus
        a) Light-colored ring surrounding the iris
        b) May be normal finding in an older adult patient (called *arcus senilis*)
        c) Abnormal in younger patients; associated with hyperlipidemia
     3) Exophthalmos: may be seen in advanced HF with pulmonary hypertension
  d. Ears
     1) Diagonal bilateral earlobe creases (referred to as *McCarty sign*): may indicate CAD if seen in individuals younger than 45 years of age
  e. Neck
     1) Jugular vein distention (JVD)
        a) To evaluate JVD (Fig. 3.30)
           i) Place patient at a 45-degree angle.
           ii) Identify the sternal angle, a raised notch that is created where the manubrium and the body of the sternum join; also called the *manubriosternal junction* or *angle of Louis*.
           iii) Measure the height of neck vein distention above the level of the sternal angle.
           iv) Normal the height of neck vein distention is 1 to 3 cm above the sternal angle.
        b) Neck vein distention of greater than 3 cm above the sternal angle is indicative of any of the following:
           i) RVF
           ii) Hypervolemia
           iii) Tension pneumothorax
           iv) Cardiac tamponade
        c) To estimate CVP
           i) The angle of Louis is assumed to be approximately 5 cm above the right atrium, so 5 cm is added to the height of neck vein distention above the angle of Louis to estimate CVP.
           ii) Normal CVP is approximately 3 to 8 cm of H_2O pressure.
        d) To evaluate hepatojugular (or abdominojugular) reflux

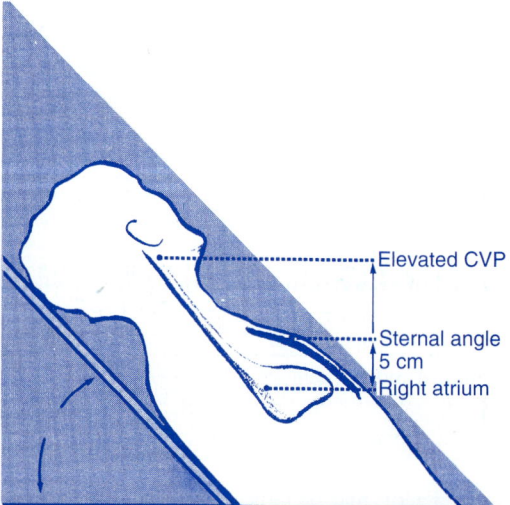

Fig. 3.30 Jugular venous distention and estimation of central venous pressure: assess jugular venous distention with patient in 45-degree angle, determine height of jugular venous distention above the sternal angle, and add 5 cm to this measurement to estimate central venous pressure in cm of water pressure. (From Guzzetta, C. E., & Dossey, B. M. [1992]. *Cardiovascular nursing: Holistic practice*. St. Louis: Mosby.)

i) The test is performed by applying pressure over right upper quadrant for 30 to 60 seconds while evaluating an increase in neck vein distention.
ii) A positive result is a sustained increase in neck vein distention of 4 cm or more or a decrease of 4 cm or more after release of pressure.
iii) A positive result is an indication of HF
6. Precordium: inspect and palpate entire precordium
   a. Point of maximal impulse (PMI) or apical impulse
      1) Frequently visible and usually palpable; may not be palpable in patients with obesity, muscular chest wall, or an increased anterior-posterior diameter
      2) Location
         a) Normal location of the PMI is at the fifth LICS at the MCL.
         b) Lateral displacement is associated with any of the following:
            i) LV dilation (e.g., aortic or mitral insufficiency)
            ii) Upward displacement of the diaphragm (e.g., pregnancy, ascites)
            iii) Right to left mediastinal shift (e.g., right pleural effusion or tension pneumothorax)
            iv) Left ventricular hypertrophy (LVH) or left ventricular failure (LVF)
         c) Medial displacement may occur with any of the following:
            i) Downward displacement of the diaphragm (e.g., COPD)
            ii) Left to right mediastinal shift (e.g., left pleural effusion or tension pneumothorax)
      3) Intensity
         a) Normal intensity is only a light tap.
         b) Failure may increase the intensity and cause a heave.
      4) Size
         a) Normal size is approximately 1 to 2 cm.
         b) The size is more diffuse with ventricular aneurysm.
   b. Heave
      1) Lifting of the chest wall indicative of failure
      2) LV heave felt at or near the apex
      3) RV heave (or lift) felt at or near the sternum
   c. Thrill
      1) Palpable vibration associated with murmur or bruit
      2) Felt where the murmur is heard the loudest or at location of bruit
7. Abdomen
   a. Aortic pulsation
      1) Normally visible, especially during expiration
      2) Normally palpable at midline or slightly to left of midline; feel for lateral expansion, which might be indicative of aneurysm
8. Extremities
   a. Arterial versus venous disease (Table 3.6)
   b. Temperature
      1) Coolness or coldness may indicate decreased blood flow caused by hypoperfusion or vasoconstriction.
      2) Excessive warmth may indicate hyperthyroidism or fever.
   c. Peripheral pulses
      1) Location (Fig. 3.31)
         a) Carotid: palpate only lower half and never palpate both carotids simultaneously
         b) Brachial
         c) Radial
         d) Ulnar
         e) Femoral
         f) Popliteal
         g) Posterior tibialis
         h) Dorsalis pedis
      2) Rate and rhythm
      3) Amplitude
         a) 0 = not palpable
         b) 1+ = weak and thready, easily obliterated
         c) 2+ = normal, not easily obliterated
         d) 3+ = full and bounding, cannot obliterate
      4) Capillary refill rate
         a) Color should return to blanched area within 3 seconds; delay beyond 3 seconds indicates hypoperfusion.
      5) Apical-radial pulse deficit
         a) Performed by two nurses using one watch
         b) Deficit (radial pulse rate less than apical rate) indicative of dysrhythmia (e.g., atrial fibrillation, ventricular ectopy)

Table 3.6 Comparison of Clinical Indications of Arterial and Venous Peripheral Vascular Disease

	Arterial	Venous
Pain	• Excruciating in acute occlusion • Intermittent claudication in chronic occlusion	• Crampy pain • Homans sign in thrombophlebitis
Pulses	• Diminished or absent	• Normal (but may be difficult to palpate due to edema)
Color	• Pale	• Normal or ruddy
Temperature	• Cool or cold	• Warm
Edema	• Absent	• Present; may be severe
Skin changes	• Thin, shiny, atrophic skin • Loss of hair • Thickened toenails	• Brown pigmentation at ankles
Ulcerations	• At toes or points of trauma	• At sides of ankles

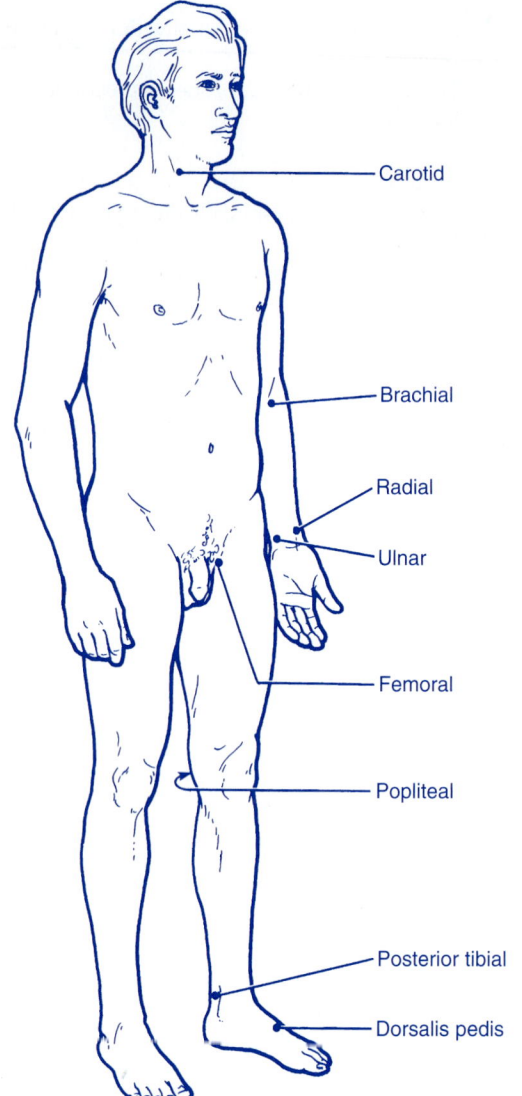

Fig. 3.31 Locations of peripheral pulses. (From Lewis, S. M., & Collier, I. C. [1992]. Medical-surgical nursing: *Assessment and management of clinical problems* [3rd ed.]. St. Louis: Mosby.)

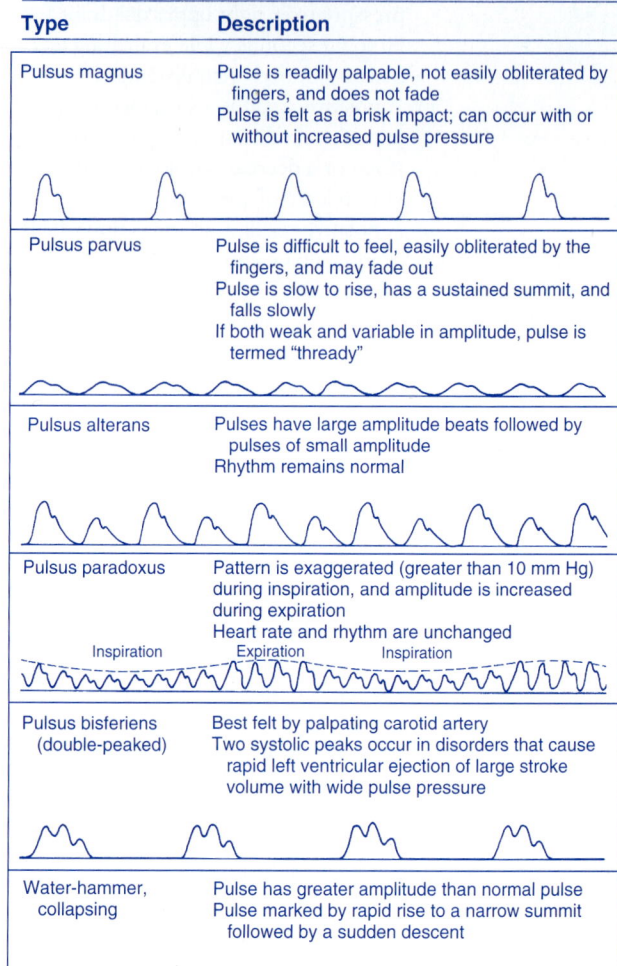

Fig. 3.32 Pulse contour. (Modified from Cannobio, M. M. [1990]. *Cardiovascular disorders*. St. Louis: Mosby.)

6) Pulse contour (Fig. 3.32)
   a) Pulsus magnus
      i) Strong, bounding pulses with rapid upstroke and downstroke
      ii) Characteristic of any of the following:
         (a) Hypertension
         (b) Thyrotoxicosis
         (c) Aortic insufficiency
         (d) Patent ductus arteriosus (PDA)
         (e) Arteriovenous fistula
   b) Pulsus parvus
      i) Small, weak pulse
      ii) Characteristic of any of the following:
         (a) Aortic stenosis: also tardus (late)
         (b) Mitral stenosis
         (c) Constrictive pericarditis
         (d) Cardiac tamponade
   c) Pulsus alternans
      i) Alternating pulse waves, every other beat being weaker than the preceding one
      ii) Characteristic of LVH
   d) Pulsus paradoxus
      i) Pulsus paradoxus is an exaggeration of normal physiologic response to inspiration
         (a) The normal decrease in BP during inspiration is 10 mm Hg or less.
         (b) BP drop of more than 10 mm Hg during inspiration is pulsus paradoxus.
      ii) Pulsus paradoxus may be characteristic of any of the following conditions:
         (a) Pericardial effusion
         (b) Constrictive pericarditis
         (c) Cardiac tamponade
         (d) Severe lung disease
         (e) Advanced HF
         (f) Hemorrhagic shock

Box 3.1	Clinical Manifestations of Acute Arterial Occlusion*
Pain	Paresthesia
Pallor	Paralysis
Pulselessness	Polar (cold)

*These 6 Ps are the format for neurovascular assessment.

   e) Pulsus bisferiens
      i) Two pulses palpated during systole with the second slightly weaker than the first
      ii) Characteristic of any of the following:
         (a) Hypertrophic cardiomyopathy
         (b) Constrictive cardiomyopathy
         (c) Aortic stenosis or regurgitation
   f) Water-hammer (or *Corrigan*) pulse
      i) Increased pulse pressure with a rapid upstroke and downstroke and shortened peak
      ii) Characteristic of aortic regurgitation or PDA
d. Homan sign
   1) Identified by dorsiflexing the foot with the knee slightly bent
   2) Homan sign is present if the patient has pain in the calf with this action.
   3) Suggestive of thrombophlebitis but not definitive
e. Petechiae or ecchymosis
f. Varicose veins
g. Neurovascular assessment
   1) Assess neurovascular status in all of the following situations:
      a) After cardiac catheterization
      b) After PCI procedure (e.g., angioplasty, atherectomy, valvuloplasty)
      c) When the patient has intraaortic balloon pump (IABP) catheter in place
      d) When the patient has a fracture of an extremity (to monitor for compartment syndrome)
      e) When the patient has a circumferential burn of an extremity
   2) Monitor for clinical indications of acute arterial occlusion: 6 Ps (Box 3.1)
h. Clinical indications of hypoperfusion (Table 3.2): because hypoperfusion is progressive, the earlier these changes are identified, the more appropriate the management and the chances for successfully reversing the changes.

Auscultation

1. Qualities of a good stethoscope
   a. Snug-fitting earplugs to eliminate extraneous sounds
   b. Tubing
      1) Two tubings are preferable for high-frequency sounds.
      2) Tubing should be no longer than 12 to 15 inches.

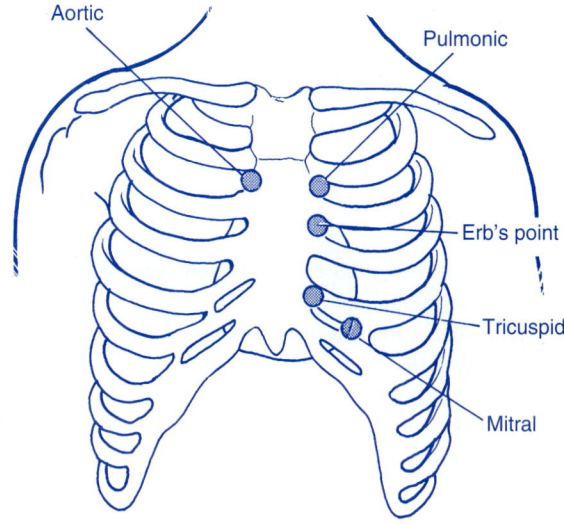

Fig. 3.33 Cardiac auscultatory areas. (From Price, S., & Wilson, L. [2003]. *Pathophysiology: Clinical concepts of disease processes* [6th ed.]. St. Louis: Mosby.)

   c. Chest piece
      1) Diaphragm
         a) Used for high-pitched sounds (e.g., S_1, S_2, splits of S_1 and S_2, pericardial friction rubs, most murmurs)
         b) Held firmly against skin
      2) Bell
         a) Used for low-pitched sounds (e.g., S_3, S_4, murmurs of AV valve stenosis)
         b) Held only tightly enough against skin to create a seal
2. Auscultatory areas (Fig. 3.33)
   a. Mitral: fifth LICS at MCL
   b. Tricuspid: fifth LICS at left sternal border (LSB)
   c. Erb point: third LICS at LSB
   d. Pulmonic: second LICS at LSB
   e. Aortic: second RICS at RSB
3. Method of cardiac auscultation
   a. Ensure a quiet room by turning off television and radio and asking others to be quiet.
   b. Listen to all four auscultatory areas with both bell and diaphragm.
   c. Concentrate on one cardiac event at a time: S_1; S_2; systole; diastole
4. Heart sounds
   a. Rules to consider
      1) Left-sided heart events precede right-sided heart events (i.e., the mitral component [M_1] precedes the tricuspid component [T_1] of S_1, and the aortic component [A_2] precedes the pulmonic component [P_2] of S_2).
      2) Left-sided heart events are normally louder than right-sided heart events (i.e., M_1 is the loudest component of S_1, and A_2 is the loudest component of S_2).
      3) Left-sided heart events are normally loudest during expiration, and right-sided heart events are normally loudest during inspiration.

b. S_1
1) Caused by closure of the AV valves: mitral and tricuspid
2) Marks the end of diastole and the beginning of systole
3) Loudest at the apex
4) Note if a single sound or split.
5) Note any increase in intensity (closing snap).
c. S_2
1) Caused by closure of the semilunar valves: aortic and pulmonic
2) Marks the end of systole and the beginning of diastole.
3) Loudest at the base
4) Note if a single sound or split.
5) Note any increase in intensity.
d. Splits
1) Split S_1
a) Both components (M_1 and T_1) of S_1 can be heard.
b) A split S_1 is heard best at the tricuspid area.
c) A narrowly split S_1 may be normal.
d) A split S_1 is more often abnormal than normal and associated with any of the following:
i) Right bundle branch block (RBBB)
ii) LV (epicardial) pacemaker
iii) LV ectopy
2) Split S_2
a) Both components (A_2 and P_2) of S_2 can be heard.
b) A split S_2 is heard best at the pulmonic area.
c) Inspiratory only split of S_2 is normal
i) Called a physiologic split of S_2
ii) Normal and frequently heard in individuals younger than 50 years of age
iii) Split only during inspiration
iv) Caused by changes in intrathoracic pressure related to ventilation; increased venous return to right ventricle and decreased venous return to left ventricle delay pulmonic valve closure (P_2).
d) Expiratory split of S_2 is abnormal.
i) Increased splitting during inspiration (split on expiration but split more during inspiration); associated with any of the following:
(a) RBBB
(b) LV ectopy
(c) LV (epicardial) pacemaker
(d) Severe mitral regurgitation
(e) Pulmonary stenosis
(f) Pulmonary hypertension
(g) Ventricular septal defect (VSD)
ii) Fixed splitting (split the same on inspiration and expiration); associated with atrial septal defect
iii) Paradoxical split (split on expiration but not on inspiration); associated with any of the following:
(a) Left bundle branch block (LBBB)
(b) RV (endocardial) pacemaker
(c) RV ectopy
(d) Severe aortic stenosis or regurgitation
(e) PDA
e. Extra heart sounds (Table 3.7 is a summary of extra heart sounds.)
1) S_3
a) Also called a ventricular gallop
b) Dull, low-pitched sound occurring early in diastole after S2; may sound like "Ken-tuc-ky" with the "ky" being the S3
c) Caused by rapid rush of blood into a dilated ventricle; considered abnormal in patients older than 30 years of age
d) Heard best with bell, with the patient lying on the left side
i) Left-sided S_3
(a) Heard best at apex
(b) Heard best during expiration
ii) Right-sided S_3
(a) Heard best at sternum
(b) Heard best during inspiration
e) Associated primarily with failure
f) May also be associated with any of the following:
i) Fluid overload
ii) Cardiomyopathy
iii) VSD or PDA
iv) Mitral or tricuspid regurgitation
2) S_4
a) Also called an *atrial gallop*
b) Dull, low-pitched sound occurring late in diastole before S_1; may sound like "Ten-nes-see" with the "Ten" being the S_4
c) Caused by atrial contraction of blood into a noncompliant ventricle; abnormal in adults
d) Heard best with bell with patient lying on the left side
i) Left-sided S_4: heard best at apex
ii) Right-sided S_4: heard best at sternum
e) Associated with any of the following:
i) Myocardial ischemia or infarction
ii) Hypertension
(a) Systemic: left-sided S_4
(b) Pulmonary: right-sided S_4
iii) Ventricular hypertrophy
iv) AV blocks
v) Severe aortic or pulmonic stenosis
3) Quadruple rhythm: all four heart sounds heard
4) Summation gallop
a) All four heart sounds with tachycardia
b) Merging of S_3 and S_4 causes a louder mid-diastolic sound
5) Pericardial friction rub
a) High-pitched "to-and-fro" scratchy sound; usually triphasic including systolic, early diastolic, and late diastolic components

Table 3.7 Extra Sounds

Sound	Cause	Timing	Location	Pitch	Position	Respiratory Effect
S_3 (also called ventricular gallop)	Rapid ventricular filling into dilated ventricle	Early diastole (rapid filling subphase of diastole)	Mitral if LV; tricuspid if RV	Low	Heard best in left lateral position	LV S_3 increases with expiration; RV S_3 increases with inspiration
S_4 (also called atrial with gallop)	Atrial contraction into noncompliant ventricle	Late diastole (atrial contraction subphase of diastole)	Mitral area if LV; tricuspid area if RV	Low	Heard best in left lateral position	LV S_4 increases with expiration; RV S_4 increases with inspiration
Quadruple rhythm	All four heart sounds are heard	S_3 heard in early diastole, and S_4 heard in late diastole	Apex	Low	Heard best in left lateral position	As for S_3, S_4
Summation gallop	S_1, S_2 heard along with merged S_3 and S_4; occurs with tachycardia	Mid-diastole	Apex	Low	Heard best in left lateral position	As for S_3, S_4
Pericardial friction rub	Inflammation of the pericardium	Systolic, early diastolic, and late diastolic components	Lower left sternal border	High	Heard best with patient leaning forward	Heard best if patient holds breath after expiration
Pericardial knock	Constriction of the pericardium	Early diastole	Lower left sternal border	Low	Heard best with patient leaning forward or in left lateral position	Heard best if patient holds breath after expiration
Ejection click	Opening of defective semilunar valve	Early systole	Aortic or pulmonic	High	Heard best with patient leaning forward	Aortic: not affected by respiratory phase Pulmonic: increased with expiration
Midsystolic click	Prolapse of mitral valve leaflet	Midsystole	Mitral	High	Heard best in left lateral position	Increased with expiration
Opening snap	Abrupt recoil of stenotic AV valve	Early diastole	Mitral	High	Heard best in left lateral position	Mitral: increased with expiration Tricuspid: increased with inspiration
Mediastinal crunch	Pneumomediastinum; heart movements displacing air that is present in the mediastinum	Random	Apex or lower left sternal border	High	Heard best in left lateral position	Increased with inspiration

AV, Atrioventricular; *LV*, left ventricle; *RV*, right ventricle; S_1, first heart sound; S_2, second heart sound; S_3, third heart sound; S_4, fourth heart sound.

      b) Heard best at the fourth-fifth ICS at lower LSB with patient leaning forward
      c) Differentiate between pericardial and pleural friction rubs: ask the patient to hold breath; if the rub persists, it is a pericardial friction rub
      d) Caused by inflammation of the pericardium; commonly heard after MI or cardiac surgery
  6) Pericardial knock
      a) Loud, early-diastolic sound heard best at lower LSB
      b) Caused by constrictive pericarditis
  7) Snaps
      a) Opening snap
          i) Short, high-pitched sound heard early in diastole at third-fourth LICS at LSB; earlier, sharper, higher pitched than S_3
          ii) Caused by either of the following:
              (a) Opening of stenotic AV valve; usually precedes a diastolic murmur
              (b) Increased flow (e.g., VSD, PDA)
      b) Closing snap
          i) Really a loud S_1
          ii) Caused by closure of AV valve
  8) Clicks: high-pitched sounds heard during systole
      a) Aortic ejection click
          i) High-pitched sound heard early in systole over aortic area to apex; may precede systolic ejection murmur
          ii) Caused by aortic valve disease or dilated aorta (e.g., aortic aneurysm or coarctation)
      b) Pulmonic ejection click
          i) High-pitched sound heard early in systole over pulmonic area

ii) Caused by pulmonic valve disease, PE, pulmonary hypertension, hyperthyroidism
- c) Midsystolic click
  - i) High-pitched sound heard best at apex or lower left sternal border
  - ii) May occur alone or before a late systolic murmur
  - iii) Caused by mitral valve prolapse (MVP) or mitral regurgitation
- d) Prosthetic valve click: metallic click caused by opening and closing of prosthetic valve
9) Mediastinal crunch
- a) Crunching sound heard best at apex or along LSB in left lateral position
- b) Caused by air in mediastinum

f. Murmurs
1) Causes of turbulence (referred to as a *murmur* if intracardiac or referred to as a *bruit* if extracardiac) (Fig. 3.34)
  - a) Increased flow across a normal valve (e.g., flow murmur)
    - i) May also be called *functional* (as opposed to structural); always soft (not louder than grade II/VI) and systolic (but never holosystolic)
    - ii) Caused by any of the following:
      - (a) Hyperthermia
      - (b) Anemia
      - (c) Pregnancy
      - (d) Hyperthyroidism
  - b) Forward flow through a stenotic valve
  - c) Backward flow through a regurgitant (also called *insufficient* or *incompetent*) valve
  - d) Flow through an AV fistula or septal defect
  - e) Flow into a dilated chamber or a portion of a vessel
2) Description
  - a) Timing
    - i) Systolic
      - (a) Holosystolic: AV regurgitation or VSD
      - (b) Ejection (midsystolic): semilunar stenosis
      - (c) Late: papillary muscle dysfunction, mitral valve prolapse, hypertrophic cardiomyopathy (previously called *idiopathic hypertrophic subaortic stenosis*)
    - ii) Diastolic
      - (a) Early diastolic: semilunar regurgitation
      - (b) Mid-diastolic or late diastolic: AV stenosis
  - b) Location: place at which the murmur is loudest
  - c) Radiation: direction in which the murmur radiates
  - d) Intensity: Levine scale
    - i) Grade I/VI: barely audible, difficult to detect
    - ii) Grade II/VI: clearly audible but quiet

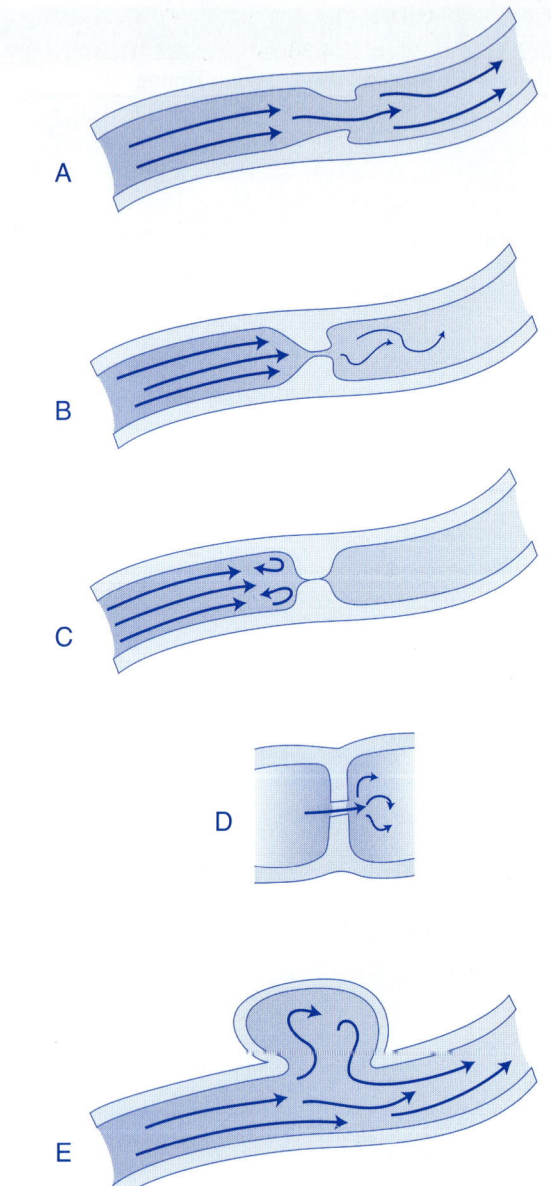

Fig. 3.34 Causes of turbulence. **A,** Increased flow across a normal valve. **B,** Forward flow through a stenotic valve. **C,** Backward flow through an incompetent valve. **D,** Flow through a septal defect or an AV fistula. **E,** Flow into a dilated chamber or a portion of a vessel.

- iii) Grade III/VI: moderately loud, without a thrill
- iv) Grade IV/VI: loud; with or without a thrill
- v) Grade V/VI: very loud, thrill present, audible with stethoscope partially off the chest
- vi) Grade VI/VI: loudest possible, thrill present, audible with stethoscope off the chest
- e) Configuration
  - i) Crescendo: gets louder
  - ii) Decrescendo: gets softer
  - iii) Crescendo-decrescendo: louder then softer
  - iv) Plateau: even intensity throughout

                f) Pitch
                    i) High pitched (heard best with diaphragm)
                        (a) Mitral and tricuspid regurgitation
                        (b) Aortic and pulmonic stenosis
                        (c) Aortic and pulmonic regurgitation
                    ii) Low pitched (heard best with bell): mitral and tricuspid stenosis
                g) Quality
                    i) Soft
                    ii) Harsh
                    iii) Blowing
                    iv) Musical
                    v) Rumbling
                    vi) Rough
            3) Differentiation of murmurs (Fig. 3.35)
    5. Vascular sound
        a. Bruit
            1) Turbulent sound
            2) May be heard over carotids, aorta, renals, iliacs, femorals
            3) Associated with plaque or aneurysm
        b. Doppler pulse
            1) A Doppler stethoscope is used to identify presence of pulse if the pulse is not palpable and may be used to confirm that the pulse palpated is the patient's and not the nurse's.
        c. Doppler pressure
            1) A Doppler stethoscope is used to measure the BP distal to vascular lesions or surgery.
            2) Apply sphygmomanometer on the calf or below the graft site and inflate to a pressure above the patient's systolic brachial pressure; allow pressure to decrease and note pressure when pulse is audible again; note posterior tibial pressure and dorsalis pedis pressures.
            3) Use the best pressure (posterior tibial or dorsalis pedis) to calculate the ankle-brachial index (ABI).
                a) Divide the systolic pressure from the leg by the brachial systolic pressure (ankle/brachial) to calculate the ABI.
                b) Evaluation
                    i) Unreliable: greater than 1; consider using toe/brachial index (TBI) described later
                    ii) Normal: 0.95 to 1
                    iii) Mildly abnormal: 0.95 to 0.75
                    iv) Moderately abnormal: 0.75 to 0.5
                    v) Ischemia: 0.50 to 0.25
                    vi) Severe ischemia: less than 0.25
                    vii) Clinically significant: decrease of 0.15 or more
                c) Some recommend TB, using the great toe's systolic pressure and dividing it by the brachial systolic pressure; normal and abnormal values are the same as for ABI.

Diagnostic Studies
1. Serum chemistries
    a. Sodium: normal 136 to 145 mEq/l
    b. Potassium: normal 3.5 to 5 mEq/l
    c. Chloride: normal 96 to 106 mEq/l
    d. Calcium: normal 8.5 to 10.5 mg/dl
    e. Phosphorus: normal 3 to 4.5 mg/dl
    f. Magnesium: normal 1.5 to 2.2 mEq/l or 1.8 to 2.4 mg/dl
    g. Glucose: normal 70 to 110 mEq/l
    h. Hgb A1C (HbA1C): measures serum glucose over time
        1) Normal values
            a) People without DM: 4.0% to 5.6%.
            b) Higher risk for developing DM: 5.7% to 6.4%
            c) DM is present: 6.5% or higher
    i. BUN: normal 5 to 20 mg/dl
    j. Creatinine: normal 0.7 to 1.5 mg/dl
    k. Enzymes
        1) Total creatine kinase (CK): normal 55 to 170 U/l for males; 30 to 135 U/l for females
        2) Creatine kinase-muscle/brain (CK-MB): 0% of total CK
        3) Lactate dehydrogenase (LDH): 90 to 200 IU/l
        4) LDH-1: 17% to 25% of total LDH
    l. Muscle proteins
        1) Myoglobin: normal less than 110 ng/ml
        2) Troponin I: normal less than 1.5 ng/ml
        3) Troponin T: normal less than 0.1 ng/ml
    m. Lipid profile
        1) Cholesterol: normal 150 to 200 mg/dl
        2) Triglycerides: normal 40 to 150 mg/dl
        3) Lipoprotein-cholesterol fractionation
            a) HDL: normal 29 to 77 mg/dl
            b) LDL: normal 62 to 130 mg/dl
    n. Homocysteine: normal less than 15 μmol/l
    o. C-reactive protein: normal less than 1 mg/dl
    p. BNP: normal less than 100 pg/ml
        1) HF
            a) Mild: 100 to 300 pg/ml
            b) Moderate: 300 to 700 pg/ml
            c) Severe: more than 700 pg/ml
        2) May also be earlier indicator of acute MI than either CK-MB or troponin I
2. Arterial blood gases (ABGs)
    a. pH: normal 7.35 to 7.45
    b. $PaCO_2$: normal 35 to 45 mm Hg
    c. HCO_3: normal 22 to 26 mM
    d. Base excess: −2 to +2
    e. PaO_2: normal 80 to 100 mm Hg
    f. SaO_2: greater than 95%
    g. Arterial lactate: less than 1 mmol/l
3. Hematology
    a. Hematocrit (Hct): normal 42% to 52% for males; 37% to 47% for females
    b. Hgb: normal 14 to 18 g/dl for males; 12 to 16 g/dl for females
    c. White blood cell (WBC) count: normal 4000 to 11,000/mm^3
    d. Erythrocyte sedimentation rate (ESR): normal up to 15 mm/hr for males; up to 20 mm/hr for females
4. Clotting profile
    a. Prothrombin time (PT): normal 12 to 15 seconds; therapeutic 1.5 to 2.5 times normal
    b. Partial thromboplastin time (PTT): normal 60 to 90 seconds; therapeutic 1.5 to 2.5 times normal

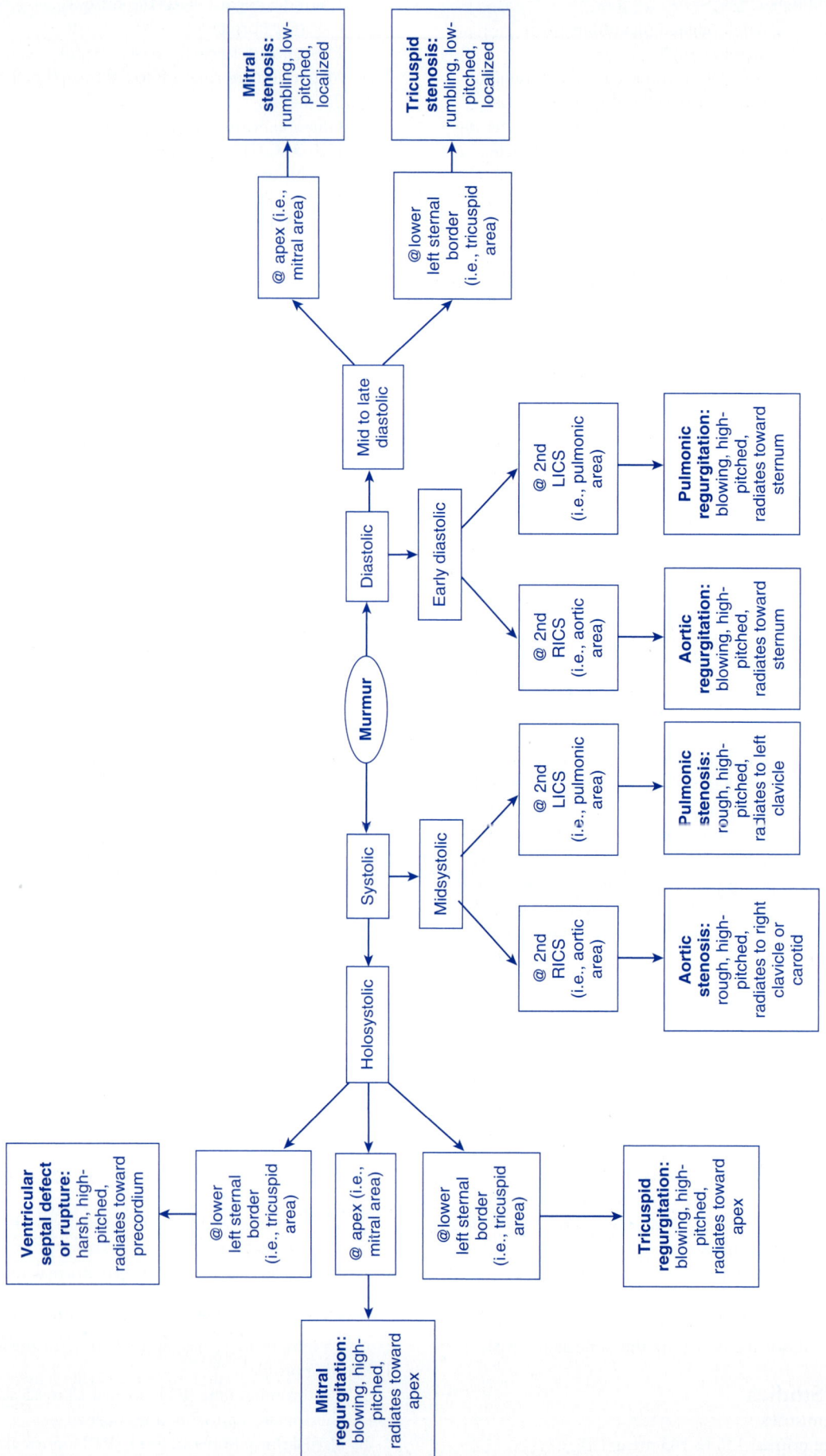

Fig. 3.35 Murmurs. *LICS*, Left intercostal space; *RICS*, right intercostal space.

c. Activated partial thromboplastin time (aPTT): normal 25 to 38 seconds; therapeutic 1.5 to 2.5 times normal
d. Activated clotting time (ACT): normal 70 to 120 seconds; therapeutic 150 to 190 seconds
e. Thrombin time: normal 10 to 15 seconds
f. Bleeding time: normal 1 to 9.5 minutes
g. International normalized ratio (INR): normal less than 2
   1) Therapeutic range for atrial fibrillation: 1.5 to 2.5
   2) Therapeutic range for deep vein thrombosis (DVT) or PE: 2 to 3
   3) Therapeutic range for prosthetic valves: 2.5 to 3.5
h. Platelets: normal 150,000 to 400,000/mm^3
5. Urine
   a. Glucose: normal negative
   b. Ketones: normal negative
   c. Specific gravity: 1.005 to 1.03
   d. Osmolality: 50 to 1200 mOsm/l
6. Other diagnostic studies (Table 3.8)

Table 3.8 Cardiovascular Diagnostic Studies

Study	Evaluates	Comments
Aortography	• Aortic valve insufficiency • Aneurysms or dissection of ascending aorta • Coarctation of the aorta • Injuries to the aorta and major branches	• Contrast medium used: check for allergy to iodine, shellfish, dye; ensure hydration after procedure • Monitor for clinical indications of anaphylaxis (e.g., flushing, urticaria, stridor) • Monitor puncture site
Cardiac biopsy	• Effect of cardiotoxic drugs • Evidence of cardiac transplant rejection • Inflammatory heart disease • Tumors • Cardiomyopathy	• Observe closely for signs of cardiac perforation and cardiac tamponade

Cardiac catheterization and coronary angiography	• Severity of coronary artery stenosis
	• Cardiac muscle function
	• Pressures within the heart
	• Cardiac output and ejection fraction
	• Blood gas analysis within chambers
	• Allows angioplasty, atherectomy, intracoronary stents, or lasers to reduce coronary artery obstruction
		• Before the test:
		  • Check for allergy to iodine, shellfish, dye (contrast medium used)
		• After the test:
		  • Ensure hydration after procedure (contrast medium used)
		  • Keep extremity in which catheter was placed immobilized in a straight position for 6–12 hr
		  • Monitor arterial puncture point for hemorrhage or hematoma; collagen (e.g., AngioSeal) or stitch device (e.g., Perclose) may be used
		  • Monitor neurovascular status of affected limb
		  • Note complaints of back pain and vital sign changes (may indicate retroperitoneal hemorrhage)

Chest radiography	• Cardiac size and shape and chamber size • Abnormalities of the lungs, ribs, pleura, pulmonary vasculature • Presence of pleural effusions • Presence of thoracic aneurysm or calcification of the aorta • Presence and location of catheters, pacemaker and AICD leads	• Inquire about possibility of pregnancy
CT, EBCT: high speed imaging provides improved view of vascular structures, including calcification	• Left ventricular wall motion • Cardiac tumors • Myocardial infarction • Pericardial effusion • Aortic aneurysm • Aortic dissection	• May be done with or without contrast medium • If contrast medium used: check for allergy to iodine, shellfish, dye; ensure hydration following procedure
Digital subtraction angiography	• Vascular disease and degree of occlusion	• Contrast medium used: check for allergy to iodine, shellfish, dye; ensure hydration after procedure • Monitor for clinical indications of anaphylaxis (e.g., flushing, urticaria, stridor) • Monitor puncture site
Doppler ultrasonography Duplex ultrasonography	• Vascular disease and degree of occlusion	

Continued

Table 3.8 Cardiovascular Diagnostic Studies—cont'd

Study	Evaluates	Comments

Echocardiography
• M-mode: single ultrasound beam
• 2D: planar ultrasound beam; wider view of heart and structures
• Doppler: addition of Doppler to demonstrate flow of blood through the heart
• Color flow: Doppler blood flow superimposed on 2D echocardiogram
• Stress echocardiography: images before, during, and after exercise or pharmacologic stress
• TEE: transducer placed in esophagus
	• Chamber size and wall thickness
	• Valve functioning
	  • Papillary muscle functioning
	  • Prosthetic valve functioning
	• Ventricular wall motion abnormalities
	• Intracardiac masses
	• Presence of pericardial fluid
	• Intracardiac pressures (Doppler)
	• Ejection fraction and cardiac output (Doppler)
	• Valve gradients (Doppler)
	• Intracardiac shunts (Doppler)
	• Thoracic aneurysm (transesophageal)
		• Transesophageal echocardiography is particularly better if patient is obese, has COPD, chest wall deformity, chest trauma, or thick chest dressings
		• Monitor for methemoglobinemia if local anesthetic is used
		• If TEE, monitor for clinical indications of esophageal perforation (i.e., sore throat, dysphagia, epigastric or substernal pain)

ECG	• Dysrhythmias • Conduction defects, including intraventricular blocks • Electrolyte imbalance • Drug toxicity • Myocardial ischemia, injury, infarction • Chamber hypertrophy	• List what drugs the patient is receiving on ECG request • Be alert to electrical safety hazards
EPS	• Dysrhythmias under controlled circumstances • Best therapy for control of dysrhythmia: drug, required dosage of therapy; pacemaker; catheter ablation	• Patients may have near-death experience during EPS; encourage expression of fears, concerns, anxieties • Monitor puncture site
Holter monitor	• Suspected dysrhythmias over 24- to 48-hr period • Pacemaker function • Silent ischemia	• Instruct patient regarding importance of diary keeping
IVUS	• Coronary artery size and patency • Structure of vessel wall • Coronary artery stent position and patency • Aorta and presence of aneurysm, aneurysm dissections	• As for cardiac catheterization
MRI	• 3D view of the heart • Anatomy and structure of the heart and great vessels including: cardiomyopathy; congenital defect; masses; aneurysm • Changes in chemistry of tissues before structural changes occur	• Does not involve radiation or dyes • Cannot be used in patients with any implanted metallic device, including pacemakers, implantable defibrillators, metallic heart valves, intracranial aneurysm clips
MUGA scan (radionuclide angiography)	• Ventricular size and ventricular wall motion • Cardiac output, cardiac index, end-systolic volume, end-diastolic volume, and ejection fraction • Intracardiac shunts	• Assure patient that amount of radioactive material is minimal
Pericardiocentesis and pericardial fluid analysis	• Presence of blood, pus, pathogens, or malignancy • Also used for emergency relief of cardiac tamponade	• Observe closely for signs of cardiac tamponade

Peripheral angiography	• Atherosclerotic plaques, occlusion, aneurysms, or traumatic injury	• Before the test:
		  • Contrast medium used: check for allergy to iodine, shellfish, dye
		• After the test
		  • Contrast medium used, ensure hydration postprocedure
		  • Keep extremity in which catheter was placed immobilized in a straight position for 6–12 h
		  • Monitor arterial puncture point for hemorrhage or hematomaMonitor neurovascular status of affected limbMonitor for indications of systemic emboli

Table 3.8 Cardiovascular Diagnostic Studies—cont'd

Study	Evaluates	Comments
Plethysmography: arterial or venous	Arterial: • Patency of peripheral arteries and presence of occlusive vascular disease Venous: • Patency of peripheral venous system and presence of deep vein thrombosis	• Requires one normal extremity because one extremity is compared with the other
PET (cardiac PET scan)	• Severity of coronary artery stenosis • Collateral circulation • Patency of bypass grafts • Size and location of infarcted tissue	• Assure patient that amount of radioactive material is minimal
Sestamibi exercise testing and scan Sestamibi-dipyridamole stress test (for patients with physical limitation preventing exercise)	• Myocardial ischemia during exercise (ischemic areas show increased uptake of radioactivity [hot spots])	• Monitor for myocardial ischemia
Signal-averaged ECG	• Presence of late electrical potentials which may be responsible for malignant ventricular dysrhythmias; may be performed before and after ablation	• Patient must lie still for 10 min
Stress electrocardiography (also referred to as *exercise tolerance test*)	• Persons with high risk for CAD, patients with known CAD, or post-CABG patients for ischemia with exercise or pharmacologic agents (e.g., adenosine, dipyridamole, dobutamine) if patient cannot tolerate exercise • Exercise-induced dysrhythmias	• ≥1 mm transient ST-segment depression 80 msec after the J point is suggestive of CAD • Monitor closely for exercise-induced hypotension or ventricular dysrhythmias • Adenosine is the preferred agent for pharmacologic stress test because it has a short half-life and does not require reversal agent
Technetium-99 pyrophosphate scan	• Size, location of acute MI (infarcted areas show increased uptake of radioactivity ["hot spots"] 1–7 d after MI)	• Assure patient that amount of radioactive material is minimal • Peak accuracy at 12–48 hr after initial symptoms
Thallium stress electrocardiography	• Myocardial ischemia during exercise (ischemic areas show decreased uptake of radioactivity [cold spots])	• Assure patient that amount of radioactive material is minimal
Thallium-201 scan	• Myocardial ischemia (ischemic areas show decreased uptake of radioactivity [cold spots])	• Assure patient that amount of radioactive material is minimal
Vectorcardiography	• Chamber hypertrophy • Bundle branch blocks and hemiblocks • Myocardial ischemia or infarction	
Venography (ascending contrast phlebography)	• Deep leg veins • Presence of DVT • Competence of deep vein valves • May be used to locate suitable vein for arterial bypass graft	• Contrast medium used: check for allergy to iodine, shellfish, dye; ensure hydration postprocedure • Monitor for clinical indications of anaphylaxis (e.g., flushing, urticaria, stridor) • Monitor puncture site
Ventriculography	• Ventricular wall motion • Wall thickness • Ventricular aneurysm • Mitral valve motion • LV end-diastolic volume, end-systolic volume, stroke volume, ejection fraction • Intracardiac shunt	• Contrast medium used: check for allergy to iodine, shellfish, dye; ensure hydration postprocedure • Monitor for clinical indications of anaphylaxis (e.g., flushing, urticaria, stridor) • Monitor puncture site

AICD, Automatic implantable cardiac defibrillator; *CAD*, coronary artery disease; *CABG*, coronary artery bypass graft; *COPD*, chronic obstructive pulmonary disease; *CT*, computed tomography; *DVT*, deep vein thrombosis; *EBCT*, electron beam computed tomography; *ECG*, electrocardiography; *EPS*, electrophysiologic studies; *IVUS*, intravascular ultrasound; *MRI*, magnetic resonance imaging; *MUGA*, multiple-gated acquisition; *PET*, positron emission tomography; *TEE*, transesophageal echocardiography; *3D*, three dimensional; *2D*, two dimensional.

Electrocardiography

General Information
1. The electrocardiograph measures and records the electrical activity of the heart by measuring electrical potential at the skin surface; the ECG is a recording of that activity.
2. An ECG is used to detect or demonstrate any of the following:
   a. Rhythm disturbances
   b. Conduction defects
   c. Electrolyte imbalances
   d. Drug effects and toxicity
   e. Chamber enlargement or hypertrophy
   f. Myocardial ischemia, injury, or infarction
3. ECG paper (Fig. 3.36)
   a. Horizontal axis measures time
      1) Each small (1-mm) box is equal to 0.04 seconds.
      2) Each large (5-mm) box is equal to 0.2 seconds.
      3) Small marks at the top of the paper identify 3-second intervals.
   b. Vertical axis measures voltage.
      1) Useful only if standardized, as on multiple-lead ECG; rhythm strips are not generally standardized because the size (i.e., gain) can be changed
      2) If standardized
         a) Each small (1-mm) box is equal to 0.1 mV.
         b) Each large (5-mm) box is equal to 0.5 mV.
4. Rule of electrical flow
   a. Impulses traveling toward the positive pole of a lead cause a positive deflection.
   b. Impulses traveling toward the negative (or away from the positive) pole of a lead cause a negative deflection.

Rhythm Strip Analysis
1. Monitoring leads
   a. Standard electrode placement with five-lead system (Fig. 3.37)
      1) White (right arm): just below right clavicle
      2) Black (left arm): just below left clavicle
      3) Brown
         a) For V_1: fourth ICS at right sternal border
         b) For V_6: fifth ICS at left midaxillary line
      4) Green (right leg): lower chest, above and to right of umbilicus
      5) Red (left leg): lower chest, above and to left of umbilicus
      6) NOTE: Remember "white on the right, snow over grass, smoke over fire, brown on the ground" (Barill, 2003)
      7) Available leads: I, II, III, aVR, aVL, aVF, or V (which V lead depends on placement of the brown lead)
   b. Typical leads monitored in three-lead system (Fig. 3.38)
      1) Lead II: positive (red) at lower left torso; negative (white) under right clavicle; ground (black) under left clavicle (NOTE: Remember "white to the right. Smoke over fire" [Barill, 2003])

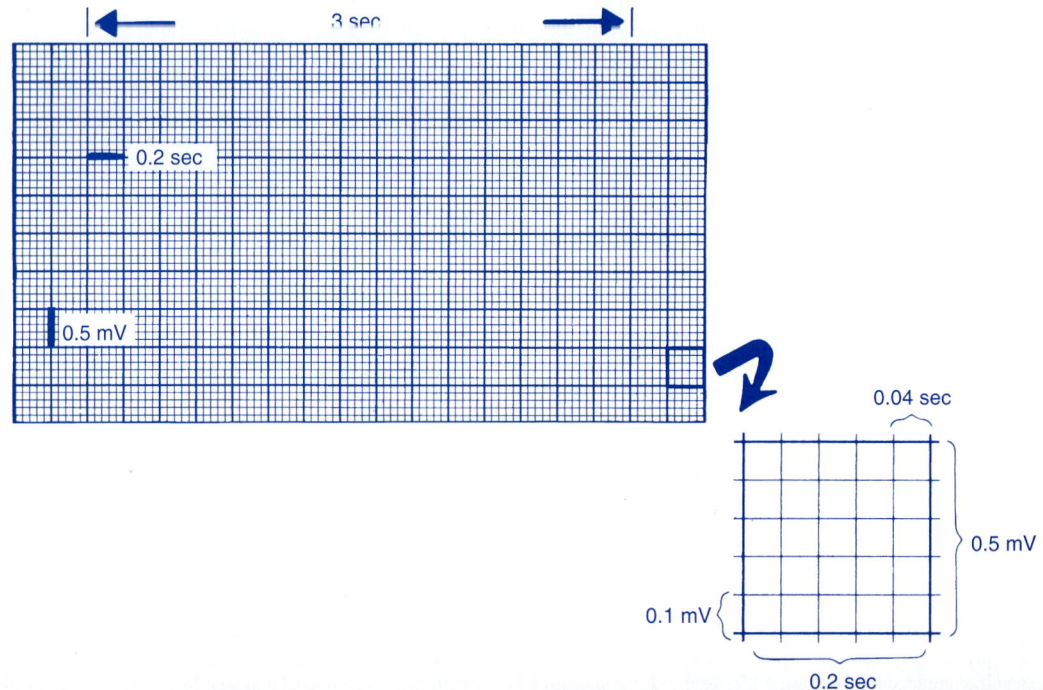

Fig. 3.36 Electrocardiogram paper: horizontal axis represents time with each small block equal to 0.04 second and each large block equal to 0.2 second with 3-second intervals marked off at top of paper; vertical axis represents voltage when standardized with each small block equal to 0.1 mV and each large block equal to 0.5 mV. (From Kinney, M. R., Dunbar, S., & Brooks-Brunn, J. A. [1998]. *AACN's clinical reference for critical-care nursing* [4th ed.]. St. Louis: Mosby.)

2) Modified chest leads (MCLs)
    a) MCL₁
        i) Monitor: set at lead I
        ii) Lead placement: positive (black) at fourth ICS at RSB; negative (white) under left clavicle; ground (red) under right clavicle
    b) MCL₆
        i) Monitor: set at lead II
        ii) Lead placement: positive at fifth ICS at left midaxillary line (MAL)
    c) Note that the difference between MCLs and true V leads is that V leads are unipolar and preferred if available and MCLs are bipolar
c. Lead placement for continuous derived 12-lead ECG (EASI)
    1) E (brown): lower part of the sternum at the fifth ICS
    2) A (red): right midaxillary line at fifth ICS
    3) S (black): upper part of the sternum
    4) I (white): left midaxillary line at fifth ICS
    5) Fifth electrode (green) can be placed anywhere on the torso; it serves as a ground.
d. Lead selection
    1) Lead II
        a) Advantages
            i) Upright P and QRS waves
            ii) Normal appearance
        b) Disadvantage: ectopy and aberrancy look-alike
        c) Clinical indication: atrial dysrhythmias

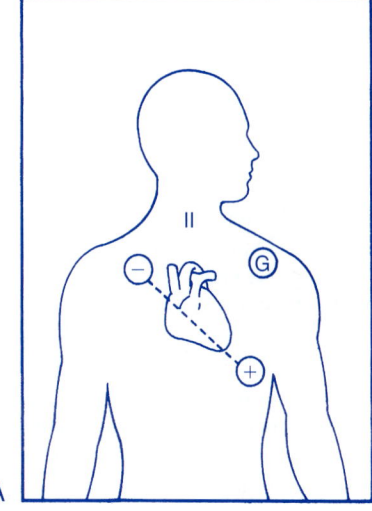

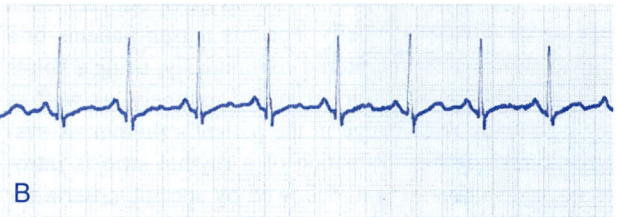

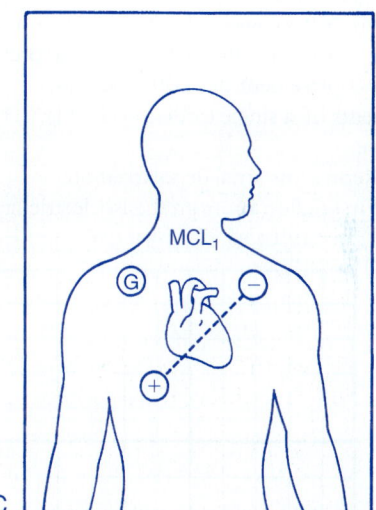

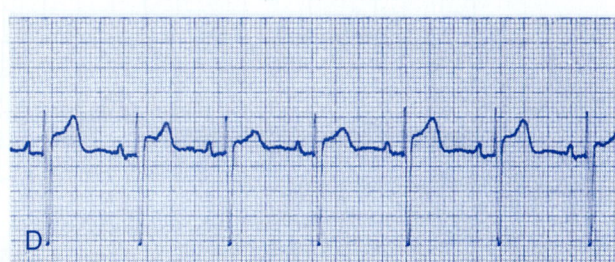

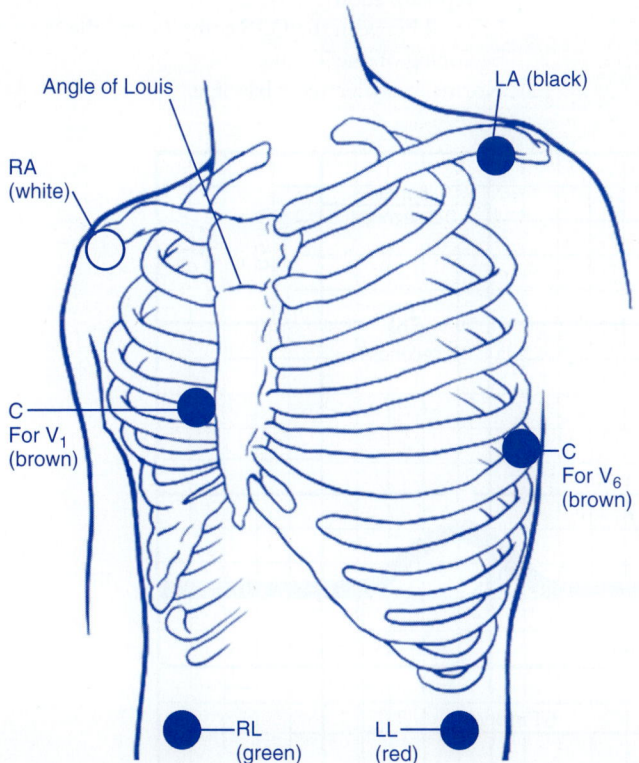

Fig. 3.37 Standard electrode placement for monitoring with a five-lead system. (From Drew, B [2002]. *Philips—AACN cardiac monitoring pocket reference*. Philips PN #5990-0487. Aliso Viejo, CA: American Association of Critical-Care Nurses.)

Fig. 3.38 Monitoring leads. **A**, Electrode placement for lead II. **B**, Representation of appearance of electrocardiogram in lead II. **C**, Electrode placement for MCL₁. **D**, Representation of appearance of ECG in MCL₁. (From Urden L. D., Lough M. E., & Stacy K. M. [1995]. *Priorities in critical care nursing*. St. Louis: Mosby.)

2) V_1 or MCL_1
    a) Advantages
        i) Better differentiation of ectopy from aberrancy
        ii) Differentiation of LBBB from RBBB
        iii) Differentiation of LV ectopy from RV ectopy
    b) Disadvantages
        i) Diphasic P wave
        ii) Negative QRS
    c) Clinical indications
        i) Diagnosis of wide QRS complexes (e.g., differentiation of ventricular ectopy from supraventricular tachycardia (SVT) with aberrancy, differentiation of RBBB or LBBB): V_1 and/or V_6
        ii) Ischemia, injury, infarction: however, two leads are best
            (a) Second lead is determined by lead with significant ST segment elevation (patient's ischemic fingerprint).
            (b) If the patient's ischemic fingerprint is not known: second lead should be lead III or V_3
        iii) Pacemaker: V_1
        iv) HF or cardiomyopathy to monitor for the development of bundle branch block: V_1
3) V_6 or MCL_6
    a) Advantages as for V_1; may be especially helpful if incision or dressing prevents placement of lead at sternum

2. Components of a single cardiac cycle (Fig. 3.39)
    a. P wave
        1) Represents atrial depolarization
        2) First deflection from the isoelectric line
        3) Normal P wave: no more than 2.5 mm tall and no more than 0.11 seconds wide
    b. PR segment
        1) Represents the delay in AV node
        2) Isoelectric line between P wave and QRS complex
    c. PR interval
        1) Represents atrial depolarization + delay in AV node
        2) Measured from beginning of P wave to beginning of QRS complex
        3) Normal PR interval: 0.12 to 0.2 seconds
    d. Q wave: the first negative wave after the P wave but before the R wave
    e. R wave: the first positive wave after the P wave
    f. S wave: the negative wave after the R wave
    g. QRS complex
        1) Represents ventricular depolarization
        2) May have one, two, or all three: Q, R, S
            a) Case indicates size; for example, qRS indicates a small q and large R and S
            b) A prime sign (') after an R indicates that it is a second R (i.e., R') as in bundle branch blocks; so, for example, rSR' indicates small R, large S, large second R.
        3) Measured from beginning of the first wave of complex to the end of last wave of complex
        4) Normal QRS interval: 0.06 to 0.11
        5) Normal QRS amplitude: less than 30 mm in chest leads
    h. ST segment
        1) Represents the time during which the ventricles have completely depolarized and the beginning of repolarization
        2) Located between the QRS complex and the beginning of the T wave
        3) Normally isoelectric at baseline

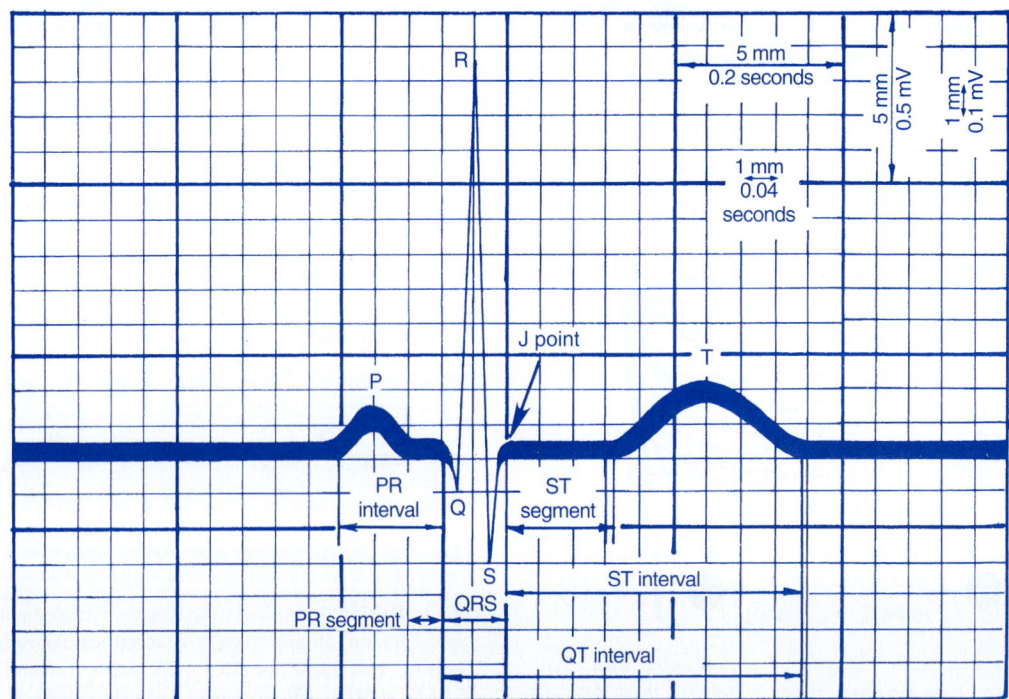

Fig. 3.39 Components of a single cardiac cycle. (From Seidel, J. C. [1986]. *The Methodist Hospital: Basic electrocardiography: a modular approach*. St. Louis: Mosby.)

i. J point
   1) The angle at which the QRS complex ends and the ST segment begins
   2) The J point deviates from the isoelectric line if the ST segment is elevated or depressed.
j. T wave
   1) Represents ventricular repolarization
   2) Wave after the QRS; may be positive or negative
   3) Normal T wave: less than 5 mm in limb leads and less than 10 mm in chest lead
k. U wave
   1) May represent repolarization of the Purkinje fibers
   2) Small wave after the T wave; often not seen because of its low voltage
   3) Normal U wave: less than or equal to 1 mm
l. QT interval
   1) Represents time of ventricular depolarization and repolarization
   2) Measured from first wave of QRS complex to the end of the T wave
   3) Normal QT interval based on HR; the slower the HR, the longer the normal QT; the faster the HR, the shorter the normal QT
      a) For HRs 60 to 100 beats/min, the normal QT interval is less than half of the RR interval.
   4) To correct for changes in HR (especially for HRs not 60–100 beats/min), calculate the QTc
      a) Formula: QT ÷ Square root of the R-R interval
      b) Normal QTc: 0.32 to 0.44

5) Indications for monitoring of QT interval
   a) Congenital long QT syndrome
   b) Significant bradycardia (less than 50 beats/min)
   c) Antidysrhythmics that are known to prolong the QT interval
      i) IA: quinidine, procainamide, disopyramide
      ii) IC: flecainide, propafenone
      iii) II/III: sotalol
      iv) III: ibutilide, dofetilide
   d) Electrolyte imbalances
      i) Hypokalemia
      ii) Hypomagnesemia
      iii) Hypocalcemia
   e) TCAs (e.g., amitriptyline, nortriptyline)
   f) Antibiotics: fluoroquinolones (e.g., gemifloxacin, moxifloxacin), macrolides (e.g., azithromycin), erythromycin
   g) Cerebrovascular disease (e.g., intracranial or subarachnoid hemorrhage, stroke, intracranial trauma)
   h) Hypothermia
   i) Hypothyroidism
   j) Hypoglycemia
   k) Myocardial ischemia or MI
   l) HF or cardiomyopathy
3. Steps in analysis of a rhythm strip (Table 3.9)
4. Criteria for basic dysrhythmias and blocks (Table 3.10)

Table 3.9 Rhythm Strip Analysis

Component	Assessment
Regularity (rhythm)	• Is it regular? • Is it irregular? • Are there any patterns to the irregularity? • Are there any ectopic beats; if so, are they early (premature) or late (escape)? • Is regularity of P waves and QRS complexes the same? (If there is only one P wave for each QRS, only one regularity needs to be recorded)

Rate	• Methods
	  • Count dark lines between P waves or QRS complexes as 300, 150, 100, 75, 60, 50, 43, 38, 33, 30.
	  • Count number of QRS complexes in a 6-second strip and multiply by 10.
	  • Use a rate ruler.
	• Are atrial and ventricular rates the same? (If there is only one P wave for each QRS, only one rate needs to be recorded.)

P waves	• Are the P waves regular? • Is there one P wave for every QRS? • Is there a P wave in front of the QRS or behind it? • Is the P wave normal and upright in lead II? • Are there more P waves than QRS complexes? • Do all P waves look alike? • Are irregular P waves associated with ectopic beats? If so, are they early (premature) or late (escape)?
PR intervals	• Is PRI measurement within normal range? • (normal interval: 0.12–0.2 sec) • Are all PRIs constant? • If PRI varies, is there a pattern to the changing measurements?
QRS complexes	• Is QRS measurement within normal limits? (normal interval: 0.06–0.11 sec) • Are all QRS complexes of equal duration? • Do all QRS complexes look alike? • Are unusual QRS complexes associated with ectopic beats? If so, are they early (premature) or late (escape)?
QT interval	• Is the QT measurement within normal limits? (measured QT less than half of previous R-R interval or QTc of 0.32–0.44)
Patient presentation	• Is the patient symptomatic? • Are there clinical indications of hypoperfusion such as hypotension, syncope, or chest pain?

Table 3.10 Criteria for Basic Dysrhythmias and Blocks

Rhythm	Rate	Regularity	P Waves	PR Interval	QRS Duration
Normal sinus rhythm	60–100 beats/min	Atrial and ventricular rhythms regular	Normal	0.12–0.2 sec and constant	<0.12 sec
Sinus bradycardia	<60 beats/min	Atrial and ventricular rhythms regular	Normal	0.12–0.2 sec and constant	<0.12 sec
Sinus tachycardia	>100 beats/min (usually 100–160/min)	Atrial and ventricular rhythms regular	Normal	0.12–0.2 sec and constant	<0.12 sec
Sinus dysrhythmia	Usually 60–100 beats/min but may be slower or faster	Atrial and ventricular rhythms regularly irregular; rate increases with inspiration (so R-R interval shortens) and decreases with expiration (so R-R interval lengthens); difference between shortest and longest R-R <0.12 sec	Normal	0.12–0.2 sec and usually constant; may vary slightly with rate variation	<0.12 sec
Sinus block (sinus exit block)	Dependent on underlying rhythm	Atrial and ventricular rhythms regular with an irregularity; R-R interval at block measures an exact multiple of the normal R-R interval	One or more entire cardiac cycle is absent; P wave absent during block	None during block	QRS absent during block
Sinus arrest	Dependent on underlying rhythm	Atrial and ventricular rhythms regular with an irregularity (a pause); R-R interval at pause measures more or less than an exact multiple of the normal R-R interval	Indefinite period of time without an entire cardiac cycle; P wave absent during arrest	None during arrest	QRS absent during arrest
Premature atrial contractions	Dependent on underlying rhythm	Dependent on underlying rhythm; PAC interrupts underlying rhythm	P wave of this early beat differs from sinus P; the ectopic P wave is early and may be flattened, notched, or lost in preceding T wave	Usually 0.12–0.2 sec but may be >0.2 sec	<0.12 sec
Wandering atrial pacemaker	Usually 60–100 beats/min	Atrial and ventricular rhythms usually slightly irregular	P waves look different beat to beat; at least three different-looking P waves	0.12–0.2 sec and may vary	<0.12 sec
Supraventricular tachycardia*	>100 beats/min; usually 150–250 beats/min	Atrial and ventricular rhythms regular	P waves are impossible to distinguish; may be lost in QRS or preceding T wave	Cannot measure	<0.12 sec
Atrial tachycardia	150–250 beats/min	Atrial and ventricular rhythms regular	P wave differs from sinus P; may merge with preceding T wave	0.12–0.2 sec	<0.12 sec
Multifocal atrial tachycardia (also called chaotic atrial rhythm)	Usually 100–150 beats/min	Atrial and ventricular rhythms usually slightly irregular	P waves look different beat to beat; at least three different-looking P waves	0.12–0.2 sec and may vary	<0.12 sec

Table 3.10	Criteria for Basic Dysrhythmias and Blocks—cont'd				
Rhythm	**Rate**	**Regularity**	**P Waves**	**PR Interval**	**QRS Duration**
Atrial flutter	Atrial rate ≈300 beats/min; ventricular rate varies with conduction through the AV node; 2:1 atrial flutter has a ventricular rate of ≈150 beats/min, 4:1 atrial flutter has a ventricular rate of ≈75 beats/min	Atrial flutter waves regular; ventricular rhythm (response) usually regular	No true P waves; flutter waves have characteristic sawtooth appearance	No true P waves	<0.12 sec
Atrial fibrillation	Atrial rate >350 beats/min; ventricular rate varies greatly depending on conduction through AV node	Atrial fibrillatory waves irregular; ventricular rhythm irregularly irregular	No true P waves; fibrillatory waves manifested by quivering baseline	No true P waves	<0.12 sec
Premature junctional contraction (PJC)	Dependent on underlying rhythm	Dependent on underlying rhythm; PJC interrupts underlying rhythm	P wave if visible will be inverted; may be in front of, in, or after the QRS complex	Can be measured only if P wave is in front of QRS; PR will be <0.12 sec if measurable	<0.12 sec
Junctional escape rhythm	40–60 beats/min	Atrial and ventricular rhythms regular	If visible, P wave inverted; may be in front of, in, or after the QRS complex	Can be measured only if P wave is in front of QRS; PR will be <0.12 sec if measurable	<0.12 sec
Accelerated junctional rhythm	60–100 beats/min	Atrial and ventricular rhythms regular	If visible, P wave inverted; may be in front of, in, or after the QRS complex	Can be measured only if P wave is in front of QRS; PR will be <0.12 sec if measurable	<0.12 sec
Junctional tachycardia	>100 beats/min; usually 100–180 beats/min	Atrial and ventricular rhythms regular	If visible, P wave inverted; may be in front of, in, or after the QRS complex	Can be measured only if P wave is in front of QRS; PR will be <0.12 sec if measurable	<0.12 sec
First-degree AV nodal block	Dependent on underlying rhythm	Dependent on underlying rhythm	P wave normal	>0.2 sec	<0.12 sec
Second-degree AV nodal block type I[†] (Wenckebach)	Atrial rate dependent on underlying rhythm; ventricular rate dependent on conduction ratio; atrial rate greater than ventricular rate	Atrial rhythm regular, ventricular rhythm irregular (P-P is regular, but R-R is irregular); groupings identifiable between P waves that were not conducted	P waves normal, but some P waves not followed by a QRS	Normal PR interval progressively lengthens until a P wave is not followed by a QRS; entire cycle begins again with normal PR interval	<0.12 sec
Second-degree AV nodal block type II[†]	Atrial rate dependent on underlying rhythm; ventricular rate dependent on conduction ratio but usually <60 beats/min; atrial rate >ventricular rate	Atrial rhythm regular, ventricular rhythm regular or irregular depending on whether conduction ratio varies or is constant; P-P regular, but some R-Rs may be twice normal	P waves normal, but there are P waves not followed by a QRS without preceding progressive lengthening	Usually 0.12–0.2 sec of conducted P waves but may be longer; constant for each conducted QRS	≥0.12 sec
Third-degree (or complete) AV block	Atrial rate dependent on underlying rhythm; ventricular rate dependent on focus of escape rhythm (40–60 beats/min if escape focus is junctional, 20–40 beats/min if escape focus is ventricular)	Atrial rhythm regular, ventricular rhythm usually regular; P-P regular; R-R usually regular	Normal but P waves not followed by (associated with) QRS	No consistent PR interval; no relationship between the P waves and the QRS complexes	<0.12 sec if escape focus is junctional; 0.12 sec or longer if escape focus is ventricular

Continued

Table 3.10 Criteria for Basic Dysrhythmias and Blocks—cont'd

Rhythm	Rate	Regularity	P Waves	PR Interval	QRS Duration
Left bundle branch block	Dependent on underlying rhythm	Dependent on underlying rhythm	P wave normal	0.12–0.2 sec as long as no coexisting AV nodal block	≥0.12 sec; QRS is negative in V_1
Right bundle branch block	Dependent on underlying rhythm	Dependent on underlying rhythm	P wave normal	0.12–0.2 sec as long as no coexisting AV nodal block	≥0.12 sec; QRS is positive in V_1
Premature ventricular contraction	Dependent on underlying rhythm	Dependent on underlying rhythm; PVC interrupts underlying rhythm	No associated P wave	No associated P wave; cannot measure PR	≥0.12 sec; QRS of PVC looks different than normal QRSs
Monomorphic ventricular tachycardia (VT)	100–250 beats/min *VT is usually ~150 beats/min; VT at 200–250 beats/min may be called ventricular flutter	Ventricular rhythm usually regular; if dissociated P waves are identifiable, atrial rhythm regular	No associated P waves but may have dissociated P waves scattered through the rhythm	No associated P waves; cannot measure PR	≥0.12 sec; QRS of VT looks different than normal QRSs
Polymorphic ventricular tachycardia (torsades de pointes)	150–250 beats/min	Ventricular rhythm may be regular	None	None	≥0.12 sec with QRS that seems to twist around a center line; gradual alteration in the amplitude and direction of the QRS
Ventricular fibrillation	None	Irregular; chaotic baseline	None	None	None
Idioventricular rhythm	20–40 beats/min	Ventricular rhythm usually regular; no atrial activity	None	None	≥0.12 sec
Accelerated idioventricular rhythm	40–100 beats/min	Ventricular rhythm usually regular; no atrial activity	None	None	≥0.12 sec
Asystole	None	No atrial or ventricular activity	None	None	None

*Supraventricular tachycardia refers to any narrow QRS tachycardia with a focus that cannot be definitely identified; the term should be used only when a more definitive diagnosis cannot be made.
†2:1 block is a second-degree block but may be either type I or II; the QRS width may be helpful in differentiating between the two; if the QRS is of normal width, it is probably type I; and if the QRS is 0.12 or greater, it is probably type II.
AV, Atrioventricular; *PAC*, premature atrial contraction.

    a. The pacemaker rule: the fastest rate will control the heart.
        1) This is usually the SA node unless an irritable focus (e.g., atrial, junctional, or ventricular) is faster; this is called *irritability*.
        2) If an upper pacemaker (e.g., SA node) fails, it is up to lower pacemakers (e.g., junctional or ventricular) to assume control: this is called *escape*.
5. ECG changes in electrolyte imbalance
    a. Hypokalemia
        1) If 3 mEq/l or less
            a) Flat T with prominent U wave
            b) T wave and U wave of approximately the same amplitude
            c) ST segment flattening and/or depression
        2) If 2 mEq/l or less
            a) U wave taller than T wave
            b) Prolongation of QT interval
            c) ST segment depression
        3) If 1 mEq/l or less
            a) U wave fuses with T wave.
    b. Hyperkalemia
        1) If greater than 6 mEq/l
            a) ST segment disappears, and T waves become tall, narrow, and peaked.
            b) QRS complex widens.
        2) If 6.5 mEq/l or greater
            a) QRS complex widens more.
            b) P wave widens and flattens.
        3) If 7.5 mEq/l or greater
            a) Sinus arrest with disappearance of P waves
        4) If 10 to 12 mEq/l or greater
            a) Wide QRS merged with T wave
            b) VF or asystole
    c. Hypocalcemia
        1) Prolonged QT
        2) Prolonged ST segment
    d. Hypercalcemia
        1) Shortened QT
        2) Shortened ST segment
    e. Hypomagnesemia
        1) Prolonged QT
        2) Broad, flattened T wave

f. Hypermagnesemia
   1) PR, QT prolonged
   2) Prolonged QRS
6. Drug effects on the ECG
   a. Digitalis
      1) Scooping of ST-T wave (known as *digitalis effect*)
      2) Shortened QT
      3) PR interval may be prolonged
   b. Type IA antidysrhythmics (e.g., procainamide, quinidine, disopyramide)
      1) QT prolongation
      2) T wave flattening

Multiple-Lead Electrocardiogram Analysis

1. ECG leads (Fig. 3.40)
   a. Limb leads: frontal plane
      1) Lead I: + at LA (left arm); - at RA (right arm)
      2) Lead II: + at F (foot); - at RA
      3) Lead III: + at F (foot); - at LA
      4) Lead aVR: unipolar RA
      5) Lead aVL: unipolar LA
      6) Lead aVF: unipolar F
   b. Chest leads: horizontal plane
      1) Lead V_1: 4ICS at right sternal border (RSB)
      2) Lead V_2: 4ICS at left sternal border (LSB)

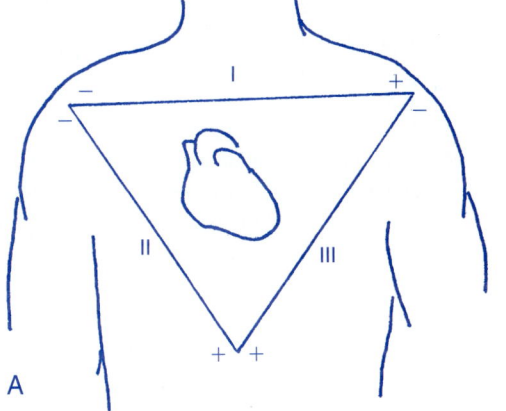
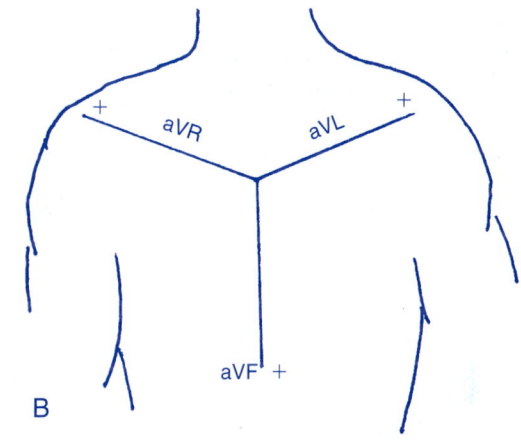
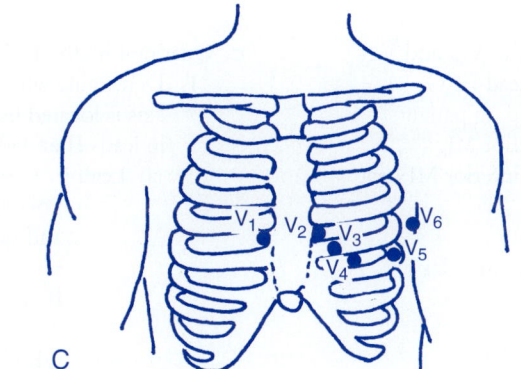
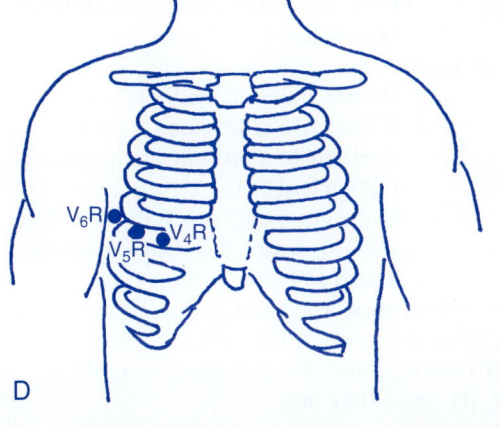
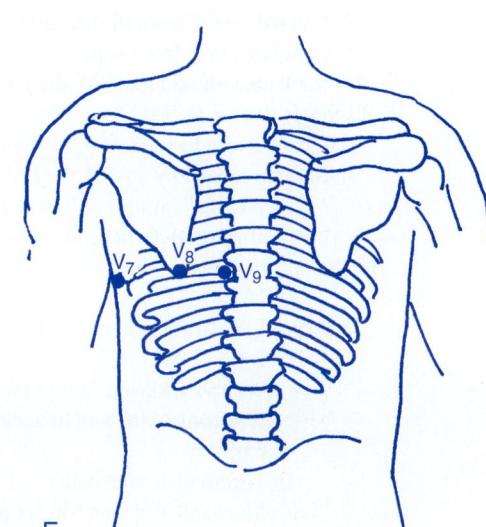

Fig. 3.40 Electrocardiogram leads. **A,** Bipolar limb leads: I, II, III. **B,** Unipolar limb leads: aVR, aVL, aVF. **C,** Standard chest leads: V_1 to V_6. **D,** Right ventricular leads: V_{4R} to V_{6R}. **E,** Posterior leads: V_7 to V_9.

3) Lead V_3: halfway between V_2 and V_4
4) Lead V_4: 5ICS at left midclavicular line (LMCL)
5) Lead V_5: 5ICS at left anterior axillary line (LAAL)
6) Lead V_6: 5ICS at left midaxillary line (LMAL)
7) R wave gets taller across the precordium from V_1 to V_6 (referred to as *normal progression of the R wave across the precordium*); the S wave gets smaller across the precordium (V_1 to V_6).
8) Conditions associated with poor R wave progression across the precordium include the following:
   a) Anterior MI
   b) LBBB
   c) Emphysema
9) Conditions associated with low voltage across the precordium include the following:
   a) Emphysema
   b) Pericardial effusion
   c) MI
   d) Obesity
   c. Specialty leads
      1) Posterior leads
         a) Lead V_7: 5ICS at left posterior axillary line (LPAL)
         b) Lead V_8: halfway between V_7 and V_8
         c) Lead V_9: 5ICS next to vertebral column
      2) RV leads
         a) Lead V_{4R}: 5ICS at RMCL
         b) Lead V_{5R}: 5ICS at RAAL
         c) Lead V_{6R}: 5ICS at RMAL
         d) The standard 12 leads plus V_{4R}-V_{6R} and V_{7-9} make the 18 leads of an 18-lead ECG
         e) RV leads routinely performed on patients with ECG indicators of inferior MI (33%–50% of patients with inferior MI have concurrent RV infarction)
2. Mean QRS axis
   a. Represents the average direction of ventricular depolarization
   b. Described on a 360-degree circle
      1) Normal axis
         a) Downward and to the left (0–90 degrees)
         b) Caused by the normal direction of depolarization from superior to inferior and the larger muscle mass of the left ventricle
      2) Left axis deviation (LAD)
         a) Upward and to the left (0 to -90 degrees)
         b) May be caused by any of the following:
            i) Normal variant: only considered abnormal if more negative than -30 degrees
            ii) LVH
            iii) Left anterior hemiblock
            iv) Inferior MI
            v) Wolff-Parkinson-White (WPW) syndrome with a right accessory pathway
            vi) Ventricular pacemaker
            vii) Mechanical shift of heart to more horizontal: ascites; pregnancy; abdominal tumor
      3) Right-axis deviation (RAD)
         a) Downward and to the right (+90 to ±180 degrees)
         b) May be caused by any of the following:
            i) Normal variant: only considered abnormal if more positive than +110 degrees
            ii) Right ventricular hypertrophy (RVH)
            iii) PE
            iv) Left posterior hemiblock
            v) Lateral MI
            vi) WPW syndrome with a left accessory pathway
            vii) Dextrocardia
            viii) Mechanical shift of heart to more vertical: emphysema
      4) Indeterminate axis
         a) Upward and to the right (-90 to ±180)
         b) Although this axis deviation is frequently referred to as *no-man's land* or *extreme right axis deviation,* it could be extreme RAD or extreme LAD; therefore, indeterminate is more appropriate.
         c) May be caused by any of the following:
            i) VT
            ii) Ventricular pacemaker
            iii) Multiple infarctions
            iv) Hyperkalemia
            v) Severe RVH (e.g., severe pulmonary disease)
   c. Quadrant method (Fig. 3.41)
      1) Determine which quadrant where the mean QRS axis is located by using the direction of the QRS in leads II and aVF.
         a) Lead I
            i) Positive pole is at the left arm, and negative pole is at the right arm.
            ii) If the mean QRS axis is to the left, there will be a predominantly positive QRS in lead I.
            iii) If the mean QRS axis is to the right, there will be a predominantly negative QRS in lead I.
         b) Lead aVF
            i) Positive pole is at the foot.
            ii) If the mean QRS axis is downward, there will be a predominantly positive QRS in lead aVF.
            iii) If the mean QRS axis is upward, there will be a predominantly negative QRS in lead aVF.
      2) If QRS is positive in I and positive in aVF, mean QRS axis is normal (0 to +90).
      3) If QRS is positive in I and negative in aVF, a LAD exists (0 to -90).
      4) If QRS is negative in I and positive in aVF, a RAD exists (+90 to ±180).
      5) If QRS is negative in I and negative in aVF, an indeterminate axis deviation exists (-90 to ±180)

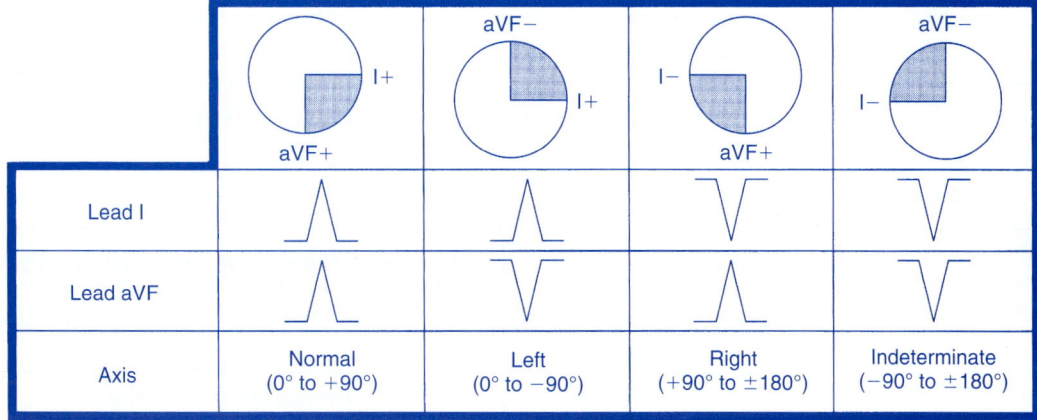

Fig. 3.41 Quadrant method of axis determination. (Modified from Kinney, M. R., Dunbar, S., & Brooks-Brunn, J. A. [1998]. *AACN's clinical reference for critical-care nursing* [4th ed.]. St. Louis: Mosby.)

3. Bundle branch blocks (Fig. 3.42)
    a. Block of either bundle branch causes the following:
        1) A delay in the conduction through the ventricles and a prolongation of the QRS interval
        2) Branching (commonly referred to as *rabbit ears*) or slurring of the QRS complex also usually occurs, indicating that the two ventricles are depolarized out of sync.
        3) T-wave deflection in the opposite direction of the QRS
    b. LBBB is a bifascicular block (loss of both major hemibundles) and is manifested by:
        1) QRS of 0.12 secs or more
        2) QRS which is positive in V_6 and negative in V_1
            a) Monophasic QRS or rsR' complex in V_6
            b) rS or QS in V_1
    c. RBBB is a unifascicular block and is manifested by:
        1) QRS of 0.12 secs or more
        2) QRS that is positive in V_1 and negative in V_6
            a) rSR' in V_1
            b) Wide terminal S wave in leads I and V_6
4. Chamber enlargement and/or hypertrophy
    a. Atrial enlargement is manifested by changes in the P wave; the two best P wave leads are lead II and lead V_1 (Fig. 3.43).
        1) In lead II: look for tall or wide P waves.
        2) In lead V_1 or MCL_1: the first half of the normally diphasic P wave represents the right atrium, and the second half of the normally diphasic P wave represents the left atrium; look for a more dominant initial or terminal phase of the diphasic P wave in V_1 or MCL_1.
        3) Right atrial enlargement is manifested by the following ECG changes:
            a) Tall (greater than 2.5 mm), peaked P wave in II (sometimes referred to as *P-pulmonale*)
            b) Larger initial phase of the diphasic P wave normally seen in V_1

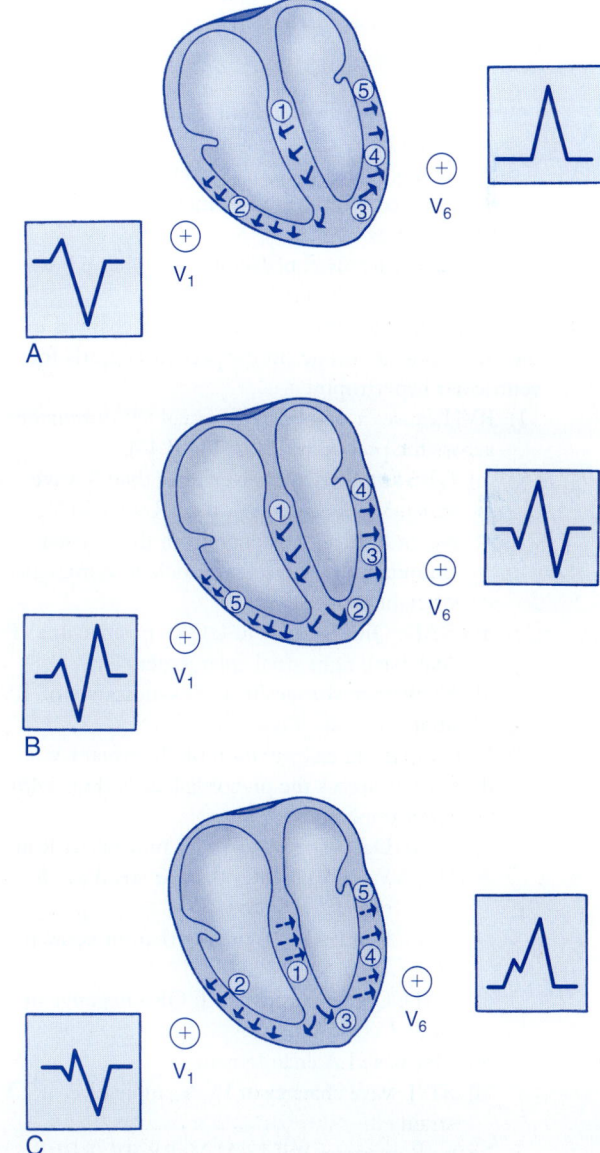

Fig. 3.42 A, Normal ventricular depolarization. **B,** Right bundle branch block. **C,** Left bundle branch block. (From Urden, L., Stacy, K., & Lough, M. [2018]. *Critical care nursing: Diagnosis and management* [8th ed.]. St. Louis: Mosby.)

Condition	P wave appearance		Mnemonic features
	Lead II	Lead V$_1$	
Normal sinus rhythm (NSR)	⋀	⋁ or ⋀⋁	• The P should be upright in lead II if there is sinus rhythm • The P may be upright, negative or biphasic in lead V$_1$ with sinus rhythm
RAE (=P Pulmonale)	⋀ 2.50		• **P**rominent (greater than or equal to 2.5 mm tall) **p**eaked P waves in the **p**ulmonary leads (II, III, and aVF)
LAE (=P Mitrale)	⋀⋀ 0.12	⋁ or ⋁▯	• **M**-shaped, widened (greater than or equal to 0.12 sec) P waves in one or more of the **m**itral leads (I, II, or aVL) • Deep, negative component to the P wave in lead V$_1$

Fig. 3.43 Atrial enlargement. *LAE*, Left atrial enlargement; *RAE*, right atrial enlargement. (From Grauer, K. [1998]. *A practical guide to ECG interpretation* [2nd ed.]. St. Louis: Mosby.)

4) Left atrial (LA) enlargement is manifested by the following ECG changes:
   a) Wide (greater than or equal to 0.12 sec), notched P wave in II (sometimes referred to as *P-mitrale*)
   b) Larger terminal phase of the biphasic P wave normally seen in V$_1$
b. Ventricular hypertrophy is manifested by changes in the QRS; look at changes in the precordial leads for ventricular hypertrophy.
   1) RVH causes a change in the usual LV dominance across the precordial leads (Fig. 3.44).
      a) QRS amplitude: R wave larger than S wave in V$_1$, V$_2$; S wave larger than R wave in V$_5$, V$_6$ (indicative of change from the normal dominance of the left ventricle to dominance of right ventricle)
      b) RAD: QRS negative in I; QRS positive in aVF
      c) May have right atrial enlargement
      d) ST-T wave changes in V$_1$, V$_2$ indicative of RV strain
   2) LVH causes an exaggeration of the usual LV dominance across the precordial leads (Fig. 3.45)
      a) QRS amplitude
         i) Deepest S in V$_1$ or V$_2$ plus tallest R in V$_5$ or V$_6$ greater than or equal to 35 mm
         ii) R in lead aVL greater than or equal to 12 mm
      b) LAD: QRS is positive in I; QRS negative in aVF
      c) May have LA enlargement
      d) ST-T wave changes in V$_5$, V$_6$ indicative of LV strain
   3) NOTE: Remember WiLLiaM MaRRoW (RBBB, 2010)
      a) In LBBB, there is a W in V1 and an M in V$_6$.
      b) In RBBB, there is an M in lead V1 and a W in lead V$_6$.

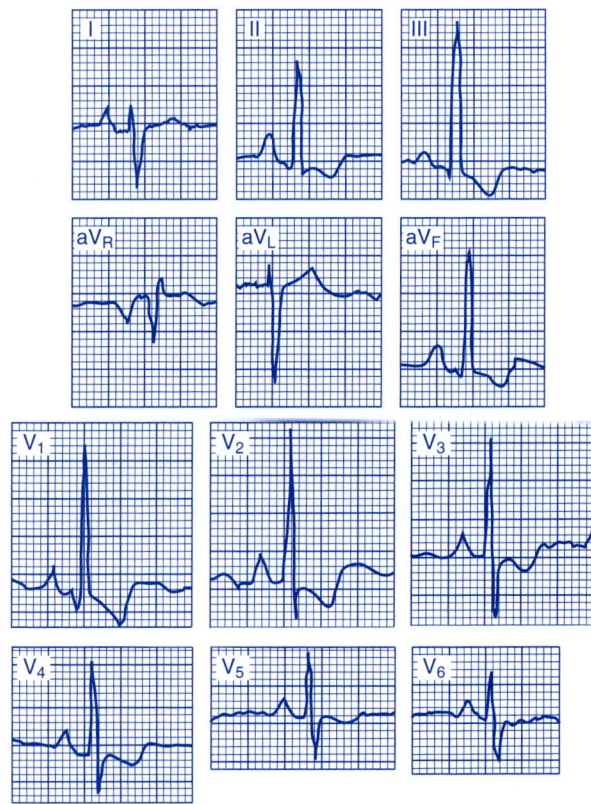

Fig. 3.44 Right ventricular hypertrophy with right atrial enlargement. Note tall, peaked P waves in lead II with dominant initial component of the P wave in V$_1$ as evidence of right atrial enlargement. Note dominant R wave in V$_1$ and reverse progression of the R wave across the precordium along with right axis deviation and right ventricular strain (ST-segment depression and asymmetrical T-wave inversion in V$_1$, V$_2$) as evidence of right ventricular hypertrophy. (From Conover, M. B. [2003]. *Understanding electrocardiography*. [8th ed.]. St. Louis: Mosby.)

5. Myocardial ischemia, injury, infarction
   a. ECG indicators (Fig. 3.46)
      1) Ischemia is manifested by T-wave changes; these are the earliest changes in the evolution of MI.

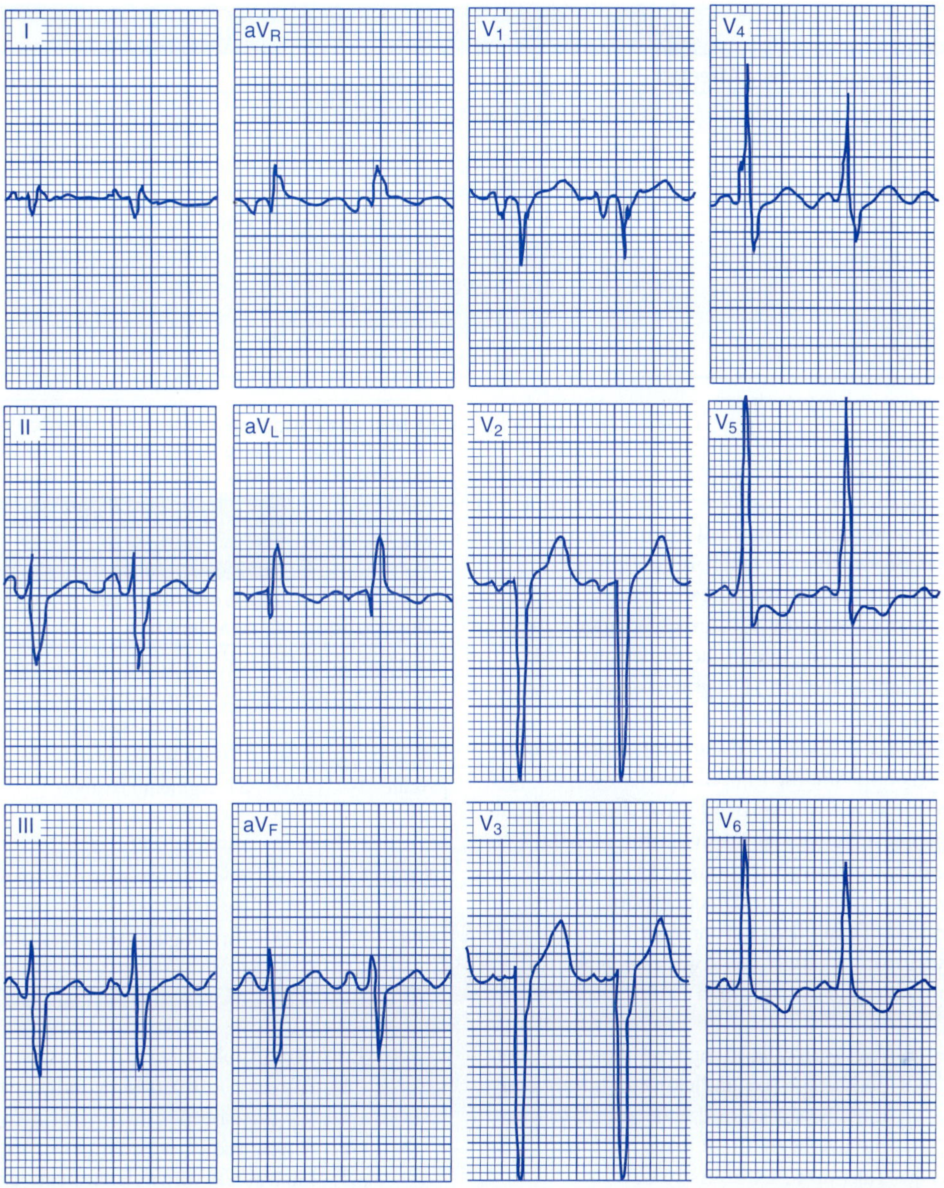

Fig. 3.45 Left ventricular hypertrophy with left atrial enlargement. Note wide, notched P waves in lead II with dominant terminal component of the P wave in V_1 as evidence of left atrial enlargement. Note deep S wave in V_2 and tall R wave in V_5 with left axis deviation and left ventricular strain (ST-segment depression and asymmetrical T-wave inversion in V_5, V_6) as evidence of left ventricular hypertrophy. (From Conover, M. B. [2003]. *Understanding electrocardiography* [8th ed.]. St. Louis: Mosby.)

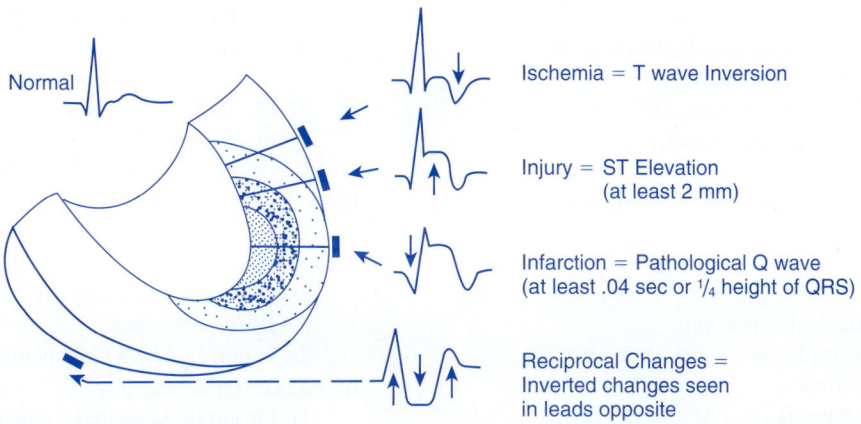

Fig. 3.46 Electrocardiogram indicators of ischemia, injury, infarction, and reciprocal changes. (From Harvey, M. [2000]. *Study guide to core curriculum for critical care nursing* [3rd ed.]. Philadelphia: Saunders.)

Table 3.11 Electrocardiogram Lead Correlation with Myocardial Infarction Locations*

Location	Coronary Artery Affected	Indicative Leads	Reciprocal Leads
Anterior	LAD	(V_2), V_3, V_4	V_7, V_8, V_9
Septal	LAD	V_1, V_2	$V5$, V_6
Anteroseptal	LAD	V_1, V_2, V_3, (V_4)	I, aVL
Lateral	LCA	I, aVL (high lateral), V_5, V_6 (low lateral)	II, III, aVF
Anterolateral	LCA	V_3, V_4, V_5, V_6, (I, aVL)	II, III, aVF
Inferior	RCA	II, III, aVF	I, aVL
RV	RCA	V_{4R}, V_{5R}, V_{6R} may be transient	I, aVL
Posterior	RCA and/or LCA	V_7, V_8, V_9 or reciprocal in V_1, V_2, V_3	V_1, V_2, V_3

*Changes may also be seen in leads in parentheses.
LAD, Left anterior descending coronary artery; *LCA*, left circumflex artery; *RCA*, right circumflex artery; *RV*, right ventricle.

   a) Indicative change: symmetrically inverted T waves in leads facing the ischemic area
   b) Reciprocal change: tall T waves in leads opposite the ischemic area
 2) Injury is manifested by ST-segment changes; these are intermediate changes in the evolution of MI.
   a) Indicative change: ST-segment elevation in leads facing the injured area
   b) Reciprocal change: ST-segment depression in leads opposite the injured area
 3) Infarction is manifested by Q wave changes; these are the latest changes in the evolution of MI.
   a) Indicative change: pathologic Q wave (0.04 second wide and/or 25% height of R wave) in leads facing the necrotic area
   b) Reciprocal change: tall R waves in leads opposite the necrotic area
   c) Q waves
     i) Are normal in many leads; to be pathologic (i.e., indicative of infarction) must be 0.4 second wide and 25% of the height of the R wave
     ii) Take up to 24 hours to develop
     iii) Relate to mass loss of myocardium
     iv) Prevented by successful reperfusion therapies (e.g., fibrinolytics, PCI)
 4) Some conditions may make ECG diagnosis of MI difficult by changing the morphology of the QRS, the ST segment, and/or the T waves; some examples include the following:
   a) Unstable angina (e.g., Wellens syndrome)
   b) Ventricular pacemakers
   c) LBBB: chance of acute MI is more likely if the following are present:
     i) New onset
     ii) ST segment depression of 1 mm in leads V_1, V_2
     iii) ST segment elevation of more than 5 mm
   d) Ventricular hypertrophy
   e) WPW syndrome
   f) Pericarditis
   g) Hypothermia
   h) Hemorrhagic stroke
   i) Electrolyte imbalances

Table 3.12 Determination of Age of Myocardial Infarction

Description	Electrocardiogram Characteristics	Time from Onset of Pain
Hyperacute	• ST-segment elevation • Tombstone-shaped T waves or T-wave inversion	Minutes to hours
Acute	• ST-segment elevation • T-wave inversion • Pathologic Q waves	Hours to days
Recent	• T wave inversion • Pathologic Q waves	Weeks to months
Old	• Pathologic Q waves	After several months

  b. Location (Table 3.11)
    1) Anterior left ventricle: indicative changes in V_3, V_4 (possibly V_2)
    2) Septal: indicative changes in V_1, V_2
    3) Lateral left ventricle: indicative changes in I, aVL and/or V_5, V_6
      a) I, aVL are considered high lateral leads
      b) V_5, V_6 are considered low lateral leads
    4) Inferior left ventricle: indicative changes in II, III, aVF
    5) Posterior left ventricle
      a) Reciprocal changes in V_1, V_2
      b) Indicative changes in V_7, V_8, or V_9
        i) V_8 and V_9 are the most significant.
    6) RV: indicative changes in V_{4R}, V_{5R}, V_{6R}; V_{4R} are the most significant.
  c. Determination of age of MI (Table 3.12)
6. ECG changes in angina
  a. Variant (also referred to as *Prinzmetal* or *vasospastic*) angina
    1) Angina at rest caused by spasm of the coronary artery or arteries
    2) Manifested by ST segment elevation with pain
  b. Wellens syndrome (Fig. 3.47)
    1) Group of signs that are associated with occlusion of proximal LAD artery and high risk of sudden cardiac death in a patient with unstable angina

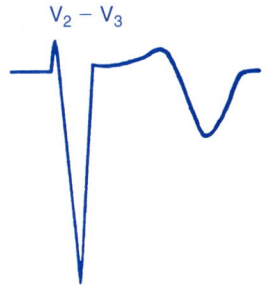

Fig. 3.47 Wellens syndrome. (From Conover, M. [2003]. *Understanding electrocardiography* [8th ed.] St. Louis: Mosby.)

     a) Symmetrical, deeply inverted T waves in V_2 and V_3 that persist even when the patient is pain free
     b) Little or no ST segment elevation
     c) Little or no enzyme elevation
     d) No development of Q waves or loss of precordial R waves
    2) Cardiac catheterization with PCI is indicated
7. ECG changes in pericarditis
  a. ST segment normal in V_1 and aVR, but all other leads show ST segment elevation
  b. Depression of PR interval in limb leads and left chest leads (V_5, V_6)
  c. Decrease in QRS voltage if pericardial effusion present
8. ECG changes in myocardial trauma (e.g., myocardial contusion)
  a. Nonspecific ST and T wave changes; infarction pattern if necrosis
  b. High risk of dysrhythmias and AV nodal blocks
9. ECG changes in hypothermia (seen when temperature less than 30°C)
  a. J wave (also referred to as an *Osborne wave*): rounded waves above the isoelectric line between the QRS complex and the early part of the ST segment; usually seen best in lead II and V leads
  b. ST segment elevation
  c. Prolonged intervals
10. ECG changes in hypothyroidism
  a. ST segment depression
  b. Prominent T waves with T wave inversion
  c. May have LVH

ST-Segment Monitoring

1. Continuous monitoring of ST segment for changes associated with ischemia because the ischemia may not cause chest pain (referred to as *silent* ischemia)
2. Indications
  a. Acute coronary syndrome
  b. MI
  c. After PCI: optional depending on clinical indications such as chest pain, dysrhythmias
  d. During and after cardiac surgery
  e. During and after noncardiac surgery in patients at risk of myocardial ischemia
3. Lead choice
  a. Choose a lead that best demonstrates ST changes during ischemia, evolving MI, or at the time of balloon occlusion at the time of PCI (referred to as the patient's *ischemic fingerprint*).
  b. If information regarding the ischemic fingerprint is not available, use lead III and V_3.
4. Note significant changes in the ST segment: ST segment elevation or depression of at least 1 mm for at least 60 seconds is considered significant.
  a. ST-segment elevation represents more severe, usually transmural, ischemia.
  b. ST-segment depression represents less severe, usually subendocardial, ischemia or reciprocal changes of ischemia.
  c. Other causes of ST-segment deviation include electrolyte imbalances, pericarditis, hypothermia, ventricular aneurysm, hypothyroidism, hyperventilation, pulmonary infarction, and drugs such as digoxin.

Hemodynamic Monitoring

General Information Regarding Hemodynamic Monitoring

1. Definition: monitoring of blood flow generally through the use of invasive catheters
2. Uses
  a. Measure hemodynamic pressures and record waveforms
    1) Arterial catheter: systemic arterial BP including systolic, diastolic, and mean
    2) CVP catheter: CVP measured as a mean
    3) PAC
     a) Allows measurement of the following:
      i) RAP measured as a mean
      ii) PAP, including systolic, diastolic, and mean
      iii) PAOP measured as a mean as an indirect reflection of LAP
      iv) CO usually measured by thermodilution technique
     b) Lumens of a typical PAC (Fig. 3.48)
      i) Proximal lumen opens in the right atrium and allows measurement of RAP and administration of infusions; this port is also used for bolus injections for the thermodilution measurement of CO.
      ii) Proximal infusion lumen: many catheters have another right atrial port to be used for central infusions.
      iii) Distal lumen: opens at the distal tip of the catheter; PAP is measured at this port with the balloon deflated, and PAOP is measured at this port with the balloon inflated
      iv) Balloon lumen: allows inflation of the balloon at the distal tip of the catheter for measurement of PAOP; a 1.5-ml capacity balloon is attached to the port and there is a gate-valve that can be opened and closed

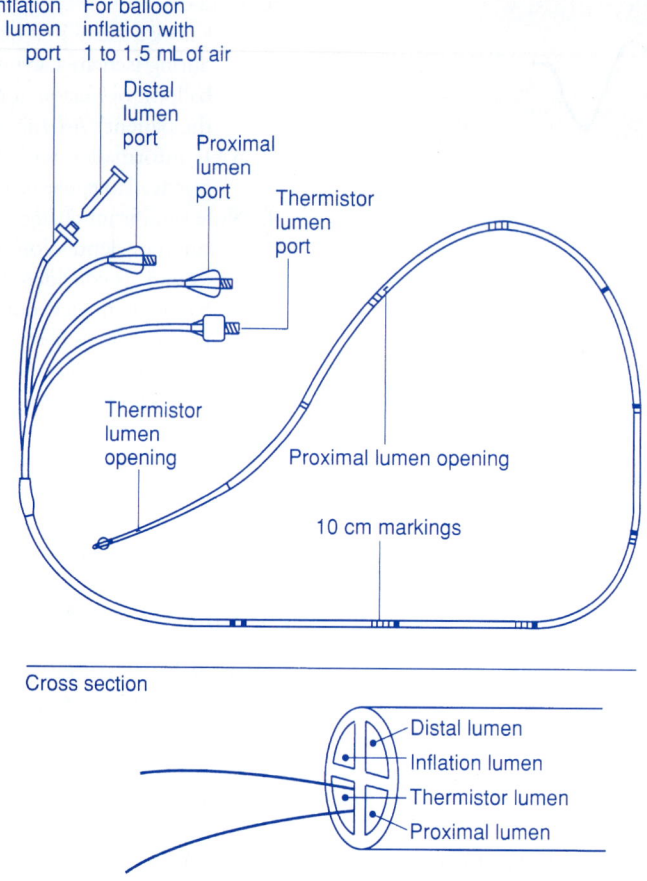

Fig. 3.48 Pulmonary artery catheter. (From Visalli, F., & Evans, P. [1981]. The Swan-Ganz catheter: A program for teaching safe effective use. *Nursing* 81[11],1.)

      v) Thermistor: located 4 cm proximal to the balloon, the thermistor measures core body temperature and temperature changes that occur with injectates during thermodilution CO measurements
      vi) There are black lines on the catheter every 10 cm; each thin line indicates 10 cm; a thick line indicates 50 cm.
    c) Specialized catheters also allow the evaluation of the following:
      i) Continuous CO (CCO)
      ii) SvO_2: oxygen saturation of mixed venous blood
      iii) $ScvO_2$: oxygen saturation of venous blood in the superior vena cava
      iv) REF: RV end-systolic volume, RV end-diastolic volume, RV SV, and RVEF
  b. Obtain blood samples.
    1) Arterial catheter
      a) Intermittent arterial samples for ABGs and serum arterial lactate
      b) Continuous intraarterial blood gas monitoring allows measurement of pH, PaO_2, and $PaCO_2$ through the use of fiberoptic and electrochemical sensors in an intraarterial catheter.
    2) Central venous catheter: venous
    3) Pulmonary artery catheter
      a) Right atrial (proximal port): venous
      b) Pulmonary artery (distal port): mixed venous
  c. Provide central venous access for administration of fluids or drugs.
    1) Central venous catheter: usually triple lumen
    2) PAC
      a) Right atrial (proximal) port
      b) Pulmonary artery (distal) port: saline flush solution to ensure patency; heparin may be added to flush solution (though still controversial), but this port should not be used for fluid or drug administration
      c) VIP (i.e., venous infusion port) catheters: provide an extra right atrial port
  d. Perform intracardiac pacing via specialized PAC
3. Common indications for hemodynamic monitoring
  a. Shock of any etiology
  b. MI especially with:
    1) Acute left or RVF
    2) Refractory pain
    3) Significant hypotension or hypertension
    4) RV infarction
    5) Mechanical complications (e.g., papillary muscle rupture, rupture of interventricular septum)
  c. High-risk surgical patient

d. Acute RVF (e.g., after PE)
e. Severe valvular disease
f. Cardiac tamponade
g. Pulmonary edema of uncertain etiology: used to differentiate between cardiac and noncardiac pulmonary edema
h. Pulmonary hypertension
i. Acute respiratory failure (e.g., acute respiratory distress syndrome [ARDS])
j. Need for evaluation of fluid status and guide fluid resuscitation (e.g., burns, multiple trauma, complex surgical procedures especially in patients with preexisting cardiopulmonary disease)
k. Need for evaluation of hemodynamic response to potent pharmacologic agents (e.g., hypertensive crisis treated with nitroprusside)
4. Relative contraindications of invasive hemodynamic monitoring
   a. Severe coagulopathy
   b. Severe pulmonary hypertension
   c. Presence of a prosthetic tricuspid or pulmonic valve
   d. Presence of an endocardial pacemaker
   e. Lack of trained physicians and nurses
5. Controversies regarding invasive hemodynamic monitoring
   a. It is unclear which patients actually benefit from invasive hemodynamic monitoring (i.e., benefits outweigh risks), but research efforts to link hemodynamic monitoring with improvement in outcomes continue.
   b. A retrospective observation study (i.e., no controls of confounding variables) showed an association between invasive monitoring and an increase in mortality (Connors et al., 1996).
      1) There was a 65% reduction in the use of PACs between 1993 and 2004 with a significant drop after this 1996 publication (Wiener & Welch, 2007).
   c. Some significant issues to consider include the following:
      1) There is an institutional and human tendency to "routinize" technology (Benner, 2003) such as invasive monitoring.
      2) Studies suggest that nurses' and physicians' knowledge regarding hemodynamic waveforms and data interpretation is limited.
      3) Interrater variability and lack of reproducibility continue to be problematic in evaluating values.
   d. Vincent et al. (2008) recommend that rather than abandoning invasive hemodynamic monitoring, the following should be ensured:
      1) Correct measurement
      2) Correct interpretation
      3) Correct application
6. Components of a pressure monitoring system (Fig. 3.49)
   a. Physiologic signal: intravascular pressure carried to the transducer by a catheter (inserted into the cardiovascular circuit) and fluid-filled tubing
      1) Static pressure is produced by the volume of blood in the vascular system at zero flow
      2) Dynamic pressure is produced by the heart; equal to flow × resistance
      3) Hydrostatic pressure is related to the density of the fluid, gravity, and the height of the column of blood between the heart and the vessels
         a) "Zeroing" the pressure monitoring system by leveling the air-fluid interface of the transducer at the phlebostatic axis (which correlates to the atrial level), turning the stopcock to open the system to air, and ensuring that the digital display and the graphic representation both indicate zero corrects for the hydrostatic gradient.
   b. Transducer: converts the mechanical signal to an electrical signal
   c. Monitor
      1) Amplifier: device that increases the magnitude of the electrical signal and filters out electrical interference
      2) Oscilloscope: device that displays the resultant signal as a pressure waveform and as a numerical value
      3) Recorder: device that records the pressure waveform on paper for analysis

Hemodynamic Parameters (Table 3.13)

1. Arterial and ventricular pressures measured as systolic/diastolic while atrial pressures measured as a mean
2. Systemic arterial BP
   a. Pressure in a systemic artery; reflects systemic arterial BP
   b. BP = CO × SVR; changes in BP are caused either by a change in CO or SVR.
   c. Measured by a catheter in a peripheral artery or the second lumen of an intraaortic balloon catheter (central aortic arterial line)
      1) Radial artery site is the preferred peripheral site because of collateral circulation provided by the ulnar artery.
         a) Allen test must be performed before any radial artery puncture to assess patency of radial-ulnar arch; this test is performed by compressing both the radial and ulnar artery to blanch the hand; when the ulnar artery is released, evaluate the time until return of color; if longer than 7 seconds, this radial artery should not be punctured (for ABGs or for radial artery cannulation).
      2) Neurovascular assessment of the limb distal to any arterial line is essential; thrombosis or embolization may cause acute arterial occlusion and loss of limb.
   d. Systolic arterial pressure: maximal pressure with which the blood is ejected from the left ventricle
   e. Diastolic arterial pressure: reflects the rapidity of flow of the ejected blood through the arterial system and the vessel's elasticity
      1) Diastolic pressure is expected to be higher (and pulse pressure to be narrowed) if there is endogenous catecholamine release or the patient is receiving sympathomimetic agents (e.g., epinephrine, dopamine, or norepinephrine).
      2) Diastolic pressure is expected to be lower (and pulse pressure to be widened) if there are excessive vasodilatory mediators (e.g., septic shock, anaphylactic shock).

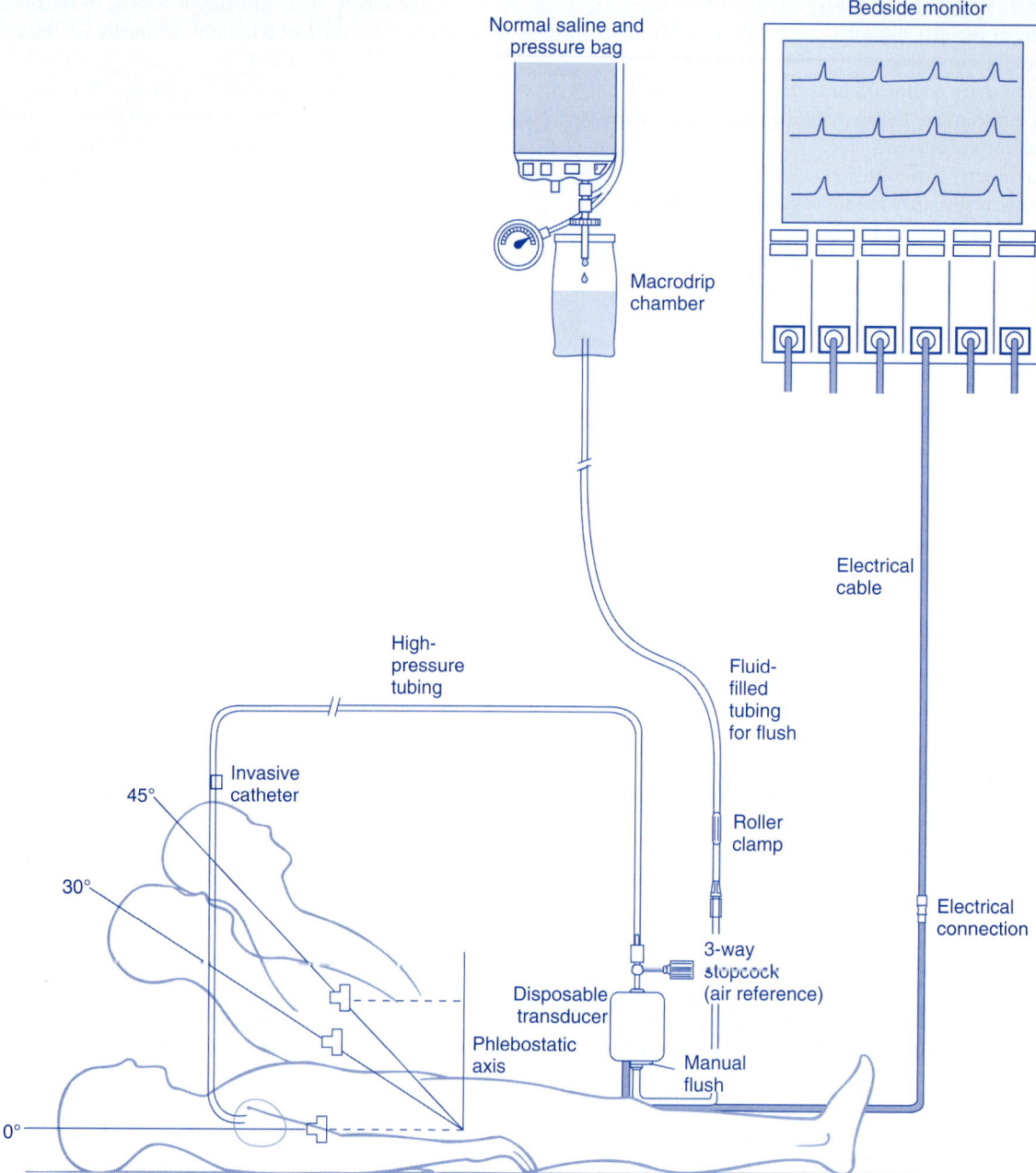

Fig. 3.49 Components of a pressure monitoring system. (From Urden, L., Stacy, K., & Lough, M. [2018]. *Critical care nursing: Diagnosis and management* [8th ed.]. St. Louis: Mosby.)

    f. MAP: average pressure occurring in the aorta and its major branches during the cardiac cycle; MAP of at least 60 mm Hg is necessary to perfuse the vital organs

    g. Normal pressure values
        1) Systolic: 90 to 140 mm Hg
        2) Diastolic: 60 to 90 mm Hg
        3) Mean: 70 to -105 mm Hg

    h. Causes of abnormal pressures (Table 3.14)
        1) Arterial catheter versus cuff pressures
            a) Arterial catheters are a direct measurement and therefore more accurate (assuming proper zeroing, leveling, and dynamic response), especially in shock states, severe hypertension, vasoconstriction, and obesity.

                i) Indirect BP measurements, including auscultation and oscillometric methods, tend to underestimate systolic pressure and overestimate diastolic pressure.
                ii) MAPs tend to be the same even in these situations and is a more consistent evaluation of perfusion pressure.
            b) Expect radial artery catheters to show a pressure slightly higher (~10 mm Hg) than brachial cuff measurement because the radial artery is smaller than the brachial artery.

Table 3.13 Hemodynamic Parameters, Methods of Measurement or Calculation, and Normal Values

Parameter	Method of Measurement or Calculation	Normal
Heart rate (HR)	Measured: Count rate at apex or number of R waves by ECG monitor	60–100 beats/min
Mean arterial pressure (MAP)	Calculated: [BP systolic + (BP diastolic × 2)] ÷ 3 Systolic and diastolic pressures can be obtained by direct (arterial line) or indirect (auscultated using a sphygmomanometer)	70–105 mm Hg (Normal systolic BP is 90–140 mm Hg; normal diastolic BP is 60–90 mm Hg)
Cardiac output (CO)	Measured: Usually by thermodilution technique	4–8 l/min
Cardiac index (CI)	Calculated: CO ÷ BSA	2.5–4 l/min/m^2
Stroke volume (SV)	Calculated: CO ÷ HR	60–120 ml/beat
Stroke index (SI)	Calculated: SV ÷ BSA	30–65 ml/m^2/beat
Central venous pressure (CVP)	Measured: At the tip of a catheter (frequently multilumen) in the superior vena cava; may be measured with a transducer or a water manometer	2–6 mm Hg (transducer) 3–8 cm H$_2$O (water manometer)
Right atrial pressure (RAP)	Measured: At the proximal port of the PAC; this port is located in the right atrium	2–6 mm Hg 3–8 cm H$_2$O
Pulmonary artery pressure (PAP)	Measured: At the distal port of the PAC with the balloon deflated; the tip is located in a pulmonary arteriole	Systolic (PAs): 15–30 mm Hg Diastolic (PAd): 5–15 mm Hg Mean (PAm): 10–20 mm Hg
Pulmonary artery occlusive pressure (PAOP)	Measured: At the distal port of the PAC with the balloon inflated; because right heart pressures are blocked by the inflated balloon, PAOP indirectly reflects left atrial pressure, LVEDP, and left ventricular preload	8–12 mm Hg (Note: Although 8–12 mm Hg is "normal," many patients require a higher pressure [as high as 15–20 mm Hg] to achieve optimal stretch on the myofibrils and optimal preload.)
Systemic vascular resistance (SVR)	Calculated: [(MAP − RAP) × 80] ÷ CO	800–1400 dynes/sec/cm^{-5}
Systemic vascular resistance index (SVRI)	Calculated: [(MAP − RAP) × 80] ÷ CI	2000–2400 dynes/sec/cm^{-5}/m^2
Pulmonary vascular resistance (PVR)	Calculated: [(PAm − PAOP) × 80] ÷ CO	100–250 dynes/sec/cm^{-5}
Pulmonary vascular resistance index (PVRI)	Calculated: [(PAm − PAOP) × 80] ÷ CI	225–315 dynes/sec/cm^{-5}/m^2
Left ventricular stroke work index (LVSWI)	Calculated: [SI × (MAP − PAOP)] × 0.0136	45–65 g•m/m^2
Right ventricular stroke work index (RVSWI)	Calculated: [SI × (PAm − RAP)] × 0.0136	5–12 g•m/m^2
Coronary artery perfusion pressure (CAPP)	Calculated: Diastolic BP|PAOP	60–80 mm Hg
Right ventricular end-diastolic volume (RVEDV)	Measured: By thermodilution method with REF PAC	100–160 ml
Right ventricular end-diastolic volume index (RVEDVI)	Calculated: RVEDV ÷ BSA	60–100 ml/m^2
Right ventricular end-systolic volume (RVESV)	Measured: By thermodilution method with REF PAC	50–100 ml
Right ventricular end-systolic volume index (RVESVI)	Calculated: RVESV ÷ BSA	30–60 ml/m^2

Continued

Table 3.13 Hemodynamic Parameters, Methods of Measurement or Calculation, and Normal Values—cont'd

Parameter	Method of Measurement or Calculation	Normal
Right ventricular ejection fraction (REF)	Measured: By thermodilution method with REF PAC	40%–60%
Arterial oxygen saturation (SaO_2)	Measured: By pulse oximetry or by arterial blood gas analysis	95%–100%
Mixed venous oxygen saturation (SvO_2)	Measured: By SvO_2 port of a fiberoptic oximetric PAC or by mixed venous blood gas analysis	60%–80%
Central venous oxygen saturation ($ScvO_2$)	Measured: By fiberoptic oximetric central venous catheter or by venous blood gas analysis	65%–85%
Arterial oxygen content (CaO_2)	Calculated: $1.34 \times Hgb \times SaO_2$	18–20 ml/dl
Venous oxygen content (CvO_2)	Calculated: $1.34 \times Hgb \times SvO_2$	12–16 ml/dl
Oxygen delivery (DO_2)	Calculated: $CO \times CaO_2 \times 10$	900–1100 ml/min
Oxygen delivery index (DO_2I)	Calculated: $CI \times CaO_2 \times 10$	550–650 ml/min/m²
Oxygen consumption (VO_2)	Calculated: $CO \times Hgb \times 13.4 \times (SaO_2 - SvO_2)$	200–300 ml/min
Oxygen consumption index (VO_2I)	Calculated: $CI \times Hgb \times 13.4 \times (SaO_2 - SvO_2)$	110–160 ml/min/m²
Oxygen extraction ratio (O_2ER)	Calculated: $CaO_2 - CvO_2/CaO_2$	22%–30%
Oxygen extraction index (O_2EI)	Calculated: $SaO_2 - SvO_2/SaO_2$	20%–27%

BP, Blood pressure; *BSA*, body surface area; *CI*, cardiac index; *CO*, cardiac output; *ECG*, electrocardiogram; *LVEDP*, left ventricular end-diastolic pressure; *PAC*, pulmonary artery catheter; *PAd*, pulmonary artery diastolic pressure; *PAm*, pulmonary artery mean pressure; *PAs*, pulmonary artery systolic pressure *RAP*, right atrial pressure.

Table 3.14 Causes of Abnormal Hemodynamic Pressures

Parameter	Increased	Decreased
Systemic arterial blood pressure Normals: • Systolic: 90–140 mm Hg • Diastolic: 60–90 mm Hg • Mean: 70–105 mm Hg	• Increase in systemic vascular resistance (e.g., hypertension, SNS innervation) • Increase in CO (e.g., hyperthyroidism)	• Decrease in systemic vascular resistance (e.g., sepsis, anaphylaxis) • Decrease in CI (e.g., MI, tachydysrhythmias)

Right atrial pressure (RAP)
Normals:
• 2–6 mm Hg mean
• 3–8 cm H_2O
	• Hypervolemia
	• Tricuspid valve dysfunction: stenosis or regurgitation
	• Right ventricular failure or infarction
	• VSD with left-to-right shunt
	• Pulmonic stenosis
	• Pulmonary hypertension
	  • Active: hypoxemic pulmonary vasoconstriction (PaO_2 <60 mm Hg)
	    • PE
	    • COPD
	    • ARDS
	  • Passive: mitral valve dysfunction (stenosis or regurgitation)
	• Positive-pressure ventilation
	• Constrictive pericarditis
	• Cardiac tamponade
	• Mitral valve dysfunction: stenosis or regurgitation
	• Chronic left ventricular failure (RAP would be a late indication of LVF)
		• Hypovolemia
		• Vasodilation
		  • Venous vasodilators (e.g., nitroglycerin, morphine)
		  • Endogenous systemic vasodilation (e.g., septic shock, anaphylactic shock, neurogenic shock)

Table 3.14	Causes of Abnormal Hemodynamic Pressures—cont'd	
Parameter	Increased	Decreased
Right ventricular pressure Normals: • Systolic: 15–30 mm Hg • End-diastolic: 0–8 mm Hg	• Right ventricular failure or infarction • VSD with left-to-right shunt • Pulmonary hypertension • Mitral valve dysfunction: stenosis or regurgitation • Constrictive pericarditis • Cardiac tamponade • Chronic LVF	• Hypovolemia • Excessive vasodilation (e.g., vasodilators, septic shock, anaphylactic shock, neurogenic shock)
Pulmonary artery pressure (PAP) Normals: • Systolic: 15–30 mm Hg • Diastolic: 5–15 mm Hg • Mean: 10–20 mm Hg	• Hypervolemia • VSD with left-to-right shunt • Pulmonary hypertension • Positive-pressure ventilation • Mitral valve dysfunction: stenosis or regurgitation • Constrictive pericarditis • Cardiac tamponade • Left ventricular failure	• Hypovolemia • Excessive vasodilation (e.g., vasodilators, septic shock, anaphylactic shock, neurogenic shock)
Pulmonary artery occlusive pressure (PAOP) Normal: • 8–12 mm Hg	• Positive-pressure ventilation especially with PEEP • Hypervolemia • Mitral valve dysfunction: stenosis or regurgitation • Constrictive pericarditis • Cardiac tamponade • Left ventricular failure • Severe aortic stenosis	• Hypovolemia • Excessive vasodilation (e.g., vasodilators, septic shock, anaphylactic shock, neurogenic shock)
Cardiac output and cardiac index Normals: • CO: 4–8 l/min • CI: 2.5–4 l/min	• SNS innervation (endogenous catecholamines) (e.g., stress, exercise) • Exogenous catecholamines (e.g., epinephrine, isoproterenol, dobutamine, dopamine) • Other positive inotropes (e.g., digitalis, amrinone) • Infection, early sepsis • Hyperthyroidism • Anemia	• Decreased contractility (e.g., MI, cardiomyopathy, beta-blockers) • Increased afterload (e.g., systemic or pulmonary hypertension, aortic or pulmonic stenosis, polycythemia) • Alteration in preload: excessively increased (e.g., hypervolemia, HF) or decreased (e.g., hypovolemia, cardiac tamponade, mitral or tricuspid valve disease) • Significantly increased or decreased heart rate (e.g., bradydysrhythmias, tachydysrhythmias)

SvO_2
Normal: 60%–80%
$ScvO_2$
Normal: 70%–80%
	• Increased oxygen supply and delivery
	  • Increased SaO_2 (e.g., increased FiO_2, CPAP, or PEEP)
	  • Increase in CO or IA (inotropes, IABP, ventricular assist device, decrease in excessive afterload, hyperdynamic [i.e., early] stage of septic shock)
	  • Increased hemoglobin (e.g., blood administration)
	• Decreased oxygen demand
	  • Anesthesia, analgesics, or both
	  • Muscle paralysis or sedation
	  • Hypothermia
	  • Sleep
	  • Hypothyroidism
	  • Beta-blockers
	• Decreased oxygen extraction at tissue level
	  • Early sepsis
	  • Cyanide toxicity
	• Shift of oxyhemoglobin dissociation curve to the left (e.g., alkalosis, hypothermia, decreased levels of 2,3-DPG)
	• Technical problems
	  • PAC in occluded position
	  • Deposits of fibrin on the tip of the catheter
		• Decreased oxygen supply and delivery
		  • Decrease in SaO_2 (e.g., decreased FiO_2, CPAP, or PEEP, suctioning, acute respiratory failure, pulmonary edema)
		  • Decrease in CO or CI (e.g., shock, HF, hypovolemia, dysrhythmias, excessive CPAP or PEEP, negative inotropes, excessive afterload)
		  • Decrease in Hgb (e.g., anemia, hemorrhage) or abnormal hemoglobin (e.g., methemoglobinemia, sickle cell anemia)
		• Increased metabolic needs (e.g., seizures, shivering, restlessness, pain, hyperthermia, increased work of breathing, increased metabolic rate, exertion [e.g., turning, bathing, active range of motion])
		• Increased oxygen extraction at tissue level (e.g., early sepsis)
		• Shift of oxyhemoglobin dissociation curve to the right (e.g., acidosis, hyperthermia)

ARDS, Acute respiratory distress syndrome; *CI*, cardiac output; *CO*, cardiac output; *COPD*, chronic obstructive pulmonary disease; *CPAP*, continuous positive airway pressure, *FiO₂*, fraction of inspired oxygen; *HF*, heart failure; *Hgb*, hemoglobin; *IABP*, intraaortic balloon pump; *LVF*, left ventricular failure; *MI*, myocardial infarction; *PAC*, pulmonary artery catheter; *PE*, pulmonary embolism; *PEEP*, positive end-expiratory pressure; *RAP*, right atrial pressure; *SaO₂*, arterial oxygen saturation; *SNS*, sympathetic nervous system; *2,3-DPG*, 2,3-diphosphoglycerate; *VSD*, ventricular septal defect.

c) If there is a significant variation between pressure measured by arterial catheter and pressure auscultated using a sphygmomanometer other than in the situations listed earlier, do the following:
   i) Check the pressure monitoring system for air bubbles, occlusions, and positioning of catheter against wall of artery.
   ii) Ensure that the air-fluid interface of the transducer is level with the phlebostatic axis.
   iii) Ensure adequate damping of the pressure monitoring system.
   i. Normal waveform (Fig. 3.24)
3. RAP
   a. Pressure in the right atrium
   b. Reflects venous return to right heart; also, reflects RV end-diastolic pressure and preload as long as RV compliance and tricuspid valve function are normal
   c. Measured through catheter in superior vena cava (central venous catheter [i.e., CVP]) or at the proximal port of PAC (i.e., RAP)
      1) Insertion of a CVP catheter or PAC
         a) Preceded by insertion of a venous introducer into the internal jugular, subclavian, or femoral vein; the right internal jugular vein is the preferred site because the risk of pneumothorax is reduced by the use of the internal jugular vein
         b) The catheter is then threaded through the introducer into place with the CVP catheter tip in the superior vena cava and the PAC tip in a pulmonary arteriole in the dependent area (West zone 3), although the RAP is measured from the proximal port, which is in the right atrium.
      2) Although these parameters (CVP and RAP) are not actually the same, they are the same in practicality and are frequently used interchangeably.
      3) CVP may be measured by a water manometer in cm H_2O pressure or by a transducer in mm Hg pressure.
      4) RAP from the proximal port of the PAC is generally measured by a transducer in mm Hg.
      5) To convert values, remember that 1 mm Hg is equal to 1.36 cm H_2O.
   d. Normal pressure value: 2 to 6 mm Hg mean (or 3–8 cm H_2O)
   e. Causes of abnormal pressures (Table 3.14)
   f. Normal waveform (Fig. 3.50)
4. RV pressure
   a. Pressure in the right ventricle
   b. Measured only during insertion of the PAC as the distal tip of the PAC is floated through the right ventricle
   c. Normal pressure values
      1) Systolic: 15 to 30 mm Hg
      2) End-diastolic: 0 to 8 mm Hg
   d. Causes of abnormal pressures (Table 3.14)
   e. Normal waveform (Fig. 3.51)
5. PAP (Box 3.2)
   a. Pressure in the pulmonary artery with the balloon *deflated*
   b. Measured from the distal tip of the PAC with the balloon *deflated*
      1) PA systolic pressure (PAs): pressure in the pulmonary artery during RV systole
      2) PA end-diastolic pressure (PAd): pressure in the pulmonary artery at the end of RV diastole; reflects LAP in the absence of pulmonary disease and left ventricular end-diastolic pressure (LVEDP) in the absence of pulmonary disease and mitral valve dysfunction
   c. Normal pressure values
      1) Systolic: 15 to 30 mm Hg
      2) Diastolic: 5 to 15 mm Hg
      3) Mean: 10 to 20 mm Hg
   d. Causes of abnormal pressures (Table 3.14)
   e. Correlation between PAd and PAOP
      1) PAd is normally 2 to 4 mm Hg greater than PAOP
      2) PAd 5 mm Hg or more greater than PAOP can be caused by any of the following:
         a) Tachycardias greater than 125 beats/min
         b) Pulmonary hypertension
            i) Active: hypoxemic pulmonary vasoconstriction with PaO_2 less than 60 mm Hg (e.g., ARDS, COPD, PE)
            ii) Passive: mitral valve dysfunction (stenosis or regurgitation)

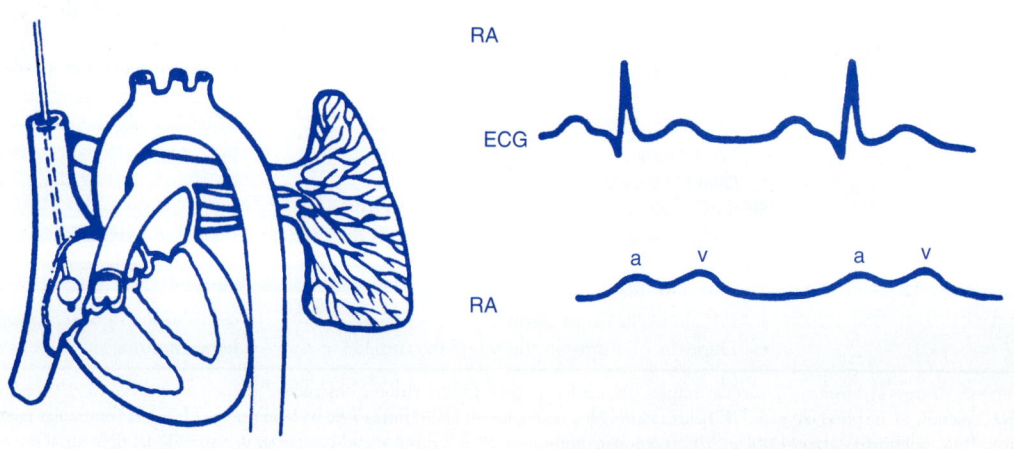

Fig. 3.50 Right atrial waveform. (Courtesy of Baxter Healthcare, Irvine, CA.)

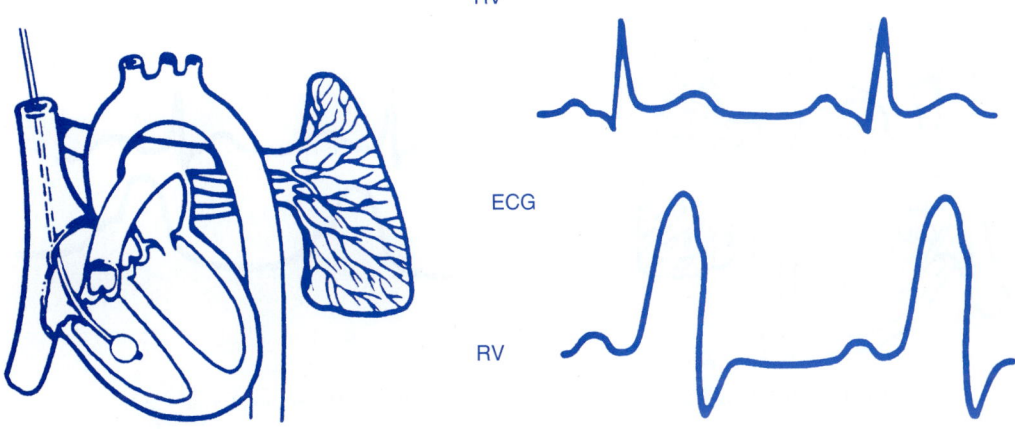

Fig. 3.51 Right ventricular waveform. (Courtesy of Baxter Healthcare, Irvine, CA.)

> **Box 3.2 Hemodynamic Parameters' Reflection of Cardiac Status***
>
> RAP = right heart
> PAd = pulmonary vascular bed
> PAOP = left heart

* One of the ways to remember causes of abnormal pressures is to consider that pressure behind the problem will be increased, while pressure in front of the problem will be decreased. For example, in massive pulmonary embolism and acute cor pulmonary, the pulmonary artery occlusive pressure (PAOP) would be decreased (in front of the problem), and the pulmonary artery diastolic pressure (PAd) and right atrial pressure (RAP) will be increased (behind the problem).

    3) The difference between the PAd and the PAOP is sometimes referred to as the *R-to-L gradient* and is most helpful in differentiating cardiogenic from noncardiogenic (e.g., ARDS) pulmonary edema.
        a) If the PAd is elevated but the PAOP is normal (R-to-L gradient of greater than 5 mm Hg): this is an indication of pulmonary hypertension, and pulmonary edema is noncardiogenic pulmonary edema caused by an increase in alveolocapillary membrane permeability with leaking of fluid into the pulmonary interstitium and alveolus.
        b) If the PAd and the PAOP are both elevated (R-to-L gradient 5 mm Hg or less): this is an indication of cardiogenic pulmonary edema caused by an increase in the pulmonary capillary hypostatic pressure pushing fluid into the pulmonary interstitium and alveolus.
  f. Normal waveform (Fig. 3.52)
  g. Changes in waveform (Table 3.15)
    1) Fling (also referred to as *whip*) (Fig. 3.53)
    2) Damped (Fig. 3.54)
6. PAOP (also referred to as *PCWP* or *PAWP*)
  a. Pressure in the pulmonary artery with the balloon inflated; reflects pressure from the left atrium in the absence of pulmonary hypertension
  b. Measured from the distal tip of the PAC with the balloon inflated; the balloon blocks right heart pressures from the distal tip; LAP reflects LV end-diastolic pressure and LV preload in the absence of mitral valve disease or LA tumor
  c. Normal pressure value: 8 to 12 mm Hg (measured as a mean); remember that some patients require a PAOP as high as 15 to 20 mm Hg for optimal preload
  d. Causes of abnormal pressures (Table 3.14)
  e. Normal waveform (Fig. 3.55)
    1) The *a* wave correlates with atrial contraction: it is the first wave seen after the QRS using dual channel recording.
    2) The *v* wave correlates with ventricular contraction: it is the first wave after the T wave using dual channel recording.
  f. Changes in waveform (Table 3.15)
    1) Large *a* waves
    2) Large *v* waves
    3) Large *a* waves and large *v* waves
  g. PAOP greater than PAd caused by any of the following:
    1) PAd artificially low or PAOP artificially high
    2) Mitral regurgitation with mean of PAOP used rather than the *a* wave amplitude (because mitral regurgitation causes large *v* waves on the PAOP waveform, it increases the PAOP if the mean is used; use the mean of the *a* wave measurement when there are large *v* waves) (Fig. 3.56)
    3) Forceful atrial contraction
7. LAP
  a. Pressure in the left atrium; reflects LV end-diastolic pressure and LV preload in the absence of mitral valve disease or LA tumor
  b. Measured by a catheter placed directly in the left atrium, usually placed during cardiac surgery
  c. A PAC usually used to measure PAOP as an indirect reflection of LAP because of the risk of complications related to direct LA catheter (e.g., air embolism, cardiac tamponade)
  d. Normals, waveforms, etc., as for PAOP

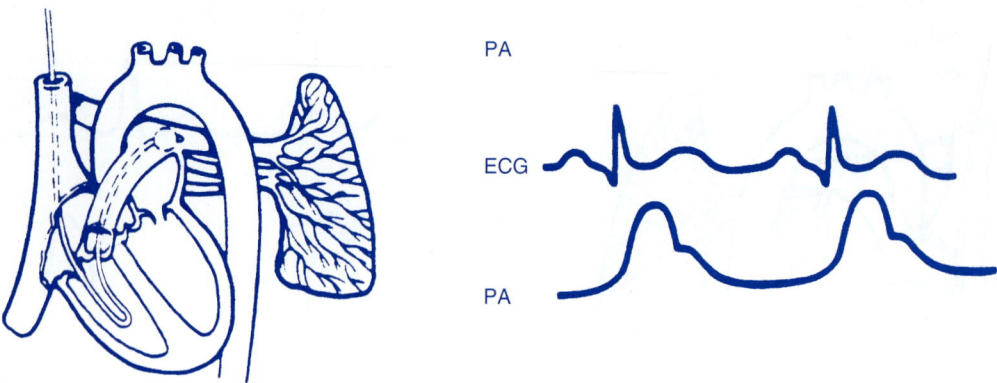

Fig. 3.52 Pulmonary artery waveform. (Courtesy of Baxter Healthcare, Irvine, CA.)

Table 3.15 Hemodynamic Waveform Abnormalities

Abnormality	Cause	Implications and Treatment
Pulmonary Artery		

Fling (or whip) (Fig. 3.53)	• Excessive catheter length in RA or RV
	• Catheter tip is located near the pulmonic valve
		• Turn patient to left side to see if catheter will float out into PA.
		• Monitor closely for indications that the catheter has flipped back into RV.
		  • Loss of dicrotic notch characteristic of an arterial waveform
		  • Decrease in diastolic pressure to close to 0 mm Hg
		  • Ventricular ectopy: PVCs, possible ventricular tachycardia
		• Inflate balloon to increase the chance that it will float distally back into position.
		• Catheter needs to be repositioned distally for fling or if catheter is in RV.

Damped (Fig. 3.54)	• Air bubbles within the pressure monitoring system • Catheter occlusion (e.g., fibrin at the tip of the catheter or catheter tip against the wall of the vessel) • Spontaneous occluded position	• Check the system for bubbles or blood; check that stopcocks are all positioned correctly and that stopcocks are covered with dead-end stopcock port covers (no holes). • Try to aspirate the catheter; DO NOT FLUSH because catheter may be in wedge position; if a clot is aspirated, discard and flush catheter. • If still damped, ask patient to take deep breaths, cough, and turn to side; if still in spontaneous occluded position, catheter needs to be repositioned proximally.
Pulmonary Artery Occlusive Pressure (PAOP) Waveform		
Large *a* waves	• Mitral stenosis • Severe aortic stenosis • Hypertension • AV block with AV asynchrony	

Large *v* waves	• Mitral regurgitation
	• VSD
		• NOTE: In patients with large V waves:
		  • The mean PAOP may be higher than PAd; do not use mean as the pressure value for PAOP.
		  • Use the measurement of the *a* wave for the pressure value for PAOP because the mitral valve is open during the *a* wave (atrial contraction), and this value has better correlation with LVEDP.

Large *a* and *v* waves (looks like M)	• Cardiac tamponade • Constrictive pericarditis • Hypervolemia • LVF	

AV, Atrioventricular; *LVEDP*, left ventricular end-diastolic pressure; *LVF*, left ventricular failure; *PA*, pulmonary artery; *PAd*, pulmonary artery diastolic pressure; *PVC*, premature ventricular contraction; *RA*, right atrium; *RV*, right ventricle; *VSD*, ventricular septal defect.

8. CO
   a. Amount of blood ejected by the ventricle each minute
   b. Invasive method using a PAC and thermodilution technique
      1) Intermittent: method
         a) Injection of a known volume of a known temperature solution into an unknown volume of blood at a known temperature
         b) The injectate solution (usually normal saline) is injected into the proximal lumen (RA) of the PAC.
         c) There is mixing of the injectate with the blood.
         d) The temperature change is sensed downstream at the thermistor located 4 cm from the distal tip of the PAC.
         e) The amount of the unknown volume of blood is deduced from the amount of change in temperature.
         f) Calculate the average of three measurements that are within 10% of a median value.

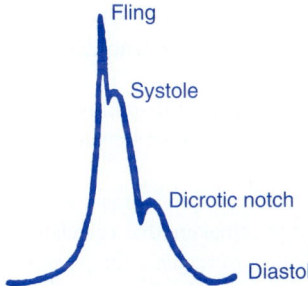

Fig. 3.53 Pulmonary artery waveform: catheter fling (or whip).

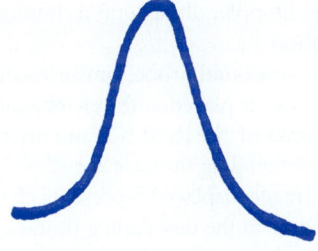

Fig. 3.54 Pulmonary artery waveform: damped waveform.

2) Continuous (referred to as *continuous cardiac output* [CCO])
   a) Method
      i) A thermal filament in the right ventricle creates a signal by warming the blood as it flows by
      ii) The thermistor at the distal tip measures the temperature of the blood downstream.
      iii) The computer produces a thermodilution curve and calculates the CO.
      iv) The CO is updated approximately every 5 minutes.
   b) Advantages over intermittent method
      i) More accurate especially in patients with low output states
      ii) Continuously updated
      iii) Decreases required nursing time
      iv) Eliminates interrater reliability caused by variability in injectate volume, rate of injection, and selection or elimination of values for averaging
      v) Reduces risks of contamination and fluid overload
   c) Disadvantage: catheter approximately three times the cost of conventional catheter
c. Minimally invasive methods
   1) Pulse contour waveform analysis method allows derivation of CO, SV, and stroke volume variability (SVV) from analysis of the arterial waveform.
   2) Method: requires a venous catheter and an arterial catheter
      a) Lithium dilution CO (PulseCO by LiDCO): requires calibration using a subtherapeutic dose of lithium to be injected into the venous catheter which is measured at the arterial sensor
         i) Requires recalibration every 4 to 8 hours
         ii) Cannot be used in patients on therapeutic lithium

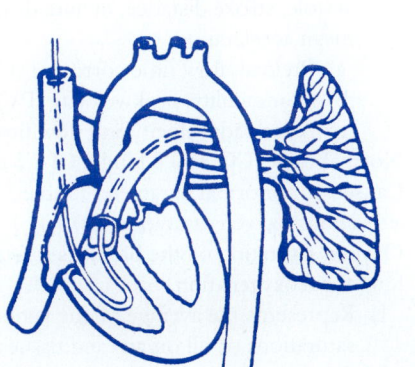 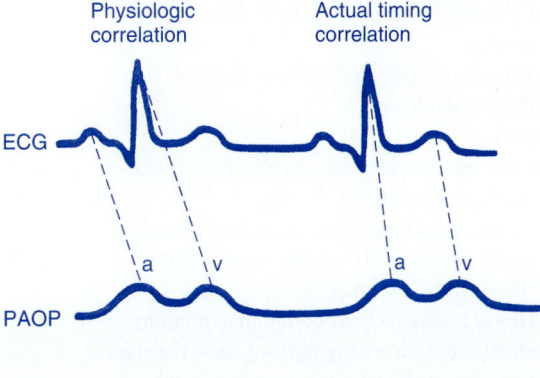

Fig. 3.55 Pulmonary artery occlusive pressure waveform. Although the *a* wave correlates physiologically to atrial depolarization and the P wave and the *v* wave correlate physiologically with the QRS and ventricular depolarization, tubing and catheter cause a time delay. In actuality, the first wave seen after the QRS is the *a* wave, and the first wave seen after the T wave is the *v* wave. (Adapted from and courtesy Baxter Healthcare, Irvine, CA.)

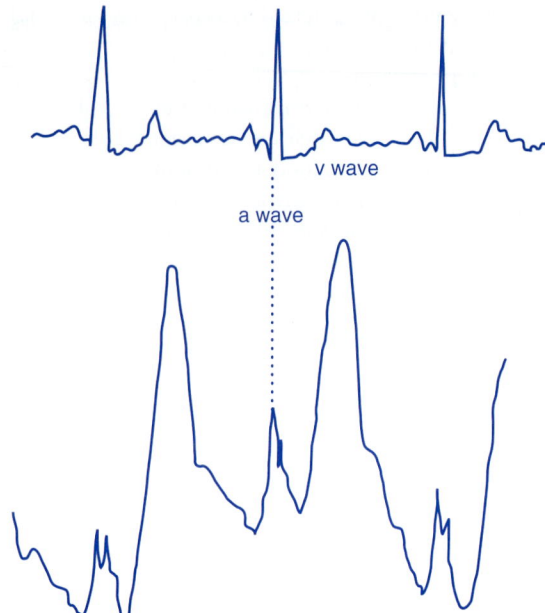

Fig. 3.56 Pulmonary artery occlusive pressure (PAOP) waveform of a patient with mitral regurgitation. Note the very large *v* waves. Use of the mean of the PAOP waveform or the *v* wave will result in an exaggerated PAOP. Because the mitral valve is open during the *a* wave, the mean of the *a* wave is a better reflection of the left ventricular end-diastolic pressure. (From Druding, M. C. [2000]. Integrating hemodynamic monitoring and physical assessment. *Dimens Crit Care Nurs*, 19[4], 25-30.)

- b) Pulse contour CO system (PiCCO by Pulsion Medical Systems) requires calibration using cold saline injected into the venous catheter, which is measured at the arterial sensor
  - i) Requires recalibration every 4 to 8 hours
  - ii) Requires femoral or axillary arterial cannulation
- c) Vigileo (Edwards Lifesciences) uses a specialized (i.e., Flotrac) sensor added to the arterial pressure monitoring system
  - i) Does not require calibration
  - ii) Provides CO, SV, SVV, and SVR
- d. Noninvasive measurement by bioimpedance
  1) Uses thoracic electrical bioimpedance technology
     a) Impedance (Z): resistance to flow of electrical current
  2) Method
     a) Four dual sensors are placed on each side of the neck and thorax.
     b) A low-amplitude, high-frequency electrical signal is emitted from the outer sensors through the thorax.
     c) Blood is an excellent conductive medium, and electricity follows the path of least resistance; the aorta is the largest, most distensible, blood-filled vessel in the thoracic cavity.
     d) Aortic blood flow is readily tracked by this method.
  3) Allows continuous measurement of the following parameters
     a) Composite parameters
        i) CO
        ii) CI
        iii) SV
     b) Thoracic fluid status: base thoracic impedance (Zo): normal 20 to 30 ohms for males and 25 to 35 for females
     c) Afterload: SVR: normal 800 to 1200 dynes/sec/cm^{-5}
     d) Contractility
        i) Change in impedance over time (dZ/dt): normal 0.8 to 2.5 ohms/second
        ii) Acceleration contractility index (ACI): normal 2 to 5 ohms/second
        iii) Left cardiac work index (LCWI): normal 3 to 5 kg/min/m^2
        iv) Preejection period: normal 0.05 to 0.12 sec
        v) Ventricular ejection time: normal 0.25 to 0.35 second
     e) Change in impedance/change in time (dZ/dt)
  4) Causes no risk or discomfort to the patient, but the patient must be supine, recumbent, and quiet
  5) Contraindicated in patients with impedance-driven pacemakers that calculate minute ventilation to regulate the pacemaker rate because the impedance current may cause the pacemaker rate to accelerate
- e. Noninvasive measurement by transesophageal Doppler
  1) Uses Doppler ultrasound technology
  2) Method
     a) Ultrasound probe, similar to an orogastric tube, is placed in the esophagus to the level of the third ICS and oriented to the descending thoracic aorta.
     b) Image displayed represents changes in blood flow in the descending thoracic aorta with each systolic cycle.
  3) Allows measurement or calculation of CO and index, SV and index, SVR and SVRI, flow time corrected for HR, peak velocity of blood during systole, stroke distance, minute distance, and mean acceleration
     a) Preload: flow time corrected (FTc)
     b) Contractility: peak velocity (PV)
     c) Afterload: velocity and flow time
- f. Normal value: CO 4 to 8 l/min; CI 2.5 to 4 l/min
- g. Causes of abnormal parameter (Table 3.14)

9. Mixed venous oxygen saturation (SvO$_2$)
   a. Oxygen saturation of the blood as it returns to the lung for reoxygenation
      1) Represents the average of the venous oxygen saturations of all organs and tissues
      2) Provides a global perspective of how well the body's demand for oxygen is met by the amount of oxygen supplied

b. Measurement
   1) Blood gas analysis of blood drawn from the distal lumen of the PAC
   2) Fiberoptic oximetric PAC
      a) Perform calibration as indicated.
         i) In vitro before the catheter is inserted
         ii) In vivo every 24 hours
      b) Monitor the signal quality indicator to ensure reliability.
      c) Note that accuracy may be affected by Hct, catheter position, blood temperature, or pH.
c. Normal SvO_2: 60% to 80%
   1) Affected by changes in DO_2 and/or VO_2
d. Causes of abnormal parameter (Table 3.14)

10. Central venous oxygen saturation ($ScvO_2$)
    a. Oxygen saturation of the blood in the superior vena cava
       1) Serves as a surrogate for SvO_2 before PAC inserted or when PAC placement is not possible such as when admission to a critical care unit is not possible or not yet necessary
       2) Although the $ScvO_2$ consistently overestimates the SvO_2 (by around 5%–15%) under shock conditions, there is a close correlation between the two parameters.
    b. Measurement
       1) Blood gas analysis of blood drawn from a catheter in the superior vena cava or right atrium
       2) Fiberoptic oximetric central venous catheter (e.g., Edwards PreSep) inserted into the jugular or subclavian vein with the tip in the superior vena cava or right atrium
          a) Femoral vein placement is not recommended; Davison et al (2010) found that more than 50% of values from a femoral catheter diverged more than 5% from $ScvO_2$ values.
    c. Normal $ScvO_2$: greater than 70%
       1) Affected by changes in DO_2 and/or VO_2
    d. Causes of abnormal parameter as for SvO_2

11. RV parameters
    a. Measured with special REF PAC
    b. Normal values for RV parameters (Table 3.14)

12. Oxygenation parameters
    a. Calculated parameters
    b. Normal values for oxygenation parameters (Table 3.14)

13. Gastric tonometry
    a. Detects regional alterations in tissue perfusion based on the concept that the splanchnic circulation is the first body system to be affected by inadequate perfusion
    b. Method
       1) A vented nasogastric tube with a tonometer balloon located a few inches from the catheter's distal tip is placed into the stomach; a three-way stopcock is at the proximal end of the tonometer port.
       2) The tonometer balloon is filled with saline and is permeable to carbon dioxide.
       3) After a period of equilibration, saline samples taken from the balloon are analyzed for CO_2 to reflect the $PiCO_2$ (intramucosal carbon dioxide) at the same time that arterial blood is drawn for bicarbonate level.
       4) The pHi is then calculated; a low pHi (<7.2) indicates perfusion abnormality.
    c. Trends are monitored and interventions evaluated by changes in pHi.

14. Sublingual capnography
    a. Detects regional alterations in tissue perfusion; developed to overcome limitations and difficulties of gastric tonometry
    b. Method: a sensor is placed under the patient's tongue and held in place for 60 to 90 seconds.
    c. Increases in $P_{sl}CO_2$ correlate with decreases in arterial BP and CI and an increase in serum lactate.

Use of Hemodynamic Monitoring for Clinical Decision Making

1. Maximize accuracy, reproducibility, and reliability of measured parameters.
   a. The transducer must be leveled and balanced to zero (i.e., *zeroed*) with each head-of-bed position change or at least every 12 hours.
      1) Level the air-fluid interface of the transducer to the phlebostatic axis at the time of setup, any time the head of bed (HOB) is changed, any time the transducer and monitoring cable are disconnected, or any time the accuracy of the pressure readings are questionable.
         a) The air-fluid interface (also referred to as the *air reference port*) of the transducer needs to be leveled using either a laser or carpenter's level with the phlebostatic axis to ensure accuracy of measurement; the phlebostatic axis correlates with the right atrium and is at the fourth ICS and midway between the sternum anterior and the spine posterior (Fig. 3.57); this reference point is used if the patient is supine.
            i) Mark the phlebostatic axis on the patient's chest so that clinicians are consistent.
            ii) Be aware of the clinical importance of having the air-fluid interface level with the phlebostatic axis (Frazier, 2008).
               (a) If transducer too high, readings will be too low (2 mm Hg lower for every 1 inch above the phlebostatic axis).
               (b) If transducer too low, readings will be too high (2 mm Hg higher for every 1 inch below the phlebostatic axis).
         b) If the patient is supine, there is no need to put the HOB flat to take pressure measurements as long as the HOB is elevated no more than 60 degrees and the air-fluid interface is at the level of the phlebostatic axis (Fig. 3.57).

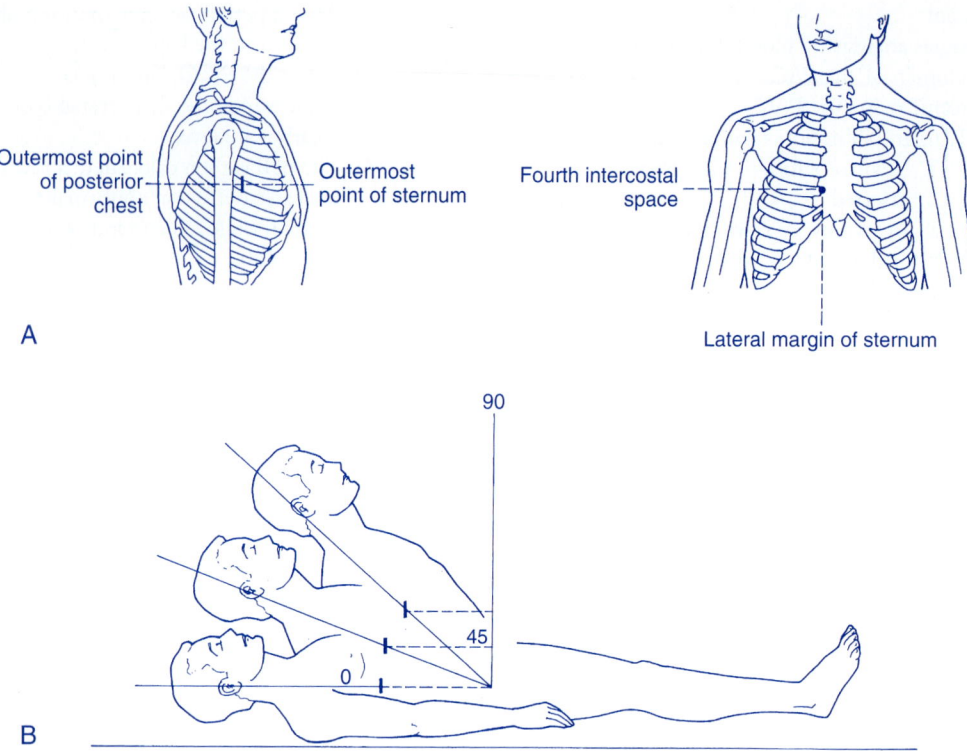

Fig. 3.57 Phlebostatic axis. **A,** Location of phlebostatic axis. **B,** Note that the measurements are accurate with head of bed elevated up to 45 degrees as long as the air-fluid interface is level with the phlebostatic axis. (From Flynn, J. B. M., & Bruce, N.P. [1993]. *Introduction to critical care skills.* St. Louis: Mosby.)

      c) Patients may also be lateral 20, 30, or 90 degrees or prone for pressure readings (Bridges, 2009).
          i) Reference point for 30 degrees: half the distance from surface of the bed to the left sternal border
          ii) Reference point for 90 degrees right: fourth ICS at midsternum
          iii) Reference point for 90 degrees left: fourth ICS at left sternal border
      d) Wait 5 to 15 minutes after any position change before obtaining pressure measurements (Bridges, 2009).
    2) Zero referencing at the time of setup, any time the HOB is changed, any time the transducer and monitoring cable are disconnected, or any time the accuracy of the pressure readings is questionable.
      a) Zero referencing the transducer requires closing the transducer to the patient, opening of the stopcock closest to the transducer to air, and ensuring that the monitor and the recorder read 0 ± 1 mm Hg.
      b) This negates the force exerted by the atmosphere so that only cardiovascular pressures are sensed, measured, and recorded.
 b. Ensure accurate calibration.
    1) Calibration ensures the accuracy of a quantitative measuring instrument.
    2) Transducer calibration
      a) To calibrate, a known pressure (e.g., using a sphygmomanometer) is exerted on the transducer to see that the monitor measures and displays it correctly.
      b) Reusable transducers require calibration before use; disposable transducers are precalibrated and only require calibration if the accuracy of the measurements is questionable
    3) Monitor calibration
      a) Some monitors require calibration.
      b) Consult the operating manual for specific instructions for the monitor in use.
    4) Oximetry calibration
      a) SvO_2 oximeters require calibration with the oxygen saturation measured from blood drawn from the distal port of the PAC (frequently referred to as *mixed venous oxygen saturation*).
      b) This calibration is done in vitro before catheter insertion and in vivo daily and anytime that the fiberoptics may have been damaged, the oximeter module is disconnected from the fiberoptic PAC, or the SvO_2 values are questionable.
 c. Analyze the graphic recording with simultaneous ECG as the most reliable means of measuring hemodynamic pressure at end-expiration (Fig. 3.58).
    1) Graphic method is more reliable than digital or cursor methods.

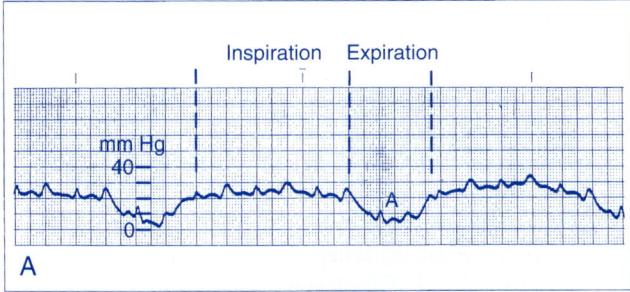

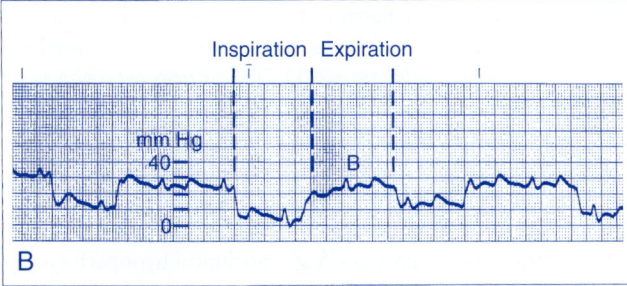

Fig. 3.58 Hemodynamic measurements are done at end-expiration. **A,** When a patient is receiving positive-pressure mechanical ventilation, inspiration is positive, and expiration is neutral. Readings should be done at the valley. Remember: volume ventilator—valley. **B,** When a patient is spontaneously breathing or on pressure-cycled ventilator, inspiration is negative and expiration is positive. Readings should be done at the peak. Remember: patient or pressure ventilator—peak. (Reprinted with permission from Schermer, L. [1998]. Physiologic and technical variables affecting hemodynamic measurements. *Crit Care Nurse*, 8[2], 33-40.)

2) Pressure readings obtained at end-expiration minimize the effects of intrathoracic pressure changes because intrathoracic pressure is closest to atmospheric pressure at the end of expiration.
   a) Spontaneously breathing patient: expiration is positive (high point of fluctuation)
   b) Mechanically ventilated patient: expiration is neutral (low point of fluctuation)
   c) Remember: ventilator valley, patient peak
d. Ensure proper PAC position in West lung zone III.
   1) PAOP pressure measurements are most accurate when the PAC tip is located in West lung zone III because pulmonary venous pressure is higher than the surrounding alveolar pressure and all capillaries are open.
   2) The PAC tip is below the level of the left atrium when the catheter is in this position.
   3) Indications that the PAC tip is in zone III (Martin, 2006; Bridges, 2006)
      a) Confirmed by chest radiography: tip is below the left atrium on frontal chest radiographs
      b) PAd greater than PAOP
      c) Normal PAOP waveform with clearly identifiable *a* and *v* waves
      d) Respiratory variation in PAd greater than respiratory variation in PAOP
      e) Change in positive end-expiratory pressure (PEEP) results in a change in PAOP of less than one half of the change in PEEP.

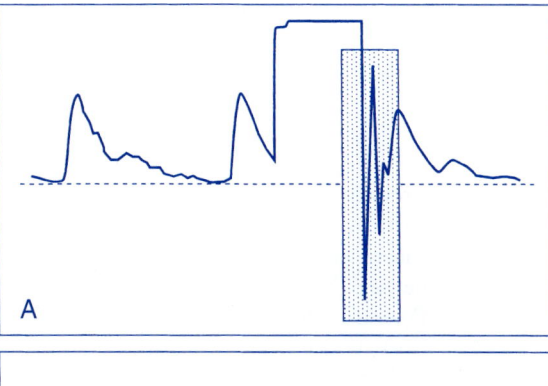

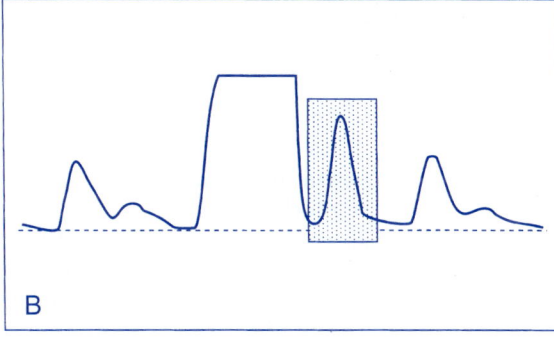

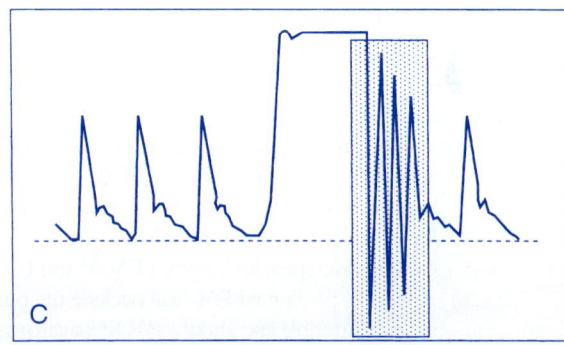

Fig. 3.59 Square wave test using the fast-flush valve. **A,** Normal test and accurate waveform. **B,** Overdamped. **C,** Underdamped.

e. Ensure adequate damping using the square wave test (also referred to as *dynamic response test* or *frequency response test*) (Fig. 3.59) on initial pressure monitoring setup, at least every 12 hours, when the system has been opened (e.g., zeroing, drawing blood, tubing change), whenever the waveform appears distorted or damped, or at any time the accuracy of the pressure readings is questionable.
   1) Fast flush the system causing the waveform to square off at the top of the screen.
   2) Analyze the waveform after the flush.
      a) One or two oscillations indicate an optimally damped system.
      b) No peaks should be more than 1 mm apart, and the second peak should be less than one third of the height of the first peak.
   3) Overdamping
      a) Evidence: there are no oscillations after the square wave.
      b) Potential effects on pressure readings: underestimation of systolic and overestimation of diastolic pressures
      c) Treatment

i) Check for occlusion (e.g., kinks, clots) or air in system.
ii) Ensure that noncompliant tubing is in place between the catheter and the transducer.
iii) Ensure tight-fitting connections.
4) Underdamping
a) Evidence: more than two oscillations after square wave or more than one to two blocks between bounces
b) Potential effects on pressure readings: overestimation of systolic and underestimation of diastolic pressures
c) Treatment
i) Restrict catheter and tubing length to 4 feet maximum.
ii) Add a damping device to absorb unwanted frequency vibration or turn a stopcock slightly.
f. Obtain chest radiographs after insertion of CVP or PAC to ensure proper positioning of the catheter.
1) The tip of a CVP catheter is positioned in the proximal superior vena cava.
2) The tip of a PAC is positioned in a pulmonary arteriole in lung zone 3.
a) When the catheter tip of the PAC is inserted in lung regions in which alveolar pressure exceeds venous pressure (zones 1 and 2), PAOP will not accurately represent LAP; also PEEP in a patient who is hypovolemic or has noncompliant lungs can convert a zone 3 into a zone 1 or 2, causing discrepancies between PAOP and LAP.
b) An ideally positioned PAC will occlude the pulmonary arteriole and show a PAOP waveform when between 1.25 and 1.5 ml of air has been used to inflate the 1.5-ml capacity balloon.
i) When a PAOP waveform is seen when less than 1.25 ml has been injected into the 1.5-ml capacity balloon, the catheter is too distal and prone to cause arteriolar occlusion without balloon inflation (referred to as *spontaneous wedge*).
ii) When the balloon is inflated to obtain a PAOP measurement, the nurse must observe the monitor and stop injecting air into the balloon as soon as the PA waveform converts to a PAOP waveform to avoid overwedging and potentially fatal pulmonary artery rupture.
g. Ensure accuracy of thermodilution CO measurements.
1) Use CCO technology if possible.
2) If intermittent methodology is used
a) Room temperature injectates for CO determination by thermodilution are adequate as long as a 12°F difference exists between blood temperature and injectate temperature; keep injectate solution and tubing away from direct sunlight and heat lamps.
b) Iced injectates may be used in low or high CO states or if the CO value obtained using room temperature is suspected to be inaccurate.
c) CO injectate must be injected within 4 seconds.
3) Enter the appropriate computation constant into the CO computer or monitor for calculation of CO; catheter size and type and injectate volume and temperature determine the computation constant.
2. Ensure patency of the catheter by maintaining a saline flush system.
a. Heparin may be added, although this is currently controversial; usual heparin concentration is 1 unit of heparin/1 ml of flush solution.
1) Heparin is contraindicated in patients with a history of heparin-induced thrombocytopenia (HIT) (also referred to as *heparin-associated thrombosis and thrombocytopenia* [HATT] or *white clot syndrome*).
b. Intermittent flush devices deliver 3 to 5 ml/hr as long as the pressure bag is maintained at 300 mm Hg
3. Correlate numerical value of parameter with the patient's clinical presentation.
a. Hemodynamic parameter changes may precede clinical presentation changes (e.g., subclinical hypoperfusion).
b. Hemodynamic parameter changes may reflect inaccurate measurements; care must be taken to be consistent in measuring techniques.
c. Note trends of change of measured parameters over time and in response to therapeutic interventions.
d. Notify the physician of significant changes from patient's normal.
1) PA systolic more than 4 to 7 mm Hg
2) PA diastolic more than 4 to 7 mm Hg
3) PAOP more than 4 mm Hg
4. Use hemodynamic parameters in clinical decision making.
a. Determination of best PEEP: PEEP that will give the best PaO_2 and SaO_2 without causing a drop in CO and CI
b. Determination of best PAOP or optimal point on Starling curve
1) PAOP that will give the best SV and CO without producing pulmonary edema
2) RV end-diastolic volume may be a more valid parameter to monitor in evaluation of best stretch and filling volumes
a) The main issue is whether pressure truly reflects volume.
b) Pressure is not a reflection of volume in patients with poor ventricular compliance.
c) These measurements require a special REF PAC.
c. Determination of true PAOP with patients on PEEP (especially important if patient is on high levels of PEEP)
1) Convert cm H_2O measurement of PEEP to mm Hg by dividing by 1.36.
2) Subtract one half of the PEEP (in mm Hg) from the measured PAOP to get a "true" PAOP when evaluating fluid status and filling volumes.
3) This is of questionable clinical value because trends, rather than absolute pressure measurements, are of the most clinical significance.
d. Utilization of the patient's clinical presentation and hemodynamic parameters to detect physiologic alterations and responses to therapy (Table 3.16)

Table 3.16 Hemodynamic Profiles for Selected Critical Care Conditions

Condition	Clinical Presentation	Hemodynamic Presentation
Cardiogenic shock	• Tachycardia, hypotension, tachypnea • S_3 • Crackles • Dyspnea • JVD • Hepatomegaly • Peripheral edema • Oliguria	• CO and CI decreased • RAP, PAP, PAOP increased • SVR, SVRI increased • LVSWI decreased • SaO_2, SvO_2 decreased • DO_2 decreased
Hypovolemic shock	• Flat neck veins • Tachycardia, hypotension, tachypnea • Oliguria	• CO and CI decreased • RAP, PAP, PAOP decreased • SVR, SVRI increased • SvO_2 decreased • DO_2 decreased
Anaphylactic shock	• Hypotension, tachypnea • Tachycardia • Angioedema • Warmth, erythema, pruritus, hives • Wheezing, stridor	• CO and CI decreased • RAP, PAP, PAOP decreased • SVR, SVRI decreased • SvO_2 decreased • DO_2 decreased
Neurogenic shock	• Hypotension, tachypnea • Bradycardia • Warm, dry, flushed skin • Hypothermia • Neurologic deficit	• CO and CI decreased • RAP, PAP, PAOP decreased • SVR, SVRI decreased • SvO_2 decreased • DO_2 decreased
Septic shock (early) (late as in hypovolemic shock)	• Tachycardia, hypotension, tachypnea • Hyperthermia • Irritability, confusion • Warm, moist, flushed skin	• CO and CI increased • RAP, PAP, PAOP decreased • SVR, SVRI decreased • SvO_2 increased • DO_2 increased; VO_2 decreased
Pulmonary hypertension (COPD, PE, mitral valve disease, hypoxemia)	• Tachycardia • JVD may occur • Dyspnea	• RAP may be increased • PVR >250 dynes/sec/cm^{-5} • PAm >20 mm Hg • PAd > 5 mm Hg greater than PAOP • SaO_2, SvO_2 decreased
Cardiogenic pulmonary edema	• Tachycardia • Dyspnea • Crackles • S_3	• CO and CI decreased • RAP, PAP, PAOP increased • SVR, SVRI increased • PVR, PVRI increased • SaO_2, SvO_2 decreased • DO_2 decreased
Noncardiogenic pulmonary edema (e.g., ARDS)	• Dyspnea • Crackles • Evidence of decreased lung compliance (e.g., increased work of breathing if patient spontaneously breathing, increased peak and plateau pressures if patient is being mechanically ventilated)	• PAP elevated, PAOP normal • PVR, PVRI increased • SaO_2, SvO_2 decreased • DO_2 decreased
Cardiac tamponade	• "Fullness" in chest • Tachycardia, hypotension, tachypnea • Muffled heart sounds • JVD • Electrical alternans	• CO and CI decreased • RAP, PAP, PAOP increased • Equalization of intracardiac pressures; RAP, PAd, PAOP will all be increased within a 5–mm Hg variation • Large *a* and *v* waves (M) on PAOP waveform • Pulsus paradoxus (drop in BP >10 mm Hg during inspiration) • SvO_2 decreased • DO_2 decreased
Papillary muscle rupture (acute mitral regurgitation)	• Tachycardia, hypotension, tachypnea • Dyspnea • Crackles • S_3 • New holosystolic murmur at apex	• CO and CI decreased • RAP, PAP, PAOP increased • Large *v* waves on PAOP waveform • SaO_2, SvO_2 decreased • DO_2 decreased

Continued

Table 3.16	Hemodynamic Profiles for Selected Critical Care Conditions—cont'd	
Condition	**Clinical Presentation**	**Hemodynamic Presentation**
Rupture of ventricular septum	• Tachycardia, hypotension, tachypnea • New holosystolic murmur at lower left sternal border	• Inaccurate CO measurement: because CO measurement by thermodilution is actually a right ventricular cardiac output, measured CO will be high, but the CO from the left ventricle is actually low • RAP, PAP increased • Large *v* waves on PAOP waveform may be seen • SvO_2 (or mixed venous oxygen saturation) increased • Increased oxygen gradient (oxygen step-up) between blood drawn from proximal port (RA) and distal port (PA) • DO_2 decreased
Left ventricular infarction	• Chest pain • S_4 at apex • ECG changes of LVMI	• Significance of hemodynamic compromise determined by amount of ventricular ischemia/injury/infarction and the wall(s) affected • CO and CI may be decreased • RAP, PAP, PAOP may be increased • LVSWI may be decreased
Right ventricular infarction	• Chest pain • S_4 at sternum • Distended jugular neck veins • Clear lungs • ECG changes of RVMI	• Significance of hemodynamic compromise determined by amount of ventricular ischemia, injury, or infarction • CO and CI may be decreased • RAP may be increased • PAP, PAOP may be decreased • RVSWI may be decreased

ARDS, Acute respiratory distress syndrome; *BP,* blood pressure; *CI,* cardiac index; *CO,* cardiac output; *COPD,* chronic obstructive pulmonary disease; DO_2, oxygen delivery to the tissue; *ECG,* electrocardiogram; *JVD,* jugular venous distention; *LVMI,* left ventricular myocardial infarction; *LVSWI,* left ventricular stroke work index; *PA,* pulmonary artery; *Pad,* pulmonary artery diastolic pressure; *PAm,* pulmonary artery mean pressure; *PAOP,* pulmonary artery occlusive pressure; *PAP,* pulmonary artery pressure; *PE,* pulmonary embolism; *PVR,* pulmonary vascular resistance; *PVRI,* pulmonary vascular resistance index; *RA,* right atrium; *RAP,* right atrial pressure, S_3, third heart sound; *S4,* fourth heart sound; SaO_2, arterial oxygen saturation; *SVR,* systemic vascular resistance; *SVRI,* systemic vascular resistance index

1) Use indexes to evaluate parameters (e.g., CI versus CO).
2) Use therapeutic manipulations (e.g., drug administration and titration, fluid therapy, IABP) to optimize CO and vital organ perfusion while minimizing myocardial oxygen consumption (Fig. 3.60).
5. Prevent, detect, and assist in management of complications of hemodynamic monitoring (Table 3.17).

Cardiopulmonary Arrest

Definition
A sudden cessation of the CO and effective circulation; cardiac arrest is followed by ventilatory cessation

Etiology
1. Dysrhythmias
2. Electrical shock
3. Drowning
4. Asphyxiation
5. Trauma
6. Hypothermia
7. Terminal phases of a chronic illness (cardiopulmonary resuscitation [CPR] may not be attempted on the patient according to advance directives and "do not resuscitate" [DNR] orders)

Pathophysiology
1. Cardiac arrest ceases delivery of oxygen and removal of carbon dioxide, causing tissue hypoxia and metabolic (i.e., lactic) acidosis.
2. Ventilatory arrest causes hypercapnia, respiratory acidosis, and hypoxemia.
3. Cerebral cortex is irreversibly damaged within 4 to 6 minutes at normal body temperature, and severe neurologic deficit or biological death occurs

Clinical Presentation
1. Loss of consciousness
2. Absence of breathing; agonal breathing may be a precursor to cardiopulmonary arrest
3. Absence of central pulses
4. Absence of auscultated or palpated BP
5. Anoxic seizures may occur
6. Urinary and bowel incontinence may occur
7. ECG
    a. Most commonly VF
    b. Less commonly VT
    c. Rarely asystole
    d. Cardiopulmonary arrest with a stable electrical rhythm (referred to as *pulseless electrical activity [PEA]*)

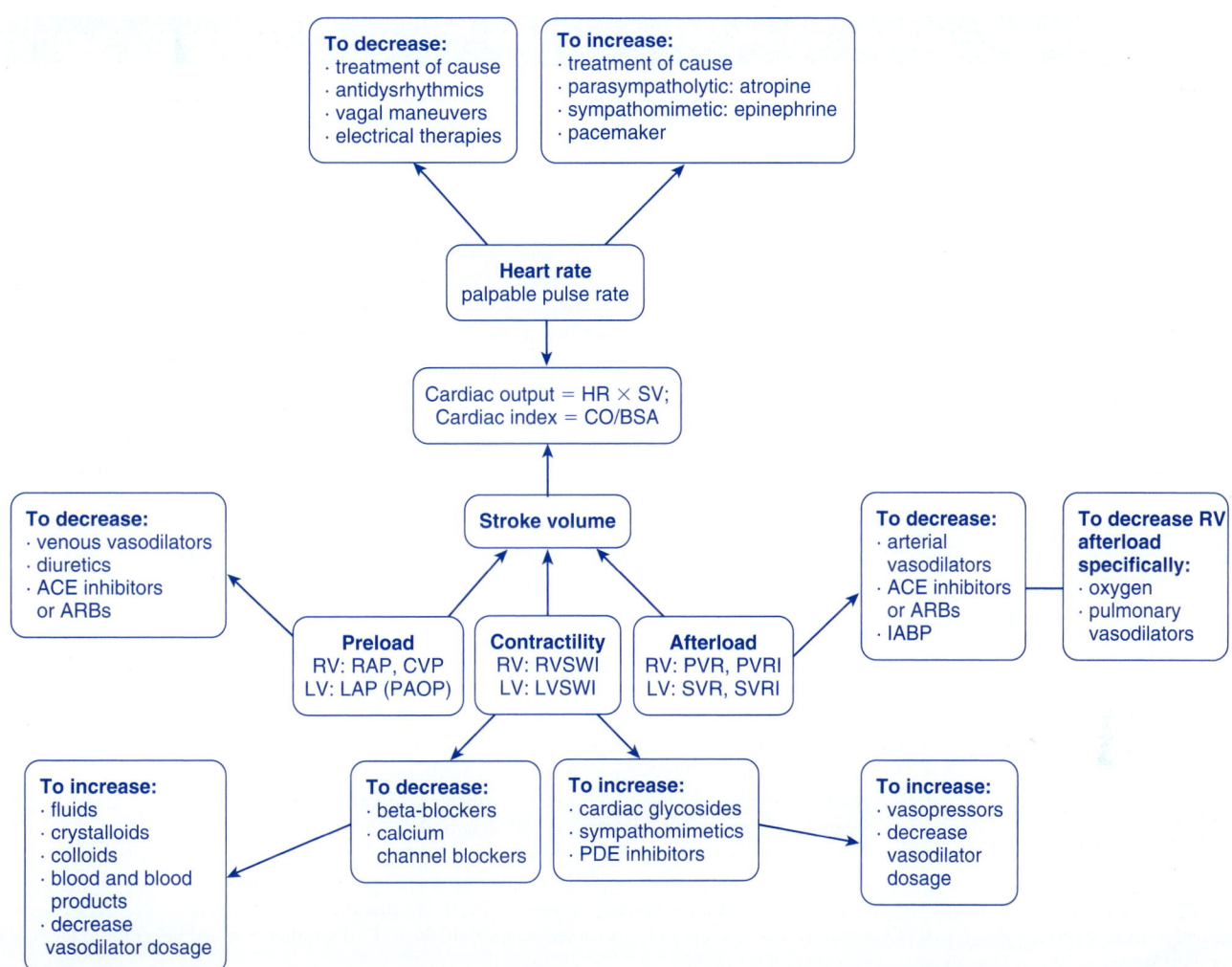

Fig. 3.60 Therapeutic manipulations to optimize cardiac output and vital organ perfusion and/or minimize myocardial oxygen consumption. *ACE,* Angiotensin-converting enzyme; *ARB,* angiotensin receptor blocker; *BSA,* body surface area; *CO,* cardiac output; *CVP,* central venous pressure; *HR,* heart rate; *IABP,* intraaortic balloon pump; *LAP,* left atrial pressure; *LV,* left ventricle; *LVSWI,* left ventricular stroke work index; *PAOP,* pulmonary artery occlusive pressure; *PDE,* phosphodiesterase; *PVR,* pulmonary vascular resistance; *PVRI,* pulmonary vascular resistance index; *RAP,* right atrial pressure; *RV,* right ventricle; *RVSWI,* right ventricular stroke work index; *SV,* stroke volume; *SVR,* systemic vascular resistance; *SVRI,* systemic vascular resistance index.

Table 3.17	Complications of Hemodynamic Monitoring
Complications	**Prevention, Detection, and Treatment**
Air emboli	• Use Trendelenburg position for insertion of deep vein catheters. • Place sterile gloved finger over needle hub with any disconnection during insertion to prevent air emboli. • Aspirate air from flush solution bag to avoid air embolus with inadvertent emptying of flush solution bag. • Flush all lumens with saline before insertion of catheters. • Monitor the pressure monitoring system for air bubbles. • Use only Luer-Lok connections. • Have the patient hold his or her breath during catheter-tubing disconnects (e.g., tubing changes or removal of deep vein catheters). • If air embolus is suspected, turn patient to left side with head down (i.e., Durant maneuver) and administer oxygen.
Arterial puncture (during venous cannulation)	• Hold pressure for at least 5–10 min; a longer time may be required for patients on anticoagulants or patients who have received fibrinolytics.

Continued

Table 3.17	Complications of Hemodynamic Monitoring—cont'd
Complications	**Prevention, Detection, and Treatment**
Balloon rupture	• Test the balloon before insertion by inflating the balloon and holding it in a basin of sterile saline and watching for bubbling. • Store catheters away from sunlight and heat. • Limit the length of time that catheter is left in (ideally <72 hr). • Limit the number of times the balloon is inflated to only when indicated (balloons are expected to last about 72 inflations); use PAd as a reflection of LVEDP in patients without pulmonary hypertension. • Do not overinflate balloon; stop injecting air as soon as the PAOP waveform is seen. • Do not aspirate air from the balloon; allow passive deflation and reattach the empty syringe to the balloon port. • Indications that the balloon has ruptured include an inability to obtain PAOP waveform and absence of resistance during inflation. • If balloon rupture has occurred, label balloon lumen accordingly so that others do not continue to try to inflate balloon; use PAd as a reflection of LVEDP in patients without pulmonary hypertension; if a PAOP is required, a new PAC must be inserted. • This complication is particularly dangerous in right-to-left shunt (e.g., neonates); adults typically shunt left to right.
Clotting and catheter occlusion	• Maintain saline drip with an intermittent flush device; heparin may be added but is currently controversial. • Monitor for any change in waveform (e.g., damping).

Dysrhythmias: usually ventricular dysrhythmias or RBBB	• Have emergency equipment (including transcutaneous pacemaker) available during insertion.
	• Inflate balloon to capacity (e.g., 1.5 ml) when the catheter is in the right atrium during insertion so that the balloon cushions the catheter tip.
	• Observe the ECG monitor closely during insertion.
	• Ensure that the catheter has been sutured in place to decrease risk of movement.
	• Assess PAP waveform for indications that the catheter has flipped back into RV.
	  • Request catheter repositioning for catheter fling or RV waveform.
	  • If RV waveform is noted, inflate balloon to capacity (e.g., 1.5 ml) to cushion the catheter tip.
	  • Turn patient to left side to encourage distal migration of catheter back into PA.
	  • Deflate balloon after successful repositioning back into the PA.
	• Observe the ECG monitor closely during removal of the PAC; the catheter should be removed in a smooth continuous movement with balloon deflated.

Emboli	• Aspirate if you suspect a small clot rather than flush.
Exsanguination	• Use only Luer-Lok connections. • Maintain alarms in ON position; pressure alarms are usually set 10–20 mm Hg above and below the patient's normal.
Fluid overload	• Limit the number of fast flushes. • Use 5 ml instead of 10 ml for COs when indicated or use continuous CO, which requires no fluid boluses for determination of CO. • Limit the frequency of COs to every 4 hr unless required more often.
Hematoma	• Maintain pressure for 5–10 min with single-thickness pressure dressing after catheter removal; a longer time may be required for patients on anticoagulants or patients who have received fibrinolytics.
Hypothermia	• Use room temperature injectate. • Apply blankets and radiant heaters as needed.
Infection	• Encourage percutaneous catheter insertion (results in a much lower incidence of infection than does cutdown). • Change the flush solution bag whenever it is empty or every 72–96 hr or according to your hospital protocol. • Change the tubing every 72–96 hr or according to your hospital protocol. • Dress and inspect the site using sterile technique every 72–96 hr or according to your hospital protocol. • Avoid clear semipermeable dressings in patients with oily skin. • Use normal saline rather than D_5W for the flush solution. • Flush well after drawing blood samples; do not allow dried blood to stay in stopcock ports or tubing. • Limit the number of stopcocks in the pressure monitoring system. • Replace all vented stopcock covers with nonvented "dead-end" caps. • Use strict sterile technique with blood sampling and cardiac outputs. • Encourage use of catheter sleeve through which the PAC is threaded; allows for sterile catheter manipulation. • Limit the length of time that catheter is left in place (ideally <72–96 hr). • Monitor for clinical indications of infection at catheter insertion site: redness, warmth, induration, purulent drainage, and pain at insertion site. • Monitor for clinical indications of catheter sepsis: fever, chills, leukocytosis, positive blood culture or catheter culture.

Table 3.17	Complications of Hemodynamic Monitoring—cont'd
Complications	**Prevention, Detection, and Treatment**
Microshock	• Recognize that this risk is caused by elimination of the skin as a protection from microshock in patients with intracardiac catheters. • Ensure that all electrical equipment is properly functioning and grounded. • Do not touch the patient and a piece of electrical equipment at the same time.
Nerve palsy	• Maintain limbs in functional position (e.g., do not keep the wrist hyperextended to prevent ulnar nerve palsy).
Pneumothorax, hemothorax, chylothorax during insertion	• Have chest radiography taken after central vein catheter cannulation. • Assist with insertion of chest tube if pneumothorax (air in pleural space), hemothorax (blood in pleural space), or chylothorax (lymph fluid in pleural space) occurs.
Pulmonary artery rupture	• Recognize patients at high risk: older adult patients; patients with pulmonary hypertension; patients receiving anticoagulant, fibrinolytic, or platelet aggregation inhibitor therapy; hypothermic patients; postcardiac surgery patients. • Inflate balloon with only enough air to cause PAOP waveform; do not overinflate and limit inflation time to a maximum of 15 sec because both prolonged inflation and excessive balloon volume put too much tension on the vessel wall. • Monitor patient for sudden onset of hemoptysis, especially after inflation of balloon, dyspnea, and hypotension as indications of pulmonary artery rupture. • If rupture of the pulmonary artery does occur: increase the FiO_2, suction the airway, position the patient with the affected lung down, assist with intubation with double-lumen endotracheal tube, use PEEP or PAC balloon inflation for tamponade effect as prescribed, monitor vital signs and oxygenation levels closely for changes, and prepare the patient for surgery if requested.
Pulmonary infarction	• Inflate balloon only long enough for graphic recording. • Continuously monitor PAP so that if catheter advances into PAOP position, it will be noted and the catheter repositioned. • Request proximal repositioning if it takes <1.25 ml to achieve occluded position because this indicates that the catheter is positioned too distal and may spontaneously occlude the pulmonary arteriole (commonly referred to as *spontaneous wedge*) and cause ischemia and infarction. • Monitor for chest pain, dyspnea, and decreased SaO_2 as an indication of pulmonary infarction.

Thrombosis	• Maintain saline drip with IFD; keep pressure bag at 300 mm Hg so that IFD is functional
	  • Heparin may be added to flush solution with usual concentration of 1 unit/ml; although this practice has been shown to improve patency, it increases the risk of HITT.
	• Limit the length of time that catheter is left in (ideally <72 hr).
	• Prevent trauma to the intima by skillful catheter insertion.
	• To prevent or detect arterial thrombosis with arterial catheters:
	  • Select the site with collateral flow (e.g., radial artery).
	  • Use the smallest catheter feasible (e.g., 20 gauge for radial artery cannulation).
	  • Perform neurovascular assessment hourly to promptly detect acute arterial occlusion.
	• If arterial occlusion occurs, assist with intraarterial fibrinolytic or embolectomy.

CO, Cardiac output; D_5W, dextrose 5% in water; *ECG*, electrocardiogram; FiO_2, fraction of inspired oxygen; *HITT*, heparin-induced thrombosis and thrombocytopenia; *IFD*, intermittent flush device; *LVDEP*, left ventricular end-diastolic pressure; *PA*, pulmonary artery; *PAC*, pulmonary artery catheter; *PAd*, pulmonary artery diastolic pressure; *PAOP*, pulmonary artery occlusive pressure; *PAP*, pulmonary artery pressure; *PEEP*, positive end-expiratory pressure; *RBBB*, right bundle branch block; *RV*, right ventricle; SaO_2, arterial oxygen saturation.

Collaborative Management

1. Recognize the factors that are crucial in survival; these are referred to as the *chain of survival* by the American Heart Association (AHA) (Hazinski et al., 2015).
   a. Immediate recognition of cardiac arrest and activation of the emergency response system
   b. Early CPR with emphasis on chest compressions; reasons for recent change from ABC to CAB
      1) Most cardiac arrests occur as a result of VF or pulseless VT in adults, and chest compressions and defibrillation are most crucial to survival.
      2) ABC sequence delayed chest compressions because the time required to look, listen, feel for airflow, open the airway, and start mouth-to-mouth ventilation or retrieve a barrier or other ventilation equipment; in the new sequence, ventilation is only delayed until after a cycle of 30 compressions.
      3) Because lay persons are reluctant to give mouth-to-mouth ventilation to a stranger, compressions are more promptly initiated with the new Hands-Only CPR for lay rescuers.
   c. Rapid defibrillation
   d. Effective advanced life support
   e. Integrated postcardiac arrest care
2. Recognize cardiac arrest and activate the emergency response system.
   a. Complete assessment: if the person is unresponsive and either not breathing or only gasping
   b. Call for help: call 911 for out-of-hospital cardiac arrest or follow specific protocol (e.g., Code Blue) for in-hospital cardiac arrest.
   c. Retrieve defibrillator.
3. Provide basic life support (BLS) as recommended by current AHA guidelines (http://circ.ahajournals.org/content/132/18_suppl_2/S444).
   a. Circulation
      1) Assess a carotid pulse for no more than 10 seconds.

2) Deliver compressions.
   a) Place heel of one hand over the lower half of sternum; place the other hand over the first hand.
   b) Compress the sternum at a depth of 2 to 2.4 inches at a rate of 100 to 120 compressions/min.
      i) New guidelines emphasize that the provider push hard and fast, allowing the chest to completely recoil after each compression.
      ii) Compression ratio is 30:2 for CPR to adults.
      iii) All rescue efforts, including defibrillation, insertion of advanced airways, intravenous (IV) access, and administration of medications, should be performed with minimal interruption of compressions.
      iv) Compressions should be maintained without pauses for ventilation.
   b. Airway and ventilation
      1) After the initial 30 compressions, open the airway using head tilt–chin lift maneuver; jaw thrust maneuver is no longer recommended in initial establishment of airway.
      2) If the patient is adequately breathing, position him or her on the left side in recovery position.
      3) If the patient is not breathing or breathing inadequately, health care providers should deliver two breaths using any of the following methods:
         a) Mouth-to-mask ventilation
         b) Manual resuscitation bag-valve-mask secured over nose and mouth
         c) Manual resuscitation bag to endotracheal (ET) tube or tracheostomy tube if already in place
      4) Note that each rescue breath does make the chest rise.
      5) Continue rescue breathing every 6 to 8 seconds (8–10 breaths/min); note that hyperventilation is associated with poor survival rates.
   c. Coordination of compressions and ventilation: Maintain a ratio of 30 compressions to 2 ventilations for one or two rescuers.
   d. Considerations
      1) CPR performed expertly provides only 25% to 30% of normal CO, but most of this goes to the upper body, including the heart and brain.
      2) Mortality rates increase despite prompt CPR if advanced cardiac life support (ACLS) is delayed beyond 12 minutes.
      3) Resistance of ventricular dysrhythmias to defibrillation occurs over time; prompt defibrillation is critical to survival.
4. Initiate rapid defibrillation.
   a. Principle: by delivering a shock of sufficient strength, a critical mass of myocardium is depolarized simultaneously, allowing emergence of a dominant normal rhythm.
   b. Uses
      1) Pulseless VT and VF
      2) Unstable or refractory VT with a pulse
      3) May also be used in asystole where the rhythm is unclear and could be fine VF
   c. Timing: should be performed *immediately* for VF or pulseless VT as soon as defibrillator is available
      1) Ideally within 3 minutes
      2) Minimal delay between cessation of CPR and defibrillation and defibrillation and resumption of CPR
   d. Method for manual defibrillation
      1) Check pulse: make sure that VF pattern is not merely artifact caused by loose ECG electrode
      2) Remove any foil-lined patches from the patient's chest (e.g., nitroglycerin patches) because they may cause arcing and patient burns; patient must be dry and not in contact with any metallic objects.
      3) Turn defibrillator on and make sure that the synchronizer switch is off so that charge is delivered as soon as buttons are pushed; most defibrillators automatically reset to nonsynchronized mode so you can immediately defibrillate if VF occurs after cardioversion.
      4) Apply defibrillation pads to chest for paddle placement or apply conductive jelly to paddles.
         a) Four pad/paddle positions are equally effective (Link et al., 2010).
            i) Anterolateral (considered the default position)
            ii) Anteroposterior: this paddle placement may be better for obese patients, patients with hyperinflated lungs (e.g., COPD), and patients with an implantable cardioverter-defibrillator (ICD).
            iii) Anterior-left infrascapular
            iv) Anterior-right infrascapular
         b) Pacemakers
            i) In patients with permanent pacemakers, the paddles should not be placed within 8 cm of the pulse generator (Link et al., 2010).
            ii) Turn temporary pacemaker pulse generator off during defibrillation.
      5) Charge to appropriate voltage for defibrillation.
         a) Biphasic: 150 to 200 J for a biphasic truncated exponential waveform or 120 J for a rectilinear biphasic waveform; if unknown, use maximum available
            i) Advantages of biphasic defibrillation is that it offers equal or better efficacy at lower energies than traditional monophasic waveform defibrillators (less than or equal to 200 J is safe and has equal or greater efficiency for terminating VF compared with higher energy monophasic shock), less risk of myocardial injury, and skin burns.
            ii) In the first phase, the current moves from one paddle to the other (as in monophasic defibrillation), and in the second phase, the current reverses direction.
         b) Monophasic: 360 J

6) Apply paddles to defibrillation pads or jellied paddles to chest using firm (~25 lb) pressure.
  7) Say the word *clear* and ensure that no one is touching the patient or the bed.
  8) Press both discharge buttons simultaneously.
  9) Resume CPR, beginning with chest compressions; note that current guidelines recommend only one shock before resuming CPR.
  10) Recheck rhythm after 5 cycles (~2 minutes).
       a) If rhythm and pulse are restored, administer antidysrhythmic drug therapy.
       b) If rhythm and pulse are not restored, continue with appropriate algorithm.
 e. Method for using an automatic external defibrillator (AED)
  1) Attach the device to the patient: put one pad to the right of the sternum below the right clavicle and the other pad lateral to the apex in the left midaxillary line.
  2) Turn on the device.
  3) Ensure that the patient is completely still and no one is touching the patient.
  4) Press the analyze button. The device will signal "stand clear" and perform a 3-second analysis.
  5) If VT or VF is detected, the AED will charge to 200 J (biphasic) and display a "shock indicated" message.
  6) Call "clear" and ensure that no one is touching the patient.
  7) Press the shock button to deliver the shock if it was indicated.
  8) If rhythm and pulse are restored, antidysrhythmic drug therapy will be administered.
  9) If rhythm and pulse are not restored, continuance of CPR and appropriate algorithm
 f. Successful defibrillation is less likely if any of the following is present:
  1) Hypoxia
  2) Severe acidosis
  3) Alkalosis
  4) Local ionic imbalance
  5) Ischemia
  6) Long VF duration
 g. Complications
  1) Dysrhythmias: asystole, bradycardia, AV blocks, VF
  2) Hypotension
  3) Myocardial damage
  4) Pulmonary edema
  5) Emboli
  6) Muscle pain
  7) Skin burns
5. Provide effective ACLS as recommended by current AHA guidelines (http://circ.ahajournals.org/content/132/18_suppl_2/S444)
 a. Utilization of ACLS algorithms to provide assistance with decision making in a cardiopulmonary arrest (Figs. 3.61 to 3.63)
 b. Identification and treatment of the cause of cardiac arrest, especially important in treatment of PEA
  1) 5 Hs: hypovolemia, hypoxia, hydrogen ion (acidosis), hyper- or hypokalemia, and hypothermia
  2) 5 Ts: tension pneumothorax, tamponade (cardiac), toxins, thrombosis (coronary), and thrombosis (pulmonary)
 c. Oxygen therapy
  1) Administer 100% oxygen during cardiopulmonary arrest with a bag-valve-mask; a reservoir bag or tubing attached to the bag-valve-mask is required to achieve as high a concentration of oxygen as possible.
  2) Remember that there is no contraindication to 100% oxygen during cardiopulmonary arrest.
 d. Vascular access
  1) Determination of patency of existing central or peripheral IV line or heparin lock; if a central vein catheter is in place when the arrest occurs, it should be used to administer drugs during the resuscitation
  2) Antecubital or external jugular veins are preferred if a venous catheter or additional venous catheters must be established.
     a) Peak drug concentrations are lower and circulation times are longer when drugs are administered by peripheral sites compared with central sites.
     b) If peripheral venous access is used for resuscitation drugs, administer bolus drugs rapidly, follow with a 20-ml saline, and elevate the extremity for 10 to 20 seconds.
  3) Central vein cannulation may be performed.
     a) The major disadvantage of central vein cannulation during cardiopulmonary arrest is the need to stop CPR.
        i) Internal jugular and subclavian sites require cessation of CPR.
        ii) Femoral vein cannulation does not require cessation of CPR.
     b) Another consideration is that unsuccessful central vein cannulation may contraindicate the use of fibrinolytics and increase the risk of bleeding with the use of glycoprotein IIb/IIIa agents (e.g., abciximab, eptifibatide, tirofiban) and anticoagulants.
  4) Distal wrist and hand veins and distal saphenous veins in the legs are the least favorable sites for drug administration during CPR.
  5) Intraosseous (IO) access may be used if IV access is not available; drugs administered by the IO route take approximately 2 minutes to reach the heart.
 e. ET intubation
  1) Attempt as soon as feasible, but defibrillation and administration of epinephrine are the first and second priorities.
  2) Hyperventilation with 100% oxygen should precede any intubation attempt.

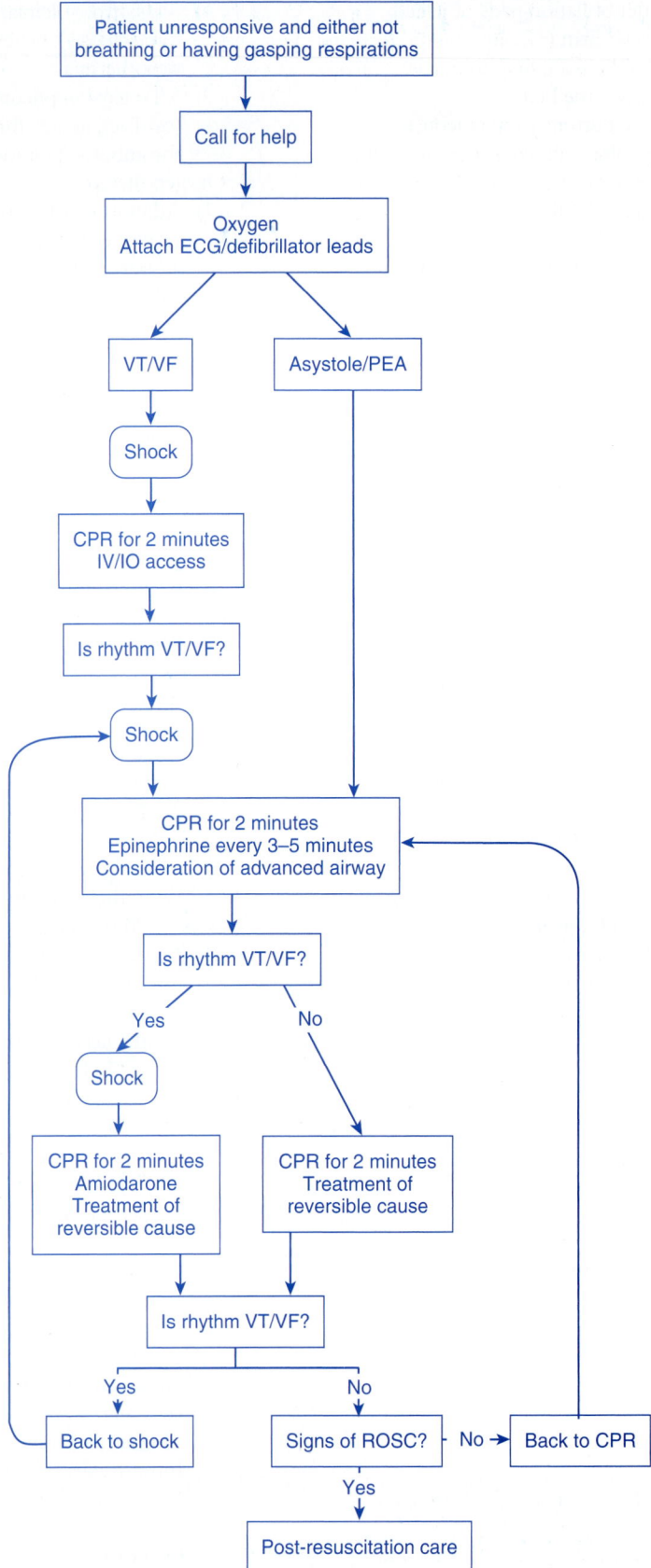

Fig. 3.61 Advanced cardiac life support (ACLS) cardiac arrest algorithm. *CPR,* cardiopulmonary resuscitation; *ECG,* electrocardiogram; *PEA,* pulseless electrical activity; *ROSC,* return of spontaneous circulation; *VF,* ventricular fibrillation; *VT,* ventricular tachycardia. (Data from American Heart Association. [2015]. Web-based Integrated Guidelines for Cardiopulmonary Resuscitation and Emergency Cardiovascular Care. Part 7 Adult Advanced Cardiac Life Support. Retrieved from https://eccguidelines.heart.org/index.php/circulation/cpr-ecc-guidelines-2/part-7-adult-advanced-cardiovascular-life-support/.)

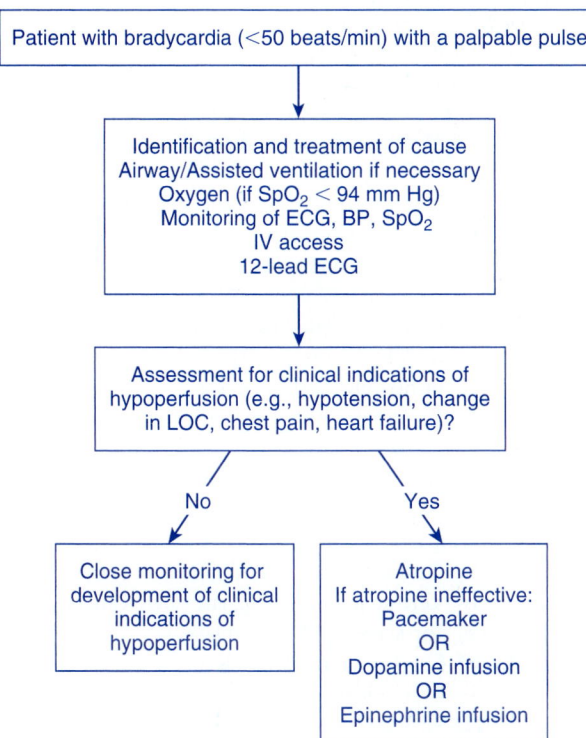

Fig. 3.62 Bradycardia algorithm. *BP,* Blood pressure; *ECG,* electrocardiogram; *LOC,* level of consciousness; *SpO₂,* oxygen saturation by pulse oximetry. (Data from American Heart Association. [2015]. Web-based Integrated Guidelines for Cardiopulmonary Resuscitation and Emergency Cardiovascular Care. Part 7 Adult Advanced Cardiac Life Support. Retrieved from https://eccguidelines.heart.org/index.php/circulation/cpr-ecc-guidelines-2/part-7-adult-advanced-cardiovascular-life-support/.)

3) Confirm ET tube placement by listening for equal bilateral breath sounds along with esophageal detector device, end-tidal carbon dioxide indicator, or capnography; chest radiography is obtained after the patient is stabilized.
   a) Capnography is recommended for confirmation and monitoring of ET tube placement and the quality of CPR (Hazinski et al., 2015).
4) Advantages of ET intubation include reduction of the risk of vomiting and aspiration and provision of a relative airway seal.
5) If IV route cannot be established but ET tube placement has been achieved, some emergency drugs can be given via the ET tube; however, the IV route is preferred.
   a) Epinephrine, lidocaine, atropine, and naloxone may be administered via the ET tube.
   b) ET administration requires adjusting the dose to 2 to 2.5 times the usual dose and diluting the drug with isotonic saline to make a total volume of at least 10 ml; follow with several quick insufflations with the manual resuscitation bag.
6) Two alternative airway techniques are placed orally and are inserted past the hypopharynx but not into the trachea.
   a) Laryngeal mask airway (LMA)
   b) Esophageal-tracheal Combitube (ETC)

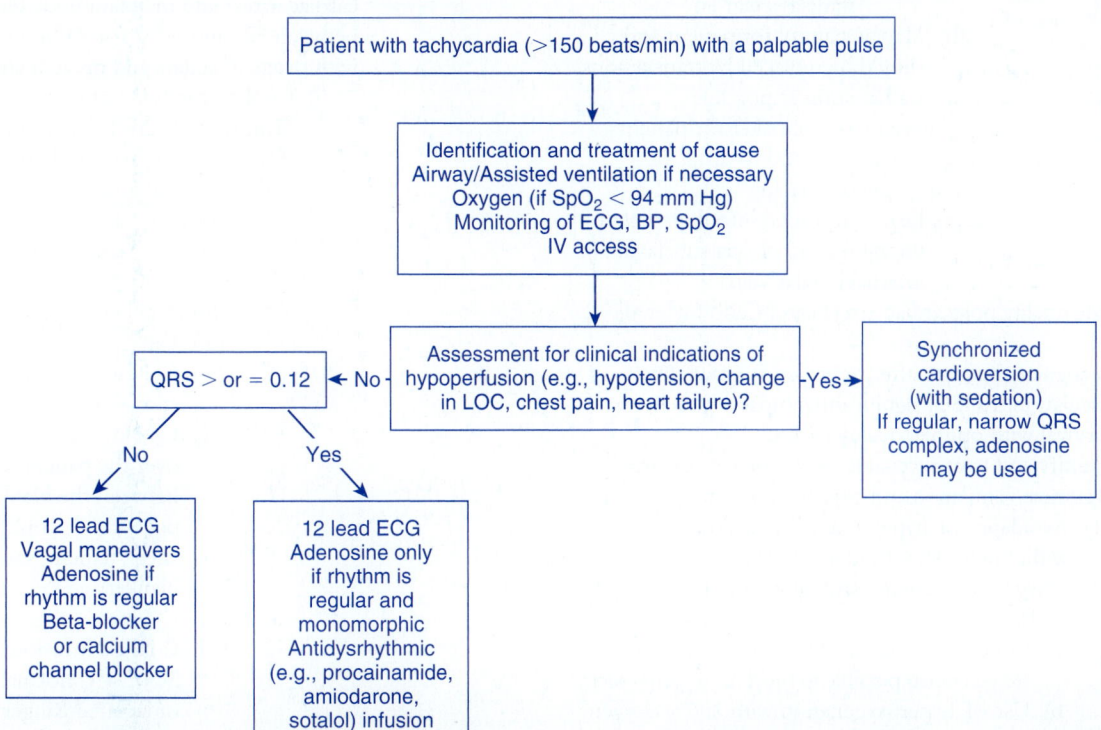

Fig. 3.63 Tachycardia algorithm. *BP,* Blood pressure; *ECG,* electrocardiogram; *IV,* intravenous; *LOC,* level of consciousness; *SpO₂,* oxygen saturation by pulse oximetry. (Data from American Heart Association. [2015]. Web-based Integrated Guidelines for Cardiopulmonary Resuscitation and Emergency Cardiovascular Care. Part 7 Adult Advanced Cardiac Life Support. Retrieved from https://eccguidelines.heart.org/index.php/circulation/cpr-ecc-guidelines-2/part-7-adult-advanced-cardiovascular-life-support/.)

f. IV fluids: normal saline is used to maintain adequate preload and to mix IV drug infusions.
g. Pharmacologic agents as indicated in algorithms (Figs. 3.61 to 3.63)
h. Electrical therapies to change an abnormal cardiac rhythm to a normal one
　1) Defibrillation for VF or pulseless VT as previously described
　2) Cardioversion for unstable SVT or VT with a pulse
　3) Temporary pacemaker: for patients who have problem with impulse formation and/or conduction
　　a) Indications
　　　i) Symptomatic bradycardia nonresponsive to drug therapy (e.g., atropine)
　　　ii) Symptomatic AV blocks
　　　iii) Note that pacing is no longer recommended for patients with asystolic cardiac arrest; it has not been shown to be effective and delays or interrupts chest compressions (Link et al., 2010).
　　b) Types
　　　i) Transcutaneous pacemaker
　　　　(a) Large surface skin electrodes applied anterior and posterior
　　　　　(i) Posterior: positive electrode applied between spine and left scapula at level of heart
　　　　　(ii) Anterior: negative electrode applied at left fourth ICS at midclavicular line
　　　　(b) May be painful for patient and should be replaced by transvenous lead as soon as possible
　　　ii) Transvenous pacemaker for patients who do not respond to drugs or transcutaneous pacing
　　　　(a) Lead is threaded into the apex of the right ventricle via subclavian or internal jugular vein.
6. Provide quality postcardiac arrest care (Calloway et al., 2015).
　a. Recognize that care after return of spontaneous circulation (ROSC) significantly impacts patient survival with optimal quality of life.
　b. Identify and treat reversible causes of cardiac arrest.
　c. Optimize ventilation and oxygenation.
　　1) Avoidance of hyperventilation; keep $PaCO_2$ within between 40 and 45 mm Hg
　　2) Oxygen to maintain SaO_2 at greater than or equal to 94%
　　　a) Close monitoring of ABGs and decrease of oxygen when possible to prevent oxygen toxicity
　　　b) Use of hyperoxygenation with 100% oxygen during suctioning to avoid hypoxemia
　　3) Advanced airways as required
　　4) Limitation of tidal volume to 6 to 8 ml/kg to prevent acute lung injury
　　5) Waveform capnography as available and indicated
　d. Treat hypotension (i.e., systolic BP less than 90 mm Hg)
　　1) Treatment of causes
　　2) IV or IO boluses
　　3) Inotropic or vasopressor agents as indicated
　　4) Antidysrhythmics as indicated
　e. Use targeted temperature management strategy of induced hypothermia if the patient is unresponsive but with an adequate BP after resuscitation; shown to improve neurologic recovery and reduce mortality rate
　　1) Indications
　　　a) Out-of-hospital cardiac arrest as the result of VF or pulseless VT; may also be used for in-hospital cardiac arrest
　　　b) Persistent change in neurologic function after ROSC
　　　c) Able to maintain BP with or without vasopressors after ROSC
　　2) Contraindications (Calloway et al., 2015)
　　　a) Coma of other etiology before cardiac arrest
　　　b) Terminal illness (e.g., late-stage cancer)
　　　c) Intracerebral hemorrhage
　　　d) Surgery within 14 days
　　　e) Systemic infection or sepsis
　　　f) Known bleeding or coagulopathy
　　3) Method
　　　a) Prepare patient for initiation of cooling.
　　　　i) Intubation and mechanical ventilation
　　　　ii) Foley catheter
　　　　iii) Temperature monitoring via use of internal temperature monitor: urinary bladder, rectal, or pulmonary artery
　　　b) Initiate cooling within 2 to 6 hours of cardiac arrest and maintain body temperature between 32° and 34°C for 24 hours along with drugs to sedate and prevent shivering.
　　　　i) Cooling methods: at least one study (Tomte et al., 2011) has found no difference in outcomes between surface and core cooling methods.
　　　　　(a) Surface
　　　　　　(i) Ice packs applied to armpits, neck, torso, groin
　　　　　　(ii) Air circulating cooling system
　　　　　　(iii) Fans
　　　　　　(iv) Cold water or alcohol sponge baths or sprays
　　　　　　(v) Cooling blanket under and over the patient with a sheet between the blanket and the patient (i.e., cooling blanket, sheet, patient, sheet, cooling blanket)
　　　　　(b) Core
　　　　　　(i) Cold IV infusions: 1 to 2 l of 4°C normal saline or lactated Ringer solution by peripheral or femoral vein access; 30 ml/kg over 30 minutes is a common protocol.
　　　　　　(ii) Gastric lavage may be used.

(iii) Endovascular cooling catheters may be used.
(iv) Extracorporeal circulation may be used.
ii) Close monitoring of vital signs, CBC, PT, aPTT, INR, serum chemistries, ABGs every 12 hours
iii) Control of discomfort and shivering
(a) Shivering causes increase in oxygen consumption.
(b) Sedation with benzodiazepines such as midazolam (Versed) is indicated; muscle paralytics, such as vecuronium or pancuronium, may be required.
(i) Drug clearance is decreased during hypothermia.
c) Rewarm gradually (0.25° to 0.5°C/hr) over 24 hours to avoid hypotension and cerebral edema.
4) Complications
a) Infection: decrease in number and function of neutrophils and decreased antibody production
b) Impaired tissue oxygenation: shift in oxyhemoglobin dissociation curve to the left impairs drop off of oxygen at tissue level
c) Coagulopathy
d) Dysrhythmias
i) Atrial fibrillation with temperature less than 32°C
ii) VF with temperature less than 30°C
e) Hyperglycemia
f) Electrolyte imbalance: hypokalemia, hypophosphatemia, and hypomagnesemia due to cold-induced diuresis
f. Facilitate coronary reperfusion as indicated for ST-segment elevation myocardial infarction (STEMI) or high suspicion of acute MI.
1) PCI (e.g., angioplasty, atherectomy, stent placement)
g. Provide advanced critical care management as required.
1) Prevention, close monitoring, or correction of electrolyte imbalance
2) Prevention, close monitoring, or correction of hypoglycemia or hyperglycemia
3) Prevention, close monitoring, and/or correction of myocardial stunning with inotropic agents, fluid management, or IABP
4) Prevention, close monitoring, or correction of acute renal injury with fluid management and renal replacement therapy
5) Prevention, close monitoring, or correction of acute brain injury
a) Avoidance of calcium, which has been shown to cause cerebral vessel spasm
b) Avoidance of dextrose in water: use isotonic normal saline rather than dextrose 5% in water (D_5W); the dextrose in D_5W is quickly metabolized to leave only hypotonic water; this contributes to hypoosmolality and potentially cerebral edema
c) Positioning: elevate HOB 30 degrees; avoid neck flexion or rotation; avoid hip flexion
d) Increased cerebral perfusion pressure: increase MAP and decrease intracranial pressure (ICP) as indicated; the following pharmacologic agents may be used:
i) Analgesics to reduce pain
ii) Anticonvulsants (e.g., phenytoin) to prevent seizures
iii) Isotonic or hypertonic solutions
iv) Sedatives and muscle paralytics (e.g., pancuronium) to decrease cerebral oxygen requirements
v) Osmotic agents (e.g., mannitol) to increase cortical circulation and reduce cerebral edema
vi) Calcium channel blockers (e.g., nimodipine) to prevent cerebral vasospasm
vii) Steroid (e.g., methylprednisolone) to reduce cerebral edema
7. Monitor for complications of CPR.
a. Fracture of sternum, ribs
b. Hemothorax
c. Pneumothorax
d. Laceration of abdominal viscera, especially the liver
e. Myocardial contusion
f. Cardiac rupture
8. Special circumstance: cardiac arrest with hypothermia
a. If body temperature is less than 95°F (35°C)
1) Initial treatment
a) Perform CPR.
b) Defibrillate for the initial series of three shocks for VF or pulseless VT.
c) Intubate and ventilate with warm, humidified oxygen.
d) Obtain IV access and administer warmed IV saline.
b. If core temperature is less than 86°F (30°C)
1) Continue CPR but withhold IV medications.
2) Continue with warm inspired oxygen and warm IV fluids.
3) Also peritoneal lavage with warm saline, extracorporeal rewarming, and esophageal rewarming tubes may be used.
c. If core temperature is greater than 86°F (30°C)
1) Continue CPR and administer IV medications but space longer than usual ACLS intervals.
2) Repeat defibrillation for pulseless VT or VF as core temperature rise above 95°F (35°C).

Psychosocial Considerations
1. The patient
a. During the resuscitation
1) Touch the patient's hand and talk to her or him during the resuscitation efforts.
2) Maintain the patient's modesty and dignity during the resuscitation efforts with drapes, curtains, and doors; ensure that all team members are respectful of the patient.

b. After the resuscitation
1) Patients frequently (~40%) have near-death experience during cardiac arrest but are frequently reluctant to discuss it.
a) As the patient regains consciousness, assure the patient that she or he is not alone; reorient the patient to person, place, and time.
b) Consider asking the patient if he or she remembers anything that occurred during the time his or her heart was stopped.
c. If the resuscitation efforts are unsuccessful: provide respectful and culturally sensitive care of the body.
2. The family
a. Need for information
1) If the patient's condition has been worsening, the family should be informed of the worsening condition.
2) If the cardiopulmonary arrest was sudden, the family should be informed about what has happened, what is being done, and an estimate of how long it may be before more information will be available.
a) If information must be conveyed by telephone, they should be told that the situation is serious but not told of a death by telephone.
b. Need for privacy
1) Escort the family to a family conference room where they can grieve apart from other visitors but do not leave them alone.
2) Ask if someone, such as a religious leader or a family member or friend, can be telephoned; offer to call someone from pastoral services or have a social worker or a volunteer to be there with them.
3) Allow the family to "tell their story" but do not give inappropriate reassurance.
4) Be honest; do not give inappropriate reassurance but be hopeful, warm, and caring.
c. Family presence during cardiopulmonary arrest is being advocated today as part of holistic care.
1) The family's wishes should be adhered to if they do not conflict with the wishes of the patient.
2) Consideration must be given to the family members' coping abilities.
3) If a family member (generally limited to one member) desires to be present during resuscitation efforts:
a) Prepare the family members for what to expect.
b) Drape the patient appropriately.
c) Set limits before entering the room; explain where they may stand and if they may touch the patient, such as hold the patient's hand.
d) If the patient is not responding to resuscitation efforts and death is imminent, allow the family member time to talk to the patient.
e) If the code team asks the family member to leave, escort him or her out and make sure that someone stays with the family member.
d. If resuscitation efforts are successful, allow family visitation as soon as possible.
e. If the resuscitation efforts are unsuccessful:
1) The family is usually informed of the patient's death by the physician.
2) Express your sympathy.
3) Answer whatever questions the family asks.
4) Ask the family members if they desire to see the body and prepare them for what they will see.
5) Prepare the body for visitation by discarding trash and removing clutter; remove the ET tube if legally acceptable (i.e., not a coroner's case) and remove any blood from the face and hands.
6) Place a couple of chairs close to the body and escort the family to the bedside; stay with them.
7) Contact the organ transplant coordinator.
3. Other patients
a. Screen the patient being resuscitated from other patients.
b. Make sure that other patients are being cared for during resuscitation efforts on a patient.
4. The staff
a. Ensure constructively critical multidisciplinary debriefing of the resuscitation efforts aids in quality improvement, team building, and stress reduction.
1) Performance of the team as a team; critique of the poor performance of an individual member should not occur in a group setting
2) Adequacy of supplies and equipment
b. Counseling services should be available for staff.

Evaluation
1. Patient airway, adequate oxygenation (i.e., normal PaO_2, SpO_2, SaO_2) and ventilation (i.e., normal $PaCO_2$)
2. Absence of clinical indications of respiratory distress
3. Stable cardiac rate and rhythm
4. Stable hemodynamic status
5. Alert and oriented with no neurologic deficit
6. Control of chest pain, discomfort, or dyspnea

Dysrhythmias and Blocks

Definitions
1. Dysrhythmia: any cardiac rhythm other than sinus rhythm at a normal rate
a. Sinus
b. Atrial
c. Junctional
d. Ventricular
2. Block: failure of an intrinsic impulse to be conducted through the conduction system
a. AV blocks: differentiation of degrees and types of blocks (Fig. 3.64)
b. Bundle branch blocks
1) LBBB
a) Hemiblocks: blockage of one of the two major branches of the LBB; these are diagnosed by axis deviation and exclusion of other causes
i) Left anterior hemiblock
ii) Left posterior hemiblock
2) RBBB

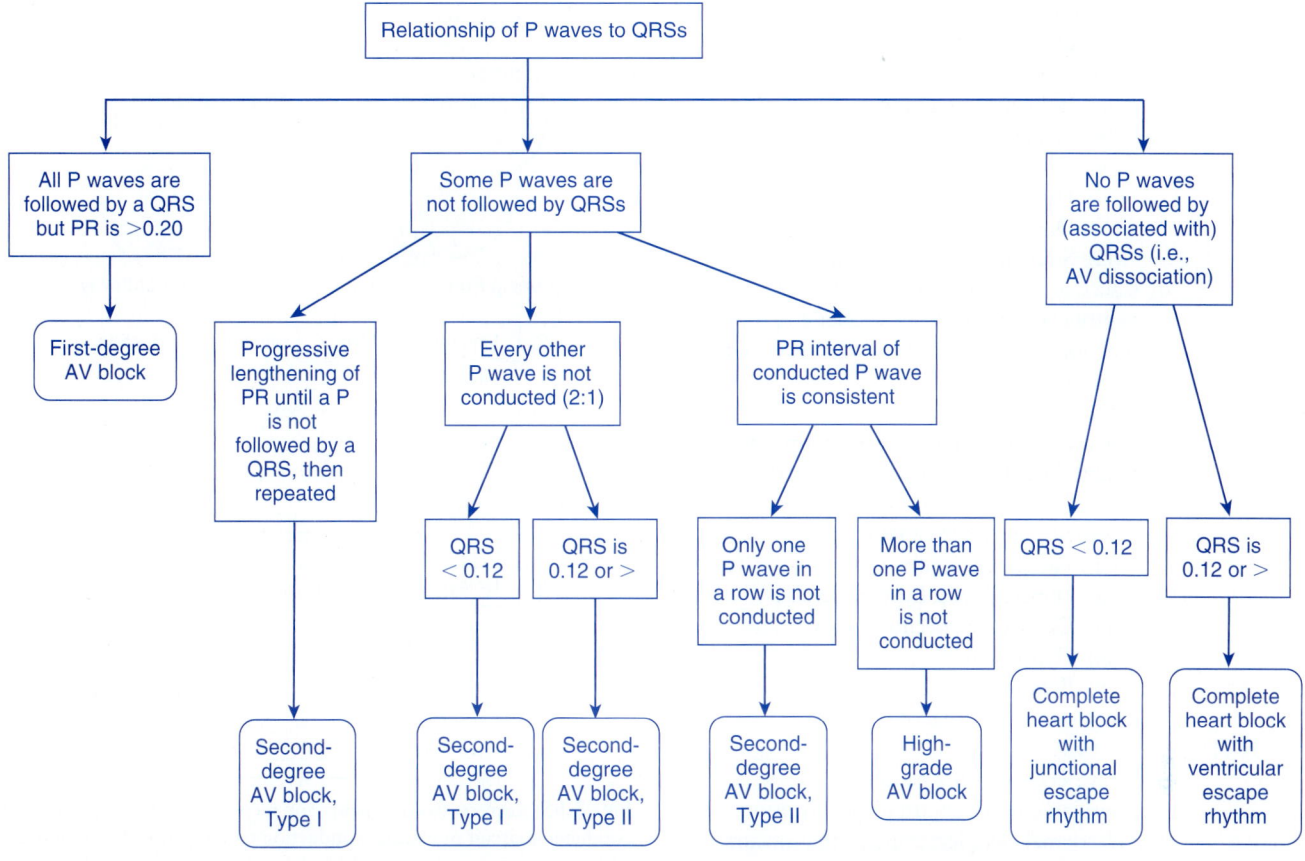

Fig. 3.64 Differentiation of degrees and types of atrioventricular block.

Etiology
1. General
   a. Congenital
      1) Long QT syndrome
         a) Two types with separate gene affected
            i) Romano-Ward syndrome
            ii) Lange-Nielsen syndrome: associated with deafness
         b) Manifestations
            i) ECG characteristics: prolonged QT interval; sustained or nonsustained torsades de pointes
            ii) Loss of consciousness, seizures, or cardiac arrest
      2) Brugada syndrome
         a) Autosomal dominant pattern in 50% of cases; more common in Southeast Asians and Japanese
         b) Manifestations
            i) ECG characteristics
               (a) ST-segment elevation and negative T wave in leads V_1 and V_2
               (b) RBBB
               (c) Prolonged PR interval
            ii) Sudden cardiac arrest may occur as a result of polymorphic VT and VF; dysrhythmias may be triggered by antidysrhythmics (IA, IC, or III) which prolong the QT interval; antimalarials; antidepressants (e.g., tricyclics such as amitriptyline); fever; hyperglycemia; cocaine; or lithium.
      3) Accessory pathways
         a) WPW syndrome
         b) Long-Ganong-Levine syndrome
         c) Mahaim fibers
   b. Myocardial ischemia or infarction
   c. Hypoxemia or hypoxia
   d. Electrolyte imbalance
   e. Acid–base imbalance
   f. SNS stimulation via endogenous catecholamines or sympathomimetic drugs (e.g., epinephrine, dopamine)
   g. Parasympathetic (i.e., vagal) stimulation
   h. Drug effects or toxicity
      1) "Holiday heart" syndrome caused by excessive alcohol consumption; this binge drinking may cause acute dysrhythmias, usually a SVT
2. Etiology Specific to Each Dysrhythmia (Appendix D)

Pathophysiology: Arrhythmogenic Mechanisms
1. Problems with impulse formation
   a. Altered automaticity
      1) Enhanced automaticity
         a) Abnormal condition of latent pacemaker cells in which their firing rate is increased beyond their inherent rate (even nonpacemaker cells may depolarize spontaneously)
         b) Resting membrane potential is less negative, or threshold potential is lower, increasing the chance of depolarization.

c) Caused by:
   i) Hypoxia
   ii) Hypercapnia
   iii) Ischemia, infarction
   iv) Hypokalemia, hypocalcemia
   v) Catecholamines
   vi) Hyperthermia
   vii) Digitalis toxicity
   viii) Stretching of the heart muscle
d) Cause of most atrial, junctional, and ventricular ectopic beats; accelerated junctional rhythm; accelerated idioventricular rhythm; and some VT

2) Depressed automaticity
   a) Resting membrane potential is more negative or threshold potential is higher, decreasing the chance of depolarization.
   b) Caused by any of the following:
      i) Vagal stimulation
      ii) Hyperkalemia, hypercalcemia
      iii) Decreased catecholamines
      iv) Hypothermia
      v) Beta-blockers
   c) Cause of bradycardia or blocks

b. Triggered activity
   1) Repetitive ectopic firing caused by afterdepolarizations; an afterdepolarization is an abnormal electrical impulse that occurs during or after repolarization of an action potential
   2) If an afterdepolarization is strong enough to reach threshold, a triggered beat or rhythm occurs.
   3) This activity is not self-generating but is dependent on the preceding beat.
   4) They may be early or late.
      a) Early: occur when the QT is prolonged
         i) Caused by: prolongation of repolarization and effective refractory period
         ii) Example: torsades de pointes
      b) Delayed: the result of elevated intracellular calcium
         i) Caused by
            (a) Electrolyte imbalances
            (b) Catecholamines
         ii) Cause of tachycardias of digitalis toxicity

2. Problems with impulse conduction
   a. Reentry (Fig. 3.65): the most common mechanism for tachydysrhythmias
      1) An impulse travels through an area of the myocardium and depolarizes it, but then reenters the same area to depolarize it again.
      2) Requirements
         a) An available circuit: reentry can occur in areas of the heart where conduction velocity is abnormally slow.
         b) Unequal responsiveness of two segments of the circuit (i.e., delay in one limb of the circuit)

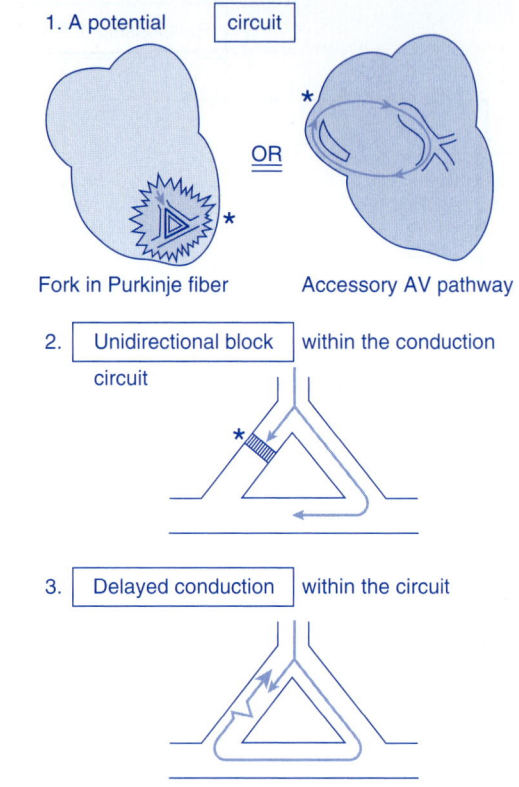

Fig. 3.65 Reentry. Requirements for reentry include (1) a potential conduction circuit or circular conduction pathway, (2) a block or delay within part of the circuit, and (3) delayed conduction within the remainder of the circuit. *AV*, Atrioventricular. (From Aehlert, B. [2011]. *ECGs made easy* [4th ed.]. St. Louis: Mosby.)

   c) An area of slowed conduction or unidirectional block
      i) Conduction must be slow enough to allow time for the previously stimulated area to recover the ability to conduct.
      ii) The area of unidirectional block provides a return pathway for the original stimulus to reenter a previously stimulated area and time to repolarize.
   3) Caused by:
      a) Myocardial ischemia or infarction
      b) Electrolyte imbalance
      c) Antidysrhythmic drugs
   4) Cause of any of the following:
      a) Some ectopy
      b) Some VTs
      c) Most SVTs
      d) Tachycardias seen with accessory pathways

b. Accessory pathways (Fig. 3.66)
   1) Lown-Ganong-Levine syndrome
      a) Caused by:
         i) AV nodal bypass tract
         ii) AV node smaller than normal
         iii) Fibers running through AV node that do not have the built-in delay feature that nodal fibers have

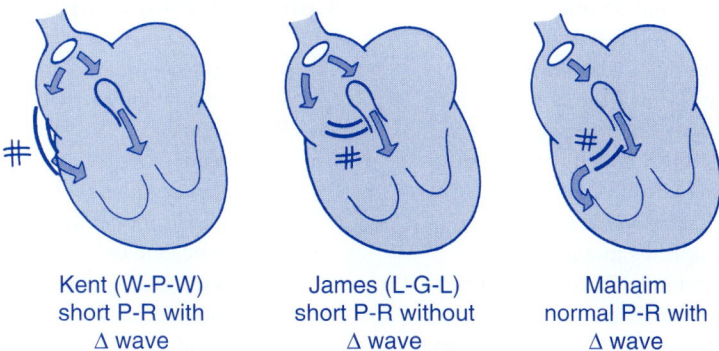

Fig. 3.66 Accessory pathways. Location of accessory pathways and corresponding electrocardiogram characteristics. *L-G-L*, Lown-Ganong-Levine; *W-P-W*, Wolff-Parkinson-White. (From Aehlert, B. [2009]. *ECGs made easy* [3rd ed.]. St. Louis: Mosby.)

b) Cause of:
   i) History of palpitations
   ii) Tachydysrhythmias with short PR, normal QRS
2) WPW syndrome
   a) Caused by Kent bundle, which bypasses the AV node
      i) Type A: Kent bundle on left; R wave in V_1 with inverted T wave and depressed ST
      ii) Type B: Kent bundle on right; QS in V_1 with upright T wave and elevated ST
   b) Cause of:
      i) Tachydysrhythmias
         (a) History of palpitations
         (b) Short PR, wide QRS with slurring of first portion of QRS (referred to as a *delta wave*) (Fig. 3.67)
         (c) QRS morphology during tachycardia
            (i) Wide QRS: sinus impulse may take accessory pathway around the mandatory delay in the AV node (referred to as *preexcitation*) causing severe SVTs with a wide QRS
            (ii) Narrow QRS: impulse may also take AV node but reenter via accessory pathway; narrow QRS
         (d) Treatment
            (i) Antidysrhythmics: amiodarone, flecainide, procainamide, propafenone, or sotalol
            (ii) Cardioversion if drugs fail to convert
            (iii) Avoid adenosine, calcium channel blockers, and digoxin.
            (iv) Long-term treatment: ablation via catheter or surgically

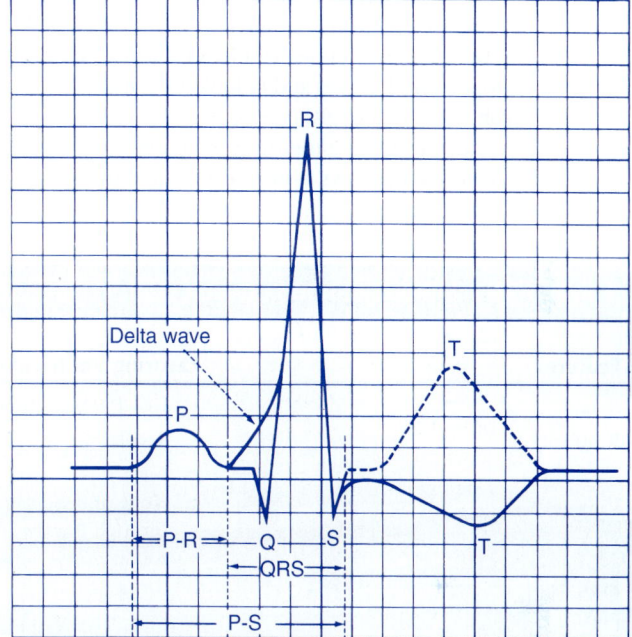

Fig. 3.67 Wolff-Parkinson-White syndrome. Note the short PR interval, the delta wave, widened QRS complex, and T-wave inversion characteristic of preexcitation. (From Kinney, M. R., Dunbar, S., & Brooks-Brunn, J. A. [1998]. *AACN's clinical reference for critical-care nursing* [4th ed.]. St. Louis: Mosby.)

3) Mahaim fibers
   a) Caused by nodoventricular or fasciculoventricular fibers
   b) Cause of:
      i) Tachydysrhythmias
         (a) History of palpitations
         (b) Normal PR interval with LBBB pattern
      ii) Normal PR, narrow QRS with rS in lead III when in sinus rhythm
c. Aberrant conduction
   1) Aberrant conduction occurs most often when:
      a) Rate is rapid.
      b) Very premature atrial contractions
      c) There are changes in cycle length (e.g., atrial fibrillation [QRS that ends a short cycle length after a long cycle length is likely to be conducted aberrantly is referred to as *Ashman phenomenon*]).

2) Because one of the bundle branches (usually the right) is still refractory when a supraventricular impulse reaches it, the impulse must travel down the nonrefractory bundle and across to the other ventricle; this causes a wide QRS which is frequently mistaken for a premature ventricular contraction (PVC) if a single complex or VT if several complexes in a row
3) Unlike ectopy, aberrancy is no more serious than the supraventricular mechanism that caused it (e.g., atrial fibrillation with aberrancy is no more clinically significant than atrial fibrillation).
4) QRS morphology is the most important criterion in the differentiation between ectopy and aberrancy, but other criteria may also be helpful (Table 3.18); multiple-lead ECG is often helpful to identify P waves and in looking at the morphology of the QRS.
5) Ectopy is more common than aberrancy; if in doubt, always assume ectopy and treat accordingly.

Clinical Presentation
1. Anxiety, restlessness
2. Vertigo, syncope
3. Weakness, fatigue, activity intolerance
4. Palpitations
5. Chest pain
6. Clinical indications of LVF: dyspnea; S_3; crackles
7. Clinical indications of hypoperfusion (Table 3.2)
8. Diagnostic studies
   a. Electrocardiography: multiple-lead ECG
   b. Serum electrolyte levels
   c. Drug levels
   d. ABGs

Collaborative Management
1. Assess for clinical manifestations of hypoperfusion (Table 3.2): follow ACLS algorithms for lethal dysrhythmias (see Cardiopulmonary Arrest section of this chapter).
2. Treat cause of the dysrhythmia; some examples include the following:
   a. Decrease psychological and physical stress.
   b. Correct ischemia or infarction if possible with reperfusion therapies such as PCI or fibrinolytics.

Table 3.18 Differentiation between Ventricular Ectopy and Aberrancy

Features	Favoring Ventricular Ectopy	Favoring Supraventricular Origin with Aberrancy
Rate	• 130–150 beats/min	• >150 beats/min
Regularity	• Regular	• Irregular (because most likely to be atrial fibrillation)
P wave	• None or dissociated (AV dissociation) • Inverted P wave after QRS (retrograde conduction to atria)	• Premature
QRS width	• >0.14 sec	• 0.12–0.14 sec
QRS morphology	• Initial vector opposite normal beats • Precordial concordance (all QRSs V_1–V_6 positive or all QRSs V_1–V_6 negative) • QRS morphology similar to previously seen PVCs	• Initial vector same as normal beats
QRS morphology in V_1 NOTE: Upper case letters indicate large waves; lower case letters indicate small waves.	• Monophasic R • Rr′ with left peak taller • Biphasic qR • Biphasic Rs or rS	• Monophasic QS • Biphasic rS • Triphasic rSR′ or rR′
QRS morphology in V_6 NOTE: Upper case letters indicate large waves; lower case letters indicate small waves.	• Monophasic QS • Biphasic qR • Biphasic rS	• Monophasic R • Triphasic qRs
Fusion beats	• Yes	• No
Compensatory pause after single beat or at end of run	• Yes	• No
Axis	• Indeterminate or LAD of −30 or greater	• Normal or RAD
Patient history	• History of PVCs • History of heart disease	• History of PACs, atrial fibrillation • History of preexisting bundle branch block
Response to carotid massage	• No effect on ventricular rate	• Often causes at least temporary slowing of ventricular rate
BP	• Usually very low or absent (but may be normal)	• Moderately low or normal
Consciousness	• Frequently unconscious (but may be conscious)	• May complain of lightheadedness
Seizures	• Frequently present (but may be absent)	• Absent

AV, Atrioventricular; *LAD, BP*, blood pressure; left anterior descending coronary artery; *PVC*, premature ventricular contraction; *RAD*, right-axis deviation.

c. Correct hypoxemia and hypoxia with oxygen.
d. Correct electrolyte imbalance with electrolyte replacement or restriction or dialysis.
e. Correct acid–base imbalance by treating the cause.
   1) Improve oxygen delivery to the tissues if lactic acidosis is present.
   2) Insulin and fluid administration for diabetic ketoacidosis
   3) Dialysis for renal failure with metabolic acidosis
f. Correct drug toxicity by withholding the suspected drug and antidote (e.g., digoxin immune fab) or dialysis if appropriate.
g. Administer beta-blockers for hyperthyroidism.
3. Correct ischemia if possible.
   a. Coronary artery vasodilators and/or antispasmodics: nitrates, calcium channel blockers
   b. Fibrinolytics
   c. PCI
4. Correct hypoxemia or hypoxia
   a. Improve SaO₂ (e.g., oxygen, ET intubation, mechanical ventilation, PEEP).
   b. Improve CO (e.g., inotropes, vasodilators, IABP).
   c. Improve Hgb (e.g., blood).
5. Correct electrolyte imbalances.
   a. Replace deficient electrolytes.
   b. Decrease excessive electrolyte levels (e.g., electrolyte restriction, diuretics, ion exchange resins, dialysis).
6. Correct acidosis.
   a. Improve perfusion to correct metabolic acidosis caused by lactic acid.
   b. Initiate dialysis for patients with renal failure.
   c. Provide hydration and insulin therapy for patients in diabetic ketoacidosis.
   d. Improve ventilation to correct respiratory acidosis.
7. Eliminate cause of catecholamine release or block effects.
   a. Treat pain.
   b. Decrease anxiety with relaxation techniques and anxiolytics.
   c. Administer beta-blockers for cardioprotection as prescribed.
8. Initiate standing orders (e.g., IV, oxygen, multiple-lead ECG)
9. Initiate antidysrhythmic therapy as indicated by standing orders or as prescribed.
   a. Vaughan-Williams classification system (Table 3.19)

Table 3.19 Vaughan-Williams Antidysrhythmic Classification System

Class	Effect	Examples
IA	• Blocks sodium influx, which depresses the rate of depolarization • Delays repolarization and prolongs action potential duration • Decreases contractility (negative inotrope) • Prolongs QT (torsades de pointes potential) and QRS duration	• Quinidine • Procainamide • Disopyramide
IB	• Blocks sodium influx during phase 0, which depresses the rate of depolarization • Accelerates repolarization and shortens action potential duration • Suppresses ventricular automaticity in ischemic tissue	• Lidocaine • Mexiletine • Phenytoin
IC	• Blocks sodium influx, which depresses the rate of depolarization • Does not change repolarization and action potential duration • Has pronounced proarrhythmogenic potential	• Flecainide • Propafenone

II	• Depresses SA node automaticity
	• Increases refractory period of atrial and AV junctional tissue to slow conduction velocity
	• Shortens action potential duration
	• Inhibits sympathetic activity (i.e., blocks beta receptors)
	• Reduces atrial and ventricular contractility
		• Beta-blockers
		  • Propranolol
		  • Esmolol
		  • Acebutolol
		  • Sotalol (both II and III)

III	• Blocks potassium movement during phase III • Delays repolarization and increases action potential duration • Prolongs effective refractory period	• Amiodarone • Sotalol (both II and III) • Ibutilide • Dofetilide

IV	• Blocks calcium movement during phase II
	• Depresses automaticity in the SA and AV nodes
	• Prolongs the conduction time in the AV junction and increases the refractory period at the AV junction
	• Decreases contractility
		• Calcium channel blockers
		  • Verapamil
		  • Diltiazem

Misc.	• Blocks reentry mechanism • Shortens action potential of atrial tissue with little or no effect on action potential of ventricle • Prolongs AV nodal refractory period • Decreases SA node automaticity and slows sinus rate	• Adenosine
Misc.	• Blocks parasympathetic nervous system effects to increase SA node firing rate and improve AV nodal conduction	• Atropine
Misc.	• Slows conduction through AV node • Prolongs AV nodal refractory period • Decreases SA node automaticity and slows sinus rate	• Digoxin

AV, Atrioventricular; *SA*, sinoatrial.

b. Drugs and treatments of choice for each dysrhythmia (Appendix D)
    1) Information regarding indications, actions, dosage, contraindications, and adverse effects of selected antidysrhythmic agents (Table 3.20)
c. Monitor closely for adverse effects of antidysrhythmic agents.
10. Use electrical therapies as indicated.
    a. Cardioversion
        1) Uses
            a) Urgent cardioversion is used for tachydysrhythmias (other than sinus) that is rapid enough to cause hemodynamic compromise or that has not responded to antidysrhythmic drug therapy.
            b) Elective cardioversion is performed for tachydysrhythmias that are reasonably well-tolerated hemodynamically but have not responded to antidysrhythmic drug therapy.
        2) Contraindications
            a) Tachydysrhythmias that result from digitalis toxicity
            b) Nonsustained tachydysrhythmias
            c) Long-standing atrial fibrillation
            d) Atrial fibrillation with normal or slow ventricular rate in the absence of AV nodal blocking drugs
            e) Multifocal atrial tachycardia
        3) Method: as for defibrillation except:
            a) Conscious patients should be sedated with diazepam, lorazepam, or midazolam.
            b) Elective procedures should be preceded by at least a 6-hour fast.
            c) Anterior-posterior electrode placement is preferable for cardioversion of atrial fibrillation.
            d) Emergency equipment and drugs must be available.
            e) Synchronizer switch is on so that charge is delivered only during QRS, avoiding the descending limb of the T wave.
            f) Voltage is from 50 to 200 J (Neumar et al., 2010).
                i) Narrow and regular: 50 to 100 J
                ii) Narrow and irregular: 120 to 200 J biphasic or 200 J monophasic
                iii) Wide and regular: 100 J
                iv) Wide and irregular: defibrillate with 120 to 200 J biphasic or 360 J monophasic rather than synchronized cardioversion.
            g) Antidysrhythmic drug therapy is used after sinus rhythm is restored.
        4) Complications: as for defibrillation
    b. Defibrillation: see Cardiopulmonary Arrest
11. Use pacemaker therapies for patients who have problem with impulse formation or conduction.
    a. Definition: an electronic device that delivers an electrical stimulus to the heart to cause depolarization of the myocardium and increase or decrease the HR
        1) Terminology used to discuss pacemakers (Table 3.21)
    b. Indications for pacemaker
        1) Sick sinus syndrome with syncope
            a) Symptomatic bradydysrhythmias
            b) Sinus block or sinus arrest with ventricular asystole
            c) Alternating tachycardia and bradycardia (called *tachy-brady syndrome*)
        2) Hypersensitive carotid sinus syndrome
        3) AV blocks
            a) Second-degree AV block type I with symptomatic bradycardia
            b) Second-degree AV block type II
            c) Third-degree AV block
        4) Bundle branch block with AV block
        5) Bifascicular block (i.e., LBBB or RBBB with hemiblock) with acute MI
        6) Trifascicular block (e.g., bilateral bundle branch block)
        7) Refractory tachydysrhythmias unresponsive to drug therapy or cardioversion (referred to as *tachycardia overdrive*); an important treatment modality for torsades de pointes
        8) Hypertrophic cardiomyopathy or HF are indications for biventricular pacing.
        9) Prophylactic use during cardiac surgery in patients with acute coronary syndrome or cardiac dysrhythmias
        10) Note that pacemakers are not currently recommended for cardiac arrest with ventricular asystole.
    c. Components
        1) Pulse generator
            a) Components
                i) Battery
                    (a) Lithium-iodide batteries in permanent pacemakers last approximately 7 to 10 years
                ii) Microprocessor that controls pacing (voltage) and sensing
            b) Types
                i) Single chamber atrial
                ii) Single chamber ventricular
                iii) Dual-chamber AV
                iv) Dual-chamber biventricular
        2) Lead(s)
            a) Atrial
            b) Ventricular
        3) Electrode(s)
            a) Unipolar
                i) Negative only
                ii) Metal of pulse generator acts as positive
            b) Bipolar
                i) Positive: proximal; sensing
                ii) Negative: distal; pacing
    d. Types of pacemakers
        1) Temporary or permanent
            a) Temporary (external pulse generator): hours to weeks
                i) Transthoracic epicardial
                    (a) Electrodes attached to epicardium of atrium, ventricle, or both during cardiac surgery and brought through the chest wall

Table 3.20 Selected Antidysrhythmic Agents

Drug	Classification and Actions	Indications	Administration	Adverse Effects	Nursing Implications
Procainamide hydrochloride	Class IA antidysrhythmic • Increases atrial refractoriness • Decreases automaticity, conductivity, contractility • Causes peripheral vasodilation	• Supraventricular dysrhythmias • Ventricular dysrhythmias	• PO 0.5–1 g every 4–6 hr • IM 250–500 mg every 4–6 hr • IV injection: 50–100 mg every 5 min • Stop injections and start maintenance infusion when suppression of dysrhythmia; widening of QRS by 50%; hypotension; or a total of 17 mg/kg occur • IV infusion: mix 2 g in 500 ml (4 mg/ml) and infuse at 1–4 mg/min • Therapeutic blood level 3–10 mcg/ml	• Bradycardia • Hypotension with IV administration • AV block • Dysrhythmias, including torsades de pointes • Anorexia, nausea, vomiting, abdominal pain, diarrhea • Hepatic dysfunction • Bitter taste • Rash, urticaria • Fever • Mental depression • Hallucinations • Seizures • Bone marrow depression, thrombocytopenia • Worsening HF • Lupus-like syndrome	• Monitor BP, HR, ECG • ECG effects include increased PR interval, QRS width, and QT interval • Note contraindications: known hypersensitivity, myasthenia gravis, AV block • Use cautiously in renal disease, liver disease, HF, respiratory depression, patient receiving digitalis • Administer PO drug with food • Instruct patient to report fever, rash, muscle pain, bruising or bleeding, diarrhea, chest pain
Lidocaine hydrochloride	Class IB antidysrhythmic • Decreases ventricular automaticity and excitability • Increases ventricular fibrillation threshold	• Ventricular dysrhythmias	• IV injection: VF: 1.5 mg/kg repeated every 3–5 min VT: 1 mg/kg repeated every 5–10 min • Maximum: 3 mg/kg • IV infusion: mix 2 g in 500 ml (4 mg/ml) and infuse at 1–4 mg/min • Therapeutic blood level: 2–5 mcg/ml	• Hypotension • SA arrest • AV block • Nausea, vomiting • Tremors • Restlessness • Lightheadedness • Anaphylaxis • Clinical indications of toxicity (in relative order of occurrence) • Perioral paresthesias • Feelings of dissociation • Dizziness • Drowsiness • Euphoria • Mild agitation • Dysarthria • Hearing impairment • Disorientation • Confusion • Muscle twitching • Seizures • Respiratory arrest	• Monitor BP, HR, ECG • Note contraindications: known hypersensitivity, AV block, supraventricular dysrhythmias, sick sinus syndrome • Use cautiously in liver disease, HF, respiratory depression, and malignant hyperthermia and in older adults • Note that toxicity incidence is increased if patient has HF or liver disease, has low lean body mass or is elderly, or is concurrently taking cimetidine or beta-blocker • Note that the administration of prophylactic lidocaine after MI is no longer recommended; although the incidence of VF is decreased, the incidence of asystole is increased

Continued

Table 3.20 Selected Antidysrhythmic Agents—cont'd

Drug	Classification and Actions	Indications	Administration	Adverse Effects	Nursing Implications
Mexiletine	Class IB antidysrhythmic • Decreases ventricular automaticity and excitability • Increases ventricular fibrillation threshold	• Life-threatening ventricular dysrhythmias	• PO: initial dose of 200–400 mg followed by 200–400 bid, tic, or qid; maximum: 1200 mg/day	• Proarrhythmia, including PVCs, ventricular tachycardia, torsades de pointes, PACs, supraventricular tachycardia, bradycardia, AV block, bundle branch block • Hypotension • Nausea, vomiting • Diarrhea or constipation • Elevated liver enzymes • Palpitations • Chest pain • Dyspnea • Headache • Paresthesia, tremors, nystagmus, ataxia, dysarthria • Tinnitus • Blurred vision • Dizziness • Drowsiness, insomnia • Confusion • Seizures	• Monitor HR, BP, ECG • Note contraindications: second- or third-degree block or sick sinus syndrome without pacemaker, cardiogenic shock • Administer with meals to decrease GI adverse effects • Note that risk of toxicity is greater if patient is concurrently receiving cimetidine or beta-blocker; dosage is adjusted in heart failure and liver disease • Monitor closely for clinical indications of toxicity: tremor; dizziness; ataxia; nystagmus
Flecainide	Class IC antidysrhythmic • Blocks sodium influx during phase 0, which depresses the rate of depolarization • Does not change repolarization and action potential duration	• Life-threatening or refractory ventricular dysrhythmias • Atrial or ventricular dysrhythmias that do not respond to other drugs	• PO: 50–200 mg twice daily; maximum dose 400 mg/day	• Proarrhythmia including PVCs, VT, torsades de pointes, PACs, supraventricular tachycardia, bradycardia, SA block or arrest, AV block, bundle branch block • Nausea, vomiting, abdominal pain, constipation • Dyspnea • Chest pain • Headache • Drowsiness • Dizziness • Blurred vision • Tremor • Dry mouth	• Monitor HR, BP, ECG • Report widening of QRS of >25% • Monitor closely for heart failure • Note contraindications: known hypersensitivity, second- or third-degree AV block, cardiogenic shock • Use cautiously in heart failure, SA or bifascicular blocks or sick sinus syndrome without a pacemaker, renal disease, liver disease, myasthenia gravis • Use cautiously in patient also receiving another negative inotropic agent (e.g., verapamil, procainamide, beta-blocker) • Correct electrolyte imbalance before therapy if possible

Drug	Action	Uses	Dosage	Side/Adverse Effects	Nursing Considerations
Propafenone	Class IC antidysrhythmic • Blocks sodium influx during phase 0, which depresses the rate of depolarization • Does not change repolarization and action potential duration	• Life-threatening or refractory ventricular dysrhythmias • Atrial fibrillation	• PO: 150–300 mg tid; maximum: 900 mg/day	• Proarrhythmia, including PVCs, VT, torsades de pointes, PACs, supraventricular tachycardia, bradycardia, SA block or arrest, AV block, bundle branch block • AV block • Nausea, vomiting, constipation • Heart failure • Dyspnea, bronchospasm • Dizziness • Diplopia • Paresthesia • Headache • Bitter or metallic taste • Leukopenia, agranulocytosis, thrombocytopenia, anemia • Bruising	• Monitor HR, BP, ECG • Report widening of QRS of >25% • Monitor closely for clinical indications of heart failure • Note contraindications: heart failure, cardiogenic shock, SA, AV, bifascicular blocks or sick sinus syndrome without a pacemaker, myasthenia gravis, COPD, hypotension • Use cautiously in patients with renal or liver disease; dosage may be adjusted • Use cautiously if the patient is also receiving another negative inotropic agent (e.g., verapamil, procainamide, beta-blocker) • Use cautiously in patients receiving digitalis because this drug can increase plasma concentration • Use cautiously in patients receiving oral anticoagulants because propafenone can increase plasma concentration • Administer with food to diminish GI adverse effects • Correct electrolytes before therapy • Instruct patient to report recurrent or persistent infection

Continued

Table 3.20 Selected Antidysrhythmic Agents—cont'd

Drug	Classification and Actions	Indications	Administration	Adverse Effects	Nursing Implications
Propranolol	Noncardioselective beta-blocker Class II antidysrhythmic • Decreases heart rate, contractility, automaticity, excitability, conductivity • Depresses sinus node automaticity • Increases AV nodal refractoriness and decreases conduction velocity • Decreases myocardial oxygen consumption	• Supraventricular and ventricular dysrhythmias • Hypertension • Angina • Pheochromocytoma • Hyperthyroid crisis • MI (primary prevention and secondary prevention of extension and reinfarction) • Hypertrophic cardiomyopathy	• PO: 10–80 mg tid or qid • IV injection: 0.1 mg/kg in three divided doses at rate not to exceed 1 mg/min • IV infusion: mix 20 mg in 250 ml (0.08 mg/ml); usual dose: 3–8 mg/hr • Therapeutic blood level: 0.04–0.90 mcg/ml	• Bradycardia • AV block • Hypotension • Nausea, vomiting, diarrhea • Fatigue, lethargy • Rash • Syncope • HF • Bronchospasm, especially in patients with asthma • Mental depression • Hyperglycemia in type 2 DM • Asymptomatic hypoglycemia in type 1 DM • Impotence • Emotional lability • Insomnia • Agranulocytosis, thrombocytopenia	• Monitor HR, BP, ECG • Monitor for clinical indications of HF • Note contraindications: known hypersensitivity, sinus bradycardia, AV block >first degree, HF, shock, asthma, Raynaud syndrome • Use cautiously in DM, renal disease, hyperthyroidism, COPD, liver disease, myasthenia gravis, peripheral vascular disease, hypotension • May potentiate the hypoglycemic effects of insulin and prevents sympathetic symptoms of hypoglycemia • Note that this drug limits cardiac reserve and exercise capacity because heart rate cannot increase • Note that this drug masks sympathetic clinical indications of shock because receptors are blocked
Esmolol	Cardioselective beta-blocker Class II antidysrhythmic • Decreases heart rate, contractility, automaticity, excitability, conductivity • Depresses sinus node automaticity • Increases AV nodal refractoriness and decreases conduction velocity • Decreases myocardial oxygen consumption	• Supraventricular tachycardia • Intraoperative or postoperative tachycardia or hypertension	• IV injection: loading dose of 500mcg/kg over 1 min followed by maintenance dose of 50 mcg/kg/min for 4 min • If desired effect does not occur, repeat the loading dose of 500 mcg/kg over 1 min and follow with a dose increased by 50 mcg/kg/min for 4 min (e.g., 500 + 100, 500 + 150, 500 + 200) • IV infusion: when desired effect is achieved, no additional loading doses are needed and the maintenance dose is increased by 50 mcg/kg/min and maintained	• Bradycardia • Hypotension • AV block • Nausea, vomiting • Fatigue, lethargy • HF • Bronchospasm, especially in patients with asthma • Urinary retention • Inflammation and induration at injection site	• Monitor HR, BP, ECG • Monitor for clinical indications of HF • Note contraindications: known hypersensitivity, bradycardia, AV block >first degree, HF, shock, asthma • Use cautiously in DM, renal disease, hyperthyroidism, COPD, liver disease, myasthenia gravis, peripheral vascular disease, hypotension • May potentiate the hypoglycemic effects of insulin and prevent sympathetic symptoms of hypoglycemia; masks sympathetic clinical indications of shock because receptors are blocked

Metoprolol	Cardioselective beta-blocker Class II antidysrhythmic • Decreases heart rate, contractility, automaticity, excitability, conductivity • Depresses sinus node automaticity • Increases AV nodal refractoriness and decreases conduction velocity • Decreases myocardial oxygen consumption	• Hypertension • Angina • Myocardial infarction (primary prevention and secondary prevention of extension and reinfarction)	• PO: 100–450 mg/day in one or two doses • IV injection: 5 mg IV slowly at 5-min intervals to a total of 15 mg	• Bradycardia • AV block • Hypotension • Nausea, vomiting, diarrhea, constipation • Fatigue, lethargy • Rash • Syncope • HF • Dyspnea, wheezing • Mental depression • Hyperglycemia in type 2 DM • Asymptomatic hypoglycemia in type 1 DM • Impotence • Emotional lability • Agranulocytosis, thrombocytopenia	• Monitor HR, BP, ECG • Monitor for clinical indications of HF • Note contraindications: known hypersensitivity, sinus bradycardia, AV block >first degree, HF, shock, asthma, Raynaud syndrome • Use cautiously in DM, renal disease, hyperthyroidism, COPD, liver disease, myasthenia gravis, peripheral vascular disease, hypotension • May potentiate the hypoglycemic effects of insulin and prevents sympathetic symptoms of hypoglycemia • Note that this drug limits cardiac reserve and exercise capacity because heart rate cannot increase • Note that this drug masks sympathetic clinical indications of shock because receptors are blocked
Sotalol (NOTE: Class II and III)	Class II and III antidysrhythmic • Depresses SA node automaticity • Increases refractory period of atrial and AV junctional tissue to slow conduction • Shortens action potential duration • Inhibits sympathetic activity • Blocks potassium movement during phase III • Increases action potential duration • Prolongs effective refractory period	• Life-threatening or refractory ventricular dysrhythmias	• PO: initial 80 mg bid followed by 160–320 mg/daily divided into two to three doses • IV injection: 100 mg (1.5 mg/kg) over 5 min	• Proarrhythmia including torsades de pointes, sinus bradycardia; second- or third-degree AV block • Heart failure • Hypotension • Dyspnea • Bronchospasm (especially in patients with history of asthma) • Headache	• Monitor HR, BP, ECG • Report prolongation of QT interval to more than half of RR interval or hypotension • Monitor serum glucose in patients with DM • Monitor closely for clinical indications of HF • Note contraindications: second- or third-degree AV block, SA block without pacemaker, QT prolongation • Do not administer concurrently or within 4 hr of class IA antiarrhythmics or other class III antiarrhythmics; do not administer with other drugs that prolong the QT interval such as phenothiazines, tricyclic antidepressants • Correct electrolytes before therapy • Warn patient not to discontinue abruptly

Continued

Table 3.20 Selected Antidysrhythmic Agents—cont'd

Drug	Classification and Actions	Indications	Administration	Adverse Effects	Nursing Implications
Amiodarone hydrochloride	Class III Antidysrhythmic • Prolongs the action potential and effective refractory period	• Life-threatening or refractory ventricular dysrhythmias • Refractory supraventricular dysrhythmias especially those caused by WPW syndrome	• PO: loading dose of 800–1600 mg/day for 1–3 wk; then 600–800 mg/day for 1 month; then 200–800 mg/day • IV injection (loading dose): 150 mg over 10 min followed by: • IV infusion: mix 900 mg in 500 m (1.8 mg/ml); usual dose is 1 mg/min for the next 6 hr followed by 0.5 mg/min • Use central venous catheter if more concentrated solution is used • Use solutions diluted in PVC containers within 2 hr; solutions diluted in glass or polyolefin containers within 24 hr • Administer through PVC tubing because dosing has taken into account adsorption to tubing • Therapeutic blood level: 1.5–2.5 mcg/ml	• Hypotension • Proarrhythmia, including PVCs, ventricular tachycardia, torsades de pointes, PACs, supraventricular tachycardia, bradycardia, SA block or arrest, AV block, bundle branch block • HF • Nausea, vomiting • Dizziness • Headache • Fatigue, malaise, muscle weakness • Corneal microdeposits • Rash, photosensitivity • Altered liver enzymes, hepatotoxicity • Hyperthyroidism, hypothyroidism • Blue-gray skin discoloration • Tremors, peripheral neuropathies, extrapyramidal symptoms • Cough, progressive dyspnea, pulmonary fibrosis	• Monitor HR, BP, ECG, breath sounds, electrolytes, liver function studies, thyroid function studies, pulmonary function studies, chest radiography, neurologic symptoms • Monitor for clinical indications of HF, pulmonary fibrosis • Note contraindications: known hypersensitivity, marked sinus bradycardia, second- or third-degree AV block unless functioning pacemaker, cardiogenic shock • Use cautiously in patients with sinus node disease, conduction disturbances, severely depressed ventricular function, and marked cardiomegaly • Do not confuse amiodarone (an antidysrhythmic agent) with amrinone (an inotropic agent) • Advise methylcellulose ophthalmic solution and annual eye examinations for patients on long-term therapy • Advise use of SPF 15 sunscreen and sunglasses for patients on long-term therapy • Monitor for drug interactions: interacts with digitalis, anticoagulants, beta-blockers, calcium channel blockers, phenytoin, and class I antidysrhythmics • If used concurrently with digitalis, monitor closely for indications of digitalis toxicity • Administer PO drug with food to decrease GI adverse effects

Ibutilide	Class III antidysrhythmic • Blocks potassium movement during phase III • Increases action potential duration • Prolongs effective refractory period	Recent onset atrial fibrillation or atrial flutter	IV infusion: mix 1 mg in 50 ml and infuse over 10 min for patients weighing >60 kg (0.01 mg/kg in patients weighing <60 kg); may be repeated after 10 min if needed • Discontinue if atrial fibrillation or flutter terminates, a new dysrhythmia occurs or if prolongation of the QT occurs	• Proarrhythmia, including PVCs, ventricular tachycardia, torsades de pointes, PACs, supraventricular tachycardia, bradycardia, AV block, bundle branch block • Hypotension	• Monitor HR, BP, ECG • Report widening of QRS by >25% or prolongation of QT interval to more than half of RR interval or hypotension • Correct electrolyte imbalances (especially hypokalemia) before initiating ibutilide • Administer anticoagulants for 2–3 wk as prescribed for patients with atrial fibrillation of more than 2–3 d duration • Note contraindications: patients with second- or third-degree AV block, SA block without pacemaker, hypersensitivity to ibutilide, congenital or acquired long QT syndrome, in patient receiving verapamil or drugs that prolong the QT interval • Use cautiously in patients receiving digitalis because this drug may mask the cardiotoxicity associated with excessive digoxin levels • Do not administer concurrently or within 4 hr of class IA antiarrhythmics or other class III antiarrhythmics; do not administer with other drugs that prolong the QT interval such as phenothiazines, TCAs

Continued

Table 3.20 Selected Antidysrhythmic Agents—cont'd

Drug	Classification and Actions	Indications	Administration	Adverse Effects	Nursing Implications
Dofetilide	Class III antidysrhythmic • Blocks potassium movement during phase III • Increases action potential duration • Prolongs effective refractory period	• Recent onset of atrial fibrillation or atrial flutter • Maintenance of sinus rhythm in patients with highly symptomatic atrial flutter or atrial fibrillation of >1 wk duration	• PO: 500 mcg twice daily • Initiation of this oral therapy requires hospitalization for monitoring of QT interval while dosage is adjusted • Dosage is also adjusted according to creatinine clearance	• Proarrhythmia, including PVCs, ventricular tachycardia, torsades de pointes, PACs, supraventricular tachycardia, bradycardia, AV block, bundle branch block • Hypotension • Nausea • Syncope • Chest pain	• Monitor HR, BP, ECG • Report widening of QRS by >25% or prolongation of QT interval to more than half of RR interval or hypotension • Correct electrolyte imbalances (especially hypokalemia or hypomagnesemia) before initiating dofetilide • Note contraindications: patients with second- or third-degree AV block, SA block without pacemaker, hypersensitivity to dofetilide, in patient receiving verapamil or drugs that prolong the QT interval • Do not administer concurrently or within 4 hr of class IA antiarrhythmics or other class III antiarrhythmics; do not administer with other drugs that prolong the QT interval such as phenothiazines, TCAs
Verapamil	Calcium channel blocker Class IV antidysrhythmic • Depresses rate of SA node • Increases refractoriness of AV node • Relaxes vascular smooth muscle decreasing SVR, BP	• Supraventricular dysrhythmias • Angina • Hypertension • Hypertrophic cardiomyopathy	• PO: 40–120 mg every 6 hr • IV injection: 0.075–0.15 mg/kg (5–10 mg); may be repeated in 15–30 min at 5–10 mg Maximum: 20 mg • IV infusion: mix 50 mg in 250 ml (200 mcg/ml); usual dose is 1–5 mcg/kg/min Therapeutic blood level: 0.1–0.15 mcg/ml	• Bradycardia • AV block • Hypotension • Nausea • Constipation or diarrhea • Elevated liver enzymes • Headache • Dizziness • HF	• Monitor HR, BP, ECG, liver function studies, breath sounds, heart sounds • Note contraindications: known hypersensitivity, AV block, sick sinus syndrome, WPW syndrome, advanced HF, cardiogenic shock • Use cautiously in HF, hypotension, liver disease, renal disease, patients receiving digitalis or beta-blockers • Do not give concurrently with IV beta-blockers • Administer calcium (500 mg–1 g IV over 10 min) as prescribed before IV verapamil to prevent hypotension
Diltiazem	Calcium channel blocker • Relaxes vascular smooth muscle, decreasing preload and afterload • Relieves coronary artery spasm • Slows SA and AV nodal conduction times	• Angina • Coronary artery spasm • Mild HF • Hypertension • Hypertrophic cardiomyopathy • Supraventricular tachycardia	• PO: 30–60 mg every 6 hr • IV injection: 0.15–0.25 mg/kg (20 mg average) over 2 min, may be repeated in 15 min at 0.35 mg/kg (25 mg average) over 2 min • IV infusion: mix 125 mg in 100 ml for a total volume of 125 ml (1 mg/ml) and infuse at 5–15 mg/hr	• Bradycardia • Dysrhythmias • AV block • Hypotension • Nausea • Headache • Flushing • Fatigue • Drowsiness • Edema • Rash • Renal failure • Transient elevation in liver enzymes	• Monitor HR, BP, ECG • Note contraindications: known hypersensitivity, severe hypotension, second- or third-degree AV block, SSS, WPW syndrome, acute MI, pulmonary edema • Use cautiously in HF, hypotension, liver disease, renal disease, older adults

Drug	Action	Indications	Dosage/Administration	Side/Toxic Effects	Nursing Considerations
Digitalis	Cardiac glycoside • Increases cardiac contractility to increase CO • Increases the refractory period of the AV node • Decreases sinus node firing rate • Decreases atrial automaticity • Increases ventricular automaticity • Increases GFR and urine output	• HF • Supraventricular tachycardias, especially in patients with HF	• IV, PO • Digitalizing dose: 0.75–1.5 mg dose over 24 hr, usually in 4 doses of 0.25 mg • Administer IV dose over 5 min • Maintenance dose: 0.125–0.5 mg qd • Therapeutic blood level 0.5–2 ng/ml	Toxic effects • Anorexia, nausea, vomiting, diarrhea • Fatigue, muscle weakness • Agitation • Hallucinations • Visual disturbances • SA and AV blocks • Junctional and ventricular dysrhythmias Treatment of toxicity • Discontinue drug • Correct hypoxemia, ischemia, acid-base or electrolyte imbalance • Treat tachydysrhythmias as prescribed: usually lidocaine • Treat bradydysrhythmias as prescribed: usually atropine or pacemaker • Administer Digibind as prescribed for life-threatening dysrhythmias or blocks • Correction of hypokalemia is recommended before digoxin immune fab • Average dose is 400–800 mg over 30 min or IV bolus if cardiac arrest • Administered through inline filter • Reversal of digitalis toxicity occurs within 30–60 min, but digoxin levels remain elevated	• Monitor apical HR, ECG, serum electrolytes, especially potassium, calcium, magnesium • Note contraindications: known hypersensitivity, SSS, SA or AV block, ventricular tachycardia, hypertrophic cardiomyopathy, WPW • Use cautiously in patients with acute MI, hypothyroidism, liver disease, renal disease, hypothyroidism, older adults • Assess patient for clinical indications of digitalis toxicity • Withhold for 1–2 d before elective electrical cardioversion
Adenosine	Endogenous nucleoside Unclassified antidysrhythmic • Slows conduction through the AV node • Interrupts the reentry pathways through the AV node to restore normal sinus rhythm	• Supraventricular tachycardias, including those associated with WPW syndrome • Not effective in atrial fibrillation or atrial flutter but may slow rate so that fibrillatory or flutter waves can be identified	• IV injection: 6 mg IV; must be given within 6 sec; repeat at 12 mg IV if conversion is not achieved within 1–2 min; 12-mg dose may be repeated once • Must be administered as quickly as possible (referred to as IV "slam") because of very short half-life (10 sec); administer as quickly as possible into NS flush or insert Y connector into line to push NS flush as quickly as possible after pushing adenosine as quickly as possible	• Transient dysrhythmias at the time of conversion (including short asystolic pause) • Pause may be prolonged, especially in patients with SSS • Hypotension if large doses are used • Nausea • Facial flushing • Headache • Dyspnea • Bronchospasm • Chest pressure • Recurrence of dysrhythmias	• Monitor HR, BP, ECG, BP and depth, breath sounds • Note contraindications: known hypersensitivity, second- or third-degree AV block, SSS, ventricular dysrhythmias • Use cautiously in patients with asthma or older adults • Decrease initial dosage as prescribed in patients receiving dipyridamole, diazepam, phenobarbital, or carbamazepine; initial dose may be prescribed as 3 mg • Increase initial dosage as prescribed in patients receiving aminophylline or another xanthine; initial dose may be prescribed as 12 mg • Store at room temperature; solution must be clear at time of use

Continued

Table 3.20 Selected Antidysrhythmic Agents—cont'd

Drug	Classification and Actions	Indications	Administration	Adverse Effects	Nursing Implications
Atropine sulfate Ipratropium	Anticholinergic (also called parasympatholytic) • Decreases vagal tone • Increases sinus rate • Slightly increases conduction through the AV node • Relaxes smooth muscle; prevents bronchospasm • Decreases GI, tracheobronchial secretions	• Symptomatic sinus bradycardia • Asystole • Preoperative preparation for surgery • Anticholinesterase (i.e., organophosphate) insecticide poisoning • Bronchospasm; asthma	• IV injection: 0.5–2 mg (0.5 mg given as initial dose in sinus bradycardia, 1 mg given as initial dose in asystole, 2 mg given as initial dose in organophosphate poisoning); repeated as needed at 3- to 5-min intervals • Maximum: 0.04 mg/kg (usually ≈3 mg) • Nebulizer: 0.025 mg/kg diluted with 3–5 ml of normal saline every 6–8 hr • Handheld inhaler: 2 puffs every 6–8 hr	• Tachycardia, palpitations • Bradycardia if given slowly or in dose of <0.5 mg • Hypotension • Dry mouth • Blurred vision, dilated pupils • Urinary retention • Constipation, paralytic ileus • Headache • Dizziness • Restlessness • Increased myocardial oxygen consumption and chest pain in patients with CAD NOTE: Ipratropium (by inhalation) causes virtually no systemic adverse effects	• Monitor HR, BP, ECG, urine output, bowel sounds • Note contraindications: known hypersensitivity to belladonna, glaucoma, GI obstruction, myasthenia gravis, thyrotoxicosis, ulcerative colitis, prostatic hypertrophy, tachydysrhythmias • Use cautiously in renal disease, HF, hyperthyroidism, hepatic disease, hypertension • Use cautiously in acute MI: do not administer atropine for bradycardia unless the patient is symptomatic; increasing heart rate increases myocardial oxygen consumption and can increase infarction size • Do not use pupils as a reflection of brain status after atropine: pupils will be dilated and nonreactive • Use hard candy to help alleviate side effect of dry mouth unless contraindicated
Isoproterenol	Unclassified antidysrhythmic; beta-selective adrenergic agent • Increases heart rate, contractility, conductivity • Shortens repolarization and QT interval • Causes bronchodilation	• Bradycardia refractory to other drugs • Torsades de pointes	• Mix 1 mg in 250 ml (4 mcg/ml); infuse at 2–20 mcg/min	• Tachycardia, palpitations • Hypotension • Ventricular dysrhythmias • Chest pain • Flushing • Headache • Nausea, vomiting • Anxiety, tremor • Hyperglycemia	• Monitor BP, HR, ECG • Note contraindications: tachydysrhythmias, digitalis toxicity, angina, narrow-angle glaucoma • Use cautiously in older adults and those with hyperthyroidism, chest pain, hypertension, psychoneurosis, diabetes mellitus

AV, Atrioventricular; *bid*, twice a day; *BP*, blood pressure; *CAD*, coronary artery disease; *CO*, cardiac output; *COPD*, chronic obstructive pulmonary disease; *DM*, diabetes mellitus; *ECG*, electrocardiogram; *GFR*, glomerular filtration rate; *GI*, gastrointestinal; *HF*, heart failure; *IM*, intramuscular; *IV*, intravenous; *MI*, myocardial infarction; *NS*, normal saline; *PAC*, pulmonary artery catheter; *PO*, oral; *PVC*, premature ventricular contraction; *qid*, four times a day; *SA*, sinoatrial; *SPF*, sun protection factor; *SSS*, sick sinus syndrome; *SVR*, systemic vascular resistance; *TCA*, tricyclic antidepressant; *tid*, three times a day; *VF*, ventricular fibrillation; *VT*, ventricular tachycardia; *WPW*, Wolff-Parkinson-White;

Table 3.21 Pacemaker Terminology

Artifact	The spike recorded on the ECG depicting the electrical energy discharge from the pulse generator
A-V interval	In a dual-chamber pacemaker, the period of time between an atrial event (sensed or paced) and a paced ventricular event
Blanking period	The interval of time during which the pacemaker cannot sense any events
Burst pacing	The delivery of rapid, multiple electrical stimuli; typically used to interrupt a fast heart rate
Capture	Depolarization of the atria and/or ventricle by an electrical stimulus delivered by an artificial pacemaker; one-to-one capture occurs when each electrical stimulus causes a corresponding depolarization
Committed (DVI) operation	A characteristic of some DVI pacemakers whereby a ventricular stimulus always follows an atrial stimulus regardless of intrinsic ventricular activity
Cross talk	The phenomenon that can occur in dual-chamber pacemakers in which a stimulus from the atrial lead is sensed by the ventricular lead or vice versa, resulting in an inappropriate pacemaker response such as inhibiting or resetting of the refractory period.
Demand pacemaker	A pacemaker that only discharges when the patient's heart rate drops below the pacemaker's preset rate
Dual-chamber pacing (i.e., AV sequential)	The pacing in both the atria and the ventricles to artificially restore the natural contraction sequence of the heart; also called *physiologic pacing*
Electrode	The uninsulated conductive portion of a pacing lead that makes electrical contact with tissue
Electromagnetic interference (EMI)	Radiated or conducted energy—either electrical or magnetic—that can interfere with or disrupt the function of a pulse generator
End of life	The point at which a pacemaker signals that it should be replaced because its battery is nearing depletion
Escape interval	The time between a paced or sensed cardiac event and the subsequent pacing stimulus of a pulse generator
Fusion beat	A spontaneous cardiac depolarization that occurs coincidentally with a paced depolarization; the paced and natural depolarization waveforms fuse
Hysteresis	A pacing parameter that allows a longer escape interval after a sensed event, allowing perpetuation of the patient's intrinsic rhythm
Inhibited	A common type of pacemaker that does not pace when its output is suppressed by sensed spontaneous cardiac events occurring at a rate more rapid than the pacing rate
Intrinsic	Inherent; belonging to or originating from the heart itself
Lead	The insulated wire or wires that carry electrical signals to and from the heart, a connector pin, and stimulating, sensing electrode(s)
Milliamperage (mA)	The unit of measurement used for electrical stimulus (i.e., output) generated by a pacemaker
Multisite pacing	The ability of a pacemaker to stimulate more than one site, such as biventricular pacing
Myopotentials	Electrical signals that originate in body muscles; these signals may be sensed by the pacemaker and falsely interpreted as depolarization
Output	An electric stimulus delivered by the pulse generator; measured in mA
Pacemaker syndrome	A collection of signs and symptoms related to the adverse hemodynamic effects of ventricular pacing, usually attributed to the absence of synchrony between the atrial and ventricular contractions
Pacing mode	The manner in which a pacemaker provides artificial rate and rhythm support in the presence of dysrhythmia; identified by a three- or five-letter code
Programmable	A pulse generator with a pacing mode and/or parameters that can be changed noninvasively at any time by means of an external programmer
Pulse generator	The portion of the pacing system that produces electrical pulses and contains the power supply and electronic circuit
Pulse width	The duration of the pacing pulse expressed in millisecond; also called *pulse duration*
Rate responsive or rate modulated pacing	The ability of a pacemaker to increase or decrease its rate in response to the heart's intrinsic rate or detected changes in the body (i.e., body activity, atrial activity, respiratory rate)
Refractory period	The time during which the pacemaker's sensing mechanism becomes nonresponsive to cardiac activity
Safety pacing	In some DVI and DDD pacemakers, following atrial pacing, the pacemaker is designed to trigger a ventricular pacing output if ventricular sensing occurs during the first portion of the programmed A-V interval; this ensures a ventricular depolarization if the event sensed was electrical interference
Sensing	The ability of the pacemaker to detect the patient's intrinsic activity and respond appropriately by either triggering or inhibiting output

Continued

Table 3.21 Pacemaker Terminology—cont'd

Sensing threshold	The minimum atrial or ventricular intracardiac signal amplitude required to inhibit or trigger a demand pacemaker
Sensitivity	The degree to which a pacemaker is responsive to levels of electrical activity in the heart
Stimulation threshold	The minimum electrical stimulus needed to obtain consistent capture
Telemetry	The ability of the pacemaker to send information (i.e., programmed status, measurements, signals to the programmer)
Tracking	When ventricular pacing is synchronized to sensed atrial activity
Triggered	To deliver an electrical stimulus upon detecting a spontaneous depolarization
V-A interval	With dual-chamber pacemakers, the period of time elapsing from a ventricular event (sensed or paced) to the next scheduled atrial pace

AV, Atrioventricular; *ECG*, electrocardiogram.

From Medtronic. (2005). *Pacing Glossary*. https://wwwp.medtronic.com/medtronicconnect/resources/presentationtools//1332879501392/MedtronicPacingGlossary2007.pdf.

Table 3.22 The NASPE/BPEG Generic (NBG) Pacemaker Code

Position I	Position II	Position III	Position IV	Position V
Chamber(s) paced	Chamber(s) sensed	Response to sensing	Rate modulation	Multisite pacing
O = None	O = None	O = None	R = Rate modulation	O = None
A = Atrium	A = Atrium	T = Triggered		A = Atrium
V = Ventricle	V = Ventricle	I = Inhibited		V = Ventricle
D = Dual (A+V)	D = Dual (A+V)	D = Dual (T + I)		D = Dual (A+V)

BPEG, British Pacing and Electrophysiology Group; *NASPE*, North American Society of Pacing and Electrophysiology.

From Bernstein, A. D., Daubert, J. C., et al. (2002). The revised NASPE/BPEG generic code for antibradycardia, adaptive-rate, and multisite pacing. North American Society of Pacing and Electrophysiology/British Pacing and Electrophysiology Group. *PACE, 25*(2), 260-264.

      ii) Transvenous endocardial
         (a) Pacing lead(s) inserted percutaneously via internal jugular or subclavian vein and advanced into the right atrium, right ventricle, or both
      iii) Transcutaneous
         (a) Percutaneous leads applied to chest and back; used during cardiac arrests until transvenous pacer can be inserted
   b) Permanent (internal pulse generator): months to years
      i) Transvenous endocardial: lead inserted into cephalic vein and advanced into the right atrium or right ventricle; pulse generator implanted in subcutaneous fat under clavicle
      ii) Epicardial: electrodes sewn onto epicardium (thoracotomy required); pulse generator implanted in subcutaneous fat of abdomen
  2) Asynchronous vs synchronous
   a) Asynchronous
      i) Also called fixed rate
      ii) The pacemaker delivers a pacing stimulus at a fixed rate regardless of the heart's intrinsic activity.
      iii) Will cause competition with the heart's intrinsic activity, and the pacing stimulus may land during the descending limb of the T wave
      iv) Rarely seen today
   b) Synchronous
      i) Also called *demand*
      ii) The pacemaker delivers a pacing stimulus only when the heart's intrinsic pacemaker fails to function at a predetermined rate.
      iii) The pacing stimulus will be either inhibited or triggered when the intrinsic activity is seen.
  e. North American Society of Pacing and Electrophysiology (NASPE) generic code (Table 3.22)
  f. Pacemaker modes (Table 3.23)
   1) Atrial: AOO, AAI
     a) Pacing stimulus occurs before the P wave
     b) Requires an intact AV nodal conduction
   2) Ventricular: VOO, VAT, VVI, VVT, VDD
     a) Pacing stimulus occurs before the QRS complex
   3) AV sequential: DOO, DVI, DDD
     a) Maintains AV synchrony and the hemodynamic benefit of the atrial kick
     b) Pacing stimulus before both or either P wave or QRS complex
     c) Sufficient AV delay set to allow atrial depolarization and contraction to complete ventricular filling
   4) Multisite: atriobiventricular (also referred to as *cardiac resynchronization therapy*)
     a) Used in severe HF in patients with ventricular depolarization asynchrony

Table 3.23 Pacemaker Modes

Code	Description	Indications	Advantages	Disadvantages
AOO	Fixed-rate atrial pacer	• Consistently slow sinus rate with intact AV nodal conduction	• Single lead • Maintains AV synchrony	• Atrial competition • No protection in case of AV nodal block
AAI	Demand atrial pacer	• Sick sinus syndrome • Sinus arrest • Sinus bradycardia • Must have intact AV nodal conduction	• Single lead • Maintains AV synchrony	• No protection in case of AV nodal block
VOO	Fixed-rate ventricular pacer	• Complete heart block with slow idioventricular rhythm • Rarely used today	• Single lead • Protection from ventricular asystole	• Ventricular competition with possible stimulation of ventricular dysrhythmias
VAT	Atrial-triggered ventricular pacer	• Complete heart block with intact sinus node	• Synchronized AV conduction with atrial "kick" optimizes cardiac output • Ventricular rate increases with atrial rate, so more exercise responsive	• Two leads • May cause pacemaker-mediated tachycardia: rapid ventricular response in sinus or atrial dysrhythmias • May cause pacemaker-mediated tachycardia
VVI	Demand ventricular pacer	• Sick sinus syndrome • Sinus bradycardia • Sinus arrest • Complete heart block	• Single lead • Simple and reliable • Inexpensive • Protection from ventricular asystole • Little chance of competitive rhythms	• Loss of synchronized AV conduction and atrial "kick" may reduce cardiac output • Not rate responsive • (NOTE: VVIR is a VVI with rate responsiveness)
VVT	Pacing stimulus delivered if needed or not; stimulus depolarizes ventricle if no intrinsic depolarization; stimulus lands harmlessly in QRS if intrinsic depolarization	• Sick sinus syndrome • Sinus bradycardia • Sinus arrest • Complete heart block	• Single lead • Can evaluate pacer function even if intrinsic activity faster than pacer rate	• Loss of synchronized AV conduction and atrial "kick" may reduce cardiac output • Not rate responsive • Difficult to evaluate QRS morphology
VDD	Ventricular pacer that can be atrial triggered or inhibited by intrinsic ventricular depolarization	• Sick sinus syndrome • Sinus bradycardia • Sinus arrest • Complete heart block	• Maintains AV synchrony • If atrial activity is present as pacer functions in atrial triggered mode; if no atrial activity, paces the ventricle in demand mode with inhibition to intrinsic ventricular depolarization	• Two leads • May cause pacemaker-mediated tachycardia • Does not pace the atria, so loss of atrial contraction if no intrinsic atrial activity
DOO	Fixed rate AV sequential pacer	• Consistently slow atrial and ventricular rate	• Synchronized AV conduction with atrial "kick" optimizes cardiac output	• Two leads • Not rate responsive • Atrial and ventricular competition
DVI	Fixed rate atrial pacer with demand ventricular pacer	• Sick sinus syndrome • Sinus bradycardia • Sinus arrest • Complete heart block	• Synchronized AV conduction with atrial "kick" optimizes cardiac output	• Two leads • Not rate responsive • Blind to intrinsic atrial activity, so atrial competition and even atrial fibrillation may occur
DDD	Demand atrial and ventricular pacer; ventricular pacing may be atrial triggered or ventricular inhibited	• Sick sinus syndrome • Sinus bradycardia • Sinus arrest • Complete heart block	• Synchronized AV conduction with atrial "kick" optimizes cardiac output • Near-normal physiologic function	• Two leads • Most expensive • May cause pacemaker-mediated tachycardia • Difficult troubleshooting • Is not used in atrial fibrillation

AV, Atrioventricular.

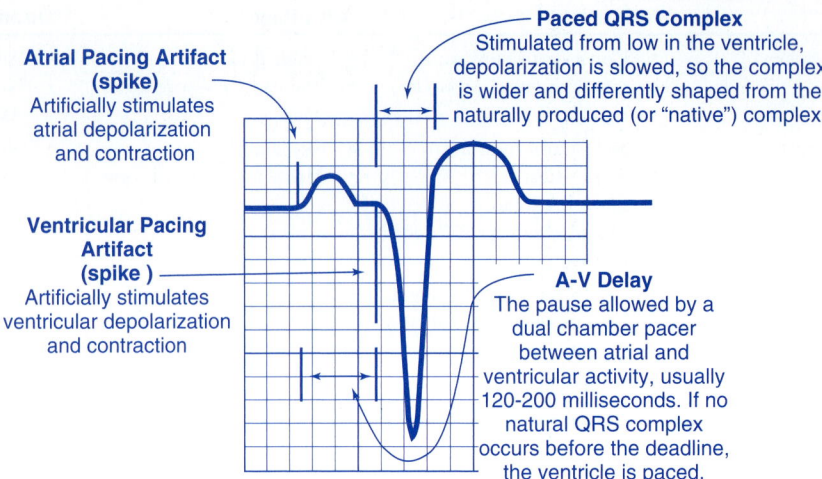

Fig. 3.68 Electrocardiogram evidence of pacing. (From Witherall, C. [1990]. Questions nurses ask about pacemakers. *Am J Nurs*, 90 [12], 20.)

b) Placement of a LV lead (either placed directly on the left ventricle [epicardial] by thoracotomy approach or endocardially via the coronary sinus) along with RV and right atrial leads
c) An AV delay adequate to allow atrial contraction to contribute optimally to ventricular filling
d) Optimal timing of stimulation of both ventricles; this may be with one ventricle stimulated slightly before the other rather than simultaneous,
e) May or may not include an implantable cardioverter-defibrillator
5) Rate-responsive: the HR is adjusted according to demands for CO
   a) HR changes are stimulated by changes in muscle activity, minute ventilation, or blood changes in temperature or pH
   b) Rate-responsive modes: AAIR, VVIR, DDDR
g. Collaborative management
  1) Assess for proper functioning
    a) Determination of the type of pacemaker
    b) ECG evidence of pacing (Fig. 3.68 and 3.69)
      i) Spike before paced event
      ii) Wide QRS if ventricular pacer
      iii) Presence of T wave confirms ventricular depolarization
      iv) Presence of fusion beats
    c) Determination of settings
      i) Rate: usually set at 70 to 90 beats/min but higher than the intrinsic rate for tachycardia overdrive
      ii) Mode (Table 3.23)
      iii) Output: usually set at 1.5 to 2 times the pacing threshold
        (a) The pacing threshold is determined by decreasing the mA until capture is lost and then increased until capture is again obtained; typical pacing threshold is 1 to 1.5 mA so the mA is usually set at 1.5 to 3.
      iv) Sensitivity: usually set at approximately 2 to 5 mV
      v) AV interval: like a PR interval for AV sequential pacemakers
    d) Systematic assessment of rhythm strip in patient with pacemaker (Aehlert, 2011)
      i) Identify the patient's intrinsic rate and rhythm.
      ii) Determine if there is evidence of paced activity (i.e., pacing artifact).
        (a) If there is evidence of atrial pacing, evaluate the paced interval to determine rate and regularity.
        (b) If there is evidence of ventricular pacing, evaluate the paced interval to determine rate and regularity.
      iii) Evaluate the escape interval.
        (a) Compare the escape interval with the paced interval; these should be the same unless there is hysteresis.
      iv) Analyze the rhythm strip for electrical complications of failure to fire, failure to capture, failure to sense, or oversensing (Table 3.24).
  2) Specific to temporary pacemaker
    a) Maintain electrical safety.
      i) Ensure proper grounding of equipment.
      ii) Touch side rails before touching patient to discharge static electricity.
      iii) Wear rubber gloves when making adjustments.
      iv) Keep patient and linens dry.
      v) Avoid sources of electromagnetic interference (EMI) (e.g., electrocautery, defibrillation, magnetic resonance imaging [MRI], transcutaneous electrical nerve stimulation [TENS] units, radiation therapy, lithotripsy).

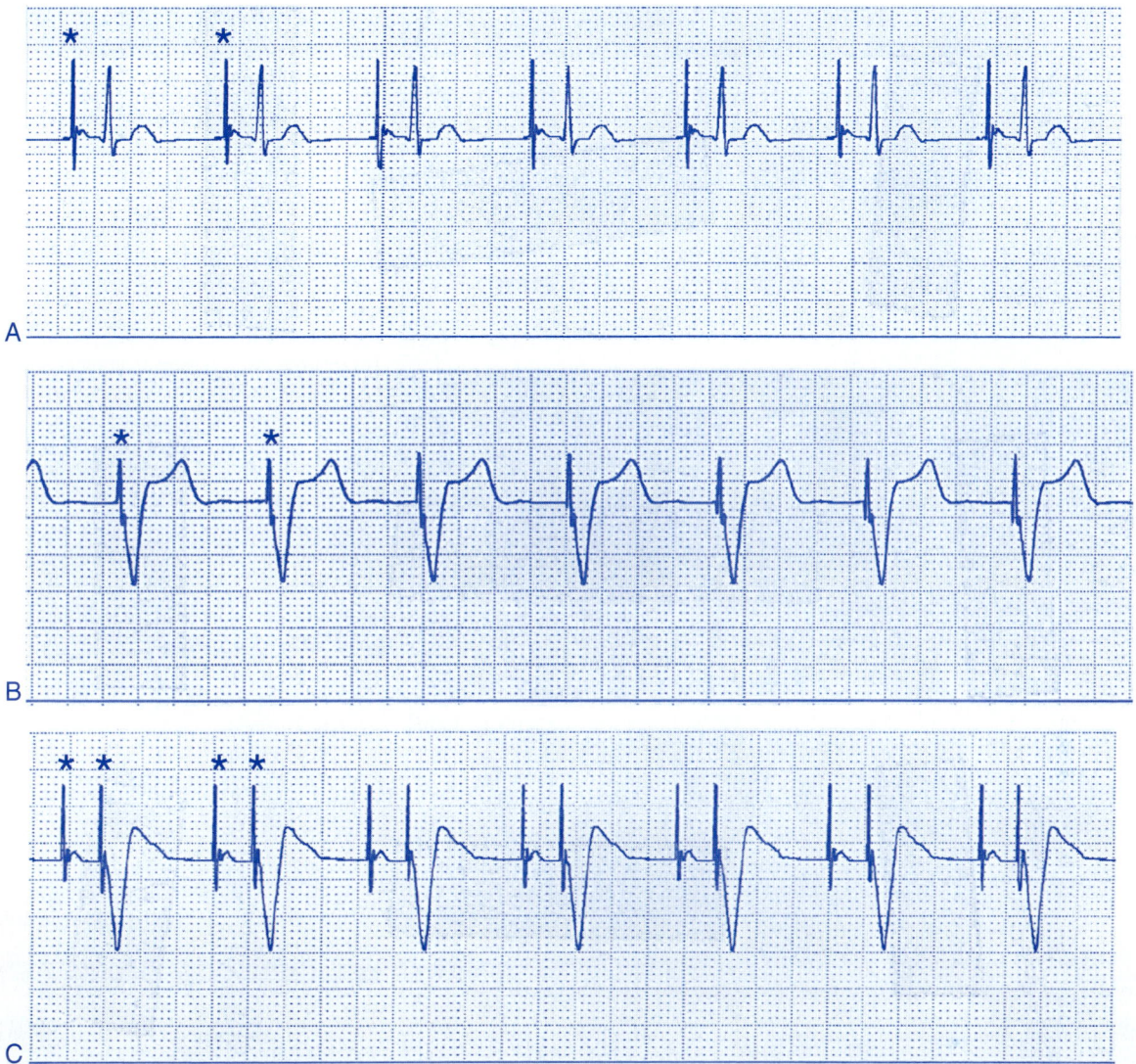

Fig. 3.69 Pacing examples. **A,** Atrial pacing. **B,** Ventricular pacing. **C,** Dual-chamber pacing. Each asterisk represents a pacemaker artifact (i.e., spike). (From Urden, L., Stacy, K., & Lough, M. [2018]. *Critical care nursing: Diagnosis and management* [6th ed.]. St. Louis: Mosby.)

  b) Prevent complications.
    i) Cover dial to prevent accidental changes in settings.
    ii) Limit mobility of affected extremity to prevent accidental catheter dislodgement.
    iii) Observe catheter site for signs of infection.
    iv) Assist with establishment of pacing threshold and set mA slightly above this; usually initially set at between 3 and 5 mA depending on pacing threshold.
    v) Observe cardiac monitor for pacemaker malfunction.
  3) Specific to permanent
    a) Prevent complications.
      i) Limit mobility of affected upper extremity for 48 hours to prevent lead dislodgement.
      ii) Encourage arm exercise after 48 hours to prevent frozen shoulder (i.e., ankylosis).
      iii) Observe incision for signs of infection.
      iv) Observe cardiac monitor for pacemaker malfunction.
    b) Provide patient and family instruction.
      i) How to take pulse, symptoms to report
      ii) Sources of EMI to avoid (e.g., MRI, metal detectors, radio transmitters, electrical generating plants)
      iii) Avoidance of lifting anything over 5 pounds with the arm closest to the pacemaker for 1 to 2 months
      iv) Avoidance of lifting arm closest to the pacemaker above the head for 1 to 2 months
      v) Clinical indications of pacemaker malfunction (e.g., dyspnea, syncope, chest pain, fatigue, peripheral edema, persistent hiccups)

Table 3.24 Pacemaker Electrical Malfunctions

Malfunction	Causes	Interventions
Failure to fire (pace): pacemaker does not fire when it is physiologically indicated for it to fire • Recognized by pauses longer than the automatic interval and absence of pacer spike at end of escape interval	• Loose connections • Battery depletion • Lead displacement • Lead fracture • Sensing malfunction (e.g., EMI)	• Tighten connections if temporary • Replace battery or pulse generator • Lead repositioning or replacement may be needed • Evaluate patient's own rhythm and patient's response; if inadequate, administer atropine and/or apply external transcutaneous pacemaker; CPR may be required • May be caused by sensing malfunction; to identify a sensing malfunction, convert pacemaker to asynchronous by placing a magnet over an implanted pacemaker or switching to asynchronous on an external pacemaker; if pacer spikes seen in asynchronous mode, sensing malfunction exists • Remove source of EMI
Failure to capture: pacemaker fires but depolarization does not occur • Recognized by spike not followed by depolarization (e.g., P wave if atrial pacer or QRS if ventricular pacer)	• Displacement of lead • Lead fracture • Increased pacing thresholds (e.g., electrolyte imbalance, drug toxicity, acid-base imbalance, ischemia) • Fibrosis or scar tissue at the lead tip • Battery failure • Chamber perforation • Complexes not visible	• Position patient on left side or to whatever position patient was in when capture was last seen • Increase mA • May require lead repositioning, lead replacement • Replace battery or pulse generator • Check chest radiography for lead fracture and lead placement • Correct metabolic or electrolyte imbalance • Consider drug levels and toxicity • Check for diaphragmatic pacing and monitor or cardiac tamponade if catheter perforation is suspected • May require external transcutaneous pacing or CPR
• Undersensing or failure to sense: pacemaker fails to recognize intrinsic activity (e.g., P wave or QRS) • Recognized by pacer spikes falling closer to the intrinsic beats than the escape interval; spikes land indiscriminately throughout the cardiac cycle including potentially on the descending limb of the T wave	• Displacement of lead • Lead fracture • Sensitivity set too low or set on asynchronous • Disconnection of sensing circuit • Inadequate signal (e.g., low P or QRS voltage) • Battery failure • Increased sensing threshold (e.g., edema or fibrosis at lead tip) • Chamber perforation	• Position patient on left side or to whatever position sensing was last seen • Lead repositioning or replacement may be necessary • Make sure that pacer is not set on asynchronous • Increase sensitivity (i.e., turn down the mV) • Check connections on temporary pacemaker • Administer lidocaine if the QRSs that are not sensed are PVCs • Check chest radiography for lead placement or lead fracture • Replace battery or pulse generator • If patient's own rhythm adequate, turn pacer off or heart rate down to minimum • If patient's own rhythm inadequate, increase pacer rate to override patient's own rhythm
Oversensing pacemaker recognizes extraneous electrical activity or the wrong intrinsic electrical activity as the inhibiting event • Recognized by absence of pacer spikes and failure to fire	• Sensitivity set too high • EMI • Oversensing of P waves or T waves • Myopotentials • Crosstalk (no ventricular pacing)	• Decrease sensitivity (i.e., turn up the mV) • Remove from EMI; ensure that all equipment is properly grounded • Decrease atrial output, decrease ventricular sensitivity, increase ventricular blanking period • May require external transcutaneous pacing or CPR

CPR, Cardiopulmonary resuscitation; *EMI*, electromagnetic interference; *PVC*, premature ventricular contraction.

vi) Wound care (e.g., keeping clean and dry until healed)
vii) Importance of carrying pacemaker identification card and informing healthcare providers of presence of pacemaker
4) Monitor for complications.
a) Frozen shoulder
b) Infection
c) Pneumothorax
d) Myocardial perforation
e) Catheter or lead displacement
f) Hematoma
g) Dysrhythmias
i) Pacemaker-mediated tachycardia: a rapid paced rhythm that can occur with atrial tracking pacemakers; it begins with and is sustained by ventricular events that are conducted retrogradely to the atria; the pacemaker senses this retrograde atrial depolarization and then delivers a stimulus to the ventricle, causing a ventricular depolarization, which again is conducted retrogradely to the atria; the cycle repeats itself to produce a tachycardia.
h) Electrical malfunction (Table 3.24)
12. Prepare and care for the patient with an ICD.
a. Definition: implantable device to provide for immediate termination of VT or VF in patients in whom these dysrhythmias cannot be pharmacologically or surgically controlled
b. Tiered therapy (also called *third generation*) devices have all of the following (Morton & Fontaine, 2009):
1) Bradycardia pacing: VVI, DDD, VDD
2) Antitachycardia pacing: burst
3) Low-energy cardioversion: 1 to 8 J
4) High-energy cardioversion: 15 to 36 J
5) Defibrillation: 30 to 36 J
c. Indications
1) One or more episodes of spontaneous VT or VF in a patient in whom EPS or spontaneous ventricular dysrhythmias cannot be used to accurately predict the efficacy of other treatment
2) Recurrent episodes of sustained VT or VF in a patient in whom antidysrhythmic therapy is suboptimal because of intolerance or noncompliance
3) Persistent inducibility of sustained VT or VF during EPS despite antidysrhythmic therapy or ablation
4) VF in a patient with no evidence of structural heart disease and no detectable suppressing triggering factors
d. Contraindications
1) Frequent episodes of VT or VF (more than 2 events/month)
2) Uncontrolled HF
3) Less than 6 to 12 months of productive life expectancy
4) History of noncompliance
5) Extreme psychological barriers to use of the device
e. Components
1) Generator
a) Processes information from the lead system and delivers the electrical impulses
b) Stores information about the patient's heart rhythm and therapy delivered
c) Placed in the left upper quadrant of abdomen or under the clavicle
d) Usually lasts about 3 to 5 years before replacement required
2) Leads record heart rhythm and carry pulses and shocks from the generator to the heart
a) Atrial lead
b) Ventricular lead
f. Method
1) System evaluates HR and probability density function (PDF).
a) PDF diagnoses the amount of time the QRS spends away from the isoelectric baseline.
2) System is turned on and off by using a donut-shaped magnet.
a) Device is usually not turned on during early postoperative period because of frequent occurrence of sinus tachycardia during this period.
3) When VT is sensed, the ICD will first initiate antitachycardia pacing.
4) If the VT is not successfully pace terminated, the ICD will cardiovert the rhythm with low-energy synchronized shocks.
5) If the rhythm deteriorates to VF or if VF is the initial rhythm, the ICD will defibrillate at a higher energy level.
6) When a shock is delivered, the device senses the rhythm.
7) If sinus rhythm is not restored, up to five shocks of 25 to 35 J are delivered.
8) If the electrical rhythm deteriorates to bradycardia or asystole, the bradycardia back-up pacing function is activated.
g. Collaborative management
1) Provide postprocedure management as for pacemaker insertion
2) Monitor for dysrhythmias and evaluate effectiveness of ICD if firing occurs; administer antidysrhythmic agents as prescribed.
3) If cardiopulmonary arrest occurs, do the following:
a) Obtain emergency equipment and prepare to cardiovert or defibrillate.
b) Treat this patient as you would any patient in cardiopulmonary arrest; do not wait for the device.
c) Do not place defibrillator paddles within 8 cm of the generator.
d) Anterior-posterior paddle placement may be more effective.
4) Deactivate the ICD using a magnet as requested by the physician.

                5) Monitor for complications.
                    a) Observe incision for signs of infection.
                    b) Observe for clinical indications of cardiac tamponade.
                6) Encourage the patient to express fears and concerns about being shocked; consider referral to support group.
                7) Monitor for complications.
                    a) Atelectasis
                    b) Pneumonia
                    c) Pneumothorax
                    d) Lead migration
                    e) Lead fracture
   13. Prepare and care for the patient having ablation therapy.
        a. Use: to eradicate dysrhythmia in patients who experience frequent, disabling, or life-threatening dysrhythmias that are not suppressed with pharmacologic therapy or in whom pharmacologic therapy is not well tolerated
        b. Types
            1) Radiofrequency catheter ablation
                a) A catheter is placed in the heart via cardiac catheterization.
                b) Radiofrequency energy is applied to the area in which the dysrhythmia originates or an accessory pathway (e.g., WPW).
                c) Controlled, localized necrosis occurs
                d) Postprocedure care is as for cardiac catheterization or angioplasty; monitor closely for dysrhythmias.
            2) Surgical ablation: the area in which the dysrhythmia originates is either excised or eliminated by cryosurgery or laser.
   14. Prepare for and care for the patient having maze procedure for atrial fibrillation.
        a. Performed either by cardiothoracic surgery or PCI
        b. A maze of carefully planned sutures or laser-created cuts create an electrical conduction route through atrial myocardium, corralling and herding chaotic atrial impulses from the SA node to the AV node.
        c. Provide postoperative management as for cardiothoracic surgery or PCI, depending on procedure performed.

Acute Coronary Syndrome

Definitions
1. Arteriosclerosis: a group of diseases characterized by thickening and loss of elasticity (calcification) of arterial walls
    a. Atherosclerosis: the most common form of arteriosclerosis; a chronic disease process characterized by the build-up of fatty plaque along the subintimal layer of arteries leading to a decrease in arterial lumen
    b. Progression (Fig. 3.70)
2. CAD: a progressive disease of the coronary arteries that results in narrowing and obstruction of the vessels and eventually myocardial ischemia; may also be referred to as *ischemic heart disease, coronary heart disease,* or *atherosclerotic heart disease*
3. Acute coronary syndrome: the group of clinical symptoms compatible with myocardial ischemia and differentiated by ECG findings; includes the following (Fig. 3.71):
    a. Unstable angina: patient presenting with chest pain, no ST-segment elevation, and normal cardiac biomarkers
        1) De novo angina: new-onset angina
        2) Crescendo angina: angina that has increased in frequency, intensity, or duration
        3) Preinfarction: angina of prolonged duration that occurs even at rest
        4) Wellens syndrome: angina with deep T-wave inversion in V_2, V_3 indicative of critical proximal LAD stenosis
        5) Variant (also called *Prinzmetal* or *vasospasm tic*): angina with ST-segment elevation related to coronary artery spasm
    b. MI: electrical and mechanical death of a portion of the myocardium
        1) ST elevation
            a) STEMI: patient presenting with chest pain, elevated cardiac biomarkers, and ST-segment elevation
            b) Non–ST-segment elevation MI (NSTEMI): patient presenting with chest pain and elevated cardiac biomarkers but no ST-segment elevation
        2) Location: Table 3.25 describes wall of MI along with coronary artery affected, indicative ECG leads, and anticipated complications
            a) Left ventricular MI (LVMI): most MIs are LV
                i) Anterior LV: 42%
                ii) Septal LV: 10%
                iii) Lateral LV: 10%
                iv) Inferior LV: 33%
                v) Posterior LV: 5%
            b) Right ventricular MI (RVMI)
                i) Concurrent with inferior LVMI; one third of all inferior MIs have concurrent RV infarction
                ii) Rarely isolated: isolated RVMI more common in patients with RVH (e.g., COPD)
                iii) Smaller infarct because of decreased oxygen requirements of right ventricle
                iv) Almost always transmural

Etiology
1. Etiology of arteriosclerosis or atherosclerosis
    a. Nonmodifiable risk factors
        1) Heredity: when siblings or parents develop CAD before 55 years of age
            a) Maternal history of CAD before 65 years conveys greater risk than paternal history in women.
            b) Several risk factors have genetic predisposition (e.g., hypertension, hyperlipidemia, DM).
        2) Advancing age: older than 45 years for men and older than 55 years for women
        3) Gender: men have twice the risk of premenopausal women; risk increases in women after menopause.

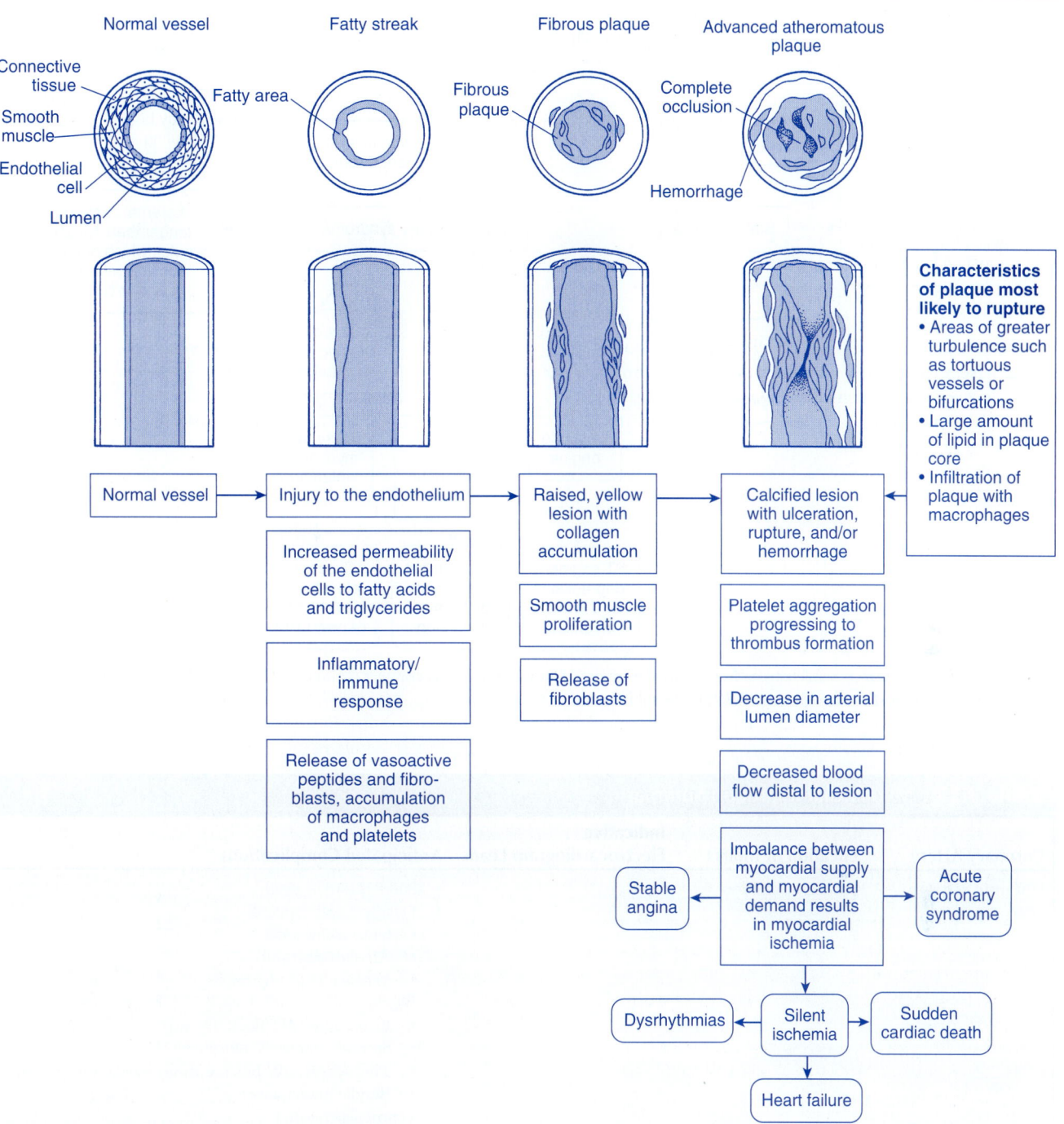

Fig. 3.70 Progression of atherosclerosis. (Modified from Thelan, L. A., Urden, L. D., Lough, M. E., & Stacy, K. M. [1998]. *Critical care nursing: Diagnosis and management* [3rd ed.]. St. Louis: Mosby.)

b. Modifiable risk factors
1) Hypertension: BP greater than 120/<80 mm Hg or requiring antihypertensive agents to achieve BP less than 120/<80 mm Hg
2) Hyperlipidemia: elevated levels of cholesterol, triglycerides, or low-density lipoproteins (LDLs) or decreased levels of high-density lipoproteins (HDLs); desirable levels of lipids are the following:
   a) Cholesterol level less than 200 mg/dl
   b) LDL level less than 100 mg/dl for patients with heart disease or DM; less than 130 mg/dl for patients with two or more risk factors; or less than 160 mg/dl for patients with only one risk factor
   c) HDL level greater than 40 mg/dl
   d) Triglyceride level less than 150 mg/dl
3) Smoking: increases LDL level, platelet aggregation, and fibrinogen level and may cause vasospasm; elevated carbon monoxide levels decrease the oxygen-carrying capacity of Hgb; complete smoking cessation is desired
4) DM or glucose intolerance
   a) Control of blood glucose in patients with DM is advocated to control risk of sequelae, including CAD; desirable fasting glucose level is less than 150 mg/dl.
   b) DM is also associated with increased levels of LDL and triglycerides and obesity.

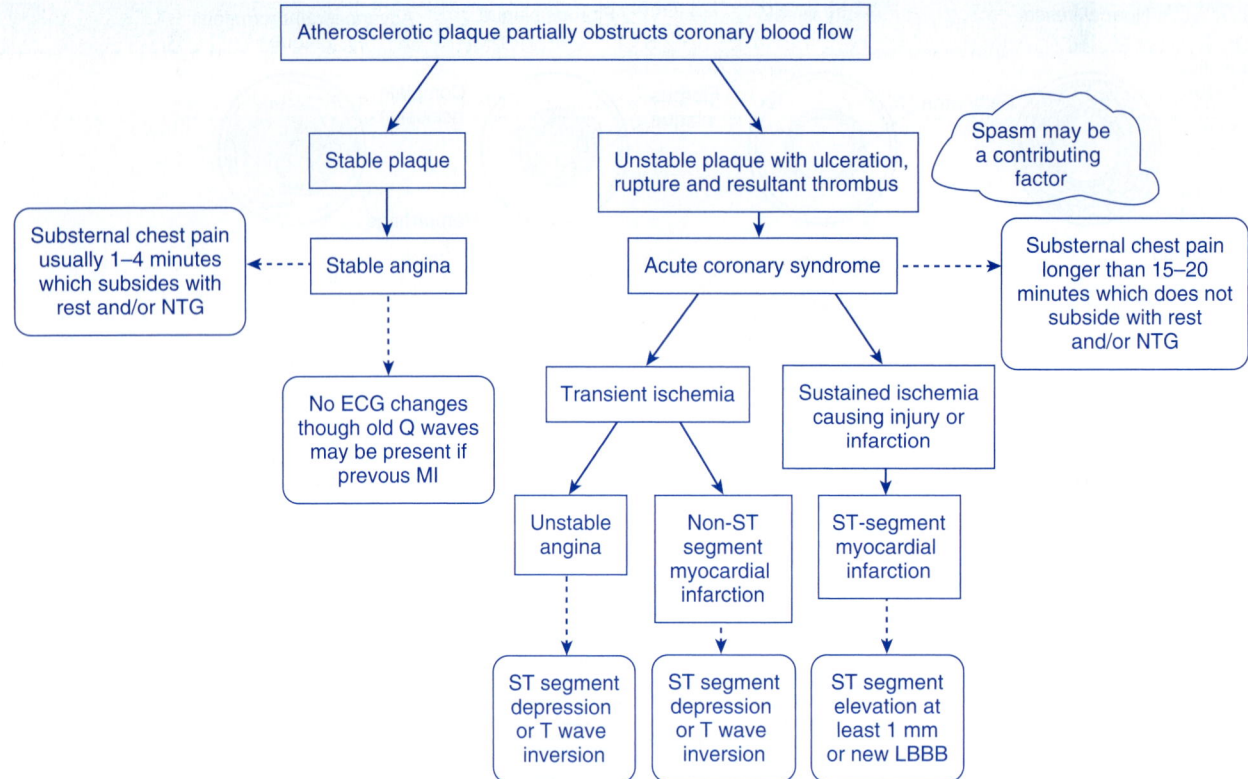

Fig. 3.71 Differentiation of stable angina from acute coronary syndrome. *Dotted lines* connect pathology to the clinical presentation. *LBBB,* Left bundle branch block; *NTG,* nitroglycerin; *MI,* myocardial infarction.

Table 3.25 Myocardial Infarction Summary

Coronary Artery	Location of Infarct	Indicative Electrocardiogram Leads	Anticipated Complications

Left main coronary artery	Extensive anterior	V_1–V_6	• Sudden cardiac death
			• Dysrhythmias especially:
			  • Sinus tachycardia
			  • Atrial dysrhythmias
			  • Ventricular dysrhythmias
			• Blocks
			  • First-degree AV block
			  • Second-degree AV block type II
			  • Third-degree AV block with ventricular escape
			  • Bundle branch block
			• Ventricular rupture
			• Ventricular septal defect
			• Ventricular aneurysm
			• Heart failure
			• Cardiogenic shock

Left anterior descending artery	Septal	V_1, V_2	• Dysrhythmias, especially:
			  • Sinus tachycardia
			  • Atrial fibrillation
			  • Ventricular dysrhythmias
			• Blocks
			  • First-degree AV block
			  • Second-degree AV block type II
			  • Third-degree AV block with ventricular escape
			  • Bundle branch block
			• Ventricular septal rupture

Table 3.25	Myocardial Infarction Summary—cont'd		
Coronary Artery	**Location of Infarct**	**Indicative Electrocardiogram Leads**	**Anticipated Complications**

	Anterior	V_3, V_4	• Dysrhythmias, especially:
			  • Sinus tachycardia
			  • Atrial fibrillation
			  • Ventricular dysrhythmias
			• Blocks
			  • First-degree AV block
			  • Second-degree AV block type II
			  • Third-degree AV block with ventricular escape
			  • Bundle branch block
			• Ventricular aneurysm
			• Heart failure
			• Cardiogenic shock

Left circumflex artery	Lateral	High: I, aVL Low: V_5, V_6	• Dysrhythmias • Heart failure

Right coronary artery	Inferior	II, III, aVF	• Dysrhythmias, especially:
			  • Sinus bradycardia
			  • Sinus arrest
			  • Junctional rhythms
			  • Ventricular dysrhythmias
			• Blocks
			  • SA blocks
			  • First-degree AV block
			  • Second-degree AV block type I
			  • Third-degree AV block usually with AV junctional escape
			  • Bundle branch block
			• Papillary muscle rupture
			• Heart failure

	Posterior	Reciprocal changes in V_1, V_2
		Indicative changes in V_7-V_9 (especially V_8, V_9)
			• Dysrhythmias, especially:
			  • Sinus bradycardia
			  • Sinus arrest
			  • Junctional rhythms
			  • Ventricular dysrhythmias
			• Blocks
			  • First-degree AV block
			  • Second-degree AV block type I
			  • Third-degree AV block usually with AV junctional escape
			• Papillary muscle rupture with acute mitral regurgitation

	Right ventricular	V_{4R}–V_{6R} (especially V_{4R})	• Dysrhythmias, especially:
			  • Sinus bradycardia
			  • Sinus arrest
			  • Junctional rhythms
			  • Ventricular dysrhythmias
			• Blocks
			  • First-degree AV block
			  • Second-degree AV block type I
			  • Third-degree AV block usually with AV junctional escape
			  • Bundle branch block
			• Papillary muscle rupture with acute tricuspid regurgitation
			• Right ventricular failure

AV, Atrioventricular; *SA*, sinoatrial.

5) Hyperhomocysteinemia: homocysteine level greater than 14 µmol/l
   a) Homocysteine is an essential sulfur-containing amino acid formed during the processing of dietary protein; elevated levels are toxic to the vascular endothelium and increase coagulability.
   b) Deficiencies of folate, vitamin B_{12}, and vitamin B_6 have all been implicated in elevated levels of homocysteine; elevated levels of homocysteine may be successfully reduced by folate, vitamin B_{12}, or pyridoxine therapy.
6) Sedentary lifestyle: exercise is inversely related to cardiovascular mortality; sedentary people are also more likely to be obese, hypertensive, and diabetic.
7) Stress
   a) Chronic stress promotes the long-term development of CAD.
   b) Acute stress increases catecholamine levels, myocardial oxygen consumption, and dysrhythmia potential.
   c) Personality type A with aggression may also contribute.
8) Obesity: body weight greater than 120% of ideal body weight; ideal body weight is desirable
   a) Obesity also contributes to hypertension, hyperlipidemia, glucose intolerance, and sedentary lifestyle.
   b) Midline fat is of greater risk than hip and thigh fat (i.e., apple versus pear).
   c) BMI greater than 30 is considered obese and increases cardiac risk.
   d) Metabolic syndrome (i.e., combination of BMI >30 kg/m², elevated triglycerides and reduced HDL, hypertension, and fasting serum glucose >110 mg/dl or type 2 DM) increases the risk of CAD.
9) Oral contraceptives: increase risk of MI especially in smokers; increases BP; smoking cessation is desirable for all people but especially in women who use oral contraceptives

c. Protective factors
   1) Exercise: elevates HDL, decreases BP and resting HR, decreases body fat, and increases endogenous tissue plasminogen activator (tPA) levels
      a) Intensity: sufficient to increase HR to 50% to 80% of predicted maximal HR
      b) Duration: 20 to 30 minutes
      c) Frequency: at least three times per week
      d) Type of exercise: recommendation is to vary the type of exercise to prevent boredom, but walking is an excellent form of exercise for almost all patients.
   2) Stress management: reduces catecholamine levels, decreases BP, and reduces muscle tension
      a) Methods include daily stretching, breathing exercises, meditation, prayer, and yoga.
   3) High-fiber, low fat diet: reduces total cholesterol
   4) Alcohol (1–2 beverages per day): increases HDL and may decrease platelet aggregation; overall health benefit diminishes after 1 or 2 alcoholic beverages per day
   5) Aspirin (ASA) (81–325 mg/day): prevents platelet aggregation and decreases inflammation (one postulated contributor to CAD)
   6) Omega-3 fatty acids: decrease platelet aggregation, increase HDL levels, decrease triglyceride levels
      a) Alpha linolenic acid found in canola oil, walnuts, flaxseeds
      b) Eicosapentaenoic acid (EPA) and docosahexaenoic acid (DHA) found in salmon, trout, sardines
   7) Flavonoids: antioxidant effect, induce nitric oxide formation, may inhibit platelet aggregation; found in tea and cocoa
   8) Loving relationships
      a) Decrease the overall incidence of CAD, although mechanisms are unclear; loneliness and depression have been identified as contributing factors to CAD
      b) Pets also have a beneficial effect by decreasing stress and depression.

2. Etiology of MI
   a. Arteriosclerosis or atherosclerosis
   b. Coronary artery thrombosis
   c. Coronary artery spasm
   d. Cocaine induced: excessive sympathetic stimulation causes tachycardia, hypertension, and arterial vasoconstriction and spasm; coronary artery spasm may cause MI, especially non–Q-wave infarction.
   e. Combination of these factors: most MIs are caused by atherosclerosis and thrombosis.
   f. Other less commonly seen causes
      1) Severe prolonged hypotension
      2) Sudden, severe anemia
      3) Chest trauma (e.g., myocardial contusion)
      4) Trauma to coronary artery or arteries
      5) Aortic stenosis or insufficiency
      6) Thyrotoxicosis
      7) Blood dyscrasias
      8) Aortic dissection
      9) Arteritis
      10) Carbon monoxide poisoning

Clinical Presentation

1. Subjective
   a. Pain: 75% to 85% of all patients with MI have pain
      1) Provocation: emotional or physical stress; may occur at rest
      2) Palliation: not relieved by oxygen, rest, or nitrates; relieved by narcotics or reperfusion (e.g., fibrinolytics or PCI)
      3) Quality
         a) Frequently described as pressure on the chest
         b) May also be described as knifelike, stabbing, burning, or indigestion
         c) May feel like usual anginal pain but more severe

           d) Atypical pain common in women
           e) If described as tearing or ripping, consider dissecting the aortic aneurysm.
        4) Region and radiation
           a) Primary location is usually chest but may be epigastric (especially with inferior MI).
           b) Radiation is usually to the left arm, left elbow, left shoulder, both arms, or jaw.
           c) If radiating to back, consider dissecting the aortic aneurysm.
        5) Severity: from vague, slight discomfort to severe pain; more intense than the patient's typical anginal pain
        6) Timing
           a) Most MIs occur within 3 hours of awakening.
           b) The pain is continuous from onset with a duration of 20 minutes or more.
           c) Pain that comes and goes for as long as several days before the actual MI is referred to as a *stuttering MI pattern*: intermittent pain before continuous pain is preinfarction angina.
     b. Silent MI: as many as 25% of all patients with MI have no pain.
        1) More likely in patients who are older or have diabetes
        2) Clues suggesting possible silent MI: new-onset HF or acute change in mental status, unexplained abdominal pain, unexplained dyspnea or fatigue
     c. Associated symptoms
        1) Nausea and vomiting: seen more often in inferior or posterior MI
        2) Dyspnea or orthopnea: seen more often in anterior MI
        3) Diaphoresis
        4) Palpitations
        5) Apprehension
  2. Objective
     a. HR and rhythm
        1) Tachycardia: seen more often in anterior MI
        2) Bradycardia: seen more often in inferior MI
     b. Normotension, hypotension, hypertension
        1) Hypertension: seen more often in anterior MI
        2) Hypotension: seen more often in inferior MI
        3) Equality in arms: inequality in arms indicates possible dissecting thoracic aortic aneurysm.
     c. Tachypnea
     d. Elevated temperature: may occur 48 to 72 hours after MI
     e. Levine sign: clenched fist held over sternum
     f. May have JVD: indicative of RVF; commonly seen in RV infarction
     g. May have abnormal PMI: downward and lateral displacement
     h. Heart sound changes
        1) May have diminished heart sounds: related to decreased contractility
        2) May have S_4: indicative of LV noncompliance; common for first 24 hours
        3) May have S_3: early sign of LVF
        4) May have pericardial friction rub: indicative of pericarditis
        5) May have systolic murmur of mitral regurgitation (high-pitched, blowing, holosystolic murmur loudest at apex which radiates to the axilla); may indicate LVF or papillary muscle dysfunction or rupture
        6) May have murmur of ventricular septal rupture (high-pitched, harsh, holosystolic murmur loudest at lower left sternal border)
     i. May have carotid, aortic, or femoral bruits
     j. May have clinical indications of hypoperfusion (Table 2.2)
     k. May have clinical indications of HF
        1) LVF (e.g., S_3, crackles, dyspnea) in LV infarction
        2) RVF (e.g., JVD, hepatomegaly, peripheral edema) in RV infarction
  3. Serum
     a. Leukocyte count: increased (usually 12,000–15,000/mm^3) at 48 to 72 hours in acute MI
     b. ESR: increased at 48 to 72 hours in acute MI
     c. C-reactive protein: increased in acute MI
     d. Interleukin-6: increased in acute MI; marker of increased risk of mortality in acute MI
     e. Cardiac biomarkers (Table 3.26)
        1) Positive serum isoenzymes
           a) CK: positive CK-MB (>3%) is indicative of MI; highly specific test for MI
           b) LDH: normally LDH_2 is greater than LDH_1; LDH_1 greater than LDH_2 (referred to as *flipped LDH*) is indicative of MI; does not occur until 48 to 72 hours after the onset of pain
        2) Increased serum muscle proteins
           a) Myoglobin: muscle protein; high sensitivity but low specificity; excellent early negative predictive value
           b) Troponin: contractile protein
              i) Cardiac troponin I (cTnI): found only in cardiac muscle; more specific but later rise and peak
              ii) Cardiac troponin T (cTnT): found in cardiac muscle as well as skeletal muscle; less specific than I, especially in patients with renal failure but earlier rise and peak
              iii) High sensitivity troponin assays, both cTNI and cTNT, detect concentrations of the same proteins but in much lower concentrations
  4. ECG
     a. ST segment depression in unstable angina
     b. ST segment elevation in variant angina
     c. As a diagnostic tool for acute MI: most helpful when clearly abnormal
        1) If initial ECG nondiagnostic, repeat ECGs should be done every 30 minutes until pain cessation or the ECG is clearly diagnostic and definitive therapy can be initiated.
        2) The typical criteria for prompt reperfusion therapies (e.g., PCI, fibrinolytics) in acute MI include either of the following:
           a) ST segment elevation of greater than or equal to 1 mm in at least two continuous leads
           b) New LBBB

Table 3.26 Cardiac Biomarkers for Acute Myocardial Infarction

Test	Normal Values	Abnormal Values Consistent with MI	Time to Rise (after Injury)	Peak (after Injury)	Return to Normal (after Injury)
CK-MB	0% of total CK	>3%	6–10 hr	12–24 hr	2–3 d
LDH_1	17%–25% of total LDH	>40%	8–24 hr	72 hr	8–14 d
Myoglobin	Men: 20–90 ng/ml	Men: >90 ng/ml	1–4 hr	6–12 hr	1–2 d
	Women: 10–75 ng/ml	Women: >75 ng/ml			
Cardiac troponin I (cTnI)	<1.5 ng/ml	>4 ng/ml	4–6 hr	18 hr	1–2 wk
Cardiac troponin T (cTnT)	<0.1 ng/ml	>0.2 ng/ml	3–4 hr	24 hr	2–3 wk

CK-MB, Creatine kinase-muscle/brain; *LDH*, lactate dehydrogenase.

3) There are multiple problems with ECG diagnosis of MI.
   a) Lag time of hours (or even days) may exist before diagnostic ECG changes become evident; first ECG diagnostic only 50% of the time.
   b) Changes may be subtle.
   c) Previous ECG may not be available for comparison.
   d) Changes may be obscured by a competitive condition.
      i) LBBB or ventricular pacemaker obscures anterior MI.
      ii) WPW obscures anterior MI.
      iii) Left anterior hemiblock obscures inferior MI.
      iv) Left posterior hemiblock obscures lateral MI.
      v) Ventricular hypertrophy may obscure anterior or lateral MI.
   e) 15 or 18 leads are used to prevent missing an infarction in a traditionally "electrically silent" area of the heart; sensitivity and inclusion for reperfusion therapy are increased through the use of RV and posterior lead
      i) 18-lead ECG: 12 standard, 3 RV leads, 3 posterior leads
      ii) 15-lead ECG: 12 standard + V_{4R} + V_8 + V_9
  d. ECG indicators (see Electrocardiography section and Fig. 3.46)
  e. Locations, indicative leads, coronary artery affected (see Electrocardiography section and Table 3.11)
  f. Determination of the age of the MI (see Electrocardiography section and Table 3.12)
5. Echocardiography
  a. Normal wall motion: strong predictor of nonischemic pain
  b. Reduced wall motion: strong predictor of ischemia or infarction
  c. May show mechanical complications (e.g., VSD, papillary muscle rupture)
6. Chest radiography: may show cardiomegaly, indications of HF
7. Cardiac catheterization: will likely show coronary artery occlusion; PCI may be performed after diagnosis
8. Radionuclide studies
  a. Technetium-99 pyrophosphate scan: infarcted areas show up as "hot spots"
  b. Thallium-201 scan: ischemic or infarcted areas show up as "cold spots"

Pathophysiology (Fig. 3.72)
1. LVMI (Fig. 3.72)
2. RVMI (Fig. 3.73)
3. Factors affecting mortality rate
  a. Age
  b. LVEF
  c. Number of occluded vessels
  d. Previous history of MI
  e. Presence of cardiogenic shock: associated with loss of 40% of LV muscle mass; may be from one MI or several cumulative MIs
  f. NOTE: Women have twice the mortality rate of men, probably related to the fact that they tend to be older and have more significant risk factors (e.g., DM, hypertension) when they develop MI.

Collaborative Management
1. Provide care according to national guidelines (Fig. 3.74).
2. Manage cardiopulmonary arrest if required.
  a. VF frequently occurs within 1 hour: early identification of clinical indications of MI and hospitalization is very important.
  b. Manage airway, oxygenation, and circulation using BLS and ACLS.
3. Monitor ECG, vital signs, physical examination, and hemodynamic parameters for changes.
  a. Safely and accurately monitor the patient's hemodynamic parameters as indicated; hemodynamic monitoring is likely to be useful in the following situations in acute MI.
    1) Persistent chest pain
    2) Persistent tachycardia
    3) Significant hypertension or hypotension
    4) Significant LVF or RVF
    5) IV inotropic or vasoactive agents
    6) New systolic murmur
  b. Use hemodynamic parameters in evaluating clinical status for changes and responses to prescribed therapies.

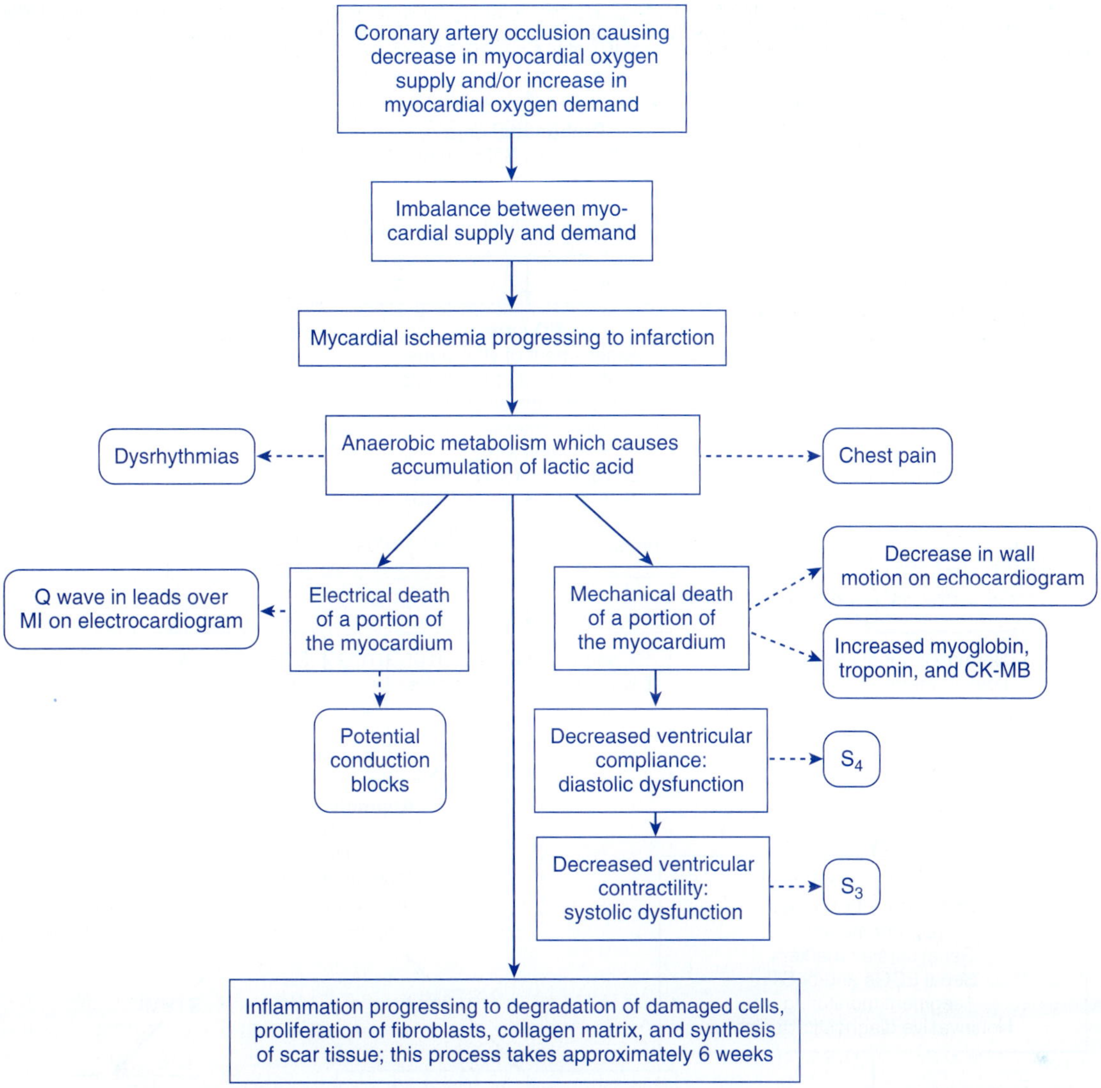

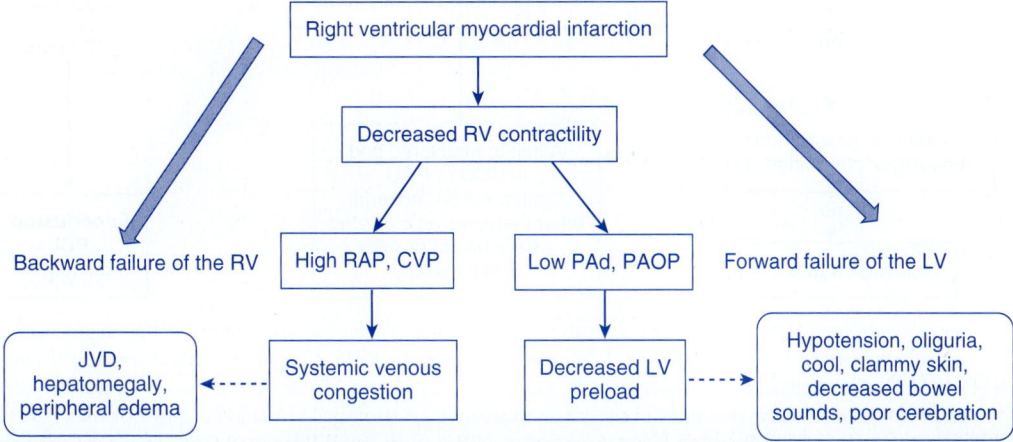

Fig. 3.72 Pathophysiology of myocardial infarction. *Dotted lines* connect pathology to the clinical presentation.

Fig. 3.73 Pathophysiology of right ventricular myocardial infarction. Dotted lines connect pathology to the clinical presentation. *CVP*, central venous pressure; *JVD*, jugular venous distention; *LV*, left ventricular; *PAd*, pulmonary artery diastolic pressure; *PAOP*, pulmonary artery occlusive pressure; *RAP*, right atrial pressure; *RV*, right ventricular.

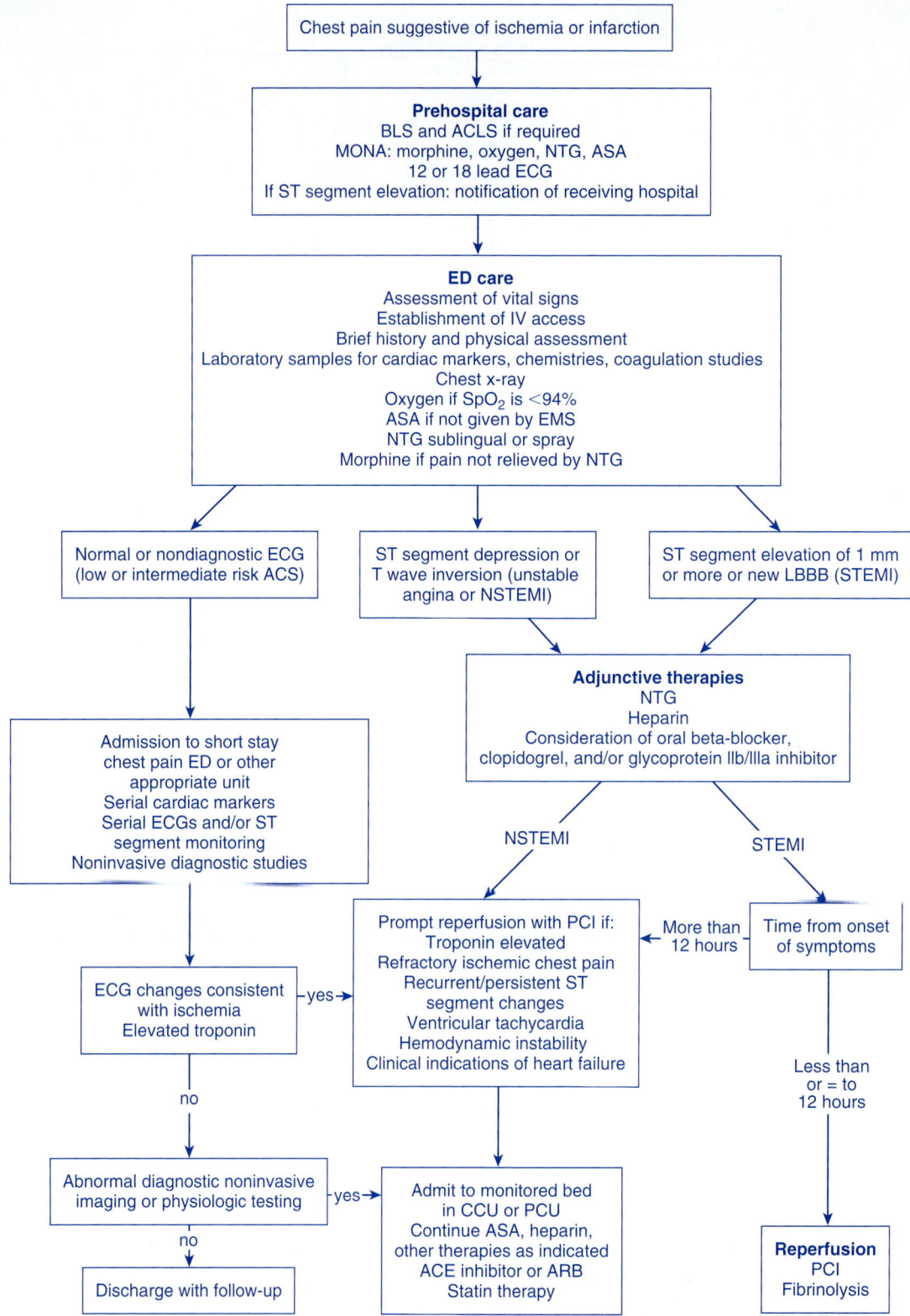

Fig. 3.74 Acute coronary syndrome (ACS) management algorithm. *ACLS*, advanced cardiac life support; *ARB*; angiotensin receptor blocker; *ASA*, aspirin; *BLS*, basic life support; *CCU*, critical care unit; *ECG*, electrocardiogram; *EMS*, emergency medical services; *IV*, intravenous; *LBBB*, left bundle branch block; *MONA*, morphine, oxygen, nitroglycerin, aspirin; *NSTEMI*, non–ST-segment elevation myocardial infarction; *NTG*, nitroglycerin; *PCI*, percutaneous coronary intervention; *PCU*, progressive care unit; *SpO2*, oxygen saturation by pulse oximetry; *STEMI*, ST-segment elevation myocardial infarction. (Data from American Heart Association. [2015]. Web-based Integrated Guidelines for Cardiopulmonary Resuscitation and Emergency Cardiovascular Care. Part 9 Acute Coronary Syndrome. Retrieved from https://eccguidelines.heart.org/index.php/circulation/cpr-ecc-guidelines-2/part-9-acute-coronary-syndromes.)

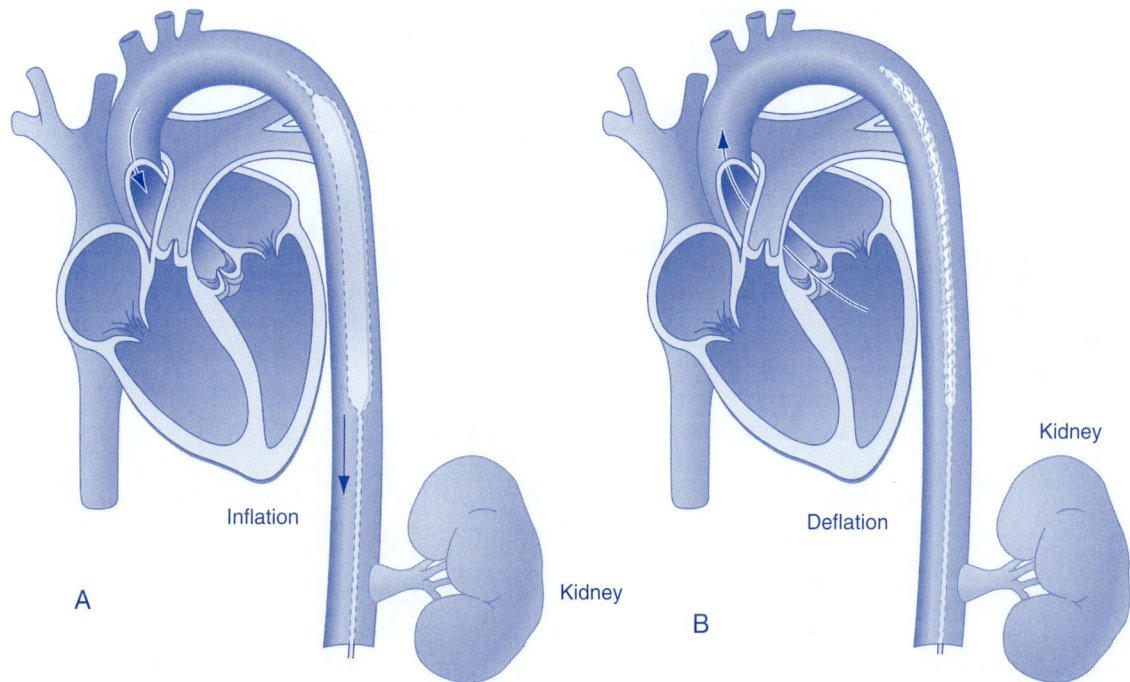

Fig. 3.75 Intraaortic balloon pump movement. **A,** Inflation during diastole moves blood toward the heart to increase coronary artery perfusion pressure. **B,** Deflation during systole moves blood away from the heart to decrease afterload. (From Carlson, K. K. [Ed.]. [2009]. *AACN Advanced critical care nursing*. St. Louis: Saunders.)

4. Reduce size of MI: myocardial salvaging techniques
   a. Treat pain promptly and adequately: decreases catecholamine release and myocardial oxygen demand
      1) Morphine sulfate: 2 to 4 mg IV every 5 minutes pain relief
         a) Actions: decreases preload; decreases catecholamine release via pain relief, which decreases HR and afterload; decreases anxiety and restlessness
         b) Cautions: inferior MI; RV MI
      2) Nitroglycerin: usually given initially sublingually; may be given prophylactically at 25 to 100 mcg/min IV for 24 to 48 hours
         a) Actions
            i) Decreases preload to decrease myocardial oxygen demand
            ii) Dilates epicardial coronary vessels to increase myocardial oxygen supply
            iii) Augments the analgesic effect of morphine
         b) Caution: may cause reflex tachycardia; beta-blockers may be needed
      3) Calcium channel blockers (e.g., nifedipine); especially for variant angina
      4) Reperfusion therapies (e.g., fibrinolytics, PCI): relieve pain by reestablishing blood flow and aerobic metabolism
      5) IABP: may be used for intractable pain as it increases CAPP (Figs. 3.75 to 3.77 and Table 3.27)
   b. Increase myocardial oxygen supply
      1) Administer oxygen at 2 to 6 l/min per nasal cannula for 24 to 48 hours.
         a) Probably has little effect on the myocardial arterial oxygen content of otherwise normal individuals but may significantly improve oxygenation of an ischemic myocardium, especially in patients with hypoxemia from pulmonary edema
         b) Even in the absence of pulmonary edema or other complications, it seems that some patients develop modest hypoxemia early during the course of acute MI.
      2) Provide either emergent PCI or fibrinolytics to reestablish patency of the infarct-related artery (IRA) within the benchmark time frame.
         a) Assist with decision making regarding reperfusion therapies.
            i) When PCI facilities are available, PCI is preferred over fibrinolytics for the majority of patients (O'Connor et al., 2010).
            ii) When PCI facilities are not available, prompt transport to a facility with PCI capability is preferred over fibrinolytics if transfer to PCI time is less than 120 minutes (O'Connor et al., 2010).
         b) Assist in prompt preparation of the patient for emergent PCI if PCI is determined to be the appropriate method of reperfusion for this specific patient; the goal is to achieve a door-to-balloon time (DTBT) of 90 minutes or less (Table 3.28)
            i) Strategies to reduce STEMI DTBT (Hammond, 2010; Farwell, 2010)
               (a) Establish protocols that define the process and facilitate crucial assessment studies (e.g., ECG, troponin) and interventions (IV, ASA).

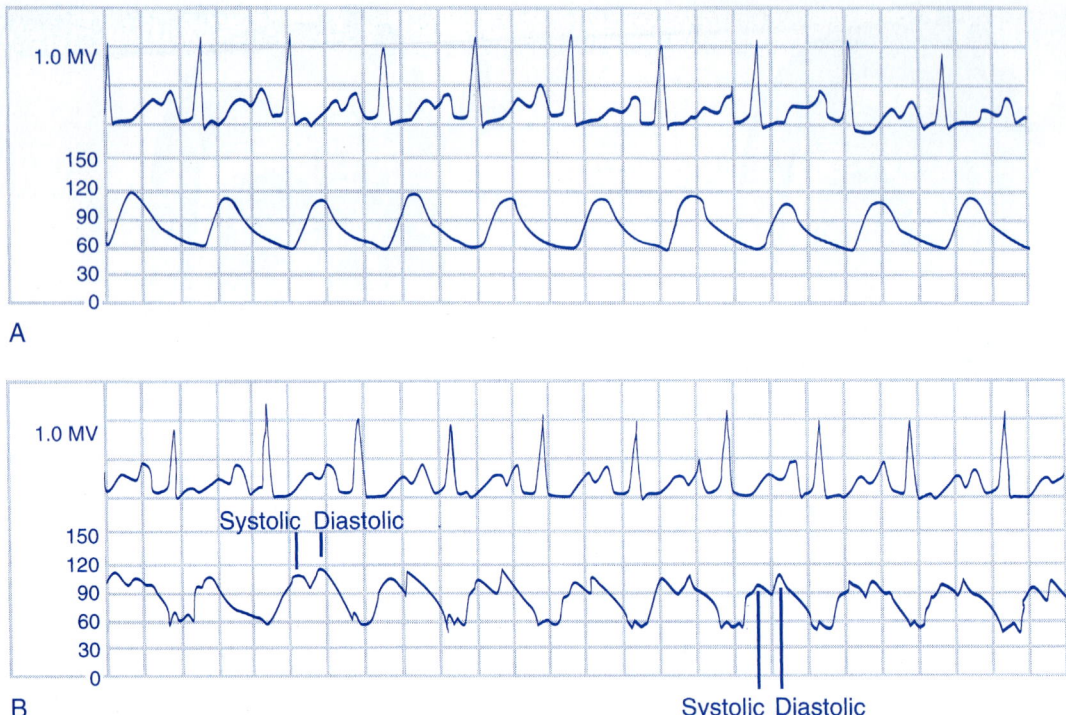

Fig. 3.76 Simultaneous electrocardiographic and arterial blood pressure recordings before *(panel A)* and during *(panel B)* intraaortic balloon counterpulsation. The peak diastolic (coronary perfusion) pressure is increased, and the peak systolic pressure is decreased during counterpulsation. (From Darovic, G. O. [2002]. *Hemodynamic monitoring: Invasive and noninvasive clinical application* [3rd ed.]. Philadelphia: Saunders.)

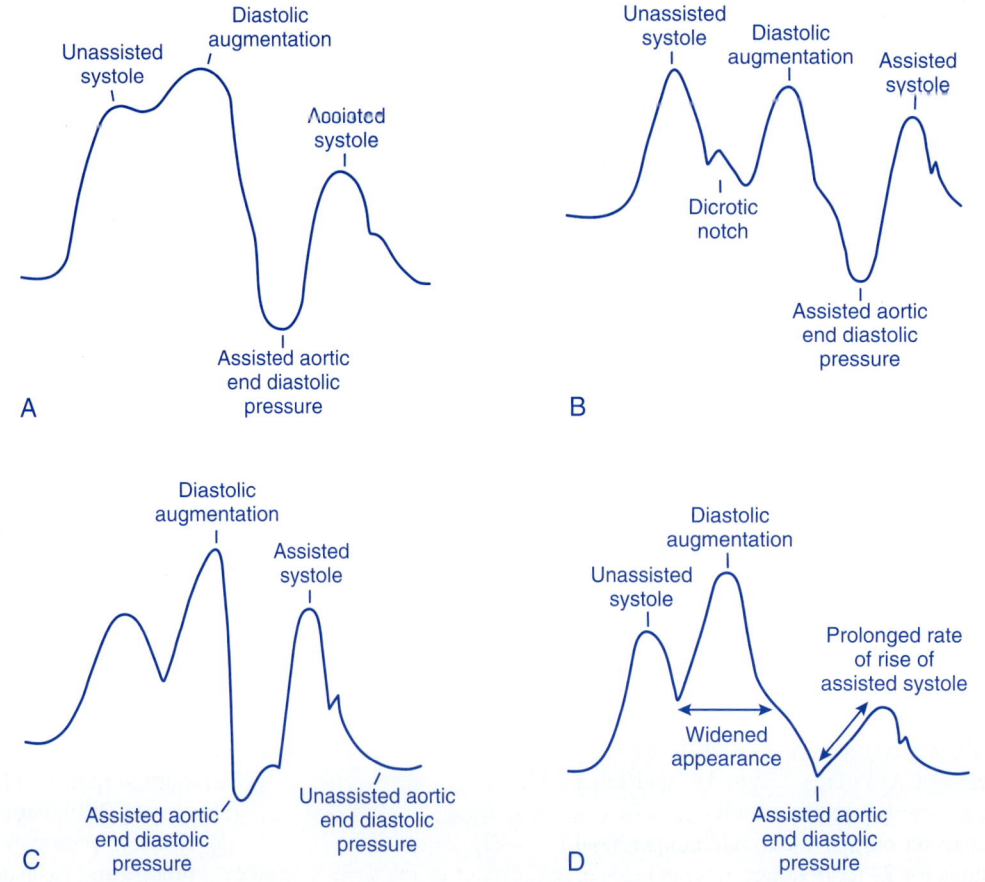

Fig. 3.77 Inaccurate intraaortic balloon pump timing. **A,** Early inflation. **B,** Late inflation. **C,** Early deflation. **D,** Late deflation. (From Datascope Corporation [1989]. *Mechanics of intraaortic balloon counterpulsation*. Montvale, NJ: Datascope.)

Table 3.27	Intraaortic Balloon Pump
Indications	• Unstable angina refractory to medical therapy • Impending MI or MI • Cardiogenic shock or severe LVF • HF, as a bridge to LVADA or transplant • Mechanical complications of acute MI (e.g., ruptured papillary muscle with acute mitral regurgitation, acute ventricular septal rupture) • Ischemia-related intractable ventricular dysrhythmias • High-risk patient undergoing PCI • Preoperative, perioperative, and/or postoperative support before coronary artery bypass graft or other major surgery • Difficulty weaning from cardiopulmonary bypass • Myocardial contusion • Septic shock

Contraindications	• Absolute
	  • Aortic valve regurgitation
	  • Aortic dissection
	  • Patients with chronic end-stage heart disease who are not awaiting a cardiac transplant
	  • Patients with irreversible brain damage or terminal condition
	• Relative
	  • Aortic aneurysm
	  • Uncontrolled sepsis
	  • Severe bilateral peripheral vascular disease (e.g., absent femoral pulse); if patient has had bilateral femoropopliteal bypass grafts, the balloon may be placed via the left axillary artery into the ascending aorta
	  • Coagulopathy
	  • Tachydysrhythmias

Actions (Fig. 3.75)	• Balloon is inflated during diastole to increase myocardial oxygen supply
	  • Increases coronary artery blood flow by displacing blood retrograde toward the aortic arch and increasing diastolic blood pressure
	  • Increases blood flow to the renal arteries and lower extremities by displacing blood antegrade toward the renal and lower extremities arteries
	  • Increases MAP to improve tissue perfusion
	• Balloon is deflated immediately before systole to decrease myocardial oxygen demand
	  • Decreases left ventricular afterload by decreasing systolic BP

Insertion and mechanics	• Catheter with balloon is inserted via femoral artery (NOTE: The catheter may be inserted via iliac, subclavian, or axillary artery if the femoral artery is not an option.)
	• Balloon is positioned in descending thoracic aorta between left subclavian and renal arteries
	  • The tip of the catheter should be at the second to third ICS, 1–2 cm from the left subclavian artery and above the renal arteries by chest radiography
	  • The balloon occludes 80% of the aortic diameter when inflated
	• Helium to inflate the balloon is shuttled into and out of the balloon by a pump which is housed in a console at the bedside

Timing (Fig. 3.76)	• By ECG
	  • Inflated after the T wave
	  • Deflated before QRS
	• By arterial waveform (NOTE: Newly IABP catheters have fiberoptic pressure sensors in the tip that provide real-time pressure signals because the signal travels at the speed of light rather than assuming a delay with fluid-filled transducer systems.)
	  • Inflated at the dicrotic notch
	  • Deflated at the end-diastolic dip immediately before systole
	• Inflation and deflation are usually triggered by ECG, but fine timing is done by the nurse using the arterial waveform
	• Frequency may be 1:1, 1:2, or 1:3, but timing is always adjusted in 1:2 setting

Assessment	• HR: a normalization of heart rate is desirable • BP: a decrease in systolic BP, an increase in diastolic BP, and an increase in MAP is desirable • CO/CI: an increase in CO/CI is desirable • PAP/PAOP: a decrease in PAP and PAOP is desirable • A decrease in the amplitude of v wave on the PAOP waveform is desirable in patients with mitral regurgitation or ventricular septal rupture • SaO_2: an increase in SaO_2 is desirable • SvO_2: an increase in SvO_2 is desirable • Urine output: an increase in urine output is desirable • Complaints of chest pain: a decrease in chest pain is desirable • ECG: a decrease in the presence or frequency of dysrhythmias is desirable • Neurovascular status of affected limb: the presence of palpable pulses and a warm limb with normal capillary refill is desirable

Continued

Table 3.27 Intraaortic Balloon Pump—cont'd

Brief summary of nursing management	• Assess the parameters described earlier • Ensure optimal timing of balloon inflation and deflation • Titrate pharmacologic therapies to augment the mechanical therapy of the IABP • Ensure positioning of the patient with head of bed elevation >30 degrees and avoidance of hip flexion • Observe for complications and provide appropriate management for the prevention of complications

Complications: prevention and treatment	• Thrombosis causing lower extremity ischemia
	  • Insertion precautions
	    • Use the smallest sheath that will allow the catheter to be advanced through it
	    • Select the limb with the best pulse
	  • Dextran 40 as prescribed as an antiplatelet aggregation agent
	  • Restraint of affected leg to prevent displacement of the balloon and trauma to intima of artery
	  • Neurovascular assessment of the affected limb every hour
	  • If limb ischemia is noted: treatment may include any of the following:
	    • Removal of catheter with placement of the sheath and catheter in the other femoral artery if the IABP is still needed
	    • Catheter thrombectomy
	    • Femorofemoral graft
	    • Lidocaine or papaverine: to decrease arterial spasm
	• Catheter displacement causing renal or left upper extremity ischemia
	  • Elevation of head of bed no more than 20–30 degrees to prevent displacement of the balloon
	  • Restraint of affected limb to prevent displacement of the balloon
	  • Close monitoring of urine output
	  • Notification of physician of significant changes in urine output
	  • Neurovascular assessment of left arm every hour
	• Emboli
	  • Dextran 40 as prescribed as an antiplatelet aggregation agent
	  • Heparin may be prescribed
	  • Avoidance of allowing the balloon to remain static (noninflating) for >30 min; clots may form in the folds of the balloon and be embolized when the balloon is then reinflated
	• Infection
	  • Sterile dressing changes daily or every other day
	  • Close monitoring of the site for erythema, edema, induration, warmth
	• Aortic dissection
	  • Attention to complaints of back pain, vital sign changes
	  • Removal of catheter and repair of aorta if dissection occurs
	• Anemia
	  • Attention to presence of petechiae or ecchymosis, platelet counts
	  • Discontinuance of heparin
	  • Blood and/or blood products may be prescribed
	• Balloon complications
	  • Leak
	    • Attention to increase in volume or frequency of refilling
	    • Replacement of catheter if leak occurs to prevent gas embolism
	  • Rupture
	    • Attention to blood in catheter
	    • Replacement of catheter if rupture occurs to prevent entrapment
	• Inaccurate timing (Fig. 3.77)
	  • Inflation is too early: aortic valve closes too early and stroke volume is decreased
	  • Inflation is too late: diastolic augmentation is decreased
	  • Deflation is too early: less increase in coronary artery perfusion pressure and less of a decrease in afterload
	  • Deflation is too late: increase in afterload
	• Inadequate pumping: usually due to dysrhythmias
	  • Timing method changed from ECG to arterial line

Weaning	• Indications
	  • CI >2.0 l/min
	  • PAOP <18 mm Hg
	  • MAP >70 mm Hg
	  • SVR <1400 dynes/sec/cm^{-5}
	  • SpO$_2$ >94%
	  • Absence of anginal pain
	  • Urine output at least 0.5 ml/kg/hr
	  • Absence of clinical indicators of hypoperfusion
	• Methods
	  • May be done by decreasing the frequency (e.g., from every cardiac cycle to every other cardiac cycle to every third cardiac cycle)
	  • May be done by decreasing the volume in the balloon with each inflation (e.g., decreased by 25% with each weaning step)

Table 3.27	Intraaortic Balloon Pump—cont'd
Balloon removal	• Gown, mask, eye protection must be used • Pump is turned off, sutures are removed, catheter is removed and inspected to ensure that the entire catheter has been removed • Firm pressure is applied to the insertion site for at least 15 min but may be required for more than 30 min if the patient has been receiving anticoagulants; a vascular hemostasis device may be used • Pressure dressing to insertion site for 2–4 hr • Monitor site frequently for the next 4–8 hr for bleeding or hematoma formation

BP, Blood pressure; *CI*, cardiac index; *CO*, cardiac output; *ECG*, electrocardiogram; *HF*, heart failure; *HR*, heart rate; *IABP*, intraaortic balloon pump; *ICS*, intercostal space; *LVAD*, left ventricular assist device; *LVF*, left ventricular failure; *MAP*, mean arterial pressure; *MI*, myocardial infarction; *PAOP*, pulmonary artery occlusive pressure; *PAP*, pulmonary artery pressure; *PCI*, percutaneous coronary intervention; SaO_2, arterial oxygen saturation; SvO_2, saturation of venous blood; *SVR*, systemic vascular resistance.

Table 3.28	Percutaneous Coronary Interventions

Procedures	• Percutaneous transluminal coronary angioplasty (PTCA): inflation of a balloon-tipped catheter in an area of coronary artery stenosis from plaque; plaque is pushed back against the wall of the vessel and fractured (controlled trauma)
	  • Cutting balloon microsurgical dilation catheter system: microsurgical blades mounted longitudinally on an angioplasty balloon to open narrowed artery; as the balloon expands radially, the blades are exposed and incise plaque in the arteries; claimed to facilitate maximum dilatation of the target lesion with more precision and less trauma than conventional angioplasty
	• Coronary artery stent: use of a metal mesh tube that acts as a scaffolding device to support a coronary artery and maintain patency after PTCA; previously used only in case of acute closure, most PTCA procedures include planned stent placements
	  • Stents are usually stainless steel but may be nitinol, tantalum, or another metal
	  • Stents have usually been thought of as a coil, but they may be a mesh, slotted tube, ring, or another design
	  • Stents are either deployed by balloon expansion or they may be self-expanding
	  • Stents may be drug eluting (i.e., drug-eluting stent) to reduce the risk of neointimal hyperplasia and restenosis rates
	    • Sirolimus, an immunosuppressive agent, to prevent proliferation of normal tissue and inflammation
	    • Paclitaxel, an antineoplastic agent, to inhibit cell proliferation and migration
	• Brachytherapy: use of intracoronary irradiation to reduce risk of restenosis; combined with PTCA or stent placement
	• Coronary atherectomy: removal of plaque from a coronary artery by a high-speed diamond-tipped (rotational) or shaving (directional) device
	  • Directional coronary atherectomy (DCA): a directional device shaves pieces of the atheroma into the catheter tip
	  • Coronary rotational ablation (Rotablator): a diamond-coated burr drills through the atheroma and pulverizes the plaque
	  • Transluminal extraction catheter (TEC): a motorized cutting head shaves the atheroma from the arterial wall and suctions out the pieces
	  • Excimer laser coronary atherectomy (ELCA): use of a laser to vaporize the atheroma
	• AngioJet: high speed saline jet; most effective for thrombus

Indications	• Unstable or chronic angina • Acute or postacute MI • Postcoronary artery bypass graft with postoperative angina • Patient must be surgical candidate (in case of coronary artery dissection)
Contraindications	• Left main CAD (unless there is a patent bypass around it, referred to as *protected*) • Stenosis of coronary artery at orifice • Variant angina • Critical valvular disease
Action	The goal of percutaneous coronary interventions is to reduce the degree of coronary artery stenosis; the intervention is considered successful if the degree of stenosis is reduced to 20%–30% stenosis without serious complications
Assessment	• Vital signs: BP, HR, RR, T • ECG: monitor closely for ST-segment elevation • Sheath insertion site: usually femoral but may be radial • Neurovascular status of affected limb • Any complaints of chest pain • Any complaints of back pain

Continued

Table 3.28	Percutaneous Coronary Interventions—cont'd

Brief summary of specific nursing management	• Monitor for myocardial ischemia: note any new chest pain, ST-segment elevation especially if PCI performed for acute ischemia or infarction
	• Assess puncture site frequently to detect bleeding and/or hematoma formation
	  • Control systolic BP to <150 mm Hg and diastolic BP <90 mm Hg with antihypertensives as prescribed
	  • Monitor platelet count and aPTT (patient will receive platelet aggregation inhibitors and either unfractionated or low-molecular-weight heparin to prevent reocclusion)
	  • Immobilize groin by restraining with sheet stretched over knee on affected side and tucked on each side of bed rather than restraining ankle
	  • Perform neurovascular checks to detect peripheral ischemia related to femoral artery thrombosis
	• Monitor for clinical indications of retroperitoneal hemorrhage: postural tachycardia and/or hypotension; back and/or flank pain; Grey-Turner sign; decrease in hemoglobin and hematocrit (unfortunately there are no early indications)
	• Keep affected limb straight and immobile; HOPB should be elevated no more than 30 degrees as long as the sheath is in place and for 4–8 hr after removal
	• Assist with removal or remove sheath (depending on hospital protocol) if not completed in the cardiac catheterization laboratory; Perclose, VasoSeal, or Angio-Seal may be used when the sheath was removed in the cardiac catheterization laboratory
	  • If IV heparin has been infusing, it will be discontinued and the ACT needs to be <150 sec; if unfractionated heparin is to be restarted, it will be restarted several hours after sheath removal; LMWH subcutaneously may be used
	  • Pain control and sedation (e.g., local infiltration with lidocaine or IV morphine and/or midazolam or lorazepam)
	  • Pressure to where the sheath entered the artery which is about 1 inch above the skin entry site
	  • Manual pressure or mechanical pressure devices (e.g., C-clamp, FemoStop) may be used
	  • Pressure is held for at least 30 min or until hemostasis achieved
	  • Control of bleeding must be maintained while peripheral pulses are still palpated

Complications: prevention and treatment	• Acute reocclusion or closure due to:
	  • Trauma to intima initiating clotting cascade
	    • ASA and heparin are used to prevent thrombosis
	    • GP IIb/IIIa platelet receptor blockers (e.g., abciximab, eptifibatide, or tirofiban HCl) are used for PCI in ACS patients who have not been receiving clopidogrel
	    • ASA and clopidogrel are maintained after the procedure
	    • Prasugrel is another platelet receptor blocker that may be used but should not be used for ACS patients with stroke or transient ischemic attack
	    • Monitor aPTT; usually maintained at 50–70 sec
	    • Proton pump inhibitor is recommended with dual antiplatelet therapy
	  • Coronary artery spasm
	    • Nitroglycerin infusion and/or calcium channel blockers are frequently used
	    • NOTE: New onset chest pain or ST-segment changes should be reported immediately
	• Coronary artery dissection: caused by catheter trauma; necessitates placement of stent or, in severe cases, emergent coronary artery bypass graft
	• Cardiac tamponade: due to cardiac perforation
	• Dysrhythmias: caused by ischemia or reperfusion
	• Pseudoaneurysm: due to catheter dissection of artery
	• Hemorrhage or hematoma: due to anticoagulated state
	  • Retroperitoneal hemorrhage or hematoma
	  • Femoral artery puncture site hemorrhage or hematoma
	• Embolic complications (e.g., myocardial infarction, cerebral infarction, peripheral emboli)
	• Chronic restenosis: due to intimal hyperplasia
	• Hypotension, bradycardia (i.e., vagal reaction): caused by increased parasympathetic nervous system during sheath removal; atropine is effective

Postprocedure education	• Information about devices placed: give the patient a stent identification card with date, facility, type, and site of implant • Care of site used for catheter insertion (e.g., femoral or radial) • Need for drugs to maintain stent patency: usually aspirin and clopidogrel • Avoid MRI scans within 8 wk of stent placement • Symptoms to report: site pain, chest pain, bleeding

ACS, Acute coronary syndrome; *ACT*, activated clotting time; *aPTT*, activated partial thromboplastin time; *ASA*, aspirin; *BP*, blood pressure; *CAD*, coronary artery disease; *ECG*, electrocardiogram; *GP*, glycoprotein; *HOB*, head of bed; *HR*, heart rate; *IV*, intravenous; *LMWH*, low-molecular-weight heparin; *MI*, myocardial infarction; *MRI*, magnetic resonance imaging; *PCI*, percutaneous coronary intervention; *RR*, respiratory rate; *T*, temperature.

(b) Empower emergency medical services or emergency department (ED) physician to activate the STEMI team; eliminate unnecessary consults.
(c) Facilitate sharing of information through computerization.
(d) Provide feedback to participants so that improvements can continue.

c) Administer fibrinolytics if they are determined to be the appropriate method of reperfusion for this specific patient; the goal is to achieve door-to-needle time of 60 minutes or less (Table 3.29).
d) Either primary PCI or fibrinolytics are preceded by platelet aggregation inhibitors or anticoagulants.
  i) Platelet aggregation inhibitors
    (a) ASA (160–325 mg initially and daily) and/or another antiplatelet drug (e.g., clopidogrel, prasugrel) to decrease platelet aggregation and clot extension
    (b) Glycoprotein (GP) IIb/IIIa platelet receptor blockers (e.g., abciximab, eptifibatide, tirofiban HCl) (Table 3.30)
  ii) Anticoagulants (Table 3.30)
    (a) Unfractionated heparin (UFH) may be prescribed for 24 to 48 hours to maintain an aPTT of 45 to 60 seconds
      (i) Indirect thrombin inhibitor
      (ii) Initial dosing should be weight based; then infusion is adjusted by aPTT results
      (iii) Usual dose of UFH: bolus of 60 units/kg; then infusion of 12 units/kg/hr
    (b) Subcutaneous low-molecular-weight heparin
      (i) Indirect thrombin inhibitor
      (ii) Lower incidence of heparin-induced thrombocytopenia (HIT) than UFH
    (c) Bivalirudin (Table 3.30)
      (i) Direct thrombin inhibitor
      (ii) Most frequently used after PCI
    (d) Warfarin (Table 3.30) is usually prescribed for at least 3 months in patients with any of the following:
      (i) Anterior Q-wave MI
      (ii) HF
      (iii) Severe LV dysfunction
      (iv) Atrial fibrillation
      (v) Previous embolic event
3) Prepare patient for coronary bypass grafting as indicated; CABG (Table 3.31) is used to provide arterial or venous conduits to redirect coronary blood flow around occluded coronary arteries

Table 3.29	Fibrinolytic Therapy

Actions	• Activate plasminogen to plasmin, the active agent that breaks down clots (speeds up the normal fibrinolytic process to allow early reperfusion)
	• Limit cellular necrosis and decrease infarction size
	• Decrease mortality, morbidity
	  • Short term: reestablishing arterial patency
	  • Long term: maintaining ejection fraction

Fibrinolytic agents (Table 3.30)	• Streptokinase (SK) (rarely used today)
	• Recombinant tissue plasminogen activator (rt-PA)
	  • Alteplase: short-half life so administered as a bolus followed by infusion
	  • Tenecteplase: longest half-life so administered as a one-time bolus
	• Recombinant plasminogen activator (r-PA)
	  • Reteplase: intermediate half-life so administered as two boluses 10 min apart
	• Urokinase (rarely used in acute MI but may be used in peripheral arterial occlusion)

Indications	• History strongly suggestive of MI • ST-segment elevation of more than 1 mm in at least two contiguous leads or new LBBB • Pain of <6 hr or still having pain (NOTE: As long as the patient is having pain, salvageable myocardium is assumed because dead myocardium does not metabolize aerobically or anaerobically, and neither lactic acid or pain would be produced.)
Absolute contraindications	• Active internal bleeding • History of hemorrhagic stroke, intracranial neoplasm, AVM, or aneurysm • Intracranial or intraspinal surgery or trauma within 2 months • Known bleeding disorder (e.g., thrombocytopenia, hemophilia) • Suspected aortic aneurysm or acute pericarditis • Systolic BP >or equal to 200 mm Hg and/or diastolic BP >or equal to 120 mm Hg • Prolonged (more than 10 min) or traumatic CPR • Pregnancy • Streptokinase is contraindicated if the patient has received streptokinase or had a streptococcal infection within the last 6–9 mo but t-PA can still be used

Continued

Table 3.29	Fibrinolytic Therapy—cont'd
Relative contraindications	• Major surgery or trauma within 10 days • Recent GI or GU bleeding • Cerebrovascular disease • Oral anticoagulant therapy • Systolic BP ≥or 180 mm Hg and/or diastolic BP ≥110 mm Hg • Significant liver dysfunction • Septic thrombophlebitis • Subacute bacterial endocarditis • High likelihood of left heart thrombus (e.g., mitral stenosis with atrial fibrillation, ventricular aneurysm, left atrial myxoma) • Diabetic hemorrhagic retinopathy • Advanced age (older than 70–75 yr) with consideration of physiologic age, severity of concomitant diseases, mental status • Any condition when bleeding would be a significant hazard or would be difficult to manage (e.g., recent femoral artery puncture or sheath)

Clinical indications of reperfusion	• Pain cessation
	• ST-segment return to baseline
	• Reperfusion dysrhythmias
	  • Sinus bradycardia
	  • Idioventricular rhythm, accelerated idioventricular rhythm
	  • AV blocks
	  • Ventricular irritability: PVCs, ventricular tachycardia, ventricular fibrillation
	• CK washout: early or markedly elevated CK peak

Assessment	• Heart rate • BP • ECG rhythm; note reperfusion dysrhythmias • Clinical indications of reperfusion • Bleeding (e.g., puncture points, gums, saliva, sputum, gastric secretions, stools, urine) • Complaints of chest pain, back pain, or headache

Brief summary of nursing management	• Administer adjuvant therapy: t-PA is followed by ASA, heparin (SK causes significant fibrinogen depletion, and heparin is not indicated due to increased bleeding risk)
	• Monitor for clinical indications of reperfusion; notify physician if these are not seen so that emergent PCI can be scheduled
	• Avoid punctures: arterial; IV, IM,
	  • Apply pressure until hemostasis is achieved if punctures are required after fibrinolytics initiated
	  • Insert multiple (i.e., two or three) IV catheters before initiation of fibrinolytic therapy; one of these catheters may be used for venous sampling
	• Monitor stools, urine, emesis, sputum, saliva for blood
	• Monitor for complications

Complications	• Hemorrhage
	  • At site of vascular puncture: 80% incidence
	  • GI or GU bleeding: 15%–20% incidence
	  • Intracranial bleed: 1% incidence
	• Reocclusion: monitor for new pain and/or ST-segment changes
	• Allergic reactions to streptokinase
	  • Monitor for urticaria, fever, bronchospasm, dyspnea, stridor, or dysrhythmias
	  • Administer diphenhydramine and/or hydrocortisone as prescribed in attempt to prevent allergic reaction
	• Reperfusion dysrhythmias: usually transient
	  • Administer antidysrhythmics or perform cardioversion or defibrillation as indicated for sustained ventricular tachycardia or ventricular fibrillation (prophylactic antidysrhythmics are no longer recommended with fibrinolytic therapy)
	  • Administer atropine or apply transcutaneous pacemaker for symptomatic bradycardia or block

ASA, Aspirin; *AV*, atrioventricular; *AVM*, arteriovenous malformation; *BP*, blood pressure; *CK*, creatine kinase; *CPR*, cardiopulmonary resuscitation; *ECG*, electrocardiogram; *GI*, gastrointestinal; *GU*, genitourinary; *IM*, intramuscular; *IV*, intravenous; *LBBB*, left bundle branch block; *MI*, myocardial infarction; *PCI*, percutaneous coronary intervention; *PVC*, premature ventricular contraction; *SC*, subcutaneous; *t-PA*, tissue plasminogen activator.

Table 3.30 Drugs that Affect Clotting Used for Patients with Myocardial Infarction

Drug	Classification and Actions	Indications	Administration	Adverse Effects	Nursing Implications
Abciximab	Platelet aggregation inhibitor (GP IIb/IIIa platelet receptor blocker) • Inhibits platelet aggregation and platelet-mediated thrombosis	• ACS with or without PCI • PCI when risk for thrombosis is high	• IV injection: 0.25 mg/kg administered between 10 min and 1 hr before the start of the PTCA or atherectomy followed by infusion • IV infusion: 0.125 mcg/kg/min (10 mcg/min maximum) for 12 hr	• Bleeding • Intracranial hemorrhage • Hematuria • Hematemesis • Bleeding at sheath site or other puncture point • Thrombocytopenia • Hypotension • Bradycardia • Nausea, vomiting, abdominal pain • Chest pain • Back pain • Headache • Pain at injection site • Allergic reaction, anaphylaxis (especially with repeat administration)	• Monitor PT, aPTT, or ACT, platelet count • Administer with aspirin and heparin therapy as prescribed • Note contraindications: patients with active internal bleeding, clinically significant bleeding in the GI or GU tract within the past 6 wk, bleeding diathesis, history of CVA within the past 2 yr or CVA with significant residual neurologic deficit, intracranial neoplasm, aneurysm, or AV malformation, severe uncontrolled hypertension, oral anticoagulants within 7 d unless prothrombin time is <1.2 × control, thrombocytopenia, presumed or documented history of vasculitis, major surgery or trauma within the past 6 wk, pericarditis, known hypersensitivity to abciximab or murine proteins • Use cautiously in patients who weigh <75 kg, patients older than 65 yr of age, patients with a history of GI disease, patients receiving fibrinolytics • Do not administer with dextran • Monitor oral secretions, sputum, vomitus, NG aspirate, stool, urine for blood • Limit venipuncture and urinary catheterization as possible; use IV catheter with saline lock for blood sampling; avoid noncompressible IV sites • Avoid nasotracheal and NG tubes if possible • Avoid automatic BP cuffs • Administer platelets as prescribed for thrombocytopenia • Store refrigerated, do not shake (should be clear), administer through filter

Continued

Table 3.30 Drugs that Affect Clotting Used for Patients with Myocardial Infarction—cont'd

Drug	Classification and Actions	Indications	Administration	Adverse Effects	Nursing Implications
Eptifibatide	Platelet aggregation inhibitor (GP IIb/IIIa platelet receptor blocker) • Inhibits platelet aggregation and platelet-mediated thrombosis	• ACS with or without PCI • PCI when risk for thrombosis is high	For acute coronary syndrome • IV injection: 180 mcg/kg over 1–2 min followed by: • IV infusion: 2 mcg/kg/min for up to 72 hr; decreased to 0.5 mcg/kg/min during PCI and continued for 24 hr after PCI For PCI without ACS • IV injection: 135 mcg/kg over 1–2 min before procedure followed by: • IV infusion: 0.5 mcg/kg/min for 24 hr	• Bleeding • Intracranial hemorrhage • Hematuria • Hematemesis • Bleeding at sheath site • Hypotension	• Monitor PT, aPTT, or ACT, platelet count • Note contraindications: active internal bleeding, clinically significant bleeding in the GI or GU tract within the past 6 wk, bleeding diathesis, history of CVA within the past 2 yr or CVA with significant residual neurologic deficit, intracranial neoplasm, aneurysm, or AV malformation, severe uncontrolled hypertension, oral anticoagulants within 7 days unless prothrombin time is <1.2 × control, thrombocytopenia, presumed or documented history of vasculitis, major surgery or trauma within the last 6 wk, pericarditis, known hypersensitivity to eptifibatide, renal failure, thrombocytopenia • Administer with aspirin and heparin therapy as prescribed • Monitor oral secretions, sputum, vomitus, NG aspirate, stool, urine for blood • Limit venipuncture and urinary catheterization as possible; use IV catheter with saline lock for blood sampling; avoid noncompressible IV sites • Avoid nasotracheal and nasogastric tubes if possible • Avoid automatic BP cuffs • Administer platelets as prescribed for thrombocytopenia • Store refrigerated

| Tirofiban HCl | Platelet aggregation inhibitor (GP IIb/IIIa platelet receptor blocker) • Inhibits platelet aggregation and platelet-mediated thrombosis | • Acute coronary syndrome with or without PCI | • IV infusion: premixed as 25 mg in 500 ml; usual dose is 0.4 mcg/kg/min for 30 min and then continued at 0.1 mcg/kg/min (dosage is decreased in renal failure) | • Bleeding
• Intracranial hemorrhage
• Hematuria
• Hematemesis
• Bleeding at sheath site
• Hypotension
• Bradycardia
• Pelvic pain | • Monitor PT, aPTT, or ACT, platelet count
• Note contraindications: active internal bleeding, clinically significant bleeding in the GI or GU tract within the past 6 wk, bleeding diathesis, history of CVA within the past 2 yr or CVA with significant residual neurologic deficit, intracranial neoplasm, aneurysm, or AVM, severe uncontrolled hypertension, oral anticoagulants within 7 days unless prothrombin time is <1.2 × control, thrombocytopenia, presumed or documented history of vasculitis, major surgery or trauma within the last month, pericarditis, known hypersensitivity to tirofiban
• Use cautiously in patients who weigh <75 kg, patients older than 65 yr of age, patients with a history of GI disease, patients receiving fibrinolytics, patients with thrombocytopenia
• Administer with aspirin and heparin therapy as prescribed
• Limit venipuncture and urinary catheterization as possible; use IV catheter with saline lock for blood sampling; avoid noncompressible IV sites
• Monitor oral secretions, sputum, vomitus, NG aspirate, stool, urine for blood |

Continued

174 Chapter 3 The Cardiovascular System

Table 3.30 Drugs that Affect Clotting Used for Patients with Myocardial Infarction—cont'd

Drug	Classification and Actions	Indications	Administration	Adverse Effects	Nursing Implications
Recombinant tissue plasminogen activator (rt-PA) alteplase	Fibrinolytic • Converts plasminogen to plasmin at fibrin surface • Causes clot-specific lysis	• Acute MI (chest pain strongly suggestive of acute MI; ST segment of at least 1 mm in at least two leads) • Massive PE (with RVF or refractory hypoxemia) • Thrombotic stroke	For acute MI • IV injection: 15 mg followed by: • IV infusion: 0.75 mg/kg (not to exceed 50 mg) over next 30 min, followed by 0.5 mg/kg (not to exceed 35 mg) over the next 60 min • Heparin started within 1 hr of initial dose For ischemic stroke • Total dose: 0.9 mg/kg with maximum dose of < or equal to 90 mg • IV injection: 10% of this total dose over 1 min followed by: • IV infusion: remaining 90% of this total dose administered over 60 min • Anticoagulants and platelet aggregation inhibitors are not used for at least 24 hr For acute PE • IV infusion: 100 mg at 50 mg/hr for 2 hr For acute arterial occlusion • 0.05–0.1 mg/kg/hr by local intraarterial infusion • Reconstitution in sterile water only	• Severe, spontaneous bleeding including potential cerebral, retroperitoneal, GU, GI bleeding, surface bleeding • Reperfusion dysrhythmias	• Monitor aPTT, PT, thrombin time, fibrinogen, neurologic status, and for signs of hemorrhage • Note contraindications: active bleeding; history of cerebral hemorrhage, intracranial neoplasm, AVM or aneurysm; recent (within 2 mo) intracranial or intraspinal surgery or trauma; known bleeding disorder; severe uncontrolled hypertension; prolonged CPR • Use cautiously in recent (within 10 d) major surgery, GI, GU bleeding, or trauma; hypertension with SBP >180 mm/Hg or DBP >110 mm/Hg; high likelihood of left heart thrombus; acute pericarditis; significant liver dysfunction; pregnancy; retinopathy; septic thrombophlebitis; advanced age (>70–75 yr); patients receiving oral anticoagulants; any condition in which bleeding constitutes a significant hazard or would be particularly difficult to manage because of its location • Monitor for indications of reperfusion in MI • Cessation of pain • ST segments descending back to baseline • Reperfusion dysrhythmias (ventricular ectopy including PVCs, VT or VF, accelerated idioventricular rhythm, junctional escape rhythms, bradycardia) • Early CK peak • Note that signs of reperfusion are much more subtle in PE and thrombotic stroke • Limit venipuncture and urinary catheterization as possible; use IV catheter with saline lock for blood sampling; avoid noncompressible IV sites • Administer all drugs through existing IVs started before initiation of fibrinolytic therapy or by mouth • Avoid nasotracheal and NG tubes if possible • Avoid automatic BP cuffs • Monitor oral secretions, sputum, vomitus, NG aspirate, stool, urine for blood • Bleeding precautions are maintained for 12–24 hr

Recombinant tissue plasminogen activator (rt-PA) tenecteplase	Fibrinolytic
	• Converts plasminogen to plasmin at fibrin surface
	• Causes clot-specific lysis
		• Acute MI (chest pain strongly suggestive of acute MI; ST segment of at least 1 mm in at least two leads)	• IV injection over 5 sec
			• <60 kg: 30 mg
			• ≤60–<70 kg: 35 mg
			• ≥70–<80 kg: 40 mg
			• ≥80–<90 kg: 45 mg
			• ≥90 kg: 50 mg
			• Heparin administered concurrently
				• Severe, spontaneous bleeding, including potential cerebral, retroperitoneal, GU, GI bleeding, surface bleeding
				• Reperfusion dysrhythmias
					• Monitor aPTT, PT, thrombin time, neurologic status, and for signs of hemorrhage
					• Note contraindications: active bleeding; history of cerebral hemorrhage, intracranial neoplasm, AVM or aneurysm; recent (within 2 mo) intracranial or intraspinal surgery or trauma; known bleeding disorder; severe uncontrolled hypertension; prolonged CPR
					• Use cautiously in recent (within 10 days) major surgery, GI, GU bleeding, or trauma; hypertension with SBP >180 mm/Hg or DBP >110 mm/Hg; high likelihood of left heart thrombus; acute pericarditis; significant liver dysfunction; pregnancy; retinopathy; septic thrombophlebitis; advanced age (>70–75 yr); patients receiving oral anticoagulants; any condition in which bleeding constitutes a significant hazard or would be particularly difficult to manage because of its location
					
					Identify indications of reperfusion in MI:
					• Cessation of pain
					  • ST segments descending back to baseline
					  • Reperfusion dysrhythmias (ventricular ectopy including PVCs, VT or VF, accelerated idioventricular rhythm, junctional escape rhythms, bradycardia)
					  • Early CK peak
					• Limit venipuncture and urinary catheterization as possible; use IV catheter with saline lock for blood sampling; avoid noncompressible IV sites
					• Avoid nasotracheal and NG tubes if possible
					• Avoid automatic BP cuffs
					• Administer all drugs through existing IVs started before initiation of fibrinolytic therapy or by mouth
					• Monitor oral secretions, sputum, vomitus, NG aspirate, stool, urine for blood
					• Bleeding precautions are maintained for 12–24 hr

Table 3.30 Drugs that Affect Clotting Used for Patients with Myocardial Infarction—cont'd

Drug	Classification and Actions	Indications	Administration	Adverse Effects	Nursing Implications

Recombinant plasminogen activator (r-PA) reteplase	Fibrinolytic
	• Converts plasminogen to plasmin at fibrin surface
	• Causes clot-specific lysis
		• Acute MI (chest pain strongly suggestive of acute MI; ST segment of at least 1 mm in at least two leads)	• IV injection of 10 units over 2 min initially followed by 10 units over 2 min after 30 min
			• Heparin administered concurrently
				• Severe, spontaneous bleeding including potential cerebral, retroperitoneal, GU, GI bleeding, surface bleeding
				• Reperfusion dysrhythmias
					• Monitor aPTT, PT, thrombin time, neurologic status, and for signs of hemorrhage
					• Note contraindications: active bleeding; history of cerebral hemorrhage, intracranial neoplasm, AVM or aneurysm; recent (within 2 mo) intracranial or intraspinal surgery or trauma; known bleeding disorder; severe uncontrolled hypertension; prolonged CPR
					• Use cautiously in recent (within 10 d) major surgery, GI, GU bleeding, or trauma; hypertension with SBP >180 mm/Hg or DBP >110 mm/Hg; high likelihood of left heart thrombus; acute pericarditis; significant liver dysfunction; pregnancy; retinopathy; septic thrombophlebitis; advanced age (>70–75 yr); patients receiving oral anticoagulants; any condition in which bleeding constitutes a significant hazard or would be particularly difficult to manage because of its location
					• Identify indications of reperfusion in MI
					  • Cessation of pain
					  • ST segments descending back to baseline
					  • Reperfusion dysrhythmias (ventricular ectopy, including PVCs, VT or VF, accelerated idioventricular rhythm, junctional escape rhythms, bradycardia)
					  • Early CK peak
					• Limit venipuncture and urinary catheterization as possible; use IV catheter with saline lock for blood sampling; avoid noncompressible IV sites
					• Avoid nasotracheal and NG tubes if possible
					• Avoid automatic BP cuffs
					• Administer all drugs through existing IVs started before initiation of fibrinolytic therapy or by mouth
					• Monitor oral secretions, sputum, vomitus, NG aspirate, stool, urine for blood
					• Bleeding precautions are maintained for 12–24 hr

| Heparin sodium | Anticoagulant
- Prevents conversion of prothrombin to thrombin
- Prevents conversion of fibrinogen to fibrin
- Prevents extension of existing clots
- Decreases platelet aggregation | - Unstable angina or MI
- Maintenance of arterial patency after PCI or fibrinolytic therapy
- Prevention of thrombus formation during periods of inactivity
- DVT
- PE
- Peripheral arterial emboli
- Transient ischemic attacks or reversible ischemic neurologic deficit
- DIC (controversial)
- Maintenance of arterial line patency | - SC: usually prophylactic, dose is 5000 units every 12 hr (also called mini-heparin)
- IV injection: usually 80 units/kg (maximum: 10,000 units) followed by infusion (only 60 units/kg recommended if patient is receiving fibrinolytics or GP IIb/IIIa inhibitors)
- IV infusion: mix 25,000 units in 500 ml (50 units/ml) and infuse at 18 units/kg/hr (maximum: 1000 units/hr) (only 12 units/kg recommended if patient is receiving fibrinolytics or GP IIb/IIIa inhibitors); dose is adjusted to achieve aPTT of 1.5–2.5 times the laboratory control
- NOTE: The trend in IV weight-dosed heparin is to decrease the amount of heparin (60 units/kg for injection followed by 12 units/kg/hr for infusion) and desirable aPTT (45–60 sec) Maximum: 40,000 units/d | - Hemorrhage with excessive aPTT
- Hypertension or hypotension
- Hypersensitivity reaction including bronchospasm
- Fever
- Hepatitis
- Hyperkalemia especially in patients with renal failure
- Thrombocytopenia (caused by immune response referred to as HIT | - Monitor aPTT and platelet count and for signs of hemorrhage
- Note petechiae and request platelet count if petechiae noted; heparin usually discontinued if platelet count is <100,000/mm^3
  - Administer lepirudin (Refludan) or argatroban as prescribed for HIT
- Note contraindications: known hypersensitivity, active bleeding, blood dyscrasias (except DIC), suspected intracranial hemorrhage, severe hypertension, peptic ulcer disease, open wounds, recent surgery, endocarditis, shock, threatened abortion
- Use cautiously in alcoholism, liver disease, renal disease, older adults
- Monitor oral secretions, sputum, vomitus, NG aspirate, stool, urine for blood
- Ensure that protamine sulfate (antidote) is available
- Avoid IM, arterial, or venous punctures if at all possible
- Hold pressure for longer than usual if punctures necessary
- Do not discontinue suddenly: warfarin will usually have already been started and the PT within therapeutic range before heparin is discontinued
- Do not aspirate before SC administration and do not massage after administration
- Note that nitroglycerin interacts with heparin, causing more heparin to be required to achieve therapeutic aPTT; monitor aPTT closely with significant nitroglycerin dosage changes or discontinuance |

Continued

Table 3.30 Drugs that Affect Clotting Used for Patients with Myocardial Infarction—cont'd

Drug	Classification and Actions	Indications	Administration	Adverse Effects	Nursing Implications

Heparin: low-molecular-weight enoxaparin dalteparin sodium	Anticoagulant
	• Inhibits thrombin activity
	• Prevents DVT
	• Does not prevent platelet aggregation
		• High risk for DVT
		• ACS
			• Enoxaparin
			  • SC: 30 mg bid
			• Dalteparin sodium
			  • SC: 2500 international units daily starting 1–2 hr before surgery and repeated qd for 5–10 d postoperatively
			• Ardeparin
			  • SC: 50 antifactor Xa IU/kg every 12 hr beginning the evening before surgery and continued until the patient is ambulatory
			• Tinzaparin sodium
			  • SC: 175 factor antifactor Xa IU/kg daily for ≈6 days or until adequate anticoagulation with warfarin
				• Bleeding
				• Epidural or spinal hematoma (especially when used with patients with epidural or spinal anesthesia)
				• Fever
				• Elevation of liver enzymes
				• Thrombocytopenia
				• Chest pain
					• Note that LMWH does not require routine laboratory monitoring because it does not usually alter PT or aPTT
					• Note that contraindications and cautions are as for heparin
					• Obtain baseline platelet count; monitor for petechiae
					• Monitor oral secretions, sputum, vomitus, NG aspirate, stool, urine for blood
					• Ensure that protamine sulfate (antidote) is available
					• Avoid IM, arterial, or venous punctures if at all possible
					• Hold pressure for longer than usual if punctures necessary
					• Administer deep subcutaneously but avoid IM injection

Bivalirudin	Anticoagulant: direct thrombin inhibitor • Prevents conversion of prothrombin to thrombin including both free and clot-bound thrombin	• Unstable angina in patients undergoing PCI	• IV injection: 0.75–1 mg/kg followed by IV infusion • IV infus on: mix 250 mg in 250 ml of normal saline (1 mg/ml) and infuse at 1.75–2.5 mg/kg/hr for 4 hr then decrease infusion to 0.2 mg/kg/hr for an additional 14–20 hr if needed	• Bleeding • Back pain • Generalized pain • Headache • Nausea • Hypotension	• Monitor PT, aPTT, CBC, and for signs of bleeding • Note that contraindications and cautions are as for heparin • Obtain baseline platelet count and aPTT; monitor aPTT every 4 hr; ACT may also be used • Anticoagulant effects are increased in patients receiving platelet aggregation inhibitors, fibrinolytics, or other anticoagulants • Monitor oral secretions, sputum, vomitus, NG aspirate, stool, urine for blood • Avoid IM, arterial, or venous punctures if at all possible • Hold pressure for longer than usual if punctures necessary • Protect infusion from direct sunlight

| Warfarin | Anticoagulant
• Depresses synthesis of prothrombin by the liver
• Prevents extension of clot and secondary thromboembolic complications | • DVT
• Valvular heart disease
• Atrial dysrhythmias
• Postvalve replacement | • PO: 2–10 mg/day depending on PT and INR
• INR 2–3
  • MI
  • DVT prophylaxis or treatment
  • PE
  • Valvular heart disease
  • Atrial fibrillation
  • Tissue heart valve
• INR 2.5–3.5
  • Mechanical heart valve | • Hemorrhage with excessive PT
• Agranulocytosis, leukopenia
• Hepatitis
• Diarrhea
• Fever
• Rash
• Skin necrosis: occurs during the first several days of warfarin therapy; lesions occur on extremities, breasts, trunk, penis
• Cholesterol microemboli causing purple toe syndrome | • Monitor PT and for signs of hemorrhage
• Note contraindications: known hypersensitivity, bleeding disorders, leukemia, peptic ulcer disease, liver disease, severe hypertension, endocarditis, acute nephritis, blood dyscrasias, eclampsia, suspected intracranial hemorrhage, open wounds, recent surgery, threatened abortion
• Use cautiously in alcoholism, pregnancy, lactation, during menses, during use of any drainage tube, older adult, or in any patient in whom slight bleeding is dangerous
• Ensure that vitamin K (AquaMephyton) is available
• Avoid IM, arterial, or venous punctures if at all possible
• Hold pressure for longer than usual if punctures necessary
• Monitor oral secretions, sputum, vomitus, NG aspirate, stool, urine for blood
• Do not discontinue suddenly
• Teach patient to avoid trauma and increase amounts of vitamin K (green leafy vegetables), and how to monitor for bleeding
• Teach the patient to report fever or rash; usually necessitates discontinuance |

ACS, Acute coronary syndrome; *ACT*, activated clotting time; *aPTT*, activated partial thromboplastin time; *AVM*, arteriovenous malformation; *BP*, blood pressure; *CBC*, complete blood count; *CK*, creatine kinase; *CPR*, cardiopulmonary resuscitation; *CVA*, cerebrovascular accident; *DBP*, diastolic blood pressure; *DIC*, disseminated intravascular coagulation; *DVT*, deep vein thrombosis; *GI*, gastrointestinal; *GP*, glycoprotein; *GU*, genitourinary; *HIT*, heparin-induced thrombocytopenia; *INR*, international normalized ratio; *IV*, intravenous; *LMWH*, low-molecular-weight heparin; *MI*, myocardial infarction; *NG*, nasogastric; *PCI*, percutaneous coronary intervention; *PE*, pulmonary embolism; *PT*, prothrombin time; *PTCA*, percutaneous transluminal coronary angioplasty; *PVC*, premature ventricular contraction; *RVF*, right ventricular failure; *SBP*, systolic blood pressure; *SC*, subcutaneous; *VF*, ventricular fibrillation; *VT*, ventricular tachycardia.

Table 3.31 Coronary Artery Bypass Grafting

Procedures	Types of bypasses
	• Arterial bypass (preferred because of better long-term patency rates)
	  • Internal thoracic (also called internal mammary) arteries
	  • Gastroepiploic artery
	  • Inferior epigastric arteries
	  • Radial arteries
	• Vein grafts
	  • Saphenous veins
	  • Brachial veins
	Surgical approaches
	• Median sternotomy with cardiopulmonary bypass (CPB)
	  • CPB provides a motionless heart and a bloodless field
	  • Complications of CPB include SIRS, coagulopathy, atelectasis, ARDS, cerebral microemboli, thrombotic stroke, post-CPB encephalopathy, renal insufficiency, dysrhythmias
	• Off-pump coronary artery bypass graft (OPCABG)
	  • May be performed through small median sternotomy or anterior thoracotomy
	  • Bypass is performed on a beating heart
	  • Avoids complications related to CPB
	• Minimally invasive direct (MIDCABG)
	  • Performed through anterior thoracotomy
	  • May be used for proximal LAD and select lesions of RCA or circumflex
	  • Bypass is performed on a beating heart
	  • Avoids complications related to CPB
	  • Thoracoscopy may be used

Indications	• Left main artery disease or three-vessel disease • Double-vessel disease if one of vessels is proximal LAD • Single- or double-vessel disease with angina unresponsive to medical therapy • CAD with ejection fraction <35% • Emergent conditions such as unstable angina, acute MI with persistent pain or shock, or coronary artery dissection during interventional cardiology procedures
Action	• The goal of CABG is to provide arterial or venous conduits to redirect coronary blood flow around occluded coronary arteries
Assessment	• Vital signs: HR, BP, RR, T • Hemodynamic parameters: RAP, PAP, PAOP, CO, CI, SVR, PVR, LVSWI, RVSWI • Oxygenation parameters: SaO_2, SvO_2; arterial blood gases • Serum electrolytes • Mediastinal and pleural tube drainage • Complaints of incisional pain, chest pain, dyspnea • Incision for bleeding, separation, or redness and induration

Brief summary of specific nursing management	• Relieve pain
	  • Administer narcotics and sedatives for relief of incisional pain
	  • Provide instruction regarding splinting during coughing and turning
	  • Report ischemic pain; titrate nitroglycerin for relief of ischemic pain
	• Monitor closely for hemodynamic changes: titrate drug therapy to optimize cardiac output and minimize myocardial oxygen consumption
	  • Pharmacologic support of this patient may include dobutamine, dopamine, nitroglycerin, nitroprusside
	  • Vasopressors may be used to increase coronary artery perfusion pressure and maintain patency of grafts; monitor for excessive afterload and myocardial oxygen consumption as well as excessive vasoconstriction and peripheral hypoperfusion
	  • Nitroglycerin at low dose is frequently used to reduce spasm
	• Monitor closely for hemorrhage: mediastinal tube, pleural tubes, incision
	  • Administer IV fluids, blood and/or blood products, and albumin as prescribed
	  • Maintain patency of mediastinal and pleural tubes
	  • Be alert for sudden reduction of drainage via mediastinal tube because occlusion may cause cardiac tamponade
	• Monitor closely for changes in perfusion
	  • Note any complaints of chest pain, ST-segment elevation, dysrhythmias
	  • Note any changes in appearance or volume of urine
	  • Note any changes in level of consciousness or neurologic function
	  • Note any changes in SaO_2, PAP, PVR
	  • Note any changes in bowel sounds, abdominal distention, abdominal pain
	• Monitor the ECG for dysrhythmias or blocks
	  • Replace electrolytes as prescribed; potassium and magnesium imbalances predispose to dysrhythmias
	  • Administer antidysrhythmics as prescribed; prophylactic antidysrhythmics (e.g., amiodarone) may be given to prevent atrial fibrillation
	  • Use epicardial pacing wires for symptomatic bradycardias or blocks
	• Prevent or monitor for complications

Table 3.31	Coronary Artery Bypass Grafting—cont'd

Complications: prevention and treatment	• Potential complications during surgery
	  • Cerebral or myocardial infarction
	  • Hemorrhage: greater risk with internal thoracic artery implant
	  • Inability to wean from cardiopulmonary bypass: IABP and/or VAD used
	• Potential complications during postoperative period
	  • Immediate
	    • HF with hypotension and/or pulmonary edema
	    • Hemorrhage
	    • Cardiac tamponade
	    • Dysrhythmias
	    • MI
	    • Hypertension
	    • Cerebral embolism
	    • Acute respiratory failure (e.g., atelectasis, ARDS)
	    • Renal failure
	    • Electrolyte imbalance (e.g., hypokalemia, hypocalcemia, hypomagnesemia)
	    • Graft closure
	    • Coagulopathy
	  • Intermediate
	    • Donor site infection
	    • Sternal wound infection: especially if patient has diabetes or internal thoracic (i.e., mammary) artery used for bypass

ARDS, Acute respiratory distress syndrome; *BP*, blood pressure; *CI*, cardiac index; *CO*, cardiac output; *ECG*, electrocardiogram; *HF*, heart failure; *HR*, heart failure; *IABP*, intraaortic balloon pump; *IV*, intravenous; *LAD*, left anterior descending coronary artery; *LVSWI*, left ventricular stroke work index; *MI*, myocardial infarction; *NTG*, nitroglycerin; *PAOP*, pulmonary artery occlusive pressure; *PAP*, pulmonary artery pressure; *PVR*, pulmonary vascular resistance; *RAP*, right atrial pressure; *RCA*, right coronary artery; *RR*, respiratory rate; *RVSWI*, right ventricular stroke work index; *SaO$_2$*, arterial oxygen saturation; *SIRS*, systemic inflammatory response syndrome; *SvO$_2$*, saturation of venous blood; *SVR*, systemic vascular resistance *T*, temperature; *VAD*, ventricular assist device.

    4) Treat anemia if present: maintain Hgb greater than 12 g/dl if possible.
    5) Maintain CAPP.
        a) Use caution in administration of; nitroglycerin and other vasoactive agents because they may decrease CAPP by decreasing the aortic root pressure.
        b) Nitroprusside is contraindicated during ischemic pain because it may cause coronary artery steal and decrease CAPP.
    6) Control dysrhythmias.
        a) Tachydysrhythmias decrease the time for coronary artery filling and may decrease CO.
        b) Bradydysrhythmias increase the time for coronary artery filling but may decrease CO.
    7) Administer calcium channel blockers or nitroglycerin for coronary artery spasm.
        a) Especially important in cocaine-induced MI
    8) Use IABP as prescribed (Table 3.27).
  c. Decrease myocardial oxygen consumption.
    1) Administer beta-blockers as prescribed to decrease HR and contractility to decrease myocardial oxygen consumption.
        a) Actions
            i) Decrease incidence of dysrhythmias and increase VF threshold.
            ii) Block the effects of catecholamines (cardioprotection).
            iii) Reduce infarct size and severity of HF.
        b) Agents: metoprolol 5 mg IV every 2 minutes × 3 is usually given, but atenolol or esmolol may be used.
        c) Contraindications
            i) HR less than 50 beats/min
            ii) Second- or third-degree AV block
            iii) Systolic BP less than 100 mm Hg
            iv) HF
            v) Bronchospasm
                (a) No beta-blockers should be given to a patient with active bronchospasm.
                (b) Cardioselective beta-blockers (e.g., metoprolol or esmolol) may be given to a patient with a history of bronchospastic lung disease (e.g., asthma), but noncardioselective beta-blockers (e.g., propranolol) should not be given.
            vi) Cocaine-induced MI: blocking beta receptors allows unopposed alpha receptors to increase vasoconstriction and vasospasm so should not be used early but should be prescribed at discharge; nitroglycerin and/or a calcium channel blocker (e.g., diltiazem) is more likely to be prescribed along with a benzodiazepine (e.g., diazepam) to reduce agitation and seizure potential.
    2) Administer ACE inhibitors (e.g., captopril, enalapril) or angiotensin blockers (e.g., losartan, valsartan) as prescribed to attenuate ventricular remodeling.
        a) Action: block the vasoconstriction and sodium and water retention associated with activation of the RAA system.

b) Indications in acute MI: anterior or large inferior MI or evidence of HF
c) ACE inhibitors block the conversion of angiotensin I to angiotensin II; angiotensin blockers block angiotensin II and do not block the breakdown of bradykinin, so they are less likely to cause cough.
d) Caution: hypotension
3) Administer vasodilators as prescribed.
a) Venous vasodilators (usually nitroglycerin) to decrease preload
b) Arterial vasodilators (usually nitroprusside) to decrease afterload
c) Caution: hypotension; careful titration necessary to decrease myocardial oxygen consumption but to prevent hypoperfusion
4) Monitor serum glucose and administer insulin as required to maintain serum glucose below 150 mg/dl.
5) Provide physical and emotional rest.
a) Maintain bed rest for 24 hours; then gradually increase in activity as long as patient is hemodynamically stable; allow rest after meals, personal hygiene, toileting, and physical therapy.
b) Prevent Valsalva maneuver.
i) Teach patient to exhale when turning in bed.
ii) Administer stool softeners as prescribed.
iii) Provide bedside commode for elimination.
c) Explain procedures thoroughly: monitor alarms; equipment; visiting hours; reasons for procedures
d) Keep family informed regarding patient's progress and status.
e) Provide for patient's comfort.
i) Provide prompt pain control: analgesics.
ii) Provide nausea control: antiemetics, mouth care.
iii) Provide for physical comfort: temperature control, lighting, noise control.
f) Instruct patient regarding relaxation techniques; encourage utilization of these techniques; use calming music, white noise, or nature sounds to aid in relaxation.
g) Provide appropriate nutrition: clear liquid to soft diet; usually low sodium
i) Caffeine: may have up to 4 to 5 caffeinated beverages/24 hr as long as dysrhythmias do not occur
ii) Iced water: no restriction
h) Administer anxiolytics as prescribed: usually diazepam, lorazepam, or alprazolam
i) Note common emotional responses seen in acute MI and treat appropriately (Table 3.32).
d. Collaborative management specific to RV infarctions
1) Assess for clinical indications of RVMI, especially in the patient with acute inferior MI.
a) ECG changes in V_{4R}, V_{5R}, V_{6R}
b) Increased RAP, decreased PAOP
c) Decreased CO, CI, and MAP; increased SVR
d) Right-sided S_4
e) Clinical indications of RVF: JVD, hepatojugular reflux, right-sided S_3, murmur of tricuspid insufficiency
f) Minimal to absent pulmonary congestion
2) Administer therapy specific to RV infarction.
a) Maintain adequate filling volumes.
i) Measure RAP and PAOP; patients with significant RV infarction usually require hemodynamic monitoring.
ii) Administer volume: usually in the form of colloids (e.g., dextran, plasma protein fraction, albumin); fluids administered until PAOP is increased by greater than 5 mm Hg but PAOP and RAP should not exceed 20 mm Hg
iii) Avoid use of diuretics or venous vasodilators; if dilators are needed, selective arterial dilators should be used (e.g., hydralazine) so that preload is not decreased.
b) Maintain contractility: inotropes (e.g., dobutamine) are frequently required.
e. Monitor for, prevent, and treat complications (Table 3.33).
f. Provide instruction and counseling regarding lifestyle modification and need for pharmacologic therapy.
1) Nonpharmacologic therapies
a) Well-balanced diet to maintain normal weight maintenance
i) Low in saturated fat and transfatty acids while including monounsaturated fats (e.g., olive oil, canola oil)
ii) High in fiber
(a) Fresh fruit and vegetables
(b) Whole grains
iii) Adequate low-fat proteins
iv) Low (2–3 g/day) sodium may be recommended.
v) American Diabetes Association (ADA) diet for control of blood glucose for patient with DM
a) Cessation of tobacco use
b) Limitation of alcohol consumption to 1 to 2 alcoholic beverages daily
c) Regular aerobic exercise in moderation
d) Adequate rest and relaxation
e) Stress reduction: relaxation; imagery, biofeedback
f) Differentiation between symptoms of angina and MI
g) Changes in sexual activity that may be helpful

Table 3.32	Emotional Responses Seen in Acute Myocardial Infarction	
Response	Indications	Collaborative Management
Anxiety	• Increased verbalization • Inability to concentrate • Restlessness, apprehension • Sleep disturbances • Tremors • Tachycardia, mild hypertension	• Be consistent with patient assignment • Provide orientation to unit, procedures, equipment, and so on • Assess usual coping mechanisms • Invite patient to ask questions • Keep family informed about patient condition • Encourage participation in rehabilitation program
Denial	• Avoidance of discussion of heart attack • Discussions kept on a social, humorous level • Minimization of severity (e.g., "little heart attack") • Noncompliance with activity and diet restrictions; smoking • Overly cheerful demeanor • Repetition of same questions to different staff members	• Listen but do not reinforce denial • Assess consequences of denial: denial decreases in-hospital mortality rate but increases incidence of sudden cardiac death after discharge • Assess the threat causing the need for denial • Provide counseling if patient still in denial at time of discharge • Encourage participation in rehabilitation program
Depression	• Listlessness, disinterest • Expressions of hopelessness, pessimism • Abbreviated verbal responses (e.g., monosyllable answers) • Slowness in movement and speech • Withdrawn behavior • Anorexia • Sad look, crying	• Voice your observations (e.g., "you look sad") • Let patient know that it is normal to feel this way • Encourage verbalization of feelings • Allow and encourage crying • Encourage participation in rehabilitation program
Anger	• Open opposition to treatment regimen • Expressions of disappointment or frustration • Passive-aggressive behavior • Sarcasm • Voices anger, screaming, cursing	• Acknowledge angry or hostile feelings • Explore cause of anger • Let patient know that these feelings are normal • Let spouse and family know that anger is normal • Be matter-of-fact about expressions of anger • Encourage participation in rehabilitation program
Aggressive sexual behavior	• Frequent seductive comments • Frequent initiation of sexually related conversion • Frequent boasts about past sexual interests and prowess • Flirtatious compliments • Attempts to hold, fondle, or kiss parts of nurse's body • Deliberate exposure of genitals	• Be honest and simply tell the patient that such behavior makes you uncomfortable if it does • Accept compliments with a simple "thank you" • Arrange sexual counseling for patient and spouse • Encourage participation in rehabilitation program

Table 3.33	Complications of Myocardial Infarction	
Complication	Clinical Indications	Prevention and Treatment
Dysrhythmias and conduction system defects	• Change in rhythm or conduction on rhythm strip or multiple-lead ECG • Indications of hypoperfusion may be evident	• Close monitoring for changes in rhythm or conduction • Beta-blocker as a cardioprotective agent as prescribed • Magnesium, potassium, or calcium to correct electrolyte imbalance as prescribed • Antidysrhythmic agents as indicated and prescribed • Application of external pacemaker or insertion of transvenous pacemaker as indicated • Cardioversion or defibrillation as indicated

Heart failure	• Tachycardia, tachypnea
	• Clinical indications of LVF
	  • Dyspnea, orthopnea, cough
	  • S_3
	  • Crackles in lung bases
	• Clinical indications of RVF
	  • Jugular venous distention
	  • Hepatomegaly, splenomegaly
	  • Peripheral edema
	• Chest radiography shows pulmonary venous congestion, cardiomegaly
	• Increased RAP, PAP, PAOP (PAOP usually >20 mm Hg)
		• Oxygen
		• Sodium and fluid restriction
		• ACE inhibitors (e.g., captopril, enalapril)
		• Beta-blockers (e.g., metoprolol, carvedilol)
		• Diuretics (e.g., furosemide, bumetanide)
		• Vasodilators (e.g., nitroglycerin)
		• Inotropic agents (e.g., dobutamine, milrinone, digoxin)

Continued

Table 3.33 Complications of Myocardial Infarction—cont'd

Complication	Clinical Indications	Prevention and Treatment
Cardiogenic shock	• Tachycardia, tachypnea, hypotension • Clinical indications of LVF • Clinical indications of RVF • Clinical indications of hypoperfusion (Table 2.2 on page 20) • Urine output <0.5 ml/kg/hr • Cool to cold skin • Diminished to absent bowel sounds • Lethargy to confusion to coma • Chest radiography shows pulmonary venous congestion, cardiomegaly • Decreased CO/CI (usually <2 l/min/m^2) • Increased PAOP (usually >18 mm Hg) • Increased SVR (usually >2000 dynes/sec/cm^{-5})	• Oxygen • Sodium and fluid restrictions • ACE inhibitors (e.g., captopril, enalapril) • Inotropic agents (e.g., digoxin, dobutamine, inamrinone or milrinone) • Diuretics (e.g., furosemide, bumetanide) • Vasodilators (e.g., nitroglycerin, nitroprusside) • IABP • Ventricular assist devices • Emergent revascularization: fibrinolytics, PCI; CABG
Papillary muscle dysfunction or rupture	• New holosystolic murmur loudest at apex • Clinical indications of LVF • Clinical indications of hypoperfusion • Increased PAP, PAOP • Large V waves on PAOP waveform • Echocardiography shows mitral regurgitation	• Vasodilators (e.g., nitroprusside, nitroglycerin) • IABP • Surgical replacement of mitral valve with concurrent CABG
Ventricular septal rupture	• New holosystolic murmur loudest at lower left sternal border • Chest pain, dyspnea • Syncope • Increased PAP, PAOP • Increased SvO$_2$ • Increased CO/CI by thermodilution method of measurement (inaccurate) • Clinical evidence of hypoperfusion • Hypotension	• Vasodilators (e.g., nitroglycerin, nitroprusside) • IABP • Surgical correction of ventricular septal defect with concurrent CABG unless rupture is small

Cardiac wall rupture	• Clinical indications of hypoperfusion
	• Clinical indications of cardiac tamponade
	  • Jugular venous distention
	  • Muffled heart sounds
	  • Hypotension
	  • Increased RAP, PAP, PAOP with equalization within 5 mm Hg
	• Sinus tachycardia or pulseless electrical activity
	• Eventual cardiopulmonary arrest with PEA
		• Pericardiocentesis
		• CPR; internal cardiac massage may be necessary
		• Surgical repair may be attempted (survival is rare)

Ventricular aneurysm	• Diffuse PMI, left ventricular heave • Atrial fibrillation or ventricular dysrhythmias • Persistent ST-segment elevation • Chest radiography shows left ventricular dilation • Echocardiography shows dyskinesis, left ventricular dilation • Clinical indications of LVF may be present • Clinical indications of systemic emboli may be present: cerebral emboli; peripheral emboli with acute arterial occlusion	• Antidysrhythmics (e.g., amiodarone) • Anticoagulants (e.g., heparin followed by warfarin) • Treatment of HF: ACE inhibitors, beta-blockers, diuretics, vasodilators, inotropes • Surgical resection may be performed • Ablative procedures may be necessary for recurrent ventricular dysrhythmias
Pericarditis	• Fever • Chest pain which worsens with deep breath and lessens sitting up and with leaning forward • Pericardial friction rub • Elevated WBC count, sedimentation rate • Diffuse ST-segment elevation across the precordial leads • Chest radiography may show pericardial effusion	• Aspirin or NSAIDs (e.g., ibuprofen, naproxen); colchicine may also be used • Discontinuance of anticoagulants • Pericardiocentesis may be required for pericardial effusion • Close monitoring for clinical indications of cardiac tamponade
Dressler syndrome (also referred to as *postmyocardial infarction syndrome*): late pericarditis which is thought to be autoimmune	• Fever • Chest pain that worsens with deep breath and lessens sitting up and with leaning forward • Pericardial friction rub • Elevated WBC count, sedimentation rate • Diffuse ST-segment elevation across the precordial leads • Chest radiography may show pericardial effusion	• Aspirin or colchicine • Corticosteroids (e.g., prednisone) may be prescribed • Pericardiocentesis may be required for pericardial effusion • Close monitoring for clinical indications of cardiac tamponade

Table 3.33	Complications of Myocardial Infarction—cont'd	
Complication	**Clinical Indications**	**Prevention and Treatment**

Sudden cardiac death	• Cardiopulmonary arrest	• Preventive measures include:
		  • Risk factor modification
		  • Antiplatelet aggregation therapy (e.g., ASA)
		  • Beta-blockers
		  • Encouragement of family members to learn CPR
		• Treatment: BLS and ACLS

ACE, Angiotensin-converting enzyme; *ACLS*, advanced cardiac life support; *ASA*, aspirin; *BLS*, basic life support; *CABG*, coronary artery bypass graft; *CI*, cardiac index; *CO*, cardiac output; *CPR*, cardiopulmonary resuscitation; *ECG*, electrocardiogram; *HF*, heart failure; *IABP*, intraaortic balloon pump; *LVF*, left ventricular failure; *NSAID*, nonsteroidal antiinflammatory drug; *NTG*, nitroglycerin; *PAOP*, pulmonary artery occlusive pressure; *PAP*, pulmonary artery pressure; *PCI*, percutaneous coronary intervention; *PEA*, pulseless electrical activity; *PMI*, point of maximal impulse; *RAP*, right atrial pressure; *RVF*, right ventricular failure; S_3, third heart sound; SvO_2, saturation of venous blood; *SVR*, systemic vascular resistance; *WBC*, white blood cell.

   2) Pharmacologic agents
      a) Prescribed medication regimen for secondary prevention of MI: aspirin, beta-blocker, ACE inhibitor (if indicated)
      b) Control of cardiac risk factors
         i) Antihypertensives for hypertension
         ii) Lipid-reducing therapy (e.g., statin) for hyperlipidemia
         iii) Oral hypoglycemics and/or insulin for DM
         iv) Thyroid hormone replacement or suppressive agents for thyroid disorders

Heart Failure

Definitions

1. HF: a clinical syndrome characterized by dyspnea, activity intolerance, and fluid overload that adversely affects the patient's functional status and quality of life (Hunt et al., 2001)
   a. Clinical indications of intravascular and interstitial volume overload (e.g., dyspnea, crackles, edema)
   b. Clinical indications of tissue hypoperfusion (e.g., fatigue, exercise intolerance)
2. Acute decompensated HF: the sudden or gradual onset of the signs or symptoms of HF that necessitate unplanned office visits, ED visits, or hospitalization; a nearly universal finding is pulmonary and systemic congestion caused by increased left- and right-heart filling pressures (Gheorghiade et al., 2005)
3. Pulmonary edema
   a. Fluid in the alveolus
   b. Impairs gas exchange and causes hypoxemia by impairing the diffusion between alveolus and capillary
   c. May be cardiac versus noncardiac; frequently differentiated using PAOP and the difference between PA diastolic pressure and PAOP
      1) Cardiac pulmonary edema
         a) Caused by acute LVF
         b) Elevated PAP, elevated PAOP; difference between PA diastolic and PAOP less than 5 mm Hg
         c) Fluid is *pushed* from the pulmonary capillary into the interstitium and finally into the alveolus because of increased pulmonary capillary hydrostatic pressure
      2) Noncardiac pulmonary edema
         a) Most common cause is ARDS; may also be caused by drowning
         b) Elevated PAP, normal PAOP; difference between PA diastolic and PAOP greater than 5 mm Hg
         c) Fluid *leaks* from the pulmonary capillary into the interstitium and alveolus because of increased permeability of the damaged alveolocapillary membrane.

Etiology

1. Risk factors
   a. #1 CAD, especially with history of MI
   b. Congenital heart disease
   c. Valvular heart disease
   d. Hypertension
   e. DM
   f. Obesity
   g. Alcoholism
   h. Smoking
   i. High or low Hct
   j. Sedentary life style
   k. High-fat, high-salt diet
2. Etiologic factors (Table 3.34)
3. Causes of decompensation in a patient with HF
   a. Progression of LV dysfunction
   b. New or worsening ischemia
   c. Hypoxemia
   d. Worsening of anemia
   e. Drugs such as nonsteroidal antiinflammatory drugs (NSAIDs), initiation of beta-blocker dosage at too high dosages
   f. Hypertension
   g. New dysrhythmia, particularly atrial fibrillation
   h. Missed or suboptimal medication
   i. Dietary indiscretion, such as high-salt foods
   j. Alcohol
4. Common comorbidities in a patient with HF
   a. CAD
   b. MI
   c. Hypertension with systolic BP greater than 140 mm Hg
   d. Renal insufficiency
   e. Hyperlipidemia
   f. DM
   g. Atrial fibrillation
   h. COPD or asthma

Table 3.34 Etiologic Factors of Heart Failure	
Left Ventricular Failure	**Right Ventricular Failure**
• CAD or LV infarction	• LVF
• Cardiomyopathy	• CAD or RV infarction
• Hypertension	• Pulmonary hypertension
• Dysrhythmias	• Passive: mitral valve disease
• Volume overload	• Active: hypoxemia; pulmonary embolism
• Valvular disease: mitral or aortic	• Dysrhythmias
• Ventricular septal defect	• Volume overload
• Coarctation of aorta	• Valvular disease: mitral or pulmonic
• Myocarditis	• Ventricular septal defect
• Cardiac tamponade	• Cardiomyopathy
	• Myocardial contusion
	• LVF
	• CAD or RV infarction
Biventricular Failure	
Increased demand	Electrolyte imbalance
• Thyrotoxicosis	• Hyponatremia
• Anemia	• Hypokalemia
• Pregnancy	• Hypocalcemia
• Systemic infection	• Hypomagnesemia
• Beriberi	• Hypophosphatemia
• Paget disease	

CAD, Coronary artery disease; *LV*, left ventricular; *LVF*, left ventricular failure; *RV*, right ventricular.

Pathophysiology

1. Adaptive compensatory processes progress to maladaptive process: in the short term, mechanisms compensate for the failing heart, but in the long term, all of these factors trigger a process of pathologic growth and remodeling (Fig. 3.78).
   a. Signal-modulating inhibitors: primary therapies are directed toward blocking dysfunctional compensatory mechanisms.
      1) SNS: beta-blockers, alpha- and beta-blockers
      2) RAA system: ACE inhibitors and angiotensin II receptor blockers (ARBs)
      3) Aldosterone: aldosterone antagonists
2. Interrelationship between LVF and RVF (Fig. 3.79)

Classifications of Heart Failure

1. Location: left or right; note that the most common cause of RVF is LVF
2. Onset: acute or chronic
3. Output state: low output (e.g., MI, cardiomyopathy) or high output (e.g., thyrotoxicosis, anemia)
4. Type of pumping defect: backward (i.e., high volume and engorgement behind the failing ventricle) versus forward (i.e., low filling volume for the ventricle in front of the failing ventricle)
5. Relationship to the cardiac cycle: systolic (60%–70%) or diastolic (30%–40%)
   a. Systolic dysfunction (pump problem): inability of the ventricle to shorten against a load; the left ventricle loses its ability to contract normally against progressive increases in afterload
      1) Possible causes: MI, myocardial contusion, myocarditis, dilated cardiomyopathy, hypertension, valvular heart disease, electrolyte imbalance, dysrhythmias
      2) Hemodynamics: decreased contractility; EF less than 40%; increased cardiac volumes and pressures
      3) Clinical indications: displaced PMI, JVD, S_3, crackles, dyspnea, peripheral edema, cardiomegaly
      4) Drug therapy: treatment of cause, diuretics if congestive symptoms; ACE inhibitor or ARB; beta-blocker or alpha- and beta-blocker but not pure alpha-blocker; inotropes may be required for diuretic-resistant congestion; antidysrhythmics and anticoagulants may be indicated
   b. Diastolic dysfunction (filling problem): an impairment in LV filling at near normal or mildly elevated LA and LV pressures; caused by a decrease in ventricular compliance; small changes in volume are associated with a disproportionate increase in pressure
      1) Possible causes: myocardial ischemia, hypertrophic cardiomyopathy, ventricular hypertrophy, constrictive pericarditis or cardiac tamponade, valvular heart disease, aging
      2) Hemodynamics: increased contractility, normal EF, increased cardiac pressures with normal or slightly increased cardiac volumes
      3) Clinical indications: S_4, crackles, dyspnea, peripheral edema, precordial heave, normal heart sound
      4) Drug therapy: treatment of cause, diuretics if congestive symptoms, ACE inhibitor or ARB, beta-blocker or alpha- and beta-blocker, calcium channel blocker, control of tachydysrhythmias
6. New York Heart Association (NYHA) functional classification
   a. Class I: patients with cardiac disease but without resulting limitation of physical activity; ordinary physical activity does not cause undue fatigue, palpitation, dyspnea, or angina
   b. Class II: patients with cardiac disease resulting in slight limitation of physical activity; they are comfortable at rest; ordinary physical activity results in fatigue, palpitation, dyspnea, or angina
   c. Class III: patients with cardiac disease resulting in marked limitation of physical activity; they are comfortable at rest; less than ordinary activity causes fatigue, palpitation, dyspnea, or angina
   d. Class IV: patients with cardiac disease resulting in inability to carry on any physical activity without discomfort; symptoms of cardiac insufficiency or angina may be present even at rest; if any physical activity is attempted, discomfort is increased

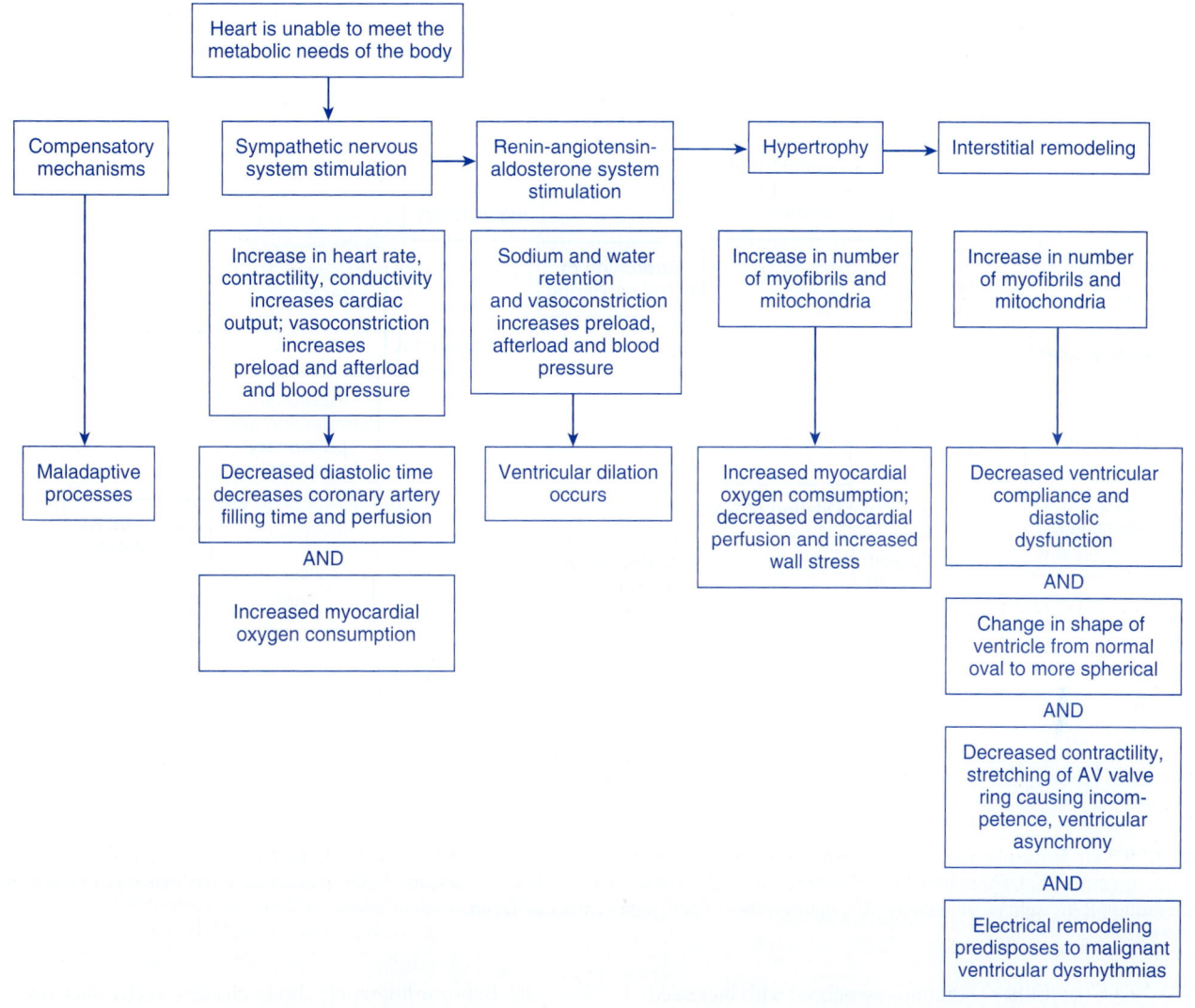

Fig. 3.78 Progression of adaptive compensatory mechanisms to maladaptive processes.

7. American College of Cardiology (ACC)/AHA staging system for HF (Hunt et al., 2001)
   a. Stage A: high risk for developing HF
      1) Hypertension
      2) CAD
      3) DM
      4) Family history of cardiomyopathy
   b. Stage B: asymptomatic HF
      1) Previous MI
      2) LV systolic dysfunction
      3) Asymptomatic valvular disease
   c. Stage C: symptomatic HF
      1) Known structural heart disease
      2) Shortness of breath and fatigue
      3) Reduced exercise tolerance
   d. Stage D: refractory end-stage HF
      1) Marked symptoms at rest despite maximal medical therapy

Clinical Presentation (Table 3.35)

1. First symptoms frequently cough, exertional dyspnea, edema, or fatigue
2. Proportional pulse pressure
   a. Calculation: (systolic BP − diastolic BP)/systolic BP
   b. Proportional pulse pressure of less than 25% is associated with a CI of less than 2.2 l/min/m^2
3. Serum
   a. Electrolyte levels: may reveal or confirm imbalances, especially hypokalemia, hypocalcemia, and hypomagnesemia
   b. Albumin levels: may show hypoproteinemia, which can contribute to edema
   c. ABGs: may show hypoxemia (especially if pulmonary edema present) and acid–base imbalances (including lactic acidosis in severe hypoperfusion states)
   d. Drug levels: may reveal abnormal levels of digoxin, antidysrhythmic agents
   e. Thyroid profile: may reveal abnormal thyroid function
   f. CBC: may show anemia or leukocytosis
   g. BUN, creatinine: may be elevated to detect renal impairment
   h. BNP
      1) Normal: less than 100 g/ml; levels greater than 100 g/ml indicate HF
      2) Elevated BNP level correlates with an increased LV end-diastolic pressure and volume and PAOP.

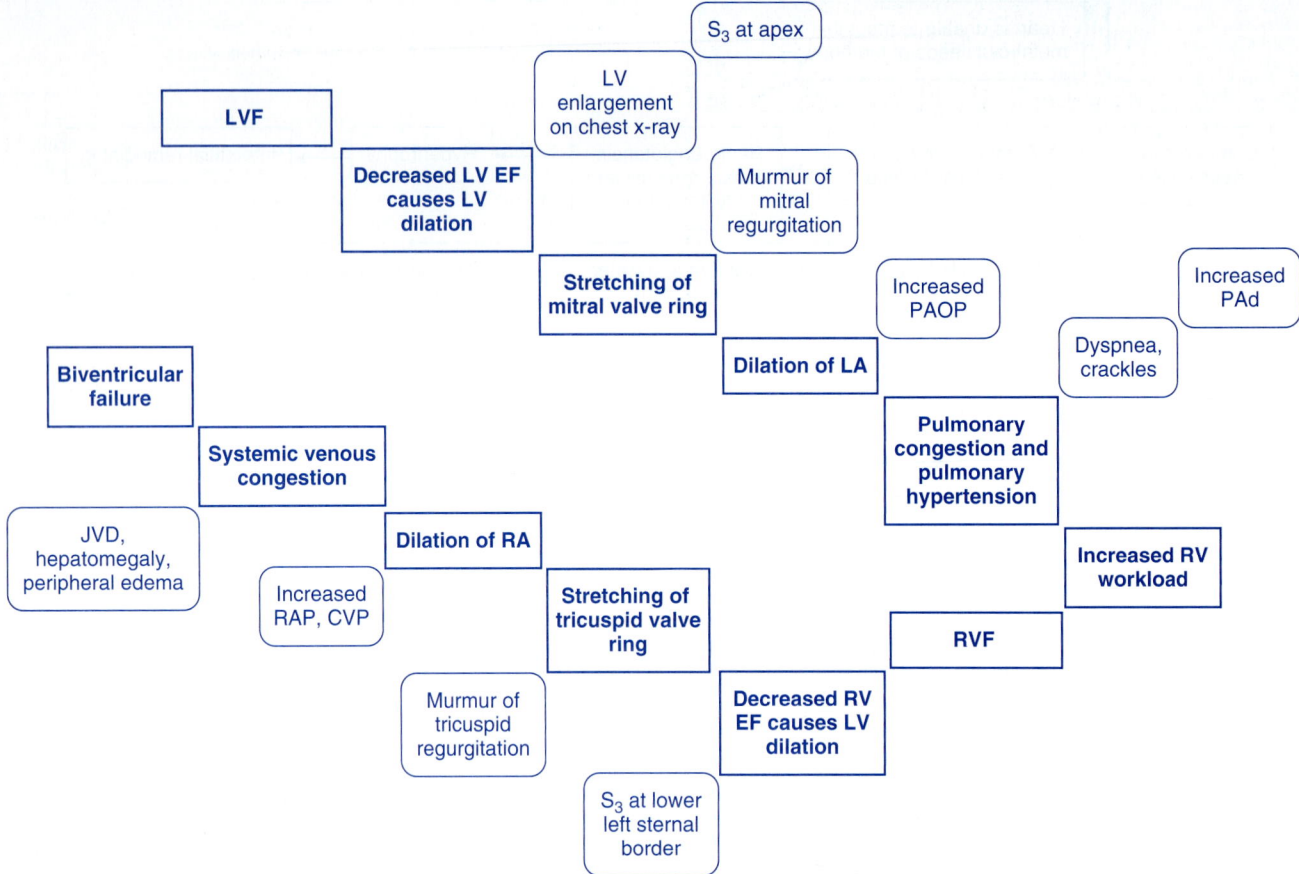

Fig. 3.79 Left ventricular failure (LVF) progressing to biventricular failure. *CVP*, Central venous pressure; *EF*, ejection fraction; *JVD*, jugular venous distention; *LA*, left atrium; *LV*, left ventricular; *PAd*, pulmonary artery diastolic pressure; *PAOP*, pulmonary artery occlusive pressure; *RA*, right atrium; *RAP*, right atrial pressure; *RV*, right ventricle; *RVF*, right ventricular failure.

  a) Other conditions associated with increased BNP levels
   i) LVF
   ii) Cardiac inflammation
   iii) Primary pulmonary hypertension
   iv) Renal failure
   v) Ascitic cirrhosis
   vi) Endocrine disorders (e.g., primary hyperaldosteronism, Cushing syndrome)
   vii) May be elevated in elderly patients
  b) May replace chest radiography as the test of choice in differential diagnosis of dyspnea in acute care setting
 i. Urine: may show proteinuria and/or presence of red blood cells (RBCs) or casts
4. Diagnostic studies
 a. Chest radiography: shows cardiac enlargement and dilation; may show pulmonary congestion
 b. Cardiac catheterization and coronary angiography
  1) May show CAD or valve abnormalities
  2) Cardiac pressures increased and EF decreased in systolic dysfunction
  3) Cardiac pressures increased and EF normal in diastolic dysfunction
 c. Computed tomography (CT): may be used to evaluate LV wall motion and detect cardiac tumors, MI, aortic aneurysm
 d. Echocardiography: shows changes in chamber size, wall thickness, and valve motion
 e. ECG
  1) May show myocardial ischemia or infarction
  2) May show atrial enlargement or ventricular hypertrophy
 f. Multiple-gated acquisition (MUGA) scan: may be used to evaluate cardiac function, determine EF, and detect wall motion abnormalities
5. Hemodynamic parameters
 a. Increase in volume indicators: RAP, PAP, PAOP
 b. Decrease in CO/index
 c. Increase in SVR
 d. Increase in pulmonary vascular resistance: PVR
 e. Hemodynamic subtypes of HF (Fig. 3.80)

Collaborative Management

1. Treat the cause or contributing factors if possible
 a. Reperfusion in acute MI along with neurohormonal antagonism with beta-blocker (or alpha or beta-blocker [e.g., carvedilol]) and ACE inhibitor
 b. Revascularization of patients with CAD
 c. Valve replacement if required, especially for acute valvular disorder such as ruptured papillary muscle with acute mitral regurgitation
 d. Treatment of symptomatic or life-threatening dysrhythmias with antidysrhythmic agents, electrical

Table 3.35 Clinical Indications of Left Ventricular, Right Ventricular, and Biventricular Failure

Left Ventricular Failure	Right Ventricular Failure
• Tachypnea, dyspnea, orthopnea, PND	• Jugular venous distention
• Tachycardia	• Hepatojugular reflux
• Left-sided S_3	• Dependent pitting edema
• Displaced PMI, heave at apex	• Heave at sternum
• Crackles, wheezes	• Hepatomegaly or splenomegaly
• Cough, frothy sputum, hemoptysis	• Anorexia, nausea, vomiting
• Diaphoresis	• Abdominal pain and bloating
• Pulsus alternans	• Ascites
• Oliguria	• Nocturia
• Weakness, fatigue	• Weakness, fatigue
• Mental confusion	• Weight gain
• Murmur of MR	• Murmur of TR
• ABGs: decreased PaO_2, SaO_2	• Right-sided S_3

• Hemodynamics
  • Elevated PA, PAOP
  • Decreased CO/CI
	• Hemodynamics
	  • Elevated CVP, RAP

• Abnormal chest radiography
  • Cardiomegaly
  • Engorged pulmonary vasculature
  • Kerley B lines
  • Pleural effusion
	• Abnormal liver function studies
	  • ALT
	  • AST
	  • LDH

• ECG
  • Left atrial enlargement
  • Left ventricular hypertrophy
  • Atrial dysrhythmias
	• ECG
	  • Right atrial enlargement
	  • Right ventricular hypertrophy
	  • Atrial dysrhythmias

ABG, Arterial blood gas; *ALT*, alanine transaminase; *AST*, aspartate transaminase; *CI*, cardiac index; *CO*, cardiac output; *CVP*, central venous pressure; *ECG*, electrocardiogram; *LDH*, lactate dehydrogenase; *MR*, mitral regurgitation; *PA*, pulmonary artery; *PaO₂*, partial pressure of oxygen in arterial blood; *PAOP*, pulmonary artery occlusive pressure; *PMI*, point of maximal impulse; *PND*, paroxysmal nocturnal dyspnea; *RAP*, right atrial pressure; S_3, third heart sound; *SaO₂*, arterial oxygen saturation; *TR*, tricuspid regurgitation.

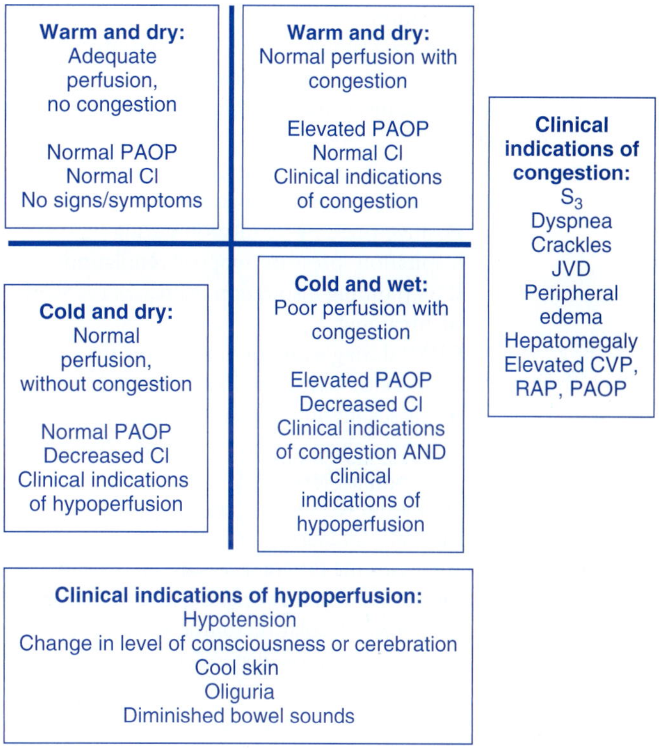

Warm and dry:
Adequate perfusion, no congestion
Normal PAOP
Normal CI
No signs/symptoms

Warm and dry:
Normal perfusion with congestion
Elevated PAOP
Normal CI
Clinical indications of congestion

Cold and dry:
Normal perfusion, without congestion
Normal PAOP
Decreased CI
Clinical indications of hypoperfusion

Cold and wet:
Poor perfusion with congestion
Elevated PAOP
Decreased CI
Clinical indications of congestion AND clinical indications of hypoperfusion

Clinical indications of congestion:
S_3
Dyspnea
Crackles
JVD
Peripheral edema
Hepatomegaly
Elevated CVP, RAP, PAOP

Clinical indications of hypoperfusion:
Hypotension
Change in level of consciousness or cerebration
Cool skin
Oliguria
Diminished bowel sounds

Fig. 3.80 Hemodynamic subtypes of heart failure. *CI*, Cardiac index; *CVP*, central venous pressure; *JVD*, jugular venous distention; *PAOP*, pulmonary artery occlusive pressure; *RAP*, right atrial pressure. (Adapted from Stevenson, L. W., & Perloff, J. K. [1989]. The limited reliability of physical signs for estimating hemodynamics in chronic heart failure. *JAMA*, 261[6], 884-888.)

therapies (e.g., cardioversion, defibrillation, pacemaker, automatic implantable cardiac defibrillator), or surgical procedures (e.g., ablation)
  e. Continuous positive-airway pressure (CPAP) for obstructive sleep apnea, which is common in patients with HF
  f. Avoidance of certain pharmacologic agents
     1) Antidysrhythmics being used to suppress asymptomatic dysrhythmias
     2) Most calcium channel blockers
     3) NSAIDs (increase resistance to diuretics)
2. Be aware of recommended medical treatment by ACC/AHA HF stage (Yancy et al., 2016).
   a. Stage A: treatment of hypertension and DM, control of metabolic syndrome, avoidance of alcohol and illicit drugs, smoking cessation, exercise, lipid control
   b. Stage B: all interventions for stage A plus the following:
      1) ACE inhibitor and ARB in appropriate patients
      2) Beta-block or alpha- and beta-blocker in appropriate patients
      3) Consideration of ICD
   c. Stage C: all interventions for stages A and B plus the following:
      1) Drugs for routine use
         a) ACE inhibitor
         b) Beta-blocker or alpha- and beta-blocker
         c) Diuretics for fluid retention
      2) Drugs for selected patients
         a) Aldosterone antagonists (e.g., spironolactone)
         b) ARB
         c) Digitalis
         d) Hydralazine or nitrates
      3) Devices in selected patients
         a) Resynchronization therapy
         b) Automatic implantable cardiac defibrillator
   d. Stage D: all interventions for stages A, B, and C plus the following:
      1) Discussion of end-of-life care
      2) Consideration of extraordinary measures
         a) Chronic inotropes
         b) Permanent mechanical support
         c) Cardiac transplantation
         d) Experimental surgeries or drugs

3. Improve oxygenation
   a. Oxygen by nasal cannula at 2 to 6 l/min to maintain SaO_2 of 95% unless contraindicated
   b. Intubation and mechanical ventilation may be required
      1) Noninvasive positive-pressure ventilation (BiPAP) may be used to avert intubation.
         a) Positive-pressure ventilation during inspiration (pressure support ventilation [PSV]) during inspiration decreases the work of breathing
         b) CPAP during expiration: increases the driving pressure of oxygen to improve oxygenation; decreases intrapulmonary shunt by opening collapsed alveoli; decreases surface tension and work of breathing
      2) PEEP may be required if patient is on mechanical ventilation.
         a) Increases the driving pressure of oxygen
         b) Decreases shunt by opening alveoli that are collapsed (alveolar recruitment) and keeps alveoli open at low distending pressure if they are still open
         c) Decreases surface tension and work of breathing
         d) Positive alveolar pressure prevents the transudation of fluid into the alveoli
   c. Elimination of accumulated fluid: diuretics
   d. Treatment of anemia: more than half of patients with HF are anemic with Hgb less than 12 g/dl and treatment of anemia improves cardiac function
      1) Packed RBCs may be required acutely if anemia is significant.
      2) Erythropoietin
      3) Iron
4. Decrease myocardial oxygen consumption.
   a. Physical and emotional rest
      1) Allow rest after meals, personal hygiene, toileting, physical therapy, etc.
      2) Prevent Valsalva maneuver.
         a) Teach patient to exhale when turning in bed.
         b) Administer stool softeners as prescribed.
         c) Provide bedside commode for elimination.
      3) Explain procedures thoroughly: monitor alarms, equipment, visiting hours, reasons for procedures
      4) Keep family informed regarding patient's progress and status.
      5) Provide for physical comfort: temperature control, lighting, noise control
      6) Instruct patient regarding relaxation techniques; encourage utilization.
      7) Provide appropriate nutrition: soft low-sodium (2–3 g/day) diet
      8) Administer anxiolytics as prescribed: usually diazepam, lorazepam, or alprazolam.
   b. Beta-blocker (or alpha- and beta-blocker) as prescribed
      1) Indications: HF as the result of systolic and diastolic dysfunction; usually used for Class II or III HF
      2) Actions
         a) Acts as a cardioprotective agent to protect the heart from excessive catecholamines
         b) Decreases LV mass and volume
         c) Changes the shape of the ventricle from spherical to elliptical
         d) Increases exercise capacity
      3) Agents
         a) Carvedilol: alpha- and noncardioselective beta-blocker
         b) Bisoprolol: cardioselective beta-blocker
         c) Sustained release metoprolol: cardioselective beta-blocker
         d) Dosages are started low and gradually increased while monitoring closely for decompensation because beta-blockers tend to decrease contractility
      4) Contraindications for the use of beta-blockers in HF
         a) Decompensated HF
         b) Cardiogenic shock
         c) Acute pulmonary edema
         d) Hemodynamic instability (requiring IV inotropic support)
         e) Bronchial asthma (cardioselective beta-blockers may be used cautiously)
         f) Second- or third-degree AV block
         g) Sick sinus syndrome
         h) Severe hepatic impairment
5. Decrease preload
   a. Positioning: low Fowler position with legs dependent
   b. Sodium and fluid restrictions acutely
      1) Fluid restriction to less than 2000 ml/24 hr
      2) Sodium restriction to less than 2 to 3 g/24 hr
      3) Daily measurement of weight to detect early fluid retention
   c. Diuretics
      1) Indication: HF with evidence of or a predisposition to fluid retention
      2) Action: eliminate symptoms as well as physical signs of fluid retention, such as JVD or edema.
      3) Agents
         a) Usually loop diuretics (e.g., furosemide, bumetanide)
            i) Continuous infusion may be superior to intermittent boluses.
         b) Aldosterone antagonists (e.g., aldosterone, eplerenone) may be used with loop diuretics or alone.
            i) Relatively weak diuretic in patients with normal renin; however, it is much more effective in patients who have edema associated with either increased production or decreased elimination of renin
            ii) Benefits are synergistic to the benefits of ACE inhibitors
            iii) Close monitoring of potassium levels is necessary, especially when patient is also on an ACE inhibitor or ARB.
            iv) Contraindicated in patients with renal insufficiency

c) Two or more diuretics may be prescribed together.
d) Short-term use of a drug that increases renal blood flow, such as fenoldopam, may be prescribed.
4) Cautions
   a) Overuse will decrease blood volume, decrease CO, and lead to organ hypoperfusion and prerenal azotemia.
   b) Diuretics may alter the efficacy and toxicity of other drugs used to treat HF (e.g., ACE inhibitors, beta-blockers).
d. ACE inhibitors and ARBs
   1) Indications: HF as the result of systolic and diastolic dysfunction
   2) Action:
      a) ACE inhibitors block conversion of angiotensin I to angiotensin II and the resultant vasoconstriction and aldosterone release.
      b) ARBs block angiotensin II and the resultant vasoconstriction and aldosterone release.
         i) ARBs are frequently used if a patient has angioedema or cough as a result of ACE inhibitors; they are also preferred with African Americans.
   3) Agents
      a) ACE inhibitors: captopril, enalapril, lisinopril, ramipril, benazepril HCl, quinapril HCl, fosinopril, moexipril HCl, trandolapril, perindopril
      b) ARBs: losartan, valsartan, telmisartan, irbesartan, candesartan, eprosartan, olmesartan
      c) If neither ACE inhibitors nor ARBs are tolerated, the combination of nitrates and hydralazine may be prescribed.
   4) Cautions
      a) Hypotension
      b) Angioedema, especially ACE inhibitors
      c) Hyperkalemia, especially when in combination with an aldosterone antagonist such as spironolactone
      d) Proteinuria and renal failure
e. Nesiritide: recombinant form of BNP
   1) Indication: decompensated HF with dyspnea at rest or with minimal activities and clinical evidence of fluid overload
      a) Systolic and diastolic dysfunction
      b) Decompensation is defined as sustained deterioration in function of at least one NYHA class, usually associated with evidence of total body salt and water overload
   2) Action: binds to the alpha-type natriuretic peptide receptor on the surface of vascular smooth muscle and endothelial cells
      a) Dilates arteries and reduces SVR
      b) Dilates veins and reduces PAOP
      c) Decreases aldosterone and norepinephrine levels
      d) Inhibits RAA system and endothelin pathways prompting the release of fluid and sodium from the body
      e) Improves symptoms of decompensated HF more than nitroglycerin with less proarrhythmogenesis and tachycardia than dobutamine
   3) Contraindications
      a) Hypovolemia
      b) Profound hypotension (e.g., cardiogenic shock)
      c) Aortic stenosis
      d) Hypertrophic or restrictive cardiomyopathy
      e) Constrictive pericarditis or cardiac tamponade
   4) Controversy: recent studies indicate that nesiritide worsens renal function; its use has decreased significantly in the past 5 years.
f. Endothelin receptor antagonist: tezosentan
   1) Action: vasodilation
   2) Does not increase HR, but higher doses are associated with hypotension
   3) Recent studies results have been mixed in terms of benefit.
g. Venous vasodilators (e.g., nitroglycerin, morphine)
   1) Not recommended in diastolic dysfunction
   2) Be familiar with the effects of commonly used vasodilators (Table 3.36)
h. Dialysis: if the patient is in renal failure
i. Continuous renal replacement therapy (CRRT): may be used to manage the overhydration in HF refractory to traditional therapies such as fluid restriction and diuretics
6. Decrease afterload.
   a. Nitroprusside: particularly helpful for hypertensive patients
   b. Calcium channel blockers
      1) Most calcium channel blockers should be avoided in the treatment of HF; amlodipine and felodipine may be used in diastolic dysfunction.
   c. ACE inhibitors or ARBs: prevent activation of angiotensin II with the resultant vasoconstriction and increase in afterload
   d. Renal artery angioplasty, stents: indicated for patient with renal artery stenosis

Table 3.36	Vasoactive Effects of Selected Drugs	
Drug	**Arteries**	**Veins**
Clevidipine	Yes	No
Fenoldopam mesylate	Yes	No
Hydralazine	Yes	No
Milrinone	Yes	Yes
Minoxidil	Yes	No
Morphine sulfate	No	Yes
Nesiritide	Yes	Yes
Nicardipine	Yes	Yes
Nifedipine	Yes	Yes
Nitroglycerin	Only if >1 mcg/kg/min	Yes
Nitroprusside	Yes	Yes
Phentolamine	Yes	Yes
Prazosin	Yes	Yes

e. Pulmonary vasodilators may be used to reduce pulmonary hypertension.
f. IABP: especially helpful in patients who have very high afterload that is refractory to arterial vasodilators or who are too hypotensive to use arterial dilators to reduce afterload

7. Increase contractility.
   a. Inotropic agents
      1) Indications
         a) Temporary treatment of diuretic-refractory decompensation
         b) Stage D HF to improve quality of life
            i) Note that inotropic agents do increase myocardial oxygen consumption; they have not been shown to improve survival and are generally not recommended
      2) Hemodynamic effects (Table 3.37)
      3) Agents (Table 3.38)
         a) Cardiac glycosides (e.g., digoxin)
            i) Recommended to improve symptoms in patients with HF due to LV systolic dysfunction with dilated ventricle and should be used together with diuretics, ACE inhibitors, and beta-blockers
            ii) Actions
               (a) Improve cardiac contractility by inhibiting Na, K-ATPase; increases EF and exercise tolerance
               (b) Inhibit SNS and reduces norepinephrine and renin activity
               (c) Slow the HR in atrial fibrillation
            iii) Major drawback: the narrow therapeutic-to-toxic ratio
         b) Sympathetic stimulants (e.g., dobutamine)
            i) Used primarily if HF in presence of acute MI
            ii) Actions
               (a) Increases contractility by stimulating beta receptors so may increase ectopy potential
               (b) Dobutamine is preferred (unless patient is hypotensive) because it causes less tachycardia than dopamine and decreases afterload rather than increases afterload such as dopamine does
            iii) Parenteral only
         c) Phosphodiesterase (PDE) inhibitors (e.g., milrinone, inamrinone)
            i) Used only if no response to digitalis, diuretics, vasodilators
            ii) Actions
               (a) Increases contractility by inhibiting PDE
               (b) Causes vasodilation to decrease preload and afterload
            iii) Parenteral only
   b. Mechanical cardiac support devices
      1) The supply of acceptable donor hearts remains insufficient for the number of patients who require them; mechanical devices offer an alternative (at least temporary); devices continue to be developed and tested as a permanent alternative to cardiac transplantation.
      2) Goal: to stabilize and improve the hemodynamic condition of the patient with loss of ventricular function
      3) Complications: infection and thromboembolism are most significant; bleeding; hypertension
      4) Ventricular assist device (VAD): used in severe cases, especially if patient is a candidate for cardiac transplantation (Table 3.39)
   c. Cardiac transplantation
      1) Indications for cardiac transplantation in HF patient
         a) Class III or IV and a life expectancy of less than 24 hours
         b) Younger than 65 years of age at the time of listing; if retransplantation or heart and kidney or heart and liver, the age of 55 years is generally used
         c) Acute HF or cardiogenic shock as a result of acute MI that is refractory to medical therapy and requires mechanical support or patients who cannot be weaned from cardiopulmonary bypass are candidates unless they have contraindications

8. Manage dysrhythmias.
   a. Atrial
      1) Atrial dysrhythmias frequently resolve with treatment of HF because atrial stretch and therefore atrial irritability is decreased.
      2) Digoxin: decreases ventricular response rate by increasing refractoriness of AV node
      3) Anticoagulants: used to prevent mural thrombi and embolic events
   b. Ventricular
      1) Antidysrhythmics as prescribed
         a) Class I antidysrhythmics (e.g., procainamide, lidocaine) should not be used except for immediately life-threatening ventricular dysrhythmia.
         b) Some Class III antidysrhythmics, such as amiodarone, do not appear to increase the risk of death and are preferred over class I agents.
      2) Correction of electrolyte deficiencies that may cause dysrhythmias and alter the efficacy and safety of antidysrhythmic agents

Table 3.37 Hemodynamic Effects of Inotropic Agents

Drug	CO/CI	MAP	PAOP	SVR	Heart Rate
Digoxin	↑	⇔	⇔	⇔	↓
Dobutamine	↑	↑	↓	↓	⇔ or ↑
Dopamine	↑	↑	↑	↑	↑
Inamrinone and milrinone	↑	⇔	↓	↓	⇔

CI, Cardiac index; *CO*, cardiac output; *PAOP*, pulmonary artery occlusive pressure; *SVR*, systemic vascular resistance.

Chapter 3 The Cardiovascular System   193

Table 3.38 Inotropic Agents

Drug	Classification and Actions	Indications	Administration	Adverse Effects	Nursing Implications
Dopamine hydrochloride	Sympathomimetic • Dosage determines action • 2–5 mcg/kg/min causes beta stimulation (increases contractility) • 5–10 mcg/kg/min causes alpha and beta stimulation (increases contractility and causes vasoconstriction) • Dosages >10 mcg/kg/min cause predominant alpha stimulation (vasoconstriction)	• Low CO states (2–10 mcg/kg/min) • Vasogenic forms of shock (10 or >mcg/kg/min)	• IV infusion: mix 400 mg in 250 ml (1600 mcg/ml) and infuse at 0.5–20 mcg/kg/min depending on desired effect • Maximum: 20 mcg/kg/min • Administer through central venous catheter if possible; if administered peripherally, use a large vein • Do not administer with alkaline solutions	• Tachycardia • Ventricular ectopy • Hypertension or hypotension • Nausea, vomiting • Dyspnea • Headache • Palpitations • Chest pain in patients with CAD • Tissue necrosis with high dosages or extravasation	• Monitor HR, BP, ECG, PA, PAOP, SVR, CI, urine output • Note contraindications: known hypersensitivity, uncorrected tachydysrhythmias, ventricular fibrillation, pheochromocytoma, hypertrophic cardiomyopathy, and in patients receiving MAO inhibitors • Use cautiously in peripheral vascular disease • Consider the cause of hypotension instead of automatically initiating dopamine to increase the BP; *improve perfusion* by treating the cause of hypotension (e.g., volume replacement, inotropes, preload or afterload reduction) • Provide volume expansion during weaning; taper gradually to wean • Do not administer if discolored • Prevent extravasation because necrosis may occur; treat extravasation with phentolamine (Regitine)
Dobutamine hydrochloride	Sympathomimetic • Increases cardiac contractility and cardiac output • Decreases preload and possibly afterload	• Cardiogenic shock • Low CO states	• IV infusion; mix 250 mg in 250 ml (1000 mcg/ml) and infuse at 2–40 mcg/kg/min • Maximum: 40 mcg/kg/min • Administer through central venous catheter if possible; if administered peripherally, use a large vein • Do not administer with alkaline solutions	• Tachycardia • Ventricular ectopy • Hypertension or hypotension • Nausea, vomiting • Dyspnea • Headache • Anxiety • Paresthesia • Palpitations • Chest pain	• Monitor BP, HR, ECG, PA, PAOP, SVR, CI • Note contraindications: known hypersensitivity, hypertrophic cardiomyopathy • Use cautiously in patients with hypertension or ventricular dysrhythmias • Note that the increase in heart rate is less than with dopamine • Use with nitroprusside as prescribed in cardiogenic shock; dobutamine increases contractility and decreases preload (and to a lesser degree afterload) and nitroprusside decreases afterload and preload

Continued

Table 3.38 Inotropic Agents—cont'd

Drug	Classification and Actions	Indications	Administration	Adverse Effects	Nursing Implications
Inamrinone Note change in generic name to avoid confusion between previously named amrinone and amiodarone Milrinone	PDE inhibitor Inotrope • Increases cardiac contractility • Relaxes vascular smooth muscle to cause vasodilation of arteries and veins and decrease afterload and preload	• HF: short-term (<5 days) management of patients with HF who have not responded to traditional therapy of digitalis, diuretics, and/or vasodilators	• IV injection: 0.75 mg/kg over 2–3 min; may repeat in 30 min • IV infusion: mix 500 mg in 500 ml (1000 mcg/ml) and infuse at 5–15 mcg/kg/min • Maximum: 10 mg/kg/day • Do not reconstitute with dextrose • IV injection: 50 mcg/kg over 10 min • IV infusion: mix 30 mg in 250 ml (120 mcg/ml); usual dose 0.375–0.75 mcg/kg/min (less if renal insufficiency)	• Ventricular dysrhythmias • Hypotension • Anorexia, nausea, vomiting, abdominal pain, diarrhea • Increased liver enzymes, hepatotoxicity • Hypokalemia • Tremor • Thrombocytopenia (inamrinone more than milrinone) • Chest pain • Hypersensitivity reactions • Headache • Burning at injection site • Fever • Blurred vision (milrinone)	• Monitor heart rate, BP, ECG, PA, PAOP, CI, SVR, platelet counts, liver function studies, electrolytes (especially potassium), BUN, creatinine • Platelet count <150,000/mm³ usually requires dosage reduction • Platelet count <100,000/mm³ usually requires discontinuance • Note contraindications: known hypersensitivity to this drug or bisulfites (preservative), severe aortic or pulmonic valvular disease, hypertrophic cardiomyopathy, ventricular dysrhythmias • Use cautiously in renal disease, liver disease, atrial dysrhythmias, older adult • Use cautiously in acute MI because myocardial oxygen consumption is increased • Correct hypokalemia and hypovolemia before or during inamrinone use • Note that milrinone is more frequently prescribed than inamrinone because of the greater incidence of thrombocytopenia with inamrinone

BP, Blood pressure; *BUN*, blood urea nitrogen; *CAD*, coronary artery disease; *CI*, cardiac index; *CO*, cardiac output; *ECG*, electrocardiogram; *HF*, heart failure; *HR*, heart rate; *IV*, intravenous; *MAO*, monoamine oxidase; *MI*, myocardial infarction; *PA*, pulmonary artery; *PAOP*, pulmonary artery occlusive pressure; *PDE*, phosphodiesterase; *SVR*, systemic vascular resistance.

Table 3.39 Ventricular Assist Device

Indications	• Bridge to recovery: use of a device until the heart recovers and transplantation is not required
	  • Persistent HF despite aggressive therapy but with potential for recovery if the heart is given time to rest
	  • Inability to wean from CPB
	  • Cardiogenic shock refractory to pharmacologic or IABP therapy
	  • Stunned (may also be referred to as *hibernating*) myocardium
	• Bridge to bridge: use of a short-term device with replacement later with a long-term device
	• Bridge to transplant: use of a device to support the patient until a donor heart is available
	  • End-stage heart disease awaiting suitable donor for cardiac transplant
	• Destination therapy: use of a permanent device as an alternative to transplantation
	  • Class IV HF with EF <25%, on continuous inotropic therapy but not a candidate for cardiac transplantation
	• Physiologic indications despite pharmacologic support or IABP therapy
	  • MAP <60 mm Hg
	  • Systolic <90 mm Hg
	  • PAOP or RAP >20–25 mm Hg
	  • Urine output <20 ml/hr
	  • CI <2 l/min/m^2
	  • EF <25%
	  • May be used with IABP

Contraindications	• Irreversible, extensive heart disease; no possibility of being weaned from VAD; and patient not a candidate for cardiac transplant • Prolonged cardiac arrest with resultant neurologic damage • Multiple organ failure • Significant complications or disease (e.g., chronic renal failure, cancer with metastasis, severe hepatic disease, significant blood dyscrasias, severe COPD)
Actions	• Maintains systemic circulation and tissue perfusion with flow assistance • Decreases myocardial workload to promote ventricular recovery • Reversal of ventricular dilation, regression of left ventricular hypertrophy, reversal of ventricular remodeling
Devices	• Total artificial heart: CardioWest, Abiomed • Displacement pumps: Thoratec, ABIOMED BVS 5000, HeartMate XVE, Novacor LVAD • Rotary, continuous flow, or axial pumps: HeartMate II, MicroMed DeBakey, Jarvik 2000 FlowMaker, Impella, Berlin Heart Incor LVAD, TandemHeart Percutaneous VAD, VentrAssist LVAD, Bio-Medicus • Magnetically levitated pumps: Levitronix CentriMag • All devices have cannula, pump, and external power source

Insertion and mechanics	• Requires an extended median sternotomy
	• Left ventricular assist device (LVAD)
	  • Outflow circuit anastomosed to patient aorta or femoral artery
	  • Inflow circuit anastomosed to left atrium or ventricle
	  • Left atrium is usually used in the pending recovery patient
	  • Left ventricle is usually used in the bridge to transplant patient
	• Right ventricular assist device (RVAD)
	  • Outflow circuit anastomosed to patient's pulmonary artery
	  • Inflow circuit anastomosed to right atrium
	• Biventricular assist device (Bi-VAD)
	  • Both ventricles are supported; the main advantage here is that with either LVAD or RVAD the unassisted ventricle may fail
	• Implanted device
	  • The pump unit may be implanted into the abdominal wall
	  • Controller unit and power source are attached to the pump unit by a percutaneous lead

Assessment	• HR: a normalization of heart rate is desirable • BP: an increase in MAP is desirable • CO/CI: an increase in cardiac output/index is desirable • Thermodilution CO will not be accurate in patients with RVAD; use Fick formula (calculation of CO using mixed venous oxygen saturation and arterial oxygen saturation) • PAP/PAOP: a decrease in PAP and PAOP is desirable • SaO$_2$: an increase in SaO$_2$ is desirable • SvO$_2$: an increase in SvO$_2$ is desirable • Urine output: an increase in urine output is desirable • Complaints of chest pain: a decrease in chest pain is desirable • ECG: a decrease in the presence or frequency of dysrhythmias is desirable • Neurovascular status of affected limb: the presence of palpable pulses and a warm limb with normal capillary refill is desirable

Continued

Table 3.39	Ventricular Assist Device—cont'd
Brief summary of nursing management	• Assess the parameters described earlier • Titrate pharmacologic therapies to augment the mechanical therapy of the VAD • Adjust fluid balance by administering colloids, crystalloids, or diuretics as prescribed • Prevent hazards of immobility: turn side to side when hemodynamics are stabilized; passive range of motion; use special mattresses and beds as indicated • Observe for complications and provide appropriate management for the prevention of complications • Provide emotional support to the patient and family; utilize social services, pastoral care, and support groups as indicated

Complications: prevention and treatment	• Thromboembolism: heparin may be prescribed
	• Hemolysis
	• Bleeding
	  • Monitor ACT while on heparin
	  • Monitor for bleeding, including cardiac tamponade
	  • Administer blood and blood products as indicated
	  • Prevent tubing disconnection; all connections should be clearly visible and securely connected
	• Infection
	  • Monitor CBC, body temperature, and heart rate
	  • Monitor for pain, tenderness, heat, redness at exit site and abdominal pump pocket
	  • Assess breath sounds and chest radiography; pneumonia is common because of immobilization; ventilatory assistance is required with some VADs
	• Dysrhythmias
	• Cerebral emboli
	• Respiratory failure
	• Renal failure
	• Air embolism
	• Mechanical failure
	• Psychological complications (e.g., depression, anxiety): anxiety concerning device failure and infection

Weaning	• The following parameters with VAD off are required before weaning the patient from the VAD
	  • MAP >60 mm Hg
	  • RAP (RVAD) or PAOP (LVAD) <25 mm Hg
	  • CI >2 l/min/m^2
	• The VAD flow is decreased
	• Anticoagulation is recommended during weaning
	• VAD removal is done in the OR

ACT, Activated clotting time; *BP*, blood pressure; *CBC*, complete blood count; *CI*, cardiac index; *CO*, cardiac output; *COPD*, chronic obstructive pulmonary disease; *CPB*, cardiopulmonary bypass; *ECG*, electrocardiogram; *EF*, ejection fraction; *HF*, heart failure; *HR*, heart rate; *IABP*, intraaortic balloon pump; *MAP*, mean arterial pressure; *OR*, operating room; *PAOP*, pulmonary artery occlusive pressure; *PAP*, pulmonary artery pressure; *RAP*, right atrial pressure; *SaO$_2$*, arterial oxygen saturation; *SvO$_2$*, saturation of venous blood; *VAD*, ventricular assist device.

    c. Dual-chamber pacemaker with rate modulation
      1) Beneficial for patients with severe HF with poor activity tolerance
      2) Increases HR in response to physical activity
    d. Cardiac resynchronization therapy (CRT): atriobiventricular pacing
      1) Indications in HF patients: 30% to 50% of patients with HF have ventricular asynchrony, and the 80% of patients with advanced HF have LBBB with resultant ventricular asynchrony.
        a) EF of 35% or less
        b) QRS of at least 130 msec (0.13 sec)
        c) NYHA class III to IV
      2) Actions
        a) Restores synchronous ventricular contraction to optimize LV filling and improve CO
        b) Improved exercise tolerance
        c) Improved quality of life
        d) Reduction in mortality rate
      3) Collaborative management: as for newly implanted pacemakers and for HF
        a) Monitor for 100% ventricular capture as well as any lengthening of the QRS that might indicate loss of capture of one of the ventricles (usually the left ventricle)
        b) Restrict movement of the arm to prevent lead dislodgement or bleeding in the pacemaker pocket; give instructions regarding: avoidance of pushing, pulling, or lifting anything heavier than 5 lb for 1 to 2 weeks after surgery; what symptoms to report; and other instructions as for implanted pacemaker
        c) Monitor for complications: infection
  9. Provide collaborative management specific to RVF (cor pulmonale).
    a. Treat the cause.
      1) Hypoxemia: oxygen to maintain SaO$_2$ of at least 90%
      2) Primary pulmonary hypertension: nitric oxide or epoprostenol may be indicated depending on etiology

3) PE
    a) Anticoagulants
    b) Fibrinolytics if RVF or refractory hypoxemia
4) Dysrhythmias: cardioversion, antidysrhythmic agents, pacemaker, resynchronization therapy
  b. Ensure volume optimization.
    1) Treatment of fluid overload: sodium restriction, diuretics, CRRT
    2) Treatment of hypovolemia: fluid administration
  c. Administer inotropic agents as required; especially when poor RV contractility (e.g., RV MI)
10. Monitor for complications.
  a. DVT or PE
  b. Progressive deterioration
  c. Dysrhythmias: common cause of sudden death
  d. Complications of therapy
    1) Fluid and electrolyte imbalance: hypokalemia, hypocalcemia, or hypomagnesemia caused by diuretic therapy
    2) Digitalis toxicity
  e. Depression
  f. Anxiety
  g. Sleep disturbances
11. Provide instruction and counseling regarding lifestyle modification and need for pharmacologic therapy.
  a. Nonpharmacologic therapies
    1) Weight normalization
    2) Dietary modifications
      a) Low saturated fat
      b) Low (2–3 g/day) sodium
      c) ADA diet for control of blood glucose for patient with DM
    3) Cessation of tobacco use
    4) Limitation of alcohol consumption to 1 to 2 alcoholic beverages daily
    5) Regular aerobic exercise in moderation
    6) Complementary therapies: relaxation; imagery, biofeedback
    7) Stress reduction
    8) Yearly flu and pneumococcal vaccine
    9) Recognition of symptoms of HF and when to call the physician
    10) Measurement of body weight is the best way to monitor when to initiate and titrate diuretic therapy.
      a) Teach the patient to notify the physician if he or she gains 2 lb/day for more than 2 days or a total of 5 lb in 1 week.
  b. Pharmacologic agents
    1) Prescribed medication regimen for HF
    2) Control of hypertension, hyperlipidemia, DM, and thyroid disorders
    3) Avoidance of drugs that may worsen HF: NSAIDs

Cardiomyopathy

Definition
Disorder causing destruction of cardiac muscle fibers (i.e., myofibrils) leading to impaired contractility and CO (Fig. 3.81)

Dilated Cardiomyopathy
1. Etiology
  a. Idiopathic
  b. Infection, especially viral (e.g., coxsackievirus B, arbovirus)
  c. Toxins (e.g., doxorubicin, daunorubicin, alcohol, lead, arsenic, cobalt)
  d. Electrolyte, vitamin or nutrient deficiency
    1) Hypokalemia
    2) Hypocalcemia
    3) Hypophosphatemia
    4) Thiamine deficiency
  e. Pregnancy
  f. Neuromuscular disorders (e.g., myasthenia gravis, muscular dystrophy)
  g. Connective tissue disorders (e.g., lupus, scleroderma, rheumatoid disease)
  h. Infiltrative disorders (e.g., sarcoidosis, amyloidosis)
  i. Hyperthyroidism
2. Pathophysiology (Fig. 3.82)
3. Clinical presentation
  a. Subjective
    1) Fatigue, weakness, decreased exercise tolerance
    2) Chest pain
    3) Palpitations
    4) Syncope
    5) Symptoms of HF: dyspnea; edema

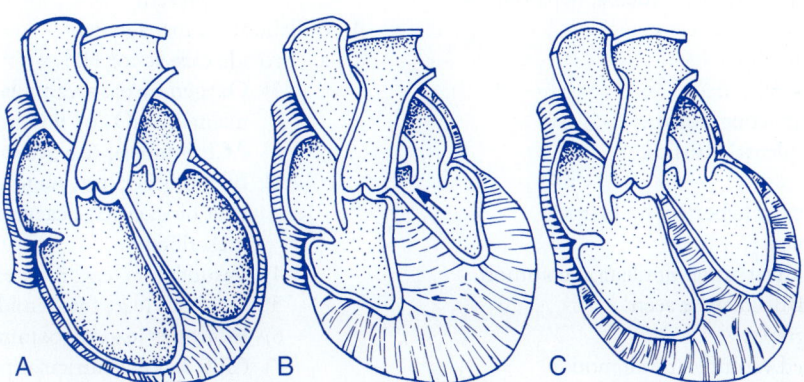

Fig. 3.81 Cardiomyopathies. **A,** Dilated. **B,** Hypertrophic. **C,** Restrictive. (From Kinney, M. R., Packa, D. R., & Dunbar, S. B. [1993]. *AACN's clinical reference for critical-care nursing* [3rd ed.]. St. Louis: Mosby.)

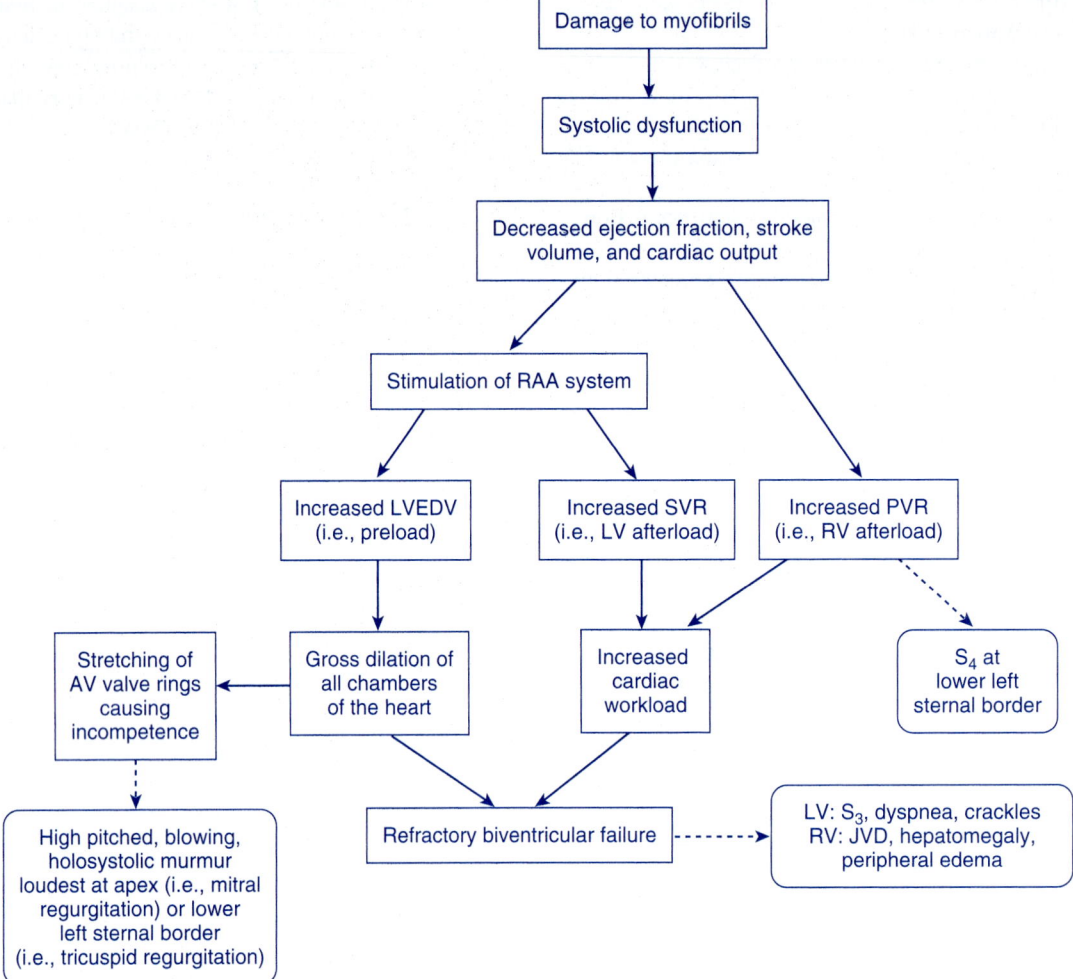

Fig. 3.82 Pathophysiology of dilated cardiomyopathy. *Dotted lines* connect pathology to the clinical presentation. *AV,* Atrioventricular; *JVD,* jugular venous distention; *LV,* left ventricular; *LVEDV,* left ventricular end diastolic volume; *PVR,* pulmonary vascular resistance; *RAA,* renin-angiotensin-aldosterone; *RV,* right ventricular; *SVR,* systemic vascular resistance.

    b. Objective
       1) Orthostatic BP changes
       2) May have murmurs of tricuspid or mitral regurgitation
       3) Signs of biventricular failure
          a) LVF: S_3; crackles; PMI displaced laterally
          b) RVF: JVD; peripheral edema; hepatomegaly
    c. Diagnostic studies
       1) Chest radiography
          a) Cardiomegaly
          b) Pulmonary congestion
          c) Possibly pleural effusion
       2) ECG
          a) Biventricular hypertrophy, biatrial enlargement
          b) Dysrhythmias: atrial fibrillation common
          c) Blocks: BBB may be seen
       3) Echocardiography
          a) Decreased ventricular wall motion
          b) Decreased EF
          c) Enlarged chamber size
          d) Abnormal wall motion
       4) Cardiac catheterization
          a) Elevated PAP, LAP, LVEDP
          b) Decreased CO
          c) Decreased EF
          d) Mitral and/or tricuspid regurgitation
          e) RAP, RVEDP may be elevated if RVF present
  4. Collaborative management
    a. Provide care as for HF.
       1) Oxygen by nasal cannula at 2 to 6 l/min to maintain SaO_2 of 95% unless contraindicated
       2) ACE inhibitor (e.g., captopril)
       3) Beta-blocker (e.g., metoprolol) or alpha- and beta-blocker (e.g., carvedilol) may be prescribed
       4) Vasodilators (e.g., nitrates)
       5) Diuretics (e.g., furosemide)
       6) Inotropes (e.g., digoxin) may be required
       7) CRT: atriobiventricular pacing
    b. Decrease myocardial oxygen consumption.
       1) Activity restrictions
       2) Sodium restrictions

3) Physical comfort: temperature; lighting; noise control
4) Anxiolytics as prescribed and indicated: usually diazepam, lorazepam, or alprazolam
c. Monitor for complications.
1) Dysrhythmias
a) Atrial fibrillation: digoxin
b) Ventricular dysrhythmias: antidysrhythmic agents (e.g., amiodarone), ICD
2) Systemic emboli: anticoagulation frequently prescribed, especially for patients with EFs less than 30%
d. Assist in preparation of the patient for mitral valve replacement or cardiac transplantation as requested.

Hypertrophic Cardiomyopathy

1. Types
   a. Nonobstructive: ventricular free wall hypertrophied
   b. Obstructive: both ventricular free wall and interventricular septum are hypertrophied; genetically transmitted
2. Etiology
   a. Heredity: genetically transmitted autosomal dominant trait
   b. Idiopathic
   c. Neuromuscular disorders (e.g., Friedreich ataxia)
   d. Hypoparathyroidism
3. Pathophysiology (Fig. 3.83)
4. Clinical presentation
   a. Subjective
      1) Dyspnea, orthopnea, paroxysmal nocturnal dyspnea (PND)
      2) Chest pain
      3) Palpitations
      4) Syncope
   b. Objective
      1) PMI displaced laterally
      2) Crackles
      3) S_4
      4) Murmurs
         a) Subaortic stenosis: systolic ejection murmur loudest along left sternal border; increases with Valsalva maneuver, decreases with squatting position
         b) Mitral regurgitation: holosystolic blowing murmur loudest at apex radiates to axilla
   c. Diagnostic studies
      1) Chest radiography
         a) LA dilation
         b) Cardiomegaly
         c) Pulmonary congestion
      2) ECG
         a) LA enlargement and LVH
         b) ST- and T-wave abnormalities

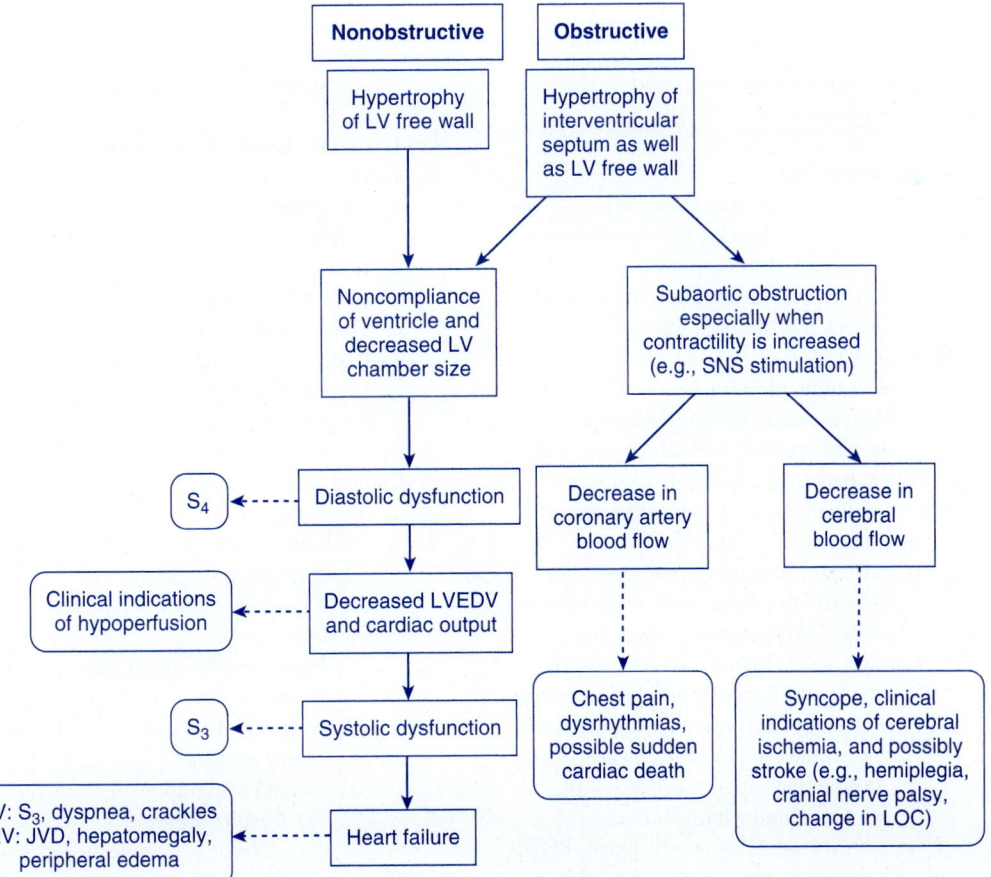

Fig. 3.83 Pathophysiology of hypertrophic cardiomyopathy. *Dotted lines* connect pathology to the clinical presentation. *AV,* Atrioventricular; *JVD,* jugular venous distention; *LV,* left ventricular; *LVEDV,* left ventricular end-diastolic volume; *PVR,* pulmonary vascular resistance; *RAA,* renin-angiotensin-aldosterone; *RV,* right ventricular; *SNS,* sympathetic nervous system; *SVR,* systemic vascular resistance.

c) Dysrhythmias
  i) Atrial fibrillation frequently seen
  ii) Ventricular dysrhythmias may be seen
d) Blocks: left anterior hemiblock frequently seen
3) Echocardiography
  a) LA enlargement
  b) Increased thickness of the LV free wall and interventricular septum causing narrowing of the LV outflow tract
  c) Abnormal wall motion, especially of septum
  d) Mitral regurgitation possible
4) Cardiac catheterization
  a) Elevated LVEDP
  b) Mitral regurgitation may be evident
  c) LV outflow pressure gradient
5. Collaborative management
  a. Prevent obstruction of the LV outflow tract
    1) Administer beta-blockers and/or calcium channel blockers as prescribed to decrease contractility and myocardial oxygen consumption; these agents also decrease the HR to improve ventricular filling.
    2) Avoid inotropic agents that would increase the outflow tract obstruction.
    3) Prepare patient for percutaneous or surgical procedures as requested.
      a) Ventricular septal myectomy: recommended for LV outflow obstruction if symptoms continue despite optimal medical therapy
        i) Surgical removal of a portion of the hypertrophied septum
        ii) Requires thoracotomy and cardiopulmonary bypass
        iii) Mitral valve usually replaced concurrently
        iv) Complications include septal perforation, blocks, and dysrhythmias along with the complications of cardiac surgery with cardiopulmonary bypass
      b) Percutaneous transluminal septal myocardial ablation (PTSMA)
        i) Recommended for LV outflow obstruction if symptoms continue despite optimal medical therapy and the patient is a suboptimal surgical candidate or the patient prefers it after a discussion of options
        ii) Percutaneous coronary intervention to isolate the septal perforator branch of the LAD coronary artery and inject 98% ethanol to cause selective infarction of a portion of the septum to prevent movement of the septum toward the LV free walls to keep the outflow tract open
          (a) Contraindications include inadequate septal thickness, RBBB, mitral valve disease, and greater than 50% occlusion of RCA.
        iii) Temporary pacemaker is usually in place for 24 to 48 hours
        iv) CK-MB and troponin should peak 7 hours after ablation.
        v) IV or oral analgesics may be required.
        vi) Care as for any other PCI along with monitoring for dysrhythmias, heart blocks, stroke, cardiac tamponade, and hypotension
      c) Dual-chamber pacing
        i) Shortening of the AV interval minimizes contraction of the septum and decreases the outflow tract obstruction.
        ii) Usually used in conjunction with pharmacologic agents
  b. Maintain adequate filling volumes.
    1) Administer IV fluids as prescribed.
    2) Administer beta-blockers and calcium channel blockers to decrease the HR, allowing more time for filling.
    3) Use caution or avoid drugs that decrease preload such as venous vasodilators and diuretics.
  c. Monitor for complications.
    1) Dysrhythmias
      a) Atrial: digoxin is not used because it may increase outflow tract obstruction; diltiazem or verapamil may be used.
      b) Ventricular: antidysrhythmics (e.g., amiodarone)
    2) Systemic emboli: anticoagulants are frequently prescribed, especially for patients with EFs less than 30%.
  d. Assist in preparation of the patient for cardiac transplantation as requested.

Restrictive: Least Common

1. Etiology
   a. Idiopathic
   b. Infiltrative disorders (e.g., sarcoidosis, amyloidosis)
   c. Endomyocardial fibrosis
   d. Glycogen deposition
   e. Hemochromatosis
   f. Radiation
   g. Lymphoma
   h. Connective tissue disorders (e.g., scleroderma)
2. Pathophysiology (Fig. 3.84)
3. Clinical presentation
   a. Subjective
     1) Chest pain
     2) Fatigue, weakness
     3) Dyspnea, orthopnea, PND
   b. Objective
     1) Signs of RVF: JVD, hepatomegaly, peripheral edema, right-sided S_3
     2) May also have signs of LVF: left-sided S_3, crackles
   c. Diagnostic studies
     1) Chest radiography
       a) Cardiomegaly
       b) Pulmonary congestion
       c) Possibly pleural effusion
     2) ECG
       a) Low QRS voltage
       b) AV blocks are common

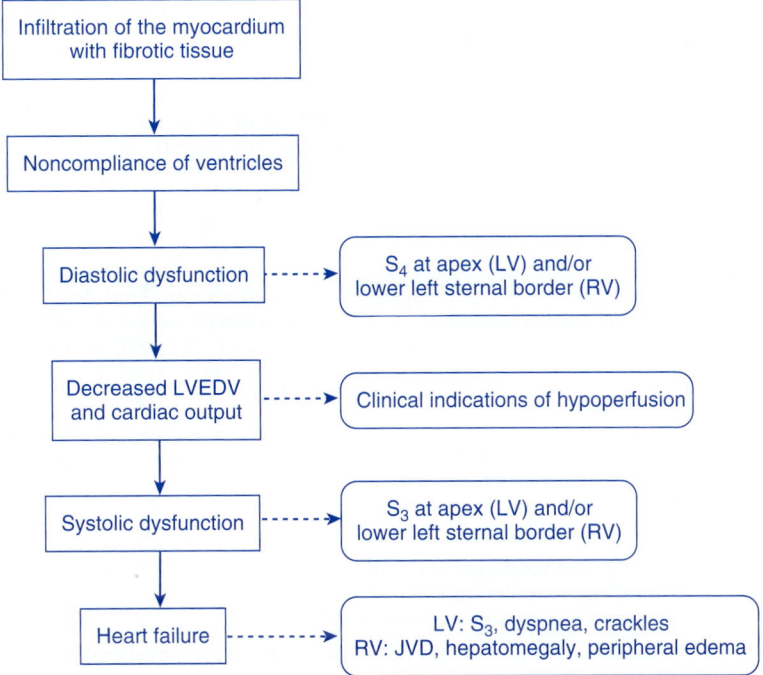

Fig. 3.84 Pathophysiology of restrictive cardiomyopathy. *Dotted lines* connect pathology to the clinical presentation. *JVD,* Jugular venous distention; *LV,* left ventricular; *LVEDV,* left ventricular end-diastolic volume; *RV,* right ventricular.

    3) Echocardiography
       a) Atrial enlargement
       b) Enlarged ventricular outside dimension but small ventricular chamber
       c) Pericardial effusion may be evident
    4) Cardiac catheterization: elevated RAP, RVEDP, PAP, LAP, LVEDP
  4. Collaborative management
    a. Treat the cause: may include steroids
    b. Provide care as for HF
      1) Oxygen by nasal cannula at 2 to 6 l/min to maintain SaO_2 of 95% unless contraindicated
      2) ACE inhibitors (e.g., captopril)
      3) Beta-blockers (e.g., metoprolol)
      4) Vasodilators (e.g., nitrates)
      5) Diuretics (e.g., furosemide)
      6) Inotropes (e.g., digoxin)
    c. Monitor for complications
      1) Dysrhythmias
        a) Atrial fibrillation: digoxin
        b) Ventricular dysrhythmias: antidysrhythmic agents (e.g., amiodarone)
      2) AV blocks: pacemaker may be needed
      3) Systemic emboli: anticoagulants frequently prescribed, especially for patients with EFs less than 30%
    d. Assist in preparation of the patient for cardiac transplantation as requested.

Indications for Cardiac Transplantation

1. Heart disease
    a. Severe functional limitations
    b. Poor prognosis
    c. Not surgically correctable
    d. Unresponsive to medical therapy
    e. PVR normal or reversible with therapy (if pulmonary hypertension is severe and irreversible, the patient may be a candidate for a heart–lung transplant)
2. Age of 70 years or less
3. Lack of intrinsic disease in other organ systems that would limit long-term survival or be worsened by immunosuppressive therapy
4. Favorable psychosocial profile
5. Blood negative for HIV and hepatitis B virus

Valvular Heart Disease

Definition

An acquired or congenital disorder of a cardiac valve; characterized by stenosis (obstruction) or regurgitation (backward flow) of blood

Mitral Regurgitation (Insufficiency, Incompetence)

1. Etiology
    a. Trauma
    b. Rheumatic heart disease (RHD) or other form of infective endocarditis
    c. Papillary muscle dysfunction or rupture, rupture of chordae tendineae
    d. Congenital malformation of mitral valve
    e. MVP (also referred to as *Barlow syndrome* or *floppy mitral valve syndrome*)
    f. LV dilation from LVF
    g. Hypertrophic cardiomyopathy
    h. Marfan syndrome
    i. Calcification of mitral valve leaflets
    j. Scleroderma
    k. Prosthetic valve dysfunction

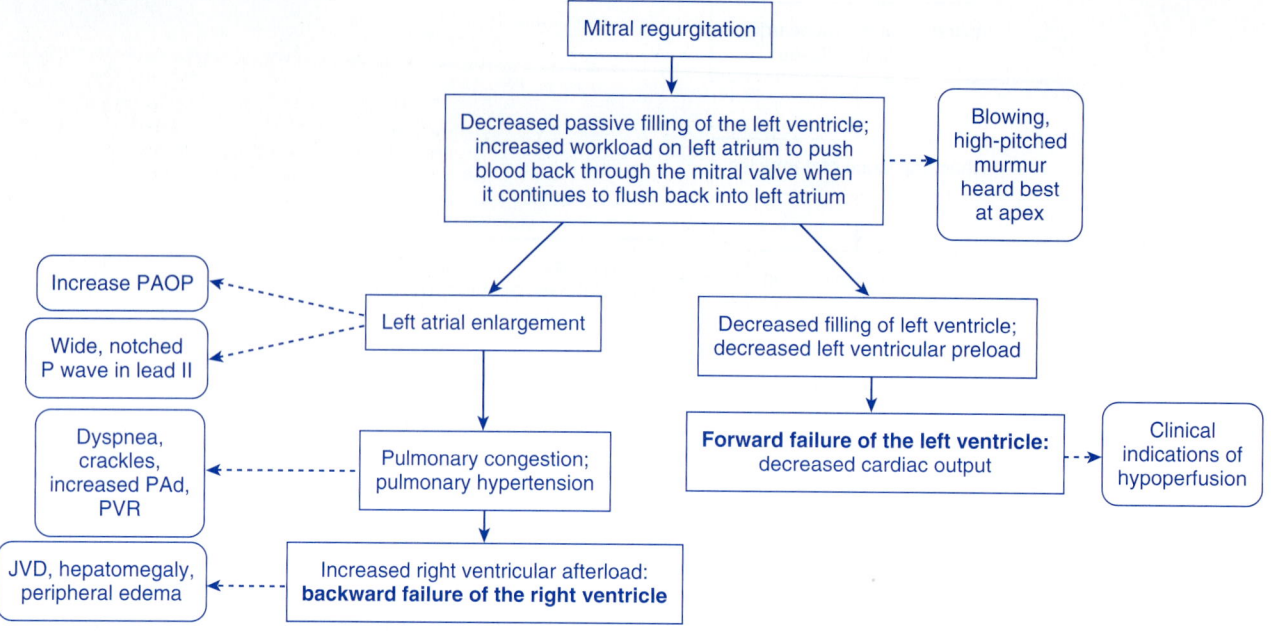

Fig. 3.85 Pathophysiology of mitral regurgitation. *Dotted lines* connect pathology to the clinical presentation. *JVD*, Jugular venous distention; *PAd*, pulmonary artery diastolic pressure; *PAOP*, pulmonary artery occlusive pressure; *PVR*, pulmonary vascular resistance.

2. Pathophysiology (Fig. 3.85)
3. Clinical presentation
   a. Subjective
      1) Dyspnea, orthopnea, PND; may have cough
      2) Chest pain may occur but is not common
      3) Palpitations may occur
      4) Weakness, fatigue
      5) Anxiety
   b. Objective
      1) Tachycardia
      2) Diaphoresis
      3) Confusion
      4) PMI displaced laterally; may be more diffuse
      5) Crackles may be present
      6) Heart sound changes
         a) S_2 may be widely split
         b) Right-sided S_3, S_4 may be heard
      c) Holosystolic murmur: high-pitched, blowing, loudest at apex, and radiates to axilla
      7) Signs of RVF: JVD, hepatomegaly, peripheral edema
   c. Diagnostic studies
      1) Hemodynamic monitoring: PAOP waveform shows large *v* waves
      2) Chest radiography
         a) Cardiomegaly
         b) LA enlargement
         c) LVH
         d) Pulmonary congestion may be present.
      3) ECG
         a) LA enlargement
         b) LVH, RVHH, or both
         c) Dysrhythmias: most frequently atrial fibrillation
      4) Echocardiography
         a) Thickening, prolapse, and calcification of mitral valve
         b) RV, LA, and LV enlargement
      5) Cardiac catheterization
         a) Increased LA and LV pressures
         b) Regurgitation of blood from the left ventricle to the left atrium

Mitral Stenosis

1. Etiology
   a. RHD
   b. Endocarditis
   c. Congenital
   d. Tumors of left atrium (e.g., atrial myxoma)
   e. Calcification of mitral annulus
2. Pathophysiology (Fig. 3.86)
3. Clinical presentation
   a. Subjective
      1) Dyspnea, orthopnea, PND, crackles
      2) Cough, hemoptysis
      3) Fatigue, weakness
      4) Palpitations
      5) Dysphagia
      6) Hoarseness
      7) Syncope may occur.
      8) Chest pain may occur but is rare.
   b. Objective
      1) Ruddy face (mitral facies)
      2) RV heave palpable at sternum
      3) Heart sound changes
         a) Loud S_1: referred to as *closing snap*
         b) Loud P_2
         c) Right-sided S_3, S_4
         d) Opening snap
         e) Mid-diastolic murmur: harsh, rumbling, loudest at apex; may have associated thrill
      4) Signs of RVF: JVD; hepatomegaly; peripheral edema
   c. Hemodynamic parameters: PAOP waveform shows large *a* waves

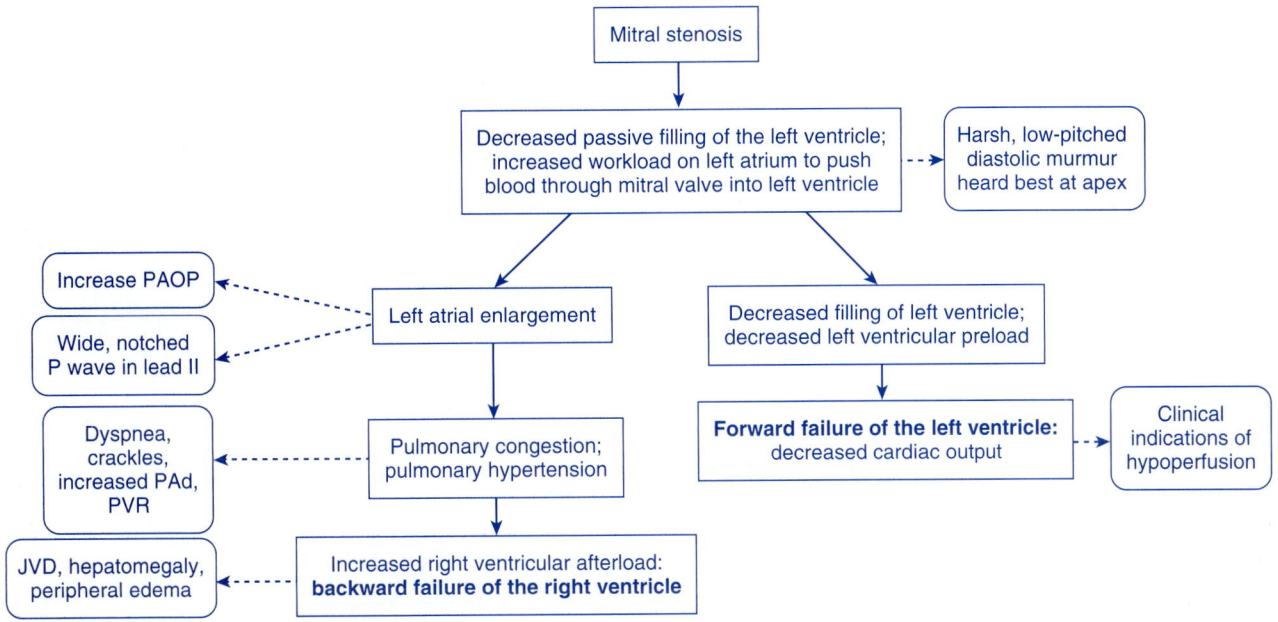

Fig. 3.86 Pathophysiology of mitral stenosis. *Dotted lines* connect pathology to the clinical presentation. *JVD*, Jugular venous distention; *PAd*, pulmonary artery diastolic pressure; *PAOP*, pulmonary artery occlusive pressure; *PVR*, pulmonary vascular resistance.

    d. Diagnostic studies
        1) Chest radiography
            a) LA enlargement
            b) Pulmonary congestion
            c) RVH
            d) Mitral valve calcification
        2) ECG
            a) LA enlargement (frequently referred to as *P-mitrale*)
            b) RVH
            c) Dysrhythmias: most frequently atrial fibrillation
        3) Echocardiography
            a) Abnormal movement and thickening of valve leaflets and narrowing of mitral valve orifice
            b) LA enlargement
            c) RVH
        4) Cardiac catheterization
            a) Elevated pressure gradient across mitral valve
            b) Elevated RAP, PAP, LAP

Aortic Regurgitation (Insufficiency, Incompetence)

1. Etiology
    a. RHD
    b. Calcification
    c. Congenital malformation (e.g., bicuspid aortic valve)
    d. Endocarditis
    e. Syphilis
    f. Marfan syndrome
    g. Hypertension
    h. Connective tissue disease (e.g., lupus erythematosus)
    i. Aortic dissection
    j. Trauma
2. Pathophysiology (Fig. 3.87)
3. Clinical presentation
    a. Subjective
        1) Fatigue
        2) Cough
        3) Symptoms of HF: dyspnea, orthopnea, PND
        4) Exertional chest pain
        5) Syncope
        6) Palpitations
    b. Objective
        1) Musset sign: nodding of the head with each systole
        2) Widened pulse pressure
        3) Water-hammer (also called *Corrigan*) pulse: rapid rise that collapses suddenly
        4) PMI displaced laterally and downward
        5) Hill sign: popliteal is greater than brachial BP by 40 mm Hg or more.
        6) Quincke sign: visible capillary pulsation of nailbeds when fingertip is pressed
        7) Signs of HF: S_3, crackles, JVD, hepatomegaly, peripheral edema
        8) Heart sound changes
            a) Diastolic murmur: high-pitched, blowing, decrescendo, loudest at base, may radiate to the apex; may have associated thrill
            b) May have aortic ejection click
            c) Systolic murmur: may have systolic ejection murmur
    c. Diagnostic studies
        1) Chest radiography
            a) LA enlargement
            b) LVH
            c) Pulmonary congestion
        2) ECH
            a) Sinus tachycardia
            b) LVH
            c) LA enlargement

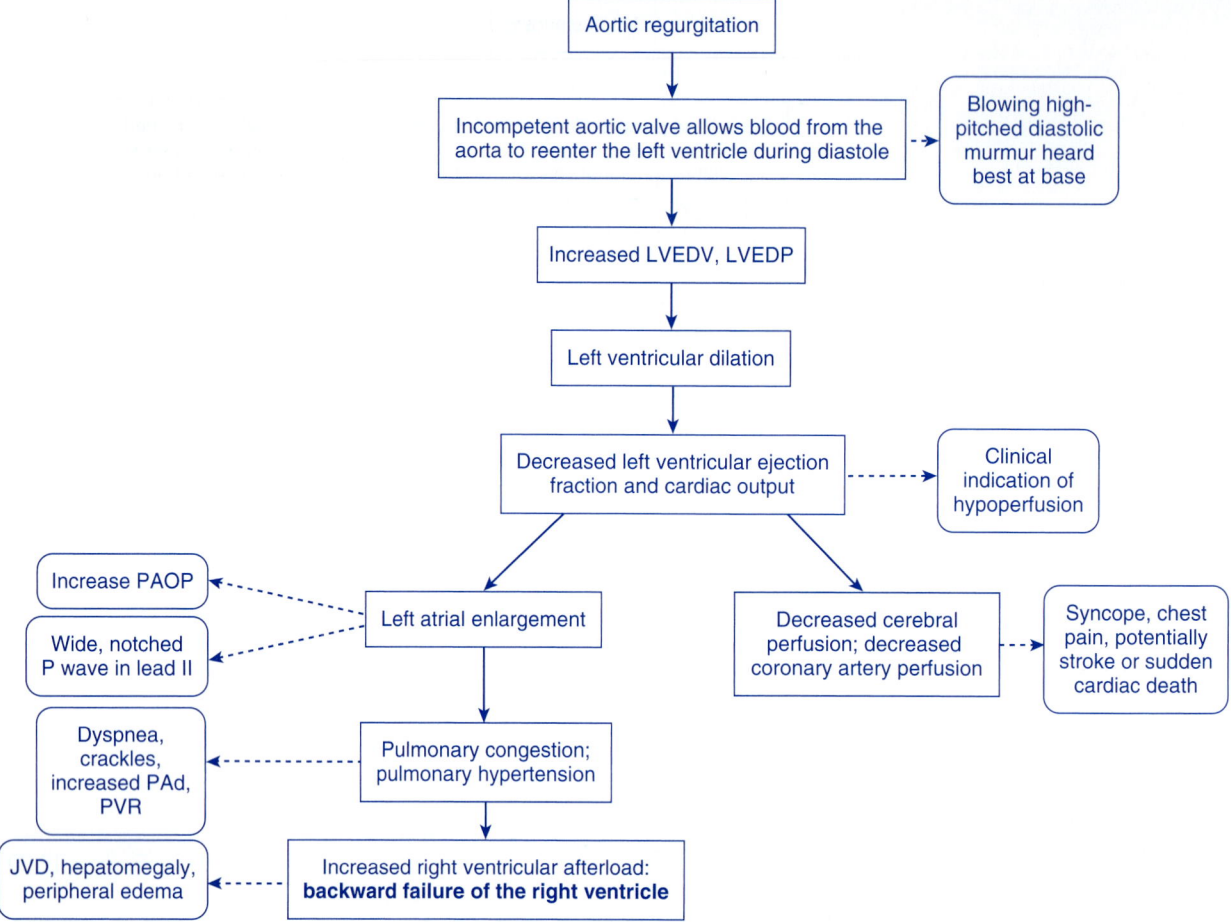

Fig. 3.87 Pathophysiology of aortic regurgitation. *Dotted lines* connect pathology to the clinical presentation. *JVD*, Jugular venous distention; *LVEDP*, left ventricular end-diastolic pressure; *LVEDV*, left ventricular end-diastolic volume; *PAd*, pulmonary artery diastolic pressure; *PAOP*, pulmonary artery occlusive pressure; *PVR*, pulmonary vascular resistance.

    3) Echocardiography
        a) Poor aortic valve motion
        b) Thickening of aortic valve
        c) LVH
        d) LA enlargement
    4) Cardiac catheterization
        a) Elevated LAP, LVEDP
        b) Regurgitation from aorta to left ventricle

Aortic Stenosis

1. Etiology
   a. RHD
   b. Calcification
   c. Congenital bicuspid valve
   d. Aortic coarctation
2. Pathophysiology (Fig. 3.88)
3. Clinical presentation
   a. Subjective
      1) Chest pain, especially on exertion
      2) Syncope, especially on exertion
      3) Symptoms of LVF: dyspnea; orthopnea; PND
      4) Fatigue, weakness
      5) Palpitations
   b. Objective
      1) Narrow pulse pressure
      2) PMI displaced laterally and/or downward
      3) Signs of LVF: S_3; crackles
      4) Heart sound changes
         a) May have split S_1
         b) Paradoxical split of S_2
         c) Systolic ejection murmur: harsh, crescendo/decrescendo, loudest at aortic area radiating to the neck
         d) May have aortic ejection click
   c. Diagnostic studies
      1) Chest radiography
         a) Calcification of aortic valve may be seen.
         b) Cardiomegaly
         c) LA enlargement
         d) LVH
         e) Pulmonary congestion
         f) RVH
      2) ECG
         a) LA enlargement (P-mitrale)
         b) LVH
         c) Dysrhythmias: most frequently atrial fibrillation
         d) Blocks: AV blocks; LBBB
      3) Echocardiography
         a) Aortic valve leaflet thickening and decreased movement of the leaflets
         b) Calcification of aortic valve

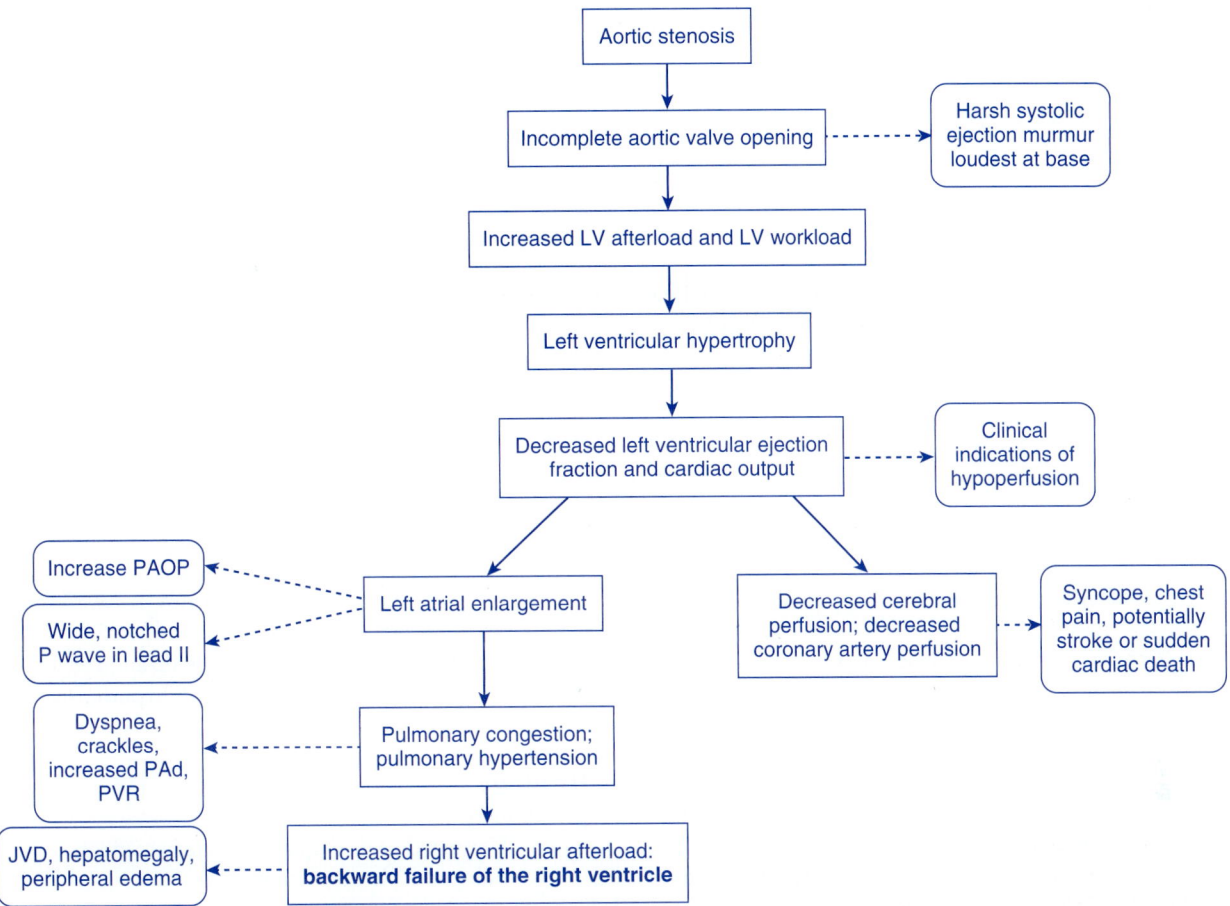

Fig. 3.88 Pathophysiology of aortic stenosis. *Dotted lines* connect pathology to the clinical presentation. *JVD*, Jugular venous distention; *LV*, left ventricular; *LVEDP*, left ventricular end-diastolic pressure; *LVEDV*, left ventricular end-diastolic volume; *PAd*, pulmonary artery diastolic pressure; *PAOP*, pulmonary artery occlusive pressure; *PVR*, pulmonary vascular resistance.

      c) High-pressure gradient between left ventricle and aorta
      d) LVH
      e) Possibly RVH
    4) Cardiac catheterization
      a) Significant pressure gradient
      b) Elevated LAP, LVEDP

Collaborative Management for Valvular Heart Disease

1. Decrease myocardial oxygen consumption.
   a. Oxygen by nasal cannula at 2 to 6 l/min to maintain SaO_2 of 95% unless contraindicated
   b. Sodium restrictions
   c. Physical comfort: temperature, lighting, noise control
   d. Anxiolytics as prescribed: usually diazepam, lorazepam, or alprazolam
2. Provide care for HF.
   a. ACE inhibitors (e.g., captopril)
   b. Beta-blockers (e.g., metoprolol) may be prescribed.
   c. Vasodilators (e.g., nitrates) but should be avoided in severe AS
   d. Diuretics (e.g., furosemide) but should be used with caution in severe AS
   e. Inotropic agents: digitalis may be used, especially if supraventricular tachydysrhythmias are present.
3. Monitor for complications.
   a. Dysrhythmias: usually atrial fibrillation
   b. Blocks: permanent pacemaker may be necessary.
   c. Emboli (mural thrombi): potential for pulmonary, cerebral, renal, splenic, mesenteric embolus; antiembolic measures, including anticoagulation
   d. Endocarditis: prophylactic antibiotics before any invasive procedures, dental procedures for prevention
4. Prepare patient for surgical repair or replacement of the affected valve as requested.
   a. Valvuloplasty: percutaneous coronary intervention to repair a valve using a balloon-tipped intracardiac catheter; considered palliative because restenosis rate is high
   b. Commissurotomy: surgical separation of the thickened adherent leaves of a stenosed valve (usually mitral)
   c. Valve repair
      1) Open commissurotomy: fused commissures are incised to reestablish mobility.
      2) Valve leaflet reconstruction: fibrous pericardium is frequently used for patches.
      3) Annuloplasty: insertion of a ring to correct the dilation of the valve annulus
      4) Repair of elongated chordae tendineae by suturing within or to the side of a papillary muscle

d. Valve replacement: replacement of the native valve with a mechanical or biological prosthetic valve
   1) Types of valve replacement
      a) Bioprosthetic valves: last approximately 5 to 10 years
         i) Types
            (a) Homografts: human cadaver valves that have been specially treated for surgical use
            (b) Heterograft: valve from an animal, usually a pig or cow, which has been prepared for surgical use
         ii) Anticoagulation
            (a) Short-term (~3 months after valve replacement) anticoagulation (INR, 2–3) is recommended.
            (b) Long-term anticoagulation is recommended if atrial fibrillation or LA thrombus.
      b) Mechanical valves: last approximately 10 to 15 years
         i) Stainless steel, carbon, or other durable material
         ii) Anticoagulation: long-term anticoagulation is recommended (INR is 2–3.5 depending on type of valve)
      c) Pulmonary autograft (also referred to as *Ross procedure*)
         i) The patient's own pulmonic valve is used to replace the diseased aortic valve with a homograft or heterograft implanted into the pulmonic position.
   2) Traditional valve replacement surgery requires cardiopulmonary bypass, and postoperative management as for CABG with close monitoring for AV nodal blocks
   3) Transcatheter aortic valve replacement (TAVR)
      a) Minimally invasive procedure done in a cardiac catheterization lab; a collapsible prosthetic valve is placed directly over the native diseased valve using either a percutaneous approach or a small incision in the chest wall.
         i) Percutaneous approaches: transfemoral, transaxillary/subclavian
         ii) Open approaches: transapical or transaortic; require small surgical incisions.
      b) Percutaneous access nursing care
         i) Monitor circulation distal to the puncture.
         ii) Perform neurovascular assessment of the affected extremity.
         iii) Assess the insertion site for signs of bleeding, hematoma, and infection.
         iv) Keep dressings clean, dry, and intact.

Hypertensive Crises

Definitions

1. Hypertension: elevation in BP above normal on at least three separate occasions
2. Hypertensive crisis: rapid rise in BP and occurs when BP elevation is severe enough to cause the threat of immediate vascular necrosis and end-organ damage; BP usually greater than 180/120 mm Hg or MAP greater than 150 mm Hg
   a. Hypertensive urgencies: an acute or chronic BP elevation not associated with any observable acute organ damage
      1) Do not usually require critical care unit admission.
      2) Usually safely treated with oral antihypertensive agents to reduce BP to baseline over 24 to 48 hours
   b. Hypertensive emergencies: an acute elevation of BP that is associated with acute and ongoing organ damage to the kidneys, brain, heart, eyes, or vascular system
      1) No absolute BP level but BP is usually greater than 240/140 mm Hg
      2) BP must be lowered within minutes to a few hours to reduce potential complications of new or progressive end-organ damage.
      3) Requires immediate hospitalization in a critical care unit and IV antihypertensive agents

Etiology

1. Primary
   a. Untreated or inadequately treated essential (idiopathic) hypertension
      1) Risk factors: family history, black race, obesity, hyperlipidemia, DM or glucose intolerance, tobacco use, excessive alcohol intake, high-fat or high-sodium diet, stress, sedentary lifestyle, aging, oral contraceptives
      2) Poor compliance frequently a factor in hypertensive crisis; factors closely related to poor compliance include lack of symptoms (i.e., the silent killer), side effects of pharmacologic agents, costs of pharmacologic agents
2. Secondary
   a. Cerebrovascular conditions (e.g., thrombotic or hemorrhagic stroke)
   b. CNS injuries
      1) Head injury
      2) Spinal cord injury: autonomic dysreflexia is hypertension with bradycardia that occurs in patients with spinal cord injury T6 or above in response to noxious stimuli.
   c. Aortic dissection or coarctation
   d. Renal disease
      1) Increased renin–angiotensin levels
         a) Renin-secreting tumor
         b) Renovascular disease
      2) Acute glomerulonephritis
      3) Chronic pyelonephritis
      4) Postrenal transplant
   e. Pregnancy: preeclampsia, eclampsia, HELLP (hemolysis, elevated liver enzyme levels, and low platelet count) syndrome
   f. Burns

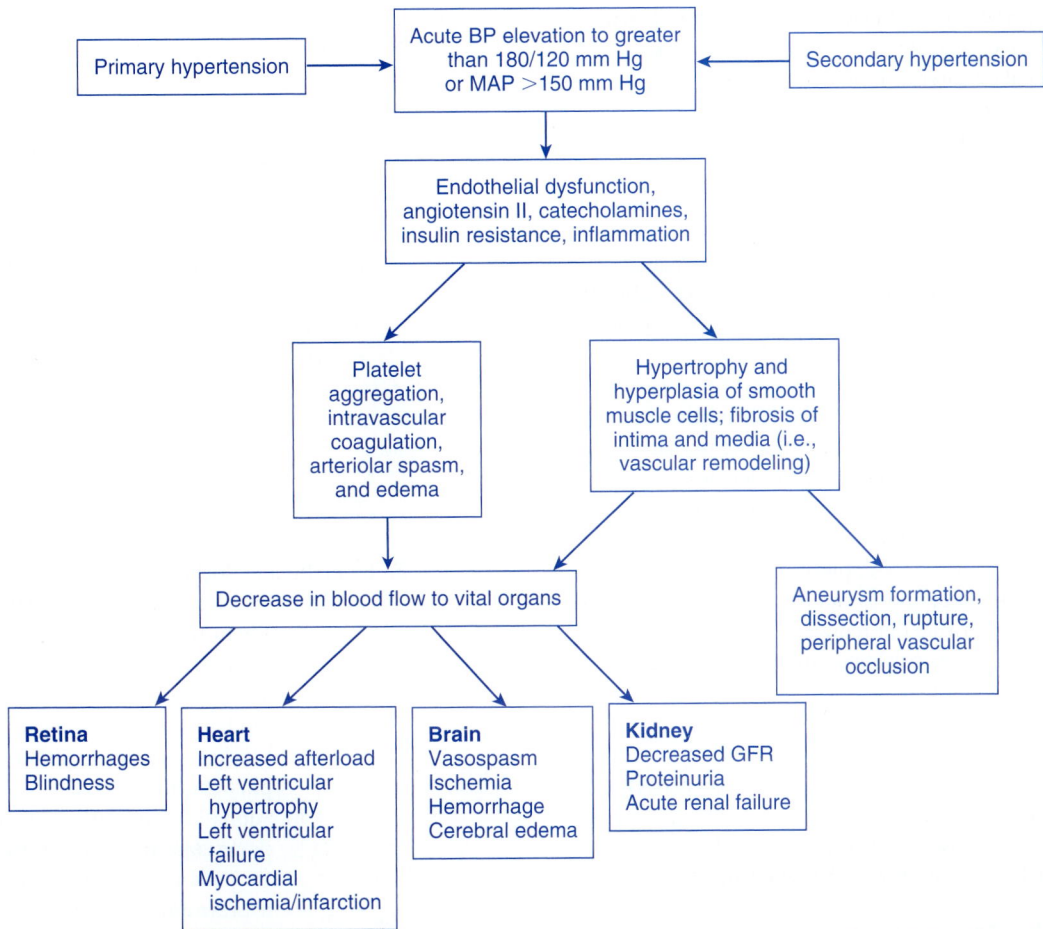

Fig. 3.89 Pathophysiology of hypertensive crisis. *BP,* Blood pressure; *GFR,* glomerular filtration rate; *MAP,* mean arterial pressure.

g. Drug side effects: oral contraceptives, steroids, cocaine, amphetamines, methamphetamine, decongestants
h. Drug interactions: monoamine oxidase (MAO) inhibitors and tyramine; disulfiram (Antabuse) and alcohol
i. Drug withdrawal: clonidine, beta-blockers, ACE inhibitors, alcohol
j. Endocrine disorders (e.g., pheochromocytoma, Cushing syndrome, primary hyperaldosteronism)
k. Vasculitis
l. Scleroderma or other connective tissue disease
m. Peri- or postoperative hypertension, especially cardiac or vascular surgery

Table 3.40 Classification of Blood Pressure Levels

Blood Pressure Category	Systolic (mm Hg)	and/or	Diastolic (mm Hg)
Normal	<120	and	<80
Elevated	120–129	and	<80
Hypertension			
Stage 1	130–139	or	80–89
Stage 2	≥140	or	≥90

Data from Whelton, P. K., & Carey, R. M. (2017). The 2017 Clinical Practice Guideline for High Blood Pressure. *JAMA, 318*(21), 2073-2074.

Pathophysiology
Fig. 3.89.

Clinical Presentation
1. General
   a. Elevation in BP above normal (Table 3.40)
   b. Epistaxis may occur.
2. Cardiovascular involvement may be present.
   a. Chest pain
   b. Signs of left LVH: PMI displaced to left, S_4, ECG indicators of LVH (i.e., deep S in V_1, V_2 and tall R in V_5, V_6)
   c. Signs of LV failure or pulmonary edema: dyspnea, orthopnea, LV heave, S_3, crackles
3. Renal involvement may be present.
   a. Nocturia
   b. Pressure-related diuresis
   c. Hematuria
   d. Elevated BUN and creatinine
4. Retinal involvement may be present.
   a. Visual disturbances (e.g., blurred vision, reduced visual acuity, photophobia, temporary loss of vision)
   b. Funduscopic changes (Keith-Wagener-Barker classification)
      1) Grade I: arteriolar narrowing
      2) Grade II: focal arteriolar spasm
      3) Grade III: hemorrhages and exudates
      4) Grade IV: papilledema

5. Neurologic involvement may be present, especially in hypertensive encephalopathy.
   a. Occipital or anterior headache especially in the morning; may be severe
   b. Nausea, vomiting
   c. Seizures
   d. Altered mental status: irritability, confusion, agitation progressing to lethargy and coma
   e. Focal neurologic signs (e.g., cranial nerve palsy, sensory or motor deficits, aphasia, positive Babinski reflex)
6. Diagnostic studies
   a. Serum
      1) Potassium: hypokalemia occurs in primary hyperaldosteronism.
      2) BUN and creatinine may be elevated.
      3) Lipid profile to evaluate additional cardiac risk
      4) Aldosterone may be elevated.
   b. Captopril challenge test: plasma renin level is measured before and 1 hour after 25 mg of captopril to confirm or rule out renovascular hypertension.
   c. Urine: hematuria or proteinuria may be present.
   d. Chest radiography
      1) Cardiomegaly may be present.
      2) Pulmonary edema may be present.
      3) Widening of mediastinum suggests dissecting thoracic aortic aneurysm.
   e. ECG: may show LA enlargement, LVH
   f. CT of brain: may show cerebral edema or hemorrhage

Collaborative Management

1. Maintain airway, ventilation, and oxygenation.
   a. Oxygen: 2 to 6 l/min via nasal cannula
   b. Airway maintenance
      1) Oropharyngeal or nasopharyngeal airway or ET intubation may be required especially if altered level of consciousness or pulmonary edema
   c. Ventilation: mechanical ventilation may be required, especially if neurologic impairment or pulmonary edema
2. Decrease myocardial oxygen consumption.
   a. Activity restriction initially
   b. Sodium restriction to less than 2 g/24 hr
   c. Smoking cessation
   d. Physical comfort: temperature control, lighting, noise control
   e. Anxiolytics as prescribed: usually diazepam, lorazepam, or alprazolam
3. Decrease BP gradually.
   a. Reduction of MAP by no more than 20% to 25% within the first hour because BP decreased too aggressively may cause neurologic damage by significantly decreasing cerebral perfusion pressure. (NOTE: If aortic dissection has occurred, BP is reduced more aggressively but reduction takes place within 5–10 minutes.)
      1) Monitor BP closely.
         a) An invasive arterial catheter is indicated in hypertensive emergency.
         b) If neurologic changes occur, BP reduction should be slowed or temporarily stopped.
   b. Antihypertensive agents (Table 3.41)
      1) Vasodilators
         a) Nitroprusside
            i) Mixed arterial and venous vasodilator but predominantly arterial
            ii) Usually first-line agent for hypertensive emergency
         b) Hydralazine: selectively arterial vasodilator
         c) Fenoldopam mesylate: selectively arterial vasodilator with dopaminergic stimulation
         d) Clevidipine: selectively arterial vasodilator
         e) Nitroglycerin: effects are dose dependent.
            i) Venous vasodilator at doses of less than 1 mcg/kg/min
            ii) Mixed arterial and venous vasodilator when dose greater than 1 mcg/kg/min
         f) Nicardipine: mixed arterial and venous vasodilator
      2) Sympathetic blockers
         a) Alpha-blockers block vasoconstriction.
            i) Phentolamine: especially helpful if hypertension is caused by autonomic dysreflexia because bradycardia contraindicates beta-blocker; also particularly helpful in pheochromocytoma
            ii) Alpha-blockers such as terazosin or doxazosin may be considered for patients with benign prostatic hypertrophy.
            iii) Alpha-blockers are associated with orthostatic hypotension.
         b) Beta-blockers block the reflex tachycardia associated with vasodilators.
            i) Esmolol: rapid acting, cardioselective beta-blocker
            ii) First line for patients with CAD and systolic HF (i.e., HF with reduced EF); metoprolol or bisoprolol is preferred for hypertension with systolic HF
            iii) Contraindicated in HF, heart block
         c) Alpha- and beta-blockers: block both vasoconstriction and tachycardia
            i) Labetalol: alpha- and noncardioselective beta-blocker
               (a) Particularly helpful in patients with intracranial hypertension because direct vasodilators would increase intracranial volume and pressure
      2) ACE inhibitors and ARBs
         a) Enalaprilat (only IV ACE inhibitor)
         b) ACE inhibitors, ARBs, and direct renin inhibitors should not be used in combination because of the significant risk of hyperkalemia.
      3) Diuretics
         a) Usually loop diuretics (e.g., furosemide, bumetanide) acutely, especially in patients with HF

Chapter 3 The Cardiovascular System

Table 3.41 Selected Drugs Used for Hypertensive Emergency

Drug	Classification and Actions	Indications	Administration	Adverse Effects	Nursing Implications
Vasodilators					
Clevidipine	Calcium channel blocker • Relaxes arteriolar smooth muscle decreasing SVR, afterload, and BP	Hypertension	• IV infusion: 1–2 mg/hr; may be doubled every 90 sec until BP approaches target; then increased by <double every 5–10 min • Maximum: 21 mg/hr for 24 hr	• Nausea and vomiting • Headache • Insomnia • Tachycardia • Rebound hypertension • Exacerbation of heart failure	• Monitor HR, BP, blood lipids • Metabolized by blood ester hydrolysis to form inactive metabolites; advantage in renal or hepatic insufficiency • Note contraindications: allergy to soybeans, soy products, eggs, or egg products, defective lipid metabolism, pancreatitis, hyperlipidemia, severe aortic stenosis • Use caution in patients with heart failure • Consider lipid calories in daily nutritional plan • Infusion must be changed every 12 hr • Use cautiously in older adults
Enalaprilat (IV), enalapril (PO)	ACE inhibitor • Inhibits conversion of angiotensin I to angiotensin II • Prevents vasoconstriction and aldosterone secretion to decrease preload and afterload	• HF • Hypertension	• PO: 5–40 mg/day • IV injection: 1.25 mg over 5 min every 6 hr	• Tachycardia • Hypotension, especially after first dose • Anorexia • Fatigue • Headache • Loss of taste • Diarrhea • Rash, angioedema • Dizziness • Photosensitivity • Proteinuria, nephrotic syndrome, renal failure • Pancytopenia • Hyperkalemia • Bronchospasm • Cough	• Monitor HR, BP, urine output, protein in urine, serum potassium, WBC count • Monitor WBC count and differential before treatment and periodically during treatment • Note contraindications: known hypersensitivity, AV block, hypotension • Use cautiously in renal disease, lupus, scleroderma, hypovolemia, leukemia, diabetes mellitus, thyroid disease, COPD, asthma, hyperkalemia and in patients on drugs that may affect WBC counts or immune response • Monitor for allergic reaction: rash, fever, pruritus, urticaria; antihistamines may be used; discontinuance may be necessary • Administer thiazide diuretics as prescribed; frequently given together • Angiotensin II blocker (e.g., losartan [Cozaar], valsartan [Diovan]) may be prescribed if cough develops • Indicated for hypertension with HF
Fenoldopam mesylate	Vasodilator Antihypertensive • Relaxes vascular smooth muscle decreasing preload (PAOP) and afterload (SVR) • Stimulates dopaminergic receptors causing diuresis	• Severe hypertension (short-term treatment) • Need to improve renal flow such as after potentially nephrotoxic dyes and contrast media	• IV infusion: mix 10 mg in 250 ml (40 mcg/ml); usual dose is 0.1–0.3 mcg/kg/min; may be increased in increments 0.05–0.1 mcg/kg/min every 15 min until target BP is reached • Maximum: 1.7 mcg/kg/min	• Tachycardia, hypotension • Ventricular dysrhythmias • Dizziness • Anxiety • Headache • Flushing • Nausea, vomiting, abdominal pain • Hypokalemia • Increased intraocular pressure • Increased intracranial pressure	• Monitor HR, BP, urine output, serum potassium, neurologic status • Note contraindications: known hypersensitivity to fenoldopam or sulfite, intracranial hypertension • Use caution in patients with glaucoma or ocular hypertension and in patients on other drugs which may cause hypotension (e.g., beta-blockers) • Indicated especially for postoperative hypertension or hypertension with renal insufficiency

Continued

Table 3.41 Selected Drugs Used for Hypertensive Emergency—cont'd

Drug	Classification and Actions	Indications	Administration	Adverse Effects	Nursing Implications
Hydralazine	Vasodilator Antihypertensive • Relaxes arteriolar smooth muscle decreasing SVR, afterload, and BP	• Hypertension • Afterload reduction	• PO: 10–50 mg every 6–8 hr • IV injection: 5–20 mg over 3–5 min every 4–6 hr • Maximum: 400 mg/day	• Tachycardia • Orthostatic hypotension • Anorexia, nausea, vomiting, diarrhea • Sodium retention • Weight gain • Palpitations • Flushing • Headache • Tremors • Dizziness • Lupus-like syndrome • Exacerbation of HF or chest pain • Leukopenia, agranulocytosis	• Monitor HR, BP, ECG • Note contraindications: known hypersensitivity to hydralazine, coronary artery disease, mitral valve disease, severe aortic stenosis • Use cautiously in renal disease, cerebrovascular disease • Administer beta-blockers as prescribed for reflex tachycardia because it may cause myocardial ischemia • Indicated for pregnancy-related hypertension (i.e., eclampsia)
Nicardipine	Calcium channel blocker • Relaxes vascular smooth muscle decreasing preload and afterload	• Hypertension • Angina pectoris	• PO: 20 mg tid initially; may be increased to 20–40 mg tid after 3 days if tolerated well • IV infusion: mix 25 mg in 240 ml (0.1 mg/ml) and infuse at 5 mg/hr (50 ml/hr); may be increased by 2.5 mg/hr (25 ml/hr) every 5 min until desired BP reduction is achieved • Do not mix in lactated Ringer solution • Maximum: 15 mg/hr	• Tachycardia • Hypotension • Nausea, vomiting, heartburn • Flushing • Headache • Chest pain • Heart failure • Hepatitis • Renal failure • Local irritation at injection site	• Monitor HR, BP • Note contraindications: known hypersensitivity, sick sinus syndrome, second- or third-degree AV block, systolic BP <90 mm Hg, severe aortic stenosis • Use caution in HF, hypotension, liver disease, renal insufficiency or failure, and in older adults • Indicated for postoperative hypertension

Drug	Class/Action	Indications	Dose	Side Effects	Nursing Implications
Nitroglycerin	Nitrates • Relaxes smooth muscle to reduce preload (PAOP) and afterload [SVR] if >1 mcg/kg/min) • Dilates coronary collateral circulation • Relieves coronary artery spasm	• Acute angina • Prophylactic use before activities that may cause angina • HF (preload reduction)	• Sublingual: 0.3–0.4 mg at 5 minute intervals to a maximum of three tablets or metered-dose sprays • PO (isosorbide): 5–40 mg every 6 hr • Transdermal: 1–4 inches every 8 hr • IV infusion: mix 50 mg in 250 ml (200 mcg/ml); initial dose 5–10 mcg/min, increase by 5–10 mcg/min every 5 min until desired results are achieved (e.g., control of chest pain, preload reduction) • Maximum: 400 mcg/min • Administer in glass bottle and via non-PVC tubing	• Tachycardia or bradycardia • Hypotension or hypertension • Palpitations • Weakness • Apprehension • Flushing • Dizziness • Syncope • Headache • Methemoglobinemia with resultant reduction in SaO_2, SpO_2, and tissue oxygen delivery	• Monitor HR, BP, urine output • Monitor RAP, PA, PAOP, SVR, CI if nitroglycerin is being administered IV and pulmonary artery catheter has been inserted • Note contraindications: known hypersensitivity, anemia, intracranial hypertension, cerebral hemorrhage, hypertrophic cardiomyopathy, right ventricular infarction, sildenafil or vardenafil within the past 24 hr • Use cautiously in hypotension; IV nitroglycerin is titratable and preferred in acute situations • Decrease nitrate tolerance by scheduling oral nitrates with nitrate-free period at night and by removing transdermal nitrates at night • Administer ASA or acetaminophen for headache; usually dose related • Teach patient to protect tablets from light and moisture and replace every 3 mo • Teach patient to limit nitroglycerin to three tablets every 5 min and if no relief is obtained, to go to the ED • Teach patient to apply NTG paste to any relatively hairless area between the knees and shoulders and to rotate sites to prevent maceration • Note that patients receiving IV nitroglycerin and heparin IV concurrently require more heparin to achieve therapeutic aPTT; monitor aPTT closely with nitroglycerin dosage changes or discontinuance • Indicated especially for hypertension with chest pain

Nitroprusside	Vasodilator
	Antihypertensive
	• Relaxes vascular smooth muscle decreasing preload (PAOP) and afterload (SVR)
		• Hypertensive crisis
		• HF (preload and afterload reduction)
		• Cardiogenic shock
		• BP control during and after vascular surgery
			• IV infusion: mix 50 mg in 250 ml (200 mcg/ml) and infuse at 0.25–10 mcg/kg/min
			• Maximum: 10 mcg/kg/min for 10 min only
			• Protect from light by wrapping aluminum foil around bag or bottle; it is not necessary to wrap foil around tubing but avoid exposure of tubing to direct sunlight
				• Nausea, vomiting, abdominal pain
				• Headache
				• Tinnitus
				• Dizziness
				• Diaphoresis
				• Apprehension
				• Hypotension
				• Tachycardia
				• Palpitations
				• Coronary artery steal causing myocardial ischemia and chest pain
				• Intrapulmonary shunt causing hypoxemia (referred to as nitroprusside-induced intrapulmonary shunt)
				• Methemoglobinemia with resultant reduction in SaO_2, SpO_2, and tissue oxygen delivery
				• Thiocyanate toxicity
					• Monitor HR, BP, urine output, neurologic status
					• Note contraindications: known hypersensitivity
					• Use cautiously in liver disease, renal disease, anemia, hypovolemia, hypothyroidism, older adult, CAD, neurologic injury
					• Discard solution after 24 hr
					• Wrap foil around bottle to protect from light
					• Discard solution if dark brown, blue, green, or red
					• Monitor for thiocyanate toxicity
					  • Thiocyanate levels should be determined daily if drugs are used longer than 72 hr
					  • Signs of thiocyanate toxicity: metabolic acidosis, confusion, hyperreflexia, seizures
					  • Treatment includes amyl nitrate, sodium nitrate, and/or sodium thiosulfate
					  • Simultaneous infusion of thiosulfate with nitroprusside may prevent thiocyanate toxicity

Continued

Table 3.41 Selected Drugs Used for Hypertensive Emergency—cont'd

Drug	Classification and Actions	Indications	Administration	Adverse Effects	Nursing Implications
Adrenergic Blocking Agents					
Esmolol (Brevibloc): Table 3.20					
Labetalol hydrochloride	Alpha- and beta-adrenergic blocker • Blocks response to alpha and beta stimulation • Causes decrease in blood pressure without reflex tachycardia • Causes decrease in HR	• Hypertension • Hypertensive crisis	• PO: 100–400 mg every 12 hr • IV injection: 20 mg over 2 min, may repeat 40 mg every 10 min • IV infusion: mix 300 mg in 250 ml for a total volume of 300 ml in 300 ml (1 mg/ml); usual dose is 1–2 mg/min until satisfactory response is achieved • Maximum: 300 mg	• Bradycardia • Orthostatic hypotension • Ventricular dysrhythmias • AV blocks • HF • Nausea, vomiting, diarrhea • Dizziness • Lethargy • Hypoglycemia without symptoms in type 1 DM • Hyperglycemia in type 2 DM • Agranulocytosis, thrombocytopenia • Bronchospasm in patients with COPD, asthma	• Monitor HR, BP, ECG, breath sounds, daily weight • Note contraindications: known hypersensitivity, shock, second- or third-degree AV block, sinus bradycardia, sick sinus syndrome, NYHA class IV HF, asthma • Note contraindications: known hypersensitivity, shock, second- or third-degree AV block, sinus bradycardia, HF, asthma • Use cautiously in DM, renal disease, hepatic disease, thyroid disease, COPD, CAD, bronchospasm, peripheral vascular disease • Keep patient supine for 3 hr after IV administration (labetalol) • Do not discontinue suddenly • Indicated for hypertension postoperatively or aortic dissection
Phentolamine	Alpha-adrenergic blocker • Blocks response to alpha stimulation • Causes decrease in blood pressure without reflex tachycardia	• Hypertension, especially autonomic dysreflexia, pheochromocytoma, MAO inhibitor-tyramine interaction • Infiltration of vasopressor agents	• IV injection: 5–15 mg; may be repeated every 5–15 min • Maximum: 15 mg	• Tachycardia • Flushing • Headache	• Monitor HR, BP • Use cautiously in CAD • Beta-blocker may be given concurrently to control tachycardia

ACE, angiotensin-converting enzyme; *aPTT*, activated partial thromboplastin time; *ASA*, aspirin; *AV*, atrioventricular; *BP*, blood pressure; *CAD*, coronary artery disease; *CI*, cardiac index; *COPD*, chronic obstructive pulmonary disease; *DM*, diabetes mellitus; *HF*, heart failure; *HR*, heart rate; *IV*, intravenous; *NTG*, nitroglycerin; *NYHA*, New York Heart Association; *PA*, pulmonary artery; *PAOP*, pulmonary artery occlusive pressure; *PO*, oral; *PVC*, premature ventricular contraction; *RAP*, right atrial pressure; SaO_2, arterial oxygen saturation SpO_2 oxygen saturation by pulse oximetry *SVR*, systemic vascular resistance; *WBC*, white blood cell.

b) Chlorthalidone is preferred diuretic long-term because of long half-life and reduction of cardiovascular risk.
c) Amiloride or triamterene may be used in patients with lower potassium and normal GFR.
4. Assist in preparation of patient for surgical procedures to treat cause of hypertension if appropriate.
   a. Angioplasty may be done for renovascular disease.
   b. Adrenalectomy is done for pheochromocytoma after tachycardia and hypertension have been adequately controlled.
5. Monitor for complications.
   a. Cerebral infarction
   b. MI
   c. HF and pulmonary edema
   d. Dissection of aorta
   e. Renal failure
6. Provide instruction and counseling regarding lifestyle modification and need for pharmacologic therapy.
   a. Nonpharmacologic management
      1) Weight normalization
      2) Dietary modifications
         a) Low-fat, no-added-salt (2–3 g/day) diet
         b) Fresh fruits and vegetables
         c) Fish, especially fatty fish such as salmon, trout
         d) Nuts
         e) Low-fat dairy
         f) Monounsaturated fatty acids (from extra-virgin olive oil)
         g) Increase potassium, magnesium, and calcium
      3) Aerobic exercise
      4) Alcohol moderation (e.g., one glass of wine or equivalent per day)
      5) Complementary therapies: relaxation, biofeedback, acupuncture, pets
   b. Pharmacologic management
      1) Stage 1 hypertension: first-line drugs include thiazide diuretics, calcium channel blockers, and ACE inhibitors or ARBs
      2) Choice of drug or combinations stage 2 hypertension: two first-line drugs of different classes are recommended.
         a) Improved adherence can be achieved with:
            i) Once-daily drug dosing rather than multiple dosing
            ii) Combination therapy rather than administration of the individual components

Vascular Disease

Peripheral Arterial Disease

1. Definition: partial or total occlusion of an artery by atherosclerosis or arteriosclerosis obliterans
2. Etiology
   a. Arteriosclerosis or atherosclerosis (same risk factors as referred in discussion of CAD)
      1) Atherosclerosis: most common cause
      2) Arteriosclerosis: significant cause in older patients
   b. Hypertension
   c. Arteritis
3. Pathophysiology (Fig. 3.90)
4. Clinical presentation
   a. Occlusive disease of terminal aorta and iliac

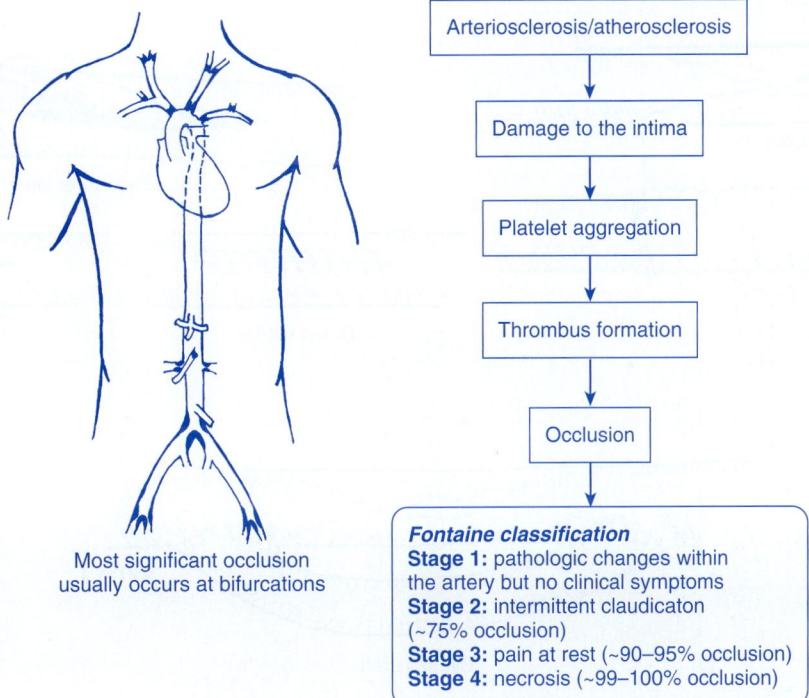

Fig. 3.90 Pathophysiology of peripheral arterial disease.

1) Subjective
    a) Intermittent claudication in thigh and hip: pain increases with exercise and decreases with rest
    b) Impotence
2) Objective
    a) Cool lower extremities
    b) Hair loss over lower extremities
    c) Decreased or absent iliac or femoral pulses
    d) Bruit or thrill over iliac area
b. Occlusive disease of femoral and popliteal arteries
    1) Subjective
        a) Intermittent claudication in lower leg progressing to pain at rest
        b) Decreased sensation or paresthesia of lower extremities
    2) Objective
        a) Coolness of lower extremities
        b) Hair loss over lower extremities
        c) Pallor and mottling of lower extremities
        d) Nonhealing ulcers on toes or points of trauma
        e) Decreased motor strength in lower extremities
        f) Decreased or absent femoral and popliteal pulses
        g) Bruit or thrill over femoral or popliteal area
    3) Diagnostic studies
        a) Arteriography: shows partial or complete arterial occlusion
        b) Doppler and duplex ultrasonography show partial to complete vascular occlusion.

5. Collaborative management
    a. Decrease peripheral oxygen requirements.
        1) Activity cessation when pain occurs
        2) Bed rest during acute occlusion
        3) Maintenance of normothermia
        4) Prevention of trauma
    b. Administer appropriate pharmacologic agents to reestablish blood flow: fibrinolytics (e.g., urokinase; streptokinase; recombinant tissue plasminogen activator [rt-PA]).
        1) These agents may be administered locally by an intraarterial infusion or systemically intravenously.
        2) Followed by an anticoagulant such as heparin
    c. Assist in preparation of the patient for percutaneous procedures aimed at decreasing occlusion (e.g., percutaneous balloon angioplasty, laser angioplasty, atherectomy); may be accompanied by insertion of flexible coil stent
        1) Postprocedure care as for PCI
        2) Catheter insertion site should be monitored closely for bleeding and hematoma formation.
        3) Peripheral perfusion should be monitored closely; any indications of arterial occlusion (i.e., 6 Ps) should be reported immediately.
        4) Anticoagulants and platelet aggregation inhibitors as prescribed
    d. Assist in preparation of the patient for surgery aimed at improving flow (Fig. 3.91) and provide postoperative management.

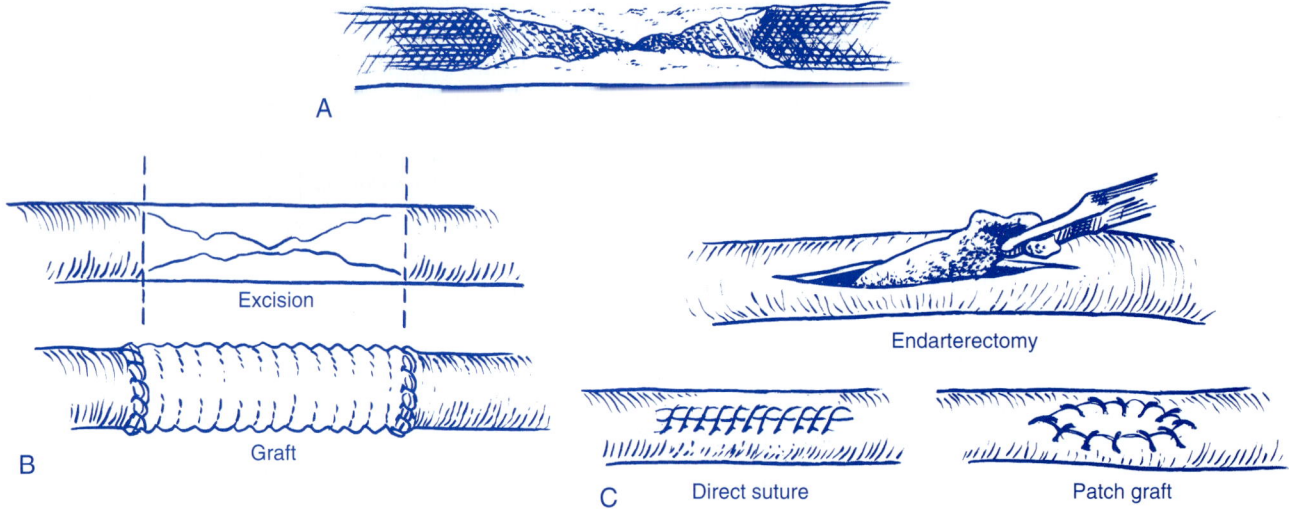

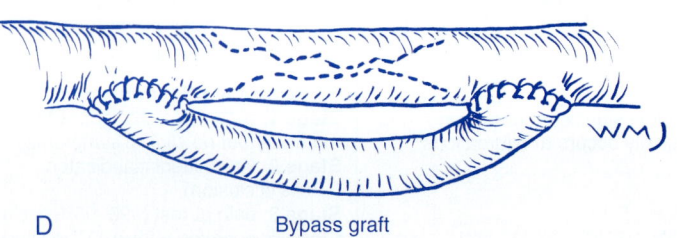

Fig. 3.91 Surgical procedures for peripheral vascular disease. **A,** Occluded vessel. **B,** Excision and circumferential graft. **C,** Endarterectomy with direct suture or patch graft. **D,** Bypass graft. (Drawing by Wendy M. Johnson.)

1) Surgical procedures
   a) Arterial embolectomy: removal of an occlusive clot from an artery; frequently accomplished with a balloon-tipped catheter
   b) Thromboendarterectomy: excision of thickened layer of artery; aortofemoral, aortoiliac, or femoral-popliteal thromboendarterectomy
   c) Bypass: graft is anastomosed proximal and distal to the occlusion.
      i) Graft may be autologous vein (usually saphenous), human umbilical vein, or an artificial graft (Dacron or polytetrafluoroethylene [PTFE]).
      ii) Commonly performed bypasses include: aortobifemoral, femoral to femoral, femoral-popliteal, and femoral-tibial.
   d) Extraanatomical bypass (EAB): prosthetic material is tunneled subcutaneously.
      i) May be used femoral to femoral or axillary to femoral
      ii) Used for patients who are high-risk for an open abdominal procedure or who have numerous previous surgical procedures or peritonitis (sometimes referred to as a *hostile abdomen*)
   e) Sympathectomy: interruption of sympathetic tract to decrease local vascular resistance to improve local blood flow
   f) Amputation: removal of limb performed only when attempts to revascularize the limb have failed
2) Postoperative management
   a) Maintain airway, oxygenation, and ventilation.
      i) Assess ventilatory status frequently: rate, rhythm, excursion, effort, use of accessory muscles, presence of stridor or other adventitious sounds, pulse oximetry.
      ii) Encourage deep breathing and incentive spirometry.
      iii) Assess frequently for edema, hematoma, tracheal deviation, and dysphagia.
      iv) Elevate HOB 30 degrees.
      v) Have equipment for artificial airway and suctioning.
      vi) Prevent aspiration: high-Fowler position while eating; nothing by mouth (NPO) until gag reflex returns; suction as necessary.
      vii) Administer oxygen at 2 to 5 l/min as prescribed.
   b) Maintain adequate flow and pressure at graft site.
      i) Maintain and control systolic BP less than 120 mm Hg.
         (a) Nitroprusside
         (b) Nicardipine
         (c) Analgesics as indicated

      ii) Prevent emboli by using antiembolic techniques.
         (a) Dextran 40 often used as platelet aggregation inhibitor.
         (b) Heparin may also be used.
      iii) Avoid pressure on incision sites.
         (a) Elevate HOB no greater than 30 degrees for first 72 hours.
         (b) Elevate legs 20 to 30 degrees.
         (c) Encourage foot and leg exercises.
         (d) Mobilize from lying to standing; avoid sitting position, flexing or crossing of legs after femoral artery revascularization
      iv) EAB specifically
         (a) Position on nonoperative side.
         (b) Prevent external pressure on graft and avoid flexion of graft.
         (c) Feel for thrill over graft.
         (d) Assess for vascular steal: clinical indications of hypoperfusion of limb from which blood was diverted
         (e) Monitor for brachial plexus injury if axillofemoral bypass.
   c) Assess for clinical indications of hypoperfusion.
      i) Perform neurovascular assessment of extremities hourly; monitor for pain, pallor, pulselessness, paresthesia, paralysis, polar (i.e., cold).
      ii) Measure Doppler pressures and calculate ABI.
         (a) Report any decrease in ABI of 0.15 or more.
         (b) Do not measure Doppler pressure if the bypass is performed to the most distal arteries of the leg because it is painful for the patient and may cause graft compression.
      iii) Maintain normal body temperature: heated blankets or automatic warming blanket, warming lights.
   d) Treat pain.
      i) Administer analgesics as indicated.
      ii) Position for comfort.
   e) Prevent skin breakdown related to ischemia and immobility.
      i) Inspect skin, bony prominences, and affected extremities frequently.
      ii) Reposition often.
      iii) Use alternating air mattress or special bed, depending on other risk factors
      iv) Keep heels elevated off bed.
   f) Maintain adequate hydration.
      i) Administer IV fluids as indicated.
      ii) Monitor urine output closely, and report urine output of less than 0.5 ml/kg/hr.

g) Monitor for postoperative complications.
    i) Hemorrhage
    ii) Infection
        (a) Assess incision and wounds for indications of infection.
        (b) Monitor WBC and body temperature.
        (c) Provide aseptic wound care.
        (d) Administer antibiotics as prescribed.
    iii) Arterial thrombosis
    iv) Cerebral embolus (i.e., blood or plaque)
    v) Peripheral ischemia, infarction, loss of limb
    vi) Graft infection
        (a) Monitor for fever, malaise, back pain, anorexia, paralytic ileus, and leukocytosis.
        (b) Administer antibiotics as prescribed.
        (c) Prepare patient for removal and replacement of graft as requested.
e. Provide instruction and counseling regarding lifestyle modification and need for pharmacologic therapy.
    1) Nonpharmacologic therapies
        a) Weight normalization
        b) Dietary modifications
            i) Low saturated fat
            ii) ADA diet for control of blood glucose for patient with DM
        c) Cessation of tobacco use
        d) Regular aerobic exercise in moderation; should not exercise to the point of pain
        e) Foot care: special attention to any lesions because healing may be impaired by decreased circulation
        f) Avoidance of constrictive clothing
        g) Complementary therapies: relaxation; imagery, biofeedback
    2) Pharmacologic agents
        a) Platelet aggregation inhibitors (e.g., ASA, clopidogrel)
        b) Agents that increase the flexibility of the RBCs: pentoxifylline
        c) Peripheral vasodilators
            i) Papaverine: rarely used today
            ii) Cilostazol: PDE III inhibitor; inhibits platelet aggregation and causes vasodilation
        d) Anticoagulants: warfarin
        e) Antihypertensives if indicated

Acute Arterial Occlusion

1. Definition: acute complete occlusion of an artery by thrombosis in an already narrowed artery, embolism, or trauma
2. Etiology
    a. Arterial embolization
        1) Atrial fibrillation
        2) Ventricular aneurysm
        3) Bacterial endocarditis
    b. Injury to arterial intima causing arterial thrombosis
        1) Postcardiac catheterization or angioplasty
        2) IABP
        3) Postarterial bypass or aneurysm
    c. Compression of artery with swelling
        1) Fracture (compartment syndrome)
        2) Circumferential burn
3. Pathophysiology (Fig. 3.92)
4. Clinical presentation
    a. 6 Ps
        1) Pain: severe and sudden
        2) Pallor, cyanosis
        3) Pulselessness
        4) Paresis or paralysis
        5) Paresthesia or anesthesia
        6) Polar

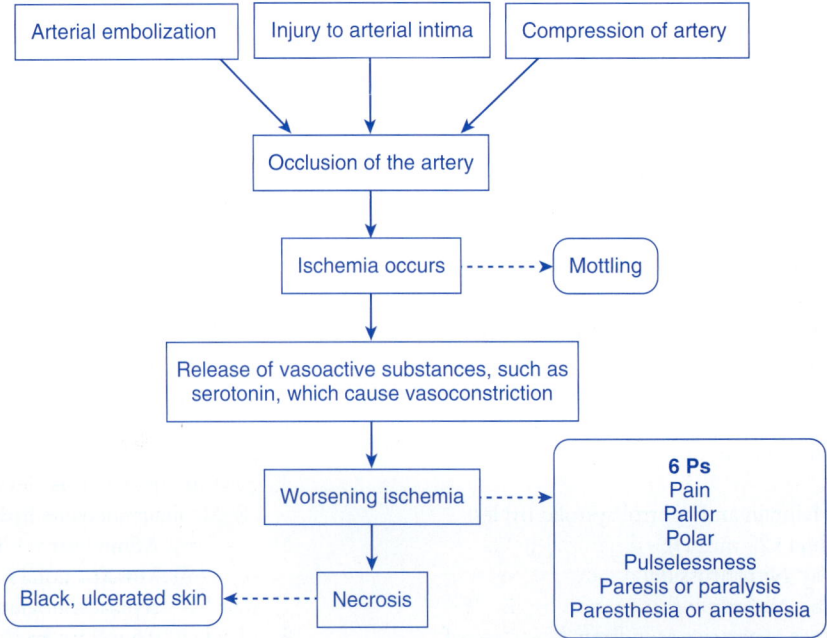

Fig. 3.92 Pathophysiology of acute arterial occlusion. *Dotted lines* connect pathology to the clinical presentation.

b. Doppler stethoscope indicates diminished or absent blood flow.
   c. Diagnostic study: angiography indicates arterial occlusion.
5. Collaborative management
   a. Initiate emergency measures immediately.
      1) Oxygen at 2 to 5 l/min to maintain SaO_2 at 95% unless contraindicated
      2) Proper positioning of limb: keep extremity straight, warm, and dependent
      3) Notification of physician immediately of perfusion defect
      4) IV infusion of normal saline at keep vein open (KVO) rate in unaffected limb
      5) Narcotics (e.g., morphine) for pain
   b. Assist in preparation of diagnostic studies: angiogram
   c. Reestablish patency of artery.
      1) Intraarterial fibrinolytic (e.g., urokinase, rt-PA) followed by anticoagulant (Table 3.30)
      2) Preparation for surgical procedures if indicated
         a) Procedures
            i) Surgical embolectomy especially for large arteries
            ii) Balloon embolectomy
            iii) Thromboendarterectomy
            iv) Bypass grafting
      3) Postoperative care as described in Peripheral Arterial Disease section
   d. Explain procedures thoroughly to minimize stress.
   e. Monitor closely for complications.
      1) Reocclusion
      2) Loss of limb
      3) Infection
   f. Provide patient teaching as for peripheral arterial disease.

Aortic Aneurysm

1. Definition: a permanent localized dilation of the aorta with an increase of at least 1.5 times its normal diameter
2. Etiology
   a. Degenerative changes caused by aging and familial predisposition
   b. Congenital weakness of the aorta
   c. Hypertension
   d. Pregnancy: especially third trimester
   e. Coarctation of the aorta
   f. Syphilis
   g. Severe systemic infection (e.g., bacterial aneurysm, mycotic aneurysm)
   h. Marfan syndrome
   i. Trauma: especially blunt trauma with acceleration-deceleration injury
   j. Arterial cannulation (e.g., PCI, IABP)
3. Pathophysiology (Fig. 3.93)
   a. Types
      1) False: does not involve all layers of the artery; pulsating hematoma that results from arterial trauma such as arterial cannulation
      2) True: involves all layers of the arterial wall; usually saccular arising from a distinct portion of the wall
      3) Saccular: outpouching from an artery that results from localized thinning and stretching of the media
      4) Fusiform: involves the total circumference of the artery with diffuse dilatation
      5) Dissecting: a cavity is formed by dissection by blood between the layers of the arterial wall
         a) Classifications
            i) DeBakey system
               (a) I: Original intimal tear begins in the ascending aorta with the dissection extending to the descending aorta.
               (b) II: Original intimal tear begins in the ascending aorta but does not extend to the descending aorta.
               (c) III: Original intimal tear begins in the descending aorta with the dissection confined in the descending aorta.
            ii) Stanford systems
               (a) A: Involves the ascending aorta
               (b) B: Involves the descending aorta
      6) Rupture: artery wall ruptures and leaks arterial blood into the mediastinum if thoracic or into abdominal cavity if abdominal.
4. Clinical presentation
   a. Subjective: usually asymptomatic until dissection or rupture occur
   b. Objective
      1) Normal to high BP; hypotension suggests cardiac tamponade or aortic rupture
      2) Pulsatile mass
      3) Increased aortic diameter on palpation
      4) Bruit over aorta
   c. Specifically ascending thoracic aorta
      1) May be asymptomatic
      2) Dyspnea
      3) Chest pain
      4) Clinical indications of aortic regurgitation: diastolic murmur, LVF, widened pulse pressure
   d. Specifically aortic arch
      1) Dyspnea
      2) Stridor
      3) Cough
      4) JVD
      5) Hoarseness
      6) Weak voice
   e. Specifically descending thoracic arch
      1) Dull chest pain and upper back pain
      2) Hoarseness
   f. Specifically dissecting thoracic aortic aneurysm
      1) Sudden, sharp, tearing or ripping pain in chest radiating to shoulders, neck, or back
      2) Hypotension
      3) Dyspnea
      4) Syncope
      5) Leg weakness, transient paralysis
      6) May have BP and pulse difference between arms or between arms and legs
      7) May have clinical indications of thrombotic stroke
      8) May have clinical indications of cardiac tamponade (see Cardiac Tamponade section)

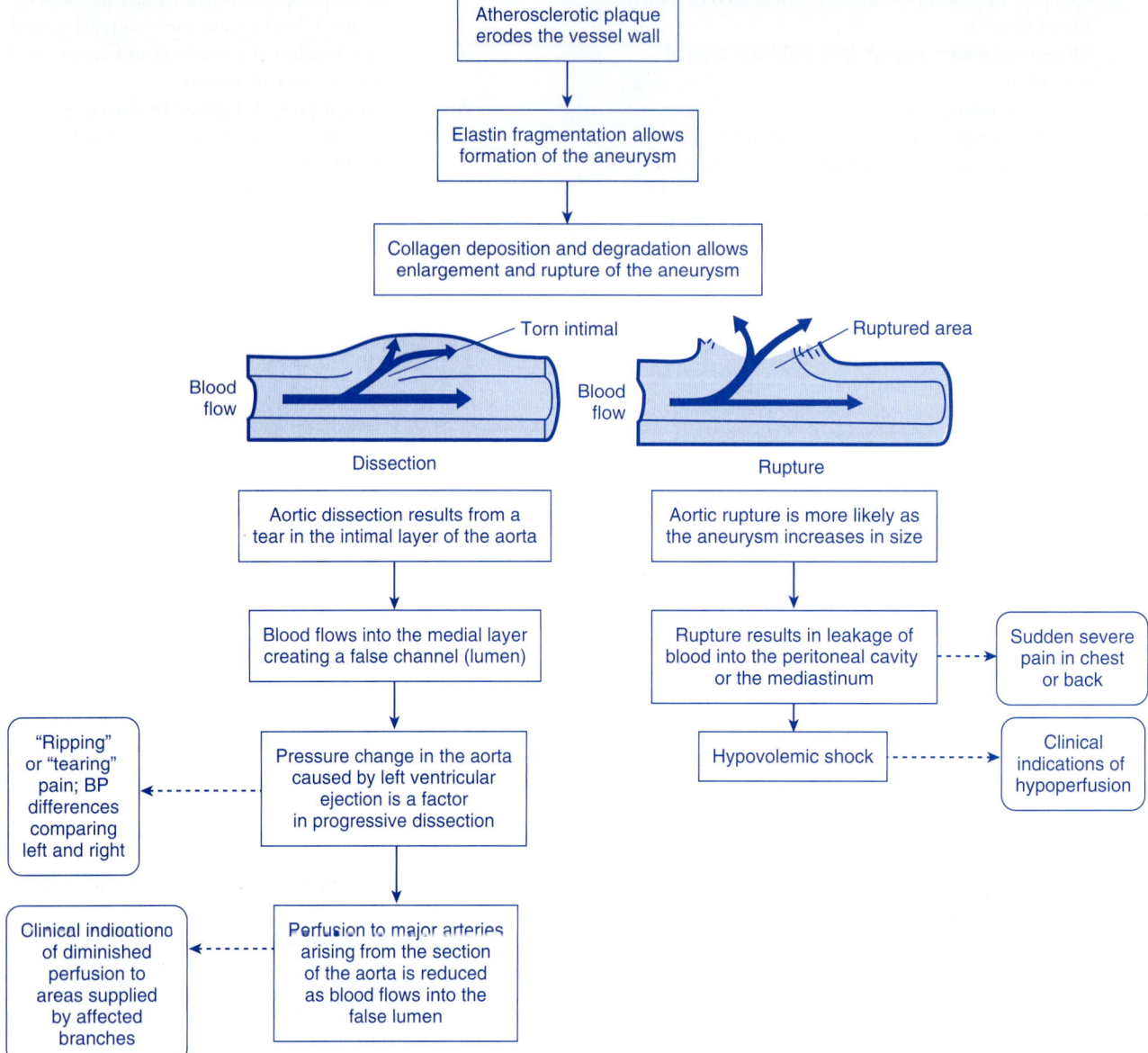

Fig. 3.93 Pathophysiology of aneurysm dissection. *Dotted lines* connect pathology to the clinical presentation. (Drawings from Urden, L. D., Stacy, K., & Lough, M. [2005]. *Thelan's critical care nursing: Diagnosis and management* [5th ed.]. St. Louis: Mosby.)

    g. Specifically abdominal aorta
        1) Dull abdominal and back pain
        2) Nausea and vomiting
        3) Abdominal bloating
        4) Pulsation in abdomen
    h. Specifically ruptured abdominal aortic aneurysm (AAA)
        1) Severe, sudden, dull, continuous abdominal pain radiating to low back, hips, scrotum; unaffected by movement
        2) Feeling of abdominal fullness
        3) Nausea and vomiting
        4) Syncope and shock
        5) Pulsation in abdomen: periumbilical area
    i. Diagnostic studies
        1) Serum: Hgb and Hct may be decreased.
        2) Chest radiography
            a) Mediastinal widening in thoracic aneurysm
            b) Aortic calcification
        3) ECG
            a) May show LVH
            b) May show nonspecific ST-T wave changes
            c) Absence of ECG indicators of MI
        4) Transesophageal echocardiography: may show aortic root dilation, intimal flap dividing true and false lumen in dissection
        5) Aortography: lumen of aneurysm; size and location of aneurysm
        6) CT scan and MRI: presence and location of aneurysm
        7) Ultrasonography: presence, size, shape, and location of aneurysm
        8) Flat plate of abdomen (KUB): outline of aneurysm
5. Collaborative management
    a. Control pain
        1) Narcotics, usually morphine, are required in rupture or dissection.
        2) Extreme caution if patient is hypotensive

b. Maintain and control MAP at approximately 60 to 75 mm Hg if dissection occurs.
   1) If patient is hypertensive
      a) Nitroprusside; may be used with propranolol (Inderal)
      b) Labetalol; decreases contractility and the pulsatile pressure on the aorta
   2) If patient is hypotensive
      a) IV access: two large-bore, short IV catheters; blood for type and crossmatch
      b) Normal saline or lactated Ringer solution by rapid infusion until blood is available; colloids (e.g., albumin, hetastarch, dextran) may also be used
      c) Blood and blood products
c. Decrease tissue oxygenation requirements.
   1) Activity restriction
   2) Oxygen by nasal cannula at 2 to 6 l/min to maintain SaO_2 of 95% unless contraindicated
   3) Intubation and mechanical ventilation may be necessary.
   4) Physical comfort: temperature control, lighting, noise control
   5) Anxiolytics as prescribed: usually diazepam, lorazepam, or alprazolam
d. Assist in preparation of patient for surgical repair.
   1) Indication for surgical repair: aneurysmal dilation of 5 to 6 cm in diameter; indications for immediate surgical repair include:
      a) Involvement of ascending aorta; aortic insufficiency
      b) Failure of drug therapy to control progression of dissection as evidenced by continued pain and progressive symptoms
      c) Cardiac tamponade
      d) Compromise of a major branch of aorta
      e) Indications of cerebral or cardiac ischemia
   2) Procedures
      a) Surgical procedure: resection of aneurysm and circumferential (fusiform aneurysm) or patch graft (saccular aneurysm)
         i) Repair of thoracic aortic aneurysm involving the ascending aorta and/or aortic arch requires cardiopulmonary bypass; concurrent aortic valve repair or replacement may be needed for ascending thoracic aneurysms.
         ii) Descending thoracic aortic aneurysms are usually repaired by thoracotomy and do not require cardiopulmonary bypass.
         iii) AAA repairs are done through abdominal incisions; a bowel preparation is performed unless surgery is emergent.
      b) Endovascular grafts for aneurysm repair
         i) Modular device that expands to fit and seal the aorta, lines the inside of the aneurysm like a sleeve providing a new path for blood flow and reducing the pressure on the aneurysm; uses either a stent or hooks to secure the sleeve
         ii) Implanted through a delivery catheter inserted through the femoral artery and positioned with the use of fluoroscopy
         iii) Advantages over traditional surgical aneurysm repair
            (a) May be used in patients at high risk for traditional aneurysm repair; originally only used for AAA but now also used for descending thoracic aneurysms as well as type B dissections
            (b) Intubation not required; may not require critical care unit stay
            (c) Fewer complications
               (i) Less blood loss than open repair
               (ii) Less hypothermia than with laparotomy
            (d) Shorter hospital stay
            (e) Lower early mortality; long-term mortality rate is comparable between the two options
         iv) Disadvantages compared with traditional surgical repair
            (a) Not all patients are candidates because the location of the aneurysm and the size of the patient's arteries above and below the aneurysm may preclude the implant.
            (b) May be more costly in the short-term and in the long-term because lifelong surveillance is required
   3) Postoperative management
      a) Maintain airway, oxygenation, and ventilation.
         i) Assess ventilatory status frequently: rate, rhythm; excursion, effort; use of accessory muscles, presence of stridor or other adventitious sounds, pulse oximetry.
         ii) Encourage deep breathing and incentive spirometry.
         iii) Assess frequently for edema, hematoma, tracheal deviation, and dysphagia.
         iv) Elevate HOB 30 degrees.
         v) Have equipment for artificial airway and suctioning.
         vi) Prevent aspiration: high-Fowler position while eating; NPO until gag reflex returns; suction as necessary.
         vii) Administer oxygen at 2 to 5 l/min as prescribed.
      b) Maintain adequate flow and pressure at graft site.
         i) Maintain and control systolic BP less than 120 mm Hg.
            (a) Nitroprusside
            (b) Nicardipine
            (c) Analgesics as indicated

ii) Prevent emboli by using antiembolic techniques.
    (a) Dextran 40 often used as platelet aggregation inhibitor
    (b) Heparin may also be used.
iii) Avoid pressure on incision sites.
    (a) Elevate HOB no greater than 30 degrees for first 72 hours.
    (b) Elevate legs 20 to 30 degrees.
    (c) Encourage foot and leg exercises.
    (d) Mobilize from lying to standing; avoid sitting position, flexing or crossing of legs after femoral artery revascularization.
c) Assess for clinical indications of hypoperfusion.
    i) Perform neurovascular assessment of extremities hourly; monitor for pain, pallor, pulselessness, paresthesia, paralysis, polar (cold).
    ii) Maintain normal body temperature: heated blankets or automatic warming blanket, warming lights
d) Treat pain.
    i) Administer analgesics as indicated.
    ii) Position for comfort.
e) Prevent skin breakdown related to ischemia and immobility.
    i) Inspect skin, bony prominences, and affected extremities frequently.
    ii) Reposition often.
    iii) Use egg crate, alternating air mattress, or special bed, depending on other risk factors.
    iv) Keep heels elevated off bed.
f) Maintain adequate hydration.
    i) Administer IV fluids as indicated.
    ii) Monitor urine output closely and report urine output of less than 0.5 ml/kg/hr.
g) Monitor for postoperative complications.
    i) Acute respiratory failure; monitor for all of the following:
        (a) Dyspnea
        (b) Hypoxemia
        (c) Tachypnea
        (d) Tachycardia
        (e) Fever
    ii) Hemorrhage, hypovolemia, and hematoma; monitor for all of the following:
        (a) Hypotension
        (b) Tachycardia
        (c) Clinical manifestations of hypoperfusion
        (d) Decreased RAP, PAP, PAOP
    iii) Myocardial ischemia and infarction; monitor for all of the following:
        (a) Chest pain
        (b) Dyspnea
        (c) Decreased CO
        (d) Dysrhythmias
        (e) ECG: ST-segment changes
    iv) Cerebral ischemia and infarction; monitor for all of the following:
        (a) Change in level of consciousness (LOC)
        (b) Pupillary change
        (c) Aphasia
        (d) Motor or sensory changes
    v) Pulmonary ischemia and infarction; monitor for all of the following:
        (a) Dyspnea
        (b) Chest pain
        (c) Pleural friction rub
        (d) Hypoxemia
    vi) Renal ischemia and infarction; monitor for all of the following:
        (a) Flank pain
        (b) Decreased urine output
        (c) Changes in BUN or creatinine
        (d) Hematuria
    vii) Mesenteric ischemia and infarction; monitor for all of the following:
        (a) Watery, bloody diarrhea
        (b) Abdominal pain
        (c) Change in bowel sounds
    viii) Splenic ischemia and infarction; monitor for all of the following:
        (a) Left upper quadrant pain radiating to the left shoulder
        (b) Abdominal rigidity
    ix) Spinal cord ischemia and infarction
        (a) Monitor for all of the following:
            (i) Paralysis of lower extremities
            (ii) Bowel and bladder paralysis
        (b) Drainage of cerebral spinal fluid (CSF) naloxone, osmotic diuretics, steroids, and/or calcium channel blockers may be prescribed to prevent or treat spinal cord hyperemia or edema.
    x) Arterial thrombosis
        (a) Sudden, painful ischemia of feet (sometimes referred to as *trash foot*) and/or lower leg
        (b) Diminished or absent peripheral pulses; decreased ABI
    xi) Complications specific to endovascular aneurysm repair
        (a) Endoleak: persistence of blood flow outside the lumen of the endoluminal graft but within the aneurysmal sac
            (i) May be managed by observation, further endovascular procedures, or open repair
            (ii) Risk for continued aneurysm expansion and risk of rupture

                    (b) Postimplant syndrome
                        (i) Back pain and fever without a leukocytosis or other signs of infection
                        (ii) May last up to 7 days
                        (iii) Cause unknown
                    (c) Graft limb thrombosis
                        (i) Thrombectomy or embolectomy may be required.
    e. Provide instruction and counseling regarding lifestyle modification and need for pharmacologic therapy as for peripheral arterial disease.

Carotid Arterial Stenosis
(May be referred to as *extracranial cerebrovascular disease*)
1. Etiology
    a. Atherosclerosis or arteriosclerosis: risk factors as for CAD and peripheral vascular disease
    b. Trauma
    c. Fibromuscular dysplasia
    d. Cervical irradiation
    e. Arteritis
2. Pathophysiology
    a. Atherosclerotic plaque accumulates at the bifurcation of the internal and external carotid arteries.
    b. Fragments of this plaque or associated thrombi may break away from the plaque causing cerebral emboli.
    c. Eventually, ischemia or infarction of the brain may occur.
        1) Ischemia
            a) Transient ischemic attack (TIA): focal neurologic deficit lasting less than 24 hours
        2) Infarction: a completed ischemic stroke
            a) Permanent neurologic deficit, although some improvement may occur over time
            b) Carotid artery stenosis is the cause of 15% to 25% of strokes.
3. Clinical presentation: literature reflects its questionable if asymptomatic carotid disease will be managed in the future.
    a. Subjective: usually asymptomatic unless TIA or completed stroke is experienced; symptoms may include:
        1) Visual changes: diplopia; ipsilateral monocular blindness (referred to as *amaurosis fugax*)
        2) Memory loss
        3) Vertigo
        4) Syncope
    b. Objective
        1) Bruit or thrill over one or both carotid arteries
        2) Signs of TIAs or stroke may include:
            a) Slurred speech or aphasia
            b) Ataxia
            c) Paresis or paralysis
            d) Temporary loss of consciousness
    c. Diagnostic studies
        1) Duplex ultrasonography of the carotid arteries: initial diagnostic test for patients with known or suspected carotid stenosis
        2) Magnetic resonance angiography or CT angiography: if sonography cannot be obtained or yields nondiagnostic results
        3) Cerebral arteriography
4. Collaborative management
    a. Administer pharmacologic agents as prescribed.
        1) Platelet aggregation inhibitors (e.g., ASA, clopidogrel *or* ASA plus dipyridamole); ASA and clopidogrel together is not recommended
        2) Agents that increase the flexibility of the RBCs: pentoxifylline
        3) Anticoagulants: warfarin for patients with atrial fibrillation or mechanical prosthetic cardiac valve to INR of 2.5
        4) Antihypertensives if indicated
    b. Prepare patient for percutaneous or surgical procedure as requested.
        1) Indications
            a) Occlusion of 70% or greater of the internal carotid artery or mild stroke within the previous 6 months
            b) No contraindications for surgery
        2) Procedures
            a) Carotid endarterectomy: removal of an atheroma at the carotid artery bifurcation
            b) Carotid artery stenting especially for patients who are high surgical risk
                i) Balloon dilation of the stenotic area and placement of a crush-resistant stent
                ii) Especially useful in patients with recurrent carotid stenosis, lesions distal in the internal carotid artery or high in the neck, or patients with history of cervical irradiation
        3) Postoperative management
            a) Maintain airway, oxygenation, and ventilation
                i) Assess ventilatory status frequently: rate, rhythm, excursion, effort, use of accessory muscles, presence of stridor or other adventitious sounds, pulse oximetry.
                ii) Encourage deep breathing and incentive spirometry.
                iii) Assess frequently for edema, hematoma, tracheal deviation, and dysphagia.
                iv) Elevate HOB 30 degrees.
                v) Have equipment for cricothyroidotomy, tracheostomy, and suction.
                vi) Prevent aspiration: high-Fowler position while eating; NPO until gag reflex returns; suction as necessary.
                vii) Administer oxygen at 2 to 5 l/min as prescribed.
            b) Monitor for or prevent alteration in cerebral perfusion related to cerebral embolism, ischemia, and infarction especially after procedures.
                i) Assess BP and HR frequently: BP is usually maintained within 20 mm Hg ± preoperative values.

ii) Report immediately clinical indications of cerebral hypoperfusion: change in level of consciousness, pupil changes, paresis or plegia, visual changes, dysphasia or aphasia, seizures, or headache.
iii) Check neurologic and cranial nerve (CN) function. (NOTE: There is no risk of injury to the cranial nerves with carotid artery stenting.)
   (a) LOC
   (b) Pupils
   (c) Motor function
   (d) Sensory function
   (e) CNs
      (i) CN VII: Ask patient to smile.
      (ii) CN IX, X: Check swallowing, speech, and gag.
      (iii) CN XI: Ask patient to shrug against your hands.
      (iv) CN XII: Ask patient to stick tongue out; check for midline position.
      (v) Recurrent laryngeal nerve: Check speech.
      (vi) Great auricular nerve: Note perception of sensation on face and ear.
iv) Administer antiplatelet aggregation drugs (e.g., ASA, clopidogrel, dextran 40) as prescribed; ASA *and* clopidogrel are recommended before and for at least 30 days after carotid artery stenting.
c) Monitor for hemorrhage or hematoma.
   i) Assess BP and HR frequently.
   ii) Assess neck dressing for hematoma or hemorrhage; check back of neck and assess drainage from drain if present.
   iii) Check for tracheal deviation.
   iv) Monitor Hgb and Hct.
   v) Administer antihypertensives (e.g., nitroprusside, labetalol) as prescribed to maintain BP: systolic 100 to 160 mm Hg, diastolic less than 100 mm Hg.
d) Monitor for complications.
   i) MI
   ii) Cerebral hemorrhage, embolism, or infarction
   iii) Carotid hemorrhage
   iv) Hematoma
   v) Cranial nerve injury
   vi) Seizures
c. Provide instruction and counseling regarding lifestyle modification and need for pharmacologic therapy as for peripheral arterial disease.

Cardiovascular Trauma

Blunt Cardiac Injury (i.e., Myocardial Contusion)

1. Definition: transient or permanent myocardial dysfunction caused by blunt trauma to the heart and may include myocardial necrosis without CAD
2. Etiology
    a. Usually acceleration–deceleration injury sustained in motor vehicle collision; sternum may hit steering wheel or dashboard; injury may also be caused by shoulder strap of seat belt
    b. Other vehicular accidents: motorcycle collisions, auto–pedestrian collisions
    c. Kicking of chest by large animal
    d. Assault with blunt instrument
    e. Industrial crush injury
    f. Explosion
    g. Vigorous CPR
    h. Projectile objects (e.g., baseball, hockey puck)
3. Pathophysiology (Fig. 3.94)
4. Clinical presentation
    a. Subjective
        1) History of events and mechanism of injury
        2) Precordial angina-like chest pain
            a) Frequently increases with inspiration, cough, and movement
            b) Unresponsive to nitroglycerin but frequently responsive to oxygen, antiinflammatory agents, or narcotics
        3) Dyspnea
        4) Palpitations
    b. Objective
        1) Tachycardia; persistent despite adequate fluid replacement
        2) Tachypnea
        3) Hypotension may occur.
        4) Ecchymosis may be present on anterior chest.
        5) Chest wall tenderness with palpation.
        6) Clinical indications of RVF: JVD, peripheral edema, hepatomegaly
        7) Clinical indications of LV noncompliance: S_4
        8) Clinical indications of hypoperfusion (Table 3.2)
        9) Cardiac arrest as a result of fatal ventricular dysrhythmias may occur.
    c. Diagnostic studies
        1) Serum: CK-MB and cardiac troponin may be positive depending on the severity of the injury.
        2) ECG with RV leads
            a) ST segment changes, T-wave inversion in V_1 to V_4; Q waves may be seen if injury is severe or if a coronary artery is lacerated or thrombosed
            b) QT interval may be prolonged.
            c) Dysrhythmias
                i) Atrial dysrhythmias: PACs, atrial fibrillation, atrial flutter
                ii) Ventricular dysrhythmias: PVCs, VT, VF
                iii) Blocks: AV blocks, RBBB
        3) Echocardiography
            a) Decreased regional wall motion (especially RV)
            b) Increased end-diastolic wall thickness
            c) Decreased RVEF
            d) May show complications (e.g., apical thrombi, pericardial effusion, cardiac tamponade)
        4) Radionuclide studies may be done: decreased RVEF.

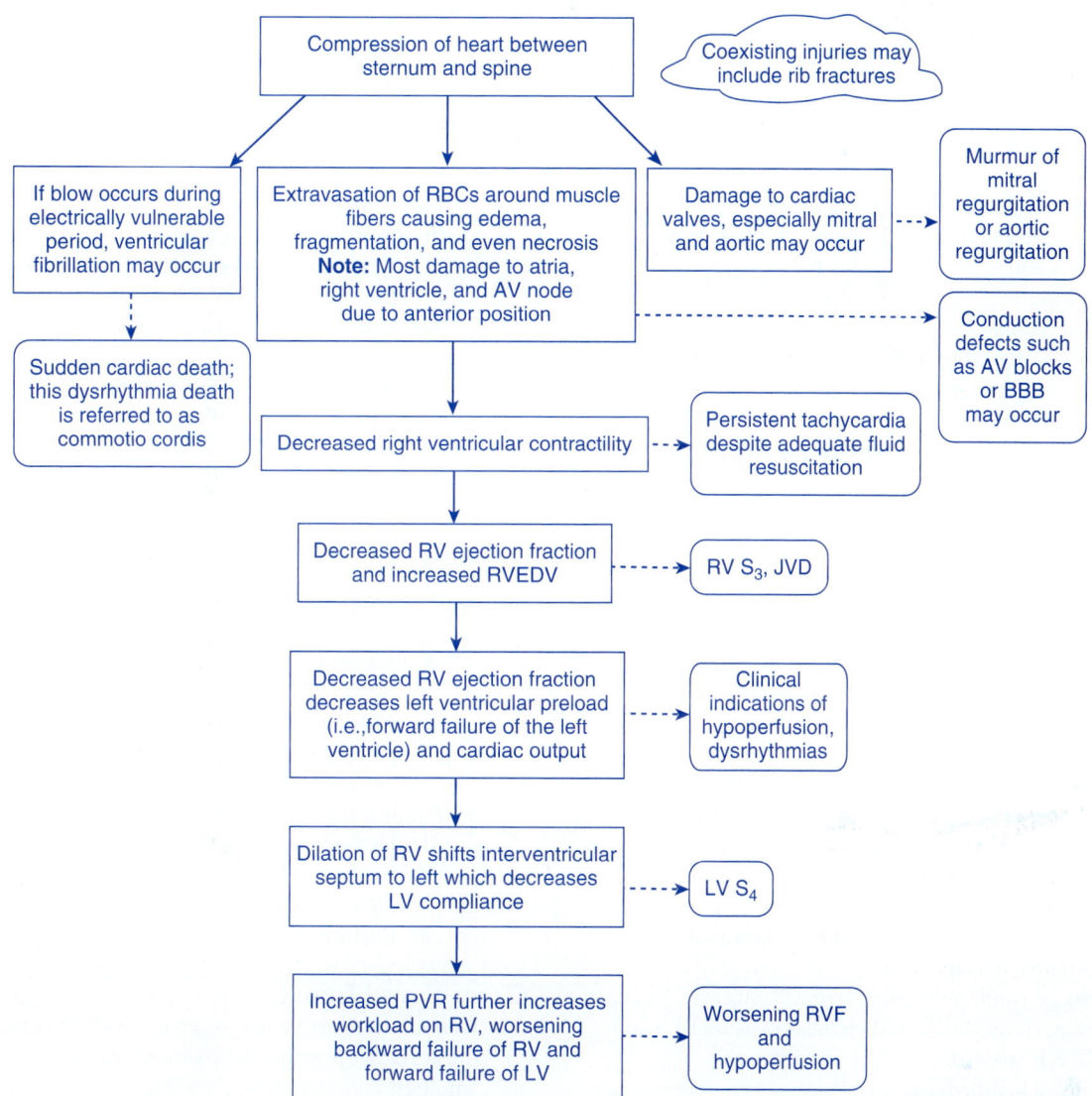

Fig. 3.94 Pathophysiology of blunt cardiac injury. *Dotted lines* connect pathology to the clinical presentation. *BBB*, Bundle branch block; *JVD*, jugular venous distention; *LV*, left ventricular; *PVR*, pulmonary vascular resistance; *RV*, right ventricular; *RVEDV*, right ventricular end-diastolic volume; *RVF*, right ventricular failure.

5. Collaborative management
    a. Treat pain.
        1) Morphine sulfate usually used.
        2) Antiinflammatory agents may also be helpful.
    b. Ensure adequate RV contractility, LV filling, and CO.
        1) Isotonic fluids as prescribed to ensure adequate LV filling; avoid venous vasodilators and diuretics
        2) Inotropes (e.g., dobutamine) as prescribed to improve RV contractility
    c. Decrease myocardial oxygen demand.
        1) Bed rest
        2) Oxygen by nasal cannula at 2 to 6 l/min to maintain SaO_2 of 95% unless contraindicated
        3) Anxiolytics as prescribed and indicated
    d. Treat dysrhythmias.
        1) Atrial: digitalis, cardioversion
        2) Ventricular: usually amiodarone
        3) Blocks: temporary pacemaker; permanent pacemaker may be necessary
    e. Assist in assessment for other thoracic injuries (e.g., fractured ribs, sternum, clavicle, pulmonary contusion).
    f. Monitor for complications.
        1) Ventricular rupture
        2) Cardiac tamponade
        3) Coronary artery thrombosis
        4) Intracardiac thrombus
        5) Valve rupture
        6) Conduction defects
        7) HF
        8) Ventricular aneurysm
        9) Cardiogenic shock: monitor for clinical manifestations of hypoperfusion.
        10) Systemic emboli
            a) Sequential compression devices may be used on the legs.
            b) Anticoagulation avoided unless there are intramural thrombi

Penetrating Cardiac Injury

1. Definition: puncture of the heart with a sharp object or rib
2. Etiology
   a. Violence (e.g., knife wound, gunshot wound, ice pick)
   b. Industrial accident (e.g., scaffolding)
   c. Motorcycle collision (e.g., handlebar impalement)
   d. Sports injury
   e. Explosion
   f. Crush injury
3. Pathophysiology (Fig. 3.95)
4. Clinical presentation
   a. Subjective
      1) History of events and mechanism of injury
      2) Chest pain
   b. Objective
      1) Visible wound; object causing penetration may be seen
      2) Bleeding from chest
      3) Hypotension
      4) Clinical indications of hypoperfusion (Table 3.2)
      5) Clinical indications of cardiac tamponade (see Cardiac Tamponade section)
   c. Hemodynamic parameters
      1) Decrease in RAP, PAP, PAOP if hemorrhage; increase in RAP, PAP, PAOP if cardiac tamponade
      2) Decrease in CO, CI
      3) Decrease in SvO_2
   d. Diagnostic studies: Hgb and Hct decreased
5. Collaborative management
   a. Manage cardiopulmonary arrest if indicated: manage airway, oxygenation, and circulation using BLS and ACLS if needed.
   b. Control hemorrhage.
      1) Do not remove an impaled object; objects may be stabilized with IV bags and dressings.
      2) Apply pressure to site if the object has been removed and there is a bleeding wound.
      3) Apply pressure around site if the object has not already been removed and there is bleeding around the wound.
      4) Assist in insertion of chest tube for hemothorax or pneumothorax.
      5) Assist with pericardiocentesis for cardiac tamponade.
   c. Improve oxygen delivery.
      1) Oxygen by nasal cannula at 2 to 6 l/min to maintain SaO_2 of 95% unless contraindicated
      2) Intubation and mechanical ventilation may be necessary.
      3) IV access: two large-bore, short IV catheters; blood for type and crossmatch
      4) Normal saline or lactated Ringer solution by rapid infusion until blood is available; colloids (e.g., albumin, hetastarch, or dextran may also be used)
      5) Blood and blood products
   d. Assist in preparation of the patient for exploratory thoracotomy.
   e. Control pain and discomfort.
      1) NSAIDs
      2) Narcotic analgesics in doses adequate to allow patient to deep breathe and cough as indicated
      3) Anxiolytics
   f. Monitor for complications.
      1) Hemorrhagic shock
      2) Cardiac tamponade
      3) Hemothorax
      4) Pneumothorax

Great Vessel Injury

1. Definition: injury or tear to great vessel or vessels, usually the aorta but possibly the pulmonary artery
2. Etiology
   a. Acceleration–deceleration injury (e.g., motor vehicle collision)
   b. Compression injury
   c. Penetrating trauma

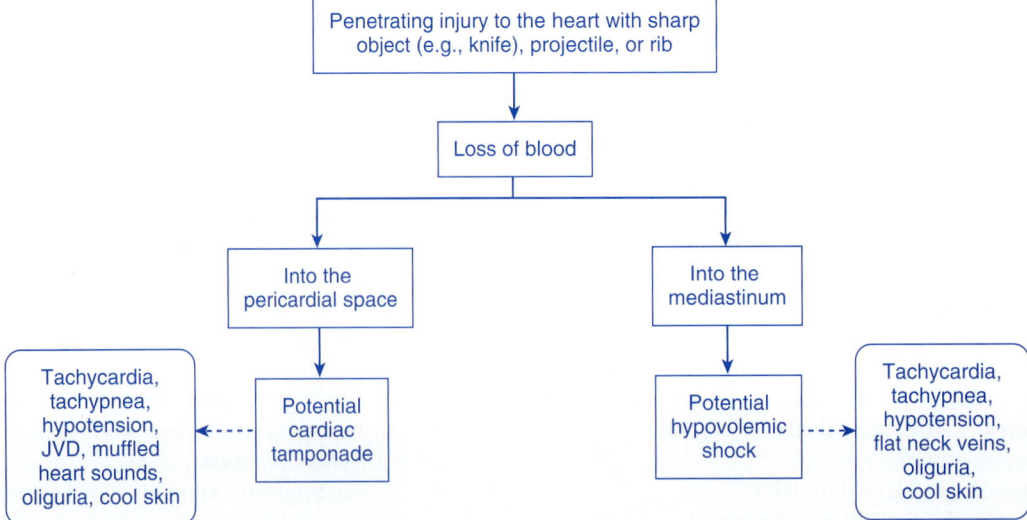

Fig. 3.95 Pathophysiology of penetrating cardiac injury. *Dotted lines* connect pathology to the clinical presentation. *JVD*, Jugular venous distention.

3. Pathophysiology: disruption of major vessel integrity causes loss of effective circulating blood volume, leading to shock.
4. Clinical presentation
    a. Subjective
        1) History of events and mechanism of injury
        2) Chest pain frequently radiating to back or back pain
        3) Dyspnea
        4) Dysphagia or hoarseness
        5) Sensory or motor changes in lower extremities
    b. Objective
        1) Tachycardia
        2) BP changes
            a) Hypertension or hypotension
            b) Difference between left and right arms
            c) Difference (greater than normal) between upper and lower extremities
        3) Tracheal shift
        4) Clinical indications of hypoperfusion
        5) Harsh systolic murmur may be audible along the precordium
    c. Hemodynamic parameters
        1) Decrease in RAP, PAP, PAOP
        2) Decrease in CO, CI
        3) Decrease in SvO_2
    d. Diagnostic studies
        1) Serum: Hgb and Hct decreased
        2) ECG: may show dysrhythmias or ST-T wave changes indicative of ischemia
        3) Chest radiography
            a) Mediastinal widening
            b) Loss of aortic knob shadow
        4) Transesophageal echocardiography or spiral CT
        5) Aortogram: will show extravasation of dye
5. Collaborative management
    a. Manage cardiopulmonary arrest if needed: manage airway, oxygenation, and circulation using BLS and ACLS if needed.
    b. Improve oxygen delivery.
        1) Oxygen by nasal cannula at 2 to 6 l/min to maintain SaO_2 of 95% unless contraindicated
        2) Intubation and mechanical ventilation may be necessary.
        3) IV access: two large-bore, short IV catheters; blood for type and crossmatch
        4) Normal saline or lactated Ringer solution by rapid infusion until blood is available; colloids (e.g., albumin, hetastarch, or dextran may also be used)
        5) Blood and blood products
    c. Control bleeding: antihypertensive may be needed to keep MAP less than 90 mm Hg.
    d. Assist in preparation of the patient for exploratory thoracotomy as soon as possible; it is not possible to truly stabilize this patient except in the operating room with vascular repair.
    e. Control pain and discomfort.
        1) NSAIDs
        2) Narcotic analgesics in doses adequate to allow patient to deep breathe and cough as indicated
        3) Anxiolytics
    f. Monitor for complications.
        1) Hemorrhagic shock
        2) Cardiac tamponade
        3) Hemothorax
        4) False aneurysm

Cardiac Tamponade

Definition
1. When fluid (blood, effusion fluid, pus) in the pericardial space compromises cardiac filling and CO
2. Tamponade is not dependent on the amount of fluid in the pericardial space but on the presence of hemodynamic consequences of pericardial fluid.

Etiology
1. Blunt or penetrating injury to heart
2. Postcardiotomy
    a. If mediastinal tube is occluded or after removal of mediastinal tube
    b. After removal of epicardial pacing wires
3. After MI
    a. Pericarditis, especially in anticoagulated patients
    b. Cardiac rupture
4. Iatrogenic causes: perforation of the myocardium by transvenous pacemaker wires, invasive catheters, intracardiac injection, cardiac needle biopsy
5. Transmyocardial revascularization
6. After CPR, electrical cardioversion
7. Fibrinolytic or anticoagulant therapy
8. Rupture of great vessels
9. Dissecting aortic aneurysms
10. Malignancy or radiation therapy
11. Connective tissue disease: rheumatoid arthritis, systemic lupus erythematosus, scleroderma
12. Metabolic disease: renal failure, hepatic failure, myxedema
13. Inflammation: pericarditis
14. Infection: viral, bacterial, fungal
    a. Tuberculosis
15. Drugs: procainamide, hydralazine, minoxidil, phenytoin, daunorubicin, methyldopa, sulfasalazine, isoniazid, methysergide, sargramostim, tetracycline derivatives

Pathophysiology
Fig. 3.96.

Clinical Presentation
1. Subjective
    a. Precordial fullness or pain
    b. Dyspnea with improvement when sitting upright
    c. Anxiety or feeling of impending doom
2. Objective
    a. Early sign is usually tachycardia but as the impairment in ventricular filling progresses, the patient may be pulseless (i.e., pulseless electrical activity [PEA]).
    b. Hypotension, narrowed pulse pressure
        1) Pulsus paradoxus: systolic pressure decrease of 10 mm Hg or more with inspiration
    c. Increased JVD: may not be seen if patient is hypotensive
    d. Absent PMI

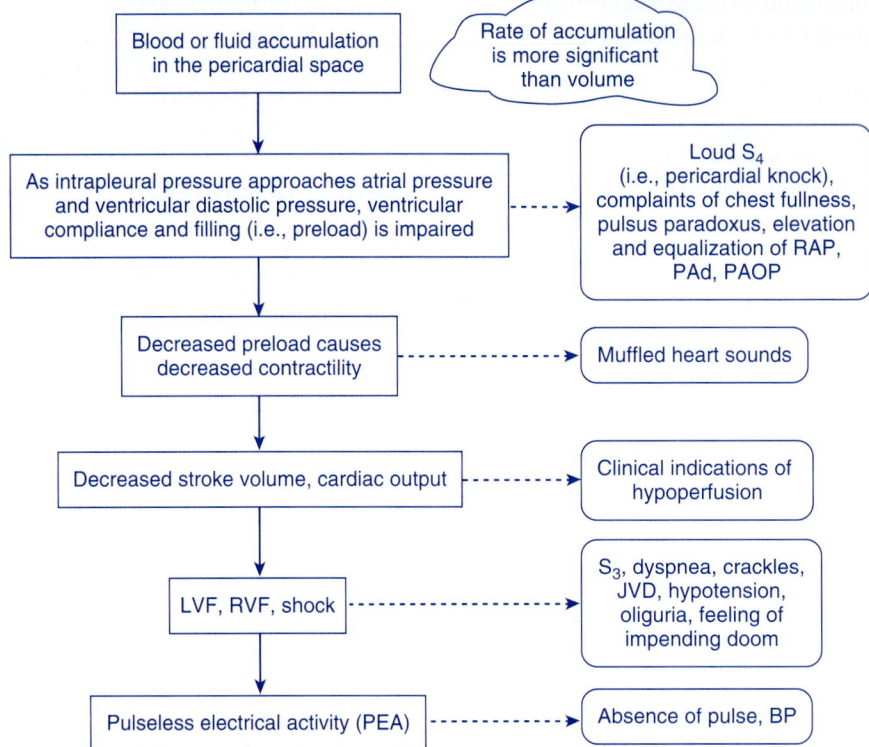

Fig. 3.96 Pathophysiology of cardiac tamponade. *Dotted lines* connect pathology to the clinical presentation. *BP*, Blood pressure; *JVD*, jugular venous distention; *LVF*, left ventricular failure; *PAd*, pulmonary artery diastolic pressure; *PAOP*, pulmonary artery occlusive pressure; *PEA*, pulseless electrical activity; *RAP*, right atrial pressure; *RVF*, right ventricular failure.

    e. Dullness to percussion below the left scapula (i.e., Ewart sign)
    f. Heart sound changes
       1) Pericardial friction rub may be heard especially if tamponade associated with pericarditis
       2) Distant, muffled, or absent heart sounds
    g. Beck triad: hypotension; distended neck veins; muffled heart sounds
    h. Excessive mediastinal tube drainage that suddenly stops in a cardiac surgery or trauma patient
3. Hemodynamic parameters
    a. Increased CVP and RAP
    b. Pulsus paradoxus on arterial waveform
    c. Equalization of left- and right-heart filling pressures with hemodynamic monitoring: RAP, PAd, and PAOP within 5 mm Hg of each other
    d. Change in PAOP waveform: large *a* wave, large *v* wave (M sign)
    e. Decrease in CO or CI
    f. Decrease in SvO_2
4. Diagnostic studies
    a. CBC with differential: assess for anemia.
    b. Type and crossmatch in preparation for blood administration if necessary
    c. Chest radiography
       1) Widened mediastinum
       2) Dilated superior vena cava
       3) Enlarged heart (i.e., water-bottle silhouette)
    d. ECG
       1) Diffuse ST-segment elevation across the precordial leads
       2) Decrease in the amplitude of the QRS or electrical alternans (i.e., alternating tall and small QRSs) across the precordial leads
       3) Bradycardia may indicate impending PEA.
       4) Ventricular dysrhythmias
    e. Echocardiogram: two dimensional (2D) or transesophageal
       1) Echo-free space will be evident between the pericardium and epicardium.
       2) RA and RV collapse
       3) Respiratory variation in cardiac chamber dimension and transvalvular flow velocities
       4) Transesophageal echocardiogram or CT imaging may be required
    f. FAST (focused assessment with sonography)
    g. CT of chest
    h. Fluoroscopy of chest: may be used during pericardiocentesis

Collaborative Management

1. Maintain airway, ventilation, oxygenation, and perfusion.
    a. Airway, oxygenation, and circulation support using BLS and ACLS if needed
    b. 100% oxygen by face mask; intubate and mechanically ventilate as indicated
    c. Circulating volume replacement
       1) Initiate two large-bore IVs: replace vascular volume as necessary
          a) Normal saline: 200 to 500 ml over 10 to 15 minutes

            b) Fresh-frozen plasma, dextran, or albumin may also be used.
            c) Blood replacement may also be necessary.
        d. Inotropes (e.g., dobutamine) as prescribed
        e. Atropine or transcutaneous pacing may be necessary for bradydysrhythmias.
    2. Prepare to assist with pericardiocentesis for emergency cardiac tamponade.
        a. Place patient in semi-Fowler position; subxiphoid or left parasternal approach are most commonly used.
        b. Apply ECG machine and electrodes.
            1) Apply limb leads.
            2) Attach chest lead wire to the exploring needle with an alligator clamp if requested; this technique is used to assess needle position because when the needle touches epicardium, ST-segment elevation is seen, and PVCs may occur.
        c. Have an echocardiography technician available to assist with 2D echo guidance if requested; fluoroscopy may also be used.
        d. Have emergency equipment available, including a transcutaneous pacemaker.
        e. Assist with administration of local anesthetic.
        f. Administer sedation if the patient is anxious.
        g. Assist with slow aspiration of the fluid and send it to the laboratory department for analysis.
        h. Assist with placement of pericardial catheter if indicated; may be used for injection of sclerosing agents, corticosteroids, fibrinolytics, or chemotherapeutic agents.
        i. Monitor for complications.
            1) Laceration of coronary artery or conduction system
            2) Myocardial perforation
            3) Pneumothorax
            4) Dysrhythmias
            5) Hypotension (usually reflexogenic)
    3. Administer drugs or therapies related to cause.
        a. Discontinuance of drug that contributed to the tamponade
        b. Protamine or vitamin K if patient is on anticoagulants
        c. Dialysis for patients with renal failure
        d. Antibiotics if purulent effusion
        e. Thyroid hormone replacement for myxedema
        f. Corticosteroids may be prescribed in drug-related pericardial effusions, uremia, and pericarditis.
    4. Assist in preparation of patient for surgical intervention.
        a. Pericardiocentesis may not resolve the tamponade if effusion is posterior; surgical drainage is indicated if purulent or hemorrhagic effusion.
        b. Subxiphoid pericardiotomy or thoracoscopic procedures may be necessary.
    5. Monitor or assist with treatment of recurrent pericardial effusion or tamponade.
        a. Monitor for recurrence of clinical indications of tamponade.
        b. Prepare the patient for the selected procedure.
            1) Percutaneous balloon pericardiotomy
            2) Intrapericardial instillation of sclerosing agent
            3) Pleuropericardial or peritoneal-pericardial window

Hypovolemic Shock

Included under Cardiovascular on the CCRN Test Plan but is covered in Chapter 11: Multisystem

Cardiogenic Shock

Included under Cardiovascular on the CCRN Test Plan but is covered in Chapter 11: Multisystem

LEARNING ACTIVITIES

CHAPTER 3

NOTE: Remember that you won't see questions like these on the CCRN examination, but these activities allow you to approach the content from a different perspective to remember it better. Multiple-choice questions (like on the CCRN examination) are available on the Elsevier website.

1. Complete the following crossword puzzle dealing with cardiovascular anatomy and physiology.

228

Chapter 3 The Cardiovascular System

ACROSS

6. The term used to describe the effect on contractility
10. These receptors are located in the renal and mesenteric artery bed, and stimulation causes vasodilation of those vascular beds
15. The type of disks that lie between myocardial cells to allow rapid transmission of the cardiac impulse
16. The interatrial pathway is frequently referred to as _____ bundle
17. The calculated parameter used to evaluate left ventricular contractility (abbrev.)
20. This innermost layer of the heart which lines the heart chamber and the heart valves
22. The left bundle branch is divided into left anterior and left posterior _____
23. During this refractory period, the cardiac muscle cell cannot respond no matter how strong the impulse is
24. This calculated parameter is used to evaluate left ventricular afterload (abbrev.)
25. The term used to describe the effect on heart rate
26. Rapid depolarization that allows cardiac muscle to contract in concert as if it were one muscle; this is referred to as a functional _____
29. Crossbridging of actin and _____ causes muscle shortening
31. Calcium is necessary for _____ which causes muscle shortening
33. The muscles which contract to close the atrioventricular valves
36. The type of pressure that pushes (such as out of the capillary and into the interstitium)
38. This layer of the serous pericardium is synonymous with the epicardium
40. The ability of the cardiac cells to respond to a stimulus
42. Another term for antidiuretic hormone
43. The valve that lies between the right ventricle and the pulmonary artery
45. A mineralocorticoid secreted by the adrenal cortex which causes sodium and water retention
47. These receptors are located in the right atrium and are sensitive to increased venous pressure
49. This refractory period is frequently referred to as the vulnerable period
51. The relaxation phase of the cardiac cycle
54. A neurotransmitter for the sympathetic nervous system that causes an increase in heart rate and contractility along with vasoconstriction
56. The pressure against which the ventricle must pump to open the semilunar valve
57. These fibers penetrate the ventricle to transmit the electrical impulse through to the endocardium
61. Pulse _____ is the difference between systolic and diastolic blood pressure
62. Elevation of this level in the blood is an indication of hypoxia and anaerobic metabolism
64. Occurs when sodium rushes into the cell causing it to become less negative
66. The fluid in the pericardial space acts as a _____
68. This layer of the pericardium acts as a barrier against infection and neoplastic invasion
73. This reflex causes an increase in heart rate with inspiration and a decrease in heart rate with expiration
75. The relationship between filling volume and contractility is frequently referred to as _____ law of the heart
78. The type of receptors that are located in the carotid and aortic bodies which are sensitive to PaO_2, $PaCO_2$, and pH
79. The basic contractile unit of the myocardium
80. The valve between the left atrium and the aorta
82. DO_2 is a calculated parameter representing the _____ of oxygen to the tissues
86. A precursor of angiotensin
89. An increase in epicardial fat is associated with _____
90. The type of vessel that forms the nutrient bed for the tissues
91. High-pressure lower cardiac chambers
92. Vasoconstrictive peptide produced by endothelial cells
93. Phase 1 of the action potential may be referred to as the _____ channel

DOWN

1. The portion of the cardiac wall that includes fibrous and serous layers
2. Fluid accumulation in spaces outside the intracellular and intravascular spaces is referred to as _____ spacing
3. The amount of blood that is ejected by the left ventricle per minute (abbrev.)
4. This peptide is associated with increased intravascular volume and is increased in heart failure (abbrev.)
5. The atrial contraction is frequently referred to as the atrial _____
7. The valve that lies between the right atrium and the right ventricle
8. The outermost layer of the artery
9. VO_2 is a calculated parameter representing the _____ of oxygen by the tissues
11. The ability of the cardiac cells to initiate electrical impulses regularly and spontaneously
12. Parameter used to evaluate right ventricular preload (abbrev.)
13. Cell layer that lines heart and blood vessels
14. The natural pacemaker of the heart is this node (abbrev.)
18. The function of these structures is to maintain unidirectional blood flow through the heart
19. A rupture of this innermost layer of the artery caused by plaque triggers the intrinsic pathway of clotting in atherosclerosis
21. Parameter used to evaluate right ventricular afterload (abbrev.)
26. The branch of the autonomic nervous system that is frequently referred to as the "fight or flight" system
27. The contraction phase of the cardiac cycle
28. The type of pressure that pulls (e.g., into the capillary from the interstitium)
30. The coronary artery that supplies the anterior left ventricle and the anterior two thirds of the septum (abbrev.)
32. Recovery; return to predominance of intracellular potassium and extracellular sodium
34. Vascular resistance is dependent upon the length and radius of the vessel and the viscosity of the blood is referred to as _____ formula
35. A cardiac contractile protein used in the diagnosis of myocardial infarction
37. The coronary artery that supplies the right atrium, right ventricle, and inferior wall of the left ventricle
39. A cardiac muscle fiber
41. These receptors are located in the heart and stimulation increases heart rate, contractility, and conductivity
43. The two important factors in coronary artery perfusion are time and _____
44. The coronary artery that supplies blood to the left atrium and the lateral left ventricle (abbrev.)
46. The outmost layer of the cardiac wall
48. Diastolic BP or PAOP (abbrev.)
50. Term for the contractile state of the heart, irrespective of preload
52. Jugular venous distention is an indication of increased preload of the _____ ventricle
53. The _____ fraction is the percentage of blood that was in the ventricle at the end of diastole that was pumped out during systole
55. The substance secreted by the kidney in response to hypoperfusion of the kidney
58. Pressure receptors

59. The valve that lies between the left atrium and the left ventricle
60. This type of cardiac cell has automaticity
61. Phase 3 of the action potential may be referred to as the ____ channel
63. Low pressure upper cardiac chambers
65. The branch of the autonomic nervous system that maintains a steady state
67. Parasympathetic stimulation is frequently referred to as _____ stimulation
69. The "powerhouse" of the cell, which uses nutrients and oxygen to make ATP
70. The effect on conductivity
71. The measured parameter used to evaluate left ventricular preload
72. These receptors are located in the vessels, and stimulation causes vasoconstriction
74. The _____ potential must be met for depolarization to occur
76. The effect of venous return on the heart which stretches the myofibrils and therefore determines the force of the next contraction
77. During this subphase of diastole and systole, no blood is moving
81. This middle layer of the artery becomes calcified in arteriosclerosis limiting the ability of the artery to dilate
83. The branches of the intraventricular conduction system are referred to as ____
84. Cellular energy (abbrev.)
85. This circulation consists of interarterial vessels that anastomose with each other as the result of gradual coronary artery occlusion
87. Phase 2 of the action potential is referred to as the ____ channel
88. Inflammation or infarction of this layer of the heart is associated with contractility problems

2. Identify the coronary artery that usually supplies the following structures. Identify the coronary artery as LAD (left anterior descending artery), LCA (left circumflex artery), or RCA (right coronary artery).

Structure	Coronary Artery
Anterior left ventricle	
AV node	
Bundle branches	
Inferior left ventricle	
Lateral left ventricle	
Left atrium	
Posterior left ventricle	
Right atrium	
Right ventricle	
SA node	
Septum	

3. Identify the determinants of myocardial oxygen supply and myocardial oxygen demand.

Myocardial Oxygen Supply	Myocardial Oxygen Demand

4. Identify the *primary* factor or factors affected in each condition and the primary effect or effects of each treatment; indicate increase or decrease of heart rate, preload, afterload, or contractility by appropriate arrows (↑ or ↓). (NOTE: Sympathetic nervous system responses may be seen in any of these conditions, but they are secondary, not primary.)

Conditions				
Aortic stenosis	___Heart rate	___Preload	___Afterload	___Contractility
Bradydysrhythmias	___Heart rate	___Preload	___Afterload	___Contractility
Cardiac tamponade	___Heart rate	___Preload	___Afterload	___Contractility
Cardiogenic shock	___Heart rate	___Preload	___Afterload	___Contractility
Cardiomyopathy	___Heart rate	___Preload	___Afterload	___Contractility
Heart failure	___Heart rate	___Preload	___Afterload	___Contractility

Conditions—cont'd				
Hypertension	___Heart rate	___Preload	___Afterload	___Contractility
Hypovolemia	___Heart rate	___Preload	___Afterload	___Contractility
Left ventricular myocardial infarction	___Heart rate	___Preload	___Afterload	___Contractility
Neurogenic shock	___Heart rate	___Preload	___Afterload	___Contractility
Pulmonary hypertension	___Heart rate	___Preload	___Afterload	___Contractility
Right ventricular myocardial infarction	___Heart rate	___Preload	___Afterload	___Contractility
Septic shock—early	___Heart rate	___Preload	___Afterload	___Contractility
Septic shock—late	___Heart rate	___Preload	___Afterload	___Contractility
Tachydysrhythmias	___Heart rate	___Preload	___Afterload	___Contractility
Treatments				
Aminophylline	___Heart rate	___Preload	___Afterload	___Contractility
Digoxin	___Heart rate	___Preload	___Afterload	___Contractility
Dobutamine	___Heart rate	___Preload	___Afterload	___Contractility
Dopamine (3–5 mcg/kg/min)	___Heart rate	___Preload	___Afterload	___Contractility
Dopamine (5–10 mcg/kg/min)	___Heart rate	___Preload	___Afterload	___Contractility
Dopamine (>10 mcg/kg/min)	___Heart rate	___Preload	___Afterload	___Contractility
Fluid challenge	___Heart rate	___Preload	___Afterload	___Contractility
Furosemide	___Heart rate	___Preload	___Afterload	___Contractility
Intraaortic balloon pump	___Heart rate	___Preload	___Afterload	___Contractility
Isoproterenol	___Heart rate	___Preload	___Afterload	___Contractility
Milrinone	___Heart rate	___Preload	___Afterload	___Contractility
Nesiritide	___Heart rate	___Preload	___Afterload	___Contractility
Nitroglycerin	___Heart rate	___Preload	___Afterload	___Contractility
Nitroprusside	___Heart rate	___Preload	___Afterload	___Contractility
Phenylephrine	___Heart rate	___Preload	___Afterload	___Contractility
Propranolol	___Heart rate	___Preload	___Afterload	___Contractility
Vasopressin	___Heart Rate	___Preload	___Afterload	___Contractility

5. Match the receptor of the sympathetic nervous system with its physiologic effect.

____ 1.	Increase in heart rate, contractility, conductivity	a. Alpha$_1$
____ 2.	Dilation of the renal and mesenteric arteries	b. Beta$_1$
____ 3.	Vasoconstriction	c. Beta$_2$
____ 4.	Vasodilation and bronchodilation	d. Dopaminergic
		e. Vasopressin$_1$

6. Identify which of these sympathomimetic (adrenergic) drugs cause the most powerful stimulation of each of these receptors.

____ 1.	Alpha$_1$	a. Albuterol
____ 2.	Beta$_1$	b. Fenoldopam
____ 3.	Beta$_2$	c. Phenylephrine
____ 4.	Dopaminergic	d. Dobutamine

7. Identify the formula for each of these parameters.

Parameter	Formula
a. Cardiac output (CO)	
b. Stroke index (SI)	
c. Blood pressure (BP)	
d. Coronary artery perfusion pressure (CAPP)	
e. Mean arterial pressure (MAP)	
f. Systemic vascular resistance (SVR)	
g. Delivery of oxygen to the tissues (DO_2)	

8. Match the heart sound to possible cause.

Heart Sound	Possible Causes
___ 1. S_1 ___ 2. S_2 ___ 3. Physiologic split of S_2 ___ 4. Paradoxical split of S_2 ___ 5. Fixed, wide split of S_2 ___ 6. S_3 ___ 7. S_4 ___ 8. Pericardial friction rub ___ 9. Midsystolic click ___ 10. Holosystolic murmur ___ 11. Systolic ejection murmur ___ 12. Early diastolic murmur ___ 13. Mid- to late-diastolic murmur	a. Changes in intrathoracic pressure created by ventilation b. Atrial septal defect; acute pulmonary hypertension; pulmonic stenosis c. Pericarditis d. Aortic stenosis; pulmonic stenosis e. Mitral stenosis; tricuspid stenosis f. LBBB; right ventricular pacemaker or ectopy; severe aortic valve disease; patent ductus arteriosus g. Mitral regurgitation; tricuspid regurgitation; ventricular septal defect h. HF; fluid overload; cardiomyopathy; ventricular septal defect; patent ductus arteriosus i. Closure of aortic and pulmonic valves j. Mitral valve prolapse; mitral regurgitation k. Closure of mitral and tricuspid valves l. Aortic regurgitation; pulmonic regurgitation m. Myocardial ischemia or infarction; hypertension; ventricular hypertrophy; AV block; severe aortic or pulmonic stenosis

9. Complete the following table describing common murmurs.

Condition	Timing	Location	Pitch
Mitral regurgitation			
Mitral stenosis			
Aortic regurgitation			
Aortic stenosis			
Mitral valve prolapse			
Papillary muscle dysfunction or rupture			
Ventricular septal defect or rupture			

10. Match the dysrhythmia to the appropriate characteristic.

____	1. Normal sinus rhythm	a.	PR interval greater than 0.2 second
____	2. Sinus bradycardia	b.	Early P wave which looks different from other P waves followed by normal QRS
____	3. Sinus tachycardia	c.	Sawtooth waves on baseline, no clearly identifiable P waves, normal QRS
____	4. Premature atrial contraction	d.	QRS is early, greater than 0.12 sec, with T wave in opposite direction of QRS
____	5. Atrial fibrillation	e.	Regular rhythm, normal P waves, normal QRS complexes, rate less than 60 unit/min
____	6. Atrial flutter	f.	Quivering baseline, irregularly irregular occurring QRSs.
____	7. Supraventricular tachycardia	g.	QRS complex is early with inverted P wave immediately (less than 0.12 sec) before the QRS, in the QRS or immediately after the QRS
____	8. Premature junctional contraction		
____	9. Junctional escape rhythm	h.	Regular rhythm with rate of 40 to 60 unit/min with narrow QRS with inverted P wave immediately (<0.12 sec) before the QRS, in the QRS or immediately after the QRS
____	10. Accelerated junctional rhythm		
____	11. Junctional tachycardia	i.	Flat line, no QRS complexes
____	12. Premature ventricular complex	j.	Regular rhythm, normal P waves, normal QRS complexes, rate greater than 100 unit/min
____	13. Accelerated idioventricular rhythm	k.	Regular rhythm, normal P waves, normal QRS complexes, rate 60 to 100 unit/min
____	14. Ventricular tachycardia	l.	Progressive PR lengthening until a P wave is not followed by a QRS
____	15. Ventricular fibrillation	m.	Regular rhythm with rate of 60 to 100 unit/min with narrow QRS with inverted P wave immediately (<0.12 sec) before the QRS, in the QRS or immediately after the QRS
____	16. Asystole		
____	17. First-degree AV block	n.	Wide QRS (>0.12 sec) rhythm with rate of 40 to 100 unit/min
____	18. Second-degree AV block, type I	o.	Regular rhythm with rate of greater than 100 unit/min with narrow QRS with inverted P wave immediately (<0.12 sec) before the QRS, in the QRS or immediately after the QRS
____	19. Second-degree AV block, type II		
____	20. Third-degree AV block	p.	Regular rhythm with rate 150 to 250/min without clearly discernible P waves with narrow QRS
		q.	P wave not followed by QRS without preceding progression of PR interval
		r.	No relationship between P waves and QRS complexes; escape rhythm established by AV junction or ventricle
		s.	Irregular baseline, absence of QRS complexes
		t.	Wide QRS (>0.12 sec) rhythm with rate greater than 100/min

11. Analyze the following ECG rhythm strips. All strips are 6 seconds.
    a.

    Interpretation

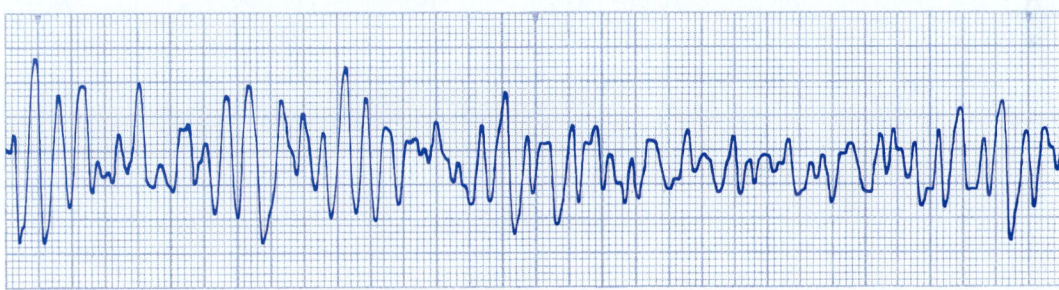

   b.

   Interpretation

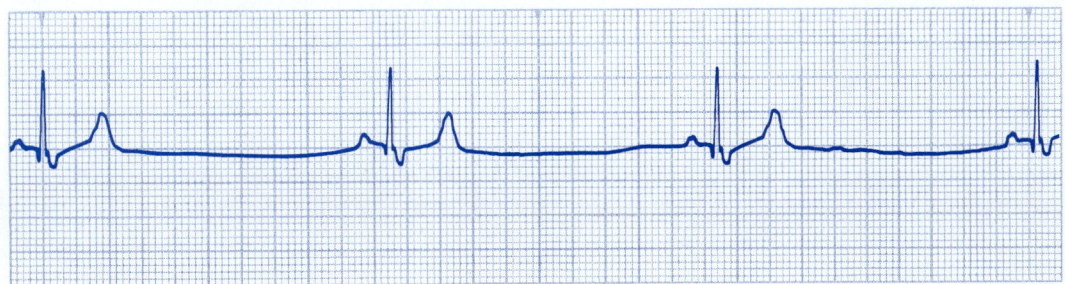

c.

Interpretation

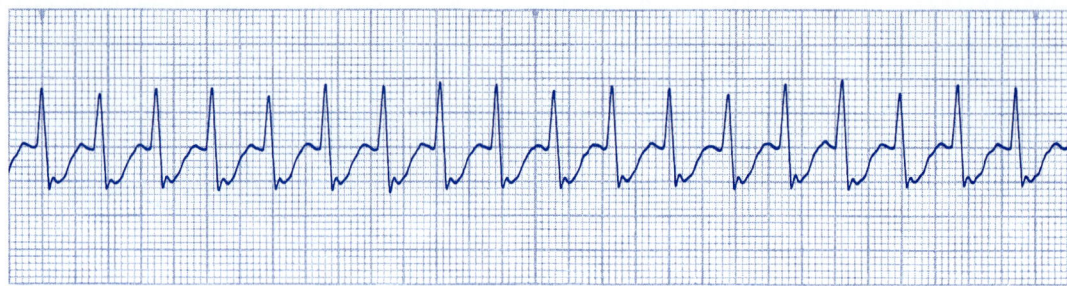

d.

Interpretation

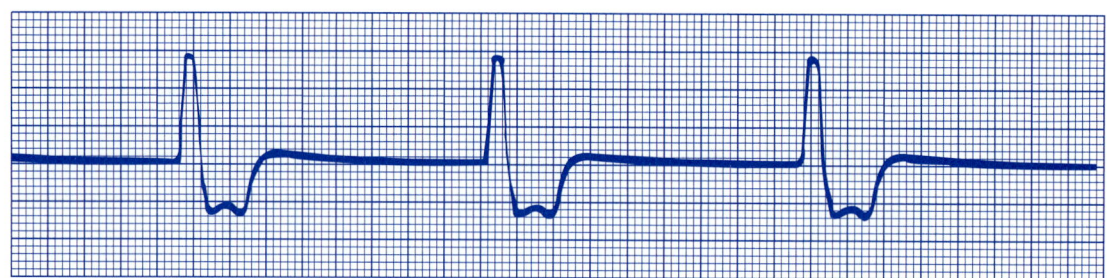

e.

Interpretation

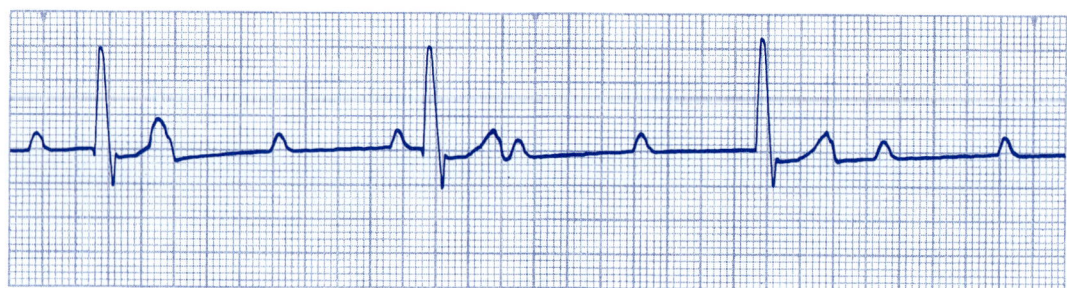

f.

Interpretation

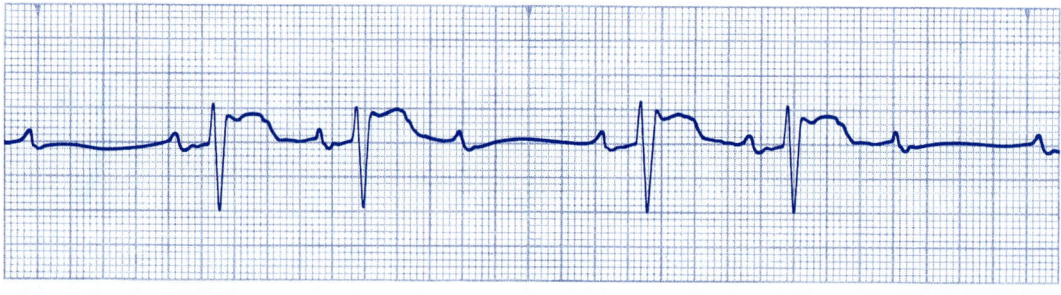

g.
Interpretation

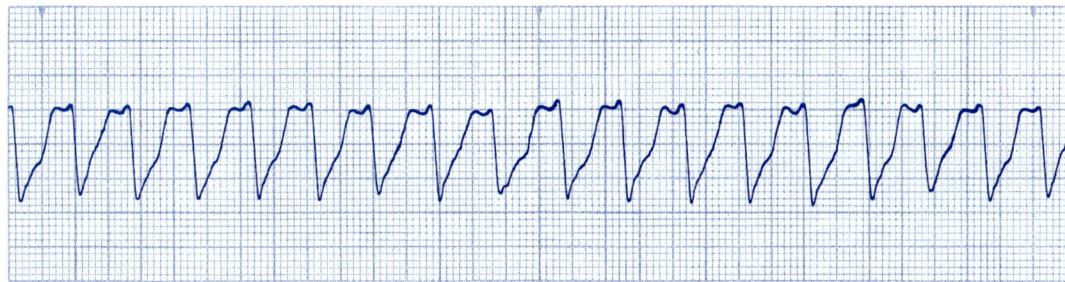

h.
Interpretation

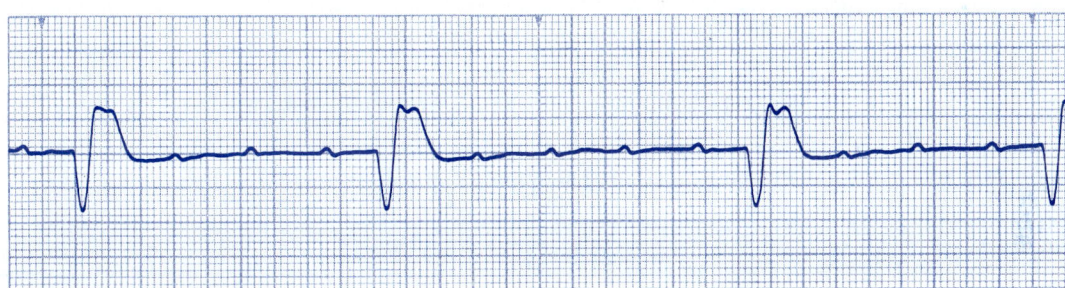

i.
Interpretation

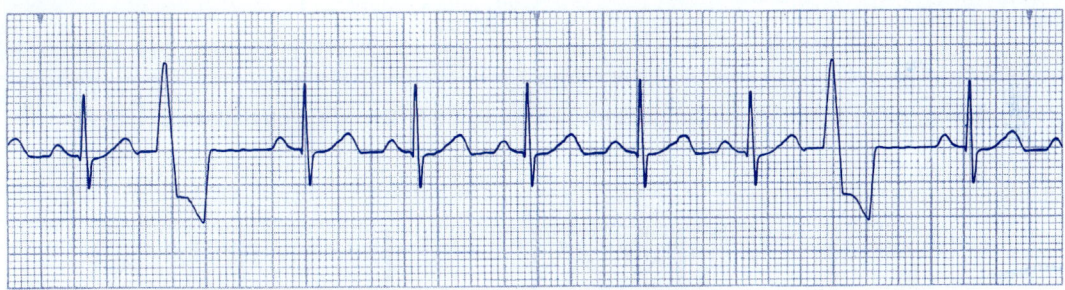

12. Match the following cardiovascular conditions to their major ECG diagnostic features.

Condition	ECG Diagnostic Features
____ 1. Acute myocardial infarction	a. Symmetrically, deeply inverted T waves in V_2, V_3 with little or no ST-segment elevation
____ 2. Hypercalcemia	b. Prolonged QT, prolonged ST segment
____ 3. Hyperkalemia	c. R wave larger than S wave in V_1, V_2, S wave larger than R wave in V_5, V_6, right axis deviation, ST-T wave changes in V_1, V_2
____ 4. Hypocalcemia	
____ 5. Hypokalemia	d. Diffuse ST-segment elevation across the precordium
____ 6. Left atrial enlargement	e. Wide (>0.11 second), notched P wave in lead II, dominant terminal component of P wave in V_1
____ 7. Left bundle branch block	f. Wide (0.12 sec or greater than) QRS below the baseline in V_1
____ 8. Left ventricular hypertrophy	g. Q waves at least 0.04 second wide and/or ¼ height of R wave along with ST-segment elevation and symmetrically inverted T waves
____ 9. Pericarditis	
____ 10. Variant angina	h. Increased QRS amplitude, left axis deviation, ST-T wave changes in V_5, V_6
____ 11. Right atrial enlargement	i. Wide (0.12 sec or greater than) QRS above the baseline in V_1
____ 12. Right bundle branch block	j. Tall (>2.5 mm) peaked P wave in lead II, dominant initial component of P wave in V_1
____ 13. Right ventricular hypertrophy	k. Shortened QT, shortened ST segment
____ 14. Wellens syndrome	l. Flat T waves, prominent U wave, ST segment depression
	m. ST-segment elevation with pain
	n. Tall peaked T waves, widening of QRS complex, atrial asystole

13. Match the cardiac wall to the lead grouping that is used to evaluate that wall.

Lead Groupings	Cardiac Wall
____ 1. II, III, aVF	a. Anterior
____ 2. V_{4R}	b. Lateral (high)
____ 3. I, aVL	c. Lateral (low)
____ 4. V_1, V_2	d. Posterior
____ 5. V_3, V_4	e. Right ventricular
____ 6. V_5, V_6	f. Septal
____ 7. V_8, V_9	g. Inferior

14. Analyze the following 12-lead ECGs for bundle branch block. Identify if left or right bundle branch block.
    a.

    Interpretation:

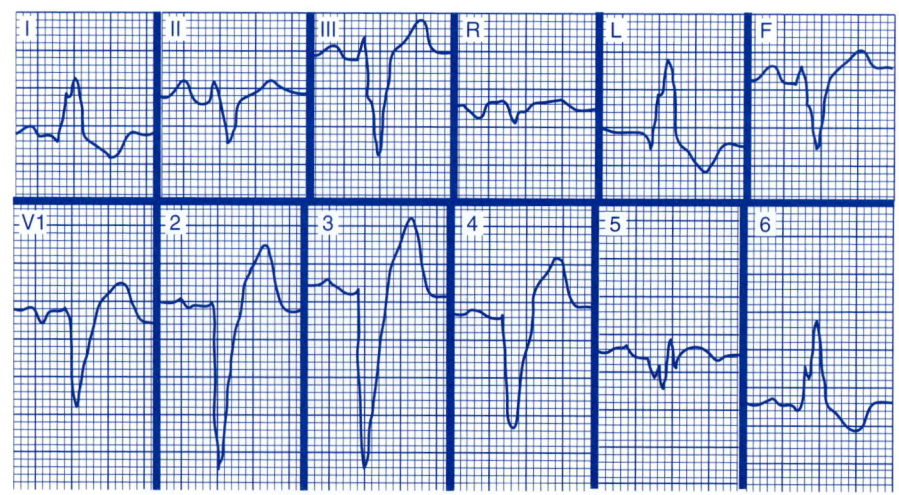

b.

Interpretation:

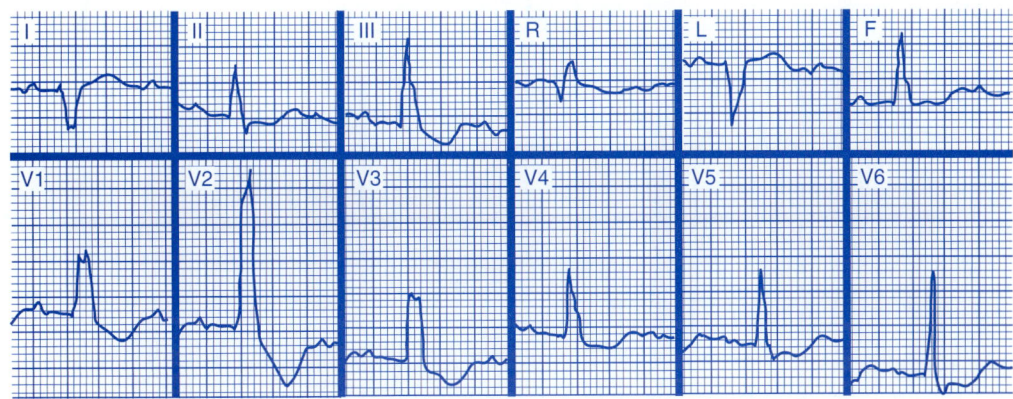

15. Analyze the following 12-lead ECGs for atrial enlargement or ventricular hypertrophy.

    a.

    Interpretation

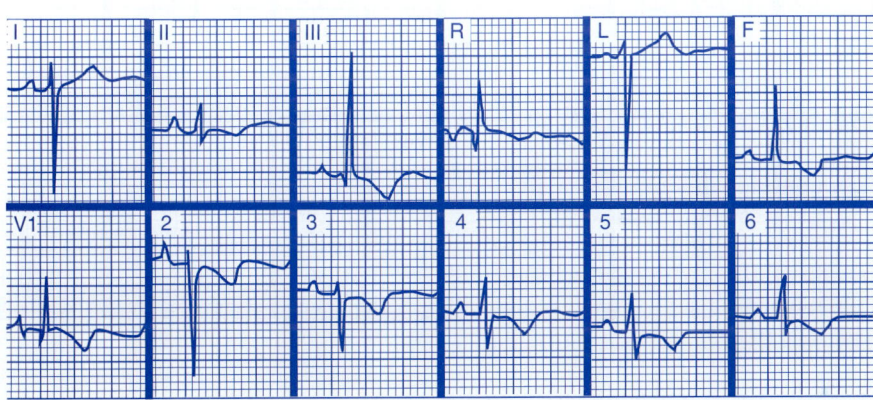

    b.

    Interpretation:

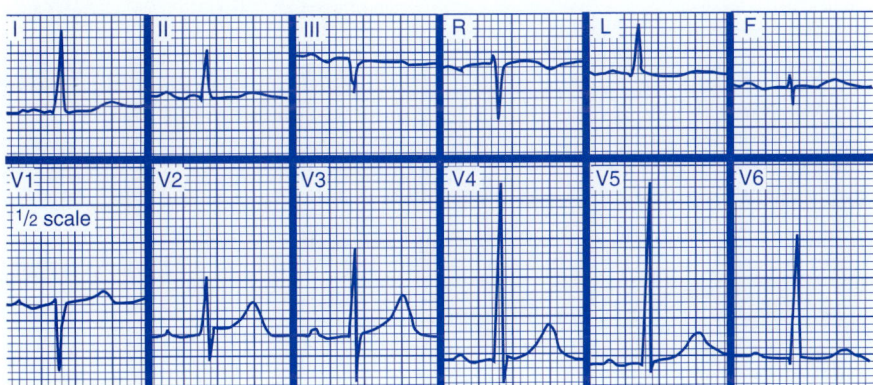

16. Analyze the following 12-lead ECGs from patients with acute chest pain for indications of MI. Identify location and age of MI if present.

    a.

    Interpretation:

    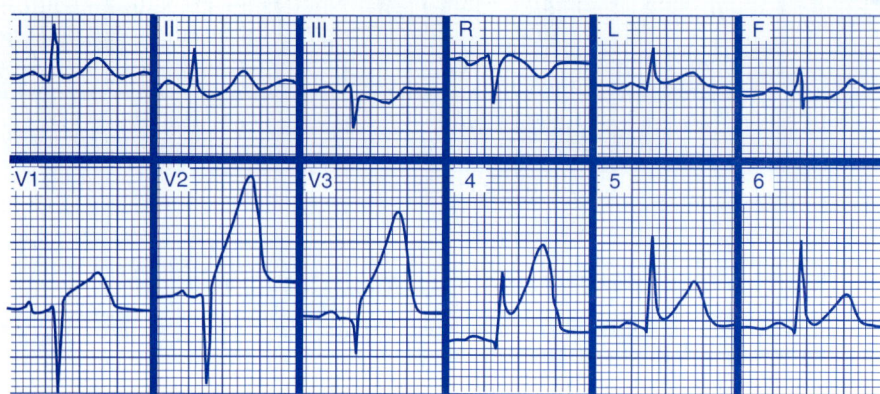

b.

Interpretation:

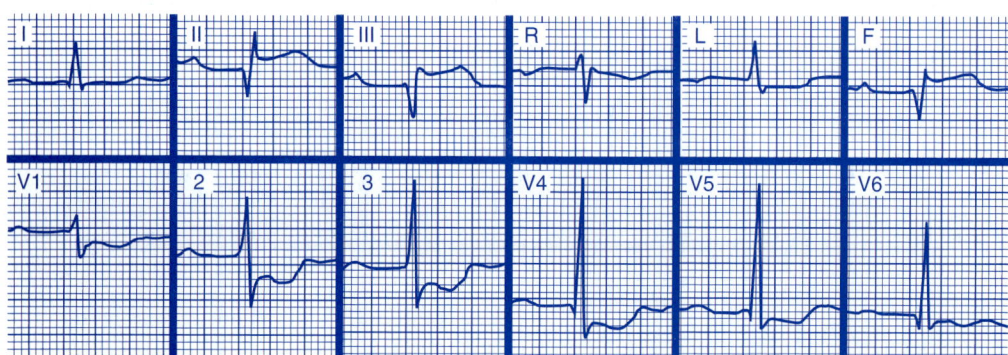

17. Complete the following crossword puzzle dealing with hemodynamic monitoring.

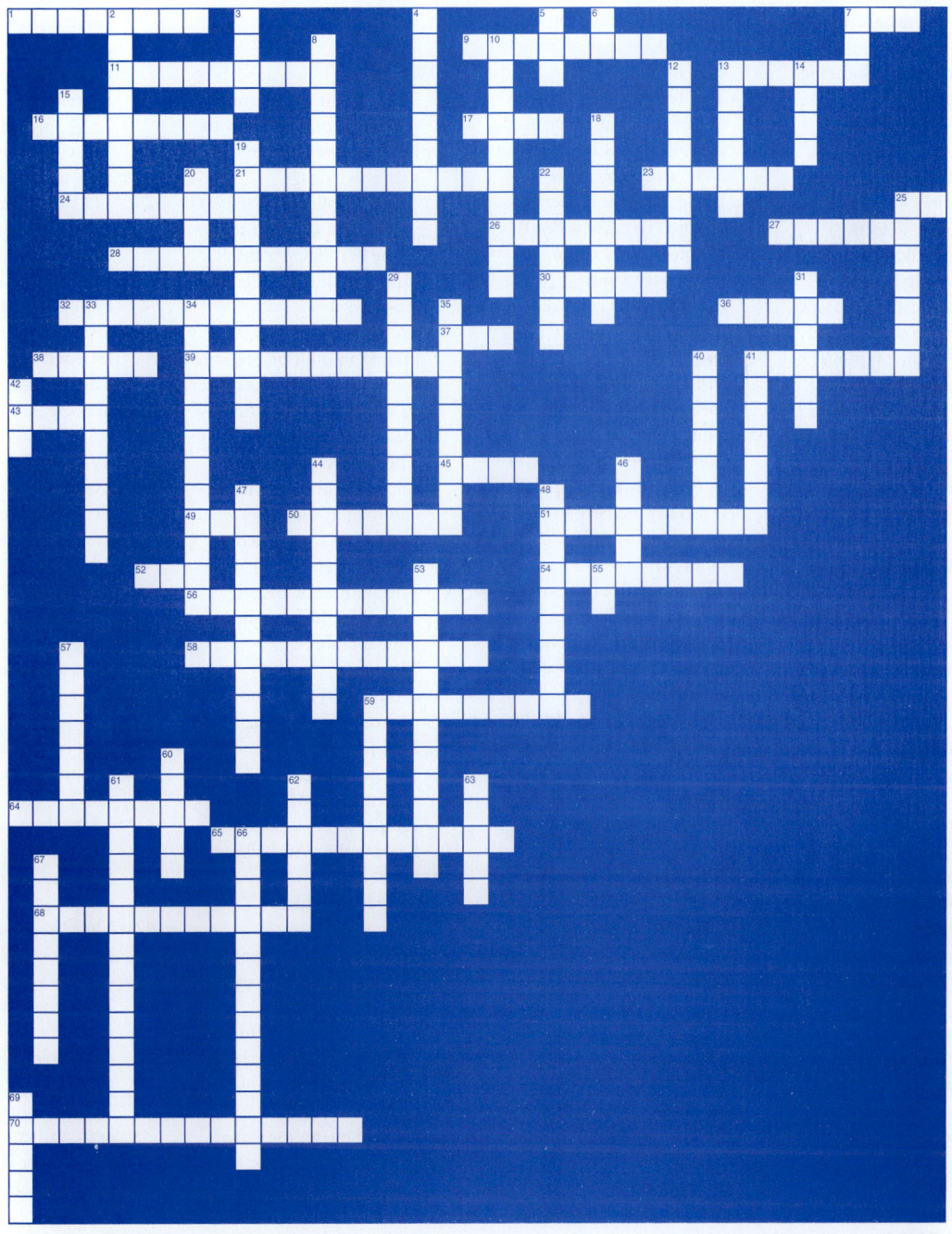

Chapter 3 The Cardiovascular System

ACROSS

1. PAP is measured with the balloon at the distal end of the PAC _____
7. Right ventricular volumetric monitoring is performed using this type of catheter (abbrev.)
9. The relaxation phase of the cardiac cycle
11. Gastric _____ detects regional alterations in tissue perfusion using gastric intramucosal carbon dioxide
13. Oxygen ___ is when the O_2 saturation in the pulmonary artery is higher than in the right atrium; indication of ventricular septal rupture
16. The ___ notch of the PA waveform represents closure of the pulmonic valve
17. Diastolic BP minus PAOP (abbrev.)
21. This type of monitoring is the monitoring of blood flow generally through the use of invasive catheters
23. The most common site for arterial catheters for monitoring of blood pressure
24. DO_2 is an abbreviation for oxygen ___
25. The amount of blood ejected from the heart each beat (abbrev.)
26. Rupture of the ventricular septum results in an _____ in SvO_2
27. Indications of PAC migration back into the right ventricle include loss of dicrotic notch, decrease in diastolic pressure, and ___
28. This type of shock results in decreased CO, decreased RAP, PAP, PAOP, increased SVR and tachycardia
30. The *a* wave of the PAOP waveform represents contraction of the ___
32. Air in the pleural space; a potential complication of central venous catheter insertion
36. ___ nerve palsy occurs when the wrist is maintained in hyperextended position
37. The pressure in the superior vena cava (abbrev.)
38. An intermittent ___ device maintains patency of a catheter by delivering a minimal amount of solution each hour
39. This type of shock results in decreased CO, increased RAP, PAP, PAOP, increased SVR, and tachycardia
41. Using more air than required to cause a PAOP waveform may cause pulmonary artery ___ manifested by massive hemoptysis
43. In-___ calibration of a SvO_2 catheter is done with the catheter inside the body
45. This therapy is particularly useful when a patient with significantly elevated SVR is too hypotensive to safely use arterial vasodilators (abbrev.)
49. This type of cardiac output monitoring allows for less risk of contamination and frequently updated values (abbrev.)
50. This drug may be added to flush solution to prevent catheter occlusion
51. The *v* wave of the PAOP waveform represents contraction of the ___
52. The average blood pressure over time (abbrev.)
54. This device records the pressure waveform on paper for analysis
56. ___ of pressures (RAP, PAd, PAOP) is an indication of cardiac tamponade
58. Pulmonary ___ is evidenced by PVR greater than 250 dynes/sec/cm^{-5}, PA mean greater than 20 mm Hg, and difference between PAd and PAOP is 5 mm Hg or greater
59. This device increases the magnitude of an electrical signal and filters out electrical interference
64. The phlebostatic axis is at the fourth ICS and ___; correlates with the location of the right atrium
65. This type of shock results in decreased CO, decreased RAP, PAP, PAOP, decreased SVR, and tachycardia
68. Zeroing the transducer negates the effect of ___ pressure
70. This fatal complication can result from disconnection of an arterial line

DOWN

2. This type of monitoring is indicated for patients with hypertensive crisis or on vasoactive drugs
3. The determination of best ____ is the ___ that results in the best SaO_2 without dropping the CO/CI (abbrev.)
4. To ___ a transducer, a known amount of pressure is exerted on the transducer to see that the pressure is measured correctly
5. The derived parameter calculated by using height and weight; used in calculation of indexed parameters (abbrev.)
6. The amount of blood ejected by the heart in 1 minute (abbrev.)
7. The parameter that is measured from the proximal port of the PAC (abbrev.)
8. The major cause of a decrease in RAP, PAP, and PAOP
10. Leaving the PAC balloon inflated or a spontaneous wedge may cause pulmonary ___
12. PAOP is measured with the balloon at the distal end of the PAC _____
13. $ScvO_2$ is advocated to be used in this type of shock to evaluate the optimization of oxygen delivery
14. The parameter measured from the distal tip of the PAC with the balloon inflated; indirectly measures LAP (abbrev.)
15. SvO_2 may be evaluated by drawing a ___ venous blood gas
18. This type of calibration of an SvO_2 catheter ensures that the oximeter values are consistent with mixed venous oxygen saturation
19. Lymph fluid in the pleural space; a potential complication of central venous catheter insertion
20. To ___ the transducer, it is opened to air and the baseline on the monitor and the numeric value is adjusted
22. Elevated blood levels of _____ indicate hypoxia
25. The contraction phase of the cardiac cycle
29. The device that converts a mechanical signal to an electrical signal
31. When the dicrotic notch on the PA waveform is lost and the amplitude is lessened
33. This type of shock results in decreased CO, decreased RAP, PAP, PAOP, decreased SVR, and bradycardia
34. This device displays the electrical signal as a pressure waveform and a numerical value
35. Inflation of the balloon at the distal tip of the PAC causes ___ and blocks right heart pressures to allow measurement of left heart pressure
40. This type of response test ensures adequate damping of a pressure monitoring system using the square wave test
41. SvO_2 is a reflection of oxygen ___
42. The calculated parameter indicative of left ventricular afterload (abbrev.)
44. The lumen of the PAC that measures the temperature of the blood in the pulmonary artery
46. In-___ calibration of an SvO_2 catheter is done with the catheter outside the body
47. VO_2 is an abbreviation for oxygen ___
48. To ___ a PAC is to use more air than is required to cause a PAOP waveform
53. This type of technology allows for the noninvasive measurement of cardiac output through cutaneous sensors
55. The amount of blood ejected by the heart in 1 minute and indexed to body size (abbrev.)
57. The stretch on the myofibrils that determines the force of the next contraction

59. Represents the pressure required to open the semilunar valve
60. The calculated parameter indicative of left ventricular contractility and indexed to body size (abbrev.)
61. Technique for measuring cardiac output
62. This early stage of this type of shock results in increased CO, decreased RAP, PAP, PAOP, decreased SVR, and tachycardia
63. Excessive artifact on the PA waveform caused by excessive movement of the catheter
66. _____ assessment of the limb with an arterial line is important in the detection of acute arterial occlusion
67. The original brand name of PAC (2 words)
69. The air-fluid interface of the transducer must be ___ with the phlebostatic axis

18. Match the pathologic condition with its hemodynamic profile.

___ 1. Cardiac tamponade	a. ↑RAP, ↓PAOP, ↓CO/CI, SvO_2, DO_2
___ 2. Noncardiogenic pulmonary edema	b. ↑PAP and PAOP, ↑SvO_2, large v waves on PAOP waveform, falsely ↑CO/CI, new systolic murmur at lower left sternal border
___ 3. Cardiogenic pulmonary edema	c. ↑PAP and PAOP, large v waves on PAOP waveform, new systolic murmur at apex
___ 4. Rupture of interventricular septum	d. PAd, PVR, PAm are all ↑ and the difference between PAd and PAOP is greater than 5 mm Hg
___ 5. Pulmonary hypertension	e. ↓RAP, PAP, PAOP, ↑SVR, ↓CO/CI, SvO_2, DO_2
___ 6. Papillary muscle rupture	f. ↑RAP, PAP, PAOP, ↑SVR, ↓SaO_2, SvO_2, DO_2
___ 7. Right ventricular MI	g. ↑PAP and PAOP, crackles, ↓SaO_2, SvO_2, DO_2
___ 8. Cardiogenic shock	h. ↑PAP, normal or decreased PAOP, crackles, ↓SaO_2, SvO_2, DO_2
___ 9. Hypovolemic shock	i. RAP, PAd, and PAOP are all ↑ and within 5 mm Hg of one another, large a and large v waves on PAOP waveform, ↓CO/CI, SvO_2, DO_2

19. Identify whether the parameters in these case studies are decreased, normal, or increased. Discuss implications and treatment goals.
    a. Patient A is a 44-year-old man who was transported to the emergency department (ED) after having chest pain for 6 hours. He had ST segment elevation from V_2 to V_6. He also has a history of two previous MIs, and the ECG shows a previous inferior MI. The next day, Q waves are noted from V_2 to V_6 despite fibrinolytic therapy administered in the ED. He is now hypotensive with an S_3 audible at his cardiac apex and crackles audible in his lung bases. Urine output has been marginal for the past 2 hours. The physician inserts a PAC to allow better evaluation of current status as well as response to therapy. The patient's BSA is 1.7 m²

Parameter	↑, ↓, or Normal	Parameter	↑, ↓, or Normal
BP: 88/70 mm Hg		SV: 23 ml/beat	
MAP: 76 mm Hg		SI: 14 ml/m²/beat	
HR: 128 beats/min		SVR: 1813 dynes/sec/cm⁻⁵	
RAP: 8 mm Hg		SVRI: 3022 dynes/sec/cm⁻⁵	
PAP: 42/26 mm Hg		PVR: 240 dynes/sec/cm⁻⁵	
PAm: 31 mm Hg		PVRI: 400 dynes/sec/cm⁻⁵	
PAOP: 22 mm Hg		LVSWI: 10.3 g m/m²	
CO: 3.0 l/min		RVSWI: 2.7 g m/m²	
CI: 1.8 l/min/m²		SvO_2: 51%	
SaO_2: 88% on 5 l/min via nasal cannula		DO_2I: 318 ml/min/m²	

b. Patient B is a 52-year-old being admitted to the critical care unit after surgery for repair of hemothorax after a gunshot wound. The postanesthesia care unit nurse gives you a report of massive blood loss before surgery; estimated blood loss in the operating room was 1 l. He has had 5 l of lactated Ringer solution and 2 units of packed red blood cells. Past medical history includes MI 5 years ago and angioplasty 2 years ago for intractable angina. A PAC was inserted before surgery to evaluate fluid status and cardiac function and to aid in fluid resuscitation. The patient's BSA is 1.9 m².

Chapter 3 The Cardiovascular System

Parameter	↑, ↓, or Normal	Parameter	↑, ↓, or Normal
BP: 92/70 mm Hg		SV: 24 ml/beat	
MAP: 77 mm Hg		SI: 13 ml/m^2/beat	
HR: 122 beats/min		SVR: 2097 dynes/sec/cm^{-5}	
RAP: 1 mm Hg		SVRI: 4053 dynes/sec/cm^{-5}	
PAP: 20/6 mm Hg		PVR: 221 dynes/sec/cm^{-5}	
PAm: 11 mm Hg		PVRI: 427 dynes/sec/cm^{-5}	
PAOP: 3 mm Hg		LVSWI: 13.1 g m/m^2	
CO: 2.9 l/min		RVSWI: 1.8 g m/m^2	
CI: 1.5 l/min/m^2		SvO$_2$: 50%	
SaO$_2$: 98% on 5 l/min via nasal cannula		DO$_2$I: 138 ml/min/m^2	
Hgb: 7 g/dl			

20. Match the dysrhythmia with the most appropriate treatment summary. You may choose an answer more than once.

____ 1. Ventricular fibrillation	a. BLS, epinephrine
____ 2. Stable monomorphic ventricular tachycardia	b. Treatment of cause, beta-blockers or sedatives
____ 3. Asystole	c. Cardioversion or amiodarone or ibutilide
____ 4. Symptomatic bradycardia	d. Vagal maneuvers and adenosine, calcium channel blocker, beta-blocker
____ 5. Pulseless electrical activity	e. Magnesium, overdrive pacing, isoproterenol
____ 6. Stable SVT	f. BLS, defibrillation, epinephrine, amiodarone
____ 7. Acute onset atrial fibrillation	g. Procainamide, amiodarone, or lidocaine
____ 8. Pulseless ventricular tachycardia	h. Transcutaneous pacing or atropine
____ 9. Junctional tachycardia	i. BLS, assess for possible causes, epinephrine
____ 10. Complete heart block with ventricular escape rhythm	j. Vagal maneuvers, withhold digoxin, administration of adenosine, calcium channel blocker, or beta-blocker
____ 11. Sinus tachycardia	
____ 12. Torsades de pointes	

21. Complete the following table by identifying the Vaughn-Williams antidysrhythmic classification of the following drugs. Some drugs are of more than one class.

Drugs	Classification
Adenosine	
Amiodarone	
Atropine	
Digoxin	
Diltiazem	
Dofetilide	
Esmolol	
Flecainide	
Ibutilide	
Lidocaine	
Metoprolol	
Procainamide	
Propranolol	
Quinidine	
Sotalol	
Verapamil	

22. Complete the following calculations.
    a. Drug: dobutamine
       Dose: 5 mcg/kg/min
       Concentration: 500 mg/500 ml
       Patient's weight: 80 kg
       Rate: _____
    b. Drug: sodium nitroprusside
       Dose: _____
       Concentration: 50 mg/250 ml
       Patient's weight: 70 kg
       Rate: 45 ml/hr
    c. Drug: dopamine
       Dose: _____
       Concentration: 400 mg/250 ml
       Patient's weight: 70 kg
       Rate: 14 ml/hr
    d. Drug: dopamine
       Dose: 2 mcg/kg/min
       Concentration: 400 mg/500 ml
       Patient's weight: 70 kg
       Rate: _____
    e. Drug: nitroglycerin
       Dose: 50 mcg/min
       Concentration: 50 mg/500 ml
       Rate: _____
    f. Drug: lidocaine
       Dose: 3 mg/min
       Concentration: 2 g/500 ml
       Rate: _____

23. Complete the following table to identify the NAPSE code for the pacemaker that would have the capabilities of the others together.

AOO		VVI		a.
VVI		VAT		b.
AAI	VAT	VVI		c.

24. Complete the following puzzle on pacemaker terminology.

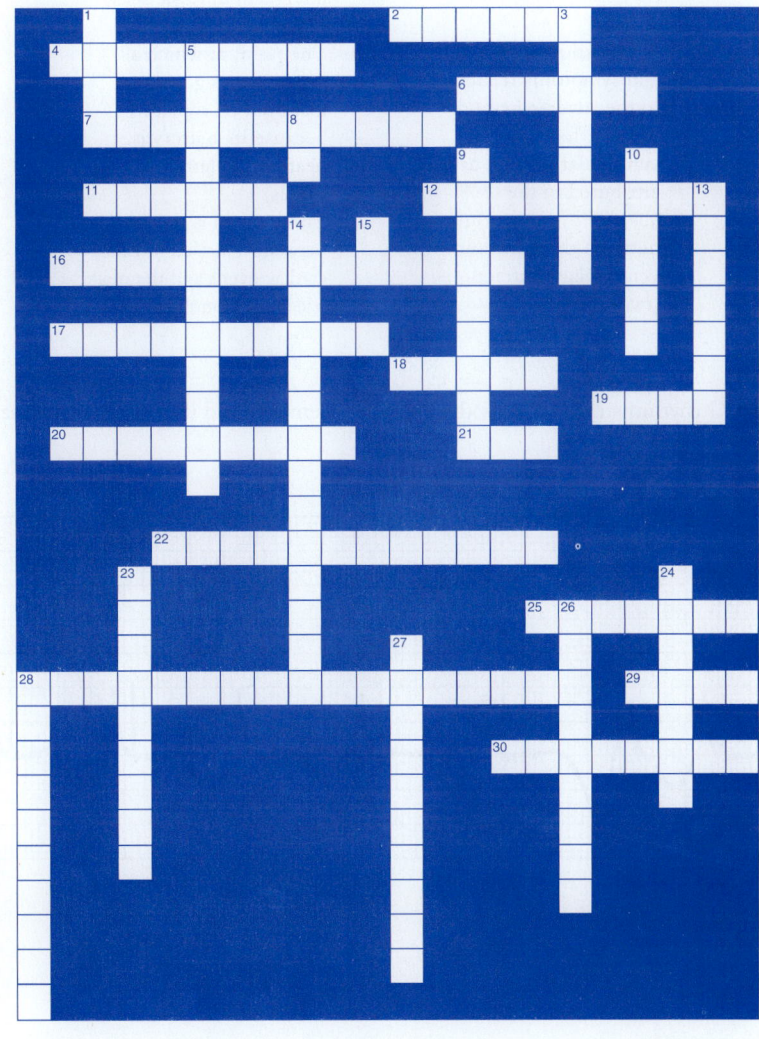

ACROSS

2. The electrical stimulus delivered by a pacemaker's pulse generator
4. The ability of the pacemaker to send information, (i.e., programmed status, measurements, signals) to the programmer
6. This type of pacemaker only discharges when the patient's heart rate drops below the preset rate for the pacemaker
7. This type of pacemaker is capable of stimulating the atria and ventricles (two words)
11. This type of beat results when an intrinsic depolarization and a paced depolarization occur simultaneously so both contribute to the depolarization
12. Inherent; belonging to or originating from the heart itself
16. The ability of a pacemaker to increase the pacing rate in response to physical activity and physiologic demand (two words)
17. A pacing parameter that allows a longer escape interval after a sensed event, allowing perpetuation of the patient's intrinsic rhythm
18. Another term for pacemaker artifact
19. This rate is the rate at which the pulse generator discharges when no intrinsic activity is detected
20. To deliver an electrical stimulus upon detecting a spontaneous depolarization
21. Radiated or conducted energy, either electrical or magnetic, that can interfere with or disrupt the function of a pulse generator (abbrev.)
22. A pulse generator with a pacing mode or parameters that can be changed noninvasively at any time by means of an external programmer
25. The ability of the pacemaker to detect the patient's intrinsic activity and respond appropriately by either triggering or inhibiting output
28. A collection of signs and symptoms related to the adverse hemodynamic effects of ventricular pacing, usually attributed to the absence of synchrony between the atrial and ventricular contractions (two words)
29. The manner in which a pacemaker provides artificial rate and rhythm support in the presence of dysrhythmia; identified by a three- or five-letter code
30. The spike recorded on the ECG depicting the electrical energy discharge from the pulse generator

DOWN

1. The wire or wires which carry electrical signals to and from the heart, a connector pin, and stimulating, sensing electrode(s)
3. When ventricular pacing is synchronized to sensed atrial activity
5. The unit of measurement used for electrical stimulus (i.e., output) generated by a pacemaker
8. This interval in dual-chamber pacing is analogous to the PR interval in intrinsic activity (abbrev.)
9. The point at which a pacemaker signals that it should be replaced because its battery is nearing depletion (three words)
10. This interval is the time between a sensed intrinsic cardiac event and the next pacemaker output
13. Successful depolarization of the atria or ventricles by an artificial pacemaker
14. This portion of the pacemaker system houses the power source and the circuitry for regulating the pacemaker (two words)
15. This interval in dual-chamber pacing is the interval between a sensed or ventricular paced event and the next atrial paced event (abbrev.)
23. The minimum amount of voltage, expressed in mA, required to obtain consistent capture
24. The lead has both positive and negative electrodes
26. The uninsulated conductive portion of a pacing lead which makes electrical contact with tissue
27. This mode of response to sensing indicates that the pacemaker output is suppressed when an intrinsic event is sensed
28. The duration of the pacing pulse expressed in millisecond; also called pulse duration (two words)

25. Analyze the following ECG rhythm strips. Identify the type of pacemaker and if there is a pacemaker malfunction.
    a.
    Interpretation

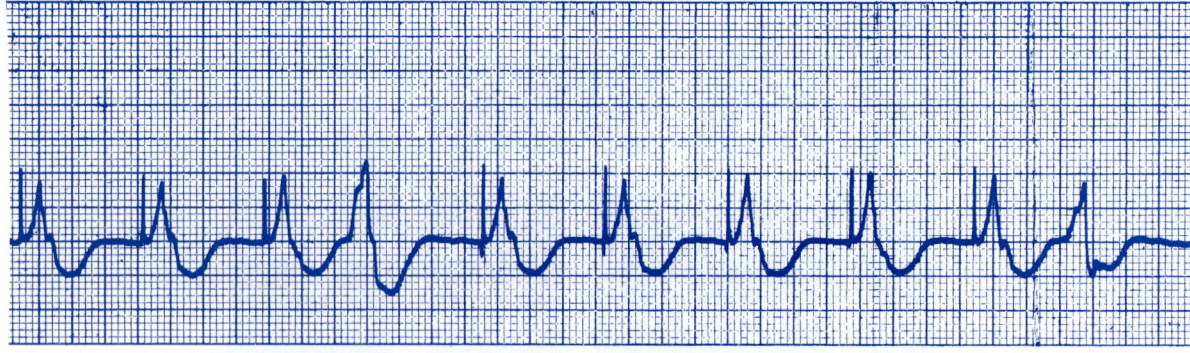

b.
Interpretation

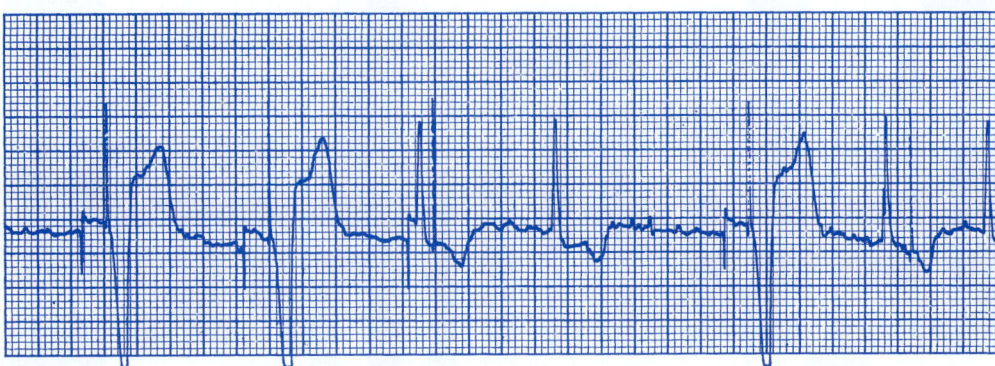

c.
Interpretation

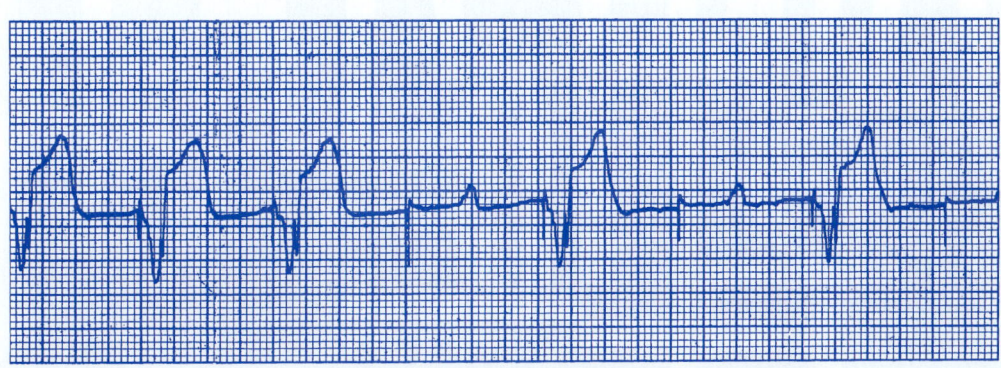

26. Complete the following table differentiating cardiac risk factors as nonmodifiable or modifiable.

Nonmodifiable	Modifiable

27. Match the following treatments for acute MI with rationales for use. More than one may apply.

___ 1. Fibrinolytics	a. Increases myocardial oxygen supply by reestablishing patency of the infarct-related artery
___ 2. Percutaneous coronary interventions (PCIs)	b. Decreases myocardial oxygen demand by blocking the effects of catecholamines
___ 3. ACE inhibitors	c. Increases myocardial oxygen supply by reducing spasm
___ 4. Nitroglycerin	d. Decreases myocardial oxygen demand by reducing preload
___ 5. Calcium channel blockers	e. Prevents extension of a clot by decreasing platelet aggregation
___ 6. Beta-blockers	f. Prevents extension of a clot by preventing the conversion of prothrombin to thrombin
___ 7. ASA	g. Prevents ventricular dilation and adverse remodeling of the myocardium
___ 8. Heparin	h. Used for secondary prevention after MI.
___ 9. Glycoprotein IIb/IIIa inhibitors	i. Decreases myocardial oxygen consumption by decreasing afterload
___ 10. Intraaortic balloon pump (IABP)	j. Increases myocardial oxygen supply by increasing coronary artery perfusion pressure

28. Complete the following crossword puzzle dealing with coronary artery disease and acute myocardial infarction.

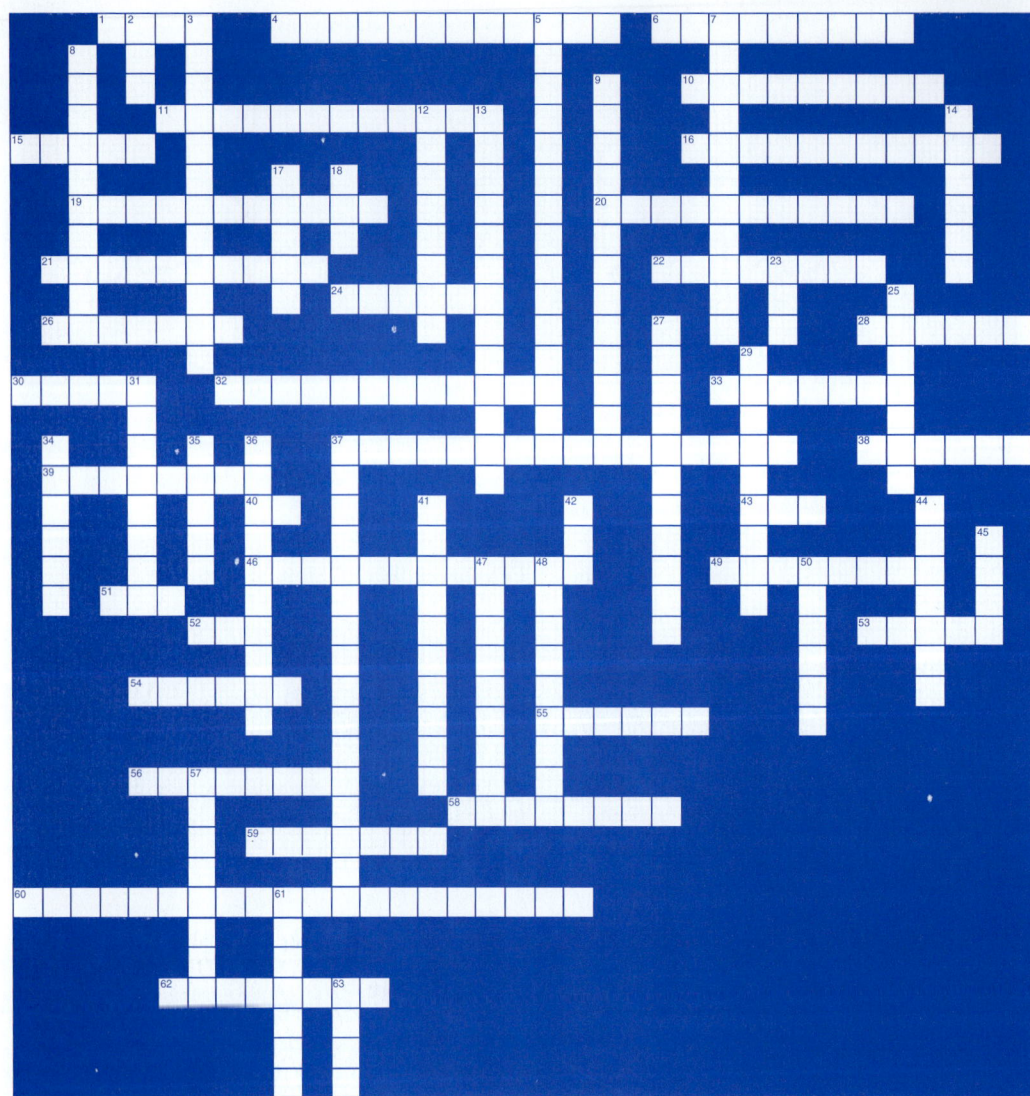

ACROSS

1. This device used to decrease afterload and increase myocardial perfusion in cardiogenic shock (abbrev.)
4. This tPA has a longer half-life than others and is administered as a single bolus
6. A GP IIb/IIIa inhibitor frequently used after PCI (generic)
10. Indicative leads for this cardiac wall are V_8 and V_9
11. The dysrhythmia most likely to cause death in MI patient is ventricular _____
15. Initial therapy for hemodynamic consequences of right ventricular MI
16. This drug is a direct thrombin inhibitor used as an alternative to heparin
19. This PCI procedure opens an occluded artery using a shaving device
20. This percutaneous coronary intervention (PCI) procedure opens an occluded artery using balloon dilation
21. This calcium channel blocker used for coronary artery spasm
22. The analgesic of choice for acute MI
24. The artery sometimes used for CABG that has a high spasm potential
26. An indirect thrombin inhibitor used to prevent extension of a clot or reocclusion
28. A new holosystolic murmur at lower sternum, increase SvO_2, and shock indicates rupture of the ___
30. Format for chest pain description
32. These drugs are used to prevent ventricular dysrhythmias post-MI and for secondary prevention
33. Indicative leads for this cardiac wall or I and aVL and/or V_5 and V_6
37. A group of diseases characterized by thickening and loss of elasticity (calcification) of arterial walls
38. Evidenced on ECG by ST-segment elevation
39. An activity that is likely to decrease body weight, BP, lipids, and stress
40. Death of myocardial tissue (abbrev.)
43. S_3, dyspnea, and crackles indicate what complication of acute MI (abbrev.)
46. The most common complication of MI
49. _____ syndrome is a late pericarditis that is thought to be an autoimmune response
51. The preferred method of reperfusion for acute MI (abbrev)
52. Bad cholesterol (abbrev.)

Chapter 3 The Cardiovascular System 247

53. These drugs are used to treat pericarditis (abbrev.)
54. Patients with diabetes mellitus are more likely to have this type of MI
55. Clenched fist held over the sternum with description of chest pain is referred to as _____ sign
56. Indicative leads for this cardiac wall are V_3 and V_4
58. Indicative leads for this cardiac wall are II, III, and aVF
59. Acute chest pain and/or ST-segment elevation after PCI may indicate acute ___
60. This risk factor for CAD treated with folic acid
62. New onset, crescendo, and variant are all categorized as this type of angina

DOWN

2. This platelet aggregation inhibitor is an important aspect of initial treatment of acute MI (abbrev.)
3. Elevated temperature, chest pain, and pericardial friction rub after MI indicates this complication
5. The most likely cause of acute MI
7. This oral platelet aggregation inhibitor frequently used for after PCI
8. The inotropic agent most likely to be used for cardiogenic shock with MI
9. This type of hemorrhage is a complication of fibrinolytics with dire consequences
12. Evidenced on ECG by T-wave inversion
13. Nitrate used for acute chest pain
14. CABG done through small thoracotomy incision used for LIMA-LAD anastomosis (abbrev.)
17. Device used during PCI to prevent closure
18. A value of greater than 30 if considered obese (abbrev.)
23. Good cholesterol (abbrev.)
25. This syndrome is characterized by chest pain with deep T-wave inversion in V_2, V_3 and associated with critical proximal LAD stenosis
27. This is evidenced by cessation of pain, ST-segment return to baseline, and dysrhythmias
29. Rupture of the ___ muscle causes acute mitral regurgitation; serious complication of acute MI
31. The internal mammary is now referred to as the internal ___
34. A major cause for delay in seeking assistance for chest pain
35. This coronary artery supplies RA, RV, and the inferior wall of LV
36. ACE inhibitors are used after MI to prevent this
37. A group of diseases characterized by thickening and loss of elasticity (calcification) of arterial walls
41. This cardioselective beta-blocker is often used for acute MI
42. The general term used for undifferentiated acute ischemic chest pain (abbrev.)
44. This type of angina is caused by spasm
45. Isolated right ventricular MI may be seen in patients with _____ (abbrev.)
47. A muscle protein measurement that is sensitive but not specific for MI
48. A tPA with short half-life so must be given as bolus followed by infusion
50. Indicative leads for this cardiac wall are V_1 and V_2
57. Measurement of this cardiac muscle protein is the most specific test for acute MI
61. Use of this drug may cause MI by stimulating SNS (increasing oxygen demand) and causing spasm (decreasing oxygen supply)
63. New-onset occurrence of this type of block may indicate acute MI (abbrev)

29. Identify the physical findings from the following list that are seen in these pathologic conditions. More than one physical finding may be listed for each pathologic condition.

___ 1. Right ventricular failure	a. Jugular venous distention
___ 2. Left ventricular failure	b. Displaced PMI
___ 3. Left ventricular MI	c. S_3 at apex
___ 4. Right ventricular MI	d. S_3 at sternum
___ 5. Cardiac tamponade	e. S_4 at apex
___ 6. Valvular dysfunction	f. S_4 at sternum
___ 7. Chronic arterial insufficiency	g. Murmur
	h. Muffled heart sounds
	i. Intermittent claudication
	j. Peripheral edema
	k. Peripheral pallor
	l. Crackles in lung bases
	m. Hepatomegaly
	n. Pulsus paradoxus

30. Identify whether the following causes or clinical findings are associated with left or right ventricular failure. Some may be associated with biventricular failure.

Causes	Left	Right
Aortic stenosis		
Cardiac tamponade		
Cardiomyopathy		
Mitral stenosis		

248   Chapter 3   The Cardiovascular System

Causes	Left	Right
Myocardial infarction (left)		
Myocardial infarction (right)		
Pulmonary embolism		
Pulmonary hypertension		
Systemic hypertension		

Sign or Symptom	Left	Right
Abnormal liver function studies		
Ascites		
Atrial dysrhythmias		
Crackles audible over lungs		
Dyspnea		
Elevated PAOP		
Elevated RAP		
Hepatomegaly		
Jugular venous distention		
Mental confusion		
Murmur of mitral regurgitation		
Murmur of tricuspid regurgitation		
Orthopnea		
Peripheral edema		
S_3, S_4 at apex		
S_3, S_4 at sternum		
Weight gain		

31.

a. List two primary effects of IABP.

b. List two major contraindications of IABP.

c. In IABP, the balloon is inflated during which phase of the cardiac cycle?

d. In IABP, the balloon is deflated immediately before which phase of the cardiac cycle?

e. List two complications caused by displacement of the balloon in the aorta.

32. Identify the labeled portions of the IABP waveform.

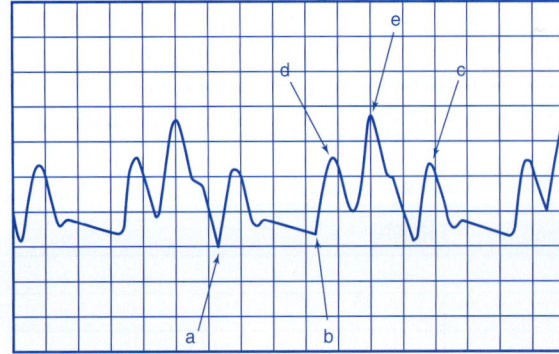

a. _____
b. _____
c. _____
d. _____
e. _____

33. Complete the questions following this case study.

    Patient A is a 75-year-old woman admitted with complaints of increasing dyspnea and fatigue. She has a past medical history of diabetes mellitus, stable angina, and CABG approximately 10 years ago. Her blood pressure is 136/82 mm Hg, and her heart rate is 92 beats/min. Her monitor shows atrial fibrillation. She has an S_3 at the apex, peripheral edema to midcalf, and JVD to 10 cm above the angle of Louis. Her current medications include captopril, carvedilol, torsemide, metformin, and warfarin. Her last measured ejection fraction was 25%.
    a. Does she meet criteria for heart failure?

    b. Is this systolic or diastolic dysfunction?

    c. What other medications might be beneficial and why?

    d. What other treatments might be helpful?

    e. What ACC stage?

34. Identify whether the following vasoactive agents are arterial or venous dilators.

Drug	Arterial Dilator	Venous Dilator
Clevidipine		
Dobutamine		
Fenoldopam		
Hydralazine		
Milrinone		
Minoxidil		
Morphine sulfate		
Nifedipine		
Nitroglycerin (<1 mcg/kg/min)		
Nitroglycerin (>1 mcg/kg/min)		
Nitroprusside		
Phentolamine		
Prazosin		

35. Complete the questions following this case study.

    Patient B is a 65-year-old man with a 10-year history of essential hypertension who came to the emergency department with complaints of headache. He rubs the back of his head and says that it has been hurting for the past several days, although he has been taking acetaminophen. He says that he had a "heart attack" 5 years ago when he started taking metoprolol and enalaprilat. He says he has "gout" and has been on allopurinol for a number of years. He recently started taking indomethacin for an acute exacerbation of gout. The only other change in his health status that he reports is a weight gain of about 20 lb over the past 2 months; he said he now weighs 80 kg.

    He denies chest pain, but he is significantly dyspneic. His BP is 220/140 mm Hg supine and 200/136 mm Hg when sitting upright. His heart rate is 62 beats/min; respiratory rate is 32/min and labored. The PMI is palpable at the anterior axillary line and the sixth left intercostal space. Cardiac auscultation reveals S_1, S_2, and an S_3. Bibasilar crackles are audible. Pulse oximeter reads 88%.

    Oxygen therapy is initiated with 5 l by nasal cannula. An IV catheter is inserted, and blood is collected for CBC, electrolytes, BUN, and creatinine. He voids only 50 ml of concentrated urine, which is sent to the laboratory for urinalysis. Chest radiography reveals cardiomegaly and pulmonary edema. Multiple-lead ECG shows left ventricular strain pattern in V_5 and V_6 and R waves in V_6 that measure 30 mm. Abnormal laboratory results included a creatinine of 3.0 mg/dl and BUN of 35 mg/dl.
    a. Identify the findings that indicate hypertensive emergency.
    b. What is the most likely cause of this abrupt increase in BP?
    c. What organs are most likely to be affected by hypertension and hypertensive crisis?
    d. Should he be admitted? PACU or critical care unit?
    e. What is the therapeutic goal for BP reduction within the next 2 hours?
    f. List a parenteral drug in each of the following categories.
        Vasodilator
        ACE inhibitor
        Alpha-blocker
        Beta-blocker
        Alpha- and beta-blocker

250 Chapter 3 The Cardiovascular System

    g. The physician prescribes nitroprusside to be started at 1 mcg/kg/min. Patient B weighs 80 kg. You reconstitute 50 mg of nitroprusside with 3 ml of sterile water and put it in 250 ml of normal saline. At what rate should infusion be started for the 1-mcg/kg/min prescription?
    h. List adverse effects of nitroprusside and how to monitor for them.
    i. Could sublingual nifedipine be used instead of the nitroprusside in this patient?
    j. Which drug would have been most appropriate if the CT had shown cerebral hemorrhage?
    k. What signs or symptoms could indicate that Patient B is experiencing thoracic aortic dissection?

36. Complete the following crossword puzzle dealing with cardiovascular pharmacology. Use only generic names.

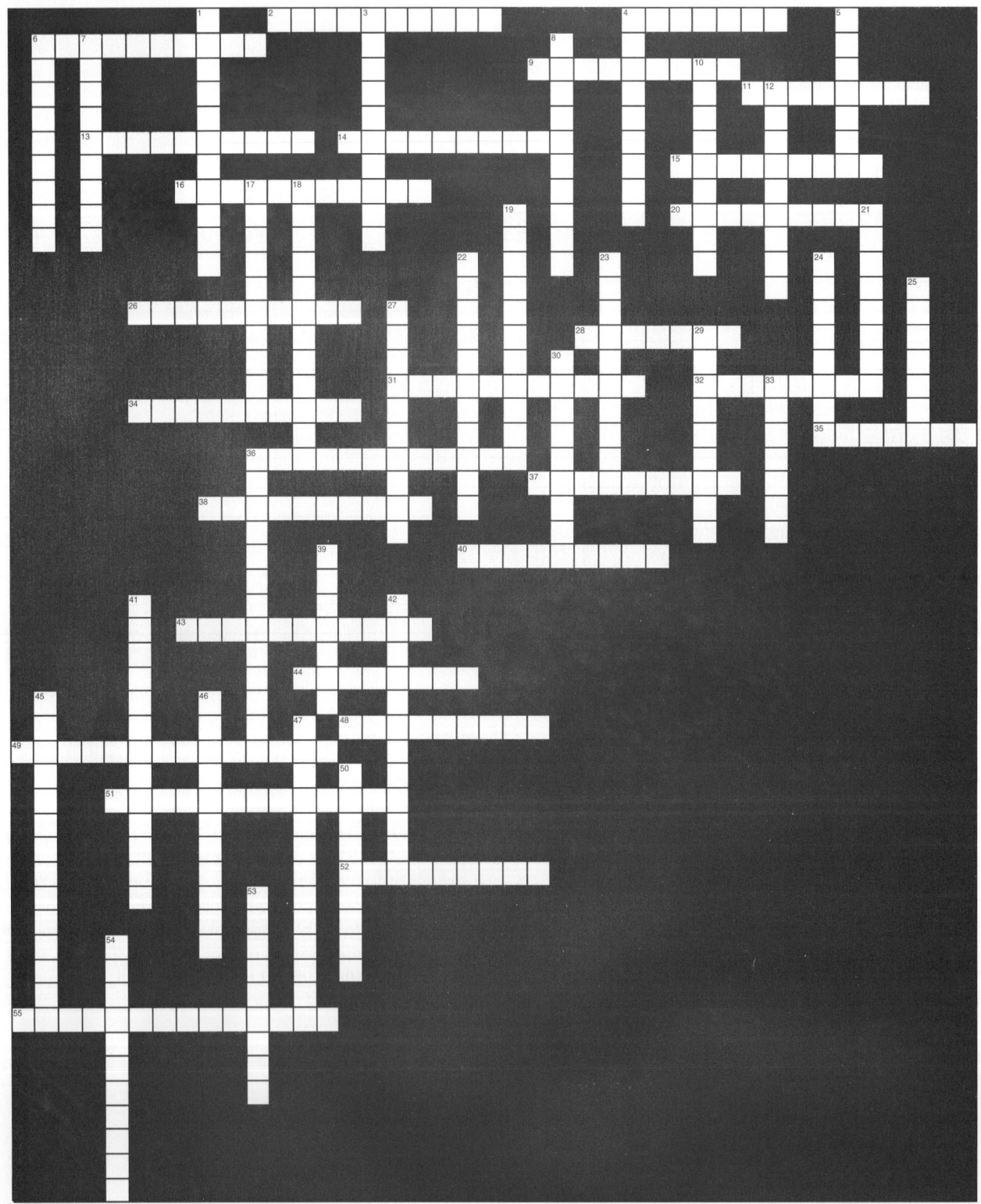

ACROSS

2. Class III antidysrhythmic; first-line antidysrhythmic agent for pulseless VT or VF
4. Electrolyte used in hyperkalemia, hypermagnesemia, hypocalcemia, and calcium channel blocker toxicity
6. Cardioselective beta-blocker; used for secondary prevention of acute MI
9. Class IV antidysrhythmic; frequently used in SVT
11. Vitamin K antagonist
13. Arterial dilator with dopaminergic stimulation used in hypertension and to improve renal flow
14. Alpha- and beta-blocker used in heart failure
15. Phosphodiesterase inhibitor; more potent and with fewer side effects than inamrinone
16. Adrenergic agent used in pulseless VT, VF, asystolic, and PEA
20. Class IV antidysrhythmic agent which decreases contractility less than verapamil
26. Beta-type natriuretic hormone used in heart failure
28. Low molecular weight form used as a platelet aggregation inhibitor, especially after vascular surgery
31. Intravenous ACE inhibitor that may be used for hypertension or heart failure
32. Adrenergic agent with dose dependent effects; may be inotropic or vasopressor
34. Loop diuretic; rapid administration may cause temporary deafness
35. Cardioselective beta-blocker with short half-life
36. Alpha-blocker; frequently used with vasopressor drug infiltration to prevent tissue necrosis
37. Alpha- and beta-blocker; used for hypertension
38. Class IC antidysrhythmic; used for refractory ventricular dysrhythmias
40. Loop diuretic that is more potent and longer duration than furosemide
43. Oral platelet aggregation inhibitor used after MI or stroke
44. Benzodiazepine anxiolytic
48. Electrolyte; usually included in postoperative fluid replacement
49. RBC colony-stimulating factor used for anemia
51. Pure beta stimulant; may be used in torsades de pointes to shorten repolarization
52. Nucleoside used to break reentrant mechanism in PSVT
55. Drug used in peripheral arterial disease to increase the flexibility of the RBCs

DOWN

1. Arterial selective IV calcium channel blocker used as an antihypertensive especially postoperatively
3. Adrenergic-type inotropic agent most frequently used in cardiogenic shock
4. Oral ACE inhibitor; may cause rash or cough
5. Indirect thrombin inhibitor
6. Electrolyte; indicated for torsades de pointes
7. Newer GP IIb/IIIa inhibitor; frequently used after PCI
8. Antihypertensive with dopaminergic qualities; also used to improve renal perfusion
10. Intravenous class III antidysrhythmic used for acute onset atrial fibrillation
12. The first IV GP IIb/IIIa inhibitor; still frequently used after PCI
17. Calcium channel blocker frequently used in variant angina
18. Class IA antidysrhythmic; may cause prolongation of the QT interval and torsades de pointes
19. Calcium channel blocker used for hypertension; available for IV use
21. Analgesic of choice in acute MI; venous vasodilator
22. Arterial dilator administered by IV injection; used in hypertension especially if pregnancy-related
23. Loop diuretic that is frequently used when patient is refractory to furosemide
24. Used in bradycardia but no longer recommended for asystole or PEA
25. This antidysrhythmic agent has both class II and class III qualities
27. Oral class III antidysrhythmic agent used for new onset atrial fibrillation; requires hospitalization and ECG monitoring during initiation of therapy
29. Aldosterone antagonist used in heart failure
30. Class IB antidysrhythmic; monitor for indications of toxicity such as paresthesia, confusion, seizures
33. Platelet aggregation inhibitor used for primary and secondary prevention of MI
36. Alpha selective adrenergic agent; used as a vasopressor especially when tachycardia is very undesirable
39. Cardiac glycoside; decreases ventricular response rate in atrial fibrillation and flutter
41. Predominantly arterial nitrate-type vasodilator
42. Tissue plasminogen activator with a longer half-life; given as a single bolus
45. Alpha dominant adrenergic agent; used as a vasopressor
46. Noncardioselective beta-blocker
47. Predominantly venous nitrate-type vasodilator; dose greater than 1 mcg/kg/min causes arterial as well venous dilation
50. ACE inhibitor available in intravenous form
53. Tissue plasminogen activator with short half-life; given as a bolus followed by an infusion
54. Hormone used in pulseless VT or VF as an alternative to the first or second dose of epinephrine; longer half-life than epinephrine

The Pulmonary System

CHAPTER 4

Selected Concepts in Anatomy and Physiology

General Information
1. The pulmonary system consists of lungs, conducting air passages, muscles of ventilation, central nervous system (CNS) control, thoracic cage, and alveoli.
2. Functions of the pulmonary system include the following:
   a. Allows interchange of gases between the atmosphere and the bloodstream
   b. Assists in maintenance of acid–base balance
   c. Contributes to phonation
   d. Acts as a reservoir for blood for the left atrium and ventricle
   e. Assists in metabolism

Functional Anatomy
1. Conducting airways: nose to terminal bronchioles
   a. Conduct airflow toward gas exchange units; no gas exchange occurs in these airways
      1) Consists of branching tubes with diminishing diameter
      2) Accounts for approximately 2 ml/kg of inspired tidal volume (V_T; this volume is referred to as *anatomical dead space*)
   b. Upper airway (Fig. 4.1): nose or mouth to external opening of vocal cords; serves as a passageway for food and inspired gas
      1) Mouth: not as effective as the nose in conditioning the inspired air
         a) Smaller surface area
         b) No ciliated epithelium to trap dust or bacteria from inspired air
      2) Nose
         a) Structure
            i) Mucous membrane lining contains cilia and mucus-producing cells.
            ii) Rich supply of blood vessels lies under the mucous membranes to provide warmth.
            iii) Skeletal rigidity maintains patency during inspiration.
            iv) Turbinates increase surface area.
            v) Four sinuses surround and drain into the nasal cavity: frontal, maxillary, ethmoid, and sphenoid.
            vi) Septum divides the nose into two fossae.
            vii) Small inlet with larger outlet allows air to have maximal contact with the nasal mucosa.
         b) Functions
            i) Warms inspired gas to body temperature
            ii) Humidifies inspired gas to relative humidity of approximately 80% to 100% at body temperature; accounts for insensible water loss of 400 ml/24 hr
            iii) Protects the lower airway from foreign material; filters inspired air of particles 5 µm or larger
            iv) Prevents inspiration of potentially dangerous environmental gases
            v) Assists in production of sound in phonation
            vi) Provides sense of olfaction: olfactory area located in the superior turbinate (sniffing directs air toward this area)
         c) More resistance (two to three times) than the mouth; this is the rationale for why dyspneic patients are more likely to breathe through their mouth
      3) Pharynx: posterior nasal cavity to esophagus
         a) Structure
            i) Nasopharynx: between posterior nasal cavity to soft palate; contains the pharyngeal tonsils and eustachian tubes
               (a) Pharyngeal tonsils (also called adenoids): dense concentration of lymphatic tissue; guard entryway into respiratory and (GI) tracts
               (b) Eustachian tubes: connection between nasopharynx to each middle ear; opens during swallowing to equalize pressure in the middle ear
                  (i) Middle ear pain or infection may develop during upper respiratory infection if eustachian tube closes.

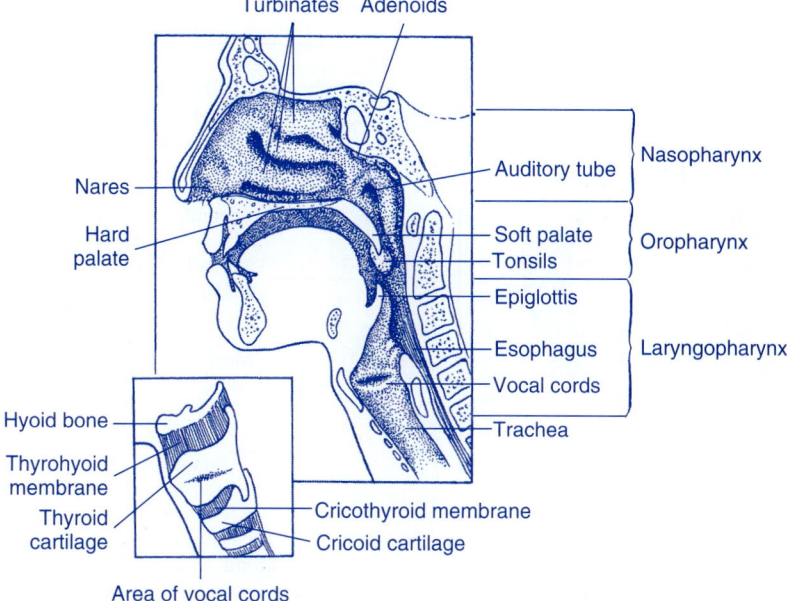

Fig. 4.1 The upper airway (lateral view). (From Luce, J. M., & Pierson, D. J. [1998]. *Critical care medicine*. Philadelphia: Saunders.)

      (ii) Nasal intubation may block eustachian tubes and cause otitis media.
   ii) Oropharynx: between the soft palate and base of tongue
      (a) Location of the palatine and lingual tonsils
      (b) Center of the gag reflex, which defends the lower airway against aspiration; gag reflex controlled by cranial nerves IX (glossopharyngeal) and X (vagus)
   iii) Laryngopharynx (also called *hypopharynx*): from base of tongue to the epiglottis
 b) Functions
   i) Swallowing: uvula and soft palate move posteriorly and superiorly to keep food and liquid from entering the nasopharynx
   ii) Protection: area is rich in lymphatic tissue
4) Larynx: upper portion of the trachea; connects the laryngopharynx with the trachea
 a) Structure: consists of thyroid cartilage, vocal cords, and cricoid cartilage
   i) Epiglottis: flexible cartilage attached to the thyroid cartilage which overhangs the larynx like a lid; prevents food from entering the larynx and trachea during swallowing
   ii) Thyroid cartilage: largest laryngeal cartilage
      (a) Contains the vocal cords
      (b) Also referred to as the *Ada*m's *apple*
   iii) Vocal folds: two pairs of membranes that protrude into the lumen of the larynx; controlled by recurrent laryngeal nerve, a branch of the vagus nerve
      (a) False vocal cords: upper pair; play no part in vocalization
      (b) True vocal cords: lower pair
        (i) Form a triangular opening between them that leads to the trachea
        (ii) Change shape and vibrate in response to contraction of muscles in the larynx to result in phonation
      (c) Glottis: passage through the vocal cords
   iv) Cricothyroid membrane: a vascular structure that connects the thyroid and cricoid cartilage; cricothyrotomy, an emergency opening of the airway, is performed at this membrane
   v) Cricoid cartilage: complete ring located below the thyroid cartilage
 b) Functions
   i) Allows speech
   ii) Prevents aspiration through the valve action of epiglottis
   iii) Allows for cough reflex and Valsalva maneuver
c. Lower airway (Fig. 4.2): below larynx; conducts air to the gas exchange surface
 1) Structure
   a) Trachea: first portion of tracheobronchial tree
      i) Consists of 16 to 20 C-shaped rings; 10 to 12 cm long
      ii) The esophagus and trachea share a common wall; erosion through this wall (tracheoesophageal fistula) may

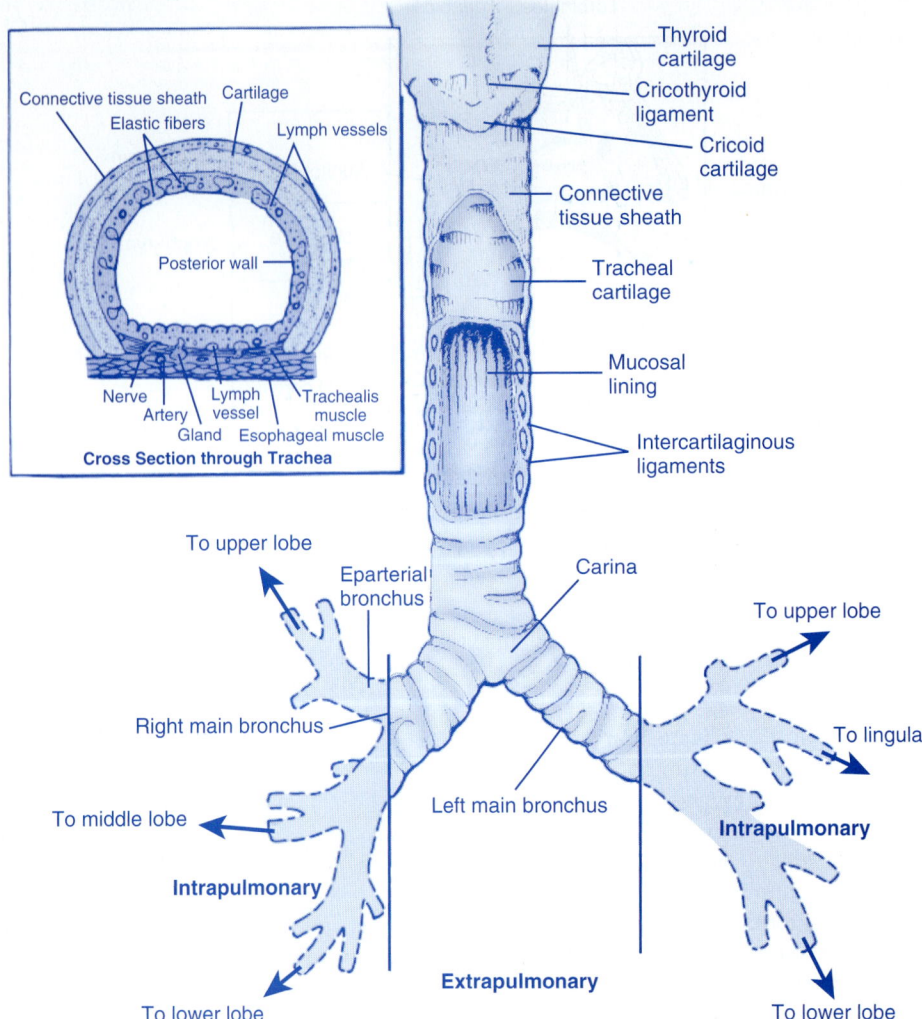

Fig. 4.2 The lower airway. (From Martin, D. E. [1988]. *Respiratory anatomy and physiology*. St. Louis: Mosby.)

be caused by an overinflated endotracheal (ET) tube or tracheostomy tube cuff.
b) Carina: bifurcation of trachea into left and right mainstem bronchi
   i) The carina is rich in parasympathetic nervous system fibers and cough receptors.
   ii) Suctioning may cause bradycardia and hypotension caused by stimulation of carina with the suction catheter.
c) Bronchi
   i) Right mainstem bronchus is almost straight (25 degrees) off trachea compared with the left (40–60 degrees) and larger in diameter than the left; aspiration of liquid or food, foreign bodies, suction catheter, and ET tube go to right preferentially.
   ii) Conducting airways branch from mainstem bronchi branch → lobar bronchi; from lobar bronchi branch → segmental bronchi; from segmental bronchi branch → subsegmental bronchi and so on
       (a) These branches are called generations or levels (Fig. 4.3): mainstem (first level), lobar (second), segmental (third), subsegmental (fourth through ninth), bronchioles (tenth through fifteenth branches).
   iii) Bronchi are supported by cartilage and smooth muscle.
   iv) Mast cells lie just beneath the bronchial epithelium near the smooth muscle and blood vessels.
d) Function
   i) The lower airway conducts, warms, cleanses, and humidifies air.
   ii) The bronchi are responsible for most of total airway resistance in a healthy person.
   iii) Mast cells secrete histamine and other mediators of the inflammatory process when stimulated by antigen–antibody response.

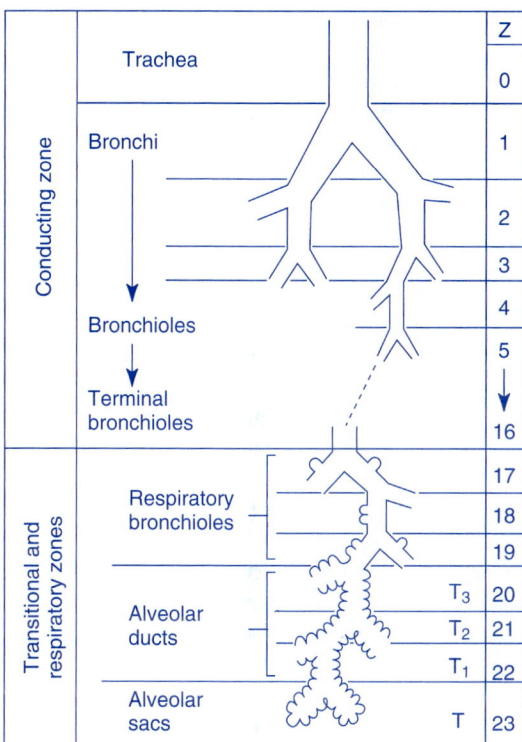

Fig. 4.3 Airway generations.

   2) Terminal bronchioles
      a) Structure
         i) 16th branch
         ii) One mm in diameter; fibrous, elastic smooth muscle with no cartilage; no mucus glands or cilia
      b) Function
         i) Terminal bronchioles are particularly sensitive to CO_2 and dilate in response to increased CO_2 levels.
         ii) Bronchospasm may significantly narrow the lumen and increase airway resistance.
2. Lung
   a. Lobes separated by fissures
      1) Right: three lobes
      2) Left: two lobes
         a) The upper left lobe is divided by a fissure.
         b) The lower portion of the left upper lobe is referred to as the *lingula*; it is approximately the same size as the right middle lobe.
   b. Segments
      1) Right: 10 segments
      2) Left: 8 segments
   c. Subsegments
   d. Lobules
      1) Primary functional units of lung
      2) Consists of terminal bronchiole, alveolar ducts, alveolar sacs, alveoli, and pulmonary circulation
   e. Gas exchange units: respiratory bronchioles to alveoli
      1) Acinus: a term used to refer to the terminal respiratory unit distal to the terminal bronchioles; has an alveolar–capillary membrane for gas exchange
      2) Respiratory bronchioles
         a) Structure
            i) Composed of the 17th through 20th branches
            ii) Less than 1 mm in diameter; bronchioles smaller than 1 mm are subject to collapse when compressed
         b) Function
            i) Increasing number of alveoli are attached.
            ii) Gas exchange takes place here.
      3) Alveolar ducts, alveolar sacs, and alveoli
         a) Structure
            i) Alveolar ducts: 20th through 22nd levels;
            ii) Alveolar sacs: level 23
            iii) Alveoli: 300 million alveoli
               (a) 1 to 2 millimicrons in size
               (b) Half of alveoli in ducts and half in alveolar sacs in grapelike clusters of 15 to 20 alveoli
               (c) Surface area is approximately 80 m^2.
               (d) Contain pores of Kohn: openings between alveoli in intraalveolar septa
                  (i) Thought to allow collateral ventilation
                  (ii) May also contribute to movement of microorganisms between alveoli and rapid transmission of infection
            iv) Lined with alveolar epithelium: site of diffusion of oxygen and carbon dioxide (CO_2) between inspired air and blood
            v) Type I pneumocytes
               (a) Cover 90% of total alveolar surface
               (b) Flat, large, squamous cells; very susceptible to injury
               (c) Responsible for integumentary air–blood barrier; cytoplasmic junctions very tight and impermeable to water under normal circumstances
            vi) Type II pneumocytes
               (a) These small, cuboidal, granular cells cover only 5% of total alveolar surface.
               (b) They produce, store, and secrete surfactant, a lipoprotein that lines the inner aspect of the alveolus.
                  (i) Surfactant decreases surface tension of the fluid lining the alveoli and prevents alveolar collapse at the end of expiration, especially at low volumes.
                  (ii) It is especially important in inferior portions of the lung where alveoli are small and distending pressures are low.
                  (iii) A deficiency of surfactant causes alveolar collapse, poorly compliant lungs, and alveolar edema.

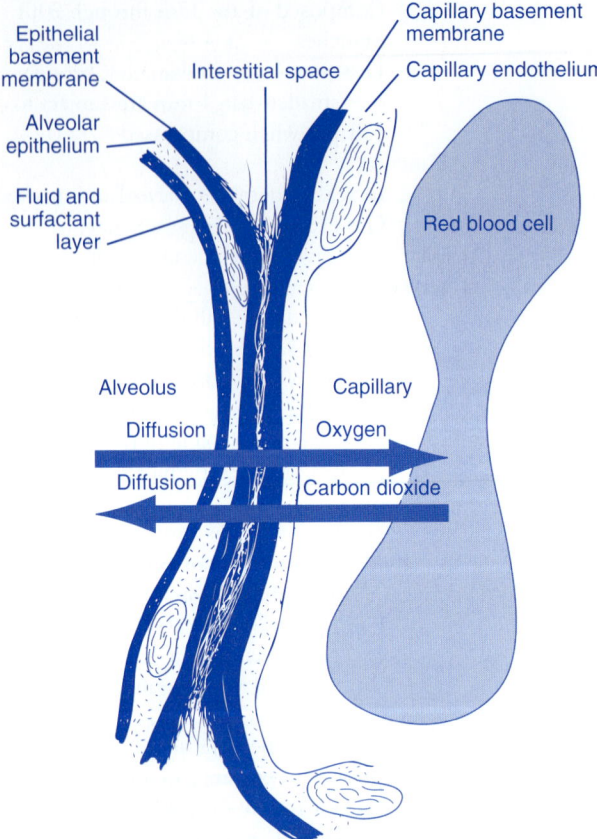

Fig. 4.4 The diffusion pathway. (From Guyton, A., & Hall, J. (2002). Textbook of medical physiology (10th ed.). Philadelphia: Saunders.)

(iv) The half-life of surfactant is only 14 hours; injury to these cells quickly results in massive atelectasis.
(c) If type I pneumocytes are injured, type II pneumocytes increase mitosis to replicate and form a cuboidal cell line and may differentiate to type I.
f. Alveolar–capillary membrane
1) Structure
a) Lines respiratory bronchioles to alveoli
b) Surface area of 1 m^2/kg of body weight and 0.5 μm in thickness
c) Diffusion pathway (Fig. 4.4): gases travel through the pathway from alveolus to blood (oxygen) or blood to alveolus (CO_2).
i) Alveolar epithelium
ii) Epithelial basement membrane
iii) Interstitial space
iv) Capillary basement membrane
v) Capillary endothelium
2) Function
a) Immense surface area and thinness of membrane allow for rapid gas exchange by diffusion.
b) Pulmonary capillary endothelial cells produce and degrade prostaglandins, metabolize vasoactive amines, convert angiotensin I to angiotensin II, and at least partly produce coagulation factor VIII.

g. Defense mechanisms
1) Upper airway
a) Nasal cilia
b) Sneeze: reaction to irritation in the nose
c) Cough: reaction to irritation in the upper airway distal to the nose
i) Vocal cords close, and intrathoracic pressure increases.
ii) Sudden opening of glottis allows propulsion of mucus.
d) Mucociliary escalator
i) Combination of mucus and cilia
ii) Particles not filtered by nasal cilia (<5 μm) are trapped in mucus and then propelled upward by the pulsatile motion of the cilia; this mucus is then coughed and expectorated or swallowed.
e) Lymphatics
2) Lower airway
a) Cough: especially at level of carina
b) Mucociliary escalator
c) Lymphatics
3) Alveoli
a) Immune system
b) Lymphatics
c) Alveolar macrophages: mononuclear phagocytes
i) Engulf and remove bacteria and other foreign substances
ii) Move from alveolus to alveolus through the pores of Kohn
4) Loss of normal defense mechanisms
a) Disease
b) Injury
c) Anesthesia
d) Corticosteroids
e) Smoking
f) Malnutrition
g) Ethanol
h) Uremia
i) Hypoxia or hyperoxia
j) Artificial airways
3. Lymphatics
a. Structure: surround lobule
b. Functions
1) Remove interstitial fluid to keep lung free of excess fluid.
a) Normal lymph drainage is approximately 20 ml/hr; may be 200 ml/hr in pulmonary edema
b) When interstitial lymphatic vessels become enlarged through increased fluid filtration such as pulmonary edema, horizontal linear opacities referred to as *Kerley-B lines* are seen on chest radiography (CXR).
2) Remove inhaled particles from distal areas of lung.
4. Circulation (Fig. 4.5)
a. Pulmonary circulation: low-pressure, low-resistance system
1) Lungs receive the full cardiac output (approximately 5 l/min).

2) RV → main pulmonary artery → left and right pulmonary arteries → arterioles → capillaries which spread over the surface of the alveoli → red blood cells (RBCs) move through in single file to allow the diffusion of gases and the attachment of oxygen to hemoglobin (Hgb)
   a) A corresponding arteriole and venule exists for every bronchiole.
   b) The network of capillaries is very dense and frequently described as a sheet of blood.
   c) The pulmonary capillaries are very small and barely accommodate erythrocyte passage.
3) Veins move out of lung toward pleura.
   a) Numerous veins gradually form four pulmonary veins that empty into the left atrium.
   b) The venous system serves as an immense reservoir of blood for the left atrium and left ventricle (LV).
4) Mean pressure in pulmonary artery: 10 to 20 mm Hg
   a) Pulmonary hypertension (PA_m >20 mm Hg)
      i) Primary pulmonary hypertension: idiopathic
      ii) Secondary pulmonary hypertension
         (a) Passive pulmonary hypertension: result of back pressure
            (i) Mitral stenosis
            (ii) Left ventricular failure
         (b) Active pulmonary hypertension
            (i) Constriction of the pulmonary circulation is caused by decreased alveolar oxygen concentration (called *hypoxemic pulmonary hypertension*); acidosis; or endogenous agents such as epinephrine, norepinephrine, angiotensin II
            (ii) Obstruction in pulmonary circuit: pulmonary embolus (PE)
      b) Dilation of the pulmonary circulation caused by:
         i) Oxygen
         ii) Pulmonary vasodilators (e.g., isoproterenol, aminophylline, epoprostenol, bosentan, nitric oxide), prostaglandins, phosphodiesterase inhibitors (e.g., sildenafil
   b. Bronchial circulation
      1) This system consists of the nutrient and oxygen circulation for the tracheobronchial tree down to terminal bronchioles, visceral pleura, interstitial and connective tissue, some arteries and veins, lymph nodes, and nerves within the thoracic cavity.
         a) Two bronchial arteries to the left lung: directly off the aorta
         b) One bronchial artery to the right lung: from the intercostal artery that originates from the right subclavian or internal mammary artery
      2) Gas exchange units are supplied with nutrients and oxygen by the pulmonary circulation.
      3) Bronchial venous blood enters the pulmonary veins and causes some desaturation of the oxygenated

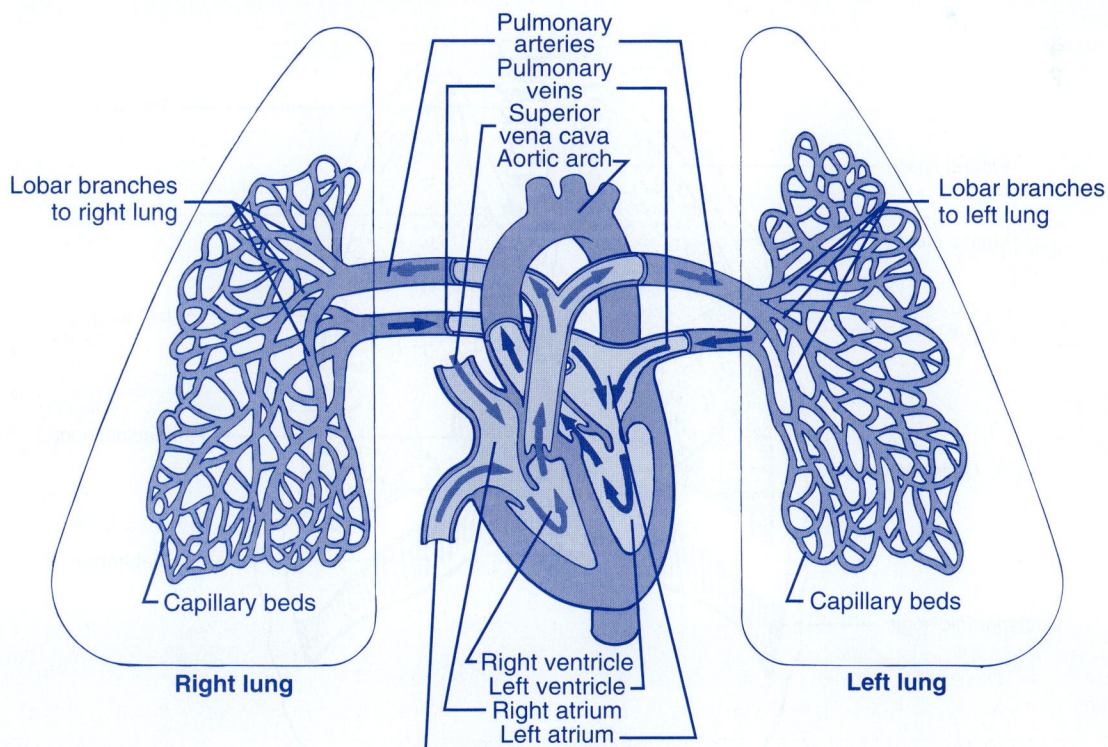

Fig. 4.5 The pulmonary circulation. (From McCance, K. L., & Huether, S. E. [2014]. *Pathophysiology: The biologic basis for disease in adults and children* [7th ed.]. St. Louis: Mosby.)

blood in the pulmonary vein; this venous blood and the blood from the thebesian veins account for the normal physiologic shunt of 3% to 5%.
5. Thoracic cage (Fig. 4.6)
   a. Muscular walls reinforced by bones
      1) Sternum anterior: three connected flat bones
         a) Manubrium
         b) Body
         c) Xiphoid

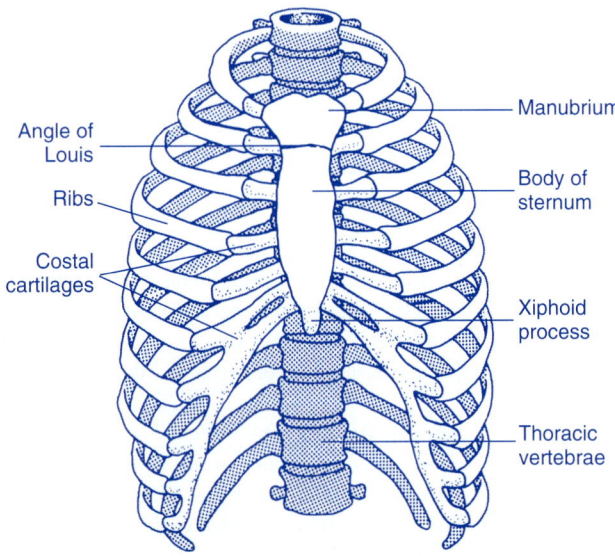

Fig. 4.6 The thoracic cage. (From Scanlan, C. L., Spearman, C. B., & Sheldon, R. L. [Eds.]. [1990]. *Egan's fundamentals of respiratory care* [6th ed.]. St. Louis: Mosby.)

2) Spine posterior: 12 pairs of ribs are attached to the vertebrae
3) Ribs anterior, lateral, and posterior
   a) Seven pairs of ribs, called *true ribs*, are attached to sternum
   b) Five pairs of ribs are attached to the rib above it
4) Clavicles superior
5) Diaphragm: inferior border of the thoracic cage
   b. Properties
      1) Rigid to protect the lungs
      2) Resilient to allow expansion and reduction of lung volume that occurs during ventilation
   c. Contents
      1) Heart
      2) Lungs
      3) Esophagus
      4) Great vessels
      5) Liver
      6) Spleen
6. Pleural cavities (Fig. 4.7)
   a. Each lung hangs in its own pleural cavity attached only at the hilum; the hilum is where the two main-stem bronchi branch and where the pulmonary vessels enter and leave the thoracic space.
   b. Pleural cavities are independent of one another.
   c. The borders of pleural cavities are as follows:
      1) Chest wall lateral
      2) Mediastinum medial
      3) Diaphragm inferior
   d. Pleural linings consist of two layers.
      1) Visceral: contiguous with lung
      2) Parietal: contiguous with chest wall

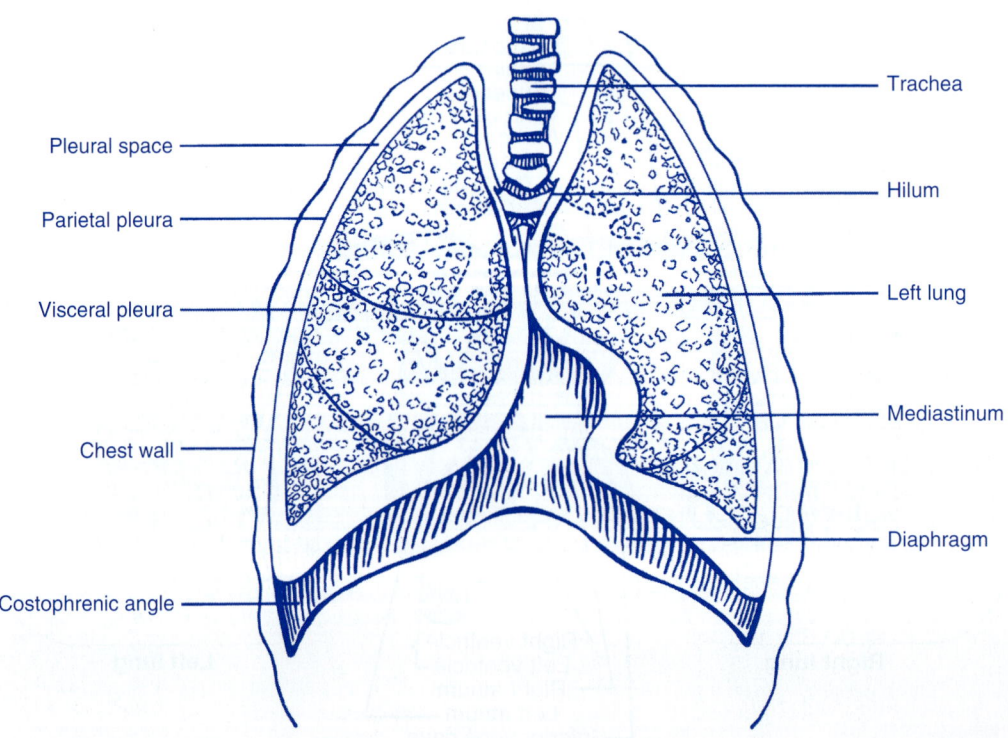

Fig. 4.7 Internal structures of the thorax, including pleural cavities. (From Dettenmeier, P. A. [1992]. *Pulmonary nursing care*. St. Louis: Mosby.)

3) Pleural space
   a) Contains a few milliliters of serous fluid, which acts as a lubricant and adhesive between the visceral and parietal pleura as they slide along each other with each ventilatory cycle
   b) Maintains a negative intrapleural pressure of approximately −5 mm Hg below atmospheric pressure; this pressure becomes more negative (−10 mm Hg) during inspiration; loss of this negative intrapleural pressure causes the lung to collapse (e.g., pneumothorax)
7. Mediastinum: center of thoracic cavity; contains the following:
   a. Heart and great vessels
   b. Trachea and mainstem bronchi
   c. Esophagus
   d. Phrenic, vagus, and other nerves
   e. Lymph nodes and ducts
   f. Thymus gland
8. Muscles of ventilation (Fig. 4.8)
   a. Inspiratory
      1) Diaphragm
         a) Innervation occurs via phrenic nerves (C3–C5)
         b) The diaphragm consists of two hemidiaphragms connected by a central membranous tendon; this tendon is contiguous with the fibrous pericardium.
         c) Contraction flattens the diaphragm.
            i) Increases size of thorax superior-inferior
            ii) Normally accounts for 70% of V_T during quiet breathing
         d) Relaxation makes the diaphragm dome shaped and decreases the volume of the thoracic cavity.
      2) External intercostals
         a) Innervation occurs from T1 to T12
         b) Contraction raises the ribs, increasing the size of thorax anteroposteriorly
      3) Accessory muscles of inspiration
         a) Scalene
            i) Located in the neck; stretch from the first cervical vertebrae to the first and second ribs
            ii) Enlarge the upper rib cage
         b) Sternocleidomastoid
            i) Located in the neck; stretch from the manubrium and clavicle to the mastoid process and occipital bone
            ii) Elevate the sternum to increase the anteroposterior and transverse diameter of the chest
         c) Not used in normal resting ventilation but used during exercise and in respiratory distress; also used in the inspiratory phase of sneeze or cough
   b. Expiratory
      1) Expiration is normally passive.
         a) It occurs when diaphragm and external intercostals relax and return to resting position.
         b) The natural tendency of the lungs is to collapse because they are made of elastic tissue; elastance is the quality of the lungs to recoil after inspiration.
      2) Accessory muscles of expiration: internal oblique, external oblique, rectus abdominis, internal intercostal, and transverse abdominis
         a) Depress the lower ribs and pull down the anterior portion of the lower chest
         b) Increase pressure in abdominal cavity and compress the abdominal viscera up against the diaphragm
         c) Used when increased levels of ventilation are needed
         d) Important in forceful expiration, coughing, and sneezing

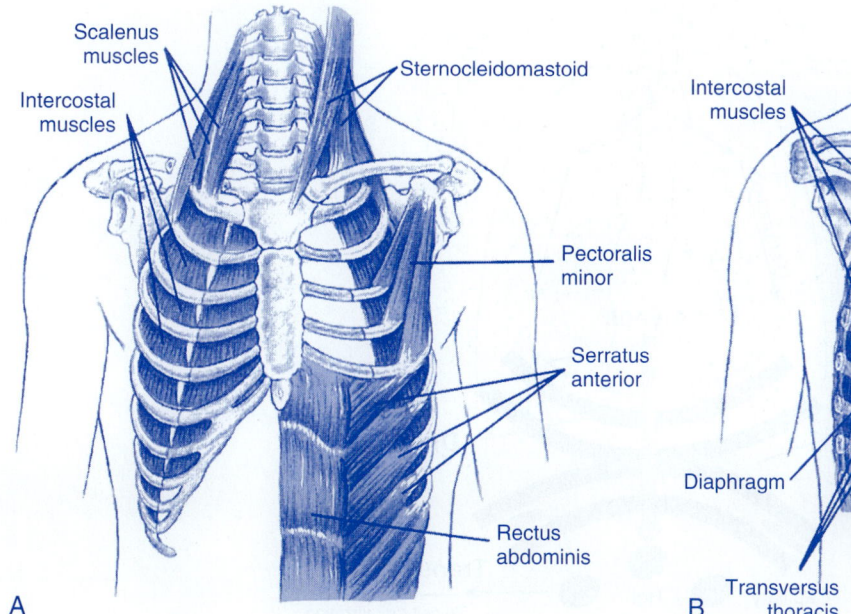
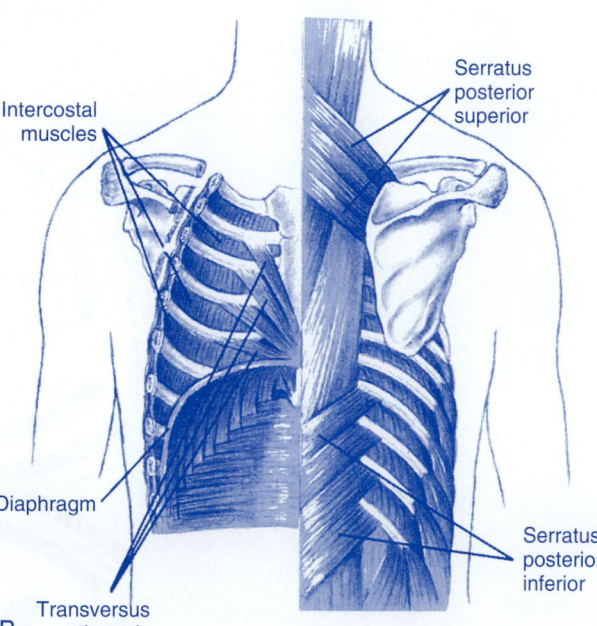

Fig. 4.8 Muscles of ventilation. **A,** Anterior. **B,** Posterior. (From Urden, L., Stacy, K., & Lough, M. [2010]. *Thelan's critical care nursing: Diagnosis and management* [6th ed.]. St. Louis: Mosby.)

9. Neuroanatomy
   a. Medulla: central chemoreceptors sensitive to cerebrospinal fluid pH (↑ $PaCO_2$ → acidosis)
      1) Primary control of ventilation is by these central chemoreceptors and $PaCO_2$ and pH levels.
      2) They respond to minimal changes in $PaCO_2$ very quickly.
      3) Adjustment of alveolar ventilation occurs.
         a) Increase in $PaCO_2$ causes an increase in the rate and depth of ventilation.
         b) Decrease in $PaCO_2$ causes a decrease in the rate and depth of ventilation.
   b. Arterial chemoreceptors in aortic arch and carotid bodies: sensitive to pH, partial pressure of oxygen in arterial blood (PaO_2)
      1) These peripheral chemoreceptors and PaO_2 levels provide secondary control of ventilation.
      2) They will not respond to $PaCO_2$ levels until a 10 mm Hg change is seen.
      3) They respond when PaO_2 falls below approximately 60 mm Hg; particularly important in patients with chronically elevated levels of $PaCO_2$.
   c. Pontine: control rhythmic ventilation
      1) Apneustic center stimulates inspiratory center.
      2) Pneumotaxic center inhibits inspiratory activity.
   d. Stretch receptors in alveoli (Hering-Breuer reflex): inhibit further inspiration to prevent overdistention of alveoli; may cause bronchodilation, tachycardia, vasodilation
   e. Proprioceptors in muscles and tendons: increase ventilation in response to body movements
   f. Baroreceptors in aortic arch and carotid bodies: increase in blood pressure (BP) inhibits ventilation
   g. Juxtacapillary receptors (also called *pulmonary J receptors*): stimulated by increase in interstitial fluid volume; may cause laryngeal constriction, hypotension, bradycardia, mucous production, dyspnea
   h. Chest wall pain receptors
      1) Lung parenchyma does not have pain receptors.
      2) Parietal pleura does have pain receptors; transmit impulses via intercostal nerves and thoracic ganglia
   i. Irritant receptors: stimulated by pulmonary edema, chemical or mechanical irritation; may cause bronchospasm, cough, mucus production
   j. Modifying influences: drugs; brain trauma, edema, or increased intracranial pressure (ICP); chronic hypercapnia

Physiology (Fig. 4.9)
1. Ventilation: movement of air between atmosphere and alveoli and distribution of air within the lungs to maintain

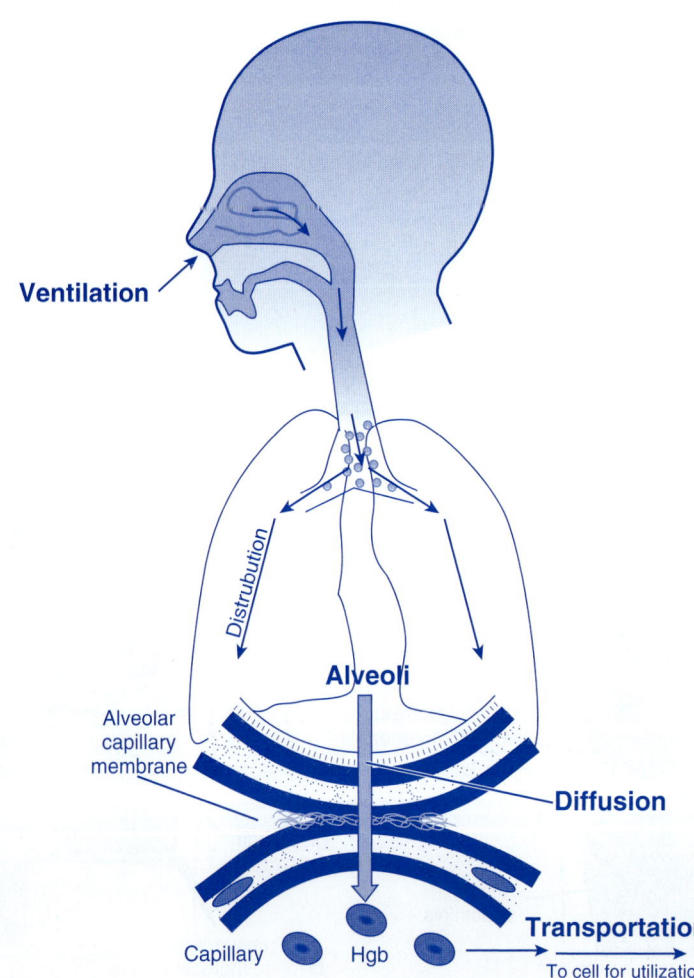

Fig. 4.9 Respiratory process: ventilation, distribution, diffusion, transportation, cellular utilization. *Hgb*, Hemoglobin.

appropriate concentrations of oxygen and CO_2 in the alveoli
  a. Process (Fig. 4.10)
    1) Inspiration (inhalation): the movement of atmospheric air into the alveoli
       a) Message from medulla travels down phrenic nerve to diaphragm.
       b) Diaphragm and external intercostals contract.
       c) Size of thorax increases.
       d) Lungs are stretched, and intrapulmonary pressure is decreased to less than atmospheric pressure (-1 cm H_2O).
       e) Air movement into lungs to equalize the difference between atmospheric and alveolar pressure
    2) Expiration (exhalation): movement of air from alveoli to the atmosphere
       a) Relaxation of diaphragm and external intercostals
       b) Recoil of lungs to their resting size and a concomitant increase in alveolar pressure above atmospheric pressure ($+1$ cm H_2O)
       c) Air movement out of lungs to equalize the pressure difference

  b. Efficiency of ventilation: evaluated by $PaCO_2$
    1) $PaCO_2$ greater than 45 mm Hg indicates hypoventilation.
    2) $PaCO_2$ less than 35 mm Hg indicates hyperventilation.
  c. Lung volumes (Fig. 4.11 and Table 4.1)
    1) Alveolar ventilation is the volume of air per minute participating in gas exchange; it is the most important portion of minute ventilation; minute ventilation minus dead space ventilation.
    2) Dead space ventilation (Fig. 4.12) is the volume of air per minute that does not participate in gas exchange.
       a) Anatomical dead space is the volume of air in conducting airways and does not participate in gas exchange; approximately 2 ml/kg of V_T
       b) Alveolar (pathologic) dead space is the volume of air in contact with nonperfused alveoli.
       c) Physiologic dead space is anatomical plus alveolar dead space.
          i) Calculated by:

$$\frac{V_D}{V_T} = \frac{PaCO_2 - P_ECO_2}{PaCO_2}$$
Normal: $0.2 - 0.4$

  d. Work of breathing = work of deforming the elastic system + work of producing airflow through the airways (Fig. 4.13)
    1) Usually the work of breathing is negligible: 2% to 3% of total energy expenditure by the body
    2) Compliance
       a) Measure of expandability of lungs, thorax, or both:
       b) $c = \dfrac{\text{change in volume}}{\text{change in pressure}}$
          i) Static compliance: affected by changes in compliance of chest wall or lung
          ii) Dynamic compliance: affected by changes in compliance of chest wall or lung or airway resistance
          iii) Calculation of static and dynamic compliance (Fig. 4.14 and Table 4.2)
       c) Factors affecting static compliance
          i) Chest wall changes
             (a) Kyphoscoliosis
             (b) Flail chest
             (c) Thoracic pain with splinting
             (d) Obesity
          ii) Lung changes
             (a) Atelectasis
             (b) Pneumonia
             (c) Pulmonary edema
             (d) Pulmonary fibrosis
             (e) Pleural effusion
             (f) Pneumothorax

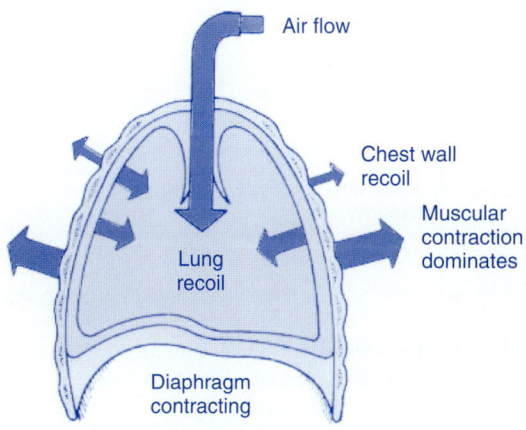
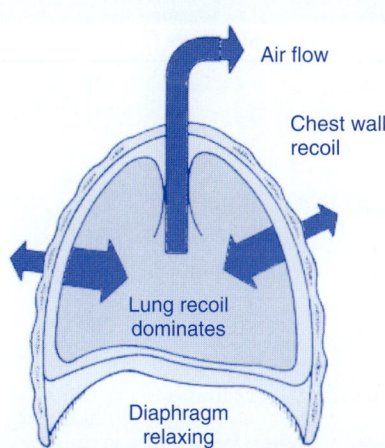

Fig. 4.10 The process of ventilation. (Modified from McCance, K. L., & Huether, S. E. [2010]. *Pathophysiology: The biologic basis for disease in adults and children* [6th ed.]. St. Louis: Mosby.)

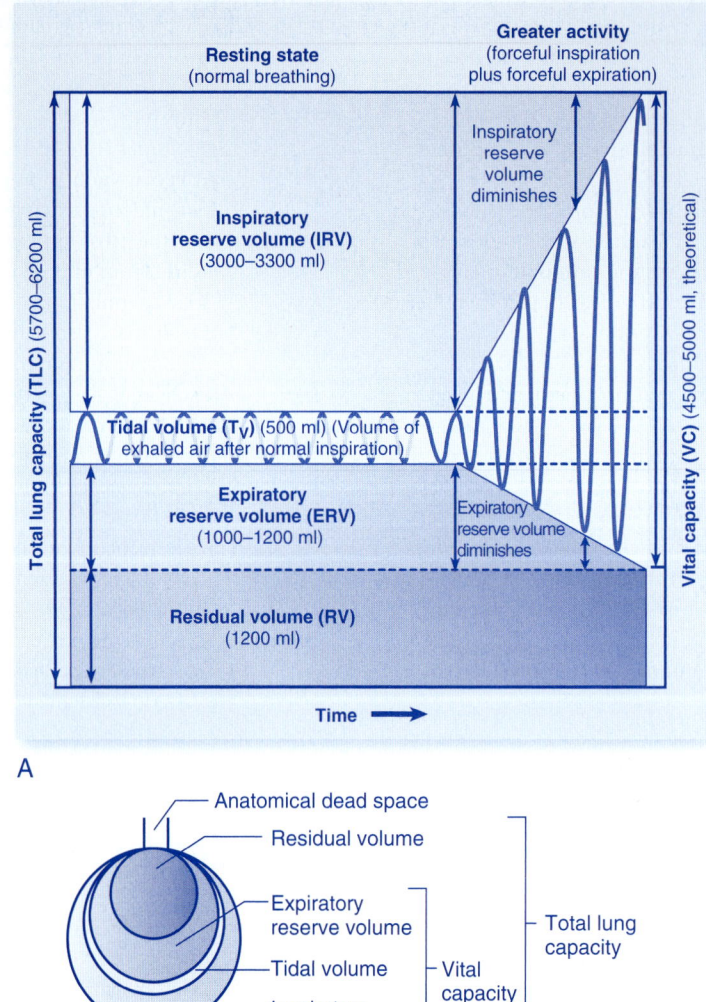

Fig. 4.11 Lung volumes and capacities. Note that upward deflection reflects inspiration and downward deflection reflects expiration. **A,** Spirometry. **B,** Lung volumes. (From Patton, K. T., & Thibodeau, G. A. [2016]. *Anatomy & physiology* [9th ed.]. St. Louis: Mosby.)

Table 4.1	Lung Volumes, Capacities, and Mechanics	
Volume	**Definition**	**Normal**
Tidal volume (V_T)	The volume of air moved in and out of the lungs with each normal breath	7 ml/kg or ≈500 ml
Inspiratory reserve volume (IRV)	The volume of air that can be maximally inspired above the normal inspiratory level	3000 ml
Expiratory reserve volume (ERV)	The volume of air that can be maximally exhaled beyond the normal expiratory level	1000 ml
Residual volume (RV)	The volume of air remaining in the lungs at the end of a maximal expiration	1000 ml
Inspiratory capacity (IC)	V_T + IRC; the volume of air that can be maximally inspired from a normal expiratory level	3500 ml
Functional residual capacity (FRC)	RV + ERV; the volume of air remaining in the lungs at the end of normal expiration	2000 ml
Vital capacity (VC)	V_T + IRC + ERV; the volume of air that can be maximally expired after a maximal inspiration	4500 ml
Total lung capacity (TLC)	V_T + IRC + ERV + RV; the volume of air that the lungs can hold with maximal inspiration	5500–6000 ml
Respiratory rate or frequency (f)	The number of breaths per minute	12–20

Table 4.1   Lung Volumes, Capacities, and Mechanics—cont'd

Volume	Definition	Normal
Minute ventilation (M_E)	$V_T \times f$; the volume of air expired per minute	5–10 l
Dead space (V_D)	$V_D/V_T = PaCO_2 - PeCO_2/PaCO_2$ $PaCO_2$ (arterial); $PeCO_2$ (exhaled) The volume or percentage of the V_T that does not participate in gas exchange; includes the volume of air in the conducting pathways (anatomical dead space) plus the volume of alveolar air that is not involved in gas exchange due to pathology (alveolar dead space)	V_D/V_T ratio is normally <0.4; V_D/V_T >0.6 is usually an indication for mechanical ventilation
Alveolar ventilation (V_A)	$V_T - V_D$; the volume of tidal air that is involved in alveolar gas exchange	350 ml
Forced vital capacity (FVC)	The volume of air in a forceful maximal expiration	Normally same as VC: 4500 ml
Forced expiratory volume (FEV)	The volume of air exhaled in a given time period; FEV_1: the volume of air exhaled in 1 second; FEV_3: the volume of air exhaled in 3 seconds	FEV_1: >75% of VC FEV_3: >95% of VC

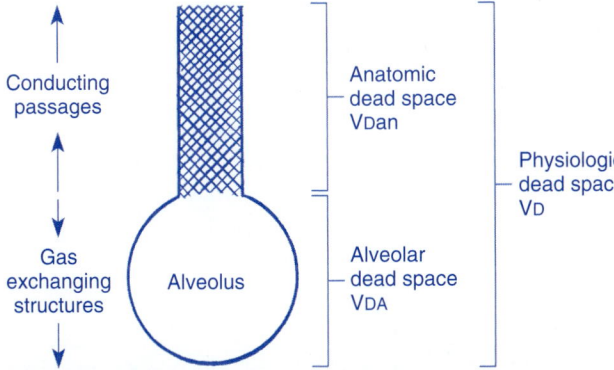

Fig. 4.12 Physiologic dead space: anatomic dead space and alveolar dead space. (Drawing by Wendy W. Johnson.)

      d) Additional factors affecting dynamic compliance
         i) As previously mentioned and airway resistance changes; the difference between static and dynamic compliance represents airway resistance
   3) Airway resistance
      a) Pressure differential required to produce a unit flow change; affected by airway caliber and length
      b) Factors affecting airway resistance (and dynamic compliance)
         i) Bronchospasm
         ii) Mucus
         iii) Artificial airways
         iv) Water condensation in ventilator tubing
         v) Mucosal edema
         vi) Bronchial tumor
2. Perfusion: movement of blood through the pulmonary capillaries
   a. Pulmonary vasculature: resistance varies to accommodate the blood flow that it receives
   b. Distribution of perfusion

      1) Related to gravity and intraalveolar pressures
         a) Gravity causes the pressure in the capillaries in the bases to be higher than the pressure in the capillaries in the apices; preferential blood flow to the gravity-dependent areas of the lungs
         b) The intraalveolar pressures are generally equal throughout the lungs.
         c) This creates the potential for intraalveolar pressure to exceed capillary hydrostatic pressure in some areas of the lung, causing absence of blood flow to these areas.
      2) Zones (Fig. 4.15)
         a) Zone 1: nondependent portion of the lung; potential for no perfusion
         b) Zone 2: middle portion of the lung; varying blood flow
         c) Zone 3: gravity-dependent area of the lung; receives constant blood flow; pulmonary artery catheters (PACs) ideally are placed in zone 3 for accurate reflection of left atrial pressure by the pulmonary artery occlusion pressure (PAOP)
      3) Hypoxemic pulmonary vasoconstriction
         a) Localized
            i) Protective mechanism that decreases blood flow to an area of poor ventilation so that blood can be shunted to areas of better ventilation
            ii) Stimulated by decreased alveolar oxygen levels
         b) Generalized
            i) If all alveoli have low oxygen levels as occurs with alveolar hypoventilation, hypoxemic pulmonary vasoconstriction may be distributed over the lungs.
            ii) Increases pulmonary vascular resistance (PVR) and pulmonary arterial pressure (PAP)
            iii) Right ventricular hypertrophy and failure (cor pulmonale) may result

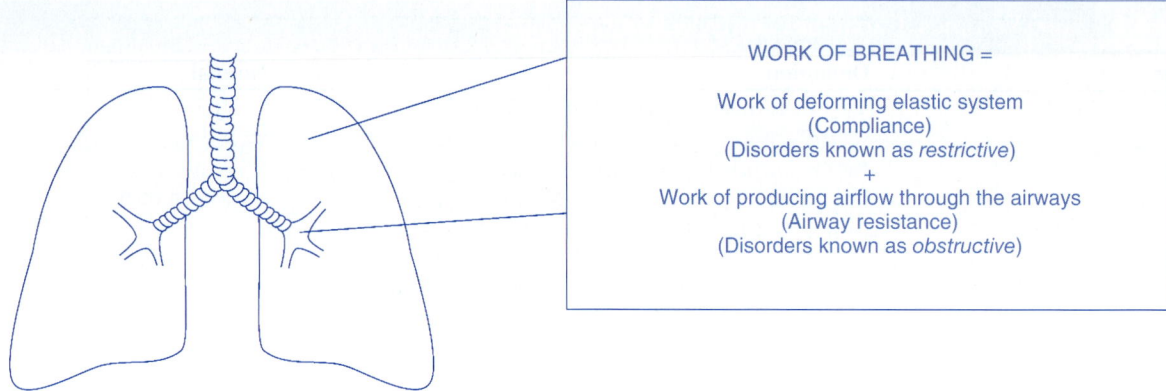

Fig. 4.13 The work of breathing.

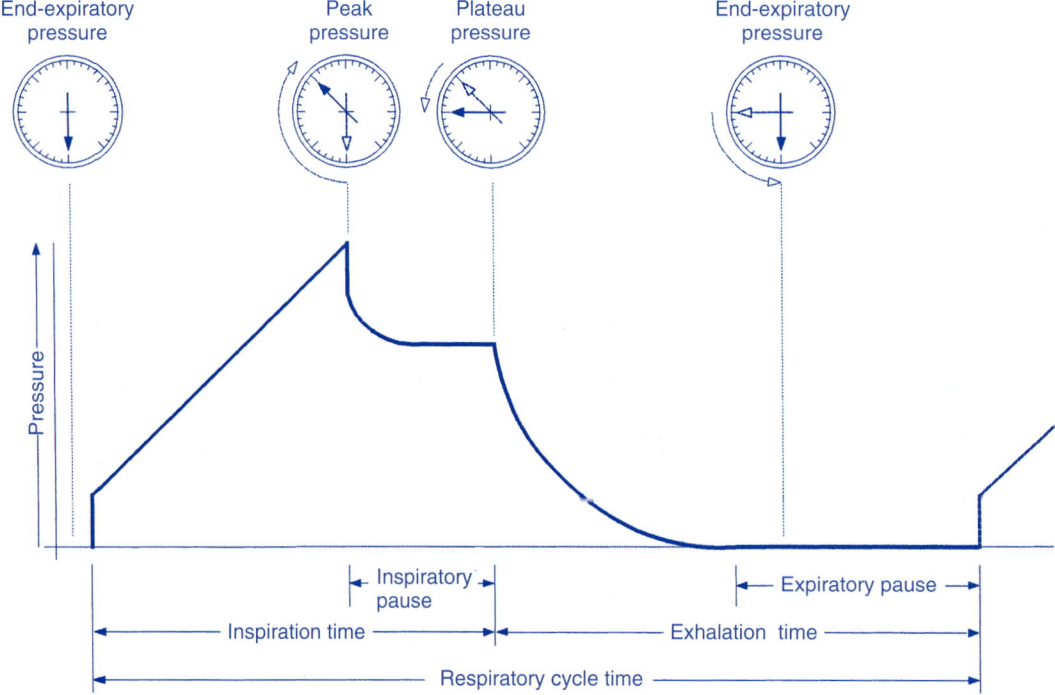

Fig. 4.14 Airway pressure in a patient on positive pressure ventilation. Plateau pressure is used to calculate static compliance. Peak pressure is used to calculate dynamic compliance. The difference between static and dynamic compliance represents airway resistance. Remember that positive end-expiratory pressure levels are subtracted from the plateau or peak pressures before calculation of compliance. (From Dupuis, Y. G [1992]. *Ventilators: Theory and clinical application* [2nd ed.]. St. Louis: Mosby-Year Book.)

Table 4.2	Types of Compliance		
Type	**Formula**	**Normal**	**Significance**
Static compliance	$\dfrac{\text{Tidal volume}}{\text{Plateau pressure} - \text{PEEP}}$	50–100 ml/cm H_2O	Affected by changes in compliance of chest wall or lung
Dynamic compliance	$\dfrac{\text{Tidal volume}}{\text{Plateau pressure} - \text{PEEP}}$	35–55 ml/cm H_2O	Affected by changes in compliance of chest wall or lung or airway resistance

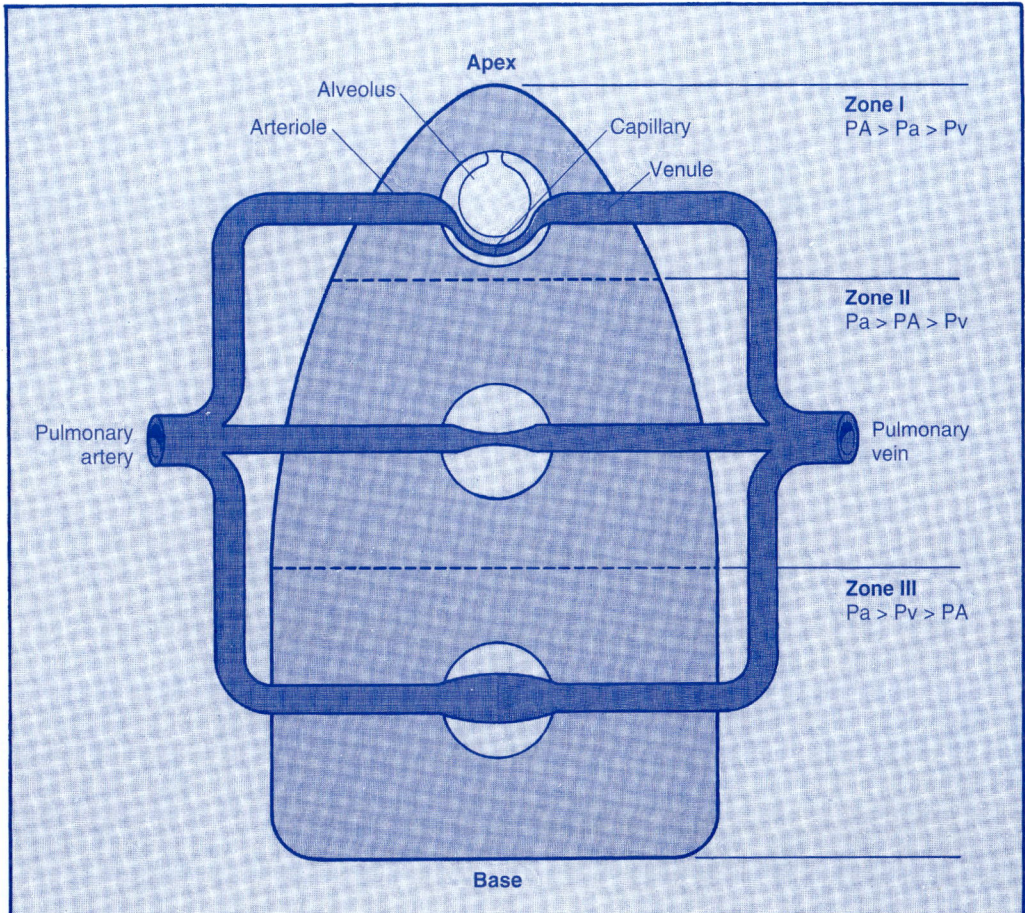

Fig. 4.15 Zones of distribution of perfusion: relationship of alveolar pressure (PA) and gravitational forces to pulmonary vascular pressures and blood flow. The upright lung can be divided into three zones. In zone I, the upper third of the lung, alveolar pressure exceeds pulmonary venous (Pv) and pulmonary arterial (Pa) pressures. In zone II, the middle third of the lung, the pulmonary artery pressure is greater than alveolar pressure, which is greater than pulmonary venous pressure. In zone III, the lower third of the lung, pulmonary artery pressure is greater than pulmonary venous pressure, which is greater than alveolar pressure. NOTE: Pulmonary artery catheters are positioned in zone III for accurate measurement of pulmonary artery occlusion pressure as a reflection of left atrial pressure. (From McCance, K. L., & Huether, S. E. [2014]. *Pathophysiology: The biologic basis for disease in adults and children* [7th ed.]. St. Louis: Mosby.)

      (a) Chronic cor pulmonale: chronic conditions such as chronic obstructive pulmonary disease (COPD)
      (b) Acute cor pulmonale: acute conditions such as PE
   c. Ventilation (V)/perfusion (Q) ratio
     1) Normal (Fig. 4.16): alveolar minute ventilation = ~4 l; normal cardiac output (100% goes to lungs) = ~5 l; normal ventilation/perfusion (V/Q) ratio = 0.8
     2) Pathologic mismatch (Fig. 4.17)
       a) Dead space: V greater than Q
         i) V/Q ratio greater than 0.8 (i.e., high V/Q ratio)
         ii) Examples include PE, shock, and decrease in perfusion to the lung caused by excessive V_T or positive end-expiratory pressure (PEEP).
       b) Shunt: Q greater than V
         i) V/Q ratio less than 0.8 (i.e., low V/Q ratio)

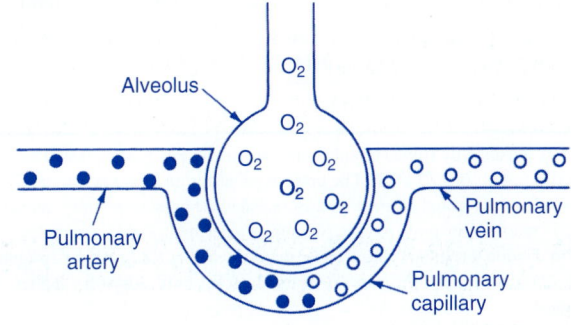

Fig. 4.16 Normal ventilation/perfusion (V/Q) ratio: normal alveolar ventilation per minute is approximately 4 l, and normal perfusion (CO) is approximately 5 l/min; normal V/Q ratio is 0.8. (From Kinney, M. R., Dunbar, S. B., Brooks-Brunn, J. A., et al. [1998]. *AACN's clinical reference for critical-care nursing* [4th ed.]. St. Louis: Mosby.)

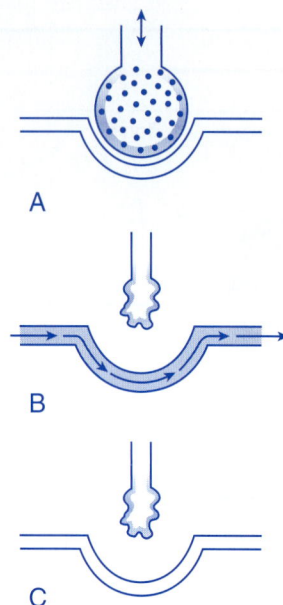

Fig. 4.17 Abnormal ventilation/perfusion (V/Q) ratio. **A,** High V/Q ratio with ventilation exceeding perfusion; also called a *dead space unit.* **B,** Low V/Q ratio with perfusion exceeding ventilation; also called a *shunt unit.* **C,** Absent ventilation and perfusion, referred to as a *silent unit.* (From Kinney, M. R., Dunbar, S. B., Brooks-Brunn, J. A., et al. [1998]. *AACN's clinical reference for critical-care nursing* [4th ed.]. St. Louis: Mosby.)

Table 4.3	Methods of Estimating Intrapulmonary Shunt*	
Parameter	**Formula**	**Normal**
a/A ratio	(PaO_2/PAO_2)	• Normal: >0.8 • Moderate: 0.5–0.8 • Significant: 0.25–0.5 • Critical: < 0.25
A:a gradient	$PAO_2 - PaO_2$	• <10 mm Hg • A:a gradient × 0.05 = approximate % shunt
PaO_2/FiO_2 (or P/F ratio)	$\dfrac{PaO_2}{FiO_2}$	• >300 • 300 = ~15% shunt • 200 = ~20% shunt
Respiratory index	$\dfrac{PAO_2 - PaO_2}{PaO_2}$	• <1

*PaO_2 is obtained by arterial blood gas measurement. PAO_2 is calculated as: FiO_2 (Pb − 47) - ($PaCO_2$/0.8). The pressure of water vapor at sea level is 47 and is subtracted from barometric pressure; 0.8 is the usual respiratory quotient. *FiO_2,* Fraction of inspired oxygen (written as a decimal); *$PaCO_2$,* arterial carbon dioxide tension; *PAO_2,* alveolar oxygen tension; *PaO_2,* arterial oxygen tension; *Pb,* barometric pressure (760 mm Hg at sea level; adjust for higher altitudes).

   ii) Examples include atelectasis, acute respiratory distress syndrome (ARDS), and pneumonia.
   iii) PaO_2 less than 60 mm Hg with a fraction of inspired oxygen (FiO_2) of 0.5 or greater suggests clinically significant shunt.
   iv) There are several methods of estimating shunt (Table 4.3).
  c) Silent: no V or Q

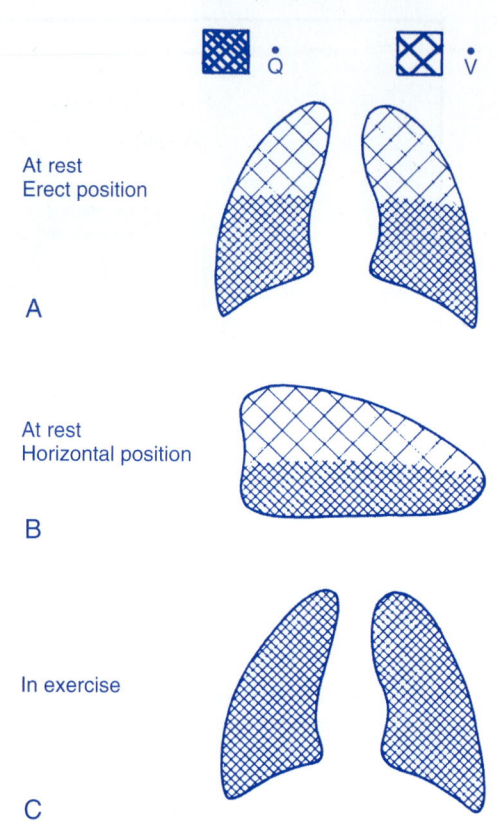

Fig. 4.18 Positional changes in ventilation and perfusion. **A,** While one is sitting or standing, the upper lobes are ventilated best, and the lower lobes are perfused best. **B,** While one is lying on one side, the superior lung is ventilated best, and the inferior lung is perfused best. **C,** In exercise, ventilation and perfusion are increased and optimally matched throughout. (From Wade, J. F. [1982]. *Comprehensive respiratory care.* St. Louis: Mosby.)

  3) Positional mismatch (Fig. 4.18)
   a) Greatest ventilation in superior areas
   b) Greatest perfusion in inferior areas
   c) This is the rationale for "good lung down" in unilateral lung conditions.
    i) Improves ventilation to the "bad lung" (e.g., atelectasis, pneumonia, pneumothorax) and optimizes perfusion to the "good lung."
    ii) Exception is pneumonectomy: patient is positioned on the operative side or back so "no lung down.
3. Distribution: movement of inspired air into lobes, segments, lobules
 a. Transpulmonary pressure or distending pressure is equal to alveolar pressure minus pleural pressure.
  1) Alveolar pressure is the pressure that reaches the alveoli after resistance has been overcome.
  2) Pleural pressure is determined by gravity.
 b. Closing volume is lung volume present when a significant number of small alveoli close.
4. Diffusion: movement of gases between the alveoli, plasma, and RBCs
 a. Gases diffuse from areas of higher concentration to areas of lower concentration regardless of medium until concentration is the same throughout the chamber.

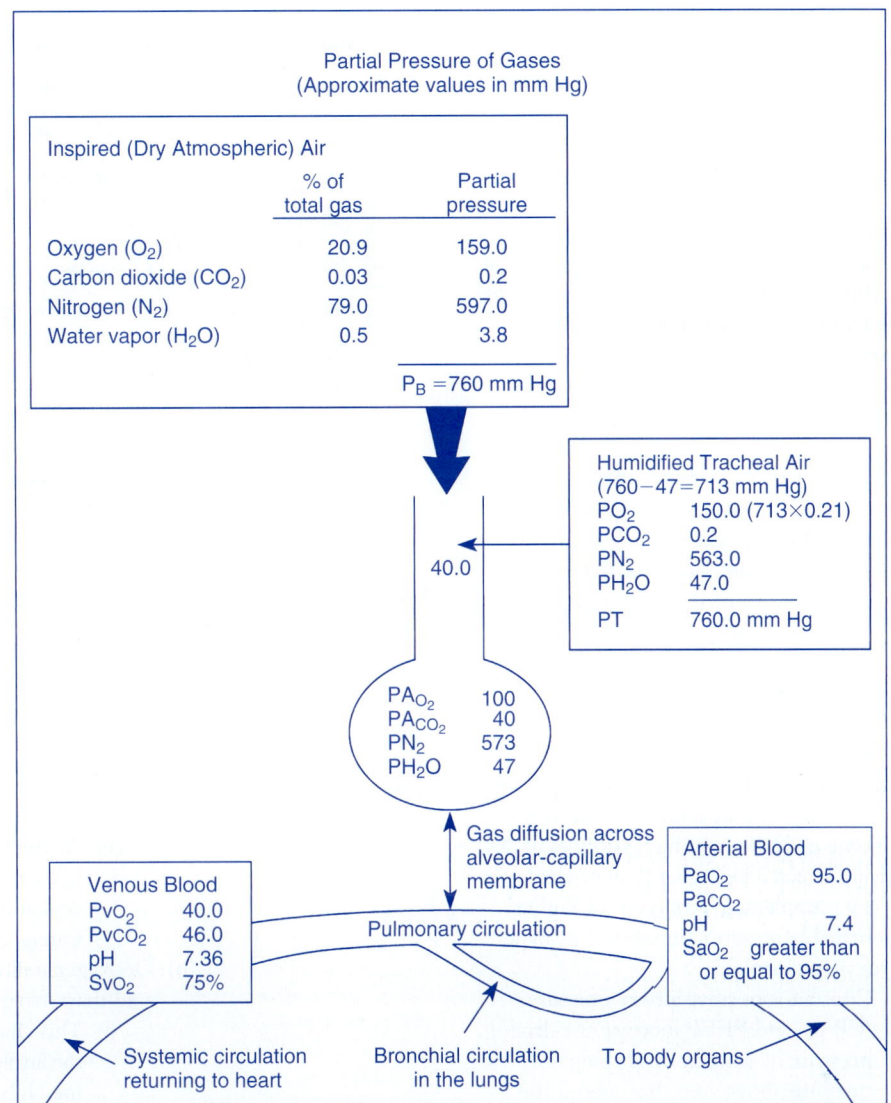

Fig. 4.19 Dalton's law of partial pressure. $PaCO_2$, Alveolar pressure of carbon dioxide; PaO_2, alveolar pressure of oxygen; PH_2O, partial pressure of water vapor; PN_2, partial pressure of nitrogen; P_T, pressure of tracheal air; PvO_2, partial oxygen pressure in mixed venous blood; $PvCO_2$, partial carbon dioxide pressure in mixed venous blood; SaO_2, arterial oxygen saturation; SvO_2, venous oxygen saturation.

b. Dalton's law of partial pressure (Fig. 4.19): in a mixture of gases the pressure exerted by each gas is independent of the other gases and directly corresponds to the percentage of the total mixture that it represents.
  1) Atmospheric (or barometric) pressure, the pressure exerted by the weight of the atmosphere, is 760 mm Hg at sea level; adjustments should be made when at high altitudes.
     a) Components and pressures in the atmosphere
        i) Oxygen represents 20.9% of 760 mm Hg and exerts 159 mm Hg.
        ii) Nitrogen represents 79% of 760 mm Hg and exerts 597 mm Hg.
        iii) CO_2 represents 0.03% of 760 mm Hg and exerts 0.2 mm Hg.
        iv) Water vapor represents 0.5% of 760 mm Hg and exerts 3.8 mm Hg.
  2) During inspiration, the upper airway warms and humidifies atmospheric air which increases the pressure of the vapor to 47 mm Hg; the partial pressures of the other gases must decrease as the total cannot exceed barometric pressure of 760 mm Hg; example:

     760 (barometric pressure at sea level)
     − 47 (pressure of water vapor at @ body temperature) × 0.21 (FiO_2 of room air)
     = 150 mm Hg

  3) As the inspired gas mixes with gas that was not expired, the concentrations of CO_2 and O_2 change again.
  4) Alveolar air is high in oxygen pressure and low in CO_2 pressure, and the pulmonary capillary blood is high in CO_2 pressure and low in oxygen pressure.

5) This differential in partial pressure of oxygen and CO_2 causes the gases to move across the alveolar-capillary membrane toward the lower side of the respective pressure gradients (e.g., oxygen moves from the alveolus to the capillary, and CO_2 moves from the capillary to the alveolus).
   c. Determinants of diffusion
      1) Surface area available for gas transfer
         a) Fick's law of diffusion: the rate of transfer of a gas through a sheet of tissue is proportional to the tissue area; alveolar surface area is normally immense
         b) Negatively affected by pulmonary resection (e.g., lobectomy or pneumonectomy) or emphysema
      2) Thickness of the alveolar-capillary membrane: negatively affected by pulmonary edema or fibrosis
      3) Diffusion coefficient of gas
         a) CO_2 is 20 times more diffusible than O_2.
            i) Diffusion problems cause hypoxemia but not hypercapnia.
            ii) Hypercapnia indicates hypoventilation (e.g., respiratory muscle fatigue).
      4) Driving pressure
         a) Fraction of the gas × barometric pressure
         b) Negatively affected by low inspired fraction of oxygen (e.g., smoke inhalation) or low barometric pressure (e.g., high altitudes)
         c) Positively affected by higher than normal FiO_2 (e.g., supplemental oxygen) or higher than normal barometric pressure (e.g., hyperbaric oxygen chamber)
            i) Continuous positive airway pressure (CPAP) and PEEP increase the driving pressure of oxygen by keeping the pressure above zero throughout the entire ventilatory cycle
5. Transport of gases in blood: movement of oxygen and CO_2 through the circulatory system; oxygen being moved from the alveolus to the tissues to be used and CO_2 being moved from the tissues to the alveolus for exhalation
   a. Oxygen
      1) Mode of transport
         a) Hgb: 97% of oxygen is combined with Hgb; represented by the oxygen saturation of arterial blood (SaO_2).
            i) One molecule of Hgb can carry four molecules of oxygen.
            ii) The amount of oxygen that the Hgb actually carries depends on the affinity of the Hgb for oxygen; there is normally more affinity at the lung level and less affinity at the tissue level due to the Bohr effect, which controls the reaction between Hgb and oxygen and CO_2.
               (a) Oxygenated Hgb is a stronger acid than deoxygenated Hgb.
                  (i) This change in pH facilitates the release of oxygen from the Hgb at the tissue level.

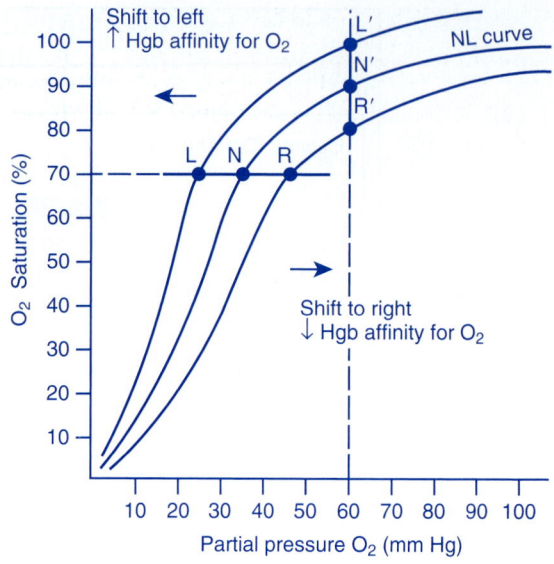

Fig. 4.20 Oxyhemoglobin dissociation curve. Normal curve(N) optimizes pickup of O_2 at the lung and drop-off of O_2 at the tissue level; left shift (L) increases the affinity between O_2 and Hgb, which optimizes pickup of O_2 at the lung level but impairs drop-off of O_2 at the tissue level; right shift (R) decreases affinity between O_2 and Hgb, which impairs pickup of O_2 at the lung level but optimizes drop-off of O_2 at the tissue level. (From Dettenmeier, P. A. [1992]. *Pulmonary nursing care*. St. Louis: Mosby.)

                  (ii) As the Hgb gives up the oxygen, it becomes a weaker acid and picks up CO_2 for transport back to the lung.
               (b) Deoxygenated Hgb is a weaker acid than oxygenated Hgb.
                  (i) This change in pH facilitates the attraction of oxygen to the Hgb at the lung level.
                  (ii) As the Hgb picks up oxygen, it becomes a stronger acid and releases CO_2 at the lung level.
                  (iii) Ability of Hgb to deliver oxygen to the tissues is negatively affected by:
                     (1) Anemia
                     (2) Abnormal Hgb (e.g., methemoglobinemia, carboxyhemoglobin, or Hgb S [sickle cell])
      b) Plasma: 3% of oxygen is dissolved in the plasma; represented by the PaO_2
   2) Oxyhemoglobin dissociation curve: shows the relationship between PaO_2 and Hgb saturation (Fig. 4.20)
      a) Critical point: PaO_2 60 mm Hg
         i) PaO_2 above 60: horizontal limb of curve; increase in PaO_2 above 60 results in minimal increases in oxygen saturation
         ii) PaO_2 below 60: vertical limb of curve; decrease in PaO_2 below 60 mm Hg results in dramatic decreases in oxygen saturation

Table 4.4	Correlation Between PaO_2 and SaO_2 with Normal Oxyhemoglobin Dissociation Curve
PaO_2 (in mm Hg)	SaO_2 (in %)
100	98
90	97
80	95
70	93
60	90
50	85
40	75
30	57
27	50

PaO_2, Alveolar oxygen tension; SaO_2, arterial oxygen saturation of arterial blood.

Box 4.1 Important Information About 2,3-Diphosphoglycerate (2,3-DPG)

What Is It?
- A substance in the erythrocyte that affects the affinity of hemoglobin for oxygen
- A chief end product of glucose metabolism and a link in the biochemical feedback control system that regulates the release of oxygen to the tissues

What Does It Do to the Oxyhemoglobin Dissociation Curve?
- Increased amounts of 2,3-DPG shift the curve to the right decreasing the affinity between hemoglobin and oxygen
- Decreased amounts of 2,3-DPG shift the curve to the left increasing the affinity between hemoglobin and oxygen

What Causes Amounts of 2,3-DPG to Increase or Decrease?
- Increased
  - Chronic hypoxemia (e.g., high altitude, congenital heart disease)
  - Anemia
  - Hyperthyroidism
  - Pyruvate kinase deficiency
- Decreased
  - Multiple blood transfusions of banked blood (i.e., total body exchange [~10 units] over minutes to hours)
  - Hypophosphatemia (e.g., malnutrition, refeeding syndrome, treatment of diabetic ketoacidosis)
  - Hypothyroidism
  - Hexokinase deficiency

---

    b) Correlation between PaO_2 and SaO_2 with a normal oxyhemoglobin dissociation curve (Table 4.4)
        i) P_{50}: the partial pressure of oxygen at which Hgb is 50% saturated with a pH of 7.4; usually PaO_2 of 27 mm Hg
    c) Shifting of the oxyhemoglobin dissociation curve
        i) Decreased P_{50} and shifting of the oxyhemoglobin dissociation curve to the left
           (a) Affinity of Hgb for oxygen is increased; therefore, Hgb is more saturated for a given PaO_2, and less oxygen is unloaded for a given PaO_2.
           (b) This means that it is easier to pick up oxygen at the lung level but more difficult to drop off oxygen at the tissue level.
           (c) Factors that shift the oxyhemoglobin dissociation curve to the left: alkalemia, hypothermia, hypocapnia, decreased 2,3-diphosphoglycerate (2,3-DPG)
           (d) Remember: there is more *left* over with a shift to the left.
        ii) Increased P_{50} and shifting of the oxyhemoglobin dissociation curve to the right
           (a) Affinity of Hgb for oxygen is decreased; therefore, Hgb is less saturated for a given PaO_2, and more oxygen is unloaded for a given PaO_2.
           (b) This means that it is more difficult to pick up oxygen at the lung level but easier to drop off oxygen at the tissue level.
           (c) Factors that shift the oxyhemoglobin dissociation curve to the right: acidemia, hyperthermia, hypercapnia, increased 2,3-DPG
           (d) Remember: it is *right* to give it away.
        iii) Discussion of 2,3-DPG (Box 4.1)
    3) Oxygen capacity
        a) Maximal amount of oxygen the blood can carry
        b) Formula: Hgb × 1.34
           i) Hgb in grams per deciliter
           ii) 1.34 represents the amount of oxygen 1 gram of Hgb can carry; it is a constant
    4) Oxygen content in arterial blood (CaO_2)
        a) Actual amount of oxygen that arterial blood is carrying
        b) O_2 capacity × O_2 saturation; amount of oxygen dissolved in the plasma (.0031 × PaO_2) may be added but is such a minute factor in most situations that it is inconsequential unless the patient is hyperoxemic (e.g., hyperbaric oxygen therapy)
        c) Formula: Hgb × 1.34 × SaO_2
           i) Hgb in grams per deciliter
           ii) 1.34 represents the amount of oxygen 1 g of Hgb can carry; it is a constant
           iii) Saturation as a decimal (e.g., 95% is 0.95)
        d) Normal 18 to 20 ml/dl (~20 ml/dl)
    5) Oxygen content in venous blood (CvO_2)
        a) Actual amount of oxygen in venous blood
        b) Formula: 1.34 × Hgb × SvO_2
           i) Hgb in grams per deciliter
           ii) 1.34 represents the amount of oxygen 1 g of Hgb can carry; it is a constant
           iii) Saturation as a decimal (e.g., 95% is 0.95)
        c) Normal 12 to 16 ml/dl (~15 ml/dl)

b. CO_2: most transported as bicarbonate
  1) Carbonic acid and water in the presence of carbonic anhydrase form bicarbonate in the erythrocyte.
  2) Five percent is dissolved in plasma ($PaCO_2$).
  3) Five percent is combined with Hgb as carbaminohemoglobin; CO_2 attaches to Hgb at a different bonding site than oxygen.
c. Diffusion between systemic capillary bed and body tissues: pressure gradients allow diffusion
  1) Haldane effect: in the tissue, as O_2 leaves Hgb, increased CO_2 is able to be picked up by Hgb; in the lungs, the binding of oxygen with Hgb tends to displace CO_2.
  2) Oxygen diffusion to peripheral tissues is affected by the following:
     a) Quantity and rate of blood flow
     b) Difference in capillary and tissue oxygen pressures
     c) Capillary surface area
     d) Capillary permeability
     e) Intracapillary distance
6. Oxygen delivery to the tissues (see Chapter 3)
7. Cellular respiration: utilization of oxygen by the cell
   a. Estimated by the amount of CO_2 produced and the oxygen consumed
      1) Respiratory quotient (RQ): ratio of these two values
         a) Normally 0.8 but changes occur according to the nutritional substrate being used; primary carbohydrate metabolism changes the ratio to 1.0 because carbohydrate metabolism produces more CO_2 than does the metabolism of protein or fat
         b) Simplified Krebs cycle: food is converted by the body to H_2O and CO_2 and cellular energy (adenosine triphosphate [ATP])
      2) Variables affecting oxygen consumption
         a) Increased oxygen consumption
            i) Increased work of breathing
            ii) Hyperthermia
            iii) Trauma
            iv) Sepsis
            v) Anxiety
            vi) Hyperthyroidism
            vii) Muscle tremors or seizures
         b) Decreased oxygen consumption
            i) Hypothermia
            ii) Sedation
            iii) Neuromuscular blockade
            iv) Anesthesia
            v) Hypothyroidism
            vi) Inactivity
   b. Oxygen is used by the mitochondria in the production of cellular energy; oxygen deficit may result in lethal cell injury if prolonged.
8. Metabolic functions of the lung
   a. Synthesis of interferon and tumor inhibiting factor
   b. Production, conversion, or removal of many vasoactive substances in the pulmonary circulation; bradykinin, serotonin, heparin, histamine, prostaglandins E and F, and certain polypeptides such as angiotensin I

Pulmonary Assessment

Interview

1. Chief complaint: why the patient is seeking help and duration of the problem; possible symptoms related to pulmonary disorders that may be identified as chief complaint may include any of the following:
   a. Dyspnea or shortness of breath
      1) Onset
      2) Duration
      3) Frequency
      4) Timing: time of day; weather or season; activity; eating; talking; deep breathing
      5) Position (e.g., orthopnea)
      6) Severity
         a) Subjective scale
            i) Grade 1: shortness of breath with mild exertion, such as running a short distance or climbing a flight of stairs
            ii) Grade 2: shortness of breath while walking a short distance at a normal pace on level grade
            iii) Grade 3: shortness of breath with mild daily activity such as shaving or bathing
            iv) Grade 4: shortness of breath while sitting at rest
            v) Grade 5: shortness of breath while lying down
         b) Effect on ability to do activities of daily living (ADLs)
         c) Frequently accentuated by anxiety
      7) Palliation: what is effective in relieving dyspnea
      8) Accompanying symptoms
         a) Cough
         b) Chest pain
         c) Wheezing
   b. Cough
      1) Onset
      2) Duration
      3) Frequency
      4) Timing: time of day, weather or season, activity, eating, talking, deep breathing
      5) Position
      6) Pattern: regular or occasional
      7) Dry or productive
      8) Accompanying symptoms
         a) Sputum production
         b) Hemoptysis
         c) Chest pain
         d) Wheezing
         e) Dyspnea
      9) Medication history: may be side effect of angiotensin-converting inhibitors (e.g., captopril, enalapril)
   c. Sputum production
      1) Duration
      2) Frequency
      3) Amount: use household measurements (e.g., teaspoons, tablespoons, shot glass, Dixie cup, iced tea glass)
      4) Color

5) Consistency
6) Odor
7) Hemoptysis
8) Usual treatment (e.g., expectorants, cough drops, a cigarette)

d. Hemoptysis
1) May be related to tuberculosis, lung cancer, bronchiectasis, pneumonia, PE
2) Character
   a) Grossly bloody
   b) Blood tinged
   c) Blood-streaked
   d) Hematest positive
3) Differentiation from hematemesis
   a) Hemoptysis: frothy, alkaline, accompanied by sputum
   b) Hematemesis: nonfrothy, acidic, dark red or brown, accompanied by food particles

e. Chest pain: (information regarding differentiation of chest pain is located in Table 3.5)
1) P
   a) Provocation: pulmonary pain is frequently provoked by trauma, coughing, deep breathing, or movement.
   b) Palliation: pulmonary pain may be relieved by sitting upright or by narcotics.
2) Q
   a) Quality: pulmonary pain is most frequently sharp and increased by coughing, inspiration, movement.
3) R
   a) Region: pulmonary pain is usually located at lateral chest.
   b) Radiation: pulmonary pain may radiate to shoulder or neck.
4) S
   a) Severity: pulmonary pain is usually moderate but may be severe.
5) T
   a) Timing
      i) Onset: pulmonary pain onset is usually gradual.
      ii) Duration: pulmonary pain duration is usually days to weeks.

f. Wheezing
1) Onset
2) Duration
3) Timing: time of day, weather or season, activity, eating, talking, deep breathing, position, inspiratory or expiratory or both
4) Identified triggers (e.g., dust, pollen, propellants)
5) Usual treatment

g. Nasal or sinus problems
1) Epistaxis
2) Nasal stuffiness
3) Postnasal drip
4) Sinus pain

h. Hoarseness: chronic hoarseness may be related to cancer of the larynx.
i. Ascites: may be related to cor pulmonale
j. Abdominal pain: may be related to cor pulmonale
k. Edema or weight gain: may be related to cor pulmonale
l. Fatigue or weakness: may be related to cor pulmonale
m. Fever: may be related to pulmonary infections
n. Night sweats: may be related to tuberculosis
o. Anorexia: may be related to cor pulmonale, dyspnea, or drug side effects (e.g., xanthine bronchodilators)
p. Weight loss: may be related to dyspnea, fatigue (preventing food preparation), or hypermetabolism
q. Sleep disturbances: may be related to dyspnea or coughing

2. History of present illness
   a. PQRST
   b. Associated symptoms

3. Past medical history
   a. Childhood diseases
      1) Frequent respiratory infections
      2) Allergies
      3) Asthma
      4) Scarlet fever
   b. Past illnesses
      1) Recurrent respiratory infections
      2) Pneumonia
      3) Cystic fibrosis
      4) Asthma
      5) COPD
         a) Possible components
            i) Chronic bronchitis: dominant reported symptom is coughing with sputum production.
            ii) Emphysema: dominant reported symptom is dyspnea.
            iii) Patients with COPD often also have asthma: dominant reported symptom is wheezing.
         b) Most patients have two, if not all three, of these components.
      6) Tuberculosis
      7) Lung cancer
      8) Pulmonary fibrosis: frequently related to occupational lung disease
         a) Pneumoconiosis (coal worker's lung disease)
         b) Asbestosis
         c) Silicosis
      9) Fungal disease (e.g., histoplasmosis)
      10) PE
      11) Pneumothorax
      12) Granulomatous diseases (e.g., sarcoidosis)
      13) Connective tissue disorders (e.g., lupus, scleroderma)
      14) Immunosuppression
      15) Cor pulmonale: right ventricular hypertrophy or failure as a result of pulmonary disease
   c. Past injury: chest trauma
   d. Past surgical procedures: thoracotomy
   e. Allergies and type of reaction
   f. Past diagnostic studies
      1) Allergy testing
      2) Tuberculin or fungal skin tests
      3) CXR
      4) Pulmonary function studies
      5) Bronchoscopy
      6) Laryngoscopy

4. Family history of genetically predisposed disease
   a. Asthma
   b. Emphysema: particularly α_1-antitrypsin deficiency-related emphysema
   c. Tuberculosis
   d. Cystic fibrosis
   e. Cancer
5. Social history
   a. Work environment
      1) Occupation
      2) Environmental hazards: chemicals, vapors, dust, pulmonary irritants, allergens
      3) Use of protective devices
   b. Home environment
      1) Allergens: pets, plants, trees, molds, dust mites
      2) Type of heating
      3) Use of air conditioner and/or humidifier
   c. Recreational habits: exposure to inhalants and allergens
   d. Exercise habits
   e. Tobacco use: present and past
      1) Type of tobacco
      2) Duration and amount
         a) Cigarettes: record as pack-years (number of packs per day times the number of years the patient has been smoking).
         b) Chewing or rubbing tobacco: type and amount per day
         c) Marijuana: joints per day
      3) Efforts to quit: previous and current desire to quit
      4) Second-hand smoke exposure
   f. Fluid consumption
      1) Volume of water per day
      2) Caffeine-containing beverages
      3) Alcohol-containing beverages: alcoholic beverages per day or per week
   g. Eating habits
      1) Quality and quantity of meals
      2) Number of meals per day
      3) Pulmonary symptoms during meals: dyspnea, cough, wheezing
6. Medication history
   a. Prescribed drug, dose, frequency, time of last dose
   b. Nonprescribed drugs
      1) Over-the-counter drugs, including herbs
         a) St. John Wort can worsen asthma symptoms if taken with theophylline or amitriptyline.
         b) Guarana can increase the likelihood of side effects if taken with respiratory medications because it contains theophylline.
         c) Ginseng reduces the effectiveness of β-blockers.
         d) Licorice elimination is reduced if taken with corticosteroids.
         e) Blue cohosh and lobelia may increase the side effects of nicotine patches.
         f) Ma hang can increase toxicity of methylxanthines in asthmatics.
      2) Substance abuse
   c. Patient's understanding of drug actions, side effects; knowledge of how to use and clean an inhaler if prescribed

Landmarks (Fig. 3.29)
1. Anatomical
   a. Clavicle
   b. Sternum
   c. Ribs
   d. Intercostal spaces
   e. Angle of Louis: sternal angle between manubrium and body of sternum
   f. Xiphoid process
   g. Costal margin
   h. Costal angle
2. Imaginary
   a. Midsternal line
   b. Midclavicular line (MCL)
   c. Anterior axillary line (AAL)
   d. Midaxillary line (MAL)
   e. Posterior axillary line (PAL)
   f. Scapular line
   g. Midspinal line
3. Location of lungs (Fig. 4.21)
   a. The apex of the lungs extends 2 to 4 cm above the inner third of the clavicle.
   b. The inferior border anteriorly is at the sixth rib at the MCL and at the eighth rib at the MAL, posteriorly at T10 on expiration and at T12 with deep inspiration.
   c. Fissure dividing upper and lower lobes is at T3 posteriorly.
   d. Upper lobes primarily anterior; lower lobes primarily posterior
   e. Trachea bifurcates at the angle of Louis anteriorly or T4 posteriorly.

Inspection and Palpation
1. Vital signs
   a. BP
   b. Heart rate
   c. Respiratory (ventilatory) rate
   d. Temperature
   e. Height
   f. Weight
2. General survey
   a. Apparent health status: compare apparent age relative with chronological age.
   b. Level of consciousness: note restlessness or confusion (frequently the first sign of hypoxia).
   c. Increased work of breathing: note use of accessory muscles.
   d. Speech pattern: note pausing midsentence to take a breath.
   e. Presence of injury, abrasion, or deformity
   f. Nutritional status
   g. Stature or posture
3. Mouth or nose
   a. Pursed-lip breathing: may be instinctive or the patient may have been taught to use this technique during times of dyspnea
   b. Artificial airway
      1) Type
      2) Size
      3) Placement (e.g., cm mark at teeth for oral ET tube)
      4) Cuff pressure (measured with a cuff pressure gauge or sphygmomanometer with three-way stopcock)

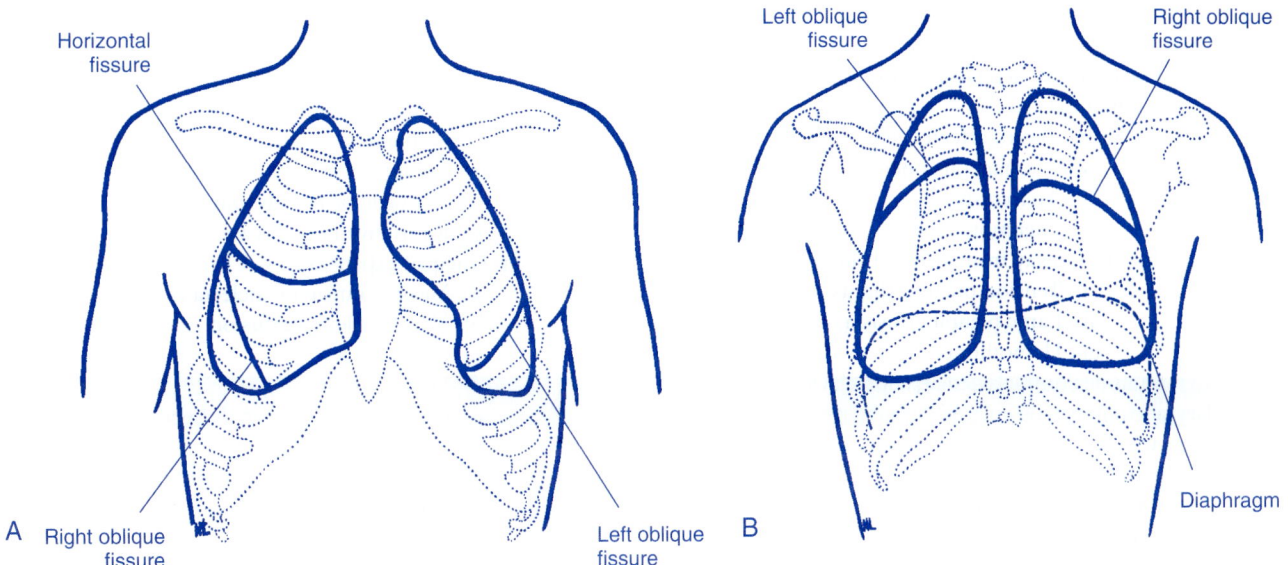

Fig. 4.21 Location of the lungs. **A,** Anterior. **B,** Posterior. (From Wilkins, R. L., Sheldon, R. L., & Krider, S. J. [1994]. *Clinical assessment in respiratory care*. St. Louis: Mosby.)

    c. Oxygen therapy
        1) Administration device and flow rate
        2) FiO_2
    d. Nasogastric (NG), nasointestinal tube, orogastric, or orointestinal tube
        1) Size
        2) Placement confirmation
            a) Aspiration of gastric (i.e., acidic) or intestinal (i.e., alkaline) contents
            b) Radiologic confirmation
    e. Condition of nasal or oral mucosa
    f. Presence of halitosis: suggests poor oral hygiene, poor dental health, or sinus infection
4. Skin, mucous membranes, and appendages
    a. Color
        1) Pallor: may indicate anemia
        2) Rubor: may indicate hypercapnia or polycythemia
        3) Cyanosis
            a) Peripheral (or cold) cyanosis
                i) Seen on fingertips and toes
                ii) Associated with peripheral hypoperfusion or vasoconstriction
            b) Central (or warm) cyanosis
                i) Seen on lips and mucous membranes
                ii) Associated with 5 g of deoxygenated Hgb
                    (a) Will be a late sign of hypoxemia in anemic patients; patients with Hgb levels of less than 5 g/dl will not be cyanotic regardless of degree of hypoxemia
                    (b) May be a relatively early sign of hypoxemia in polycythemic patients because they will be cyanotic when they have 5 g of Hgb desaturated even though they may have a normal level (~15 g) still saturated; this is why patients with chronic bronchitis are nicknamed "blue bloaters"
                    (i) Blue because of chronic cyanosis
                    (ii) Bloaters because of chronic right ventricular failure (RVF)
            c) In dark-skinned patients, cyanosis appears as an ashen color.
        4) Cherry-red: may indicate carbon monoxide intoxication
        5) Tobacco stains on fingertips
    b. Scars: especially thoracic
    c. Petechiae: may indicate any of the following:
        1) Blood dyscrasias affecting platelets
            a) Disseminated intravascular coagulation (DIC)
            b) Platelet aggregation inhibitors (e.g., aspirin [ASA], nonsteroidal antiinflammatory drugs [NSAIDs], clopidogrel)
        2) Liver disease
        3) Fat embolism
    d. Edema: may be associated with cor pulmonale
    e. Nailbeds
        1) Color: note cyanosis
        2) Clubbing
            a) Indicates chronic decrease in oxygen supply to body tissues
                i) Especially indicative of restrictive lung diseases (e.g., pulmonary fibrosis, lung cancer)
                ii) Also indicative of right-to-left cardiac shunting (e.g., cyanotic heart disease)
                iii) May be seen in late obstructive lung disease
            b) Normal angle between nailbed and nail less than 180 degrees
            c) Early clubbing angle equal to 180 degrees
            d) Late clubbing greater than 180 degrees

                a) Location
                b) Patency
                c) Rate and type of solutions
            8) Wounds
    7. Abdomen
        a. Liver
            1) May be palpable in patients with normal liver but hyperinflated lungs because liver is pushed downward
            2) May be enlarged and tender due to cor pulmonale
        b. Abdominal muscles (accessory muscles of expiration): frequently used by patients with obstructive lung disease to help push the air out of the lungs
    8. Ventilatory support
        a. Mode
        b. V_T
        c. Rate
        d. FiO_2
        e. PEEP
        f. Peak inspiratory pressure and calculated dynamic compliance
        g. Plateau pressure and calculated static compliance
    9. Clinical indications of respiratory distress (Box 4.2)
    10. Clinical indications of hypoxemia/hypoxia
        a. Hypoxemia (decreased oxygen in the blood): noted by PaO_2 less than 80 mm Hg and SaO_2 less than 95% on arterial blood gases (ABGs) or SaO_2 less than 95% by pulse oximetry
        b. Hypoxia (decreased oxygen in the tissues): noted by clinical indications of hypoxia (Box 4.3) and increased serum lactate level
    11. Clinical indications of hypercapnia (increased CO_2 in the blood): noted by increased $PaCO_2$ on ABGs and clinical indications of hypercapnia (Box 4.4)

Percussion

1. Description of percussion tones (Table 4.6)
2. Thorax
    a. Percussion tones normally heard
        1) Lung: resonance
        2) Diaphragm: flat
        3) Heart: dull
    b. Abnormal percussion tones over thorax
        1) Hyperresonant: asthma, emphysema, pneumothorax
        2) Dull: atelectasis, pneumonia, tumor
        3) Flat: pleural effusion
    c. Diaphragmatic excursion
        1) Evaluated by percussing the position of the diaphragm at expiration and then during full inspiration
        2) Normal diaphragmatic excursion is 3 to 5 cm.
        3) May be decreased by the following:
            a) Increased intrathoracic volume: emphysema
            b) Increased intraabdominal volume and pressure:
                i) Ascites
                ii) Hepatomegaly
                iii) Pregnancy
                iv) Gaseous abdominal distention
            c) Decreased chest excursion and V_T: thoracic or abdominal pain
            d) Phrenic nerve injury
3. Abdomen
    a. Liver
        1) Normal liver span in the right MCL is 6 to 12 cm

Box 4.3 Clinical Indications of Hypoxia

- Restlessness → confusion → lethargy → coma
- Tachycardia → dysrhythmias
- Tachypnea
- Dyspnea
- Use of accessory muscles
- Mild hypertension (early) → hypotension (late)
- Cyanosis may be present (depending on hemoglobin level)

Box 4.2 Clinical Indications of Respiratory Distress

- Pursed-lip breathing
- Tripod positioning
- Speaking only one or two words between breaths
- Cough
- Use of accessory muscles
- Intercostal retractions

Box 4.4 Clinical Indications of Hypercapnia

- Headache
- Irritability
- Confusion
- Inability to concentrate → somnolence → coma
- Bradypnea
- Tachycardia → dysrhythmias
- Hypotension
- Facial rubor (plethora)

Table 4.6 Percussion Tones

Tone	Intensity	Pitch	Duration	Quality	Normal Location
Tympanic	Loud	High	Medium	Drumlike	Stomach, bowel
Hyperresonant	Loud	Low	Long	Booming	Hyperinflated lungs
Resonant	Medium	Low	Long	Hollow	Normal lung
Dull	Soft	High	Medium	Thudlike	Liver, spleen, heart
Flat	Soft	High	Short	Extreme dullness	Muscle, bone

2) Hepatomegaly (i.e., liver span >12 cm in left MCL) may be seen in cor pulmonale.
   a) Assessment by percussion is necessary before specifying hepatomegaly because patients with hyperinflated lungs may have a palpable normal liver because it is pushed downward.

Auscultation

1. Method of lung auscultation
   a. Use diaphragm of stethoscope.
   b. Ask patient to take deep breaths through his or her mouth.
   c. Listen to at least one full breath at each location.
   d. Compare symmetrical areas.
2. Breath sounds
   a. Intensity
      1) Increased
         a) Hyperventilation
         b) Anything that decreases the distance between the lung and your stethoscope (e.g., thin chest wall)
      2) Decreased
         a) Hypoventilation
            i) Emphysema
            ii) Thoracic pain
            iii) Restrictive lungs (e.g., atelectasis, pulmonary fibrosis)
         b) Anything that increases the distance between the lung and your stethoscope
            i) Muscular or obese chest
            ii) Pneumothorax (may be diminished or absent)
            iii) Hemothorax (may be diminished or absent)
            iv) Pleural effusion
      3) Absent
         a) Severe bronchospasm
         b) Massive atelectasis
         c) Pneumonectomy
         d) Pneumothorax
         e) Hemothorax
         f) Malpositioned ET tube (absent breath sounds over left lung)
   b. Quality
      1) Descriptions and normal locations (Fig. 4.22 and Table 4.7)
      2) Implications
         a) Bronchial in areas other than normal location: consolidation (e.g., atelectasis, pneumonia, tumor)
         b) Bronchovesicular in areas other than normal location: partial consolidation, partial aeration
   c. Adventitious sounds (Table 4.8): pathologic extra sounds that may be heard at points in the ventilatory cycle or throughout the ventilatory cycle
   d. Voice sounds: abnormal and indicative of consolidation
      1) Bronchophony: increase in clarity of voice sounds
         a) Ask patient to say "99."
         b) Voice sounds are normally muffled.
         c) If voice sounds are clear over a particular area, bronchophony is present.
      2) Egophony: "e" to "a" conversion of voice sounds
         a) Ask patient to say "e."
         b) Muffled "e" should be heard over normal lung.
         c) If "a" is heard over a particular area, egophony is present.
      3) Whispered pectoriloquy: increase in clarity of whispered sounds
         a) Ask the patient to whisper "99."
         b) Whispered sounds are normally muffled.
         c) If whispered sounds are clear over a particular area, whispered pectoriloquy is present.

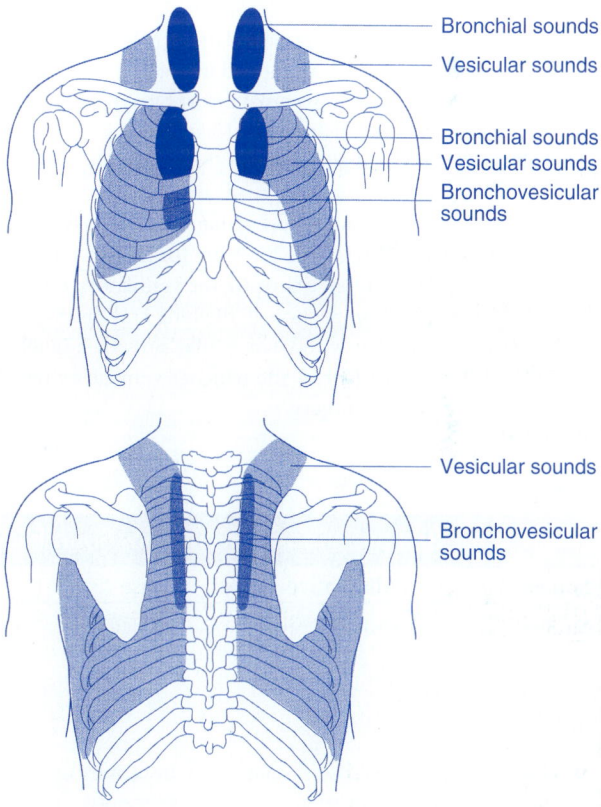

Fig. 4.22 Breath sounds: normal locations. (From Barkauskas, V. H., Baumann, L., and Darling-Fischer, C.S [1994]. *Health and physical assessment*. St. Louis: Mosby.)

Table 4.7	Breath Sounds: Quality				
Quality	I:E Ratio	Intensity	Pitch	Description	Normal Location
Bronchial	I < E	Loud	High	Hollow	Trachea
Bronchovesicular	I = E	Medium	Medium	Breezy	Mainstem bronchi
Vesicular	I > E	Soft	Low	Swishy	Peripheral lung

Bedside Assessment of Pulmonary Function

1. Bedside parameters (also referred to as *ventilatory mechanics*)
   a. Spirometry: measured with Wright respirometer
      1) V_T
         a) Amount of air moved in and out each breath
         b) Normal 7 ml/kg
            i) V_T less than 5 ml/kg indicates need for artificial airway or mechanical ventilation.
            ii) V_T greater than 5 ml/kg indicates that the patient can be weaned or extubated.
      2) Vital capacity (VC)
         a) Maximal amount of air that can be exhaled after a maximal inspiration
         b) Normal 15 ml/kg
            i) VC less than 10 ml/kg indicates need for artificial airway and/or mechanical ventilation.
            ii) VC greater than 10 ml/kg indicates that the patient can be weaned and/or extubated.
      3) Minute ventilation
         a) $f \times V_T$
         b) Normal 5 to 10 l/min
      4) Maximal voluntary ventilation (MVV)
         a) Volume of air moved into and out of the lungs with maximal effort over a short period of time (usually 10–15 seconds)
         b) Normal is 170 l/min (NOTE: One-quarter of this total is actually measured in the 15-second period; patients are not asked to ventilate at this intensity for an entire minute.)
         c) Reflects the status of the ventilatory muscles, compliance of the lung and thorax, and airway resistance; may provide a quick assessment of the patient's ventilatory reserve before surgery
   b. Maximal inspiratory pressure (MIP): measured with negative inspiratory pressure meter
      1) Also referred to as *negative inspiratory force* (NIF)
      2) Normal is greater than (more negative than) –60 to –80 cm H_2O.
         a) MIP of less than –25 cm H_2O indicates need for artificial airway, mechanical ventilation, or both.
         b) MIP of greater than –25 cm H_2O indicates that the patient can be weaned, extubated, or both.
   c. Rapid shallow breathing index (RSBI)
      1) Calculated as: f/V_T (in liters) using frequency in 1 minute and average V_T over 1 minute
      2) Provides an indication of the brain's perception of how well the respiratory muscles tolerate the work of breathing; if the brain senses that the workload is too high for the respiratory muscles to tolerate, the reflex ventilatory pattern is rapid shallow breathing
      3) RSBI of less than or equal to 105 breaths/min/l indicates readiness for weaning.
2. Capnography (may also be referred to as *end-tidal CO_2 monitoring*)
   a. Continuous noninvasive method for evaluating the adequacy of CO_2 exchange in the lungs; assesses $PaCO_2$ indirectly by detecting the level of CO_2 in the exhaled air
      1) Measurement of expired CO_2 tension
      2) Display of the CO_2 waveform from breath to breath (Fig. 4.23)
   b. Indications
      1) Verification of tracheal intubation
         a) Esophageal intubation is reflected by decreased end-tidal CO_2 ($P_{et}CO_2$) or an abnormal waveform

Table 4.8 Breath Sounds: Adventitious Sounds

Sound	Alternative Terms	Phase	Description	Cause
Stridor	Croupy	Inspiratory	High-pitched whistle audible without a stethoscope	• Upper airway obstruction • Epiglottis • Foreign body • Laryngospasm • Laryngeal edema

Wheezes	Whistles; sibilant rhonchi	Inspiratory or expiratory	High-pitched whistling sound	• Decrease in airway lumen
				  • Bronchospasm
				  • Mucus plug
				  • Tumor

Crackles	Rales	Inspiratory	Discontinuous crackling sound; similar to rubbing hair between fingers	• Pulmonary edema • Atelectasis • Pulmonary fibrosis
Rhonchi	Gurgles, sonorous rhonchi, coarse crackles	Expiratory	Continuous gurgling sound	• Fluid or mucus in airways
Pleural friction rub		Inspiratory and expiratory	Grating or scratching sound	• Pulmonary infarction • Pleurisy • Tuberculosis • Lung cancer

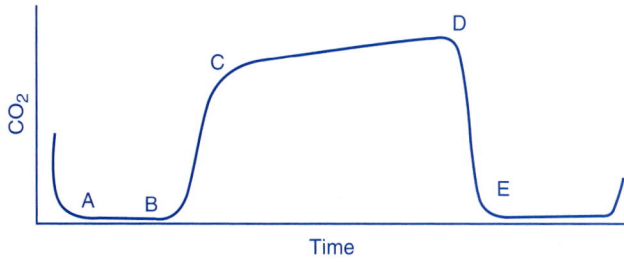

Fig. 4.23 Typical normal CO_2 waveform. *A to B*, Exhalation of CO_2-free gas from dead space. *B to C*, Combination of dead space and alveolar gases. *C to D*, Exhalation of mostly alveolar gas. *D*, Exhalation of CO_2 at maximal point (end-tidal point). *D to E*, Inspiration begins, and CO_2 concentration rapidly falls to baseline or zero. (From St. John, R. E. [2004]. Airway management. *Crit Care Nurse*, 24[2], 93-96.)

        b) Inexpensive, disposable, colorimetric CO_2 indicators are frequently used for this purpose; they do not display waveform.
     2) Verification of adequacy of chest compression during cardiopulmonary resuscitation
        a) In the absence of pulmonary blood flow, $P_{et}CO_2$ decreases rapidly because no CO_2 is being returned to the lungs.
        b) $P_{et}CO_2$ is decreased when chest compressions are inadequate, and $P_{et}CO_2$ increases when effectiveness of compression is increased.
     3) Evaluation of ventilation and $PaCO_2$
        a) This use is limited in critically ill patients because the relationship between $PaCO_2$ and $P_{et}CO_2$ is affected by changes in pulmonary dead space and perfusion.
        b) $PaCO_2 - P_{et}CO_2$ gradient may be used as an indication of changes in pulmonary dead space or a drop in cardiac output.
        c) May be used during procedural sedation to monitor for changes in ventilation
     4) Monitoring during weaning: progressive rise indicates increased work of breathing
  c. Description
     1) The CO_2 in the expired air is measured; the $P_{et}CO_2$ is assumed to represent alveolar gas and may be used to estimate the $PaCO_2$; because this relationship is dependent on the V/Q ratios throughout the lung, this assumption may be particularly erroneous in critically ill patients.
  d. Normal value: the $P_{et}CO_2$ is usually 1 to 6 mm Hg below the $PaCO_2$ or approximately 38 mm Hg.
     1) Increased $P_{et}CO_2$ assumes hypoventilation.
     2) Decreased $P_{et}CO_2$ assumes hyperventilation.
  e. Implication: changes in $P_{et}CO_2$ indicate that the patient requires prompt assessment and ABGs for analysis.
3. Pulse oximetry (SpO_2)
  a. Continuous noninvasive method of monitoring arterial oxygen saturation
  b. Indications
     1) Assessment of adequacy of oxygenation (does not adequately evaluate ventilation because $PaCO_2$ increases with hypoventilation, but PaO_2 and O_2 saturation do not decrease until much later)
     2) Recovery from anesthesia
  c. Description
     1) Sensor with light source is placed on the fingertip, toe, bridge of nose, forehead, or earlobe; care must be taken to use the appropriate sensor for the location (i.e., a finger sensor should not be attached to the earlobe).
     2) The amount of arterial Hgb that is saturated with oxygen is determined by beams of light passed through the tissue.
  d. Normal value: greater than 95%; moderate to severe hypoxemia should be suspected if less than 90%; causes of decreased SpO_2:
     1) Decrease in SaO_2 and PaO_2
     2) Decrease in cardiac output
  e. Limitations
     1) Inadequate pulsations may result from the following:
        a) Significant hypotension
        b) Vasopressor use
        c) Severe hypothermia
        d) Arterial compression
     2) Tends to overestimate SaO_2 by 2% to 5%; accuracy of SpO_2 below 70% is questionable; the lower the SaO_2, the larger the difference between it and the SpO_2
     3) Does not accurately reflect oxygen tissue delivery in patients with anemia or abnormal hemoglobins
        a) Carboxyhemoglobin
           i) Results in overestimation of oxygen saturation reading because Hgb is saturated but with carbon monoxide
          ii) Smokers may have elevated carboxyhemoglobin levels.
        b) Methemoglobin
           i) Results in overestimation of SaO_2
          ii) Methemoglobin is a form of Hgb that cannot carry oxygen.
          iii) May be related to the administration of nitroglycerin, nitroprusside, sulfonamides, or local anesthetics
        c) Hgb S: sickle cell anemia
     4) Other variables may impair accuracy.
        a) Intravenous (IV) dyes (e.g., methylene blue, indocyanine green): result in inaccurate readings
        b) Increased bilirubin (>20 mg/dl): results in inaccurately low readings
        c) Ambient light: may affect accuracy
        d) Motion artifact: may affect accuracy
        e) Edema: may result in inaccurately low readings
        f) Nail polish: blue, green, gold, black, or brown nail polish needs to be removed
        g) Pierced earlobe: results in inaccurate reading
  f. Implication: changes in SpO_2 indicate that the patient requires prompt assessment and ABGs for analysis.
4. Transcutaneous PaO_2 ($P_{tc}O_2$) monitoring
  a. Continuous noninvasive method of monitoring PaO_2
  b. Indications: as for pulse oximetry
  c. Description
     1) Sensor is placed on the skin; electrode has a heating element to warm skin and cause capillaries to dilate and increase blood flow.

d. Normal value: greater than 80 mm Hg; moderate to severe hypoxemia should be suspected if less than 60 mm Hg
e. Limitations
1) Affected by skin blood flow, thickness, temperature, skin oxygen consumption, subcutaneous emphysema, edema
2) Tends to underestimate PaO_2
3) Less reliable in adults than in infants
f. Implications
1) PaO_2 will always be equal to or greater than $P_{tc}O_2$.
2) Changes in $P_{tc}O_2$ indicate that the patient requires prompt assessment and ABGs for analysis.
5. Mixed venous oxygen saturation (SvO_2)
a. Oxygen saturation of the blood as it returns to the lung for reoxygenation; reflects how well the body's demand for oxygen is met by the amount of oxygen supplied
b. Normal SvO_2: 60% to 80%
c. Complete discussion of SvO_2 monitoring in the Hemodynamic Monitoring section of Chapter 3
6. Continuous airway pressure monitoring (CAPM)
a. Noninvasive technique for displaying the patient's airway pressure waveforms on a bedside monitoring system; provides a visual representation of the patient's own spontaneous effort and the function of the ventilator
b. Description
1) Air-filled (i.e., not primed with fluid) pressure tubing is connected to the ventilator tubing at the Y connector.
2) Tubing is connected to a transducer and the transducer is attached to a channel of the bedside monitor.
3) Zeroing is at any level.
4) Positive waveform deflections indicate positive pressure ventilation, and negative deflections indicate spontaneous inspiratory effort.
c. Implications
1) Assessment of asynchrony between patient and ventilator
2) Identification of ventilator mode
3) Detection of PEEP, including auto-PEEP
4) Improvement of accuracy of hemodynamic waveforms
5) Identification of respiratory efforts when muscle paralysis or sedation is inadequate

Basic Chest Radiography Interpretation

1. Basic principles
a. Density: denser tissues absorb more of the x-rays, and less dense tissues absorb less of the x-rays.
1) Air is radiolucent and appears black.
2) Water (e.g., heart, muscle, blood, diaphragm, liver, spleen) appears gray.
3) Fat (e.g., breasts) appears whitish-gray.
4) Bone is radiopaque and appears white.
a) Bullets, teeth, and wires are also radiopaque.
2. Initial steps
a. Check the patient's name and date on the radiographs.
b. Check for the "R" or "L" marker and orient the film appropriately on the view box.
c. Ensure the quality of the inspiratory effort: the middle of the right hemidiaphragm should be at the 10th rib posteriorly.
d. If there are previous films, view side by side with the new film.
3. Steps for interpretation (Urden et al., 2017)
a. Evaluate the different densities to determine air, fluid, tissue, and bone.
b. Evaluate the shape of each density to determine what normal anatomic structure the shape represents.
c. Compare the left and right sides to determine if there are physiologic or pathophysiologic differences (Fig. 4.24)
1) A: airway, including the large airways, lung, pleura
2) B: bones, including the clavicles, ribs, spine
3) C: circulation, including the heart, mediastinum, and vascular markings
4) D: diaphragm
d. Evaluate all structures for abnormalities.
1) Cardiomegaly: heart size more than half the lateral diameter of the chest
2) Atelectasis
a) Area of atelectasis appears whitish-gray.
b) Areas around the atelectasis appear darker than normal because of compensatory hyperinflation.
c) Elevation of the hemidiaphragm on affected side
d) Deviation of mediastinal structures toward the affected side
3) Pneumonia
a) Cloudlike infiltrates which may be localized or diffuse and may involve one or both lungs
b) May be difficult to differentiate from pulmonary edema so clinical and diagnostic (e.g., brain natriuretic peptide [BNP]) profiles are crucial
4) Hydrothorax (e.g., hemothorax or pleural effusion)
a) Upright film shows a pleural air-fluid level with air (i.e., black) on top and fluid (i.e., gray) below the level.
5) Pneumothorax
a) Area that is blacker than normal lung without vascular markings
b) Pleura may appear as a fine, white line that separates the pleural space from the aerated lung.
6) Emphysema
a) Hyperinflated (i.e., very black) lungs with flattened diaphragms
7) ARDS: depends on stage
a) Stage I: normal
b) Stage II: fine, diffuse infiltrates commonly referred to as "ground-glass infiltrates"
c) Stage III: diffuse patchy, scattered infiltrates as atelectasis progresses to "white outs."
d) Stage IV: white-out areas may appear blacker as hyaline membranes have developed.
e. If there are wires, tubes, or lines, determine if they are in the proper place (Siela, 2008).
1) ET tube: 3 to 5 cm above the carina
2) Central venous catheter: in the superior vena cava

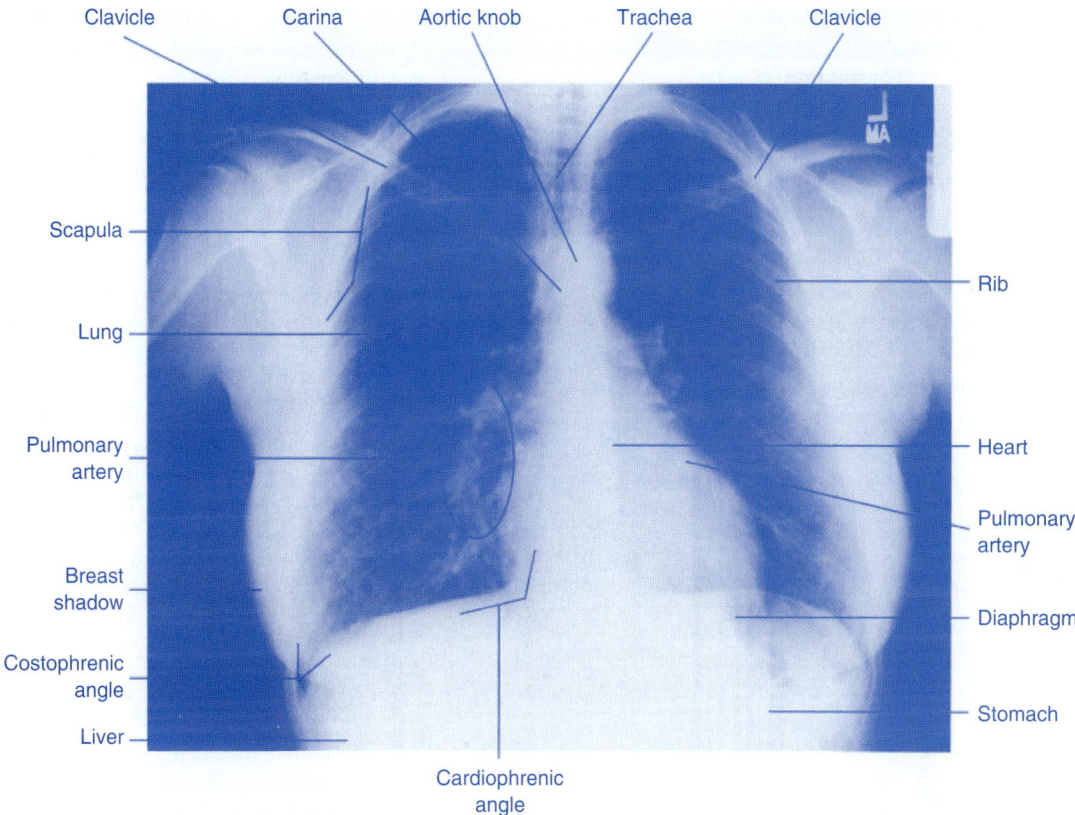

Fig. 4.24 Anatomical landmarks on chest radiographs. (From Dettenmeir, P. A. *Radiographic assessment for nurses* [1995]. St. Louis: Mosby.)

3) PAC: in the left or right pulmonary artery with tip about 2 cm from the hilum
4) IABP: tip should be distal to the origin of the left subclavian artery
5) NG tube: tip should extend to about 10 cm into the stomach
6) Dobbhoff feeding tube: tip should be in duodenum

Diagnostic Studies
1. Serum chemistries
   a. Sodium: normal 136 to 145 mEq/l
   b. Potassium: normal 3.5 to 5.0 mEq/l
   c. Chloride: normal 96 to 106 mEq/l
   d. Calcium: normal 8.5 to 10.5 mg/dl
   e. Phosphorus: normal 3 to 4.5 mg/dl
   f. Magnesium: normal 1.5 to 2.2 mEq/l or 1.8 to 2.4 mg/dl
   g. Glucose: normal 70 to 115 mEq/l
   h. Blood urea nitrogen (BUN): normal 5 to 20 mg/dl
   i. Creatinine: normal 0.7 to 1.5 mg/dl
   j. Lactate: <1 mmol/l
2. ABGs
   a. pH: normal 7.35 to 7.45
   b. $PaCO_2$: normal 35 to 45 mm Hg
   c. HCO_3^-: normal 22 to 26 mEq/l
   d. PaO_2: normal 80 to 100 mm Hg
   e. SaO_2: greater than 95%
3. Hematology
   a. Hematocrit: normal 40% to 52% for males; 35% to 47% for females
   b. Hgb: normal 13 to 18 g/dl for males; 12 to 16 g/dl for females
   c. White blood cells (WBC): normal 3500 to 11,000 mm^3
   d. D-dimer: normal negative
4. Sputum analysis: may be obtained by AM specimen by cough, induced tracheobronchial aspiration, transtracheal aspiration, or bronchoscopy
   a. Characteristics: color, odor, viscosity, presence of blood
   b. Culture and sensitivity tests: identify infecting organism and effective antibiotic agent
   c. Gram stain: differentiates between gram-negative and gram-positive bacteria
   d. Acid-fast stain: determines presence of acid-fast bacilli (tuberculosis)
   e. Cytology studies: determine presence of malignant cells
5. Pleural fluid analysis
   a. Total protein: differentiates between exudative pleural effusion and transudative pleural effusion
   b. Gram stain: differentiates between gram-negative or gram-positive bacteria
   c. Acid-fast stain: determines presence of acid-fast bacilli (tuberculosis)
   d. Cytology studies: determine presence of malignant cells
6. Skin tests
   a. Type I hypersensitivity tests ("allergy tests")
   b. Type II hypersensitivity tests: purified protein derivative (PPD) for tuberculosis
   c. Fungal diseases (e.g., *Candida*)
7. Other diagnostic studies (Table 4.9)

Table 4.9 Pulmonary Diagnostic Studies

Study	Evaluation	Comments
Bronchography	• Detects obstruction or malformation of the tracheobronchial tree	• Patient inspires radiopaque substance, and then radiographs are taken • Inquire about possibility of pregnancy
Chest radiography	• Detects lung pathology (e.g., pneumonia, pulmonary edema, atelectasis, tuberculosis) • Determines size and location of lung lesions and tumors • Verifies placement of endotracheal tube, central venous catheters, chest tubes	• Noninvasive test with minimal radiation exposure • Inquire about possibility of pregnancy • Posteroanterior and lateral films are done most commonly, but in critical care areas, anteroposterior portable films are frequently necessary because of an inability to transport patients • Lateral decubitus films aid in identification of pleural effusion
Exercise testing	• Identifies early disability • Differentiates between cardiac and pulmonary disease	• Monitor for changes in SpO_2 during exercise • Monitor closely for exercise-induced hypotension or ventricular dysrhythmias
Laryngoscopy, bronchoscopy, mediastinoscopy	• Obtain cytology specimen or biopsy • Identify tumors, obstructions, secretions, foreign bodies in tracheobronchial tree • Locate a bleeding site • May be used therapeutically to remove secretions, foreign bodies, other contaminants	• Patient is sedated before the with diazepam, midazolam, lorazepam, propofol, or dexmedetomidine • Monitor the patient for subcutaneous emphysema after study; indicates tracheal or bronchial tear • Monitor for hemoptysis; some blood in sputum is normal after biopsy but frank hemoptysis requires immediate attention
Lung biopsy Transthoracic needle lung biopsy Open lung biopsy	• Obtain specimen for cytology evaluation	• Transthoracic needle biopsy performed under fluoroscopy; inquire about possibility of pregnancy • Open lung biopsy requires thoracotomy
Magnetic resonance imaging	• Distinguishes tumors from other structures (e.g., tumor, pleural thickening, fibrosis)	• Noninvasive test • Contraindicated for patients with pacemakers or implanted metallic devices
Pulmonary angiography	• Detects changes in lung tissue (e.g., masses) • Diagnoses abnormalities in pulmonary vasculature, including thrombi and emboli • Identifies congenital abnormalities of the circulation	• Invasive test • Inquire about possibility of pregnancy • Contrast media injected into pulmonary artery; ensure adequate hydration after study • Monitor arterial puncture point for hematoma or hemorrhage
Pulmonary function studies (Table 4.1 lists lung volumes and parameters with normal values) Spirometry: volumes and capacities RV, FRC, TLC require nitrogen washout technique Ventilatory mechanics Flow-volume loop studies Diffusing capacity	• Measure lung volumes, capacities, and flow rates • Identify features of restrictive or obstructive lung disease • Evaluate responsiveness to bronchodilator therapy • Aid in evaluation of surgical risk • Document a disability or cause of dyspnea	• Noninvasive study • Frequently repeated after bronchodilator therapy
Sleep studies	• Diagnose and differentiate between obstructive sleep apnea, central sleep apnea, and cardiac sleep apnea	• Restrict caffeine before testing • Usually done during normal sleep hours
Thoracentesis (may include pleural biopsy)	• Obtain pleural fluid and/or tissue specimen • May be used therapeutically to remove pleural fluid	• Monitor patient for indications of pneumothorax • Monitor for leakage from puncture point
Thoracic computed tomography	• Defines lesions, masses, cavities, or shadows seen on a normal chest radiography • Evaluates tracheal or bronchial narrowing • Aids in planning radiation therapy	• Radiographs taken at different angles

Table 4.9	Pulmonary Diagnostic Studies—cont'd	
Study	**Evaluation**	**Comments**
Ultrasonography	• Evaluates pleural disease • Visualizes diaphragm and detects disease around diaphragm (e.g., subphrenic hematoma or abscess)	• Noninvasive test
Ventilation scan Lung perfusion scan Ventilation/perfusion (V/Q) scan	• Diagnose ventilation or perfusion abnormalities, including emphysema or pulmonary emboli	• Invasive test: radioisotope inspired and injected intravascularly • Inquire about possibility of pregnancy • Nuclear scan study: assure patient that amount of radioactive material is minimal

Acid–Base Balance and Arterial Blood Gas Interpretation

Physiology Review

1. Acid: a substance that can give up an H+ ion; acids are produced by the body as a result of cellular metabolism
    a. Volatile (e.g., carbonic acid)
        1) Exhalable
        2) Results from aerobic metabolism of glucose
        3) Eliminated by the lungs
    b. Nonvolatile (also called *fixed*) (e.g., sulfuric, phosphoric, uric)
        1) Nonexhalable and cannot be converted into a gas
        2) Results from aerobic metabolism of protein and fat and the anaerobic metabolism of glucose
        3) Eliminated by the kidney
    c. Elimination or neutralization necessary
2. Acidemia: the condition of the blood with a pH of below 7.35
3. Acidosis: the process that causes the acidemia
4. Base: a substance that can accept an H+ (the primary base in the body is bicarbonate)
5. Alkalemia: the condition of the blood with a pH of above 7.45
6. Alkalosis: the process that causes the alkalemia
7. pH
    a. Indirect measurement of hydrogen ion concentration
    b. Reflection of the balance between carbonic acid (acid regulated by the lungs) and bicarbonate (base regulated by the kidneys)
    c. Inversely proportional to hydrogen ion concentration
        1) Increase in H^+ concentration: lower pH, more acid
        2) Decrease in H^+ concentration: higher pH, more base
    d. Must be maintained within a narrow range to allow functioning of enzymatic systems in the body
        1) pH below 6.8 or above 7.8 is incompatible with life.
        2) Note that this is a 0.6 change toward acidosis but only a 0.4 change toward alkalosis. (From midline normal of 7.4); this is because the shift of the oxyhemoglobin dissociation curve caused by alkalosis affects tissue oxygenation more adversely than does the shift caused by acidosis

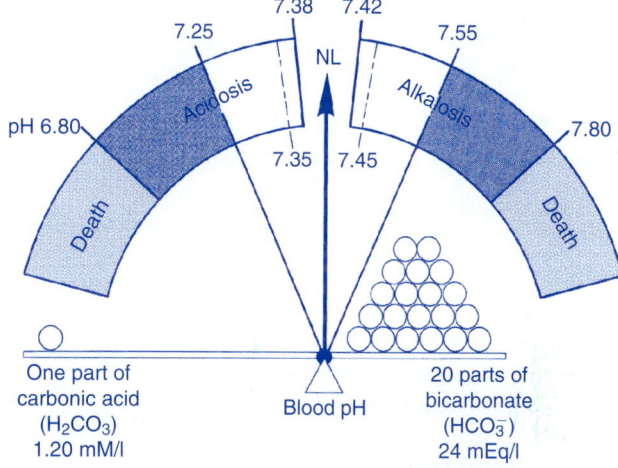

Fig. 4.25 Acid–base balance. Twenty parts of HCO_3^- is required to buffer one part carbonic acid; pH normally is maintained within the narrow range (NL) of 7.35 to 7.45; a pH below 6.8 or above 7.8 is incompatible with life. (From Price, S. A., & Wilson, L. M. [2003]. *Pathophysiology: Clinical concepts of disease processes* [6th ed.]. St. Louis: Mosby.)

8. Henderson-Hasselbalch equation
    a. pH is determined by the logarithm of the ratio of bicarbonate concentration to arterial $PaCO_2$
        1) $$pH = \frac{pK\,(Constant\,of\,6.1) + \log HCO_3^-}{PaCO_2}$$
    b. Ratio of 20 bicarbonate:1 carbonic acid maintains normal pH (Fig. 4.25)

Acid–Base Regulation

1. Physiologic buffers
    a. Weak acid and its salt
    b. Immediate response when a change in acid–base status occurs by combining with excess acid or base
    c. Buffer systems
        1) Bicarbonate–carbonic acid buffer system
            a) The most important buffer system
            b) Bicarbonate is generated by the kidney and aids in the elimination of H+

            $$CO_2 + H_2O \Leftrightarrow H_2CO_3 \Leftrightarrow H^+ + HCO_3^-$$
            Lungs $\qquad\qquad\qquad\qquad$ Kidneys

        2) Phosphate system: aids in excretion of H^+ by the kidney

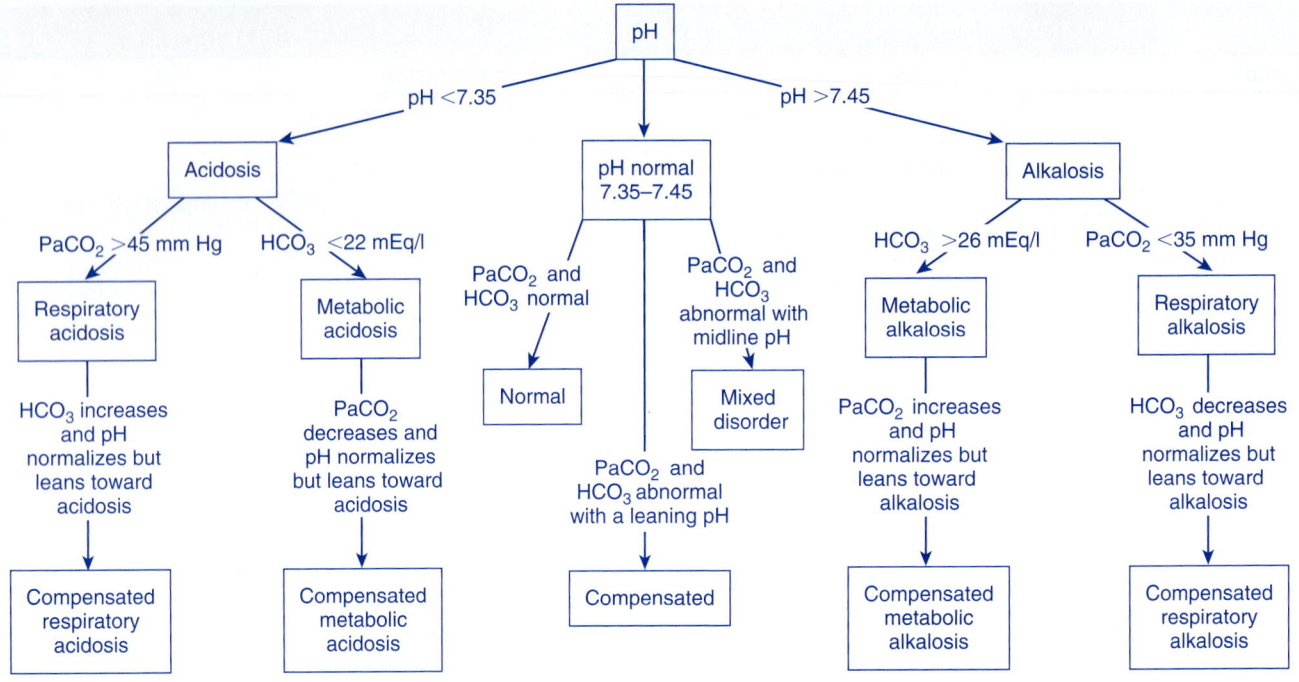

Fig. 4.26 Determination of acid–base balance or imbalance.

3) Ammonium: H⁺ is added to ammonia (NH_3) in the renal tubule to form ammonium (NH_4); allows greater excretion of H⁺ by the kidney
4) Hgb and other proteins: aid in buffering extracellular fluid

2. Respiratory system
   a. Regulates the excretion or retention of carbonic acid
      1) If pH decreases, the rate and depth of ventilation increase.
      2) If pH increases, the rate and depth of ventilation decrease.
   b. Responds within minutes: fast but weak
3. Renal system
   a. Regulates the excretion or retention of bicarbonate and the excretion of hydrogen and nonvolatile acids
      1) If pH decreases, the kidney retains bicarbonate.
      2) If pH increases, the kidney excretes bicarbonate.
   b. Responds within 48 hours: slow but powerful

Acid–Base Imbalances (Fig. 4.26)

1. Acidemia: pH below 7.35
   a. Acidosis: the process causing acidemia
      1) Caused by acid gain
         a) If acid is volatile (reflected by increase in $PaCO_2$): respiratory acidosis
         b) If acid is nonvolatile (reflected by decrease in HCO_3^-): metabolic acidosis
      2) Caused by base loss or metabolic acid gain (reflected by decrease in HCO_3^-): metabolic acidosis
      3) Anion gap is used to differentiate between metabolic acid gain or base loss as cause of metabolic acidosis
         a) Calculated: $(Na^+ + K^+) - (Cl^- + CO_2^-)$
         b) Normal 5 to 15
         c) If anion gap is normal (between 5 and 15), metabolic acidosis is due to a base loss.
         d) If anion gap is increased (>15), metabolic acidosis is due to acid gain.
            i) Memory aid for causes of increased anion gap
               (a) M: methanol or ethanol ingestion
               (b) U: uremia
               (c) D: diabetic ketoacidosis or alcoholic ketoacidosis or starvation
               (d) P: paraldehyde ingestion
               (e) I: iron or isoniazid
               (f) L: lactic acidosis
               (g) E: ethylene glycol ingestion
               (h) S: salicylate toxicity
2. Alkalemia: pH above 7.45
   a. Alkalosis: the process causing alkalosis
      1) Caused by acid loss
         a) If acid is volatile (reflected by decrease in $PaCO_2$): respiratory alkalosis
         b) If acid is nonvolatile (reflected by increase in HCO_3^-): metabolic alkalosis
      2) Caused by base gain or metabolic acid loss (reflected by increase in HCO_3^-): metabolic alkalosis
3. Compensation
   a. Respiratory acidosis
      1) The kidneys reabsorb more bicarbonate or excrete more H⁺.
      2) The bicarbonate and base excess (BE) levels increase.
      3) This change will be slow and may take as long as 2 to 3 days.
   b. Respiratory alkalosis
      1) The kidneys excrete more bicarbonate.
      2) The bicarbonate and BE levels decrease.
      3) This change will be slow and may take as long as 2 to 3 days.

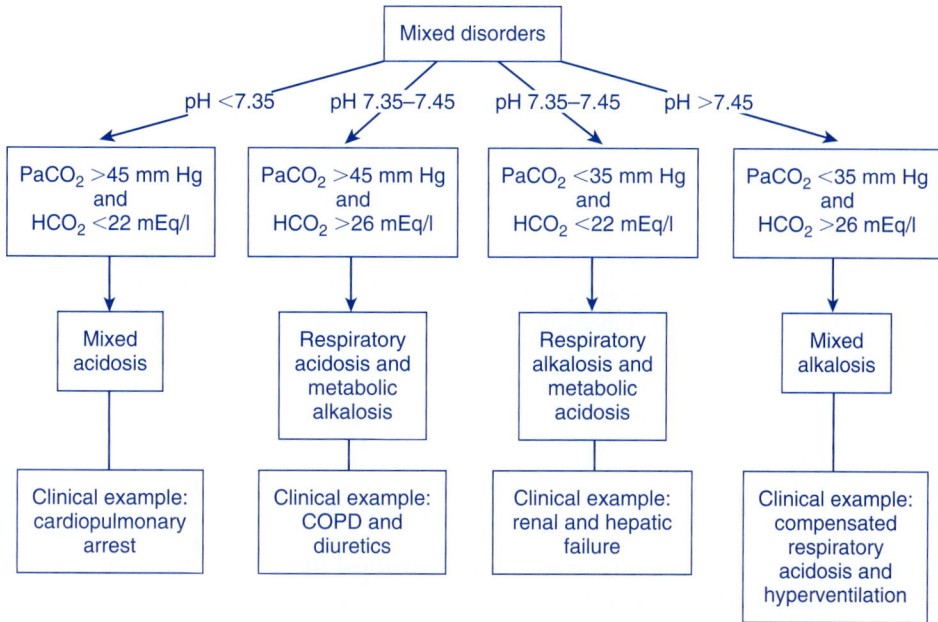

Fig. 4.27 Mixed disorders and clinical examples.

a) Because respiratory alkalosis is almost always a short-term process (e.g., hyperventilation anxiety syndrome), compensation for respiratory alkalosis is rarely seen because it takes too long, and the problem would be resolved.
c. Metabolic acidosis
  1) The lungs increase the rate and depth of ventilation.
  2) The $PaCO_2$ level decreases.
  3) This change will be rapid, usually within minutes to hours.
d. Metabolic alkalosis
  1) The lungs decrease the rate and depth of ventilation.
  2) The $PaCO_2$ level increases.
  3) This change will be rapid, usually within minutes to hours.
e. Correction versus compensation
  1) Correction may be a physiologic process or the result of appropriate therapeutic measures; correction is achieved when the pH is normal and both indicators ($PaCO_2$, HCO_3^-) are normal.
  2) Compensation is a physiologic process; the pH is normal and both indicators are abnormal.
     a) Partial compensation: pH is still abnormal, but the secondary parameter is outside normal range in the direction to move the pH toward normal.
     b) Full compensation: pH is normal, and the secondary parameter is outside normal range in the direction to move the pH toward normal.
4. Mixed disorders (Fig. 4.27)
  a. More than one disorder may coexist.
  b. The degree of respiratory component versus metabolic component can be calculated using these formulas.
     1) As the $PaCO_2$ changes by 10 mm Hg (From normal of 40), it is associated with a change in pH of .08 in the opposite direction.)

Box 4.5	Arterial Blood Gas Normal Values
pH	7.35–7.45
$PaCO_2$	35–45 mm Hg
HCO_3^-	22–26 mEq/l
PaO_2	80–100 mm Hg

  2) As the pH changes by 0.15 (from normal of 7.4), it is associated with a change in base of 10 mEq.)
  c. Compensation cannot exist in mixed disorders because each system is independently abnormal and cannot help the other.

Analysis of Arterial Blood Gases

1. Purposes of ABGs
   a. Evaluate ventilation: $PaCO_2$
   b. Evaluate acid–base status: pH; to determine the cause of the acid–base imbalance, determine which parameter is abnormal
      1) Respiratory: $PaCO_2$
      2) Metabolic: HCO_3^-
   c. Evaluate oxygenation: PaO_2
2. Parameters and normals (Box 4.5)
   a. pH: negative logarithm of hydrogen ion concentration in arterial blood
      1) Normal pH is 7.35 to 7.45
      2) Levels below 7.35 indicate an acidosis.
      3) Levels above 7.45 indicate an alkalosis.
   b. $PaCO_2$: partial pressure of CO_2 in arterial blood
      1) Normal $PaCO_2$ is 35 to 45 mm Hg
      2) Levels below 35 indicate a respiratory alkalosis or respiratory compensation for a metabolic acidosis.
      3) Levels above 45 indicate a respiratory acidosis or respiratory compensation for a metabolic alkalosis.

c. HCO_3^-: bicarbonate ion level in arterial blood
   1) Normal HCO_3^- is 22 to 26 mEq/l
   2) Levels below 22 indicate a metabolic acidosis or metabolic compensation for respiratory alkalosis.
   3) Levels above 26 indicate a metabolic alkalosis or metabolic compensation for respiratory acidosis.
d. BE: difference between acid and base levels in arterial blood
   1) Normal BE is +2 to −2.
   2) Levels below −2 (actually a base deficit) indicate a metabolic acidosis or metabolic compensation for respiratory alkalosis.
   3) Levels above +2 indicate a metabolic alkalosis or metabolic compensation for respiratory acidosis.
e. PaO_2: partial pressure of oxygen in arterial blood
   1) Normal PaO_2 is 80 to 100 mm Hg.
   2) Levels above 100 indicate hyperoxemia.
   3) Levels below 80 indicate mild hypoxemia.
   4) Levels below 60 indicate moderate hypoxemia.
   5) Levels below 40 indicate severe hypoxemia.
f. SaO_2: saturation of Hgb by oxygen
   1) Normal SaO_2 is 95% or greater.
   2) Levels below 95% indicate mild desaturation of Hgb.
   3) Levels below 90% indicate moderate desaturation of Hgb.
   4) Levels below 75% indicate severe desaturation of Hgb.
3. Steps in analysis
   a. Is pH acidotic, alkalotic, or normal?
   b. Which parameter is abnormal?
      1) $PaCO_2$: respiratory
      2) HCO_3^-: metabolic
   c. If the pH is normal, is it leaning? If so, consider compensation.
      1) Compensation causes a leaning pH; the pH leans toward the initial disorder.
         a) The body never overcompensates; a normal nonleaning pH with two abnormal indicators ($PaCO_2$ and HCO_3^-) suggests a mixed disorder (e.g., one alkalotic process + one acidotic process).
      2) For compensation to be occurring, one parameter change must help the other.
         a) Full compensation: normal pH with both indicators abnormal
         b) Partial compensation
            i) pH is still abnormal.
            ii) Both indicators ($PaCO_2$ and HCO_3^-) are abnormal with the secondary indicator moving in the direction to help normalize the pH.
   d. Assess oxygenation
      1) PaO_2 less than 80 mm Hg is hypoxemia.
      2) PaO_2 less than 60 mm Hg on room air is usually an indication for oxygen administration.
      3) Acceptable PaO_2 should be adjusted for age; one method is to subtract 1 mm Hg for each year greater than 60 years from 80 mm Hg; this gives acceptable PaO_2 on room air for a patient of that age.
4. Technical problems that may affect accuracy of ABG values
   a. Too much heparin: decrease in $PaCO_2$, decrease in HCO_3^-, increase in BE except with point of care analyzers (e.g., ISTAT)
   b. Air bubble: increase in pH, decrease in $PaCO_2$, increase in PaO_2
   c. Not chilled immediately: decrease in pH, decrease in PaO_2, increase in $PaCO_2$ except with point of care analyzers (e.g., ISTAT)
   d. Inadequate discard volume when drawing from catheter with flush solution: decreased $PaCO_2$

Discussion of Acid–Base Imbalances
Table 4.10

Airway Management

Etiology of Airway Obstruction
1. Upper airway
   a. Relaxation of tongue against hypopharynx: primary cause of obstruction in unconscious patient
   b. Foreign body aspiration
      1) Aspiration of food: primary cause of obstruction in a conscious patient
      2) Vomitus
      3) Dentures
   c. Tumor
   d. Hematoma
   e. Laryngeal spasm, edema
   f. Vocal cord paralysis
   g. Infection (e.g., epiglottis)
   h. Trauma (e.g., fractured trachea)
   i. Inflammation (e.g., angioedema, ingestion of caustic agents)
2. Lower airway
   a. Foreign bodies
   b. Secretions
   c. Hemorrhage
   d. Pneumonia
   e. Space-occupying lesions, tumors
   f. Bronchospasm

Clinical Presentation of Airway Obstruction
1. Partial obstruction
   a. Presence of air movement
   b. Restlessness, agitation, anxiety
   c. Respiratory distress: tracheal tug, intercostal retractions, use of accessory muscles
   d. Cyanosis
   e. Coughing
   f. Altered speech
   g. Inspiratory sounds: snoring, stridor
   h. Breath sound changes: wheezes, rhonchi
2. Complete obstruction
   a. Lack of air movement
   b. Extreme anxiety in conscious patient
   c. Respiratory distress: tracheal tug, intercostal retractions, use of accessory muscles
   d. Cyanosis
   e. Inability to speak, cough, or produce any sound

Table 4.10 Discussion of Acid–base Imbalances

Imbalance	Etiology	Clinical Presentation	Collaborative Management

Respiratory acidosis: pH low; PaCO$_2$ high	Hypoventilation
	• Airway obstruction
	• CNS depression from drugs, injury, or disease
	• Chest wall injury (e.g., flail chest)
	• Obstructive lung disease (e.g., chronic bronchitis, emphysema, late asthma)
	• Restrictive lung disease (e.g., kyphoscoliosis, obesity hypoventilation syndrome)
	• Oxygen-induced hypoventilation in patients with chronic hypercapnia
	• Neuromuscular abnormality (e.g., Guillain-Barré syndrome, myasthenia gravis, multiple sclerosis)
	• Atelectasis, pneumonia
	• Pulmonary edema
	• Respiratory arrest
		Initially
		• Sympathetic nervous system stimulation symptoms (e.g., tachycardia, tachypnea, diaphoresis)
		Later
		• Bradypnea
		• Hypotension
		• Dysrhythmias
		• Confusion
		• Headache
		• Blurred vision
		• Flushed face (plethora)
		• Somnolence leading to coma
		(These late symptoms are also referred to as *CO$_2$ narcosis*.)
			Increase ventilation and treat cause
			• Maintain patent airway
			• Position for optimal ventilation
			• Implement bronchial hygiene measures
			• Administer drug therapy (e.g., bronchodilators, mucolytics, antibiotics)
			• Mechanical ventilation may be necessary
			• If patient is on mechanical ventilation
			  • Increase rate
			  • Increase tidal volume

Respiratory alkalosis: pH high; PaCO$_2$ low	Hyperventilation
	• Anxiety or hysteria
	• Thoracic pain
	• Early asthma
	• Pneumothorax
	• Pulmonary embolus
	• Early salicylate intoxication
	• Hyperthyroidism
	• Hepatic failure
	• Fever
	• Gram-negative septicemia
	• CNS infection or injury
	• Excessive mechanical ventilation
		• Tachycardia
		• Palpitations
		• Dry mouth
		• Anxiety
		• Profuse perspiration
		• Paresthesia around mouth and extremities
		• Dizziness, vertigo, syncope
		• Increased muscle irritability, twitching
		• Tetany
		• Inability to concentrate
		• Seizures
		• Coma
			• Decrease ventilation and treat cause
			• Provide reassurance and maintain a calm attitude
			• Administer sedatives (frequently given intravenously)
			• Ask patient to breathe into and out of a paper bag or use a rebreathing mask
			• If patient is on mechanical ventilation
			  • Decrease rate
			  • Decrease tidal volume
			  • Change from assist-control to IMV
			  • Consider sedation
			  • Consider addition of dead space tubing

Metabolic acidosis: pH low; HCO$_3^-$ low	Acid gain (increased anion gap)
	• Tissue hypoxia (e.g., shock [lactic acidosis])
	• Ketoacidosis (i.e., diabetic ketoacidosis or starvation)
	• Renal failure
	• Drugs and toxins (e.g., salicylates; methanol, ethylene glycol)
	Bicarbonate loss (normal anion gap)
	• Bile drainage
	• Pancreatic fistula
	• Diarrhea
	• Acetazolamide therapy
		• Nausea, vomiting, abdominal discomfort
		• Weakness
		• Tremors
		• Malaise
		• Headache
		• Tachypnea progressing to Kussmaul respirations
		• Hypotension
		• Dysrhythmias
		• Confusion
		• Lethargy → coma
			• Treat cause as appropriate
			  • Improve oxygenation and/or perfusion (lactic acidosis)
			  • Give insulin for DKA
			  • Initiate dialysis for renal failure
			  • Administer antidiarrheals for diarrhea
			• Administer buffer
			  • Bicarbonate IV or orally for pH ≤7

Metabolic alkalosis: pH high; HCO$_3^-$ high	Acid loss
	• NG suction or severe vomiting
	• Potassium-wasting diuretic therapy
	• Steroid therapy
	• Cushing disease
	• Hyperaldosteronism
	• Hepatic disease
	• Hypokalemia, hypochloremia
	Bicarbonate gain
	• Bicarbonate administration
	• Excess infusion of lactated Ringer solution
	• Lactate administration in dialysis solution
		• Bradypnea
		• Nausea, vomiting, diarrhea
		• Paresthesia around mouth and extremities
		• Confusion
		• Dizziness
		• Increased muscle irritability
		• Tetany
		• Seizures
		• Coma
			• Treat cause
			  • Antiemetic
			  • Electrolyte replacement: potassium and/or chloride
			  • Discontinuance of sodium bicarbonate or lactated Ringer solution
			• Administer carbonic anhydrase inhibitor
			  • Acetazolamide
			• Administer buffer
			  • Arginine monohydrochloride
			  • Ammonium chloride
			  • Weak HCl acid solution

CNS, Central nervous system; *DKA*, diabetic ketoacidosis; *IMV*, intermittent mandatory ventilation; *IV*, intravenous.

f. Universal sign of choking: patient clutches throat with hand
g. Unconsciousness within seconds

Collaborative Management of Airway Obstruction or Respiratory Distress

1. Evaluate the patency of the airway: look, listen, feel for airflow.
2. Maintain optimal airway and thoracic position.
   a. Use head tilt–chin lift (also called *sniffing*) position for optimal airway position.
      1) True hyperextension should be avoided.
      2) Contraindicated if cervical spine fracture possible (instead use jaw thrust)
   b. Position head of bed (HOB) for optimal chest excursion: semi-Fowler to high Fowler position
3. Remove any obstruction.
   a. Inspect the mouth for blood, teeth, loose dentures, food, or anything else that may cause obstruction.
   b. Remove any visible obstruction.
      1) Use fingers to remove visible foreign bodies; blind sweeps are not recommended because of concern that the obstruction may be pushed deeper into the airway.
      2) Magill forceps may be used, but care must be taken to prevent pushing the obstruction deeper into the airway.
   c. Use abdominal thrusts (also referred to as *Heimlich maneuver*): subxiphoid thrusts to relieve upper airway obstruction
      1) Alternate five abdominal thrusts with attempts to ventilate in unconscious patient.
      2) Avoid abdominal thrusts (use chest thrusts) in any of the following situations:
         a) Patient is too obese for you to get your arms around him or her.
         b) Patient has had recent abdominal surgery.
         c) Patient is pregnant.
   d. Place in recovery position: side-lying on left side
4. Encourage deep breathing: sustained inspiratory effort
   a. Purposes of deep breathing include the following:
      1) Increases air in the alveoli, preventing atelectasis
      2) Makes coughing more effective
   b. Incentive spirometry may also be used to provide graded incentives for sustained inspiration.
5. Remove secretions as required.
   a. Cough: forceful expiration to dislodge and remove secretions from the tracheobronchial tree
      1) Indications
         a) Breath sound changes: especially rhonchi; wheezes caused by mucus plugs may also clear with coughing
         b) With PD: between position changes but never in a head-down position
         c) NOTE: Although coughing should be encouraged in the previously identified situations, routine coughing may increase the incidence of atelectasis; preventive measures (e.g., for postoperative patients) should focus on deep breathing with sustained inspiration rather than forced expiration (e.g., coughing).
      2) Technique for effective coughing
         a) Assist patient to a comfortable position.
         b) Instruct patient to do the following:
            i) Inhale deeply.
            ii) Cough two to three times with the mouth open.
            iii) Expectorate any sputum.
            iv) Inhale slowly and deeply.
      3) Special techniques
         a) Huff coughing
            i) Forced expiration with glottis open
            ii) May be helpful for patients with COPD to keep airways open
         b) Augmented coughing
            i) Includes sip ventilation (i.e., breath stacking), manual chest or abdominal thrust during expiration, or mechanical cough assist using an insufflator-exsufflator or coughalator
            ii) May be necessary for patients with abdominal muscle weakness or paralysis
         c) Use of a flutter valve
            i) Small plastic handheld device that consists of a small plastic cone containing a steel ball
            ii) Instruction to patient should include the following:
               (a) Inhaling deeply, hold the breath for 2 to 3 seconds, and then exhale into the flutter valve.
               (b) Use it three or four times daily with 10 to 15 repetitions each session.
               (c) Use any prescribed bronchodilator before use of the flutter valve.
            iii) Promotes airway clearance in the following ways:
               (a) Vibration of airways to loosen secretions
               (b) Maintenance of open airways during exhalation
               (c) Creation of mini-coughs
   b. Suctioning of oropharynx: removal of secretions from the oropharynx through the use of a suction catheter and negative pressure
      1) Performed before deflation of ET tube cuff to prevent oropharyngeal secretions from draining into tracheobronchial tree
      2) Performed routinely after suctioning of tracheobronchial tree to prevent accumulation of oropharyngeal secretions that can be silently aspirated around ET tube cuff
      3) Yankauer suction device usually used; if suction catheter that was used to suction the tracheobronchial tree is used, suction oropharynx only *after* suctioning the tracheobronchial tree and rinsing the catheter

4) Specialized ET to allow for continuous aspiration of subglottic secretions (CASS) has been shown to reduce the incidence or delay the onset of ventilator-associated pneumonia (VAP) (see Pneumonia section in this chapter)
   a) Upper airway secretions pool above the ET tube cuff and cause microaspiration and VAP.
   b) Multiple studies have established effectiveness of CASS
c. Suctioning of tracheobronchial tree: removal of secretions from the tracheobronchial tree through the use of a suction catheter and negative pressure
   1) Clinical indications for the need to suction; suctioning of the airway should not be "routine" but should be performed when indicated by the following
      a) Sympathetic nervous system stimulation (tachycardia, tachypnea)
      b) Change in BP: increased or decreased
      c) Dyspnea
      d) Noisy or shallow ventilation
      e) Rhonchi
      f) Obvious visible secretions
      g) Frequent or sustained coughing especially during inspiratory cycle of ventilator
      h) High-pressure alarm on ventilator
      i) Clinical indications of hypoxia (Box 4.3) and hypercapnia (Box 4.4)
   2) Technique for suctioning the tracheobronchial tree using principles to prevent complications
      a) Suction only if indicated and limit number of passes to minimum required.
      b) The outer diameter of the catheter should be no more than half the inner diameter of the ET tube or tracheostomy.
      c) Use a closed suction system if possible.
         i) Advantages of closed suction system include the following:
            (a) Continued oxygenation and reduction in loss of PEEP so decreased incidence of hypoxemia
            (b) Decreased cost and nursing time
            (c) Decreased chance of aerosolization of secretions, which protects the patient's and nurse's eyes
            (d) Decreased risk of introducing bacteria into airway
         ii) If closed suction system is not available, use special adaptor for patients on therapeutic PEEP because these patients frequently have significant oxygen desaturation during suctioning.
         iii) Special curved-tip catheter (Coudé catheter) is required to enter the left mainstem bronchus; it is usually adequate to use a regular suction catheter to suction the right mainstem bronchus and the trachea because the coughing stimulated effectively clears the left mainstem bronchus into the trachea.
      d) Sterile technique is used if suctioning through ET or tracheostomy; aseptic technique is used if suctioning nasotracheally
         i) Two gloves should be used.
         ii) Goggles should be worn to protect the nurse's eyes.
      e) Explain procedure to the patient; protect the patient's eyes if not using a closed suction system.
      f) Hyperoxygenation (100% oxygen) before, during, and after suctioning; ensure that SpO_2 reflects this increase in oxygen before initiating suctioning if patient experiences clinically significant oxygen desaturation during suctioning
      g) If doing nasotracheal suctioning, place patient in "sniffing" position while sitting up or place a towel roll between shoulders if patient is supine and use water-soluble lubricant to lubricate the catheter.
      h) Advance catheter to no farther than 1 cm past the end of the ET tube to avoid contact with the trachea and carina.
         i) The previous technique of advancing the catheter to the point of obstruction and then pulling back slightly before applying suction should be avoided.
         ii) Shallow suctioning decreases mucosal damage, decreases mucus production, and results in less mucosal inflammation.
      i) Limit suctioning to 10 seconds; there is no difference in patient outcomes with intermittent versus continuous suction as long as the duration is limited to 10 seconds.
      j) Avoid excessive negative pressure; keep pressure 100 mm Hg or less unless using a closed suction system; 120 mm Hg is recommended if using a closed suction system.
      k) Liquefy secretions through humidification and hydration.
         i) Instillation of saline (also referred to as *saline lavage*) has been proven ineffective and potentially harmful; contributes to hypoxemia and VAP.
         ii) If increased oral or parenteral fluids cannot be given (e.g., renal failure), either of the following may be prescribed.
            (a) Saline by inhalation (small particle size allows deeper penetration into tracheobronchial tube and liquefies mucus)
            (b) Acetylcysteine given by inhalation (breaks down disulfide bonds to liquefy mucus); concurrent bronchodilator is frequently required
      l) Rinse catheter and appropriately discard disposable catheter; if closed suction system, rinse the catheter after pulling it back to black line and then injecting saline into irrigation

port while applying suction (note that this is irrigation, not lavage) and then close irrigation port and suction valve.
- m) Monitor for complications during and after suctioning.
    - i) Keep patient on the ventilator and use a closed suction system if patient requires positive pressure to maintain SpO2.
    - ii) SpO_2 during suctioning for oxygen desaturation
    - iii) Electrocardiography (ECG) during and after suctioning for vagal stimulation (bradycardia) as well as dysrhythmias related to hypoxemia (premature ventricular contractions [PVCs])
- n) Stop suctioning if: change in heart rate, ECG rhythm, or skin color; significant change in SpO_2 or SvO_2
- o) Assess breath sounds after suctioning to evaluate effectiveness.

3) If doing nasotracheal suctioning in a patient who does not have an ET or tracheostomy tube
- a) Provide oxygen with a nonrebreathing mask before suctioning.
- b) Place patient in "sniffing" position while sitting up or place a towel roll between shoulders if patient is supine.
- c) Lubricate catheter with water-soluble lubricant before insertion.
- d) Prevent injury to the nasal mucosa.
    - i) Placement of a nasopharyngeal airway may be done to prevent injury to the nasal mucosa if frequent suctioning is required.
    - ii) Endotracheal intubation or tracheostomy may also be required if frequent suctioning is required.
- e) Ask the patient to cough and advance the catheter during that time because the glottis is open; if the patient cannot follow commands, advance the catheter during inspiration.
- f) Note indications that the catheter is in the trachea.
    - i) Patient becomes anxious
    - ii) Patient cannot speak
- g) Complete suctioning as for a patient with an ET or tracheostomy tube.

4) Advantages of closed suction system
- a) Continued oxygenation and reduction in loss of PEEP so decreased incidence of hypoxemia
- b) Decreased cost and nursing time
- c) Decreased chance of aerosolization of secretions, which protects patient's and nurse's eyes
- d) Decreased risk of introducing bacteria into airway

5) Specialized ET to allow for CASS has been shown to reduce the incidence or delay the onset of VAP (see Pneumonia section in this chapter).
- a) Upper airway secretions pool above the ET tube cuff and cause microaspiration and VAP.
- b) Multiple studies have established effectiveness of CASS, and a recent study (Speroni et al., 2011) also demonstrated cost effectiveness

6. Provide chest physiotherapy (i.e., chest PT) as indicated.
    a. Purposes
        1) To promote bronchial hygiene
        2) Improve breathing efficiency
        3) Promote physical reconditioning
    b. Postural drainage (PD): sequential positioning of the patient
        1) Purpose: use gravity to drain secretions from peripheral areas into the major bronchi or trachea so that they can be coughed and expectorated or suctioned.
        2) Indication: prevention and treatment of respiratory complications
            a) Lobar atelectasis
            b) Disorders with significant mucus production (e.g., cystic fibrosis, bronchiectasis, COPD)
        3) Technique
            a) Administer bronchodilator before PD if prescribed.
            b) Turn off enteral feedings for 30 minutes before PD; ensure that cuff of E or tracheostomy tube is inflated.
            c) Place patient in position to drain selected segment of lung or alternate through the following positions.
                i) Left side with hips higher than head
                ii) Right side with hips higher than head
                iii) Supine with hips higher than head
                iv) Prone with hips higher than head
            d) Maintain each position for 10 to 30 minutes.
            e) Cough between position changes but never in a head-down position.
            f) Avoid PD for at least 1.5 hours after meals
        4) Contraindications
            a) Obesity
            b) Spinal fracture, rib fracture, flail chest
            c) Pulmonary hemorrhage, embolism, malignancy
            d) Pneumothorax, empyema, large pleural effusion
            e) Tuberculosis
            f) Asthma, acute bronchospasm
            g) Bleeding disorder
            h) Seizures, intracranial hypertension
            i) Acute myocardial infarction (MI), heart failure (HF), hemodynamic instability
            j) Recent pacemaker insertion
            k) Increased risk of aspiration
    c. Percussion: clapping the chest with cupped hands
        1) Purpose: mechanically dislodge secretions from the bronchial walls into the major bronchi or trachea so that they can be coughed and expectorated or suctioned.
        2) Technique
            a) If using hands:
                i) Cup hands as if holding water.
                ii) Tap chest with cupped hands listening for a cupping, not slapping, sound.

b) If using vibropercussion bed function:
   i) Set timing.
   ii) May be used in conjunction with continuous lateral rotation therapy (CLRT)
c) Avoid: spine, liver, kidneys, spleen, and female patient's breasts.
3) Contraindications
   a) Known bleeding disorder
   b) Lung cancer
   c) Pneumothorax
   d) Extreme caution in older adult patients with osteoporosis after thoracotomy
d. Vibration: during expiration of areas of the chest with either an open hand or a vibrating device
   1) Purpose: loosen secretions from the bronchial walls into the major bronchi or trachea so that they can be coughed and expectorated or suctioned.
   2) Technique
      a) Hold hand flat against chest and vibrate hand during expiration.
      b) Hand vibrator may also be used.
   3) Contraindications: as for percussion
7. Turn patient at least every 2 hours; use a special bed as appropriate.
   a. Consider "good lung down" principle for patients with unilateral lung conditions (exception: pneumonectomy when the rule is "no lung down")
   b. Consider kinetic therapy through the use of continuous lateral rotational therapy bed if appropriate.
      1) Effect: promotes redistribution of ventilation, promotes redistribution of perfusion, and optimizes V/Q matching
      2) Indications
         a) ARDS or high risk for ARDS
         b) Pneumonia
         c) Prevention of VAP and lobar atelectasis
      3) Guidelines
         a) Start as early as possible.
         b) Explain the process to the patient before turning.
         c) Monitor BP and SpO_2 frequently, especially initially until acclimation.
      4) Contraindications
         a) Table rotational beds
            i) Severe claustrophobia, although most of these patients will be sedated
            ii) Uncontrolled diarrhea
            iii) Weight of greater than 500 lb
         b) Cushion-based beds and mattress replacement beds
            i) Severe claustrophobia, although most of these patients will be sedated
            ii) Uncontrolled diarrhea
            iii) Weight of greater than 300 lb
            iv) Unstable spinal cord injury
            v) Skeletal traction
   c. Consider placing the patient in prone position periodically if appropriate; frequently used ARDS
      1) Effects
         a) Improved compliance of the dorsal chest wall, which increases reexpansion of dependent lung regions which optimizes V/Q matching
         b) Reduction in the amount of lung volume compressed by the heart
         c) Lessening of the compression on the lower lobes by the pressure of the abdominal contents against the diaphragm, which improves ventilation of the lower lobes
         d) Reduction of the gradients of pleural and transpulmonary pressures, causing more even distribution of ventilation
         e) PEEP is more likely to result in more homogeneous perfusion in the lung in prone position; PEEP tends to redistribute blood flow away from well-ventilated ventral areas of the lung in supine position.
      2) Contraindications
         a) Intracranial hypertension
         b) Unstable fractures, especially cervical, thoracic, or lumbar fractures
         c) Cervical or skeletal traction
         d) Left ventricular failure
         e) Hemodynamic instability
         f) Active intraabdominal process
         g) Pregnancy
         h) Weight greater than 300 lb may be a contraindication depending on method of turning or special bed
      3) Complications
         a) Skin breakdown, particularly the face, ears, nose, eyes, mouth, shoulders, elbows, hips, knees, genitalia, and breasts
            i) Extra care must be taken with breast and penile implants
         b) Dependent edema
         c) Corneal abrasions
         d) Inadvertent extubation or removal of catheters
         e) Obstructed chest tube
         f) Nerve injury
         g) Transient supraventricular tachycardia
         h) Aspiration
      4) Methods
         a) Requires three to four personnel depending on patient size; one person should be at the head to stabilize ET, central venous catheters, and so on.
         b) Explain the procedure to the patient and administer sedation, analgesia, or both.
         c) Withhold enteral feedings for the hour before turning to prone but continue feedings once in prone position.
         d) Equipment
            i) Pillows to position patient in swimming position and elevate abdomen off the bed to prevent impairment in diaphragmatic excursion
            ii) KCI's RotoProne bed
            iii) Special bed with pronating capability (e.g., KCI's TriaDyne II with proning accessory)
            iv) The Vollman Prone Positioner

e) Monitor BP and SpO_2
f) Frequent repositioning is still required to prevent pressure ulcers.
5) Dramatic improvement in oxygenation frequently occurs, and improved survival has been demonstrated.
8. Use artificial airways safely and appropriately.
a. General principles
1) Provide humidification because natural humidification mechanisms are bypassed.
2) Use aseptic technique with upper airway artificial airways; use sterile technique with lower airway artificial airways.
3) Suction as indicated; because ETs splint the epiglottis open, effective coughing is impaired.
4) Provide method of communication; this is the most significant stressor experienced by intubated patients.
a) Picture communication board, alphabet board, magic slate, felt-tip pen or marker, and paper may be used; avoid pencils and ballpoint pens, which require more pressure.
b) Fenestrated or Passy-Muir tracheostomy tubes may be used in some patients; these allow air to leak over the vocal cords.
c) Lip reading is usually *not* an acceptable method especially if oral tube is in place.
b. Selection of appropriate artificial airway (Table 4.11)
c. Summary of artificial airways (Table 4.12)
1) Upper airway artificial airways
a) Oropharyngeal airway
b) Nasopharyngeal airway
c) Cricothyrotomy
2) Lower airway artificial airways
a) Esophageal-tracheal Combitube
b) Laryngeal mask airway (LMA)

c) ET
i) Nasotracheal tube
ii) Orotracheal tube
iii) CASS ET tube (Fig. 4.28)
d) Tracheostomy
d. Endotracheal intubation
1) Indications
a) V_T less than 5 ml/kg
b) VC less than 10 ml/kg
c) MIP less than -20 cm H_2O
d) Inability to adequately cough and clear airway
e) Loss of protective reflexes
f) Need for sealed airway (e.g., mechanical ventilation, risk for aspiration)
2) Insertion of ET tube
a) Prepare the oxygen delivery system to be used after intubation: usually T-piece with nebulizer or mechanical ventilator; manual resuscitation bag with reservoir bag with 100% oxygen may be used during cardiac arrest or until mechanical ventilator is ready.
b) Collect supplies and select tube size.
i) Tube: women, usually 7.5 to 8; men, usually 8 to 8.5
ii) Equipment to insert and secure tube: laryngoscope with straight (Miller) and curved (MacIntosh) blades with working lights, stylet, Magill forceps, lubricant, syringe, tape, or device for stabilization of tube
iii) Suction equipment including suction catheter and Yankauer suction device
c) Monitor ECG and SaO_2 during intubation.
d) Hyperoxygenate with 100% oxygen for at least 2 minutes.
e) Place patient in head tilt–chin lift position.
f) Intubation should be performed by the most qualified person available who has been trained in endotracheal intubation and frequently performs the procedure (usually physician or nurse anesthetist).
g) Intubation should be completed within 30 seconds; if not, attempts should be ceased and the patient should again hyperoxygenated.
h) Confirm placement of the ET tube.
i) Feel air movement through tube.
ii) Assess bilateral chest excursion.
iii) Auscultate bilateral breath sounds; if breath sounds are audible on the right but not on the left, right mainstem intubation has occurred; pull the tube back slightly and then recheck breath sounds.
iv) Use a capnometer to confirm consistent exhalation of CO_2.
v) Auscultate over epigastrium: air movement should not be audible.
vi) Confirm tube positioning by CXR; distal tip of tube should be 3 to 5 cm above the carina.

Table 4.11	Selection of Appropriate Artificial Airway
Problem	**Preferred Artificial Airway**
Tongue against hypopharynx	Oropharyngeal or nasopharyngeal
Need for frequent nasotracheal suctioning	Nasopharyngeal
Inability to open mouth (e.g., seizure)	Nasopharyngeal
Facial or jaw fracture	Nasopharyngeal or nasotracheal tube
Complete upper airway obstruction when endotracheal intubation is impossible (e.g., laryngeal edema or spasm, tracheal fracture)	Cricothyrotomy or tracheostomy
Need for sealed airway (e.g., mechanical ventilation or potential for aspiration)	Endotracheal tube or tracheostomy
Need for long-term lower airway access and sealed airway	Tracheostomy

Table 4.12 Summary of Artificial Airways

Type of Airway	Advantages	Disadvantages	Miscellaneous

Oropharyngeal airway	• Easy to insert
	• Inexpensive
	• Effectively holds tongue away from pharynx
		• Improper insertion technique can push tongue back and occlude airway
		• Easily dislodged
		• Poorly tolerated by conscious patients as it may stimulate gag reflex
		• Causes increased oral secretions
		• Contraindicated in patients with trauma to lower face, recent oral surgery, loose or avulsed teeth
			• Determine appropriate size: with flange at teeth, end of airway should not extend beyond the angle of the jaw
			  • Large adult: usually 100 mm (size 5)
			  • Medium adult: usually 90 mm (size 4)
			  • Small adult: usually 80 mm (size 3)
			• Insert by holding tongue down with tongue blade and sliding into place; alternative method: insert upside down and turn over when into pharynx; take care not to traumatize palate
			• Do not use as a bite block; likely to cause vomiting and potential aspiration in conscious patients
			• Remove, wash, and give mouth care every 4 hours; check mucous membranes for ulcerations

Nasopharyngeal airway (also called a nasal trumpet)	• Easy to insert
	• Inexpensive
	• Effectively holds tongue away from pharynx
	• May be used in conscious or unconscious patients
	• Prevents trauma to nasal mucosa during nasotracheal suctioning
	• May be inserted when mouth cannot be opened (e.g., during seizures, jaw fractures)
		• May cause nosebleeds, pressure necrosis, or sinus infection
		• Kinks and clogs easily
		• Contraindicated in patients predisposed to nosebleeds, nasal obstruction, bleeding disorder, and sepsis and in patients with basal skull fracture
			• Determine appropriate size: 1 inch longer than nose to earlobe; lumen smaller than naris
			  • Large adult: usually 8–9 mm internal diameter
			  • Medium adult: usually 7–8 mm internal diameter
			  • Small adult: usually 6–7 mm internal diameter
			• Insert with bevel against septum
			• Use viscous Xylocaine as a lubricant for insertion to decrease discomfort
			• Do not use in patients receiving anticoagulants
			• Provide humidification of inspired air
			• Confirm placement by visualizing the tip of the airway next to the uvula
			• Rotate naris to naris every 8 hours
			• Limit the duration of use to reduce risk of sinus infection

Esophageal-tracheal Combitube	• Allows ventilation whether the tube is inserted into the trachea or the esophagus • Reduces risk of aspiration over mask ventilation • Permits easier placement over endotracheal tube because visualization of the vocal cords is not necessary • Provides comparable ventilation and oxygenation to that achieved with an endotracheal tube	• Incorrect identification of the position of the distal lumen may result in absence of ventilation • May cause esophageal trauma • Cannot mechanically ventilate the patient with a Combitube	• Use of an end-tidal CO_2 or esophageal detector device is recommended to confirm placement as either being in the trachea or esophagus
Laryngeal mask airway (LMA)	• Permits easier placement than endotracheal tube because visualization of the vocal cords is not necessary • Provides comparable ventilation and oxygenation to that achieved with an endotracheal tube • Allows placement when there is a possibility of unstable neck injury or when appropriate positioning of the patient for tracheal intubation is impossible • Reduces risk of aspiration over mask ventilation • Permits coughing and speech	• Small proportion of patients cannot be ventilated with an LMA, so an alternative strategy is needed • Cannot prevent aspiration because it does not separate the GI tract from the respiratory tract • May cause laryngospasm or bronchospasm • May be difficult to ventilate patients who require high airway pressures to attain adequate tidal volumes	• If lubrication is required, only the posterior aspect of the airway should be lubricated • If used for mechanical ventilation, an audible air leak may occur

Continued

Table 4.12 Summary of Artificial Airways—cont'd

Type of Airway	Advantages	Disadvantages	Miscellaneous

Endotracheal tube (general)	• Provides relatively sealed airway for mechanical ventilation and prevention of aspiration
	• Permits easy suctioning
	• Prevents gastric distention with air during CPR
		• Requires skilled personnel for insertion
		• Splints epiglottis open and prevents effective cough
		• Causes loss of physiologic PEEP because epiglottis is splinted open; patient should receive 3–5 cm PEEP to reestablish physiologic PEEP
		• May kink and clog
		• Causes aphonia
		• May cause laryngeal or tracheal damage
		• Contraindicated in patients with laryngeal obstruction caused by tumor, infection, or vocal cord paralysis
			• Determine appropriate size
			  • Women: usually 7.5–8 mm internal diameter
			  • Men: usually 8–8.5 mm internal diameter
			  • Tube may need to be 0.5–1 mm smaller if to be inserted nasally
			• Provide humidification of inspired air
			• Mark tube at corner of mouth or at naris to assess any movement
			• Use minimal occlusive volume or minimal leak volume for cuff inflation; ensure that cuff pressure does not exceed 25 mm Hg (if pressure >25 mm Hg required to achieve seal, tube is too small and needs to be replaced with larger tube)
			• Confirm placement by chest radiography: tip of tube should be 3–5 cm above carina
			• Provide mouth care every 4 hours; observe oral or nasal mucosa for signs of ulcerations or necrosis
			• Position to prevent kinking; use mechanical ventilator's support arms to support ventilator tubing

Oral (specific) endotracheal tube	• Easier insertion than nasal intubation • Permits larger tube than nasal intubation	• Less stable and comfortable than nasal tube • May stimulate gag reflex • May be bitten or chewed • May cause necrosis at corner of mouth • Increases oral secretions; makes mouth care more difficult • Contraindicated in patients with acute unstable cervical spine injury because of the need for neck extension (blind nasotracheal intubation may be attempted in these patients)	• Reposition tube from one side of the mouth to the other and reapply tape when indicated; avoid unnecessary manipulation of tube
Nasal (specific) endotracheal tube	• More comfortable for patient than oral endotracheal tube • Permits good oral hygiene • Cannot be bitten or chewed	• More difficult insertion than oral intubation • May cause pressure necrosis or sinus infection • Requires smaller size • Contraindicated in patients with nasal obstruction, fractured nose, sinusitis, bleeding disorder, basal skull fracture	• Monitor for clinical indications of sinus infection: fever; increased pharyngeal drainage; halitosis; leukocytosis; sinus pain or headache
Cricothyrotomy	• Provides immediate airway access, especially helpful if complete upper airway obstruction	• May cause bleeding • Only temporary; very small opening if established with large needle; larger if airway opened with scalpel and small tracheostomy tube used	• Provide humidification of inspired air • Use large-bore over-the-needle catheter; adaptor required to attach to manual resuscitation bag • Provider may use scalpel and insert small tracheostomy tube • Monitor for bleeding, subcutaneous emphysema

Table 4.12	Summary of Artificial Airways—cont'd		
Type of Airway	**Advantages**	**Disadvantages**	**Miscellaneous**
Tracheostomy	• Provides long-term airway access • Minimizes risk of vocal cord damage from an endotracheal tube during long-term airway maintenance • Decreases dead space and decreases work of breathing • Provides a relative seal to prevent aspiration • Allows the patient to eat and swallow • Allows easier suctioning • Permits Valsalva maneuver and effective cough • Is more comfortable for patient • Is less likely to be dislodged than endotracheal tube • Bypasses upper airway obstruction	• May require surgery but may be performed percutaneously • Causes aphonia • May cause false passage anterior to trachea in patients with thick necks • May cause erosion of innominate artery with tip of tube or low stoma • Causes scar • May cause tracheocutaneous or tracheoesophageal fistula	• Usually considered if artificial airway is required longer than 2–3 weeks • Determine appropriate size: usually 5–6 • Requires humidification of inspired air • Preferred if airway obstruction (e.g., tumor or laryngeal edema or spasm) • Provide tracheostomy care that includes cleaning stoma and tube every 8 hours with saline; keep stoma dry (if 4 × 4.inch gauze used, change often if secretions present) • Keep obturator, extra tracheostomy tube, and tracheal spreader at bedside

CPR, Cardiopulmonary resuscitation; *GI*, gastrointestinal; *PEEP*, positive end-expiratory pressure.

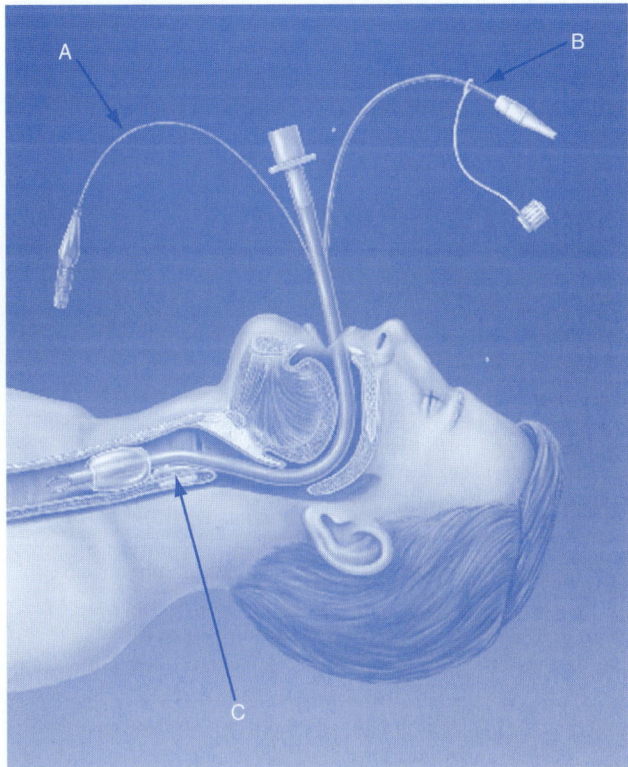

Fig. 4.28 Specialized endotracheal tube used for continuous aspiration of subglottic secretions (CASS). *A*, Lumen for inflation of cuff. *B*, Lumen for aspiration of subglottic secretions. *C*, Opening of aspiration port. (Courtesy Nellcor Puritan Bennett Inc., Pleasanton, CA.)

    i) Inflate the cuff using either minimal occlusive volume or minimal leak volume.
        i) Cuffs in current use are high-volume, low-pressure cuffs; these cuffs distribute the low pressure over a larger area of the trachea and decrease the incidence of tracheal ischemia and stenosis; laryngectomy patients may have uncuffed (and longer) laryngectomy tube.
    ii) Cuffed tubes provide *relative* seal for patients receiving mechanical ventilation and aid in prevention of aspiration; note that cuffs do not establish an absolute seal, and silent aspiration of oropharyngeal or gastric secretions is common in critically ill patients.
    iii) Inflate cuff using minimal occlusive volume or minimal leak volume.
       (a) Minimal occlusive volume
           (i) Listen over trachea with stethoscope.
           (ii) Inflate cuff until no air leak is audible during the inspiratory cycle of the ventilator.
       (b) Minimal leak volume
           (i) Listen over trachea with a stethoscope.
           (ii) Inflate cuff until no air leak is audible during the inspiratory cycle of the ventilator.
           (iii) Remove 0.1 cm of air or until a minimal leak is audible during the inspiratory cycle of the ventilator.
   j) Intracuff pressure should not exceed capillary filling pressure but should be adequate to prevent the drainage of excessive subglottic secretions.
     i) Measure and record cuff pressure every 8 hours with a cuff pressure gauge or a mercury manometer and three-way stopcock.

(a) Continuous monitoring of cuff pressure is currently being advocated because cuff pressures change over time and with some clinical activities such as endotracheal suctioning, coughing, and patient–ventilator dyssynchrony (Sole et al., 2009).
  ii) Recommended pressure is between 20 and 25 mm Hg (24-30 cm H_2O).
k) Routine deflation is not necessary with high-volume, low-pressure cuffs and may contribute to nosocomial pneumonia by allowing oropharyngeal secretions to drain into the tracheobronchial tree.
l) Tape tube in place.
  i) Secure tape to minimize pressure areas on the face; tape with tension to both sides to avoid excessive pressure on corner of mouth if oral tube.
  ii) If a commercial stabilization device is used, monitor oral mucosa carefully for evidence of excessive pressure.
m) Note the depth marking on the side of the tube.
  i) Usually at 19 to 23 cm for an average adult or three times the tube size so that a size 7 should be at ~21 cm, a size 7.5 should be at ~22.5, and so on.
  ii) Cut tube so that only 2 to 3 inches of tube extends beyond mouth or nose to decrease airway resistance and potential for kinking.
n) Attach oxygen delivery system or mechanical ventilator.
e. Extubation of intubated patients
  1) Criteria
    a) Patient awake and oriented or able to keep airway open
      i) Protective reflexes must be intact (e.g., gag).
      ii) Patient should not be paralyzed or excessively narcotized or sedated.
    b) Vital signs stable; acceptable Hgb and hemodynamics
    c) ABGs within acceptable limits after a trial of 30 minutes on nebulizer (e.g., T-piece) at 40% oxygen: PaO_2 60 mm Hg or greater, SaO_2 90% or greater, $PaCO_2$ 35 to 45 mm Hg or consistent with patient's normal values
    d) Acceptable bedside ventilatory parameters:
      i) V_T 5 ml/kg or greater
      ii) VC 10 ml/kg or greater
      iii) MIP of -20 cm H_2O or greater
  2) Technique
    a) Have postextubation oxygen delivery system ready; intubation kit should also be available.
    b) Suction trachea and then pharynx.
    c) Deflate cuff.
    d) Remove tube during expiration.
    e) Apply oxygen delivery system.
    f) Encourage patient to cough; suction if needed.
    g) Repeat blood gases 20 to 30 minutes after extubation and as indicated thereafter.
    h) Observe for laryngospasm: stridor, and dyspnea, tachypnea; treatment may include high humidity, steroids, racemic epinephrine, or reintubation.
    i) Monitor patient's tolerance to extubation by clinical observation, ventilatory measurements, and blood gas studies.
f. Weaning patients from tracheostomy tube
  1) Indications same as for ET tube extubation
  2) Techniques
    a) Progression to a smaller size uncuffed (or cuff not inflated) tracheostomy tube
      i) Allows the patient to use his or her upper airway and the opening of the tracheostomy tube
      ii) Increases airway resistance and work of breathing
    b) Change to fenestrated tube: opening at the top of tube allows air to leak upward so that the patient can use the upper airway (and can speak).
    c) Deflate cuff.
      i) Allows the patient to use his or her upper airway and the opening of the tracheostomy tube
      ii) Increases airway resistance and work of breathing
    d) Tracheostomy button
      i) Closes the opening in the trachea so that the patient uses his or her upper airway
      ii) Increases airway resistance and work of breathing
g. Complications of airway intubation
  1) Physiologic alterations created by airway diversion
    a) Inadequate humidification of inspired air
    b) Increased risk of nosocomial pneumonia caused by accumulation of secretions
      i) Increased mucus caused by tube because it is a foreign body
      ii) Impaired ciliary movement
    c) Aphonia: most significant stressor identified by patients
    d) Ineffective cough: ET tubes splint the epiglottis open, preventing effective intrathoracic pressure to achieve an effective cough; patients can cough with a tracheostomy because the epiglottis is not splinted open.
    e) Loss of physiologic PEEP
      i) ET tubes splint the epiglottis open and remove physiologic PEEP.
      ii) Physiologic PEEP is reestablished with 3 to 5 cm H_2O of PEEP for intubated patients. (NOTE: It may be contraindicated with thoracotomy patients.)

2) During placement
   a) ET tube intubation
      i) Trauma: damage to teeth, mucous membranes, perforation or laceration of pharynx, larynx, trachea
      ii) Aspiration
      iii) Laryngospasm, bronchospasm
      iv) Tube malposition: esophageal or endobronchial intubation
      v) Hypoxia or anoxia if attempts are prolonged
   b) Tracheostomy
      i) Barotrauma: pneumothorax or pneumomediastinum
      ii) Hemorrhage
      iii) Tracheoesophageal fistula
      iv) Laryngeal nerve injury
      v) Cardiopulmonary arrest
3) While tube is in place
   a) Tube obstruction or displacement
   b) Cuff rupture
   c) Disconnection between tracheal tube and ventilator, including self-extubation
   d) Pressure necrosis
      i) At corners of mouth if oral ET tube
      ii) At superior nasal concha if nasal ET tube
   e) Local infection; otitis media; sinus infection with nasotracheal tubes
   f) Bronchospasm
   g) Leaks caused by broken cuff balloon
   h) Trauma: laryngeal injury; tracheal ischemia, necrosis, dilation
   i) Transition from ET tube to tracheostomy usually occurs approximately 2 weeks after intubation, but several studies have shown benefit (e.g., decreases length of mechanical ventilation, shorter critical care and hospital stay) in earlier tracheostomy (within 3 days when it is anticipated that the patient will require prolonged mechanical ventilation).
4) Postextubation
   a) ET tube
      i) Acute laryngeal edema
      ii) Hoarseness (common)
      iii) Aspiration if swallowing is impaired
      iv) Stenosis of larynx or trachea (late complication)
   b) Tracheostomy
      i) Difficulties with decannulation of a tracheostomy
      ii) Tracheoesophageal fistula
      iii) Tracheoinnominate artery fistula
      iv) Tracheocutaneous fistula
      v) Tracheal stenosis

9. Provide oral care for patient comfort and to aid in prevention of nosocomial pneumonia.
   a. Recognize factors contributing to poor oral hygiene.
      1) Artificial airways
      2) Poor nutrition
      3) Nothing by mouth status
      4) Mouth breathing or tachypnea
      5) Oxygen administration
      6) Anxiety
      7) Drugs such as antihistamines, antiemetics, antibiotics
   b. Assess the lips, oral mucosa, tongue, gums, teeth, and soft and hard palate at least twice daily.
   c. Provide oral care periodically.
      1) Every 2 to 4 hours
         a) Use suction foam swabs over teeth, tongue, and oral mucosa followed by moisturizing swabs and water-soluble lip balm.
            i) Foam swabs stimulate the oral mucosa.
            ii) Avoid lemon glycerin swabs, which are drying to the oral mucosa.
         b) Suction oropharynx
            i) Rinse catheter (e.g., Yankauer) with sterile water or saline after each use.
            ii) Store oropharyngeal suction catheter in an unsealed bag when not in use.
            iii) Replace oropharyngeal suction device, tubing, and suction canister every 24 hours.
      2) Twice daily
         a) Brush teeth to prevent dental plaque colonization.
            i) Brushing the teeth with a toothbrush removes dental plaque and reduces the number of oral microorganisms.
            ii) A soft-bristle pediatric toothbrush should be used along with toothpaste, preferably with an alkaline pH.
            iii) Removable partial dentures should be removed and thoroughly cleaned.
         b) Administer chlorhexidine gluconate by spray or rinse as prescribed.
            i) Chlorhexidine: broad-spectrum antibacterial agent, which is not absorbed through the skin or mucous membranes
               (a) Concentration recommendations vary from 0.12% to 0.2%
            ii) Reduces risk of VAP
            iii) May be Initiated preoperatively if surgical patient

Oxygen Therapy

Definitions
1. Hypoxemia
   a. Decrease in arterial blood oxygen tension
   b. Diagnosis by ABGs
   c. Decrease in PaO_2 and SaO_2
      1) Mild hypoxemia: PaO_2 less than 80 mm Hg (~SaO_2 95%)
      2) Moderate (significant) hypoxemia: PaO_2 less than 60 mm Hg (~SaO_2 90%)
      3) Severe hypoxemia: PaO_2 less than 40 mm Hg (~SaO_2 75%)
2. Hypoxia
   a. Decrease in tissue oxygenation
   b. Diagnosis by clinical indications (Box 4.3)
   c. Affected by PaO_2 and SaO_2, Hgb, cardiac output, patent vessels, cellular demand

Etiologies of Oxygen Deficiencies

1. Hypoxemia
   a. Low inspired oxygen concentration (e.g., high altitudes, smoke)
   b. Pulmonary causes (Fig. 4.29)
      1) Hypoventilation (e.g., asthma)
      2) V/Q mismatch
         a) Low V/Q mismatch (i.e., shunt) (e.g., ARDS)
         b) High V/Q mismatch (i.e., dead space) (e.g., PE)
      3) Diffusion abnormalities (e.g., pulmonary edema, pulmonary fibrosis)
2. Hypoxia
   a. Hypoxemic hypoxia: secondary to a gas exchange problem (e.g., V/Q mismatch, shunt, diffusion abnormalities)
   b. Anemic hypoxia: secondary to reduced oxygen-carrying capacity of the blood (e.g., anemia, carbon monoxide poisoning, methemoglobinemia)
   c. Circulatory hypoxia: secondary to a reduced blood flow in the body or a reduction in cardiac output (e.g., shock)
   d. Histotoxic hypoxia: secondary to the inability of the cells to use oxygen (e.g., cyanide poisoning)

Pathophysiology

1. Decrease in PaO_2 initially stimulates the sympathetic nervous system (SNS).
2. Oxygen extraction at tissue level increases.
3. As PaO_2 becomes critically low, tissue oxygenation becomes inadequate, and hypoxia occurs.
4. Nutrient metabolism changes from aerobic to anaerobic, which results in 20 times less ATP than aerobic metabolism and lactic acid as a waste product.
5. Acidosis and decreased cellular energy results.

Assessment

1. Evidence of altered perfusion
   a. Tachycardia
   b. Hypotension
   c. Changes in skin color and temperature
2. Evidence of anaerobic metabolism: lactic acidosis (serum arterial lactate level >2 mmol/l)
3. Evidence of organ dysfunction
   a. Cerebral: altered sensorium
   b. Myocardial: decreased cardiac output or dysrhythmias
   c. Renal: decreased urine output
4. Parameters of oxygen delivery
   a. PaO_2, SaO_2, SpO_2
   b. Hgb or hematocrit
   c. CO or cardiac index (CI)

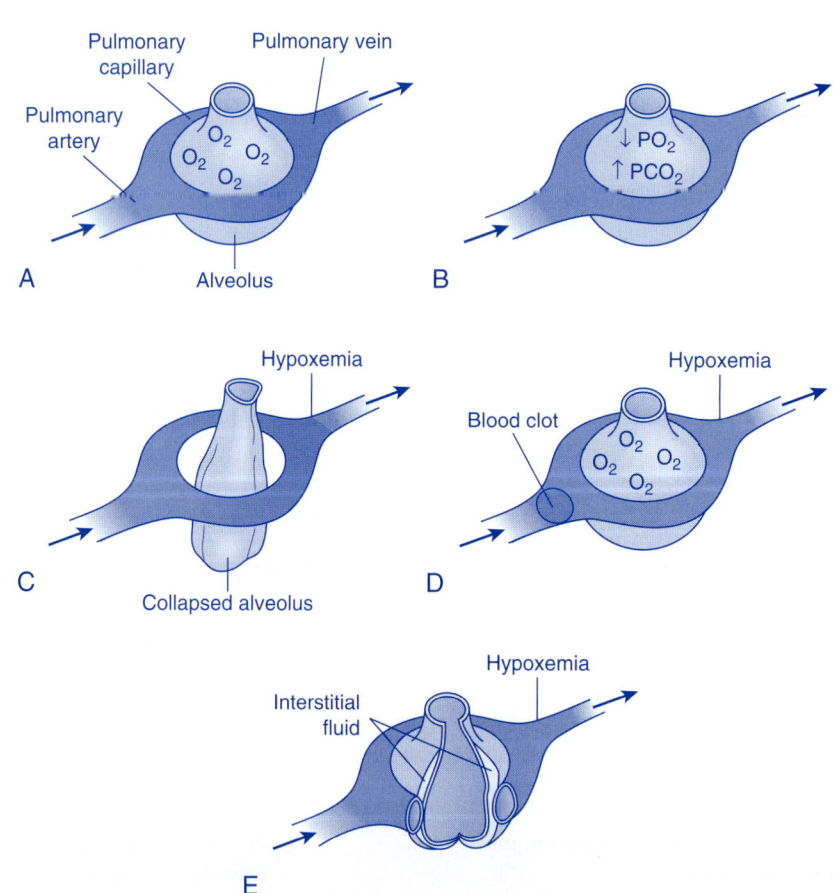

Fig. 4.29 Pulmonary causes of hypoxemia. **A,** Normal alveolar-capillary unit. **B,** Hypoventilation. **C,** Low ventilation/perfusion (V/Q) (i.e., shunt). **D,** High V/Q (i.e., dead space). **E,** Diffusion abnormality. (From Sole, M. L., Klein, D. G., & Moseley, M. J. [2017]. *Introduction to critical care nursing* [7th ed.]. Philadelphia: Saunders.)

5. Hemodynamic monitoring parameters
   a. Cardiac output
   b. Venous oxygen saturation (SvO_2)
      1) Measured by SvO_2 port of a fiberoptic oximetric PAC or by mixed venous blood gas analysis
      2) Normal 60% to 80%
   c. $ScvO_2$
      1) Measured by fiberoptic oximetric central venous catheter
      2) Normal 60% to 80%

Indications for Oxygen Therapy
1. Significant hypoxemia: PaO_2 less than 60 mm Hg; SaO_2 or SpO_2 less than 90% on room air (i.e., 21%)
2. Suspected hypoxemia (e.g., asthma, PE, aspiration, drug overdose, seizure or postictal state, pneumothorax, trauma)
3. Any acute care situation in which hypoxemia is likely
   a. Increased myocardial workload (e.g., HF, hypertensive crisis, MI)
   b. Decreased cardiac output (e.g., shock, hypotension, cardiopulmonary arrest)
   c. Increased oxygen demand (e.g., sepsis, increased ventilatory work, trauma)
   d. Before procedures that may cause hypoxemia (e.g., suctioning, during and after anesthesia, transportation of unstable patient, bronchoscopy)
4. Decreased oxygen carrying capacity (e.g., carbon monoxide or cyanide poisoning, methemoglobinemia, sickle cell disease, anemia)

Principles of Oxygen Therapy
1. Airway is always the first priority; oxygen is useless without an adequate airway.
2. Oxygen is a potent drug which is administered as prescribed; may be prescribed as flow rate, oxygen concentration (expressed as a %), or FiO_2 (expressed as a decimal)
3. The objective is to improve tissue oxygenation.
   a. Maintain PaO_2 at least 60 mm Hg and SaO_2 at 90%; serial serum lactate levels are also helpful in monitoring progression or improvement of hypoxia and degree of anaerobic metabolism.
   b. Determine the effectiveness of oxygen therapy: determined by pathology
      1) Oxygen therapy is ineffective for shunt; alveoli must be opened (also referred to as *alveolar recruitment*) to get the oxygen to the alveolar–capillary membrane; PEEP is required in these cases.
4. If high concentrations are necessary, limit duration to prevent oxygen toxicity.
   a. Frequent ABGs are mandatory if FiO_2 is above 0.4.
   b. Exact concentration of inspired O_2 should be measured with O_2 analyzer.
5. FiO_2 can be estimated by counting number of reservoirs.
   a. Nose and pharynx only (1 reservoir) less than 40%: example, nasal cannula
   b. Nose and pharynx + mask (2 reservoirs) 40% to 60%: example, simple face mask
   c. Nose and pharynx + mask + reservoir bag (3 reservoirs) 60% to 80%: example, partial rebreathing mask
   d. Nose and pharynx + mask + reservoir bag + one-way valves (3 reservoirs+ decrease in dilution) 80% to 100%: example, nonrebreathing mask
6. Safety guidelines
   a. Keep oxygen source at least 10 feet from open flame.
   b. Do not allow smoking in a room with supplemental oxygen.
   c. Do not use electrical appliances within 5 feet of oxygen source.
   d. Do not use petroleum-based products around oxygen source; use only water-soluble lubricants and creams.
   e. Turn off the oxygen when not in use.
   f. Secure the oxygen tanks to prevent accidental dropping; keep oxygen source away from heat or direct sunlight.

High-Flow versus Low-Flow Oxygen Delivery Systems
1. Low-flow oxygen delivery systems
   a. Do not provide total inspired gas; remainder of patient's inspiratory volume is met by patient breathing varying amounts of room air.
   b. FiO_2 dependent on rate and depth of ventilation and fit of device
      1) If minute ventilation increases, oxygen concentration decreases because the amount of room air (diluent) increases in relation to the amount of oxygen via the oxygen delivery system.
      2) If minute ventilation decreases, oxygen concentration increases.
   c. Does not necessarily mean low FiO_2
   d. Criteria indicating that low-flow O_2 delivery system is acceptable
      1) Normal or near-normal V_T (~7 ml/kg of ideal body weight [IBW])
      2) Respiratory rate normal or near normal (~15–25 breaths/min)
      3) Regular respiratory rhythm
      4) Specific oxygen concentration not critical to patient's care
   e. Devices
      1) Nasal cannula
      2) Reservoir systems
         a) Simple face mask
         b) Partial rebreathing mask
         c) Nonrebreathing mask
2. High-flow oxygen delivery systems
   a. Provide the entire inspired gas by high flow of gas or entrainment of room air.
   b. Provide a predictable FiO_2.
   c. Does not necessarily mean high FiO_2
   d. Criteria indicating that high-flow O_2 delivery system is needed
      1) V_T is significantly less than or more than normal (~7 ml/kg of IBW)
      2) Respiratory rate less than 15 breaths/min or more than 25 breaths/min
      3) Irregular respiratory rhythm
      4) Specific oxygen concentration is critical to patient's care
      5) Evidence of alveolar hypoventilation with hypercapnia

e. Devices
　　　　1) Venturi mask
　　　　2) T-piece: may be high or low flow depending on flow rate
　　　　3) Trach collar: may be high or low flow depending on flow rate
　　　　4) Mechanical ventilator

Oxygen Delivery Systems
Table 4.13

Hazards of Oxygen Therapy
1. Oxygen-induced hypoventilation
   a. Greatest risk if $PaCO_2$ greater than 50 mm Hg because low PaO_2 becomes primary stimulus to breathe
      1) Airway obstruction
      2) COPD
      3) Respiratory center depression
   b. Use O_2 with caution but remember low PaO_2, not FiO_2, is stimulus to breathe; use only enough oxygen to bring PaO_2 up to approximately 60 mm Hg or SaO_2 or SpO_2 up to approximately 90%.
2. Absorptive atelectasis
   a. Causes
      1) High concentrations of oxygen (an absorbable gas) wash out the nitrogen (a nonabsorbable gas) that normally holds the alveoli open at the end of expiration.
      2) Effects of oxygen on pulmonary surfactant
      3) Depression of ciliary function
   b. Prevention: do not administer oxygen that is not indicated.
3. Oxygen toxicity
   a. Cause: too high a concentration over too long a period of time (hours to days)
   b. Pathophysiology
      1) Overproduction of oxygen free radicals
      2) Large numbers of oxygen free radicals overwhelm the supply of neutralizing enzymes.
      3) Injury to capillary endothelium and increase in interstitial edema
      4) Injury to type I pneumocytes and intraalveolar edema
      5) Proliferation of type II pneumocytes
      6) Thickening of alveolar-capillary membrane
      7) Scarring and pulmonary fibrosis
   c. Clinical indications
      1) Early
         a) Substernal chest pain that increases with deep breathing
         b) Dry cough and tracheal irritation
         c) Dyspnea
         d) Upper airway changes (e.g., nasal stuffiness, sore throat, eye and ear discomfort)
         e) Anorexia, nausea, vomiting
         f) Fatigue, lethargy, malaise
         g) Restlessness
      2) Late
         a) CXR changes: atelectasis or patches of pneumonia
         b) Progressive ventilatory difficulty: decreased VC; decreased compliance; hypercapnia
         c) Increased intrapulmonary shunt: increasing A:a gradient and decreased PaO_2/FiO_2 ratio; hypoxemia
   d. Prevention
      1) Use the lowest FiO_2 possible to maintain a PaO_2 of at least 60 mm Hg (SaO_2 of 90%).
         a) Limit duration of 1 FiO_2 (i.e., 100%) to 24 hours if at all possible.
         b) Limit the use of FiO_2 above 0.6 to 2 to 3 days if at all possible.
         c) Assess ABGs frequently if FiO_2 is above 0.4 to ensure that high concentration is still required.
         d) FiO_2 of less than or equal to 0.4 is considered relatively safe.
      2) Use PEEP to increase the driving pressure of oxygen; use of PEEP achieves the following:
         a) The same PaO_2 at a lower FiO_2
         b) A better PaO_2 at the same FiO_2
      3) Remember hypoxia is far more common than O_2 toxicity and must be corrected; *actual* hypoxemia should never be allowed to persist because of concern regarding *potential* oxygen toxicity.

Hyperbaric Oxygenation
1. Definition: administration of high concentration (usually 100%) oxygen under greatly increased pressure (usually 2–3 atmospheres)
2. Indications: carbon monoxide or cyanide poisoning, air embolism, radiation therapy, gas gangrene, burns, nonhealing wounds, necrotizing fasciitis, decompression illness, osteomyelitis, intracranial abscess, anaerobic infection
3. Actions: can cause a 22-fold increase in PaO_2, which increases the amount of oxygen dissolved in the blood to enhance tissue oxygenation
4. Complications: oxygen toxicity, absorptive atelectasis, ARDS, bleeding and edema of eustachian tubes, rupture of tympanic membrane

Mechanical Ventilation

Indications for Mechanical Ventilation
1. Acute ventilatory failure with respiratory acidosis not relieved by ordinary methods, including support of cardiac function and treatment of anemia
2. Hypoxemia despite maximum oxygen therapy
3. Relief of hypoxemia causes increased CO_2 retention
4. Apnea: consideration needs to be given to the reversibility of the situation (i.e., mechanical ventilation is not indicated to prolong a terminal condition).
5. Physiologic indications
   a. VC less than 10 ml/kg or twice predicted V_T
   b. Unable to achieve maximal inspiratory force of −25 cm H_2O
   c. PaO_2 less than 60 mm Hg with FiO_2 greater than 0.6
   d. Arterial $PaCO_2$ below 30 or above 50 mm Hg
      1) Hypercapnia alone is not an indication for mechanical ventilation and must be accompanied

Table 4.13 Summary of Oxygen Delivery Systems

System	Advantages	Disadvantages	Miscellaneous
Nasal cannula 1 lpm = ~24% 2 lpm = ~28% 3 lpm = ~32% 4 lpm = ~36% 5 lpm = ~40% 6 lpm = ~44%	• Safe and simple • Comfortable • Effective for low oxygen concentration • Allows eating and talking • Inexpensive	• Contraindicated in nasal obstruction • May cause drying and irritation of nasal mucosa • May cause necrosis at ears • Cannot be used when patient has nasal obstruction • Variable concentrations of oxygen depending on tidal volume, ventilatory rate, flow rate, and nasal patency	• Ensure that flow rates do not exceed 6 l/min • Provide humidification if flow rates exceed 4 l/min • Use gauze pads under cannula at tops of ears to prevent pressure ulceration • Give oral and nasal care every 8 hours; moisten lips and nose with water-soluble lubricant
Reservoir nasal cannula; mustache style or pendant style Delivers ≥50% oxygen	• As for nasal cannula • Captures water vapor with patient exhalation and returns the moisture during inhalation, so there is no need for humidification	• As for nasal cannula • Pendant style may weigh down the ear loops	• As for nasal cannula • Must be replaced regularly • Used most often in home care • Conserves oxygen use
Simple face mask 5 lpm = ~40% 6 lpm = ~45–50% 7 lpm = ~50–55% 8 lpm = ~55–60%	• Delivers high oxygen concentration • Doesn't dry mucous membranes of nose and mouth • Can be used in patients with nasal obstruction	• Hot, confining, uncomfortable • Tight seal necessary • Frequently poorly tolerated in dyspneic patient • Interferes with eating and talking • May cause CO_2 retention if flow rate is <6 l/min • Variable concentrations of oxygen depending on tidal volume, ventilatory rate, and flow rate • Can't deliver <40% • Potential for oxygen toxicity • Impractical for long-term therapy	• Place pads between mask and bony facial parts • Wash and dry face every 4 hours • Clean mask every 8 hours • Ensure flow rate of at least 5 l/min • Check ABGs frequently • Watch for signs of oxygen toxicity
Partial rebreathing mask 6 lpm = ~35–40% 8 lpm = ~45–50% 10 lpm = ~60%	• Delivers high oxygen concentrations • Doesn't dry mucous membranes	• As for face mask • May cause CO_2 retention if reservoir bag is allowed to collapse	• Ensure that bag does not totally deflate during inhalation (increase flow rate) • Keep mask snug • Check ABGs frequently • Watch for signs of oxygen toxicity
Non-rebreathing mask 6 lpm = ~60% 7 lpm = ~70% 8 lpm = ~70% 9 lpm = ~90% 10 lpm = close to 100%	• As for other masks • One-way valves prevent rebreathing of CO_2 and increases oxygen concentrations	• As for other masks except does not cause CO_2 retention	• As for partial rebreathing mask • Check ABGs frequently • Watch for signs of oxygen toxicity
Venturi mask 4 lpm = ~24–28% 8 lpm = ~35–40% 12 lpm = ~50%	• Delivers accurate oxygen concentration depending on flow rate and diluter jet inserted despite changes in patient's respiratory pattern • Oxygen concentration can be changed • Doesn't dry mucous membranes	• FiO_2 can be lowered if mask doesn't fit snugly, if tubing is kinked, if oxygen intake ports are blocked, or if less than recommended liter flow is used • Hot, confining, and uncomfortable • Tight seal necessary • Frequently poorly tolerated in dyspneic patient • Interferes with eating and talking	• Check ABGs frequently • Watch for signs of oxygen toxicity • As for other masks
Trach collar • Delivers 21%–70% at 10 l or to provide visible mist	• Does not pull on tracheostomy • Elastic ties allow movement of mask away from tracheostomy without removing it	• Oxygen diluted by room air • Increased likelihood of infection and skin irritation around stoma because of high humidity • Condensation can collect in the tubing and drain into patient's airway, especially during turning	• Ensure that oxygen be warmed and humidified • Empty condensation from tubing frequently; empty into water trap or container for appropriate discard; do not empty water back into humidifier

Continued

Table 4.13 Summary of Oxygen Delivery Systems—cont'd

System	Advantages	Disadvantages	Miscellaneous
T-piece or tube • Delivers 21%–100% with flow rate set at 2.5 times patient's minute ventilation	• Delivers variable concentrations • Less moisture around tracheostomy than with tracheostomy collar	• May cause CO_2 retention at low flow rates • Weight of T-piece can pull on tracheostomy tube • Condensation can collect in the tubing and drain into patient's airway especially during turning	• Requires heated nebulizer • Use extension on open side to act as a reservoir and increase oxygen concentration as prescribed • Empty condensation from tubing frequently • Check ABGs frequently • Watch for signs of oxygen toxicity
Mechanical ventilation • Delivers 21%–100%	• Delivers predictable, constant concentrations of oxygen • Supports ventilation as well as oxygenation • Addition of PEEP augments the driving pressure of oxygen; this aids in the achievement of acceptable PaO_2 levels at lower oxygen concentrations	• Requires skilled personnel • Requires electricity and backup power generator (plug into red outlet) • Condensation can collect in the tubing and drain into patient's airway especially during turning	• Requires heated humidifier • Empty condensation from tubing frequently • Check ABGs frequently • Watch for signs of oxygen toxicity

ABG, Arterial blood gas; *PEEP*, positive end-expiratory pressure.

by acidosis to be an indication for mechanical ventilation: for example, a patient with COPD has chronic hypercapnia (not an indication for mechanical ventilation) but develops an even greater $PaCO_2$ level and decompensated respiratory acidosis with acute respiratory infection (a potential indication for mechanical ventilation).
   e. Dead space/V_T ratio (V_D/V_T) greater than 0.6
   f. Respiratory rate greater than 30 to 35/min
6. May also be used for the following purposes:
   a. Reduce oxygen consumption by reducing the work of breathing (e.g., shock).
   b. Stabilize the chest wall (e.g., flail chest).
   c. Allow sedation and neuromuscular paralysis.

Types of Ventilators
1. Negative-pressure ventilators
   a. Types: iron lung, chest cuirass, poncho style, body wrap
   b. Ventilatory process
      1) Negative pressure generated outside of body excluding the upper airway
      2) Negativity transmitted to intrapleural and intraalveolar spaces
      3) Pressure gradient occurs, and air moves into lungs.
      4) Expiration passively occurs by removing negative pressure around the chest wall.
   c. Uses
      1) Restricted to nonpulmonary (e.g., neuromuscular) problems
      2) Long-term ventilator support without an artificial airway
      3) Primarily in home or rehabilitation settings
   d. Advantages
      1) Artificial airway not required
      2) Normal breathing mechanics maintained so avoids harmful changes in intrathoracic pressure caused by positive-pressure ventilators
   e. Disadvantages
      1) Not helpful for patients with lung disease
      2) Not possible to precisely regulate V_T and alveolar ventilation
      3) Large size required (e.g., iron lung)
      4) Restriction of patient movement
      5) Patient care difficult because body is enclosed in ventilator.
      6) Difficulty obtaining a seal around chest
      7) May cause venous pooling in the abdomen, leading to decreased cardiac output, particularly in hypovolemic patients
2. Positive-pressure ventilators
   a. Ventilatory process
      1) Inspiration is created by positive pressure being pushed into the airway.
      2) Expiration occurs passively when the positive pressure stops.
   b. Cycling classifications
      1) Time cycled: deliver inspiratory flow until preset time interval has ended; used in neonates and children
      2) Pressure cycled: deliver inspiratory flow until preset pressure is met; pressure is set, and V_T varies
         a) Advantages
            i) Relatively inexpensive
            ii) Mobile
            iii) Run on compressed air or oxygen

b) Disadvantages
    i) V_T varies depending on compliance of the lung and the integrity of the ventilatory circuit.
    ii) Sealed airway (e.g., cuffed ET or tracheostomy tube) required
    iii) Positive intrathoracic pressure decreases venous return to the right heart and may decrease cardiac output, especially in hypovolemic patients.
    iv) Risk of ventilator-induced lung injury (VILI)
3) Volume cycled: deliver inspiratory flow until preset volume is met; V_T is set and pressure varies
    a) Advantages: deliver the set V_T regardless of changes in lung compliance
    b) Disadvantages
        i) Sealed airway required
        ii) Positive intrathoracic pressure decreases venous return to the right heart and may decrease cardiac output especially in hypovolemic patients.
        iii) Risk of VILI

Inspiratory Modes
Table 4.14
1. Volume-cycled modes end inspiration when a preset volume is achieved.
2. Pressure-cycled modes end inspiration when a preset pressure is achieved.

Expiratory Maneuvers
1. PEEP
   a. Definition: maintenance of pressure above atmospheric at airway opening at end-expiration
      1) Physiologic: 3 to 5 cm H_2O
      2) Therapeutic: greater than 5 cm H_2O
         a) Adjustment of PEEP
            i) Begin with 3 to 5 cm H_2O of PEEP
            ii) Increase in increments of 3 to 5 cm H_2O until SaO_2 (or SpO_2) of 90% is achieved
         b) Although there is no true upper limit, the higher the level, the greater the chance of barotrauma.
         c) Levels greater than 20 cm H_2O may be referred to as super-PEEP.
      3) Best (or optimal) PEEP: PEEP that provides SaO_2 of at least 90% without compromising cardiac output (remember that tissue oxygen delivery is affected by SaO_2, Hgb, and CO; if SaO_2 is increased but CO is decreased, no true gains in tissue oxygen delivery are achieved and tissue oxygen delivery may even be decreased)
      4) Auto-PEEP (also called *occult PEEP* or *intrinsic PEEP*): adds to therapeutic PEEP (Fig. 4.30)
         a) Cause: inadequate emptying of the lungs
            i) May be caused by airway obstruction or decreased compliance
            ii) May be inherent in modes with very rapid rates or short expiratory time
         b) Adverse effects
            i) Increased risk of barotrauma and volutrauma
            ii) Accentuation of hemodynamic compromise
            iii) Increased work of breathing
            iv) Patient anxiety
         c) Measurement: difference between the mean alveolar pressure and external airway pressure at end-expiration
            i) Newer ventilators may provide automated assessment
            ii) May be manually determined
               (a) Place patient on assist-control
               (b) Occlude airway at end-expiration
               (c) Observe increase in airway pressure
         d) Goal: reduce auto-PEEP to the lowest practical level
            i) Reduce bronchospasm
            ii) Adjust flow rates and I:E ratio
   b. Actions of PEEP
      1) Increases driving pressure of oxygen
         a) Improves the PaO_2 without increasing the FiO_2
         b) Allows the use of lower FiO_2 to achieve the same PaO_2, thereby decreasing risk of oxygen toxicity
      2) Decreases surface tension to prevent alveolar collapse at end-expiration
      3) Decreases intrapulmonary shunt by opening alveoli that are collapsed (referred to as *alveolar recruitment*); increases functional residual capacity
      4) Minimizes the risk of VILI by stabilizing the lung units and reducing the repeated opening and collapsing of alveoli
   c. Uses of PEEP
      1) ARDS (also referred to as *noncardiac pulmonary edema*)
      2) Cardiac pulmonary edema
      3) Acute respiratory failure with persistent hypoxemia
      4) Occasionally used to increase intrapulmonic pressure in patients with intrathoracic bleeding
      5) Physiologic PEEP is used to mimic the PEEP exerted by the closed glottis in intubated patients.
   d. Maintaining prescribed levels of PEEP
      1) Patients with an inspiratory effort pull a negative pressure and negate the level of PEEP; these patients require sedation or muscle paralysis to maintain the therapeutic effects of PEEP
   e. Adverse effects of PEEP
      1) Hemodynamic consequences of positive-pressure ventilation (PPV) are accentuated.
         a) Decreased venous return
         b) Increased right ventricular afterload
         c) Decreased left ventricular distensibility
         d) Decreased CO
      2) Barotrauma
      3) Increased ICP
   f. Contraindications of PEEP
      1) Untreated hypovolemia
      2) Extreme caution in hypotensive states
      3) Increased risk of barotrauma in patients with COPD

Table 4.14 Modes of Mechanical Ventilation

Mode	Description	Comments
Volume Modes		
Control	• Preset tidal volume and rate; the ventilator delivers the tidal volume at the rate, and the circuit is closed in between these mandatory breaths	• Patients must be apneic or paralyzed or they "fight" the ventilator • Guarantees ventilation with a specific minute ventilation • Allows ventilatory muscle rest
Assist/control (also called assisted mandatory ventilation)	• Preset tidal volume, minimum rate (control rate), and inspiratory effort required to "trigger" the ventilator to cycle to assist breaths (sensitivity); the ventilator delivers the control breaths of the specified tidal volume and responds by cycling additionally if the patient's inspiratory effort (negative pressure) is adequate	• More comfortable than control mode • Less work of breathing for patient than spontaneous breathing or IMV • Allows ventilatory muscle rest • Risk for hyperventilation because each assisted breath is delivered at same tidal volume as mandatory breaths; sedation may be necessary to decrease number of spontaneously triggered breaths
Synchronized intermittent mandatory ventilation (SIMV)	• Preset tidal volume and minimum rate; the ventilatory circuit is open between the mandatory breaths so that the patient may take additional breaths; because the ventilator does not cycle to assist these breaths, the tidal volume of these breaths varies • Mandatory breaths are synchronized so that they do not occur during the patient's ventilatory efforts	• Allows muscle reconditioning better than control or assist/control • Less potential for hyperventilation because patient-initiated breaths are at the tidal volume determined by the patient • More work of breathing for patient than assist-control because patient-initiated breaths are not assisted • Less need for sedation than assist/control or control modes • Does not decrease cardiac output as much as assist/control or control modes • Frequently used for weaning
Pressure Modes		
Pressure support ventilation (PSV)	• Preset inspiratory support pressure level; when the patient initiates a breath, this positive pressure flows to assist the patient's spontaneous breaths; tidal volume and rate is patient controlled	• Low level (5–10 cm H_2O) helps to eliminate the increased work of breathing associated with an endotracheal tube; higher levels help to augment the patient's own intrinsic tidal volume • Lessens work of breathing but also allows use of respiratory muscles to lessen muscular atrophy • Lower mean airway pressures than volume ventilation • May be used with IMV or alone; if used alone, patient must be spontaneously breathing • There is no preset ventilatory rate, and apnea occurs if the patient does not initiate a breath; newer models provide a volume ventilation backup (called *volume-assured pressure support ventilation [VAPSV]*)
Pressure-controlled ventilation (PCV)	• Preset inspiratory pressure limit, rate, and I:E ratio; the ventilator delivers air until the pressure limit is reached and maintains this pressure throughout inspiration • Tidal volumes vary because of changes in the patient's lung compliance, inspiratory time, and airway resistance	• Lower mean airway pressures than volume ventilation • Allows more even distribution of air and improves arterial oxygenation at lower FiO_2 levels • Does not provide a guaranteed tidal volume • Requires sedation
Pressure-controlled/inverse ratio ventilation (PC/IRV)	• Preset I:E ratio with inspiratory time to be greater than expiratory time; I:E ratio of ≥2:1; may be volume controlled or pressure controlled • Combination of pressure support ventilation and inverse ratio ventilation	• Improves oxygenation and allows reduction of FiO_2 • Improves distribution of ventilation • Prevents collapse of alveoli • Increases PaO_2 and SaO_2 • Increases mean airway pressure without further increases in peak inspiratory pressures • May decrease cardiac output • Makes the patient uncomfortable; patients require sedation to decrease discomfort and anxiety; muscle paralysis may be required along with sedation • May be used in ARDS with refractory hypoxemia • May cause auto-PEEP which, when added to therapeutic PEEP, increases risk of barotrauma • Do not use in patients with COPD

Table 4.14 Modes of Mechanical Ventilation—cont'd

Mode	Description	Comments
Volume-Guaranteed Pressure Modes		
VAPSV	• Preset inspiratory pressure limit, target tidal volume, and terminal flow rate • When the preset tidal volume has been achieved, inspiratory flow ends; if the preset tidal volume has not been achieved, inspiratory time is extended at the terminal flow rate until the set tidal volume is achieved • Starts as a pressure breath but ends as a volume breath if the preset tidal volume is not achieved	• Provides guarantee of adequate tidal volume lacking from PSV
Pressure-regulated volume-controlled (PRVC) (may also be referred to as *adaptive pressure ventilation* or *autoflow*)	• Preset target tidal volume and pressure limit; the ventilator automatically sets the initial flow rate and flow waveform to deliver the desired volume at the desired pressure • Inspiratory pressure changes breath to breath to augment the tidal volume delivery of subsequent breaths accounting for changes in compliance, resistance, and patient effort • Measurement of compliance at predetermined intervals and adjusts the flow rate and pressure support to deliver the set tidal volume at or below the maximal pressure	• Preferred mode for patients with high airway pressures • Produces a guaranteed tidal volume but minimizes the risk of barotrauma and volutrauma • Requires special ventilator
Airway pressure release ventilation (APRV)	• PSV with short (1–1.5 seconds) releases from higher CPAP pressure to lower CPAP pressure to allow further expiration and CO_2 elimination	• Prevents lung overdistention while maintaining inflation of newly recruited alveoli • Maintains lower mean and peak airway pressures • Less hemodynamic compromise than traditional modes
Bi-level	• CPAP with two different levels; CPAP-high and CPAP-low	• Contraindicated in patients with obstructive lung disease
High-Frequency Ventilation		
High-frequency ventilation (HFV)	• Preset (very low) tidal volumes delivered at present (very high) rates; ventilation and oxygenation are achieved by gas diffusion and convection • High-frequency positive pressure ventilation (HFPPV): 60–120 beats/min • High-frequency jet ventilation (HFJV): 120–600 beats/min • High-frequency oscillation ventilation (HFO): 500–1200 oscillations per minute	• May be used in some cases of chest trauma, bronchopleural fistula, or ARDS • Causes lower airway and intrathoracic pressures than traditional mechanical ventilation; may reduce the incidence of barotrauma and decreased cardiac output • Muscle paralysis along with sedation required • May cause increased oral secretions • Auscultation of heart and lung sounds is difficult • Requires special ventilator
Miscellaneous		
Independent lung ventilation (ILV) (also called *differential lung ventilation* or *split-lung ventilation*)	• Ventilation technique that ventilates each lung separately • Separate modes, flow rates, and PEEP may be used for each lung • May be synchronized (synchronous independent lung ventilation [SILV])	• Used for unilateral pathology or thoracic trauma • Requires double-lumen tube and separate ventilators to each lumen (and a synchronizer if SLV) • Asynchronous lung ventilation is better tolerated hemodynamically in most patients • Patient requires sedation and/or paralysis
Liquid ventilation	• Conventional ventilation along with the substitution of nitrogen with inert perfluorochemical fluids	• Perfluorochemical fluids serve as a liquid PEEP recruiting alveoli and as a local antiinflammatory • Fluids are replaced as evaporation occurs • Chest radiography interpretation is complicated by the fluid
Extracorporeal membrane oxygenation	• Transfer of blood from the patient through an artificial lung to oxygenate the blood which is then returned to the body	• Provides blood oxygenation while allowing the lung to rest and heal • Not available in all medical centers and no survival benefit shown thus far

ARDS, Acute respiratory distress syndrome; *COPD*, chronic obstructive pulmonary disease; *CPAP*, continuous positive airway pressure; FiO_2 fraction of inspired oxygen; *IMV*, intermittent mandatory ventilation *PaO_2*, partial pressure of oxygen in arterial blood *SaO_2*, Oxygen saturation of arterial blood *SILV*, synchronous independent lung *ventilation*

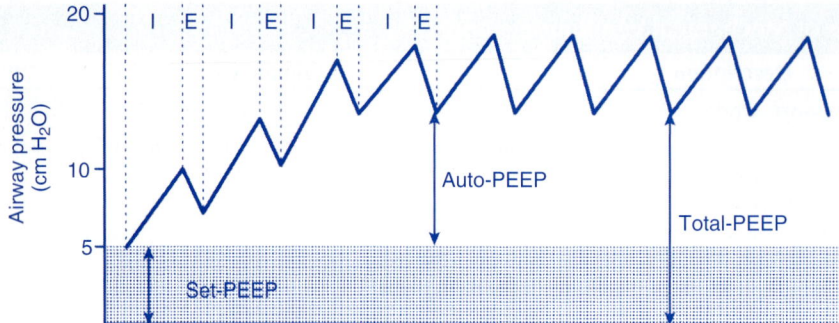

Fig. 4.30 Auto-PEEP (positive end-expiratory pressure) as frequently is seen in inverse ratio ventilation. Insufficient expiratory time permits the trapping of gases in the lung. This trapped gas creates pressure, which is known as auto-PEEP. This PEEP is added to therapeutic PEEP for total PEEP. *I*, Inspiration; *E*, expiration. (From Pierce, L. [1995]. *Guide to mechanical ventilation and intensive respiratory care*. Philadelphia: Saunders.)

Mechanical Ventilator Parameters

1. Mode
2. V_T: 5 to 10 ml/kg of ideal body weight; 4 to 8 ml/kg of ideal body weight in patients with ARDS
3. Respiratory rate: varies according to ventilator flow rate, I:E ratio, and whether ventilator is on control or assist mode; usually 4 to 20 breaths/min with slower rates used for weaning
4. FiO_2
   a. Initially 1 (i.e., 100%) for 20 minutes especially if cardiac arrest
   b. Adjusted so that PaO_2 is 60 mm Hg
   c. Use lowest FiO_2 that achieves desired PaO_2 (usually at least 60 mm Hg) and SaO_2 (usually 90%–95%).
   d. PEEP may be added to maintain acceptable PaO_2 with lower FiO_2 to reduce the risk of oxygen toxicity.
5. PEEP or CPAP
6. Sensitivity: if assist mode is used
   a. Amount of inspired effort required to initiate an assisted breath
   b. Usually set at −1 to −2 cm H_2O
7. Sigh
   a. Volume: 1.5 to 2 times the inspired V_T
   b. Frequency: 10 to 15 times/hr
   c. Although sighing was done infrequently when large V_Ts were used, they may be helpful in preventing atelectasis now that more physiologic V_Ts are being used.
8. Humidification
   a. Continuous humidification is required with inspired air warmed to body temperature; temperature is maintained at 32° to 37°C and humidity at 100%; purposes include the following:
      1) Prevent hypothermia.
      2) Thin secretions to prevent airway obstruction.
   b. Methods of adding moisture; may be active or passive
      1) Humidifiers
         a) Active
            i) Bubble humidifiers pass the inhaled gas through a water reservoir.
            ii) Passover humidifiers pass the inhaled gas over a large surface area water-soaked membrane; capillary action draws water from the reservoir.
            iii) Although active humidifiers do provide more humidification than passive systems, they allow more condensation (may be referred to as *rainout*).
               (a) Increases risk of ventilator circuit contamination and ventilation airflow obstruction
               (b) Must be emptied frequently into a water trap or container for discard
         b) Passive
            i) These devices trap the heat and humidity from the patient's exhaled air and then return some of the heat and humidity in the inhaled air.
               (a) Heat and moisture exchanger (HME)
               (b) Hygroscopic condenser humidifier (HCH)
            ii) Disadvantages of these devices
               (a) Increased mechanical dead space, which increases work of breathing
               (b) Increased the risk of obstruction because they do provide less humidity than active devices; usually used for short-term ventilation
               (c) Aerosol treatment cannot be given through an HME, so the ventilator circuit must be interrupted and risks contamination
            iii) Primary advantage is lower risk of ventilator circuit contamination.
      2) Nebulizers: high-frequency sound waves (ultrasonic) or a gas-powered airstream (pneumatic) focused on a water source produces an aerosol.
   c. Methods of adding warmth
      1) Heated wire circuit
         a) An electrically heated wire runs through the ventilator circuit to warm the inspired gas to the desired temperature.
         b) Eliminates water condensation in ventilator tubing because the wire heats the tubing so that it is the same temperature as gas leaving the ventilator

2) Servomechanism: a thermal sensor at the patient "Y" sends information to the ventilator humidity system so that the humidifier is adjusted to match the desired temperature.
9. Flow rate
   a. Usually 40 to 80 l/min but adjusted so that inspiratory volume can be completed in time allowed based on desired ventilatory rate and I:E ratio
      1) The slower the flow rate, the better distribution in the normal lung.
      2) The faster the flow rate, the better for patients with COPD so that more time is allowed for expiration.
   b. Patient comfort is also a consideration: does the patient feel like he or she is getting enough air?
10. I:E ratio
    a. Usually 1:1.5 or 1:2
    b. Inverse ratio ventilation: more time for inspiration than expiration; thought to improve distribution of inspired air, especially in ARDS
11. Alarm settings: all alarms should be on.
    a. High-pressure alarm: set alarm 10 to 20 cm H_2O above the patient's peak inspiratory pressure.
       1) Causes of high-pressure alarm
          a) Increased airway resistance: secretions, bronchospasm, kink in tubing, displacement of artificial airway, patient coughing during inspiration, patient biting on ET tube, water condensation in tubing
          b) Decreased compliance: pneumothorax (sudden increase), development of pulmonary edema, atelectasis, pneumonia, ARDS (gradual increase)
    b. Low exhaled volume alarm: set alarm at 50 to 100 ml below inspired V_T; causes of low exhaled volume alarm:
       1) Disconnection
       2) Cuff leak
       3) Leak in circuitry
       4) Overbreathing: occurs when the patient deeply inspires as the ventilator is delivering inspiration; the ventilator senses low pressure; this patient may require sedation to prevent recurrent ventilator alarms
    c. Apnea: on
       1) Patient fatigue
       2) Overmedication
       3) Decrease in level of consciousness
    d. Low FiO_2: on
       1) Oxygen disconnect
       2) Break in inspiratory circuit
12. Power: the mechanical ventilator must be plugged into a grounded electrical outlet that is backed up by the emergency generator; this outlet is usually red.

Assessment of a Mechanically Ventilated Patient

1. Pulmonary
   a. Airway: type, size, position, and cuff pressure
   b. Chest excursion and use of accessory muscles
   c. Breath sounds
   d. Secretions: amount, color, consistency, and odor
   e. Spontaneous ventilatory mechanics: at least every 24 hours without sedation (i.e., sedation vacation) though sedation withdrawal is contraindicated for some patients (e.g., neurologically injured patients)
      1) Respiratory rate
      2) Patient's own V_T
      3) VC
      4) Minute ventilation
      5) MIP
      6) Rapid shallow breathing index: best single index for assessing readiness for weaning
         a) Calculated: f/V_T
         b) RSBI less than or equal to 105 indicates readiness to wean
   f. Ventilator parameters
      1) Mode: as set
      2) V_T as set and exhaled
      3) Respiratory rate: ventilator and patient initiated
      4) FiO_2: confirmed with oxygen analyzer
      5) PEEP: airway pressure at the end of expiration (on pressure gauge not just what it is set to be)
      6) Peak inspiratory pressure: airway pressure at the peak of inspiration; calculate dynamic compliance
      7) Plateau pressure: airway pressure with an inflation hold; calculate static compliance
      8) Alarms: check that all are on.
   g. Ventilator circuitry: leaks, condensation, and temperature of inspired air
   h. Pulse oximetry: SpO_2
   i. CXR: usually done daily unless chronic situation
   j. ABGs: usually done daily and 20 to 30 minutes after any ventilator changes and as indicated by change in patient status
2. Cardiovascular
   a. Heart rate
   b. ECG rhythm
   c. Heart sounds
   d. BP: direct (arterial catheter) or indirect (auscultated)
   e. Hemodynamic parameters: right atrial pressure (RAP), pulmonary artery pressure (PAP), pulmonary artery occlusive pressure (PAOP), cardiac output (CO)/cardiac index (CI), systemic vascular resistance (SVR)/systemic vascular resistance index (SVRI), pulmonary vascular rsistance (PVR)/pulmonary vascular resistance index (PVRI), oxygen saturation of venous blood (SvO_2)
3. Neurologic
   a. Level of consciousness
   b. Airway reflexes: gag, swallowing, and corneal
   c. Sedation level
4. Renal or metabolic
   a. Urine output
   b. Urine specific gravity
   c. Serum electrolytes
5. Gastrointestinal
   a. Abdominal distention
   b. Bowel sounds
   c. Guaiac testing: NG aspirate, vomitus, stools
6. Nutritional status
   a. Daily weight
   b. Total protein, albumin, and serum transferrin levels
   c. Calorie counts and nutrient balance

7. Immunologic
    a. Temperature
    b. Sputum cultures
    c. White blood cell count
8. Psychological
    a. Complaints of pain or anxiety
    b. Clinical indicators of pain or anxiety

Collaborative Management
1. Ensure patient safety.
    a. Frequent assessment for change in status
        1) SpO_2
        2) ABGs
        3) End-tidal CO_2
        4) Breath sounds
        5) Heart sounds
        6) Neurologic status
        7) Peak inspiratory pressure and plateau pressure
        8) Cuff pressure
        9) Airway and need for suctioning
    b. Close monitoring of ventilator settings, ventilator connections, peak and plateau pressures, ventilator alarms on
    c. Empty condensation for water traps as indicated.
    d. Discontinue gastric feedings during chest physiotherapy and as indicated.
2. Assist with ventilator changes according to ABGs and patient's clinical status (Table 4.15)
    a. Note that only one change should be made at a time.
3. Reduce patient discomfort and anxiety.
    a. Communication with patient to orient to place and time, inform the patient regarding what is happening, and his or her needs using communication aids
    b. Distraction (e.g., music, television, radio)
    c. Nonpharmacologic comfort measures (e.g., massage, aromatherapy)
    d. Analgesics: morphine intermittently or infusion may be needed, especially in patients who have chest trauma or surgery.
    e. Sedatives as indicated
        1) Types of sedatives (Tables 4.16 and 4.17)
            a) Benzodiazepines (e.g., diazepam, lorazepam, midazolam)
                i) Midazolam is the benzodiazepine of choice for short-term (<24 hours) sedation of critically ill patients.
                ii) Lorazepam is benzodiazepine of choice for long-term (>24 hours) sedation of critically ill patients
            b) Sedative–hypnotics (e.g., propofol)
                i) Provides advantage of reversibility to allow for short-term breathing trial daily for patients on mechanical ventilation (i.e., "sedation vacation")
            c) α_2-Adrenoceptor agonist (e.g., dexmedetomidine): increasingly popular because of lack of respiratory depression
        2) Nursing management of pain, agitation, and delirium (Barr et al., 2013)
            a) Always treat pain first.
            b) Ensure patient safety.
            c) Talk to the patient, assess orientation, and reorient as required.
            d) Identify and treat cause of agitation (e.g., pain, anxiety, sleep deprivation, alcohol or drug withdrawal).
            e) Complement medication use with provision of comfort, control of environment, and music.
            f) Determine the need for sedation.
            g) Select and treat to a target level of sedation; use the smallest effective dose of drug.
                i) Ramsay sedation scale (Table 4.18)
                ii) Sedation-agitation scale (Table 4.19)
                iii) Motor activity assessment scale (Table 4.20)

Table 4.15 Mechanical Ventilator Parameter Changes to Make According to Arterial Blood Gases

If $PaCO_2$ is >45 mm Hg (or above the patient's normal if patient has COPD)	• Increase ventilation • Increase rate • Increase tidal volume • (if it does not currently exceed 10 ml/kg)
If $PaCO_2$ is <35 mm Hg	• Decrease ventilation • Decrease rate • Decrease tidal volume • If patient is on assist/control mode: change mode from AC to IMV • Consider sedation and/or analgesia • Mechanical dead space may be considered (tubing which acts as a rebreathing device)
If PaO_2 is <60 mm Hg	• Increase FiO_2 • Add or increase PEEP (especially if FiO_2 is already >0.6 [60%])
If PaO_2 is >100 mm Hg	• Decrease FiO_2 • Decrease PEEP (especially if FiO_2 is < 0.4 [40%])

IMV, intermittent mandatory ventilation; *COPD*, chronic obstructive pulmonary disease; *FiO₂*, fraction of inspired oxygen; *PaCO₂*, partial pressure of carbon dioxide in arterial blood; *PEEP*, positive end-expiratory pressure.

Table 4.16 Comparison of Selected Sedative Agents

	Propofol	Midazolam	Lorazepam	Diazepam	Dexmedetomidine
Elimination half-life	1–8 hours	1–12 hours	10–20 hours	20–80 hours	2 hours
Onset	1 minute	2–5 minutes	5–20 minutes	2–5 minutes	2–6 minutes
Active metabolites	No	Yes	No	Yes	No
Continuous infusion	Yes	Yes	Yes	No	Yes

Table 4.17 Selected Sedative Agents

Drug	Administration	Adverse Effects	Nursing Implications
Diazepam and other benzodiazepines	Diazepam • PO: 2–10 mg every 6–8 hours • IV injection: 1–15 mg at rate no faster than 2 mg/min; may repeat every 2–4 hours • Maximum: 60 mg • Do not mix with any other drugs or dextrose solution Other benzodiazepines Lorazepam • PO: 2–6 mg/day in divided doses • IV injection: 1–4 mg slowly every 2–4 hours • IV infusion: 1–10 mg/hr adjusted to desirable sedation level Alprazolam • PO: 0.25–0.5 mg three times daily	• Tachycardia • Hypotension (IV) • Nausea, vomiting • Urinary retention • Drowsiness • Dizziness, ataxia • Blurred vision • Slurred speech • Confusion • Respiratory depression (IV) • Drug dependence may occur	• Monitor HR, BP, ECG, respiratory rate and depth • Note contraindications: known hypersensitivity, glaucoma, psychosis • Use cautiously in liver disease, renal disease, older adults • Use large veins for IV injection • Administer flumazenil, a benzodiazepine antagonist, if necessary and prescribed
Midazolam hydrochloride	• IM injection: 0.07–0.35 mg/kg • IV injection: 0.15–0.35 mg/kg • IV infusion: mix 150 mg in 250 ml (0.6 mg/ml); usual dose is 0.05–0.25 mg/kg/hr	• Bradycardia • Dysrhythmias • Hypotension • Nausea, vomiting, hiccoughs • Headache • Agitation • Bronchospasm • Respiratory depression, apnea • Pain and tenderness at injection site	• Monitor HR, BP, respiratory rate and depth • Note contraindications: known hypersensitivity, shock, coma, acute alcohol intoxication, glaucoma • Use cautiously in COPD, HF, renal failure, older adult, debilitated person • Use large muscle mass if given IM; use large vein if given IV, avoid infiltration • Administer flumazenil, a benzodiazepine antagonist, if necessary and prescribed
Propofol	• IV injection: 5 mcg/kg initially then increase dose by 5–10 mcg/kg/min every 5–10 minutes until level of sedation is reached; followed by IV infusion • IV infusion: premixed in 10 mg/ml concentration, infuse 5–50 mcg/kg/min • Maximum: 150 mcg/kg/min • Use strict aseptic technique; discard tubing and unused solution at least every 12 hours	• Bradycardia • Hypotension • Decreased cardiac output • Nausea, vomiting • Headache • Twitching • Rash • Green urine • Respiratory depression • Reactions such as agitation, hyperactivity, combativeness may occur • Burning or pain at injection site • Hypertriglyceridemia with prolonged infusion • Metabolic acidosis with prolonged infusion • Pancreatitis • Sepsis	• Monitor HR, BP, ECG, respiratory rate • Note that this drug allows for faster weaning process and faster time to extubation than neuromuscular paralytics • Note contraindications: known hypersensitivity to propofol or lipid emulsion, hyperlipidemia and disorders of lipid metabolism, intracranial hypertension • Use cautiously in respiratory depression, dysrhythmias, pancreatitis, hypotension, hypovolemia, and in older adult • Correct hypovolemia before administration of propofol • Administer with analgesics if needed because this drug provides no analgesia • Wean by reducing the rate by 5–10 mcg/kg/min every 10–15 minutes; stop when patient reaches baseline consciousness and orientation
Dexmedetomidine HCl	• IV injection: 1 mcg/kg over 10 minutes followed by IV infusion • IV infusion: 0.2–0.7 mcg/kg/hr titrated to patient response for up to 24 hours	• Hypotension or hypertension • Bradycardia or tachycardia • Dysrhythmia especially atrial fibrillation • Nausea, vomiting • Fever • Hypoxia • Anemia	• Monitor HR, BP, SaO_2 • Arousability and alertness with stimulation does not necessarily indicate lack of efficacy in the absence of other clinical findings • Use caution in patients with advanced heart block • Coadministration with other anesthetics, sedatives, hypnotics, and opioids is likely to lead to enhancement of the effects of those drugs • Avoid contact of dexmedetomidine with rubber because it may interact with natural rubber

Continued

(c) Evaluate voltage required before paralysis if possible.
  (i) Turn voltage dial to 2 to start. Increase as necessary.
  (ii) Turn unit on and push train of four.
  (iii) Look for thumb twitch, eyelid twitch, foot dorsiflexion, or plantar flexion of great toe.
  (iv) Increase voltage if necessary.
ii) Evaluation
  (a) Desired response is one to two twitches out of four stimuli if the patient is receiving the adequate dose for neuromuscular blockade.
  (b) Underparalysis
    (i) Three or four responses of four stimuli indicates underparalysis.
    (ii) Dosage should be increased.
  (c) Overparalysis
    (i) No response even with the voltage at maximum indicates overparalysis.
    (ii) Dosage should be decreased.
4) Types of neuromuscular blockers and duration of action
  a) Depolarizing
    i) Succinylcholine: 8 to 10 minutes
  b) Nondepolarizing
    i) Mivacurium: 15 to 30 minutes
    ii) Rocuronium: 20 to 30 minutes
    iii) Atracurium: 20 to 35 minutes
    iv) Vecuronium: 25 to 30 minutes
    v) Cisatracurium: 30 to 50 minutes
    vi) Tubocurarine: 30 to 100 minutes
    vii) Pancuronium: 60 to 75 minutes
    viii) Pipecuronium: 60 to 140 minutes
    ix) Doxacurium: 100 to 150 minutes
5) Nursing management principles of neuromuscular blockage
  a) Give sedative and/or analgesics concurrently with paralytics.
    i) Clinical signs of inadequate sedation in a patient receiving neuromuscular blocking agents
      (a) Hypertension
      (b) Tachycardia
      (c) Diaphoresis
      (d) Lacrimation
  b) Explain the situation to the patient before paralysis.
  c) Protect the patient's corneas, skin, joints; deep vein thrombosis (DVT) prophylaxis is indicated.
  d) Evaluate dose by evaluating train of four and adjust accordingly.
  e) Prevent, assess for, and manage potential complications of PPV (Table 4.22).
    i) Bundles to prevent complications
      (a) Bundle concept: evidence-based interventions "bundled" together to improve patient outcomes; a small number of interventions (three to five) is recommended (Institute for Healthcare Improvement [IHI], 2012)
      (b) Interventions typically included in a "vent" bundle (IHI, 2012)
      (c) Elevation of the head of the bed
      (d) Daily "sedation vacations" and assessment of readiness to wean or extubate
      (e) Peptic ulcer disease prophylaxis
      (f) Deep venous thrombosis prophylaxis
      (g) Daily oral care with chlorhexidine

Liberation or Weaning from Ventilatory Support

1. Definition: the gradual withdrawal of ventilatory support for patients who have been mechanically ventilated more than 24 hours
2. Phases of weaning
   a. Preweaning phase: assessment to determine if the patient is capable of attempting spontaneous ventilation
      1) Respiratory factors
         a) Resolution or improvement of disease process that necessitated mechanical ventilation
         b) Oxygenation
            i) Patient does not require more than 5 cm of PEEP or FiO_2 greater than 0.5 to maintain acceptable PaO_2 (PaO_2 60 mm Hg) and SaO_2 (SaO_2 of 90%)
            ii) Perfusion/ventilation (P/F) ratio greater than or equal to 150 mm Hg
            iii) Patient has not developed ventilator-associated pneumonia (VAP) or a DVT, which may lead to venous thromboembolism (VTE).
         c) Ventilation
            i) Respiratory rate less than 30 breaths/min
            ii) $PaCO_2$ less than 45 mm Hg or equal to the patient's baseline $PaCO_2$
            iii) V_T greater than 5 ml/kg
            iv) VC greater than 10 ml/kg
            v) Minute ventilation less than 10 l/min
         d) Lung mechanics
            i) MIP greater than -25 cm H_2O
            ii) Rapid shallow breathing index less than or equal to 125 breaths/min/l
      2) Nonrespiratory factors
         a) Neurologic status: conscious
         b) Hemodynamics: stable
         c) Hgb: adequate and absence of GI bleeding
         d) Fluid and electrolytes: corrected and normal
         e) Nutrition: adequate nutritional status
         f) Psychological factors: psychologically prepared and cooperative
         g) Medications: cessation of deep sedation and muscle paralytics

Table 4.22 Complications of Mechanical Ventilation

Complication	Causes	Prevention	Clinical Presentation	Treatment
Decreased cardiac output	• Increased intrathoracic pressures that • Decrease venous return to the right heart • Increase RV afterload • Decrease LV distensibility	• Ensure adequate preload before mechanical ventilation • Avoid excessive tidal volumes • Adjust PEEP carefully	• Tachycardia, hypotension • Cool, clammy skin • Decrease in urine output • Change in level of consciousness	• Administer fluids to increase preload • Administer inotropes as prescribed
Ventilator-induced lung injury (VILI)	• Barotrauma: high inflation pressures may cause pneumothorax, pneumomediastinum, subcutaneous emphysema • Volutrauma: high inflation volumes and repeated end-expiratory collapse followed by repeated reopening during inspiration may cause release of inflammatory mediators, injury to the lung ultrastructure, and ARDS • Oxygen toxicity • High end-inspiratory lung volume, such as occurs with high levels of PEEP, auto-PEEP (e.g., IRV), and high functional residual capacity, such as older adult patients (i.e., senile emphysema) or patients with COPD	• Avoid excessive tidal volumes; now recommended to be within 5–10 ml/kg of IBW with even lower tidal volumes for patients with ALI/ARDS (~6 ml/kg of IBW) • Keep plateau pressure <30 cm H_2O • Keep FiO_2 <0.6 (60%) • Adjust PEEP carefully	• Pneumothorax: chest pain, dyspnea, sudden increase in peak inspiratory pressure, decreased breath sounds and chest movement on affected side, tracheal shift, hypotension, JVD if tension pneumothorax, clinical indications of hypoxia, decreased SpO_2, chest radiography changes • ARDS: high peak and plateau pressures, refractory hypoxemia (P/F ratio <300 mm Hg), noncardiac (PAOP <18 mm Hg) pulmonary edema, patchy atelectasis on chest radiography	• If pneumothorax is suspected: take patient off ventilator and manually ventilate with a manual resuscitation bag; assist with insertion of chest tube for pneumothorax • Decrease tidal volume or PEEP if possible to decrease mean airway pressure and prevent alveolar overdistention
Fluid retention	• Decrease in insensible loss via respiratory system • Overhydration by humidification • Decreased urine output caused by ADH and aldosterone secretion	• Avoid decrease in cardiac output, which stimulates renin–angiotensin–aldosterone system	• Weight gain • Intake greater than output • Crackles • Decreased compliance	• Use therapies above to prevent decrease in cardiac output
Atelectasis	• Airway obstruction • Small tidal volumes or lack of sighing • Infrequent turning of patient	• Use periodic sighing • Turn frequently • Provide adequate humidification • Perform tracheal suctioning as indicated • Provide chest PT as indicated • Reposition frequently	• Diminished breath sounds • Crackles • Abnormal chest radiography • Increased A:a gradient • Decreased compliance	• Provide periodic sighing • Provide chest PT
Hypercapnia; hypocapnia	• Inadequate or excessive ventilation • Hypermetabolism may contribute to hypercapnia	• Initiate ventilation with tidal volume at 10–15 ml/kg and rate of 8–12 • Make ventilator changes after initial ABGs	• Increased (>45 mm Hg) or decreased (<35 mm Hg) $PaCO_2$	• Hypercapnia: increase tidal volume (or rate) • Hypocapnia: decrease rate (or tidal volume); change to IMV or PSV
Oxygen toxicity	• Too high a concentration of O_2 over too long a time	• Maintain FiO_2 as low as possible to maintain a SaO_2 (or SpO_2) of 90% and limit duration of FiO_2 of >0.4 if possible; addition of PEEP allows reduction of FiO_2 while maintaining the same SaO_2 • **Remember:** hypoxemia is far more common than O_2 toxicity and must be corrected.	• Substernal distress • Paresthesias in extremities • Anorexia, nausea, vomiting • Fatigue, lethargy, malaise • Restlessness • Dyspnea, progressive respiratory difficulty • Decreased compliance • Increased A:a gradient	• Decrease O_2 concentration as soon as possible • Provide supportive management

Continued

Table 4.22 Complications of Mechanical Ventilation—cont'd

Complication	Causes	Prevention	Clinical Presentation	Treatment
Aspiration	• Stomach contents • Tube feedings • Oral secretions • Gastric distention • Impaired gastric emptying • Esophageal reflux	• Maintain cuff inflation using minimal occlusive volume • Keep HOB elevated 30–45 degrees • Check for gastric retention at least every 4 hours • Check NG tube placement at least every 4 hours	• Increased tracheal secretions • Fever • Rhonchi, wheezes • Signs or symptoms of hypoxemia or hypoxia • Infiltrate on chest radiography	• Provide supportive management • Administer antibiotics as prescribed • Administer steroids as prescribed
GI effects: stress ulcer, ileus, gastric dilation	• Hyperacidity • Endogenous or exogenous steroids • Gastric or mesenteric ischemia • Inadequate nutrition	• Use enteral feedings • Administer antacids; H_2 receptor antagonists (e.g., cimetidine [Tagamet]); barrier agents (e.g., sucralfate [Carafate]) as prescribed	• NG aspirate, vomitus, or stools positive for blood • Decreased bowel sounds • Gastric distention • Increased gastric retention	• Note effect of hemoglobin loss of tissue oxygenation; blood administration may be necessary • Administer antacids, sucralfate, H_2 receptor antagonists, and/or PPI, as prescribed
Infection	• Immunosuppression • Artificial airways bypass normal upper airway defense mechanisms • Ventilatory equipment: warm, moist environment is good for bacterial growth • Suctioning procedure • Silent aspiration of GI bacteria when PPIs, H_2 antagonists, or antacids used for ulcer prophylaxis; controversial issue • Cross-contamination may be cause	• Use good hand-washing techniques • Use sterile technique for suctioning • Provide aseptic airway management, tubing changes, etc • Avoid change in usual acidic gastric pH; use enteral feedings for ulcer prophylaxis if gastric mobility adequate • Keep HOB elevated during tube feedings • Keep ET tube or trach cuff inflated to 20–25 mm Hg • Drain humidifier condensation into water trap or container and not back into humidifier • Routine change of ventilator circuit is no longer indicated, but the circuit should be changed if visibly soiled or malfunctioning • Additional information in Pneumonia section of this chapter	• Tachycardia, tachypnea • Fever • Crackles, rhonchi, or wheezes • Hypoxemia • Change in color or character of sputum • Positive cultures • Infiltrate on chest radiography	• Administer antibiotic specific to culture
Patient-ventilator asynchrony (patient "fighting" ventilator)	• Incorrect ventilator setup for the patient's needs • Acute change in patient's status • Obstructed airway • Ventilator malfunction • Anxiety	• Ensure proper setup of ventilator equipment; monitor settings every hour • Monitor peak inspiratory pressure • Suction as indicated • Talk to patient; keep him or her informed • Administer anxiolytics as indicated	• Anxiety, agitation • Increase in peak inspiratory pressure • Ventilator alarm sounding • Change in pulse oximetry or ABGs	• Perform rapid check of patient and ventilator • Disconnect patient from ventilator and provide manual ventilation via manual resuscitation bag • Check vital signs, breath sounds, pulse oximetry • Assess ABGs • Suction airway • Check patency of ET or tracheostomy tube

Table 4.22	Complications of Mechanical Ventilation—cont'd			
Complication	**Causes**	**Prevention**	**Clinical Presentation**	**Treatment**
Anxiety	• Loss of autonomy over vital body function (breathing) • Inability to communicate • Sensory overload (e.g., alarms, repeated interruptions for vital signs, noise of ventilator) • Sensory deprivation (e.g., separation from family, work, meaningful activities) • Discomfort (e.g., arterial punctures, endotracheal tube, NG tube, Foley catheter)	• Explain to patient why he or she can't speak; provide method of communication • Explain all procedures thoroughly; keep patient informed regarding progress and plans • Add familiar objects to patient's environment (e.g., family photos, cards) • Have calendar and clock in room; have window shades or curtains open to orient patient to light and dark • Allow uninterrupted time for rest and sleep • Put eyeglasses and hearing aid on patient if appropriate • Encourage expression of fears • Be available; answer call bell promptly • Promote as much independence as possible • Provide emotional support to the family • Avoid uncomfortable or painful procedures if possible (e.g., arterial catheter instead of arterial punctures) • Use complementary therapies such as music, aromatherapy	• High-pressure alarm because the patient is breathing out of synch with ventilator • Tachycardia • Tachypnea, excessive triggering of ventilator is on assist/control, potentially causing hypocapnia and respiratory alkalosis • Complaints of being "nervous"	• Stay with patient during times of extreme anxiety • Use therapeutic touch (e.g., hold hand) • Use soft restraints only as necessary to prevent self-extubation • Encourage family visitation and participation if appropriate
Inability to wean or failure to liberate	• COPD: occurs when $PaCO_2$ is corrected instead of pH • Malnutrition: catabolism and muscle breakdown • Neuromuscular blocking agents: disuse syndrome • Oversedation or failure to minimize sedation • Lack of current, standardized approach or protocol for liberation from mechanical ventilation	• Correct pH instead of $PaCO_2$ in patients with COPD • Provide adequate calories to prevent catabolism; adequate protein and high calories are given; adequate calories must be given to prevent the protein from being used for energy; calories given are predominantly fat because carbohydrate metabolism produces more CO_2 • Avoid neuromuscular blocking agents if possible; limit duration of use	• Increased $PaCO_2$, increased ventilatory rate, tachycardia with weaning efforts	• COPD: allow $PaCO_2$ to increase so that the kidney will hold on to bicarbonate to compensate; keep PaO_2 close to patient's normal (e.g., 60–65 mm Hg) • Provide adequate protein and calories; avoid high carbohydrate feedings during weaning • Discontinue several days before weaning • Minimize sedation • Attempt inspiratory pressure augmentation during SBT

ABG, Arterial blood gas; *ADH,* antidiuretic hormone; *ARDS,* acute respiratory distress syndrome; *COPD,* chronic obstructive pulmonary disease; *ET,* endotracheal; *FiO₂,* fraction of inspired oxygen; *GI,* gastrointestinal; *HOB,* head of bed; *IBW,* ideal body weight; *IMV,* intermittent mandatory ventilation; *IRV,* inverse ratio ventilation; *JVD,* jugular neck vein distention; *LV,* left ventricular; *NG,* nasogastric; *P/F,* Pressure/Ventilation *PaCO₂,* Partial pressure of carbon dioxide in arterial blood *PEEP,* positive end-expiratory pressure; *PPI,* proton pump inhibitor; *PSV,* pressure support ventilation; *PT,* physical therapy; *RV,* right ventricular; *SaO₂,* Oxygen saturation of arterial blood; *SBT,* spontaneous breathing trial; *SpO₂,* Oxygen saturation of arterial blood by pulse oximetry

b. Weaning or liberation phase
  1) Methods of weaning or liberation
    a) Spontaneous breathing trial (SBT) with inspiratory pressure augmentation (5–8 cm H_2O) rather than T-piece or CPAP alone for short-term mechanical ventilation (i.e., <72 hours)
      i) Spontaneous breathing for 120 minutes through ventilator with pressure support ventilation (PSV) of 0; CPAP of up to 5 cm H_2O allowed
        (a) If successful, extubation
        (b) If unsuccessful, allow patient to rest and try again the next day; tracheostomy may also be considered. If SBT is successful and patient is at high risk for respiratory failure, consider use of preventive noninvasive ventilation (noninvasive positive-pressure ventilation [NPPV]) to avoid the need for reintubation
      ii) Advantage: may be able to liberate patient more quickly than intermittent mandatory ventilation (IMV) or PSV methods
      iii) Disadvantage: recurrent ventilatory failures discourage and frighten the patient; if recurrent failures have occurred, use of preventive NPPV may be considered.
    b) IMV
      i) Gradually reduce IMV rate.
      ii) Advantages
        (a) Provides exercise for ventilatory musculature
        (b) More physiologic $PaCO_2$ may be achieved
        (c) Large ventilator-provided breaths help to prevent atelectasis.
        (d) Safer than trial-and-error method
        (e) Good acceptance by patients
      iii) Disadvantages: may take longer than T-piece method
    c) PSV method
      i) Gradually decrease the amount of pressure support assisting the patient
        (a) Usually started at 15 to 25 cm H_2O
        (b) Gradually decreased by 3 to 6 cm H_2O every 1 to 3 days as long as maintaining a satisfactory minute ventilation
        (c) When the patient can maintain adequate ventilation with the PSV at 5 cm H_2O, extubation is considered.
      ii) Advantages
        (a) Patient comfort frequently greater with PSV
        (b) Less work of breathing than with IMV or T-piece method
    d) CPAP
      i) May be used for patients whose PaO_2 is PEEP-dependent; the patient is weaned from the ventilator by one of the previously noted methods but left on CPAP to provide the improved driving pressure needed to maintain an adequate PaO_2
  2) Criteria used to stop a weaning trial
    a) Neurologic
      i) Change in level of consciousness
      ii) Extreme anxiety
    b) Pulmonary
      i) Respiratory rate greater than 35 breaths/min or less than 10 breaths/min
      ii) Use of accessory muscle of ventilation
      iii) Paradoxical chest wall motion
      iv) Complaints of dyspnea, fatigue, or pain
      v) SaO_2 less than 90%
      vi) Increase in $PaCO_2$ of 5 to 8 mm Hg or pH of less than 7.3
    c) Cardiovascular
      i) Systolic BP greater than 180 mm Hg or less than 90 mm Hg
      ii) Heart rate greater than 140 beats/min or sustained increase 20% above baseline
      iii) PVCs greater than 6/min, couplets, or runs of ventricular tachycardia
      iv) ST-segment changes
  3) Therapies to facilitate liberation
    a) Coordination and communication among disciplines: liberation protocols, flow sheets, and communication boards
    b) Multidisciplinary liberation protocol
    c) Multidisciplinary rounds
    d) Recognition of likely reasons for failure to liberate
      i) Underlying illness has not resolved sufficiently
      ii) Oversedation or lack of ability to minimize sedation
      iii) Malnutrition
      iv) Excessive secretions
      v) Presence of auto-PEEP
      vi) Muscle weakness
      vii) Impaired muscle function secondary to electrolyte imbalance (e.g., hypokalemia, hypophosphatemia, hypomagnesemia)
      viii) Respiratory muscle fatigue
c. Weaning outcomes phase
  1) Complete weaning: the patient is able to maintain a normal respiratory rate and V_T while breathing spontaneously.
  2) Partial weaning: the patient is able to maintain spontaneous ventilation for short periods.
  3) Terminal weaning followed by death
3. General guidelines
  a. Liberation from mechanical ventilation should be done as soon as possible to avoid ventilator-associated events, including VAP and VTE.

b. Position with HOB elevated 30 to 45 degrees throughout mechanical ventilation
c. Avoid depressing the patient's ventilatory drive and muscle strength by minimizing sedation using an evidence-based protocol; treat pain without excessive use of opioids.
d. Reduce carbohydrates if indicated; equivalent calories can be provided in the form of fats.
  1) Use Pulmocare if being fed enterally: high fat and protein but low carbohydrates.
  2) Decrease glucose and increase fat (Intralipids) if being fed parenterally.
e. Begin weaning attempts in the early morning; do not attempt to wean the patient at night.
f. Begin initial SBT with inspiratory pressures augmentation (5–8 cm H_2O) rather than T-piece or CPAP alone
g. Complementary therapies such as biofeedback and music may be helpful.
h. Because the mechanical ventilator may provide security for the patient, it may be helpful to leave ventilator in room with patient for 24 hours after weaning.
i. Monitor closely for clinical indicators of fatigue and ventilatory failure and abort if necessary.
j. For patients at high risk of respiratory failure (e.g., chronic hypercapnia, COPD, HF), who have passed an SBT, consider extubation and NPPV.

Noninvasive Positive-Pressure Ventilation (NPPV)

Description
Positive-pressure ventilation (usually CPAP or bi-positive pressure ventilation [bi-PAP]) of a nonintubated spontaneous breathing patient, primarily with a face or nasal mask attached to a standard ventilator or a machine specifically for NPPV with the purpose of augmenting alveolar ventilation
1. Modes
   a. CPAP: preset positive airway pressure during spontaneous breaths
   b. Bi-PAP: preset positive pressure to be delivered during inspiration and preset pressure to be maintained during expiration; combination of PSV (I-PAP) and CPAP (E-PAP)
2. Patient–ventilator interface
   a. Types
      1) Nasal mask
      2) Facial mask
      3) Nasal prongs
      4) Helmet
   b. Considerations
      1) Patient preference
      2) Facial shape
      3) Patient acuity
      4) Patient anxiety level

Indications
1. Acute respiratory failure, especially in COPD
2. Cardiac pulmonary edema
3. After weaning or liberation from traditional mechanical ventilation or PEEP in patients at high risk for respiratory failure
4. Sleep apnea
5. Terminal care to avoid intubation, such as a patient with end-stage COPD

Advantages over Traditional Mechanical Ventilation
1. Avoidance of intubation and complications of intubation such as VAP
2. Improved patient comfort
3. Lower incidence of nosocomial pneumonia
4. Lower sedation requirements
5. Shorter critical care unit stays
6. Can be initiated, discontinued, and reinitiated if only required intermittently

Disadvantages
1. Uncomfortable because mask requires a seal
2. Seal difficult to obtain if orogastric or NG tube in place
3. Cannot eat because of a high risk of aspiration

Contraindications
1. Absolute
   a. Hemodynamic instability
   b. Problems with airway patency (e.g., copious secretions)
   c. Risk for aspiration
   d. Altered level of consciousness (i.e., patient without airway protective reflexes)
   e. Recent upper airway or esophageal surgery
2. Relative
   a. Uncooperative patient
   b. Morbid obesity
   c. Unstable angina or acute MI
   d. Inability to fit mask
   e. Agitation

Complications
1. Facial skin breakdown
2. Nasal congestion
3. Conjunctivitis
4. Gastric distention
5. Aspiration
6. Pneumothorax

Reasons to Switch to Invasive Ventilation
1. Worsening of $PaCO_2$ and respiratory acidosis
2. Worsening PaO_2 and SaO_2
3. Severe tachypnea
4. Hemodynamic instability
5. Altered level of consciousness
6. Inability to clear airway secretions
7. Inability to tolerate face mask

Chest Tubes

Purposes of Chest Tubes
Also Called *Thoracostomy Tubes* or *Thoracic Catheters*.
1. Pleural tubes
   a. To remove free air: tube placed anterior and superior (usually at second intercostal space [ICS] at MCL)

1) Pneumothorax (i.e., air in the pleural space)
    a) Chest tube is indicated if pneumothorax is greater than 15% or on mechanical ventilator.
    b) Small spontaneous pneumothorax will be resolved without a chest tube.
  b. To drain the intrapleural space: tube placed lateral and inferior (usually at fifth or sixth ICS at midaxillary line)
    1) Hemothorax (i.e., blood in the pleural space): chest tube is indicated if greater than 500 ml.
    2) Pleural effusion: liquid in the pleural space; may be transudate or exudate
      a) Transudate: occurs if there is a rise in pulmonary venous pressure (e.g., HF) or hypoproteinemia (e.g., malnutrition, cirrhosis); tends to accumulate at the base of the lungs
      b) Exudate: occurs as a result of increased capillary permeability or impaired lymphatic absorption (e.g., involvement of the pleura by inflammation or malignancy); the fluid has a higher specific gravity and protein content than a transudate
    3) Empyema (also called pyothorax): pus in the pleural space
    4) Chylothorax: chyle (i.e., lymph fluid and triglyceride fat) in the pleural space
    5) Hydrothorax: water (e.g., IV fluid) in the pleural space
  c. To reestablish negative pressure in pleural space
2. Mediastinal tubes: to drain air and blood from the mediastinum after cardiac or other mediastinal surgery

Insertion
1. Chest tubes may be inserted in surgery when the thoracic cavity must be invaded during the surgical procedure, in the interventional radiology department, or at the bedside.
2. Informed consent is required.
3. Explanation to patient and family should be given by physician and reinforced by nurse.
4. Chest drainage system is set up before insertion of tube.
5. Local anesthetic is used but pressure is felt.
6. The tube is sutured in place, the insertion site is dressed, and the tube is taped securely to avoid tugging.
7. CXR is obtained to confirm placement.

Chest Drainage System
1. Components
  a. Drainage collection bottle or chamber collects liquid drainage.
  b. Water-seal bottle or chamber provides a one-way valve to allow air to escape but does not allow atmospheric air to go into the pleural space.
  c. Suction control bottle or chamber controls the amount of suction.
2. Systems (Fig. 4.32)
  a. Three-bottle system
    1) The drainage collection bottle is the bottle closest to the patient; this bottle is connected to the water-seal bottle.
    2) The water-seal bottle is filled so that the tube from the chest tube is submerged 2 cm under the water.
    3) The water-seal bottle must have a vent open at the top of the bottle to allow air to escape.
    4) The third bottle is the suction control bottle.
      a) It has one tube to connect it to the water-seal bottle.
      b) Another tube connects it to the suction device (usually wall suction but it may be a free-standing Emerson-type suction device).
      c) The third tube is submerged under water to the prescribed suction amount in water (usually 20 cm H_2O); the other end of this tube is open to air.
      d) Suction is adjusted so that a gentle bubbling occurs in this bottle.
        i) Remember vigorous bubbling just makes it evaporate more quickly so that you must keep refilling it.
        ii) The actual amount of suction is determined by the depth that the tube is submersed minus the water seal.
        iii) Suction is not necessary to remove air and free-flowing fluid; if the pleural air or liquid does not respond to gravity water-seal drainage, suction may be applied.
  b. All-in-one system
    1) More convenient
    2) Only the water-seal and drainage collection chambers may be used, or all three will be used if suction is desired.
    3) In a wet suction control system: adjust the amount of suction by filling the water level in the suction control chamber; adjust wall suction so that gentle bubbling occurs in the suction control chamber.
      a) Again, remember the actual amount of suction is the height of the suction control chamber minus the height of the water-seal chamber
    4) In a dry suction control system: Adjust the amount of suction until the indicator appears.
  c. Portable chest drainage system
    1) Only one chamber to collect chest drainage
    2) Has a dry seal
    3) Usually used as a gravity drain only but may be used with suction; automatically regulated to -20 cm H_2O when connected to wall suction
  d. Heimlich valve (Fig. 4.33)
    1) One-way flutter valve made of rubber tubing encased in a clear, plastic chamber
    2) Used for uncomplicated pneumothorax with little or no liquid drainage
      a) May be connected to a small drainage bag to the valve but usually not used if more than 50 ml of fluid
      b) May be connected to wall suction (but is not usually)
      c) Note fluttering of the valve as air escapes from the pleural space
    3) Advantages: small and lightweight and allows the patient to move around more easily; patient may be discharged with a chest tube attached to a Heimlich valve

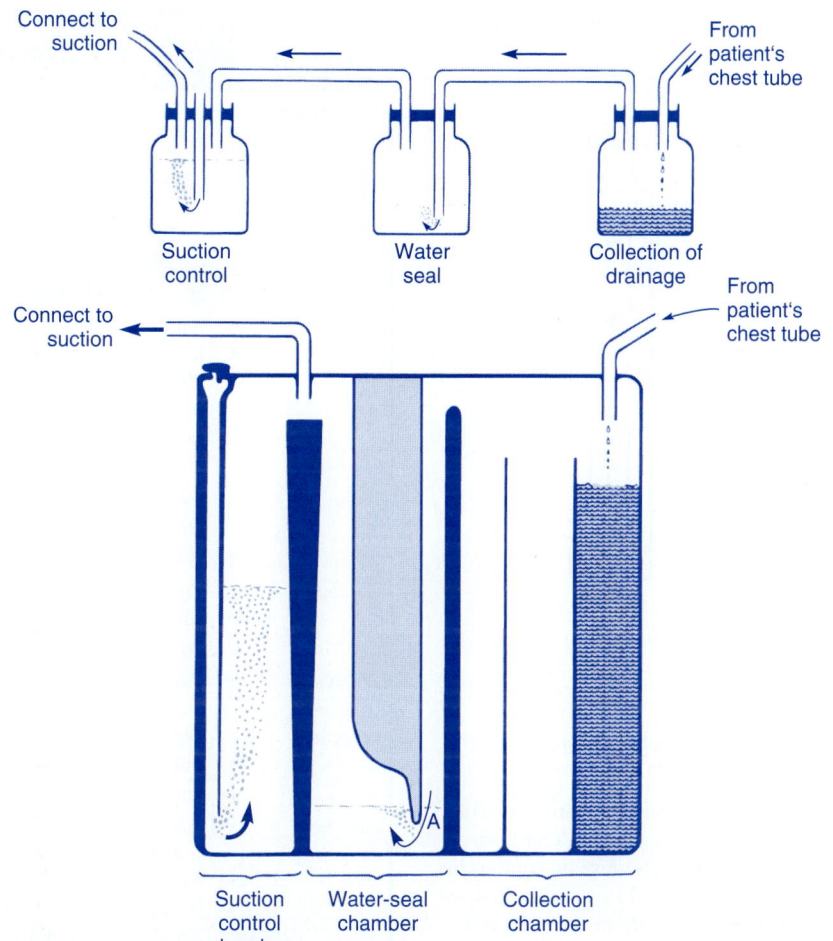

Fig. 4.32 Comparison of a commercially available chest tube drainage system with a three-bottle system. (From Urden, L. D., Stacy, K. M., & Lough, M. E. [2006]. *Thelan's critical care nursing: Diagnosis and management* [5th ed.]. St. Louis: Mosby.)

Assessment
Table 4.23
1. Patient parameters
2. Tube and drainage system

Collaborative Management
1. Control pain.
   a. Administer analgesics and/or local anesthetics as prescribed to relieve pain and encourage deep breathing.
   b. Instruct the patient how to splint chest when coughing; instruct the family how to assist.
2. Maintain airway patency and adequate oxygenation and ventilation.
   a. Position the patient for optimal V/Q matching.
      1) HOB elevated to 30 to 45 degrees
      2) "Good lung down" optimizes ventilation to encourage reexpansion of the surgical lung and optimizes perfusion to the unaffected "good" lung.
         a) Exception: pneumonectomy patients are positioned on their operative lung or back (i.e., no lung down).
   b. Assess the position of the trachea; report immediately any shift from the normal midline.
   c. Encourage deep breathing and use of the incentive spirometer.
      1) Note that air is removed from the pleural space by the positive pressure of expiration and the negative pressure of suction on the chest tube; deep breathing is *very* important in reexpansion of the lung.
   d. Maintain airway clearance.
      1) Focus on sustained inspiration maneuver; this frequently stimulates the patient to cough if coughing is needed.
      2) Suction only if the patient is unable to clear secretions.
   e. Administer oxygen as indicated by ABGs and SpO_2.
   f. Assist with weaning from mechanical ventilation and extubation as soon as possible as PPV increases risk of air leak.
3. Maintain water-seal drainage system and patency of chest tubes.
   a. Assess chest drainage system hourly.
      1) Ensure that connections are spiral taped.
      2) Position tubing to prevent kinks and dependent loops.
      3) Maintain suction level at prescribed level; water may need to be added to the suction control chamber as water evaporates in wet chest drainage systems

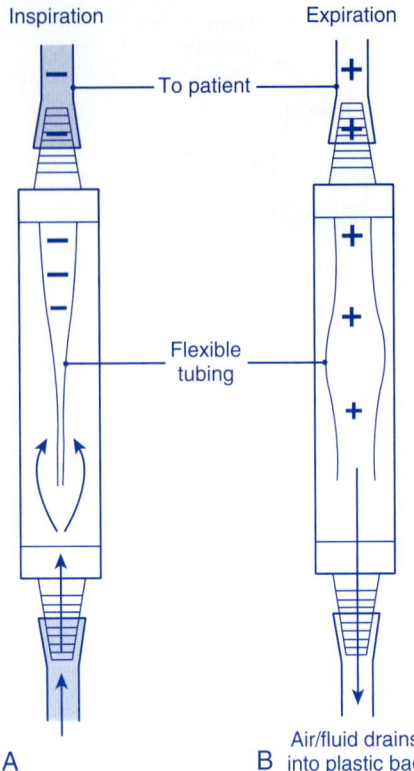

Fig. 4.33 Heimlich one-way valve. **A,** During inspiration, negative pressure collapses the flexible tubing and prevents outside air from entering the pleural space. **B,** During expiration, positive pressure opens the flexible tubing and allows air and fluid to drain into an attached plastic bag. (From Kersten, L. D. [1989]. *Comprehensive respiratory nursing: A decision-making approach.* Philadelphia: Saunders.)

Table 4.23	Assessment Parameters for the Patient with a Chest Tube
Parameter	**Note**
Patient	• Ventilatory effort • Chest discomfort or pain • Anxiety • Level of understanding • Cough • Sputum production
Breathing	• Rate • Regularity • Depth • Breath sounds (disconnection of suction from suction control chamber is required for accurate assessment of breath sounds)
Entry site	• Intactness of dressing • Drainage on dressing • Subcutaneous emphysema around insertion site
Tubing	• Tight, taped connections • Absence of kinks, compressions, or dependent loops
Drainage collection chamber	• Volume (normal 50–100 ml/hr for first few hours after thoracotomy; then 10–20 ml/hr) • Type: color; consistency; odor • Bottle below chest level
Water-seal chamber	• Filled to 2 cm or prescribed amount • Fluctuations with respirations (also referred to as *tidaling*) • Any bubbling • If not on suction: air vent open
Suction control chamber	• Filled to prescribed amount (usually −20 cm H_2O) • Gentle, continuous bubbling
Suction source	• If no control bottle: suction set at ordered level • If control bottle: suction set so gentle, continuous bubbling occurs

4) Assess the water-seal chamber for fluctuation with ventilation (also referred to as *tidaling*); if there is no tidaling, it may be caused of any of the following:
   a) The lung is reexpanded; confirm by assessment of CXR.
   b) The tube is kinked; follow the tube from chest to chest drainage system and position tube to prevent kinking.
   c) The tube is occluded.
      i) The risk of an occluded tube, especially in a patient on mechanical ventilation, is tension pneumothorax, mediastinal shift, and potential tearing of great vessels.
      ii) Although routine milking or stripping is not recommended, it may be attempted to reestablish patency of an occluded tube (and prevent tension pneumothorax).
         (a) Milk the tube first: if unsuccessful in reestablishing fluctuation in the water-seal chamber, strip short sections.
            (i) Milking is hand-over-hand squeezing of the chest tube; stripping is to clamp with the thumb and forefinger of the nondominant hand while pulling the tube between the thumb and forefinger of the dominant hand followed by release of the thumb and forefinger of the nondominant hand.
            (ii) Milking and stripping chest tubes create negative pressure within the pleural space; although it may help to move a clot along, it may also create trauma to the pleura.
         (b) If milking or stripping short sections is unsuccessful in reestablishing fluctuation in the water-seal chamber, notify the provider immediately; a new tube may be required.
5) Assess for air leak and differentiate between expected removal of air from pleural space (occasional bubble) and a break in the chest tube system.
   a) An occasional bubble indicates that the tube is still needed because air is still escaping from the pleural space.

b) Excessive bubbling indicates the need to search for a leak in the system.
 i) Brief clamping with hemostats moving from the chest drainage system to the insertion site can be helpful in identifying the location of the leak.
 ii) Ensure that all connections are connected and spiral taped.
 iii) Assess the insertion site for displacement of the tube so that the proximal eyelet is outside the skin; notify the physician so that the tube can be repositioned.
 iv) Suspect bronchopleural fistula if no external air leak can be identified.
b. Keep the chest drainage system lower than the patient's chest.
c. Avoid intentionally occluding (e.g., clamping) the tube.
 1) Clamp the tube only if one of the following occurs:
  a) The chest drainage system must be lifted above the level of the chest (e.g., putting patient in helicopter for transport) so that chest drainage does not drain back into the pleural space; clamp as briefly as possible.
   i) NOTE: Heimlich valves or portable chest drainage systems (gravity drainage) are frequently used for transports.
  b) If the drainage collection is full (e.g., large pleural effusions), have the new chest drainage system ready, clamp as briefly as possible while connecting the chest tube to the new chest drainage system.
  c) If specifically instructed to by the physician before chest tube removal
   i) This is done to see if the patient is likely to tolerate not having the chest tube.
   ii) Monitor closely for clinical indications of tension pneumothorax.
 2) If there has been a significant air leak and the chest drainage system breaks, submerse the tube about 2 cm into a bottle of sterile water or sterile saline; if a bottle of sterile water or saline is not available, put tap water into a clean Styrofoam cup and submerse the tube about 2 cm into the cup.
  a) NOTE: The patient is better off with an open pneumothorax than a tension pneumothorax.
 3) If there has been a significant air leak and the tube accidentally comes out of the chest: apply a dressing to the chest with your hand or tape it on three sides (i.e., as you would for a sucking chest wound) and notify the provider immediately.
4. Assist with removal of chest tube: usually removed when there has been no air leak from anterior tube or less than 100 ml/24 hr for posterior tube.
 a. Consider clamping chest tube before removal as requested; if done, ensure there is no air leak evident in the water seal (i.e., bubbling) before clamping the tube.
 b. Administer analgesics before chest tube removal; music may also be helpful.
  1) Recommended analgesics include the following:
   a) Ketorolac 30 mg IV 60 minutes before
   b) Morphine 4 mg IV 20 minutes before
 c. Instruct the patient to hold his or her breath when requested.
  1) There is no difference in the rate of post chest tube removal pneumothoraces using either end-inspiration or end-expiration
 d. Apply occlusive dressing after the physician removes the tube at the end of expiration.
 e. Monitor the patient for clinical indications of recurrent pneumothorax: dyspnea, chest pain, asymmetrical chest excursion, diminished breath sounds.
 f. Obtain CXR for confirmation of reexpansion.

Thoracic Surgery and Procedures

1. Bilobectomy: surgical removal of two lobes of the right lung, which may offer the most successful option for cure or effective pain control for lung cancer.
2. Bronchoplastic reconstruction (sleeve resection): removal of a mass that involves or protrudes into the airway; a section of the airway and lung is removed, and then reanastomosis of the airway proximal and distal to the resected area is performed.
3. Bronchoscopy: use of a flexible scope inserted from the mouth into the airways or lung to diagnose and treat abnormalities, including removal of masses or management of collapsed airways.
4. Bullectomy: removal of cysts or bullae in lung; may be performed with laser to avoid thoracotomy
5. Chest trauma surgery: repair of penetrating or nonpenetrating trauma; drainage of pleural cavity and control of hemorrhage
6. Closed thoracostomy: insertion of chest tube through intercostal space into pleural space; tube is connected to chest drainage system
7. Decortication of lung: removal of fibrinous membrane covering visceral and parietal pleura; used for recurrent spontaneous pneumothorax
8. Diaphragmatic hernia repair: repositioning of the abdominal contents back into the abdominal cavity and closure of diaphragm with suture or patch
9. Endobronchial ultrasound (EBUS): advanced approach to lymph node and lung nodule biopsy, offering guided access to areas not possible with a mediastinoscopy
10. Endoscopic ultrasound (EUS): technique for obtaining ultrasound images and performing biopsies within the chest, digestive tract, and surrounding tissue or organs to help stage cancer or evaluate masses in the chest
11. Esophagogastrectomy: resection of a part of the esophagus and upper portion of the stomach with end-to-end anastomosis; colon interposition using a portion of the large intestine may be performed as an alternative to end-to-end anastomosis; for cancer of esophagus or corrosive esophagitis
12. Exploratory thoracotomy: opening of the thorax to perform a biopsy or locate bleeding
13. Lobectomy: removal of one or more lobes of the lung.
14. Mediastinoscopy: the surgeon uses a small incision to insert a scope to view the mediastinum, remove and biopsy lymph nodes, evaluate middle chest tumors, or examine the outer structure of the airways.

15. Navigational bronchoscopy: advanced bronchoscopy technique using GPS-like navigation to structures deep within the lungs beyond the capacity of normal bronchoscopy, with access to mediastinal lymph nodes for diagnosis and staging; can help set borders for cyber knife or other radiosurgery
16. Open thoracostomy: insertion of chest tube during rib resection; usually used in empyema when pleural space is fixed
17. Pericardial window: procedure done to drain fluid within the mediastinum that has accumulated around the heart; sometimes, causing compression, which restricts CO
18. Pleurodesis: process of fusing the two layers of the pleura through the use of agents (e.g., doxycycline, monocycline, sterile talc), which cause a fibrotic reaction to prevent pleural fluid formation; used for recurrent malignant pleural effusion
19. Pneumonectomy: removal of an entire lung with or without mediastinal lymph node resection; indicated when tumor is centrally located at hilus or bronchus
20. Reduction pneumoplasty (lung volume reduction surgery): resection of hyperinflated areas of lung to allow more normal function of diaphragm and expansion of more normal areas of the lung
21. Removal of mediastinal masses: removal of cysts, tumors, abscesses from mediastinum
22. Robot-assisted or robotic surgery: state-of-the-art technology used to provide enhanced three-dimensional views of the surgical site and increase accuracy and minimize potential damage to the operative site.
23. Segmental resection: removal of segment(s) of a lobe
24. Segmentectomy: removal of segment(s) of a lobe contains cancer while preserving more of the surrounding healthy tissues.
25. Thoracoplasty: surgical collapse of a portion of chest wall by multiple rib resections to decrease volume in the hemithorax; may be used after pulmonary resection if lung cannot reexpand to fill thoracic space or after pneumonectomy: reduces the size of the thoracic cavity on the operative side and decreases the chance of mediastinal shift toward that side
26. Thoracotomy: opening into the thorax or pleural cavity
27. Thymectomy: removal of the thymus; frequently performed for myasthenia gravis
28. Tracheal resection: resection of a portion of the trachea with end-to-end anastomosis; removal of stenotic area of trachea or tumor
29. Tracheostomy: surgically created opening in the neck or trachea through which a hollow plastic tube is inserted to maintain a patent airway.
30. Video-assisted thoracoscopic surgery (VATS): a commonly used minimally invasive technique to avoid a thoracotomy incision
31. Wedge resection: removal of a small peripheral section of the lung without regard to segments

Collaborative Management

1. Maintain airway patency and adequate oxygenation and ventilation.
    a. Position the patient for optimal V/Q matching.
        1) HOB elevated to 30 to 45 degrees
        2) "Good lung down" optimizes ventilation to encourage reexpansion of the surgical lung and optimizes perfusion to the unaffected "good" lung.
            a) Exception: pneumonectomy patients are positioned on their operative lung or back; remember "no lung down."
        3) Frequent turning
        4) Early ambulation
    b. Encourage deep breathing and use of the incentive spirometer.
        1) Note that air is removed from the pleural space by the positive pressure of expiration and the negative pressure of suction on the chest tube; deep breathing is *very* important in reexpansion of the lung.
    c. Maintain airway clearance.
        1) Encourage sustained inspiration through deep breathing and incentive spirometry.
            a) Coughing will occur if needed, but routine coughing is not indicated because of the following:
                i) Coughing is forceful expiration that may actually increase the risk of atelectasis.
                ii) Coughing causes pain and may cause splinting and decrease in chest excursion and increase the risk of atelectasis.
        2) Suction only if the patient is unable to clear secretions by coughing.
            a) Use caution when suctioning the patient because leakage from the bronchial stump may occur (especially with pneumonectomy patients).
    d. Assess the position of the trachea.
        1) Report immediately any shift from the normal midline.
        2) If new tracheostomy is in place, ensure the device is well secured and not at risk from being dislodged.
    e. Administer bronchodilators as prescribed.
    f. Prevent gastric distention; gastric suction may be required.
    g. Administer oxygen as indicated by ABGs and SpO_2.
    h. Assist with liberation from mechanical ventilation and extubation as soon as possible
        1) PPV increases risk of air leak.
        2) Ventilator-associated events, including pneumonia, are less likely with shorter duration of intubation and mechanical ventilation.
2. Control pain.
    a. Administer analgesics and/or local anesthetics as prescribed to relieve pain and encourage deep breathing.
        1) IV analgesia: by regularly scheduled IV injection or by patient-controlled analgesia (PCA)
        2) Interpleural analgesia: local anesthetic (e.g., bupivacaine) injected into pleural space during surgery; may use chest tube with injection port for periodic lidocaine
        3) Epidural analgesia: opiate and/or local anesthetic injected into epidural space; basal rate and PCA
        4) NSAID (e.g., ketorolac) to augment the pain relief of narcotics
    b. Instruct the patient how to splint chest when coughing; instruct the family how to assist.

3. Maintain water-seal drainage system and patency of chest tubes (see Chest Tubes).
    a. Monitor drainage.
        1) Should progress from bloody to serosanguineous to serous over 2 to 3 days
        2) Expected drainage is 100 to 300 ml for the first 2 hours and then less than 50 ml/hr for the next several hours with negligible drainage within 2 days.
    b. Assess for air leak and differentiate expected removal of air from pleural space (occasional bubble) from a break in the chest tube system.
4. Monitor for common complications.
    a. Hemorrhage or shock
        1) Replace blood and fluid volume as prescribed; thoracic surgery patients generally receive less fluid than nonthoracic surgery patients in early postoperative period to prevent ARDS and pulmonary edema.
        2) Monitor for clinical indications of hypoperfusion (Table 2.2).
    b. Infection
        1) Use sterile technique while dressing the insertion site, setting up the chest drainage system, and replacing the system.
        2) Monitor for fever, purulent drainage, leukocytosis, and other clinical indications of infection.
        3) Assess the incision and the chest tube insertion site for redness, induration, and drainage; culture drainage if purulent.
        4) Monitor sputum and chest drainage for signs of infection; culture as necessary.
        5) Administer antibiotics as prescribed.
    c. Tension pneumothorax
        1) Maintain patency of the chest tube and functioning of chest drainage system.
        2) Avoid clamping the chest tube.
        3) Monitor for clinical indications of tension pneumothorax: dyspnea; chest pain; tracheal shift away from affected side; hyperresonance to percussion; decreased breath sounds on affected side
    d. Dysrhythmias: especially atrial dysrhythmias
        1) Most likely in patients undergoing more complex thoracic surgery, such as pneumonectomy
        2) Atrial fibrillation is most likely and usually resolves spontaneously
        3) Prophylactic antidysrhythmics may be initiated preoperatively
    e. Pulmonary edema: related to capillary leak and pulmonary hypertension
        1) Use caution with fluid administration.
        2) Hemodynamic monitoring may be necessary.
    f. ARDS
        1) Devastating after pneumonectomy
        2) Monitor for changes in ventilatory effort, SpO_2.
    g. PE
        1) Have patient sit on edge of bed the evening of surgery; assess activity tolerance and assist patient out of bed and into chair as soon as awake if tolerated.
        2) Ambulate as soon as possible until contraindicated by hemodynamic instability.
    h. Bronchopleural fistula: usually related to empyema
        1) Very small V_Ts used with mechanical ventilation (e.g., high-frequency jet ventilation)
    i. Empyema: treat infection with drainage and antimicrobials.
    j. Frozen shoulder: impairment in shoulder mobility
        1) Encourage range of motion to shoulder on operative side.
        2) Administer analgesics to allow movement.
        3) Encourage use of arm for self-care activities.

Acute Respiratory Failure
Definitions
1. Acute respiratory failure: failure of the respiratory system to provide for the exchange of oxygen and CO_2 between the environment and tissues in quantities sufficient to sustain life
    a. Hypoxemic respiratory failure (type I): low PaO_2 (i.e., <60 mm Hg) with normal or low $PaCO_2$
    b. Hypercapnic respiratory failure (type II): high $PaCO_2$ (> 50 mm Hg) with low PaO_2
2. COPD with acute exacerbation: acute process in a patient with a chronic condition; usually caused by respiratory infection
    a. COPD, also known as *chronic obstructive lung disease (COLD):* a disease state characterized by the presence of airflow obstruction caused by chronic bronchitis or emphysema; the airflow obstruction is progressive, may be accompanied by airway hyperactivity, and may be partially reversible (American Thoracic Society, 2007)
        1) Chronic bronchitis: defined clinically by excessive mucus secretion in the bronchi
        2) Emphysema: defined pathophysiologically by enlargement of the air spaces distal to the terminal bronchioles with destruction of alveolar walls
        3) Many of these patients have some degree of asthma.
    b. Acute exacerbation of COPD: worsening dyspnea, increase in sputum volume, and increase in sputum purulence

Etiology
1. Type I (hypoxemic) respiratory failure
    a. Pneumonia
    b. Pulmonary edema
    c. Pulmonary fibrosis
    d. Pleural effusion
    e. Pneumothorax
    f. Asthma
    g. Atelectasis
    h. Aspiration pneumonitis
    i. ARDS: early and caused by pulmonary edema; PAOP is normal
    j. HF: pulmonary edema with high PAOP
    k. Smoke inhalation
    l. PE
    m. Kyphoscoliosis
    n. Fat embolism
    o. Anemia

2. Type II (hypercapnic) respiratory failure (may also be called *acute ventilatory failure*)
   a. COPD with acute exacerbation
   b. Status asthmaticus
   c. CNS depressant drugs
   d. Anesthesia
   e. Neuromuscular blocking drugs
      1) Muscle paralytics
      2) Aminoglycosides
      3) Organophosphate poisoning
   f. Head trauma
   g. Poliomyelitis
   h. Amyotrophic lateral sclerosis
   i. Spinal cord injury
   j. Guillain-Barré syndrome
   k. Myasthenia gravis
   l. Multiple sclerosis
   m. Muscular dystrophy
   n. Morbid obesity
   o. Chest trauma
   p. Surgery: especially thoracic, abdominal, flank incision
   q. Sleep apnea
   r. Tracheal obstruction
   s. Epiglottitis
   t. Cystic fibrosis
   u. Near drowning

Pathophysiology (Table 4.24)
1. Hypoventilation
2. V/Q mismatching
3. Shunting
4. Diffusion defects

Clinical Presentation
1. Subjective
   a. History of precipitating factor
   b. Clinical indications of respiratory distress (Box 4.2)
   c. Clinical indications of hypoxia (Box 4.3)
   d. Clinical indications of hypercapnia (Box 4.4)
2. Objective
   a. Clinical indications of respiratory distress (Box 4.2)
   b. Hypoxemia: decrease in SpO_2, SaO_2, PaO_2
   c. Clinical indications of hypoxia (Box 4.3)
   d. Clinical indications of hypercapnia (Box 4.4)
3. Diagnostic studies
   a. ABG changes
      1) PaO_2 less than 50 to 60 mm Hg
      2) $PaCO_2$ greater than 50 mm Hg with a pH of less than 7.3
   b. CXR: may identify cause

Collaborative Management
1. Treat the cause.
2. Maintain patient airway and optimal ventilation.
   a. Position the patient for optimal ventilation.
      1) HOB to 30 to 45 degrees
      2) Overbed table for patient to lean on
      3) "Good lung down" if unilateral lung condition exists
      4) CLRT especially if P/F ratio is less than 250 mm Hg
      5) Prone position, especially in ARDS
   b. Maintain adequate hydration: usually 2 to 3 l/24 hr unless contraindicated by cardiac or renal disease.
      1) Oral fluids
      2) IV fluids
   c. Provide bronchial hygiene and chest physiotherapy as indicated.
      1) Inspiratory maneuvers
         a) Examples include deep breathing, incentive spirometry, and flutter valve.
         b) These methods encourage reexpansion of alveoli and generate cough if needed.
      2) Analgesics in doses adequate to allow patient to deep breathe and cough as indicated
      3) Suctioning if the patient is unable to clear airways by coughing
      4) Ambulation
      5) PD, percussion, and vibration may be necessary.
      6) Bronchoscopy may be necessary if airway clearance techniques are inadequate.
      7) Noninvasive positive-pressure ventilation (NiPPV) may be used to avert intubation.
         a) May be either CPAP or bi-PAP mode
         b) If the patient requires nocturnal CPAP or bi-PAP, the family should be asked to bring in the equipment.
      8) Intubation and mechanical ventilation may be necessary if $PaCO_2$ continues to rise and respiratory acidosis develops.
         a) The goal of mechanical ventilation is to normalize the pH, not necessarily the $PaCO_2$.
         b) It is not appropriate to normalize the $PaCO_2$ in patients with COPD and chronic hypercapnia (this causes metabolic alkalosis, eventual excretion of prolonged duration of mechanical ventilation).
   d. Administer appropriate drug therapy.
      1) Bronchodilators may be indicated.
         a) Action: smooth muscle relaxation and bronchodilation
         b) Indications
            i) Asthma (i.e., reactive airway disease)
            ii) Acute bronchospasm related to anaphylaxis
            iii) Pulmonary hypertension (specifically xanthines)
         c) Types of bronchodilators and specific actions (Table 4.25)
            i) Sympathomimetics (β-adrenergic agents) (e.g., epinephrine, isoproterenol [Isuprel], albuterol, isoetharine, metaproterenol, terbutaline sulfate, salmeterol)
               (a) $β_2$-Adrenergic agonists: these agents are preferred over nonrespiratory-selective β stimulants such as epinephrine and isoproterenol because they cause fewer cardiovascular side effects
               (b) These respiratory selective agents include albuterol, isoetharine, metaproterenol, terbutaline sulfate, salmeterol, and levalbuterol

Table 4.24	Mechanisms of Acute Respiratory Failure			
Mechanism	Pathophysiology	Etiology	Diagnosis	Treatment

Hypoventilation	Hypoventilation causes CO_2 retention and hypoxemia	Damage to or depression of the neurologic control of ventilation:
		• Head injury
		• Cerebral thrombosis or hemorrhage
		• CNS depressant drugs
		• Oxygen-induced hypoventilation
		Neuromuscular defects in the ventilatory mechanism:
		• Myasthenia gravis
		• Multiple sclerosis
		• Muscular dystrophy
		• Guillain-Barré syndrome
		• Poliomyelitis
		• Spinal cord injuries
		• Botulism
		• Tetanus
		• Neuromuscular blocking drugs
		Obstructive lung conditions
		• Asthma
		• Chronic bronchitis
		• Emphysema
		• Airway obstruction
		• Cystic fibrosis
		Restrictive lung conditions
		• Kyphoscoliosis
		• Obesity hypoventilation syndrome
		• Recent thoracic, abdominal, or flank incision
		• Lung cancer
		• Flail chest
		• Pleural effusion
		• Pneumothorax
			• Physical examination
			  • Neurologic status may be altered
			  • Abnormal chest wall motion
			  • Abnormal breath sounds
			  • Clinical indications of hypoxemia, hypercapnia
			• ABGs: hypoxemia with increased $PaCO_2$ and normal A:a gradient
			• May have abnormal chest radiography, PFT results
				• Improve oxygenation by increasing alveolar ventilation (e.g., positioning, bronchial hygiene, drug therapy)
				• Specific therapy is dependent on the specific etiology

V/Q mismatching	Low V/Q units, with perfusion in excess of ventilation, result in hypoxemia because the blood traversing these alveolar units is not fully oxygenated
	High V/Q units, with ventilation in excess of perfusion, result in ventilated alveolar units which are not perfused because of obstruction or low oxyhemoglobin
		Regional ventilation abnormalities
		• Asthma
		• Chronic bronchitis
		• Emphysema
		• Atelectasis
		• Pneumonia
		• Bronchospasm
		• Mucus plugs
		• Foreign bodies
		• Tumor
		Regional perfusion abnormalities
		• Pulmonary embolus
		• Decreased cardiac output/index
		• Excessive PEEP: anemia
			• Physical examination
			  • Abnormal chest wall motion
			  • Abnormal breath sounds
			  • Clinical indications of hypoxemia
			• ABGs: hypoxemia with a widened A:a gradient; $PaCO_2$ dependent on ventilation status
			• Abnormal chest radiography, PFTs, and/or V/Q scan
				• Oxygen
				• Specific therapy dependent on the specific etiology

Continued

Table 4.24 Mechanisms of Acute Respiratory Failure—cont'd

Mechanism	Pathophysiology	Etiology	Diagnosis	Treatment

Shunt	Blood transverses from the right heart to the left heart without being oxygenated: anatomical shunt is when the blood bypasses the alveolar-capillary unit, and physiologic shunt is when the blood goes through the alveolar-capillary unit, but it is nonfunctional	Anatomic shunts
		• Normal anatomic shunts: bronchial, pleural, thebesian veins
		• Intrapulmonary shunts: pulmonary A-V fistula
		• Intracardiac shunts: tetralogy of Fallot
		• Other pathologic shunts (e.g., shunts associated with neoplasms)
		Physiologic shunts
		• Alveolar collapse
		  • Atelectasis
		  • Pneumothorax
		  • Hemothorax
		  • Pleural effusion
		• Alveoli filled with a fluid or foreign material
		  • Cardiogenic pulmonary edema
		  • Noncardiogenic pulmonary edema
		  • Pneumonias
			• Physical examination
			  • Abnormal breath sounds
			  • Clinical indications of hypoxemia
			• ABGs: hypoxemia with a normal or decreased $PaCO_2$
			  • Widened A:a gradient
			  • Shunt >6%
			• May have abnormal chest radiography, PFT results
				• Oxygen administration has little or no effect
				• Specific therapy dependent upon the specific etiology
				• PEEP is frequently used for physiologic shunt

Diffusion abnormalities	Increased diffusion pathway: diffusion between alveolar oxygen and pulmonary capillary blood is impaired; blood exiting the gas exchange unit is hypoxemic
	
	Decreased diffusion area: decrease in alveolar-capillary membrane surface area available for diffusion and/or loss of pulmonary capillary bed
		Increased diffusion pathway
		• Accumulation of fluid
		• Pulmonary edema: cardiogenic or noncardiogenic
		• Accumulation of collagen in the pulmonary interstitium
		• Pulmonary fibrosis
		• Sarcoidosis
		• Collagen-vascular disease
		Decreased diffusion area
		• Pulmonary resection (e.g., lobectomy, pneumonectomy)
		• Destructive lung diseases
		  • Emphysema
		  • Tumor
		  • Obliterative pulmonary vascular diseases
			• History and physical examination findings are compatible with the diagnosis
			• ABGs: hypoxemia with normal or low $PaCO_2$
			  • Widened A:a gradient
			  • Further decrease in PaO_2 with exercise
			• PFTs: decreased diffusing capacity for CO
			• Chest radiography may show cause
				• Oxygen
				• Home oxygen therapy is frequently indicated

ABG, Arterial blood gas; *CNS,* central nervous system; $PaCO_2$, Partial pressure of carbon dioxide in arterial blood; *PEEP,* positive end-expiratory pressure; *PFT,* pulmonary function test; *V/Q,* ventilation/perfusion.

      ii) Anticholinergics (e.g., ipratropium)
        (a) Combivent is a combination of albuterol and ipratropium given by inhalation.
      iii) Methylxanthines (e.g., aminophylline, oxtriphylline, theophylline)
      iv) Magnesium sulfate
  2) Corticosteroids (e.g., betamethasone)
  3) Expectorants (e.g., guaifenesin, potassium iodide [SSKI]) may be used, but hydration is most important.
  4) Mucolytics (e.g., acetylcysteine) may be used to decrease the tenacity of the mucus; frequently causes bronchospasm so given with a bronchodilator
  5) Sedatives: generally avoided unless patient is very agitated and hypoxemia has been ruled out or requires mechanical ventilation
  6) Antitussives: avoid use of antitussives unless nonproductive cough is causing patient fatigue or discomfort unresolved with analgesia.
3. Optimize oxygen delivery and decrease oxygen consumption.
  a. Administer oxygen as indicated for hypoxemia.
    1) Nasal cannula or mask
    2) Flow rate or oxygen concentration to keep SpO_2 approximately 94% unless contraindicated
      a) In patients with chronic hypercapnia, adjust flow rate or oxygen concentration to keep SpO_2 approximately 90%.

Table 4.25 Bronchodilators

Drug	Administration	Adverse Effects	Nursing Implications
Short-Acting β₂-Adrenergic Agents*			
Albuterol	• PO: 2–4 mg every 6–8 hours • Handheld inhaler: 1–2 inhalations every 4.6 hours • Nebulizer: 0.5 ml (2.5 mg) in 3–5 ml of normal saline over 10–15 minutes every 6 hours	• Tachycardia • Palpitations • Nausea, vomiting • Anxiety • Tremor • Headache	• Monitor HR, BP, breath sounds • Note contraindications: known hypersensitivity, glaucoma, tachydysrhythmias; do not give with MAO inhibitors • Use cautiously in older adults and patients with diabetes mellitus, hypertension, hyperthyroidism, cardiac disease, seizure disorder, prostatic hypertrophy • Do not administer with β-blockers (they block effect)
Metaproterenol	• PO: 20 mg every 6–8 hours • Handheld inhaler: 2–3 inhalations every 3–4 hours • Nebulizer: 0.2–0.3 ml of undiluted 5% solution or 2.5 ml of a 6% solution every 6–8 hours	Tachycardia • Palpitations • Nausea, vomiting • Anxiety • Tremor • Headache	• Monitor HR, BP, breath sounds • Note contraindications: known hypersensitivity, glaucoma, tachydysrhythmias; do not give with MAO inhibitors • Use cautiously in older adults and patients with diabetes mellitus, hypertension, hyperthyroidism, cardiac disease, seizure disorder, prostatic hypertrophy • Do not administer with β-blockers (they block effect)
Anticholinergic Agents			
Ipratropium	• PO: 20 mg every 6–8 hours • Handheld inhaler: 2–3 inhalations every 3–4 hours • Nebulizer: 0.2–0.3 ml of undiluted 5% solution or 2.5 ml of a 6% solution every 6–8 hours	• Tachycardia • Palpitations • Anxiety • Restlessness • Dizziness • Headache • Cough • Blurred vision • GI distress • Dry mouth	• Monitor HR, BP, ECG, respiratory rate and rhythm, breath sounds, urine output, and fluid status • Note contraindications: known sensitivity, cardiac dysrhythmias • Use cautiously in older adults and patients with acute MI, HF, hypertension
Methylxanthines			

Aminophylline	• PO: 250–500 mg every 6–8 hours
	• IV: loading dose of 5–6 mg/kg (250–500 mg) over 20 minutes followed by infusion
	• IV infusion: mix 500 mg in 250 ml (2 mg/ml) and infuse at 0.1–0.9 mg/kg/hr
	  • HF, liver disease: ~0.1–0.2 mg/kg/hr
	  • COPD: ~0.3 mg/kg/hr
	  • Smokers: ~0.8 mg/kg/hr
	• Therapeutic blood level 10–20 mcg/ml
		• Tachycardia
		• Hypotension
		• Palpitations
		• Anxiety
		• Restlessness
		• Insomnia
		• Dizziness
		• Tremors
		• Headache
		Signs of toxicity
		• Anorexia, nausea, vomiting
		• Ventricular dysrhythmias
		• Agitation, seizures
			• Monitor HR, BP, ECG, respiratory rate and rhythm, breath sounds, urine output, and fluid status
			• Note contraindications: known sensitivity, cardiac dysrhythmias
			• Use cautiously in older adults and patients with acute MI, HF, hypertension, hepatic disease, acute peptic ulcer, hyperthyroidism, diabetes mellitus
			• Administer PO drug with meals to decrease GI adverse effects

Electrolytes			
Magnesium sulfate	• IV infusion: mix 1–2 g in 100 ml and infuse over 1–4 hours • May also be given by inhalation	• Bradycardia • Hypotension • Diaphoresis • Flushing • Hypermagnesemia resulting in respiratory muscle weakness and arrest	• Monitor HR, BP, respiratory rate, ECG, urine output, deep tendon reflexes, mental status • Note contraindications: renal disease • Use cautiously in renal insufficiency, patients on digitalis • Monitor closely for clinical indications of hypermagnesemia: hypotension, AV block, CNS depression, depressed or absent DTR, muscle weakness or paralysis, respiratory arrest • Administer calcium IV as prescribed for hypermagnesemic effects • Have intubation equipment and mechanical ventilator available

*Additional short-acting β₂-adrenergic agents include terbutaline, levalbuterol, pirbuterol, and bitolterol. Long-acting β₂ stimulants include salmeterol and formoterol.

AV, Atrioventricular; *BP*, blood pressure; *CNS*, central nervous system; *COPD*, chronic obstructive pulmonary disease; *DTR*, deep tendon reflex; *ECG*, electrocardiogram; *GI*, gastrointestinal; *HF*, heart failure; *HR*, heart rate; *IV*, intravenous; *MAO*, monoamine oxidase inhibitor; *MI*, myocardial infarction; *PO*, oral;

b. Use PEEP as necessary to maintain adequate SaO_2 and PaO_2.
   c. Ensure rest periods, especially after meals or activities.
   d. Provide a quiet, restful environment.
   e. Treat fever (controversial because pyrogens are helpful in mobilizing the immune system).
      1) Antipyretics (e.g., acetaminophen [Tylenol])
      2) Cooling blankets may be used, but shivering should be avoided because of the effect on oxygen consumption.
   f. Improve delivery of oxygen to the tissues.
      1) Improve SaO_2: oxygen, PEEP as required
      2) Improve CI: fluid administration, inotropes, intraaortic balloon pump, vasoactive agents, etc., as required
      3) Increase Hgb: packed RBCs as required
      4) Use extracorporeal membrane oxygenator as indicated and available: viewed primarily as a rescue therapy when other therapies have failed
4. Treat infection if present.
   a. Administer antimicrobials as indicated: empirically or specific to cultured microorganism
   b. Use pulmonary hygiene techniques.
5. Manage anemia
   a. Transfuse if Hgb is <7 g/dl
   b. Manage sickle cell disease
6. Monitor for or prevent complications
   a. Dysrhythmias
   b. Pulmonary infections: pneumonia
   c. Pulmonary edema: cardiogenic or noncardiogenic
   d. PE
   e. Barotrauma (e.g., pneumothorax)
   f. Pulmonary fibrosis
   g. Oxygen toxicity
   h. Renal failure
   i. Acid–base imbalance
      1) Respiratory acidosis
      2) Respiratory alkalosis occurs in patients with chronic hypercapnia when $PaCO_2$ is normalized rather than the pH because of long-term renal retention of bicarbonate.
   j. Electrolyte imbalance
   k. GI complications: abdominal distention, ileus, ulcer, hemorrhage
   l. Thromboembolism
   m. DIC
   n. Sepsis or septic shock
   o. Psychologic responses: psychosis or depression
7. Provide patient and family instruction.
   a. Smoking cessation
   b. Clinical indications of infection

Acute Respiratory Distress Syndrome

Definitions
1. A syndrome of acute respiratory failure characterized by noncardiac pulmonary edema and manifested by refractory hypoxemia caused by intrapulmonary shunt systemic inflammatory response syndrome (SIRS)
2. ARDS is defined by timing (i.e., within 1 wk of clinical insult or onset of respiratory symptoms), radiographic changes (i.e., bilateral opacities not fully explained by effusions, consolidation, or atelectasis), origin of edema (i.e., not fully explained by cardiac failure or fluid overload), and severity based on the PaO_2/FiO_2 ratio on 5 cm of CPAP.
3. Severity levels
   a. Mild ARDS
      1) Previously referred to as acute lung injury ALI: ALI was used as part of the definition of a continuum of lung inflammation and increased alveolar-capillary permeability characterized by hypoxemia resistant to oxygen therapy
      2) PaO_2/FiO_2 ratio less than 300 mm Hg with PEEP or CPAP 5 cm H_2O or greater
   b. Moderate ARDS: PaO_2/FiO_2 ratio less than 200 mm Hg with PEEP or CPAP 5 cm H_2O or greater
   c. Severe ARDS: PaO_2/FiO_2 ratio less than 100 mm Hg with PEEP or CPAP 5 cm H_2O or greater
4. Synonyms: shock lung, pump lung (postperfusion lung), wet lung, posttraumatic lung, respirator lung, congestive atelectasis, pulmonary fat embolism syndrome, alveolar-capillary leak syndrome, noncardiogenic pulmonary edema

Etiology
Risk increases if more than one occurs simultaneously
1. Direct injury
   a. Chest trauma: pulmonary contusion
   b. Near drowning
   c. Hypervolemia or pulmonary edema
   d. Inhalation of toxic gases and vapors
      1) Smoke
      2) Chemicals
      3) Oxygen toxicity
   e. Pneumonia: viral, bacterial, or fungal
   f. Aspiration pneumonitis
   g. Radiation pneumonitis
   h. PE: particularly fat or amniotic fluid
   i. Radiation
   j. Drugs: bleomycin
2. Indirect injury
   a. Sepsis: most likely cause
   b. Shock or prolonged hypotension
      1) Septic shock
      2) Hypovolemic shock
      3) Cardiogenic shock
      4) Anaphylactic shock
      5) Neurogenic shock
   c. Multisystem trauma, especially multiple fractures
   d. Blood transfusion
   e. Burns
   f. Cardiopulmonary bypass
   g. DIC
   h. Toxemia of pregnancy
   i. Acute pancreatitis
   j. Diabetic coma with ketoacidosis
   k. CNS injury
   l. Drug overdosage: heroin, methadone, barbiturates, ASA, thiazide diuretics
   m. Abdominal trauma

Pathophysiology
Fig. 4.34

Clinical Presentation
1. Phases of ARDS (Table 4.26)
2. Criteria used in ARDS diagnosis
    a. Presence of a predisposing condition
    b. Severe oxygenation defect: hypoxemia is the hallmark of ARDS.
        1) PaO_2 less than 60 mm Hg on FiO_2 greater than 0.5
        2) PaO_2/FiO_2 ratio less than or equal to 300 mm Hg with PEEP or CPAP greater than or equal to 5 cm H_2O (i.e., mild <300; moderate <200; severe <100)
    c. CXR: diffuse bilateral parenchymal infiltrates
    d. Static compliance: significantly less than the normal of 50 to 100 ml/cm H_2O (usually 15–25 ml/cm H_2O)
    e. PAOP: less than 18 mm Hg
    f. No other explanation for the previous findings
3. Table 4.27
4. Hemodynamic parameters: invasive monitoring may be used for the following:
    a. Differentiation of cardiogenic from noncardiogenic
        1) ARDS (noncardiac pulmonary edema) causes elevated PAP with normal PAOP.
        2) Cardiac pulmonary edema causes elevated PAP and PAOP.
    b. Determination of degree of pulmonary hypertension
        1) Pulmonary artery end-diastolic pressure (PAd): greater than 5 mm higher than PAOP
        2) Pulmonary artery mean pressure (Pam) greater than 25 mm Hg
        3) PVR greater than 250 dynes/sec/cm^{-5}
    c. Guide fluid management to avoid overhydration during resuscitation and fluid conservation after resuscitation.
5. Diagnostic studies
    a. May give clues to cause
    b. ABGs (Table 4.26): refractory hypoxemia (hypoxemia despite high concentration of oxygen); PaO_2 of less than 55 mm Hg despite FiO_2 0.5 or greater for 24 hours
    c. Sputum analysis: tracheal protein/plasma protein ratio greater than 0.7 (cardiac pulmonary edema <0.5)
    d. Pulmonary function studies
        1) Lung volumes decreased: V_T; VC
        2) Functional residual capacity decreased
        3) Static and dynamic compliance decreased
    e. CXR
        1) May be normal initially
        2) Bilateral diffuse interstitial and alveolar infiltrates
        3) Ground glass appearance
        4) "White-out" because of massive atelectasis
        5) Heart size is normal (one factor that differentiates ARDS from cardiac pulmonary edema).
    f. Computed tomography (CT) of thorax
        1) Gravity-dependent infiltrates
        2) Lack of homogeneity of infiltrates
    g. Bronchoalveolar lavage (BAL): prevalent polymorphonuclear leukocytes

Collaborative Management
1. Prevent ARDS or detect ARDS as early as possible.
    a. Use standard infection control measures (sepsis is the most common etiology).
    b. Treat precipitating factors (e.g., antimicrobials if infection is present).
    c. Provide nutritional support.
        1) Enteral feeding preferred
            a) Effects of enteral nutritional support significant to ARDS, SIRS, and multiple organ dysfunction syndrome (MODS)
                i) Prevents villous atrophy and increases blood flow to the GI tract
                ii) Retards transmigration (i.e., translocation) of bacteria or lipopolysaccharides, which play a significant role in sepsis and MODS
            b) Orogastric feeding with small-bore feeding tube or percutaneous endoscopic gastroscopy tube is preferred to avoid the complications of large-bore NG tubes, such as sinusitis and epistaxis.
        2) Parenteral nutrition if enteral feeding is contraindicated
            a) Dedicated IV catheter (or lumen of multilumen catheter) for parenteral nutrition
            b) Selective decontamination of the digestive tract may be used in patients who cannot be fed enterally to prevent bacterial translocation from the GI tract.
    d. Monitor patients at high risk for ARDS closely, particularly those with sepsis.
        1) Assess patient for indications of respiratory distress (e.g., tachypnea, use of accessory muscles).
        2) Monitor pulse oximetry for drop in SpO_2.
        3) Monitor static and dynamic compliance in patients on a mechanical ventilator.
2. Maintain airway, oxygenation, and ventilation; the goal is to maintain acceptable oxygenation ($SaO_2 \geq 90\%$) with nontoxic FiO_2 levels (<60%) and acceptable plateau pressures (≤ 30 ml H_2O).
    a. Position the patient for optimal ventilation.
        1) Elevate HOB 30 to 45 degrees.
        2) Turn the patient every 2 hours; kinetic therapy with 60-degree lateral rotation may be used.
        3) Position the patient in prone or semiprone position periodically.
            a) Recommended frequency has not been established, but the patient is likely to be kept prone for 4 to 8 hours with frequent repositioning to reduce pressure injury.
    b. Provide bronchial hygiene and chest physiotherapy as indicated.
        1) Encourage the patient to deep breathe to facilitate cough or suction as indicated.
        2) Chest physiotherapy may be indicated.
    c. Administer oxygen as indicated.
        1) May require high concentrations ($\leq 100\%$) with nonrebreathing mask before intubation and mechanical ventilation; high concentrations may also be necessary for a short period of time during mechanical ventilation

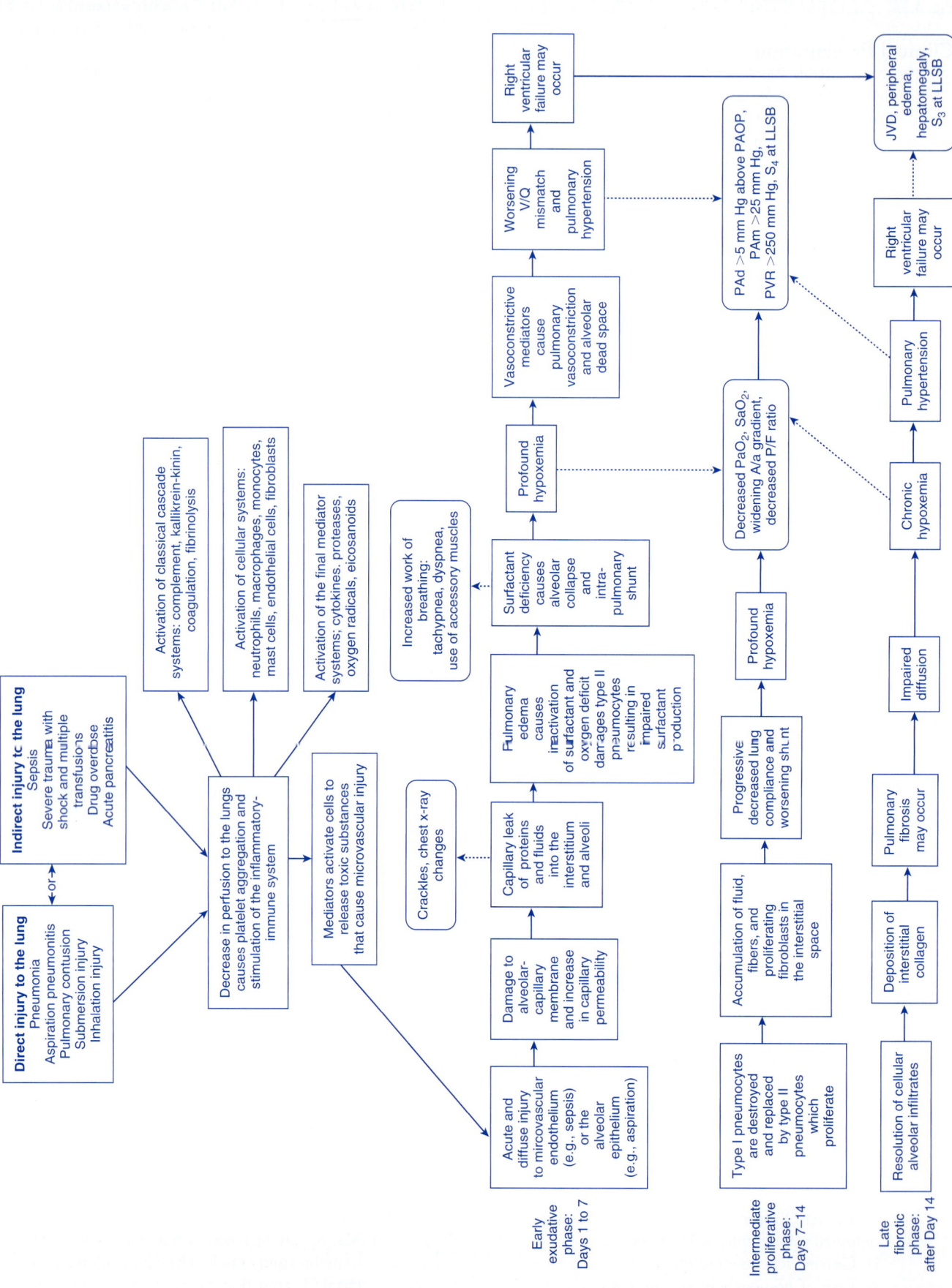

Fig. 4.34 Pathophysiology of acute respiratory distress syndrome. *Dotted lines* connect pathology to clinical presentation.

Table 4.26 Pulmonary Vasodilators

Drug	Administration	Adverse Effects	Nursing Implications
Methylxanthines			
Aminophylline: Table 4.25			
Direct Vasodilators			
Nitric oxide (NO)	• Inhalation along with inspired air delivered by mechanical ventilator: 2–80 ppm; usual dose range is 5–40 ppm; low dosages seem to have best effects	• Methemoglobinemia • Lung injury as a result of nitrogen dioxide (NO_2): NO and oxygen can combine to form nitrogen dioxide, which is injurious to the lung; risk is greatest with high levels of NO and high FiO_2 • Renal dysfunction	• Monitor heart rate, BP, ECG, SpO_2 • Monitor closely for tachycardia, pulmonary hypertension, and hypoxemia with dosage reduction; weaning usually occurs over a 24-hour period
Prostanoids			
Epoprostenol	• IV infusion by central venous catheter: 2–15 ng/kg/min titrated, based on symptoms and adverse effects • Inhalation	• Flushing • Hypotension • Headache • Nausea/vomiting • Diarrhea • Anxiety • Skeletal pain • Jaw pain • Flulike symptoms • Thrombocytopenia • Central venous catheter infections	• Monitor heart rate, BP, and for clinical indications of central venous catheter infection and/or sepsis • Requires refrigeration • Administered by central venous catheter if given IV • Do not stop abruptly; can lead to worsening of pH • Monitor for indications of platelet dysfunction (i.e., petechiae, bleeding)
Iloprost	• PO: 50–300 mcg bid • IV infusion by central venous catheter: 2–4 ng/kg/min • Inhalation: 2.5–5 mcg 6–9 times/day but not more than every 2 hours	• Flushing • Hypotension • Supraventricular tachycardia • Headache • Insomnia • Nausea and vomiting • Flulike symptoms • Cough if by inhalation • Infusion site pain	• Monitor heart rate and BP and for clinical indications of central venous catheter infection and/or sepsis • Administered by central venous catheter if given IV
Treprostinil	• IV or SC infusion: 1.25 ng/kg/min (or 0.625 ng/kg/min if it is not tolerated or the patient has mild to moderate hepatic insufficiency); dose should be increased, based on clinical response in increments of 1.25 ng/kg/min per week for the first 4 weeks of treatment and 2.5 ng/kg/min per week after that. • Inhalation: 3 breaths (18 mcg of treprostinil) per treatment session, qid	• Rash • Flushing • Headache • Nausea • Diarrhea • Jaw pain • Thrombocytopenia • Pain at infusion site • Cough, throat irritation with inhalation	• Monitor heart rate, BP, ECG • Administered IV by central venous catheter; continuous subcutaneous administration is preferred • Monitor for indications of platelet dysfunction (i.e., petechiae, bleeding) • Use cautiously in patients with hepatic insufficiency
Endothelin Receptor Antagonist			
Bosentan	• PO: start at 62.5 mg bid for 4 weeks and then increase to 125 mg bid	• Elevation of liver enzymes, hepatotoxicity • Anemia • Headache • Flushing • Hypotension • Chest pain • Syncope • Respiratory tract infections • Peripheral edema	• Monitor heart rate, BP, ECG, liver function studies • Requires liver function studies monthly and hematocrit every 3 months

Continued

Table 4.26 Pulmonary Vasodilators—cont'd

Ambrisentan	• PO: 5–10 mg/day	• Elevation of liver enzymes • Anemia • Peripheral edema • Headache • Flushing • Hypotension • Syncope	• Monitor heart rate, BP, ECG, liver function studies • Requires liver function studies monthly and hematocrit every 3 months
Phosphodiesterase Type 5 Inhibitors			
Sildenafil	• PO: 20 mg tid	• Headache • Dyspepsia • Flushing • Dyspnea • Epistaxis • Hearing loss	• Monitor heart rate, BP, ECG • Should not be administered with nitrates
Tadalafil	PO: 2.5–40 mg/day	• Headache • Flushing • Hypotension • Myalgias • Nasopharyngitis • Respiratory tract infections • Hearing or vision loss	• Monitor heart rate, BP, ECG • Should not be administered with nitrates

bid, Twice a day; *BP,* blood pressure; *ECG,* electrocardiogram; *FiO₂,* fraction of inspired oxygen; *IV,* intravenous; *PO,* oral; *qid,* four times a day; *SC,* subcutaneous; *SpO₂,* arterial oxygen saturation by pulse oximetry; *tid,* three times a day.

Table 4.27 Asthma: ABG Analysis

Stage	PaO$_2$	PaCO$_2$	pH	Acid–Base Imbalance
I	Normal	Decreased	Increased	Respiratory alkalosis
II	Decreased	Decreased	Increased	Respiratory alkalosis Mild to moderate hypoxemia
III	Very low	Normal	Normal	Significant hypoxemia
IV	Extremely low	Elevated	Decreased	Respiratory acidosis Critical hypoxemia

2) FiO_2 should be maintained as low as possible to prevent oxygen toxicity; positive pressure (i.e., CPAP or PEEP) will increase driving pressure, allowing the use of a lower FiO_2 to maintain an acceptable oxygenation.
   a) Noninvasive ventilation via mask may be used before intubation.
   b) Mechanical ventilation with PEEP; sedation and/or muscle paralysis may be necessary to maintain PEEP
   c) NOTE: These patients are usually very PEEP dependent and will quickly desaturate when PEEP is temporarily discontinued; use closed suction system or PEEP valve on a manual resuscitation bag before and after suctioning.
  d. Ensure adequate ventilation.
    1) Noninvasive positive pressure ventilation (e.g., CPAP, bi-PAP) with face mask before need for intubation as prescribed
    2) Endotracheal intubation: indicated to deliver mechanical ventilation and PEEP when FiO_2 greater than 0.50 is required to maintain acceptable oxygenation or as patient fatigues

3) Mechanical ventilation to maintain adequate ventilation and oxygenation while preventing ventilator-associated lung injury (VALI)
   a) Modes: pressure controlled-inverse ratio ventilation (PC-IRV), pressure-regulated volume-controlled (PRVC), airway airway pressure release ventilation (APRV), or high-frequency ventilation may be used.
   b) V_T: limitation of peak inspiratory pressure and reduction of regional lung overdistention by the use of low tidal volumes with permissive hypercapnia may reduce VALI and improve outcome in severe ARDS.
    i) V_T at 4.8 ml/kg (~6 ml/kg) of ideal body weight (IBW).
     (a) Large V_Ts are avoided because the ARDS lung is like a "baby lung" and large V_Ts have been shown to cause increased alveolar edema and worsening of lung injury.
      (i) Volutrauma results from large V_Ts though it is unclear as to whether the volume or the distending pressures are responsible for the lung injury.

(b) Lung injury occurs as the result of the following:
  (i) Overdistention and shearing of open alveoli
  (ii) Repeated reopening of collapsed alveoli (atelectrauma)
(c) Initially 8 ml/kg predicted body weight is recommended, and then the V_T is reduced at 1 ml/kg approximately every 2 hours until 6 ml/kg.
  (i) Predicted body weight (Appendix C)
c) Rate: 12 to 40 breaths/min to reduce the risk of dynamic hyperinflation and auto-PEEP
d) Flow rates and V_T are adjusted to keep plateau pressure at less than or equal to 30 cm H_2O:
  i) Peak inspiratory flow rate usually 70 to 80 l/min
  ii) Flow taper may be used to lower peak inspiratory flow rates.
e) Permissive hypercapnia
  i) Limitation of the V_T and minute ventilation may permit the accumulation of CO_2.
  ii) Permissive hypercapnia stems from the hypothesis that the adverse effects of alveoli overdistention is more detrimental to patient outcome than the adverse effects of respiratory acidosis
    (a) Overdistention of the alveoli causes the following:
      (i) Ventilator-associated lung injury (i.e., volutrauma and barotrauma)
      (ii) Release of inflammatory cytokines
      (iii) Decrease in surfactant production
  iii) Contraindication: intracranial hypertension
  iv) Treatment of resultant respiratory acidosis
    (a) Bicarbonate may be used if pH is less than 7.2
    (b) $ECCO_2R$: similar to extracorporeal membrane oxygenation (ECMO); used to remove CO_2
    (c) Tracheal gas insufflation: gas flow near the carina to wash CO_2 out of the large airways during expiration
4) CPAP or PEEP
  a) Effects of CPAP or PEEP in patients with ARDS
    i) Decreases surface tension, so alveoli are open at low distending pressures at the end of expiration (i.e., alveolar recruitment and the prevention of alveolar derecruitment)
    ii) Aids in reopening collapsed alveoli to reduce intrapulmonary shunt
    iii) Increases the driving pressure of oxygen to allow achievement of same PaO_2 on a lower FiO_2 or a higher PaO_2 on the same FiO_2; this effect therefore decreases risk of oxygen toxicity
    iv) Prevents shearing forces from reopening and collapsing alveoli (i.e., atelectrauma)
  b) Levels
    i) Minimum level is 5 cm H_2O
    ii) Usual level is 5 to 15 cm H_2O, but higher levels may be needed to maintain SaO_2 with moderate or severe ARDS and PaO_2 with moderate or severe ARDS; titrated upward in increments of 2 cm H_2O until oxygenation ceases to improve and/or CI is decreased despite adequate circulating blood volume
    iii) Oxygenation goal is PaO_2 of 55 to 80 mm Hg or SpO_2 of 88% to 94%.
  c) Adverse effects in the ARDS patient, particularly with high levels of CPAP or PEEP
    i) VILI
    ii) Decreased CO related to decrease in venous return
      (a) Ensure adequate preload.
      (b) Remember that a decrease in CO is more detrimental to tissue oxygenation than is borderline hypoxemia.
e. Administer aerosolized surfactant (e.g., colfosceril or beractant) as prescribed.
  1) Effects
    a) Recognition that surfactant is deficient and dysfunctional in ARDS; therefore, surfactant replacement is intended to decrease surface tension, allow more equitable distribution of V_T among the alveoli to decrease VALI, and aid in the prevention of alveolar collapse along with reinflation of already collapsed alveoli
  2) Administration by aerosolization; direct instillation into the ET being studied
  3) Although an oxygenation benefit has been demonstrated, no survival benefit has been proven in adults.
    a) Instilling surfactant directly into the lungs has shown promise but it is laborious and time consuming.
f. Use partial liquid ventilation with perfluorochemical (PFC) liquids rather than an oxygen-containing gas mixture as prescribed.
  1) Effects: PFCs are noncompressible liquid with a low surface tension and high solubility for oxygen and CO_2, which can be used instead of nitrogen as an inert carrier of O_2 and CO_2.
    a) Allows for effective gas transfer by providing a reservoir for exchange of O_2 and CO_2 with blood in the pulmonary capillaries.

- b) Opens collapsed alveoli by reducing surface tension of surfactant-deficient lung tissue which increases pulmonary end-expiratory volume and improves lung compliance; acts as a liquid PEEP
- c) Accumulates in dependent regions of the lung (because heavier than water), which concentrates their action in areas of the lung most susceptible to VALI
- d) Redistributes pulmonary blood flow to nondependent lung issues, which allows more effective gas exchange through fully aerated alveoli
- e) Reduces lung inflammation by reduction of proinflammatory cytokines
- f) Mobilizes mucus and purulent secretions from the alveoli; they float to the top of the PFC layer and can be easily removed
- g) Provides high efficiency heat exchange in the lungs

2) Method
- a) PFC is instilled via ET tube to replace all or some of the functional residual capacity, and conventional mechanical ventilation is maintained.
- b) Sedation and neuromuscular blockade are required.
- c) Complication: mucus plugging of the airways and ET tube
- d) Although an oxygenation benefit has been demonstrated, no survival benefit has been proven

g. Decrease intraalveolar fluid.
1) Administer volume as indicated by CVP readings: maintain CVP ~4 mm Hg after fluid resuscitation achieved (i.e., MAP of at least 60 mm Hg without vasopressors).
- a) Conservative fluid administration has been shown to improve lung function, shorten duration of mechanical ventilation, and reduce critical care unit stay.
- b) PAC is not routinely required for ARDS but may be required by precipitating event (e.g., trauma, shock).
- c) Overhydration, such as may occur in fluid resuscitation of trauma patients, must be avoided but conservative.
- d) Crystalloids versus colloids debate
  - i) Colloids will leak across the alveolar-capillary membrane as readily as crystalloids in this patient because of damage to the alveolar-capillary membrane.
  - ii) There is no advantage of one over the other in these patients; balanced amounts may be used or crystalloids may be used because they have a cost benefit.

2) Administer diuretics as prescribed.
- a) May be given to prevent further fluid sequestration into the alveoli
- b) May be given along with albumin in patients with hypoproteinemia with fluid retention
- c) Guided by PAOP: maintain PAOP at ~12 mm Hg.
- d) CVP may be used as an alternative to PAOP if PAC is not in use; maintain CVP at 2 to 6 mm Hg.

3) Use CPAP or PEEP to increase intraalveolar pressure and aid in prevention of further fluid sequestration into the alveoli.
4) Administer β_2 agonists as prescribed.
- a) IV albuterol has been shown to decrease alveolar-capillary permeability in patients with ARDS; although the mechanism is unclear, it may stimulate alveolar epithelial repair

h. Maintain CO and tissue oxygenation.
1) Administer volume as required to ensure adequate circulating volume but avoid overhydration, which would contribute to intraalveolar fluid and worsening diffusion defect.
2) Ensure adequate Hgb levels.
- a) Blood if Hgb is less than 7 g/dl but may be necessary at Hgb of 8 to 10 g/dl if there is impaired oxygen delivery as evidenced by SvO_2 or $ScvO_2$ (Napolitano et al., 2009)
  - i) There is a positive correlation between transfusion and ARDS, so blood transfusion should be avoided in patients at risk of ARDS after completion of resuscitation.
- b) Erythropoietin may be used.

3) Administer inotropes as indicated by left ventricular stroke work index (LVSWI) and CI.
4) Use hemodynamic monitoring, including SvO_2, to guide therapy if indicated.
- a) Volume or diuretics
- b) Inotropic therapy
- c) Best PEEP: level of PEEP to achieve SaO_2 of at ~90% but without decreasing the CI

5) Use ECMO when available and indicated.
- a) Form of cardiopulmonary bypass in which the blood is removed from the patient, passed through large membrane lungs, and then placed back into circulation; mechanical ventilation can be maintained without the high levels of FiO_2 and PEEP that may cause VALI
- b) Effects
  - i) Provides oxygenation of blood along with removal of CO_2
  - ii) Allows time for the lungs to heal
  - iii) Prevents possible VALI and oxygen toxicity
- c) May be used as a salvage therapy in patients with life-threatening respiratory failure without multiple organ dysfunction in tertiary centers with capability and experience
- d) Studies have not demonstrated a survival benefit.

6) Consider extracorporeal CO_2 removal ($ECCO_2R$) when available and indicated.
   a) Similar to ECMO and used to correct pH in patients with significant hypercapnia
   b) No survival benefit has been demonstrated.
  i. Decrease oxygen consumption.
   1) Eliminate unnecessary activity.
   2) Provide rest periods after meals and other activities that increase oxygen consumption.
   3) Decrease anxiety: initiate pain, agitation, and delirium guidelines for use of anxiolytics, sedatives, and pain management.
      a) Neuromuscular blockers may be required to reduce oxygen requirements and maintain adequate ventilation
   4) Treat fever using antipyretics (acetaminophen) and cooling blanket.
      a) Debate continues regarding the benefits of fever reduction because the pyrogens may be an essential component of the immune response
      b) Reduction of fever does reduce oxygen requirements and may help reduce the tissue oxygen deficit.
      c) Care must be taken while using cooling blanket to prevent shivering.
3. Treat pulmonary hypertension.
   a. Combine oxygen therapy with CPAP or PEEP to maintain or augment alveolar recruitment and help reduce the hypoxemia, which causes hypoxemic pulmonary vasoconstriction.
   b. Administer pulmonary vasodilators as prescribed (Table 4.26).
      1) Nitric oxide: endogenously synthesized by vascular endothelium and acts as a natural local vasodilator; exogenously administered by inhalation
         a) Nitroglycerin and nitroprusside work by a nitric oxide–activated pathway; however, these drugs given intravenously would dilate all vessels (including vessels to nonventilated alveoli), interfere with hypoxic vasoconstriction, and lead to increased intrapulmonary shunting; systemic hypotension would also likely occur.
         b) Effects of nitric oxide by inhalation
            i) Dilates vessels only to ventilated alveoli
            ii) Reduces pulmonary hypertension
            iii) Acts as a potent bronchodilator
         c) Nitric oxide is likely to have best results when used at an earlier, less severe stage of ALI; effect also augmented by prone position.
         d) Nitric oxide has not decreased mortality rates in moderate or severe ARDS patients in a systematic review of nine clinical trials (Adhikari et al., 2014).
      2) Prostacyclin (epoprostenol): existing evidence cannot support nor refute the use of aerosolized prostacyclin for ARDS (Searcy et al., 2015).
4. Modify mediator release and effect (under continuing investigation).
   a. Consider use of corticosteroids.
      1) Although not effective in preventing the onset of ARDS, they may be helpful during the fibroproliferative phase.
      2) Reduce some proinflammatory cytokines
      3) Methylprednisolone usually used
      4) No consistent improvement in outcomes has been demonstrated with high-dose, short-term therapy.
   b. Administer antioxidants as prescribed.
      1) Toxic oxygen radicals produced by activated neutrophils, macrophages, and endothelial cells play a key role in lung injury.
      2) Action: may shorten the duration of ARDS
      3) Examples: *N*-acetylcysteine (NAC) or procysteine (OTZ)
   c. Administer antiinflammatory agents: anticytokines; antiprostaglandins (e.g., ketorolac, ibuprofen, indomethacin) as prescribed.
5. Provide nutritional support to prevent respiratory muscle atrophy.
   a. Use enteral route if possible.
   b. Administer high-protein and high-calorie diet rich in omega-3 and omega-6.
      1) 1 to 2 g/kg of IBW of protein
         a) Conditionally essential amino acids glutamine and alanine may be particularly helpful in reducing endotoxemia and should be included.
      2) 20 to 25 kcal/kg of IBW of nonprotein calories to prevent exogenous protein and muscle tissue from catabolism to meet nutritional requirements
      3) Nonprotein carbohydrate calories increase CO_2 production; reduced carbohydrate formulas or elemental feedings may be preferable, especially in patients with hypercapnia
   c. Replace multivitamins and minerals: vitamins A, C, E; zinc; and selenium.
6. Monitor for complications.
   a. Secondary infections: nosocomial pneumonia
   b. Sepsis
   c. Shock
   d. MODS
   e. Airway trauma
   f. Dysrhythmias
   g. PE
   h. Pulmonary fibrosis
   i. Pneumothorax
   j. GI hemorrhage
   k. DIC
   l. HF
   m. Acute kidney injury

Pulmonary Arterial Hypertension and Pulmonary Hypertension

Definition
Abnormal elevation of the pressure in the blood vessels of the lungs

Classification and Etiology (Simonneau et al., 2009)

1. Pulmonary arterial hypertension: primary disease of small- to medium-sized arteries in the vascular bed of the lung which causes high pulmonary vascular pressures
2. World Health Organization classification
   a. Group 1: associated with abnormalities in arterioles, small pulmonary artery branches, and idiopathic pulmonary hypertension
   b. Group 2: caused by left heart disease such as cardiomyopathy, diastolic dysfunction, mitral and aortic valve disease
   c. Group 3: associated with lung diseases such as COPD, interstitial lung disease, and obstructive sleep apnea
   d. Group 4: related to chronic thromboembolic disease associated with fat, tumor, parasites, or foreign materials
   e. Group 5: pulmonary hypertension that does not fit the other categories, such as sarcoidosis, histiocytosis X, and compression of lung tissue from many reasons, including tumors

Pathophysiology
Fig. 4.35

Clinical Presentation
1. Subjective
   a. Dyspnea; initially exertional progressing to dyspnea with mild exertion to dyspnea at rest
   b. Fatigue, lethargy
   c. Chest discomfort
   d. Palpitations
   e. Syncope
   f. Cyanosis may be present.
2. Objective
   a. Tachypnea
   b. Use of accessory muscles
   c. Cough; may exhibit hemoptysis
   d. Accentuated P_2: the second component of S_2
   e. May have clinical indications of right ventricular hypertrophy (RVH): right ventricular heave; right-sided S_4
   f. May have clinical indications of RVF: JVD, peripheral edema, hepatomegaly, murmur of tricuspid regurgitation
3. Diagnostic studies
   a. Hemodynamic monitoring
      1) PA diastolic more than 5 mm Hg greater than PAOP
      2) PAP greater than 30/15 mm Hg
      3) PA mean greater than 25 mm Hg at rest or greater than 30 mm Hg with activity with a normal PAOP
      4) PVR more than 250 dynes/sec/cm^{-5}
   b. Serum
      1) Hgb and hematocrit may be elevated; polycythemia is caused by erythropoietin release triggered by hypoxemia.
      2) Liver function study results may be elevated.
      3) ABGs: may be normal at rest but hypoxemia occurs with exertion; eventually hypoxemia at rest
      4) Type B natriuretic peptide level: elevated as HF progresses.
   c. CXR: may show cardiomegaly, dilated central pulmonary vessels
   d. ECG: right atrial enlargement, right ventricular strain and hypertrophy
   e. Echocardiography: used to evaluate heart size, function, and blood flow
   f. V/Q scan: used to evaluate for presence of PE
   g. Cardiac catheterization (gold standard for definitive diagnosis): elevated right heart and pulmonary pressures
   h. Vasodilator testing for pulmonary arterial hypertension
      1) Performed in the cardiac catheterization lab with IV adenosine or epoprostenol or inhaled nitric oxide
      2) An acute response is defined as a decrease in PAm of greater than or equal to 10 mm Hg to a PAm of less than 40 mm Hg.

Collaborative Management
1. Treat cause if possible.
   a. Oxygen for hypoxemia; maintain SaO_2 greater than 90%
   b. Fibrinolytics or pulmonary embolectomy and anticoagulants if caused by PE
   c. Phlebotomy may be performed for patients with significant polycythemia.
   d. Discontinue any causative drug.
2. Decrease pulmonary vascular pressures.
   a. Drugs that affect clotting
      1) Vitamin K antagonists (VKAs), such as warfarin
      2) Direct oral anticoagulants (DOACs) such a apixaban or rivaroxaban
      3) Platelet-aggregation inhibitors, such as aspirin, may be considered
   b. Pulmonary vasodilators
      1) Action: relax the smooth muscle of the pulmonary vascular system
      2) Indications
         a) Pulmonary arterial hypertension
         b) Secondary pulmonary hypertension
            i) Remember that the most common cause of secondary pulmonary hypertension is hypoxemia; oxygen is the first treatment.
            ii) Secondary pulmonary hypertension caused by left ventricular failure requires treatment of HF.
      3) Types of pulmonary vasodilators (Table 4.26)
         a) Methylxanthines (e.g., aminophylline)
         b) Nitric oxide: administered by inhalation so that only vessels to ventilated alveoli are dilated
         c) Prostanoids (e.g., epoprostenol, iloprost, treprostinil)
         d) Endothelin receptor antagonists (e.g., bosentan, ambrisentan)
         e) Phosphodiesterase type 5 inhibitors (e.g., sildenafil, tadalafil)

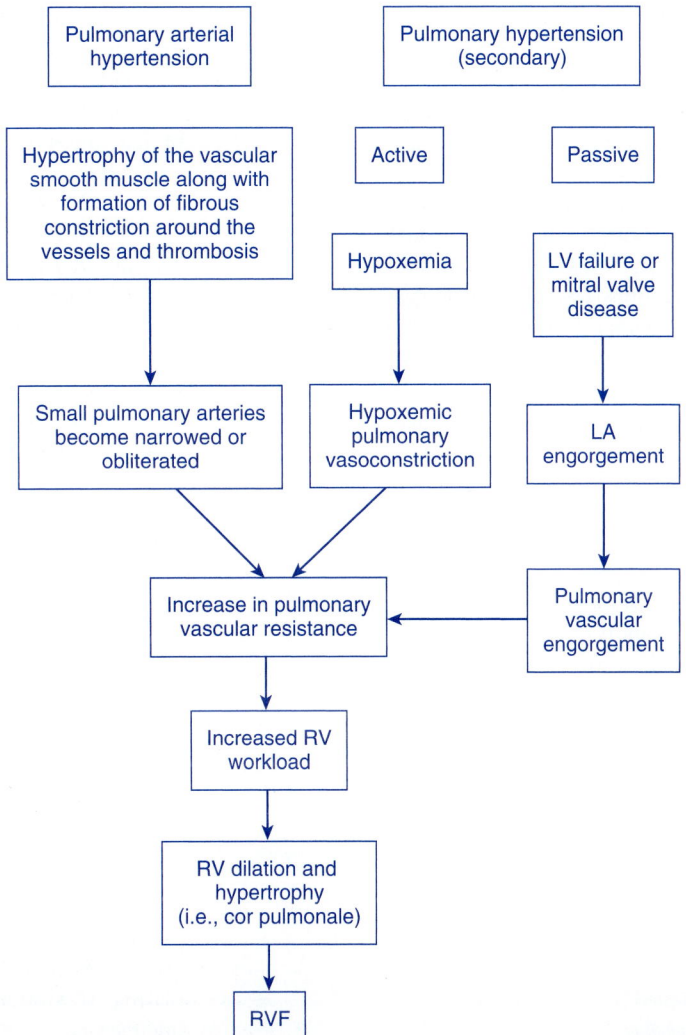

Fig. 4.35 Pathophysiology of pulmonary arterial hypertension and pulmonary hypertension. *LA,* Left atrium; *LV,* left ventricle; *RV,* right ventricle, *RVF, right* ventricular failure

  f) High-dose calcium channel blockers are also used but are effective in only a small percentage of patients.
4) Provide treatment for HF if present.
  a) Diuretics may be required for congestive symptoms.
  b) Digoxin if concurrent LVF is present
  c) Sodium restriction to 2 to 3 g/day
5) Prepare patient for surgery as requested.
  a) Surgery for treatment of cause (e.g., valve repair or replacement)
  b) Balloon dilation atrial septostomy
    i) Palliative treatment for patients with primary PH refractory to vasodilator therapy
    ii) Atrial septal defect is created; right-to-left shunting that occurs improves left ventricular filling and CO, offsetting the desaturation of the blood that bypassed the lung.
  c) Lung transplant or heart–lung transplant
    i) Single- or double-lung transplant is indicated for patients with primary PH who fail to respond to therapy.
    ii) Heart–lung transplantation is indicated for patients with left ventricular disease or congenital structural abnormalities.
6) Provide instruction and counseling regarding lifestyle modification and need for pharmacologic therapy
  a) Oxygen therapy
    i) Usually recommended for continuous use
    ii) Avoidance of high altitude, which would decrease the driving pressure of oxygen and worsen hypoxemia; oxygen should be used when flying
  b) Low (2–3 g) sodium diet
  c) Cessation of nicotine use
  d) Moderate exercise avoiding overexertion
  e) Energy conservation methods
  f) Avoidance of drugs that may accentuate PH, cause thrombogenesis, or interfere with anticoagulant therapy: oral anticoagulants (pregnancy should be avoided so another method of birth control is recommended), decongestants, aspirin and NSAIDs, herbal medications

Pneumonia

Definitions
1. Pneumonia: inflammatory process of the lung parenchyma, including alveolar spaces and interstitial tissue, produced by an infectious agent
2. Community-acquired pneumonia (CAP): infection of the lungs in individuals who have not been recently hospitalized; most commonly caused by *Streptococcus pneumoniae*
3. Health care-associated pneumonia (HCAP) or hospital-acquired pneumonia (HAP): acute infection of the lungs that develops after 48 hours of hospitalization; also referred to as *nosocomial pneumonia*
   a. Assumption of a more virulent organism; these organisms are often resistant to multiple antibiotics
   b. VAP: subtype of HCAP associated with intubation and mechanical ventilation; high concentrations may also be necessary for a short period of time during mechanical ventilation
      1) Early onset: develops within 4 days of intubation and mechanical ventilation
      2) Late onset: develops 5 or more days after intubation and mechanical ventilation

Etiology
1. Causative agents
   a. Bacteria
      1) CAP
         a) *S. pneumoniae*: most common
         b) *Haemophilus influenzae*
         c) *Staphylococcus aureus*
         d) *Enterobacter* spp.
         e) *Streptococcus pyogenes*
         f) *Chlamydia pneumoniae*
         g) *Legionella pneumophila*
         h) *Mycoplasma pneumoniae*
         i) *Moraxella catarrhalis*
         j) *Bacteroides fragilis*
         k) *Mycobacterium tuberculosis*
      2) Hospital-acquired pneumonia (HAP)
         a) *Pseudomonas* spp.
         b) *Staphylococcus aureus*
         c) *Enterobacter* spp.
         d) *Klebsiella pneumoniae*
         e) *Escherichia coli*
         f) *Haemophilus influenzae*
         g) *Serratia marcescens*
         h) *Streptococcus* spp./
         i) *Proteus mirabilis*
         j) *Acinetobacter* spp.
         k) *Legionella pneumophila*
      3) Aspiration pneumonia: occurs when oral flora are aspirated into the lower respiratory tract because of dysphagia or impaired cough mechanism. (see Aspiration Lung Disorder.)
      4) VAP
         a) Early onset
            i) *S. aureus*
            ii) *S. pneumoniae*
            iii) *H. influenzae*
            iv) *M. catarrhalis*
            v) *Proteus* spp.
            vi) *Serratia marcescens*
            vii) *Klebsiella pneumoniae*
            viii) *E. coli*
         b) Late onset: more likely to be antibiotic resistant
            i) Methicillin-resistant *S. aureus*
            ii) *P. aeruginosa*
            iii) *K. pneumoniae*
            iv) *Acinetobacter* spp.
            v) *Enterobacter* spp.
      5) Ventilator-associated events (VAEs)
         a) Term emerged in 2013 from National Healthcare Safety Network (NHSN) to more fully define conditions associated with ventilators that were not agreed upon to be VAP
         b) Includes
            i. Ventilator-associated condition (VAC)
            ii. Infection-related ventilator-associated complication (IVAC)
            iii. Possible or probable VAP
   b. Viruses
      1) Adenovirus
      2) Hantavirus
      3) Influenza types A and B
      4) Respiratory syncytium virus (RSV)
   c. Fungi
      1) *Histoplasma capsulatum*
      2) *Coccidioides immitis*
      3) *Candida* spp.
      4) *Aspergillus* spp.
   d. Parasites (e.g., *Pneumocystis carinii*)
   e. Mycoplasma: *M. pneumoniae*
2. Predisposing factors
   a. Patient related
      1) Advanced age
      2) History of smoking
      3) Periodontal disease
      4) Altered level of consciousness
      5) Chronic illness
         a) COPD
         b) Diabetes mellitus
         c) Cardiovascular disease
         d) Malignancy
      6) Severe acute illness
         a) Shock
         b) Head injury
         c) Chest trauma
      7) Malnutrition: alcoholism, malignancy, eating disorder, poverty
      8) Immunocompromise
         a) Patients with neutropenia resulting from acute leukemia or cytotoxic agents usually have gram-negative bacilli as a source.
         b) Severely immunocompromised patient may also develop pneumonia caused by
            i) Gram-negative aerobic bacteria
               (a) *H. influenzae*
               (b) *K. pneumoniae*
               (c) *L. pneumophila*
               (d) *E. coli*

(e) *P. aeruginosa*
(f) *P. mirabilis*
(g) *Enterobacter* spp.
ii) Viruses
(a) Cytomegalovirus
(b) Varicella-zoster
(c) Herpes simplex
iii) Fungi
(a) *Candida albicans*
(b) *Aspergillus fumigatus*
(c) *Cryptococcus neoformans*
iv) Protozoa: *P. carinii*
9) Chronic immobility
b. Treatment related
1) Surgery, especially if the following:
a) Thoracic, abdominal, or flank incisions
b) Craniotomy
c) Long anesthesia time
d) Prolonged hospitalization
2) Artificial airway, especially self-extubation or reintubation
3) Saline lavage during suctioning of ET tube or tracheostomy
a) Ineffective in liquefying secretions
b) Dislodges five times the number of bacterial colonies than suction catheter alone (Hagler & Traver, 1994)
c) Not completely removed with suctioning allowing colonized saline to move to dependent areas of the lung
4) Bronchoscopy
5) Mechanical ventilation
6) NG tube
7) Aspiration of colonized material related to therapies (see Aspiration Lung Disorder)
a) Oropharyngeal colonization
i) Previous or concurrent antibiotic therapy: predisposes the patient to colonization of the oropharynx
ii) Leakage of pharyngeal flora around the ET tube cuff
b) Gastric colonization
i) Gastric colonization likely with a gastric pH of greater than 4; bacteria in the stomach then migrate upward to be silently aspirated into the lungs
(a) Effects of drugs on gastric pH
(i) H_2 receptor antagonists, proton pump inhibitors (PPIs), and antacids alter the pH of the stomach (normally 1–3)
(ii) Sucralfate does not significantly alter the pH and is associated with a lower incidence of pneumonia than PPIs, H_2 receptor antagonists, or antacids.
(b) Continuous enteral feedings may also alter gastric pH.
ii) Pneumonia rates of patients receiving mechanical ventilation correlate directly with increased gastric pH levels.
8) Supine position
9) Broad-spectrum antibiotic therapy, especially cephalosporins
c. Infection control related
1) Poor hand washing
2) Failure to change gloves between contacts with patients
3) Failure to wear appropriate protective equipment, especially when antibiotic-resistant bacterial strains have been identified
4) Inadequate disinfection or sterilization of devices
5) Contaminated water for humidification
6) Contaminated respiratory therapy or anesthesia equipment
7) Changing of ventilator tubing more often than every 48 hours

Pathophysiology (Fig. 4.36)
1. Nosocomial pneumonia specifically
a. Cross-colonization
b. Altered defenses of intubated and mechanically ventilated patient
1) Normal anatomic barriers are bypassed.
2) Impairment of cough reflex
3) Increase in mucus production
4) Stagnation of mucus
5) Impairment of mucociliary apparatus
c. Contaminated aerosol generation
1) Inadequate disinfection or sterilization of devices
2) Contaminated water for humidification
3) Contaminated respiratory therapy or anesthesia equipment
4) Saline lavage during suctioning of ET tube or tracheostomy
d. Aspiration of colonized material (see Aspiration Lung Disorder)
1) Oropharyngeal colonization
a) Concurrent antibiotic therapy: predisposes the patient to colonization of the oropharynx
b) Leakage of pharyngeal flora around the ET tube cuff
2) Gastric colonization
a) Gastric colonization is likely with a gastric pH of greater than 4.
b) H_2 receptor antagonist, PPIs, and antacids contribute to alter the normal acidic pH of the stomach, allowing proliferation of bacteria in the stomach, which then migrate upward to be silently aspirated into the lungs; sucralfate is associated with a lower incidence of pneumonia than PPIs, H_2 receptor antagonists, or antacids.
c) Pneumonia rates of patients receiving mechanical ventilation correlate directly with increased gastric pH levels
d) Agents that alter gastric pH have been shown to increase the incidence of CAP, HCAP, and VAP.
e. Hematogenous spread from another site

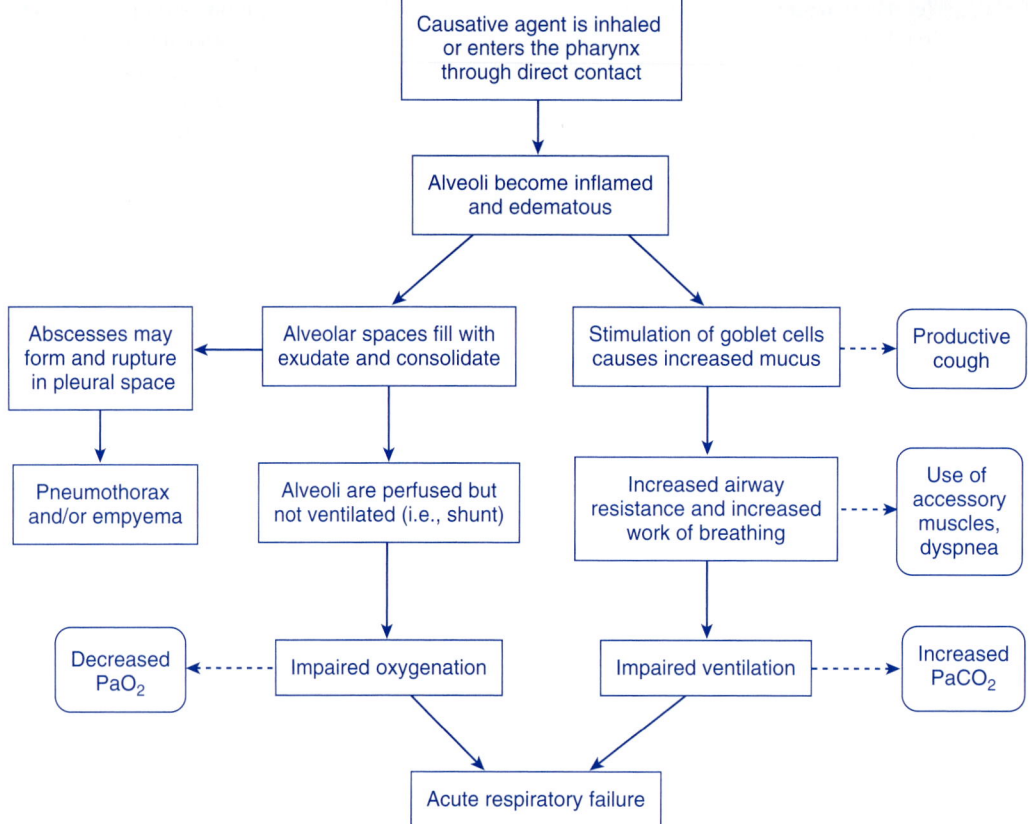

Fig. 4.36 Pathophysiology of pneumonia. *Dotted lines* connect pathology to the clinical presentation.

Clinical Presentation

1. Subjective
   a. Frequently begins with cold or flulike symptoms; infectious symptoms: chills, fever, malaise, tachycardia, headache, myalgia
   b. Chest pain (frequently pleuritic-type pain)
   c. Confusion: especially in elderly patients
2. Objective
   a. Tachycardia
   b. Tachypnea
   c. Fever though elderly patients may be hypothermic
   d. Productive cough; sputum mucoid, rusty, bloody, or purulent; may have foul odor
   e. Diaphoresis
   f. Cyanosis may be seen (dependent on Hgb and SaO_2 levels).
   g. Splinting of chest; decreased chest excursion
   h. Use of accessory muscles
   i. Increased tactile fremitus
   j. Clinical indications of dehydration
   k. Dullness to percussion over areas of consolidation
   l. Breath sound changes: diminished; bronchial breath sounds; crackles or rhonchi; rub may be audible
   m. Voice sounds: egophony, bronchophony, whispered pectoriloquy
3. Diagnostic studies
   a. Serum
      1) WBC count
         a) Elevated with shift to left if bacterial but may be normal in older patients, in immunocompromised patients, or in overwhelming infection
         b) Normal or decreased if viral
      2) ABGs: decreased PaO_2 with clinical indications of hypoxemia; $PaCO_2$ may be increased, decreased, or normal depending on ventilation
   b. Blood culture: positive for specific organism in bacteremia
   c. Sputum: may be induced or obtained through bronchoscopy with either protected specimen brush (PSB) or BAL
      1) Gram stain
      2) Acid-fast stain
      3) Culture and sensitivity to identify specific organism if bacterial
      4) Acid fast: to rule out tuberculosis
      5) *Legionella* spp.
   d. PPD skin test for tuberculosis
   e. Chest radiography
      1) Localization and pattern
         a) Bronchopneumonia: inflammation of the bronchioles and alveoli
         b) Interstitial pneumonia: inflammation of the tissue around alveoli
         c) Alveolar pneumonia: inflammation of the alveoli; usually caused by a virus
         d) Necrotizing pneumonia: necrosis of a portion of lung tissue
      2) Viral pneumonias cause diffuse changes.
      3) Pleural effusion may indicate empyema.
   f. Percutaneous needle aspiration of infiltrate: especially in immunocompromised patient not responding to antibiotics

g. Scoring systems for CAP include the Pneumonia Severity Index (PSI)/Pneumonia Patient Outcomes Research Team (PORT) score, SOAR Score, and SMART-COP score.
    1) Expanded CURB-65 scoring method for CAP (Lim et al., 2016)
        a) Criteria
            i) **C**onfusion
            ii) **U**remia (BUN >20 mg/dl)
            iii) **R**espiratory rate (≥30 breaths/min)
            iv) Low **BP** (systolic BP <90 mm Hg or diastolic BP ≤60 mm Hg
            v) Age ≥**65** years
        b) Recommendation for site of care
            i) One criterion: outpatient treatment
            ii) Two criteria: inpatient unit
            iii) Three or more criteria: often requires critical care admission

Collaborative Management

1. Prevent nosocomial pneumonia or spread of infection.
    a. Prevent cross-contamination
        1) Maintain standard precautions; use other specific precautions may be indicated depending on the type of pneumonia.
        2) Wash hands with soap and water or waterless antiseptic agent.
            a) Before and after any contact with the patient
            b) After contact with mucous membranes, respiratory secretions, or objects contaminated with respiratory secretions
        3) Wear gloves for handling respiratory secretions or any object contaminated by respiratory secretions.
        4) Avoid jewelry, artificial nails or tips, and nail polish.
            a. Implement the Institute for Healthcare Improvement Ventilator Bundle (http://www.ihi.org/resources/Pages/Tools/HowtoGuidePreventVAP.aspx).
                i) Elevation of HOB
                ii) Daily sedation interruption and daily assessment of readiness to extubate
                iii) Peptic ulcer disease (PUD) prophylaxis
                iv) DVT prophylaxis
                v) Daily oral care with chlorhexidine
    c. Prevent colonization.
        1) Avoid unnecessary antibiotics (e.g., prophylactic antibiotics in situations when not warranted).
        2) Avoid unnecessary stress ulcer prophylaxis and use sucralfate (Carafate) rather than agents that reduce the acidity of gastric secretions (Kollef, 2004); agents that alter the pH of gastric secretions, such as H_2 receptor antagonists and PPIs, may increase the risk of HAP and CAP.
        3) Provide oral care with chlorhexidine rinse.
            a) Every 2 to 4 hours
                i) Rinse followed by water-soluble lip balm.
                ii) Suction the oropharynx.
                    (a) Rinse catheter (e.g., Yankauer) with sterile water or saline after each use.
                    (b) Store oropharyngeal suction catheter in an unsealed bag when not in use.
                    (c) Replace oropharyngeal suction device, tubing, and suction canister every 24 hours.
            b) Twice daily
                i) Brush teeth to prevent dental plaque colonization.
                    (a) A soft-bristle pediatric toothbrush should be used along with toothpaste, preferably with an alkaline pH.
                    (b) Removable partial dentures should be removed and thoroughly cleaned.
                ii) Chlorhexidine gluconate 0.12% by spray or rinse as prescribed
                    (a) Has been shown to be effective in the prevention of nosocomial pneumonia
                    (b) Chlorhexidine is a broad-spectrum antibacterial agent that is not absorbed through the skin or mucous membranes.
                    (c) Initiate this oral care preoperatively for surgical patients.
        4) Consider special silver-coated ET to prevent biofilm formation
        5) Consider CLRT to prevent VAP in mechanically ventilated patients.
        6) Use aseptic preparation and maintenance of enteral feedings to prevent contamination and gastric colonization.
        7) Consider selective decontamination of the digestive tract as prescribed.
    d. Prevent aspiration of contaminated secretions and enteral feedings.
        1) Prevent accidental extubation by adequately securing ET tube.
        2) Avoid nasal tubes if possible: nasotracheal or NG, nasopharyngeal airways
            a) May cause sinusitis or potentiate gastric reflux
            b) Orotracheal tube is preferred over nasotracheal tube.
            c) Orogastric tube is preferred over NG but risk of gastric reflux is still present because it also causes incompetence of the gastroesophageal sphincter; percutaneous endoscopic gastrostomy tube is preferred if it is anticipated that the need for enteral feeding will be prolonged.
                i) Remove the NG or orogastric tube as soon as possible.
        3) Limit the duration of intubation and mechanical ventilation if possible.
            a) Interrupt sedation (i.e., "sedation vacation") daily to evaluate the patient's mental status, readiness to extubate, and level of pain control.
            b) Evaluate readiness for ventilator liberation daily using a readiness protocol.

4) Maintain endotracheal or tracheostomy cuff pressure at 20 to 25 mm Hg (25–35 cm H_2O).
5) Maintain CASS using a specialized ET (Fig. 4.28); a dorsal lumen allows continuous suctioning of pooled secretions above the cuff of the ET tube.
6) Suction only as necessary and avoid saline lavage during suctioning of ET tube or tracheostomy.
   a) Ineffective in liquefying secretion
   b) Accentuates oxygen desaturation during suctioning
   c) Dislodges five times the number of bacterial colonies than suction catheter alone
   d) Not completely removed with suctioning allowing colonized saline to lie in lungs
7) Rinse the suction catheter after suctioning (i.e., catheter pulled back to black line, saline injected into irrigation port while suction is maintained).
8) Elevate the HOB to 30 to 45 degrees; turn and reposition every 2 hours.
9) Prevent gastric distention and regurgitation.
   a) Ensure correct placement of the tube.
   b) Evaluate gastric retention for patients receiving enteral feedings; duodenal or jejunal feedings may be beneficial in prevention of aspiration.
   c) Use gastric suction if necessary.
10) Avoid ventilator circuit changes or manipulation; change ventilator circuit and closed-suction systems when contamination of the circuit with blood, emesis, or purulent secretions is noted.
    a) Empty water condensation in ventilator or nebulizer tubing into water trap, never back into humidifier reservoir.
    b) Change humidification system every week or when contaminated.
   e. Encourage the patient to breathe deeply and use incentive spirometry, especially in postoperative patients; adequate analgesia must be achieved so that the patient will breathe deeply.
2. Detect HAP and VAP.
   a. Obtain a culture for any patient with a new or changing infiltrate on CXR who also exhibits at least two of the following:
      1) Fever
      2) Leukocytosis
      3) Purulent sputum
   b. Participate in the acquisition of high quality cultures such as BAL or PSB cultures if indicated to provide the highest quality cultures; nonbronchoscopic collection of endotracheal aspirates from the lower airways or nonbronchoscopic BAL may be used but produce a lower quality culture.
3. Maintain airway and improve ventilation.
   a. Position the patient for optimal ventilation.
      1) Elevate HOB to 30 to 45 degrees.
      2) Turn from "good lung down" to back; use of a 60-degree lateral rotation bed is also advocated.
   b. Administer antimicrobials as prescribed.
      1) Antibiotics for bacterial infection
         a) CAP: should be started within 4 hours of arrival to hospital; broad-spectrum antibiotic prescribed initially empirically (i.e., most likely organism(s) as determined by experience); antibiotic prescription changed if necessary depending on patient response and/or culture
         b) Critically ill patients usually put on a β-lactam (e.g., amoxicillin, penicillin, piperacillin) and either a macrolide (azithromycin, clarithromycin, dirithromycin) or a fluoroquinolone (levofloxacin), moxifloxacin, sparfloxacin)
      2) Antivirals (e.g., amantadine, zanamivir, oseltamivir) for viral infection
      3) Other antimicrobials as prescribed
   c. Provide adequate hydration: 2 to 3 l/24 hr unless contraindicated by cardiac or renal disease
      1) Oral fluids
      2) IV fluids
   d. Maintain pulmonary hygiene and provide chest physiotherapy as indicated.
      1) Inspiratory maneuvers: deep breathing; incentive spirometry
      2) Humidified air and/or oxygen
      3) Encouragement to cough; suction only if the patient is unable to clear airways by coughing
      4) PD, percussion, vibration if necessary
      5) Bronchodilators as prescribed
      6) Expectorants (e.g., guaifenesin [Robitussin], potassium iodide [SSKI]) may be used, but hydration is most important; water is the best expectorant.
      7) Mucolytics (e.g., acetylcysteine) may be used to decrease the tenacity of the mucus.
      8) Sedatives: generally avoided unless patient is very agitated or on mechanical ventilation
      9) Antitussives: avoid use of antitussives unless the cough is nonproductive and causing fatigue.
   e. Prepare the patient for bronchoscopy as requested; may be necessary if airway clearance techniques are inadequate.
   f. Ensure intubation and mechanical ventilation as indicated.
      1) If $PaCO_2$ continues to rise and acidosis develops
      2) The goal of mechanical ventilation is to normalize the pH, not necessarily the $PaCO_2$.
4. Optimize oxygen delivery and decrease oxygen consumption.
   a. Administer oxygen.
      1) Flow rate or oxygen concentration to keep SpO_2 approximately 94% unless contraindicated; in patients with chronic hypercapnia, adjust flow rate or oxygen concentration to keep SpO_2 approximately 90%
   b. Assess activity tolerance; provide rest periods especially after meals or activities.
   c. Treat fever.
      1) Antipyretics (acetaminophen)
      2) Use cooling blankets with attention to the prevention of shivering.
5. Manage chest wall or chest muscle pain: analgesics in doses adequate to allow patient to deep breathe and cough as indicated.

6. Provide appropriate nutritional support.
7. Monitor for complications.
   a. Acute respiratory failure
   b. ARDS
   c. Pleural effusion
   d. Empyema
   e. Lung abscess
   f. Sepsis, septic shock
8. Provide instruction and counseling regarding lifestyle modification and need for pharmacologic therapy.
   a. Importance of compliance with immunization recommendations (e.g., influenza, *Pneumococcus* spp., *Haemophilus* spp.)
   b. Hydration
   c. Nutrition
   d. Smoking cessation
   e. Hand-washing techniques, disposal of tissues, prevention of cross-contamination
   f. Recognition of symptoms to report to the physician
   g. Prescribed antimicrobials and the importance of taking the entire prescription

Aspiration Lung Disease

Definitions
1. Aspiration: syndromes lung injury related to the inhalation of gastric contents, oropharyngeal secretions, food, or other foreign material into the tracheobronchial tree
   a. Chemical pneumonitis (also referred to as *Mendelson syndrome*): chemical injury of the lung caused by aspiration of gastric contents, oropharyngeal secretions, or exogenous liquids
   b. Aspiration pneumonia: lung infection caused by aspiration of colonized bacteria in oropharyngeal or gastric contents
   c. Exogenous lipid pneumonia: an unusual pneumonia resulting from aspiration of oil (mineral or vegetable)
   d. Foreign body aspiration: may cause a medical emergency if airway is obstructed; may result in bacterial pneumonia

Etiology
1. Impaired swallowing; altered consciousness or gag reflex
   a. Older age
   b. Sedation
   c. Anesthesia, especially emergency surgery when the patient has eaten recently
   d. CNS disorders
      1) Cerebral infarction or hemorrhage
      2) Seizures
      3) Neuromuscular diseases
   e. Drug or alcohol intoxication
2. Altered anatomy
   a. ET tube keeps the epiglottis splinted open.
   b. Tracheostomy tube impairs swallowing mechanism.
   c. NG or orogastric tube causes incompetence of the gastroesophageal sphincter.
   d. GI tamponade (e.g., Sengstaken-Blakemore tube)
   e. Facial, neck, or oral trauma
   f. Poor oral hygiene
3. GI conditions
   a. Esophageal abnormalities (e.g., tracheoesophageal fistula or stricture)
   b. Gastroesophageal reflux
      1) Obesity
      2) Hiatal hernia
      3) Pregnancy
   c. Decreased GI motility (e.g., diabetic gastroparesis)
   d. GI hemorrhage
   e. Vomiting
   f. Intestinal obstruction
      1) Functional (e.g., ileus)
      2) Structural (e.g., tumor, volvulus)
4. Enteral nutritional support
   a. Impaired gastric motility: a frequent problem in critically ill patients caused by perfusion deficits, sepsis, drugs (e.g., propofol, opioids)
   b. Improper positioning of patients especially if on enteral feedings
5. Drugs that decrease gastroesophageal sphincter tone: anticholinergics (e.g., atropine), adrenergics (e.g., dopamine), nitrates, caffeine, calcium channel blockers (e.g., nifedipine), estrogen

Pathophysiology
Fig. 4.37

Clinical Presentation
1. Subjective
   a. Dyspnea
   b. Cough
   c. Chest pain: pleuritic in nature
   d. Anxiety
   e. May have history of witnessed vomiting or aspiration
2. Objective
   a. Tachycardia
   b. Tachypnea
   c. Fever
   d. Increased work of breathing: use of accessory muscles; intercostal retractions
   e. Productive cough or suctioned material
      1) Foul-smelling sputum
      2) Food or stomach contents may be seen in secretions suctioned from lungs.
         a) If aspirated, enteral feedings will test positive for glucose.
      3) Pink, frothy sputum may occur with acidic aspiration.
   f. Breath sounds
      1) Stridor if obstruction of the upper airway occurs
      2) Diminished breath sounds
      3) Adventitious sounds: crackles, rhonchi, wheezing
   g. Hypoxemia (decreased SpO_2, SaO_2, PaO_2) and clinical indications of hypoxia (Box 4.3)
   h. Compliance: decreased static and dynamic compliance; increased peak inspiratory pressures
3. Diagnostic studies: guided by presentation of patient from mildly ill to critically ill
   a. Serum
      1) CBC: WBC increased
      2) ABGs

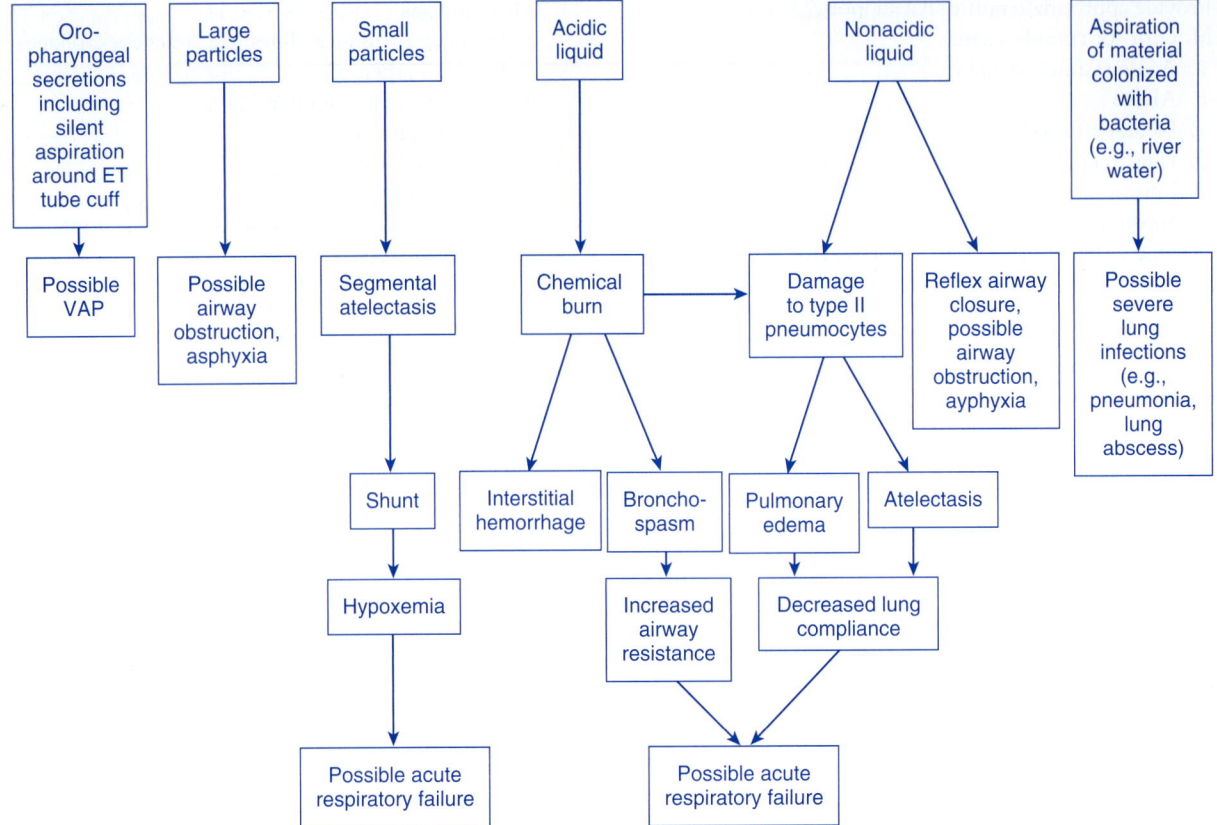

Fig. 4.37 Pathophysiology of aspiration lung disorder.

      a) PaO₂ and SaO₂ decreased
      b) PaCO₂ may be normal, decreased, or increased depending on ventilation pattern (e.g., may be low because of hyperventilation or high because of hypoventilation)
    3) Serum immunoglobulins: IgG, IgM, IgA, IgE
  b. Radiographic studies
    1) High-resolution CT scan
    2) Barium esophagram ("barium swallow")
    3) Gastroesophageal scintigraphy
    4) Chest radiography: bilateral patchy infiltrates or atelectasis; pulmonary edema may be present.
  c. Diagnostic Procedures
    1) Videofluoroscopic swallow study (VFSS)
    2) Fiberoptic endoscopic swallowing evaluation (FEES)
    3) Fiberoptic bronchoscopy
    4) Esophageal pH monitoring for 24 hours
    5) Esophagogastroduodenoscopy (EGD)
    6) Radionuclide salivagram
  d. Tracheal aspirate: visualization or analysis to determine if aspiration has occurred
    1) Pepsin: a proxy for gastric contents
      a) Likely the most sensitive indicator of aspiration
    2) pH: continuous monitoring of tracheal pH
      a) A sensitive instrument to detect acid aspirate in the trachea
    3) Glucose: use of glucose oxidase reagent strips to detect the presence of glucose
      a) More sensitive than dye method
      b) Some potential problems (Bowman et al., 2005)
        i) Blood in tracheal secretions may cause a positive test result (false positive).
        ii) Low glucose formulas may not cause a positive result.
        iii) Concerns regarding specificity because some patients not being enterally fed had positive results
        iv) Concerns about validity of using strips intended for blood or urine for tracheal aspirate
    4) Dye: visual assessment of tracheal aspirate for discoloration caused by blue dye (usually blue food coloring) that was added to enteral feeding; it is no longer recommended to add blue food coloring to enteral feedings for the following reasons:
      a) May result in generalized absorption of the dye from the GI tract; more likely in patients with multiple organ failure
        i) Discoloration of body fluids and tissues
        ii) May cause fatal liver toxicity
        iii) Causes questionable specificity because discoloration of tracheal secretions may have occurred by systemic route
      b) May result in infection caused by contamination of the food coloring

   c) Interferes with occult blood testing
   d) Causes allergic reactions in some people due to presence of FD&C Yellow No. 5
   e) Has relatively low sensitivity
  e. Sputum: presence of polymorphonuclear leukocytes
   1) Culture and sensitivity: infecting organism if pneumonia present
  f. CXR
   1) Bilateral patchy infiltrates or atelectasis
   2) Pulmonary edema may be present.

Collaborative Management

1. Prevent aspiration of gastric contents.
 a. Use appropriate positioning to reduce risk of aspiration and reduce volume of aspiration should vomiting occur.
  1) Place unconscious patient in side-lying position; endotracheal intubation may be necessary.
  2) Avoid flat position especially in patients receiving enteral feedings; keep HOB elevated to 45 degrees continuously for patients on continuous feedings and for at least 30 minutes after intermittent feedings.
   a) Stop continuous enteral feedings at least 30 minutes before any procedure that requires that the HOB must be lowered.
   b) If the HOB cannot be elevated, position the patient on his or her right side as much as possible to facilitate movement of gastric contents through the pylorus and allow drainage of emesis out of the mouth rather than be aspirated.
  3) Do not restrain in such a way as the patient cannot protect his or her airway if vomiting occurs.
 b. Maintain proper functioning of NG, orogastric, or intestinal tube used for gastric suctioning or enteral feeding.
  1) Confirm proper placement: more than one method to verify tube placement should be used.
   a) During the procedure
    i) Note any indications of respiratory distress.
    ii) Use capnography if available unless the patient is taking PPIs or other acid-suppressing medications or continuous tube feedings.
    iii) Measure pH of aspirate from tube; gastric secretions have a pH of 4 or less unless the patient is receiving acid-suppressing medications or continuous feedings; intestinal secretions have a pH of greater than 7.
    iv) Observe visual characteristics of the aspirate.
   b) Radiographic confirmation is the recommended practice for blindly inserted GI tubes; the radiography should be read by a radiologist.
   c) Auscultatory (i.e., air bolus) and water bubbling methods are unreliable.
  2) Reassess placement at least every 4 hours.
   a) Be alert to change in length of tubing outside of patient during the markings on the tube.
   b) Note change in the volume of aspirate from the tube.
   c) Obtain radiography to confirm position if location of tube is in question.
 c. Prevent aspiration in patients with artificial airways.
  1) Keep the cuff of endotracheal or tracheostomy tube inflated to 20 to 30 cm H_2O.
   a) If the patient is not on a mechanical ventilator, inflate the cuff during meals and suction mouth and oropharynx before deflating the cuff.
  2) Suction oropharynx to reduce oropharyngeal secretions that accumulate above the cuff of an ET.
   a) Subglottic suctioning is advocated to prevent pneumonia associated with this silent aspiration; involves specialized endotracheal tubing with a port above the cuff that allows continuous suction to remove accumulated secretions
 d. Select appropriate tube and site for enteral feeding.
  1) Use intragastric feedings when GI motility is normal because they are easier and less expensive to place than small intestinal tubes.
   a) Small lumen feeding tubes cause less gastroesophageal incompetence than do larger lumen NG tubes.
   b) Tubes that do not go through the gastroesophageal sphincter (e.g., percutaneous endoscopic gastrostomy [PEG] or needle jejunostomy tubes) are best for long-term enteral feeding.
  2) Use small intestinal tubes and feedings when GI motility is impaired.
   a) Because these feedings do increase gastric secretions and duodenal feedings may reflux back into the stomach, aspiration is still possible.
   b) A NG or orogastric tube may be inserted to monitor gastric volume or for gastric decompression.
 e. Monitor for gastric residual volume in patients on gastric enteral feedings.
  1) Check for residual volume before each feeding if intermittent enteral feedings are being administered and every 4 to 6 hours if continuous enteral feedings are being administered.
   a) Consensus on acceptable gastric residual volumes has not been reached; recent studies reveal the acceptable volume may need to be determined for each patient based on underlying disease processes. General guidelines include the following:
    i) If more than 400 ml are aspirated, consider the following:
     (a) Changing to continuous feedings if bolus or intermittent feedings being used

(b) Changing the enteral feeding site to the duodenum or jejunum (though this does not completely eliminate the risk)
(c) Do not hold feedings but reassess in 1 hour.
ii) If more than 500 ml, withhold feeding for 1 hour and then recheck for retention.
(a) Holding or discontinuing feedings can result in malnutrition so consider changes stated earlier.
2) Aspiration of small-lumen feeding tubes is difficult because they tend to collapse with suction; increases in abdominal girth, absent bowel sounds, and nausea are indications of retention, and causes of delayed gastric emptying need to be evaluated.
f. Monitor the secretions suctioned or expectorated: glucose testing may be performed to confirm presence of enteral feeding in sputum.
g. Keep appropriate equipment at bedside.
1) Airway suctioning equipment
2) Wire cutters for patients with wired jaws
3) Scissors for patients with Sengstaken-Blakemore tube
h. Prepare patient for surgery for intractable aspiration as requested: tracheoesophageal diversion or laryngotracheal separation
2. Maintain airway, ventilation, and oxygenation if aspiration does occur.
a. Position the bed in a slight Trendelenburg position with the patient in a right lateral decubitus position.
b. Suction the airway immediately; provide adequate oxygenation during suctioning.
1) Endotracheal intubation may be necessary.
2) Bronchoscopy for removal of large particles if indicated
c. Stop enteral feeding if being administered.
d. Monitor ABGs and pulse oximetry: a decrease in SpO_2, SaO_2, and PaO_2 may indicate the development of ARDS.
e. Administer oxygen therapy if hypoxemia is present.
1) CPAP or PEEP may be necessary to maintain adequate oxygenation.
f. Initiate mechanical ventilation as prescribed if hypercapnia develops.
g. Administer bronchodilators as prescribed.
h. Administer antibiotics as prescribed (prophylactic antibiotics are not recommended, but antibiotics specific to positive sputum or blood cultures are indicated).
i. Prepare the patient for pulmonary resection if abscess develops.
3. Monitor for complications.
a. Acute respiratory failure
b. ARDS
c. Pneumonia
d. Lung abscess
e. Empyema

Status Asthmaticus

Definitions
1. Asthma: a recurrent, reversible airway disease characterized by increased airway responsiveness to a variety of stimuli that produces airway narrowing
2. Status asthmaticus: exacerbation of acute asthma characterized by severe airflow obstruction that is not relieved after 24 hours of maximal doses of traditional therapy

Etiology
1. Extrinsic: when a specific allergy can be related to the attack
   a. Dust and dust mites
   b. Animal dander or feathers
   c. Pollen
   d. Mold
   e. Smoke
   f. Propellants
   g. Air pollution
   h. Preservatives (e.g., bisulfites)
   i. Food such as nuts, legumes (e.g., peanuts), chocolate, eggs, shellfish, and food additives
   j. Alcohol
   k. Changes in inspired air such as cold or hot air, very high or very low humidity
   l. Medications
      1) Aspirin
      2) NSAIDs
      3) β-blockers
2. Intrinsic: when the attack is seemingly unrelated to a specific allergen
   a. Infection, such as bacterial or viral pneumonia, bronchitis, or sinusitis
   b. Stress
   c. Exercise
   d. Gastroesophageal reflux disease (GERD)
   e. Aspiration
   f. Fear, anger, crying, or laughing
   g. Menstrual cycle

Pathophysiology
Fig. 4.38

Clinical Presentation
1. Subjective
   a. History of a slow, progressive worsening of airflow obstruction over the course of several days or weeks
   b. Anxiety
   c. Dyspnea
   d. Chest tightness
   e. Fatigue
   f. Insomnia
   g. Anorexia
2. Objective
   a. Tachycardia
   b. Tachypnea; inability to speak in full sentences because of dyspnea
   c. Cough with thick tenacious sputum production
   d. Use of accessory muscles

Chapter 4 The Pulmonary System 347

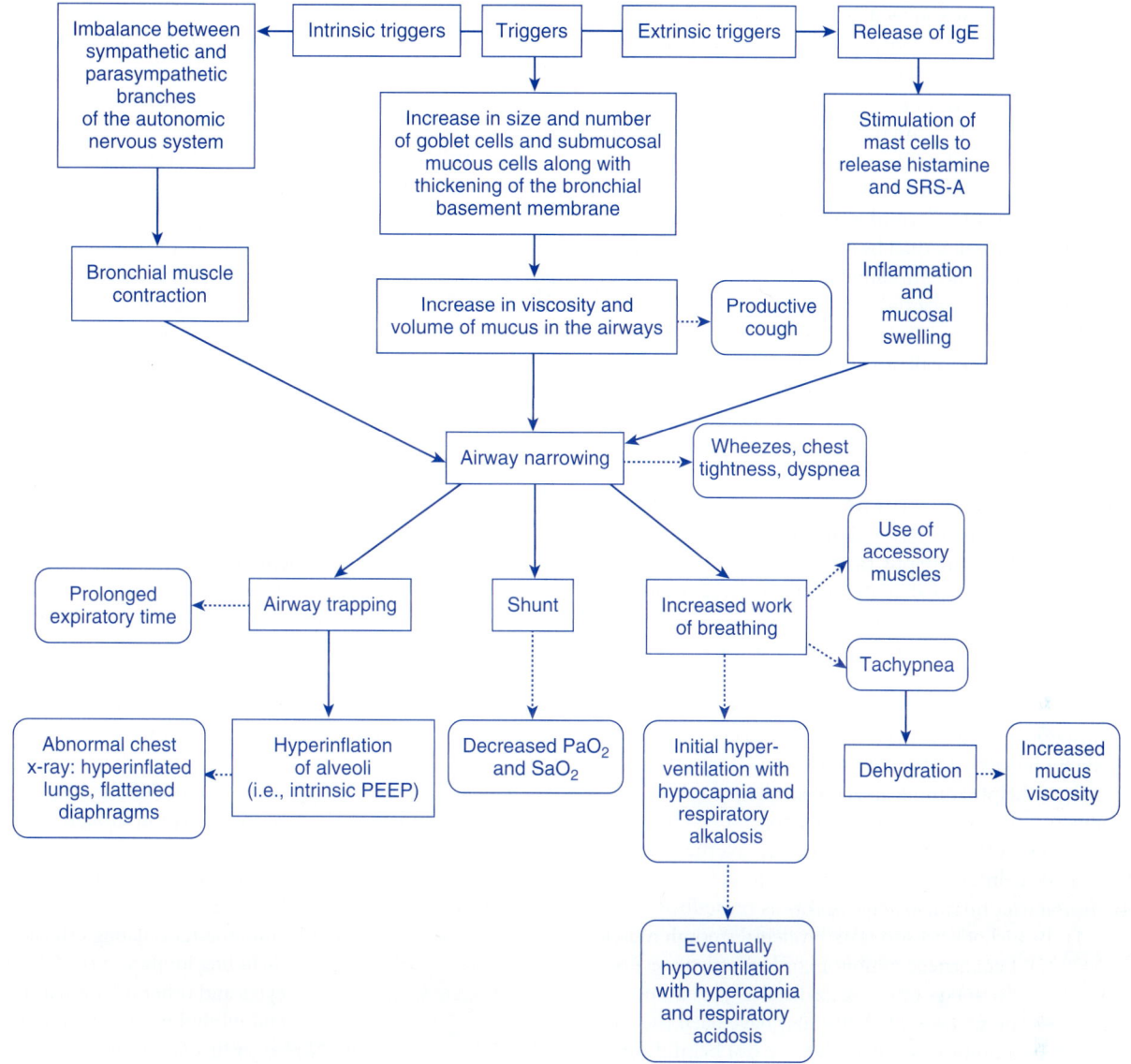

Fig. 4.38 Pathophysiology of asthma. *Dotted lines* connect pathology to the clinical presentation.

e. Intercostal retractions
f. Prolonged expiration (>1 to 3 I:E ratio)
g. Diaphoresis
h. Peak expiratory flow rate (PEFR) below 80% of patient's personal or predicted best; frequently below 50% of patient's personal best
i. Clinical indications of dehydration: poor skin turgor; dry mucous membranes; increased specific gravity of urine
j. Clinical indications of hypoxemia (Box 4.3)
k. Clinical indications of hypercapnia (Box 4.4)
l. Breath sound changes: rhonchi and wheezing
m. Indications of potential imminent respiratory arrest
   1) Change in consciousness: drowsiness or confusion
   2) Paradoxical thoracoabdominal movement
   3) Absence of rhonchi and wheezes may occur in critical stages; indication of absence of airflow
   4) Bradycardia
   5) Pulsus paradoxus greater than 20 mm Hg

3. Diagnostic studies
   a. Serum
      1) WBC count may be increased if infection is the cause.
      2) Eosinophil count may be increased if patient is not receiving steroids.
      3) Hematocrit may be increased because of dehydration.
      4) Electrolytes: potassium or magnesium may be low during an acute attack.
      5) Theophylline level: if therapeutic, 10 to 20 mcg/dl; if patient has not been taking the drug, theophylline level will be less than therapeutic
      6) ABGs (Table 4.27)
   b. Sputum
      1) Increased viscosity
      2) May have positive culture
      3) Eosinophil stain: increase in number of eosinophils indicates allergic reaction.

c. Pulmonary function studies (may be impossible to do during attack because the patient is so dyspneic)
   1) Decreased V_T and VC
   2) Increased residual volume
   3) PEF or FEV_1 are diminished with improvement after bronchodilators.
      a) A combination of best FEV_1 and patient report of symptoms is a better predictor of mortality than best peak expiratory flow in patients with asthma.
d. ECG: sinus tachycardia
e. CXR
   1) Normal or hyperinflated lungs with flattened diaphragms
   2) Helpful to rule out foreign body, aspiration, pulmonary edema, PE, pneumonia, or pneumothorax

Collaborative Management
1. Assess predisposing factors; eliminate or treat cause.
   a. Antibiotics to promptly treat infection
   b. Avoidance of exposure to pulmonary irritants and pollutants
   c. Avoidance of drugs or foods that may trigger an attack
   d. Cromolyn sodium (Intal) or nedocromil (Tilade) are inhaled mast cell stabilizers that prevent the release of histamine from the mast cells; these agents have no direct bronchodilation or antiinflammatory effect and are not helpful during an acute attack.
2. Maintain airway and improve ventilation.
   a. Elevate HOB to 30 to 45 degrees; an overbed table may be helpful for the patient to lean on.
   b. Administer pharmacologic agents as prescribed.
      1) Bronchodilators to relax bronchial smooth muscle
         a) Leukotriene inhibitors or leukotriene receptor antagonists (e.g., zafirlukast, zileuton, montelukast sodium) may have been used as a preventive agent; they are not helpful for treatment of acute bronchospasm.
         b) β_2 stimulants
            i) Action: stimulate β_2 receptors to cause smooth muscle relaxation
            ii) Long acting (e.g., salmeterol) by metered-dose inhaler will likely have been used long term by the patient with a diagnosis of asthma.
            iii) Short-acting β_2 agonists (e.g., metaproterenol, albuterol, pirbuterol, bitolterol, terbutaline, epinephrine)
               (a) Metered-dose inhaler is usually used and may be as effective as nebulizers when used with a spacing device.
               (b) Nebulizer is frequently used if the PEFR is less than 50% of the patient's personal best; the β-agonist is administered by nebulizer every 20 minutes or continuously for 1 hour.
                  (i) Continuous nebulizers have been shown as effective with no more side effects than intermittent nebulizers and require less clinician time
               (c) IV β-agonists are not recommended if inhalation therapy is possible because they do not result in better results but increase adverse effects significantly.
            iv) Monitor closely for adverse effects such as significant tachycardia, dysrhythmias, hypertension, headache, tremor, anxiety, or hypokalemia.
         c) Anticholinergic (e.g., ipratropium bromide [Atrovent]) may be used in severe attacks to augment the effects of β_2-agonists.
            i) Action: block parasympathetic stimulation (making sympathetic stimulation dominant) to cause smooth muscle relaxation
            ii) May be especially helpful for asthma stimulated by an intrinsic trigger
            iii) Administered as a metered-dose inhaler or nebulizer
            iv) May be administered as a combination agent with β-agonist (e.g., ipratropium bromide and albuterol sulfate [Combivent])
         d) Xanthines (e.g., theophylline, aminophylline) may be given intravenously for refractory attack.
            i) Actions
               (a) Smooth muscle relaxation causing bronchodilation though less effective than nebulized β-agonists; also more adverse effects than β-agonists
               (b) Immune-modulating effects, including inhibition of T lymphocytes and other inflammatory cells and inhibition of cytokine release
            ii) No longer first-line agent primarily because of the narrow therapeutic window and interactions with other commonly prescribed drugs but should be continued in patients on xanthine therapy at home
               (a) Obtain a theophylline level for patients who have been receiving xanthines at home.
               (b) Monitor closely for indications of theophylline toxicity.
                  (i) GI: anorexia, nausea, vomiting
                  (ii) Cardiac: dysrhythmias
                  (iii) Neurologic: restlessness or seizures
            iii) Administration orally for long-term therapy but usually by IV infusion in acute asthma
         e) Magnesium: used in acutely ill asthmatic patients with severe exacerbation
            i) Actions: smooth muscle relaxation, bronchodilation, improved airflow
               (a) Considered for patients who have not responded to other bronchodilators after 1 hour

ii) Administered as IV infusion: usual dose is 1 to 2 g over 20 minutes.
iii) Contraindicated in hypotension or renal failure
iv) Monitor BP during infusion; note and report significant hypotension or loss of deep tendon reflexes.
2) Corticosteroids to reduce inflammation
   a) Actions
      i) Decrease mucosal swelling and release of histamine by the mast cells
      ii) Potentiates bronchodilators
   b) Administration
      i) Patient has usually administered steroids (e.g., beclomethasone, flunisolide, triamcinolone, fluticasone) via metered-dose inhaler before hospitalization.
      ii) Steroids may be initially administered intravenously (e.g., methylprednisolone) or orally (prednisone and prednisolone) in status asthmaticus.
      iii) Steroid-resistant asthma: IV immunoglobulin may be administered.
3) Expectorants (e.g., guaifenesin, potassium iodide [SSKI]) may be used but hydration is most important; water is the best expectorant.
4) Mucolytics (e.g., acetylcysteine) are generally contraindicated because of the adverse effect of bronchospasm.
5) Antitussives: avoid use of antitussives.
6) Antibiotics: indicated only if infection
c. Maintain pulmonary hygiene.
   1) Abdominal (i.e., deep) breathing
   2) Effective coughing
   3) Suctioning only if coughing is ineffective
   4) Chest physical therapy is not generally recommended and may be unnecessarily stressful for a patient with status asthmaticus.
d. Use noninvasive ventilatory (NiPPV) methods (CPAP, Bi-PAP) as prescribed.
   1) May be used with a mask if the patient is not intubated
   2) May prevent further deterioration and intubation and mechanical ventilation by unloading the respiratory muscles and reducing the work of breathing
e. Ensure intubation and mechanical ventilation as necessary.
   1) Indicated if $PaCO_2$ continues to rise and acidosis develops
   2) The goal of mechanical ventilation is to normalize the pH, not necessarily the $PaCO_2$.
      a) Mode: usually AC or PRVC
      b) V_T: 4 to 8 ml/kg
      c) Respiratory rate: 10 to 12 breaths/min and adjust to normalize pH, although $PaCO_2$ may still be elevated
         i) Permissive hypercapnia, expected and accepted hypercapnia, results from the deliberate attempt to decrease alveolar ventilation by reducing V_Ts and alveolar pressures.
         ii) Contraindicated in intracranial hypertension or cerebral anoxia
         iii) Sedation may be required.
            (a) Morphine is avoided because it causes histamine release.
            (b) Propofol and fentanyl or ketamine (causes bronchodilation) and midazolam
         iv) Bicarbonate infusions may be used to keep the pH above 7.2 if ventilation fails to control pH.
      d) Flow rate: 60 to 100 l/min; higher inspiratory flow rate shortens inspiration to allow more time for expiration to reduce air trapping and auto-PEEP
         i) I:E ratio: 1:3 or 1:4 to allow longer expiratory times
      e) Peak inspiratory pressure should be kept under 40 cm H_2O, and plateau pressure should be kept below 35 cm H_2O if possible.
      f) FiO2: adjusted to maintain SpO2 of approximately 90%
      g) PEEP should be avoided or less than or equal to 5 cm H_2O if possible because the patient is at high risk for barotrauma.
         i) Monitor levels of auto-PEEP caused by air trapping
3. Optimize oxygen delivery and decrease oxygen consumption.
   a. Administer oxygen as indicated.
      1) Uncontrolled high-flow oxygen should be avoided in acute asthma; oxygen concentration should be adjusted to keep SpO2 ~90%.
   b. Teach and encourage relaxation techniques.
   c. Teach and encourage abdominal breathing, although it is difficult for the patient when dyspneic and tachypneic.
   d. Provide rest periods especially after meals or activities.
   e. Administer antipyretics if indicated.
   f. Use heliox as prescribed.
      1) Helium is a light gas that decreases work of breathing when it replaces nitrogen in the inspired air.
         a) Oxygen percentage is prescribed, and helium replaces nitrogen to make up the remainder (e.g., 80% helium with 20% oxygen, 70% helium with 30% oxygen, 60% helium with 40% oxygen).
      2) Actions
         a) Decreases airway resistance and work of breathing
         b) Decreases hypercapnia and need for intubation and mechanical ventilation
      3) Administration
         a) By face mask
         b) By mechanical ventilator: requires recalibration for this lighter gas
4. Provide adequate rehydration.
   a. Oral fluids
   b. IV fluids: usually D_5NS or $D_5{}^1\!/_2NS$

5. Provide instruction and counseling regarding lifestyle modification and need for pharmacologic therapy.
    a. Recognition and avoidance of triggers; allergy testing and desensitization may be needed
    b. Symptom monitoring
        1) To measure PEFR twice daily
        2) When to call the physician
            a) PEFR drops by 20% or more below its usual level
            b) Increase in symptoms such as dyspnea
            c) Indications of respiratory infection
    c. Drug therapy
        1) Inhaled bronchodilators and corticosteroids
            a) How to use and clean a metered-dose inhaler or nebulizer
            b) To use corticosteroids after the bronchodilator
            c) To rinse mouth after inhaled corticosteroids to avoid oral fungal infection (e.g., candidiasis)
        2) Cromolyn may be prescribed.
        3) Antimicrobials
    d. Breathing exercises: slow abdominal breathing and pursed-lip breathing
    e. Importance of immunizations (e.g., influenza, *Pneumococcus* spp., *Haemophilus* spp.)
    f. Control of GERD
        1) H_2 receptor antagonists or PPIs (e.g., omeprazole, lansoprazole, rabeprazole)
        2) Avoidance of large meals and supine position after eating
        3) Normalization of body weight
6. Monitor for complications.
    a. Asphyxia
    b. Acute respiratory failure
    c. Barotrauma/volutrauma (e.g., pneumothorax)
    d. Pneumonia
    e. Dysrhythmias
    f. Hypovolemia
    g. Hypotension related to hypovolemia, lung hyperinflation decreasing venous return to the heart, tension pneumothorax, oversedation

Pulmonary Embolism or Infarction

Definition
Obstruction of blood flow to one or more arteries of the lung by a thrombus lodged in a pulmonary vessel; other types of emboli include fat, air, amniotic fluid, tumor, and foreign body (e.g., catheter fragment)
1. Massive: more than 50% occlusion of pulmonary blood flow; caused by occlusion of a lobar artery or larger artery
2. Submassive: less than 50% occlusion of pulmonary blood flow; in patients with preexisting heart or lung disease, hemodynamic deterioration occurs with less than 50% pulmonary vascular obstruction

Etiology
1. Risk factors for thrombus formation (Virchow triad)
    a. Hypercoagulability
        1) Malignancy: especially breast, lung, pancreas, or GI or genitourinary tracts
        2) Estrogen, especially in smokers
            a) Oral contraceptives
            b) Postmenopausal hormone replacement therapy
        3) Pregnancy and postpartum period, especially with twin gestation or older maternal age
        4) Genetic predisposition or history of prior VTE
        5) Dehydration and hemoconcentration
        6) Sickle-cell anemia
        7) Polycythemia vera
        8) Abrupt discontinuance of anticoagulants
        9) Sepsis
        10) Protein C, protein S, or antithrombin III deficiency
    b. Alterations in the vessel wall
        1) Trauma
        2) IV drug use
        3) Aging
        4) Vasculitis
        5) Varicose veins
        6) Diabetes mellitus
        7) Atherosclerosis
        8) Inflammatory process
    c. Venous stasis
        1) Prolonged bed rest or immobilization
        2) Physical inactivity
        3) Fracture of pelvis, hip, or long bone
        4) Major orthopedic surgery
        5) Major/multiple trauma
        6) Surgery, especially involving abdomen, pelvis, or lower extremities
        7) Obesity
        8) Advanced age
        9) Burns
        10) Pregnancy
        11) HF
        12) MI
        13) Bacterial endocarditis
        14) Thrombus formation in heart (AF)
        15) Cardioversion
2. Risk factors for fat embolism
    a. Long bone (e.g., femur) fracture, pelvic fracture, multiple fractures
    b. Orthopedic surgery with intramedullary manipulation
    c. Trauma to adipose tissue or liver
    d. Osteomyelitis
    e. Sickle cell crisis
    f. Burns
    g. Acute pancreatitis
    h. Liposuction
3. Risk factors for air embolism
    a. Recent surgical procedure
    b. Insertion of deep vein catheter
    c. Cardiopulmonary bypass
    d. Hemodialysis
    e. Endoscopy

Pathophysiology (Fig. 4.39)
1. Fat emboli specifically
    a. Most likely to develop 1 to 3 days after injury but may occur up to 1 week after injury

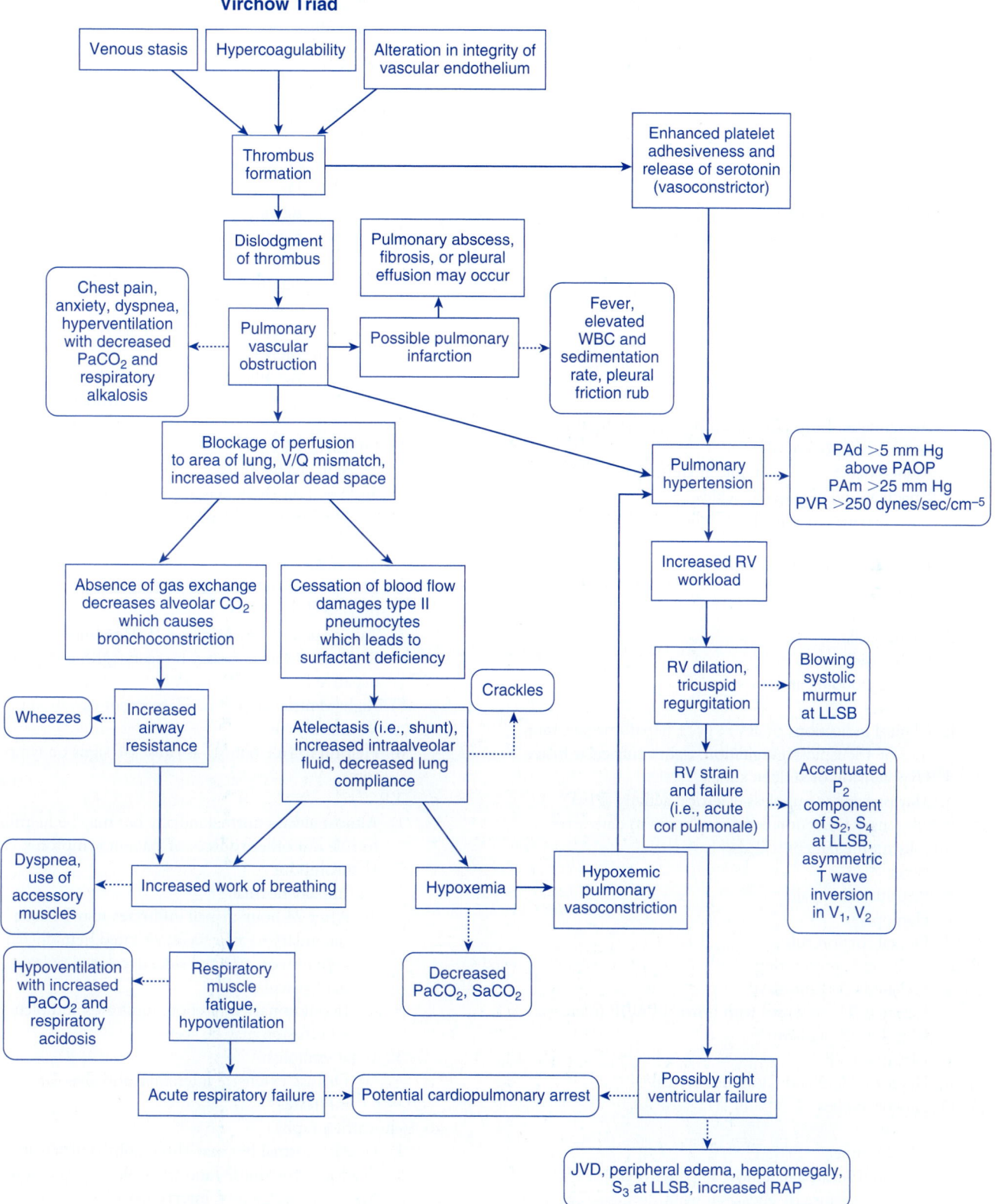

Fig. 4.39 Pathophysiology of pulmonary embolism. *Dotted lines* connect pathology to clinical presentation.

b. Fat globules enter the bloodstream and form emboli.
c. Presence of fat emboli in the bloodstream causes interactions with platelets and free fatty acids along with release of vasoactive substances.
d. Cerebral ischemia
2. Air emboli specifically
   a. Activation of the clotting cascade
   b. Interruption of circulation

Clinical Presentation
1. Small embolus: patient is asymptomatic
2. Small to medium embolus
   a. Anxiety
   b. Dyspnea
   c. Tachypnea
   d. Tachycardia
   e. Chest pain
   f. Cough
   g. Accentuated P_2 (pulmonic component of S_2; the second component of S_2)
   h. Right-sided S_3 or S_4 (audible at sternum)
   i. Breath sound changes: crackles
3. Large to massive: massive PE is when 50% of pulmonary artery bed is occluded.
   a. Feeling of impending doom
   b. Dyspnea
   c. Tachypnea
   d. Tachycardia
   e. Chest pain
   f. Mental clouding and/or syncope
   g. Cyanosis
   h. Clinical indications of RVF: JVD, hepatomegaly, murmur of tricuspid regurgitation, right ventricular heave
   i. Hypotension or sudden shock
   j. May present as pulseless electrical activity (PEA)
4. If pulmonary infarction develops (hours to days after embolism), the patient will also have
   a. Fever
   b. Pleuritic chest pain
   c. Hemoptysis
   d. Pleural friction rub
5. Hemodynamic monitoring
   a. Elevated CVP and RAP
   b. Elevated PA pressures with normal PAOP (increased PAd–PAOP gradient)
   c. Elevated PVR
   d. Decreased CO and CI in massive PE
6. Diagnostic studies
   a. Serum
      1) D-dimer
         a) Elevated in almost all patients with PE because of endogenous fibrinolysis (i.e., high negative predictive value)
         b) High sensitivity but low specificity; 99% negative predictive value
         c) Indeterminate V/Q and a positive D-dimer is an indication for pulmonary angiogram
      2) Troponin I: may be elevated; indicates right ventricular microinfarction
      3) BNP: may be elevated with right ventricular overload
   4) ABGs
      a) If thrombotic
         i) Decreased PaO_2, SaO_2, and SvO_2; PaO_2 less than 50 mm Hg in a patient with previously normal ABGs indicates greater than 50% obstruction of the pulmonary tree and that pulmonary hypertension is present
         ii) Decreased $PaCO_2$
         iii) Respiratory alkalosis initially; may have metabolic acidosis if severe hypoxemia; respiratory acidosis may develop with significant atelectasis or fatigue
      b) If fat or air embolism
         i) Decreased PaO_2 and SaO_2
         ii) Increased $PaCO_2$
         iii) Respiratory acidosis; may have metabolic acidosis if severe hypoxemia
   b. ECG
      1) Dysrhythmias
         a) Sinus tachycardia
         b) Atrial dysrhythmias, especially atrial fibrillation, are common.
         c) Ventricular dysrhythmias may occur in hypoxemia.
      2) Blocks: new right bundle branch block (RBBB) may be seen.
      3) Tall, peaked P waves in lead II (P-pulmonale)
      4) Right-axis deviation may be seen (QRS complex negative in I, positive in aVF).
      5) Right ventricular strain: ST-segment elevation in V_1 and V_2
      6) Helpful to rule out MI as cause of signs or symptoms
   c. CXR
      1) Almost always normal initially but may be helpful to rule out other sources of patient symptoms
      2) If thrombotic
         a) Initially normal
         b) After 24 hours: small infiltrates may be seen secondary to atelectasis; elevated hemidiaphragm on affected side; decreased pulmonary vascularity
         c) If pulmonary infarction: infiltrates and pleural effusion may be seen.
      3) If fat embolism
         a) Diffuse extensive interstitial and alveolar infiltrates
   d. Echocardiography
      1) Usually normal but may show right ventricular dilation, hypokinesis, and tricuspid regurgitation
      2) May show bulging of interventricular septum into the LV, which reduces LV size with D-shaped LV
      3) Also helpful to rule out cardiac tamponade, dissection of the aorta, and acute MI
   e. V/Q scan
      1) Shows perfusion defect with normal ventilation
      2) Positive predictive value of high probability V/Q scan is 96% when supported by high clinical suspicion of PE; negative predictive value of

negative V/Q scan is also excellent with a normal V/Q scan accurately ruling out PE 98% of the time; unfortunately, 75% of patients fall within the indeterminate category
    3) Intermediate- or low-probability V/Q scan with positive D-dimer is indication for pulmonary angiography.
  f. Spiral (helical) CT
    1) Easier study to obtain than a V/Q scan or pulmonary angiogram
    2) Capable of demonstrating a variety of thoracic pathologies that can mimic PE
    3) Sensitivity greatly affected by generation of scanner used; significantly better sensitivity with new scanners; excellent specificity
  g. Magnetic resonance angiography (MRA)
    1) Gadolinium-enhanced MRA allows high-resolution angiography during a single breath.
    2) Fast but accurate test that does not involve nephrotoxic contrast agents
  h. Pulmonary angiography
    1) Shows cutoff of a vessel or a filling defect within 24 to 72 hours
    2) Continues to be the "gold standard" but not without risks
    3) Indicated in patients with a high probability of having a PE and nondiagnostic noninvasive studies
    4) Excellent sensitivity and specificity
    5) Disadvantages: risk of significant bleeding, provides a relative contraindication for fibrinolytic therapy because of the risk of bleeding from the puncture site
  i. Wells criteria (Wells & Ginsberg, 1995)
    1) Scores for factors that increase likelihood that PE exists
      a) Clinically suspected VTE: 3 points
      b) The alternative diagnosis is less likely than PE: 3 points
      c) Tachycardia: 1.5 points
      d) Immobilization or surgery within previous 4 weeks: 1.5 points
      e) History of VTE or PE: 1.5 points
      f) Presence of hemoptysis: 1 point
      g) Treatment for malignancy within 6 months or palliative management: 1 point
    2) Interpretation of summative score
      a) Score greater than 6: high probability of PE
      b) Score 2 to 6: moderate probability of PE
      c) Score less than 2: low probability of PE
    3) Testing recommendations
      a) Score greater than 4: PE likely, so consider diagnostic imaging
      b) Score 4 or less: PE unlikely, so consider D-dimer to rule out PE
7. If fat embolism: may have no symptoms for 12 to 48 hours
  a. Subjective
    1) Restlessness, agitation, irritability, and confusion
    2) Dyspnea
    3) Delirium
  b. Objective
    1) Tachypnea
    2) Tachycardia
    3) Fever
    4) Petechiae on conjunctivae, anterior chest, neck, or axilla
    5) Retinal hemorrhages with emboli present on the retina
    6) Breath sound changes: stridor, wheezes, or crackles
    7) Lethargy, coma
    8) Seizures
    9) Hypoxemia: decreased SpO_2, SaO_2, and PaO_2
    10) Clinical indications of hypoxia (Box 4.3)
  c. Diagnostic studies
    1) Serum
      a) Elevated lipase
      b) Elevated triglycerides
      c) Increased free fatty acids
      d) Elevated sedimentation rate
      e) Decreased Hgb or hematocrit
      f) Thrombocytopenia
      g) Elevated fibrin split products
    2) ABGs: hypoxemia
    3) Urinalysis: fat globules in the urine
    4) Sputum: fat globules in the sputum
8. If air embolism
  a. Subjective
    1) Feeling of impending doom
    2) Lightheadedness
    3) Weakness
    4) Nausea
    5) Chest pain
    6) Dyspnea
    7) Palpitations
    8) Confusion
  b. Objective
    1) Pallor
    2) Tachypnea
    3) Tachycardia
    4) Hypotension
    5) Churning noise ("mill wheel murmur") may be audible.
    6) Hypoxemia: decreased SpO_2, SaO_2, and PaO_2
    7) Clinical indications of hypoxia (Box 4.3)
    8) Clinical indications of pulmonary edema: S_3 or crackles
    9) Seizures
  c. Diagnostic studies
    1) Serum: ABGs: hypoxemia; hypercapnia
    2) CXR: may show evidence of RVF and/or pulmonary edema
    3) V/Q scan: similar to PE but may resolve within 24 hours
    4) Echocardiography: shows air in right ventricle, right ventricular dilation, and/or pulmonary hypertension

Collaborative Management
1. Prevent emboli formation.
  a. All patients

1) Deep breathing exercises hourly for postoperative patients
2) Ambulation as soon as possible
3) Leg exercises, especially for patients who cannot be ambulated; passive range of motion of all extremities for patients who cannot do leg exercises
4) Frequent repositioning; avoid extreme knee or hip flexion; instruct patient not to cross legs
5) Adequate fluid intake to prevent dehydration and hypercoagulability
6) Careful venipuncture and IV care
   a) Avoidance of venipunctures in legs
   b) Atraumatic venipuncture; avoid multiple sticks
b. Patients with moderate risk for VTE also require elastic stockings or intermittent pneumatic compression devices.
   1) Graduated compression: care must be taken to prevent constriction and tourniquet effect of stockings; efficacy is questionable.
   2) Intermittent pneumatic compression devices: also referred to as *sequential compression devices*
      a) Stimulates endogenous fibrinolytic activity in addition to direct physical stimulation of increased venous blood return
c. Patients with high risk for VTE without an associated diagnosis of cancer, DOACs (apixaban, dabigatran, edoxaban, rivaroxaban) are recommended over VKA (warfarin) therapy; for those with cancer, subcutaneous low-molecular-weight heparin (LMWH) is recommended over VKA therapy
d. Patients with documented VTE require low-dose unfractionated heparin (UFH) or LMWH.
2. Prevent dislodgment of clot.
   a. Monitor closely for clinical indications of VTE.
      1) Low-grade fever
      2) Calf pain or tenderness
      3) Unilateral edema, erythema, warmth, or dilated collateral veins
      4) Positive venography, venous duplex, and/or compression ultrasonography
   b. Instruct the patient regarding avoidance of Valsalva maneuver.
   c. Maintain steady IV flow rates.
   d. Avoid leg massage.
   e. Avoid bed rest for VTE unless there is substantial pain and swelling
3. Maintain adequate airway, ventilation, and oxygenation.
   a. Administer oxygen to maintain SpO_2 greater than 90%.
      1) Nasal cannula at 5 l/min unless contraindicated
      2) High concentrations of O_2 via nonrebreathing mask may be required to maintain an SpO_2 greater than ~90%.
   b. Administer analgesics as prescribed to prevent splinting and encourage deep breathing.
   c. Provide quiet, restful environment.
   d. Ensure intubation and mechanical ventilation if required (e.g., massive PE).
      1) In submassive PE, the primary initial problem in PE is diffusion due to the perfusion defect; the patient is generally ventilating adequately initially (frequently even excessively as evidenced by a low $PaCO_2$) but may require intubation and mechanical ventilation as respiratory muscle fatigue occurs.
4. Arrest thrombosis and reestablish perfusion.
   a. Obtain baseline clotting profile.
   b. Administer systemic fibrinolytic therapy as prescribed.
      1) Indications
         a) Hypodynamic instability
         b) Acute RVF
         c) Significant hypoxemia despite optimal oxygen therapy
      2) Actions
         a) Dissolves recent clots promptly to speed pulmonary tissue reperfusion
         b) Reverses RVF
         c) Improves pulmonary capillary blood; systemic therapy is preferred over catheter-direct fibrinolytic therapy volume
      3) Systemic agents and typical dose; systemic therapy is preferred over catheter-direct fibrinolytic therapy
         a) Tissue plasminogen activator (tPA): alteplase 100 mg over 2 hours
         b) Streptokinase: 250,000 units IV during the initial 30 minutes; then 100,000 units/hr for 24 hours
         c) Urokinase: 4400 units/kg IV during the initial 10 minutes; then 4400 units/kg/hr for 12 hours
      4) Contraindications and nursing management as in MI section of Chapter 3
      5) Anticoagulation follows fibrinolytic therapy.
   c. Administer anticoagulants as prescribed for stable patients.
      1) Action: prevents extension of the clot and reocclusion
      2) Parenteral agents: usually maintained for 7 to 10 days
         a) Fondaparinux: a factor Xa inhibitor
            i) Dose administered subcutaneously
               (a) Body weight less than 50 kg: 5 mg
               (b) Body weight 50 to 100 kg: 7.5 mg
               (c) Body weight greater than 100 kg: 10 mg
            ii) Advantages
               (a) Lower risk of heparin-induced thrombocytopenia and thrombosis (HITT) than with heparin
               (b) Lower risk of major bleeding than with heparin
         b) LMWH: indirect thrombin inhibitor
            i) Agents
               (a) Enoxaparin (Lovenox): 1 mg/kg subcutaneously every 12 hours
            ii) Advantages
               (a) Longer plasma half-life than UFH
               (b) More predictable anticoagulant response to weight-adjusted doses than UFH

(c) No need to monitor clotting studies, although monitoring is indicated in patients who are morbidly obese, have renal insufficiency, or who weigh less than 50 kg
(d) Lower incidence of HITT
iii) Potential disadvantage: longer half-life and lesser reversibility with protamine than UFH
c) UFH: indirect thrombin inhibitor
i) Dose: bolus 70 to 80 units/kg initially followed by 15 to 20 units/kg/hr to maintain activated partial thromboplastin time at 60 to 80 seconds; higher doses may be necessary initially because of low antithrombin III levels after PE
d) For patients with HITT (also referred to as *heparin-associated thrombocytopenia* or *white clot syndrome*)
i) Lepirudin
ii) Argatroban
3) Oral agents: VKA (e.g., warfarin) or DOACs (apixaban or rivaroxaban)
a) Usually Started before parenteral anticoagulants are discontinued and continued for up to 6 to 12 months
b) Usual starting dose is 5 mg/day and adjusted to maintain INR of 2 to 3
d. Prepare patient for pulmonary embolectomy as requested: indicated for patient with massive PE with hemodynamic instability (e.g., cardiogenic shock) who cannot receive fibrinolytic therapy
1) Surgical embolectomy
a) Complication rates for pulmonary embolectomy are relatively very high
b) Requires cardiopulmonary bypass
2) Catheter embolectomy
a) Clot fragmentation using pigtail catheter
b) Rheolytic thrombectomy using high-velocity saline jet (e.g., AngioJet)
c) Clot aspiration (e.g., transluminal extraction catheter)
e. Prepare patient for insertion of inferior vena caval filter as requested; note that these are no longer recommended because of complications associated with the device.
1) Possible indications
a) Recurrent PE despite effective anticoagulation
b) Anticoagulants are contraindicated.
c) Note that these are effective in protecting the lung from successive emboli, but they do not do anything about the current PE.
2) Types
a) Simon nitinol filter
b) Greenfield filter
c) Bird nest filter
d) TrapEase filter
3) Possible complications: migration of the device into a distal blood vessel or erosion of the device into the vessel wall.
f. Provide treatment of pulmonary hypertension and acute RVF as prescribed.
1) First priority is elimination of the pulmonary vascular obstruction and reduction of PVR: fibrinolytics, embolectomy
2) Inotropes (e.g., dobutamine) and fluids may also be prescribed to ensure adequate left ventricular contractility and filling volume to maintain CO.
g. Administer antibiotics as prescribed for septic emboli (rather than fibrinolytics and anticoagulants).
5. Monitor for complications.
a. Pulmonary infarction
b. Cerebral infarction
c. Myocardial infarction
d. RVF
e. Dysrhythmias or blocks
1) Atrial dysrhythmias are common if RVF occurs.
2) Ventricular dysrhythmias may occur in hypoxemia.
3) RBBB may occur but is usually transient.
f. Hepatic congestion and necrosis
g. Pneumonia
h. Pulmonary abscess
i. ARDS
j. DIC
k. Shock
l. Complications of therapy
1) Bleeding related to fibrinolytic or anticoagulant therapy
2) Oxygen toxicity related to high concentrations of oxygen
6. Specific to fat embolism
a. Prevention: early immobilization of long-bone fractures
b. Treatment
1) Oxygen via nasal cannula at 5 l/min unless contraindicated; 100% nonrebreathing mask may be necessary to maintain SpO_2 of at least 94%
2) Intubation and mechanical ventilation may be necessary.
3) Steroids (e.g., hydrocortisone) to decrease inflammatory response (controversial)
4) Fluids to flush the fatty acids and prevent renal damage
5) Osmotic diuretics: if pulmonary edema is present
6) Red blood cells and/or platelets may be necessary
7. Specific to air embolism
a. Prevention
1) Priming of IV tubing and central catheters with fluid to remove air before connection or insertion
2) Use of IV pumps with air detectors
3) Use of twist-lock connections on central venous catheters to prevent accidental disconnections
4) Positioning of patient in Trendelenburg position for the insertion of central venous catheters or treatment of chest trauma unless contraindicated (e.g., head trauma)
5) Instruction of the patient to hold his or her breath and bear down (i.e., Valsalva maneuver) during tubing changes and catheter removal
6) Use of pressure dressing to central venous site at time of catheter removal

b. Treatment
1) Left lateral decubitus position with head down (referred to as *Durant maneuver*) if air embolism suspected
2) Attempt to aspirate the air embolus.
3) External cardiac compressions push air out of the right ventricle into the pulmonary circulation, fragmenting the air bolus into smaller air bubbles.
4) Oxygen via 100% nonrebreathing mask; hyperbaric oxygen is indicated for arterial embolization and clinical deterioration
5) Anticoagulants may be administered.

Chest Trauma

General Information
1. Types of trauma
    a. Blunt trauma leaves the body surface intact.
    b. Penetrating trauma disrupts the body surface.
    c. Perforating trauma leaves both entrance and exit wounds as an object passes through the body.
2. Etiology
    a. Motor vehicle collision
    b. Motorcycle collision
    c. Vehicle/pedestrian collision
    d. Fall
    e. Assault
    f. Explosion (i.e., blast injury)
    g. Projectiles: bullet, knives, impalement
3. Mechanisms of injury
    a. Blunt chest trauma
        1) Rapid acceleration/deceleration: shearing force causes stretching of tissue, organs, blood vessels with resultant tearing, leaking, or rupture.
        2) Direct impact: object striking chest or chest striking object causes rib, sternal, or scapular fractures or injury to the heart or lung parenchyma.
        3) Compression: force of rapid deceleration as tissues hit a fixed object, such as the sternum or rib cage; causes concussion, contusion, bleeding, or rupture of an organ
    b. Penetrating chest trauma
        1) Penetration of lung, heart, great vessel, or diaphragm causes bleeding and may cause loss of intactness of an organ or vessel.

Pulmonary Contusion
1. Definition: damage to the lung parenchyma that results in localized edema and hemorrhage
2. Etiology
    a. High-velocity blunt trauma dispersed across the chest; occurs in approximately 75% of blunt trauma patients
    b. Crush injuries
    c. Chest compressions during cardiopulmonary resuscitation
    d. Frequently associated with other chest injuries (e.g., flail chest)
3. Pathophysiology
    a. Blunt trauma causes deceleration injury to chest wall and compression of thoracic cavity.
    b. Diminished thoracic size compresses lung tissue, and decompression causes capillary rupture and subsequent hemorrhage.
    c. Initial hemorrhage caused by bruising, pulmonary tears, or lacerations
        1) Interstitial and alveolar edema at site of contusion
        2) Massive interstitial edema with general inflammation
        3) Damaged or closed alveolar-capillary units cause V/Q mismatch and shunt.
        4) Increased PVR, decreased lung compliance, and decreased pulmonary blood flow occur.
        5) Atelectasis may occur because of retained secretions and infection.
    d. Severe pulmonary lacerations may cause concurrent hemothorax.
    e. Pulmonary contusion may accompany flail chest and may be masked by the obvious ventilation difficulties seen in flail chest.
4. Clinical presentation (may be delayed 24–48 hours)
    a. Subjective
        1) Anxiety, restlessness
        2) Dyspnea
        3) Chest tenderness
    b. Objective
        1) Tachycardia
        2) Tachypnea
        3) Increased work of breathing: use of accessory muscles; tripod position
        4) Ecchymosis at site of impact
        5) Ineffective cough, guarding
        6) Hemoptysis
        7) Crepitus or deformity noted on palpation if rib fractures
        8) Subcutaneous emphysema: suggests concurrent pneumothorax or upper airway injury
        9) Dullness to percussion on affected side
        10) Breath sound changes: crackles, wheezes
    c. Diagnostic studies
        1) ABGs
            a) Decreased PaO_2
            b) $PaCO_2$ may be normal or decreased depending on ventilation pattern (e.g., may be low due to hyperventilation or high if pain or fatigue causes hypoventilation).
        2) CXR
            a) Changes may take 2 to 24 hours to develop on CXR: patchy, poorly defined areas of increased parenchymal density reflecting intraalveolar hemorrhage; linear and irregular infiltrates in the bronchioles
            b) If severe, extensive areas of increased parenchymal density within one or both lungs
            c) Diaphragm may be lower on affected side as injured lung is bigger.
            d) To differentiate ARDS from pulmonary contusion
                i) Pulmonary contusion is usually localized and occurs near the site of external trauma.
                ii) ARDS causes diffuse bilateral changes.

3) CT scan: assesses damage to pulmonary parenchyma and pleural cavity
5. Collaborative management
   a. Establish and maintain airway, ventilation, and oxygenation.
      1) Oxygen per nasal cannula at 2 to 6 l/min to achieve a SpO_2 greater than 94% unless contraindicated; if patient has history of COPD, administer oxygen to achieve an oxygen saturation of ~90% by pulse oximetry
      2) Analgesics in doses adequate to allow patient to turn and deep breathe
      3) Airway clearance
         a) Suctioning if patient cannot cough adequately to clear airways
         b) Bronchoscopy may be necessary if airway clearance techniques are inadequate.
      4) Endotracheal intubation and mechanical ventilation with PEEP may be necessary.
         a) Synchronous independent lung ventilation may be necessary to prevent the detrimental effects of PEEP on the normal alveoli (e.g., increased alveolar pressure and decreased blood flow).
            i) Requires double-lumen ET tube and two mechanical ventilators
      5) Positioning with good lung down
      6) Careful fluid administration to prevent pulmonary edema
         a) Goal is usually to maintain RAP ~4 mm Hg and PAOP ~10 mm Hg.
         b) Diuretics may also be given.
      7) Steroids were given frequently in the past but are no longer recommended because of the risk of resultant immunosuppression and infection.
   b. Control pain.
      1) Narcotics given on a regular schedule
      2) Intercostal nerve block
      3) Epidural analgesic with a basal rate and PCA
   c. Monitor for complications.
      1) Pneumonia: very common complication
         a) Prophylactic antibiotics are not recommended; antibiotics are indicated only if infection is present.
         b) Culture sputum as indicated
      2) Lung abscess
      3) Empyema
      4) Pulmonary edema
      5) PE
      6) ARDS

Closed (Noncommunicating) Pneumothorax (Fig. 4.40)

1. Definition: air enters the intrapleural space through the lung, causing partial or total collapse of the lung.
   a. Small: less than 15%
   b. Medium: 15% to 60%
   c. Large: greater than 60%
2. Etiology
   a. Primary: related to congenital bleb (common in endomorphic males, age 20–40 years)
   b. Secondary
      1) Emphysematous bullous
      2) Tuberculosis
      3) Lung cancer
   c. Traumatic
      1) Blunt trauma caused by motor vehicle collision, falls, blows to chest, blast injuries
      2) Cardiopulmonary resuscitation
      3) Positive-pressure mechanical ventilator
   d. Iatrogenic causes: central venous catheterization via subclavian or low jugular vein puncture; intracardiac injection; thoracentesis; positive pressure ventilation
3. Pathophysiology
   a. Disruption of normal negative intrapleural pressure
      1) Lung laceration by rib fracture or needle
      2) Compression of the lung at the height of inspiration when alveolar pressure is high
      3) Rupture of weak alveolus, bleb, or bullous
   b. Lung collapse
   c. Decreased surface area for exchange of gases
   d. Acute respiratory failure
4. Clinical presentation
   a. Subjective
      1) Dyspnea
      2) Chest pain: sudden, sharp, may be referred to corresponding shoulder, across chest, or abdomen
   b. Objective
      1) Tachycardia
      2) Tachypnea
      3) Cough: dry, nonproductive
      4) Asymmetrical chest excursion with limited motion of affected hemithorax
      5) Subcutaneous emphysema possible
      6) Decreased fremitus on affected side
      7) Hyperresonance to percussion on affected side
      8) Diminished to absent breath sounds on affected side
      9) Clinical indications of hypoxemia may be present
      10) If patient on mechanical ventilator
         a) Dramatic increase in peak inspiratory pressures
         b) High pressure alarm
   c. Diagnostic studies
      1) ABGs
         a) Decreased PaO_2
         b) Increased $PaCO_2$
      2) CXR
         a) Air in pleural space and lung collapse on affected side
         b) May show mediastinal shift toward unaffected side
      3) CT of thorax: better at detecting very small or anterior pneumothorax, which may be missed on CXR
5. Collaborative management
   a. Establish and maintain airway, ventilation, and oxygenation.
      1) Oxygen per nasal cannula at 1 to 6 l/min to achieve a SpO_2 greater than 94% unless contraindicated; if patient has history of COPD, administer oxygen to achieve an oxygen saturation of ~90% by pulse oximetry

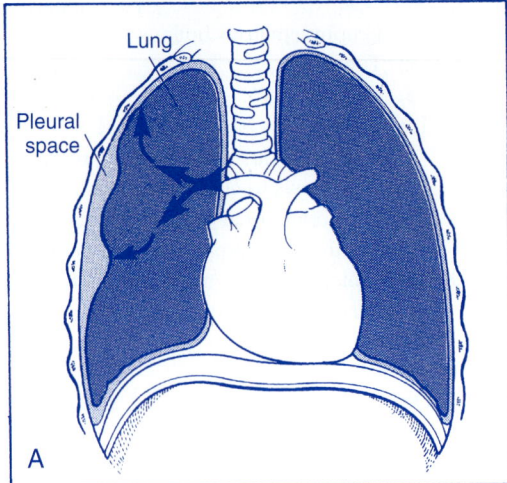
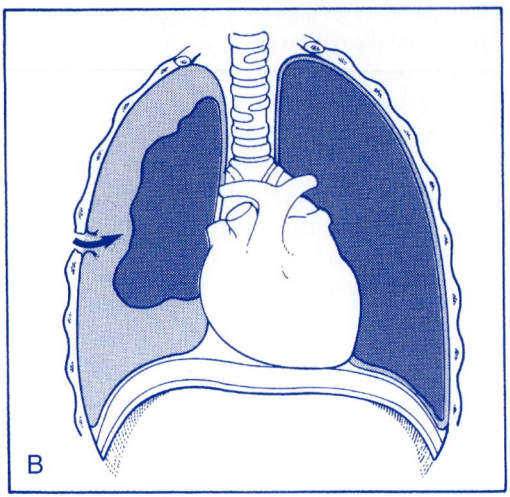
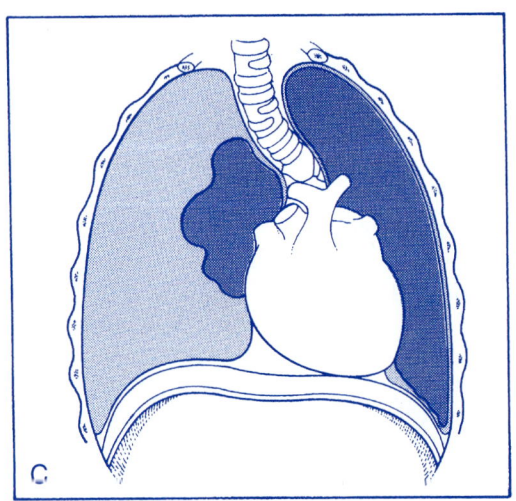

Fig. 4.40 Pneumothorax. **A,** Closed. **B,** Open. **C,** Tension. (From Wilson, T. [1990]. *Respiratory disorders [Mosby's clinical nursing series].* St. Louis: Mosby.)

      2) Analgesics in doses adequate to allow patient to deep breathe and cough as indicated
      3) Positioning for optimal ventilation: semi-Fowler or Fowler position
         a) If supine: position with good lung down.
      4) Sustained inspiratory maneuvers such as deep breathing and incentive spirometry; only necessary treatment for small (<15%) pneumothorax
      5) Chest tube (not necessary if <15% and asymptomatic)
         a) Inserted into fourth to fifth intercostal space at midaxillary line
         b) Connected to a Heimlich flutter valve or chest drainage system
  b. Control pain: narcotics given on a regular schedule
  c. Monitor for complications
      1) Recurrent pneumothorax
         a) Avoidance of intermittent positive pressure breathing (IPPB) in patients with COPD
         b) If positive-pressure mechanical ventilation: careful adjustment of V_T and PEEP; close monitoring of peak inspiratory pressures
         c) Careful placement of subclavian or jugular venous catheters
         d) Decortication may be performed for patients with recurrent spontaneous pneumothorax; involves the stripping of the parietal pleura from the apex of the lung to allow the visceral pleura to adhere to the chest wall
      2) Atelectasis
      3) Pneumonia, abscess

Tension Pneumothorax (Fig. 4.41)
1. Definition: accumulation of air in pleural space without means of escape causing complete collapse of lung and potential mediastinal shift
2. Etiology
  a. Blunt or penetrating trauma
  b. Positive-pressure mechanical ventilation, especially if patient:

1) Has emphysematous bullae or congenital blebs
2) Receiving large V_Ts and/or PEEP
   c. Nonfunctional (e.g., clotted or clamped) chest drainage system
   d. Occlusive dressing on an open pneumothorax
3. Pathophysiology
   a. Air rushes into, but not out of, the pleural space.
   b. Disruption of negative intrapleural pressure; creation of a positive pressure in the pleural space
   c. Ipsilateral lung collapses
   d. If tear does not seal, a one-way valve effect may be produced, allowing air to enter during inspiration but not to escape during exhalation.
   e. Increasing positive intrapleural pressure may cause mediastinal shift, leading to compression of the contralateral lung, thoracic aorta, vena cava, and heart.
   f. Decreased right ventricular filling, decreased CO
   g. Acute respiratory failure and shock may occur.
4. Clinical presentation
   a. Subjective
      1) Dyspnea
      2) Chest pain
   b. Objective
      1) Tachycardia
      2) Tachypnea
      3) Asymmetrical chest excursion with limited motion of affected hemithorax
      4) Subcutaneous emphysema possible
      5) Decreased fremitus on affected side
      6) Hyperresonance to percussion on affected side; may even be tympanic
      7) Diminished to absent breath sounds on affected side
      8) Clinical indications of hypoxemia may be present.
      9) If mediastinal shift:
         a) Tracheal shift away from affected side
         b) PMI shift away from affected side
         c) Jugular venous distention
         d) Hypotension
   c. Diagnostic studies
      1) ABGs
         a) Decreased PaO_2
         b) Increased $PaCO_2$
      2) CXR
         a) Absence of lung marking on the affected side
         b) Widening of the intercostal spaces on the affected side
         c) Mediastinal shift (away from the affected side) may be present.
5. Collaborative management
   a. Establish and maintain airway, ventilation, and oxygenation.
      1) Oxygen per nasal cannula at 2 to 5 l/min to achieve a SpO_2 greater than 94% unless contraindicated; if patient has history of COPD, administer oxygen to achieve an oxygen saturation of ~90% by pulse oximetry
      2) Emergency decompression with perpendicular insertion of a large-bore needle (or IV catheter [e.g., Angiocath]) into second anterior interspace at the midclavicular line on the affected side until a chest tube can be inserted; a flutter valve (e.g., Heimlich valve, finger cot with a slit cut at the end) may be placed on the needle to allow air to escape but prevent atmospheric air from entering the pleural space
      3) Chest tube and chest drainage system
      4) Analgesics in doses adequate to allow patient to deep breathe and cough as indicated
      5) Position for optimal ventilation: semi-Fowler or Fowler position
      6) If supine: position with good lung down
   b. Control pain: narcotics given on a regular schedule or by PCA
   c. Monitor for complications.
      1) Shock
      2) Cardiopulmonary arrest
      3) Atelectasis
      4) Pneumonia, abscess

Open (Communicating) Pneumothorax
Also Called *Sucking Chest Wound* (Fig. 4.41)
1. Definition: air enters the interpleural space through the chest wall.
2. Etiology: penetrating trauma

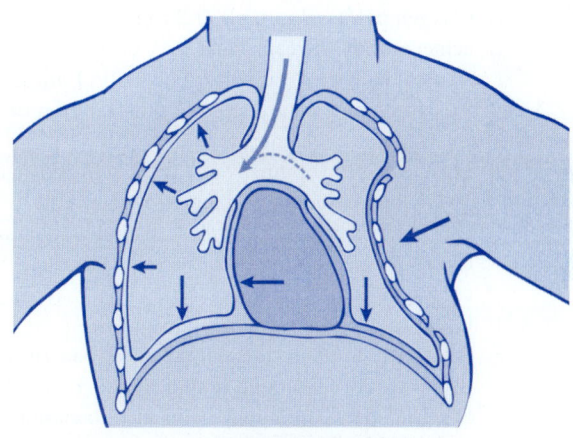

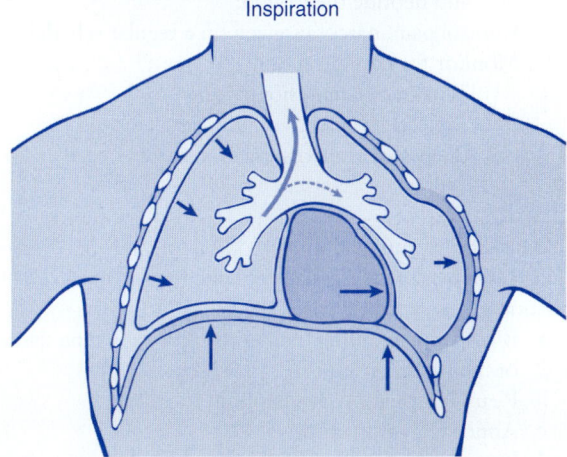

Fig. 4.41 Flail chest produces paradoxical chest excursion. On inspiration, the flail section sinks in. On expiration, the flail section bulges outward.

3. Pathophysiology
   a. Communication between the intrathoracic space and the atmosphere results in equilibrium between intrathoracic and atmospheric pressures.
   b. Air movement in and out of opening in chest wall
   c. If opening in chest wall is smaller than diameter of trachea, patient may tolerate condition well.
   d. If opening is larger, more air enters pleural space than enters lungs through trachea.
   e. During inspiration, the affected lung collapses, resulting in ineffective gas exchange.
   f. May cause tension pneumothorax
4. Clinical presentation
   a. Subjective
      1) Dyspnea
      2) Chest pain
   b. Objective
      1) Tachycardia
      2) Tachypnea
      3) Obvious wound with noise of air moving in and out of pleural space
      4) Subcutaneous emphysema is usually present.
   c. Other subjective, objective, and diagnostic findings as for closed pneumothorax
5. Collaborative management
   a. Establish and maintain airway, ventilation, and oxygenation.
      1) Oxygen per nasal cannula at 2 to 5 l/min to achieve a SpO$_2$ greater than 94% unless contraindicated; if patient has history of COPD, administer oxygen to achieve an oxygen saturation of ~90% by pulse oximetry
      2) Positioning for optimal ventilation: semi-Fowler or Fowler position, good lung down or back
      3) Closure of open sucking chest wound with gauze dressing taped on three sides so that air can escape during expiration
      4) Chest tube and water-seal drainage
      5) Analgesics in doses adequate to allow patient to deep breathe and cough as indicated
      6) Surgical intervention may be needed to explore and débride the wound.
   b. Control pain: narcotics given on a regular schedule
   c. Monitor for complications.
      1) Tension pneumothorax
      2) Atelectasis
      3) Pneumonia, abscess

Hemothorax

1. Definition: accumulation of blood in pleural space, causing compression and collapse of the lung
2. Etiology
   a. Blunt or penetrating trauma to chest wall, lung tissue, or mediastinum
   b. Pleural or pulmonary neoplasm
   c. Anticoagulant therapy
   d. Iatrogenic causes: subclavian vein puncture (e.g., insertion of deep vein catheter), lung biopsy
3. Pathophysiology
   a. Hemorrhage into pleural space compresses and collapses lung.
   b. Ventilation and oxygenation are impaired.
   c. Hemorrhage may lead to shock.
4. Clinical presentation
   a. Subjective
      1) Chest pain may be present.
      2) Dyspnea
   b. Objective
      1) Tachycardia
      2) Hypotension
      3) Asymmetrical chest excursion with limited motion of affected hemithorax
      4) Dullness to percussion on affected side
      5) Diminished or absent breath sounds on affected side
      6) May have clinical indications of shock if greater than 400 ml
   c. Diagnostic studies
      1) Serum
         a) Hgb and hematocrit: may be decreased but remember that changes may occur for up to 6 hours after blood loss
         b) ABGs
            i) Decreased PaO$_2$
            ii) Increased PaCO$_2$
      2) CXR
         a) Fluid in pleural space and lung compression
         b) Blunting of costophrenic angle if greater than 250 ml
         c) Hazy appearance over the lower chest
5. Collaborative management
   a. Establish and maintain airway, ventilation, and oxygenation.
      1) Oxygen per nasal cannula at 2 to 5 l/min to achieve a SpO$_2$ greater than 94% unless contraindicated; if patient has history of COPD, administer oxygen to achieve an oxygen saturation of ~90% by pulse oximetry
      2) Chest tube with chest drainage system may be adequate treatment if bleeding is self-limiting.
      3) Indications for surgery for isolation and repair of source of hemorrhage
         a) Initial drainage of more than 1500 ml of blood after placement of chest tube
         b) Drainage of blood at rate greater than 250 ml/hr for more than 2 hours after placement of chest tube
         c) Hemodynamic instability despite fluid resuscitation
      4) Positioning for optimal ventilation
         a) Semi-Fowler or Fowler position unless patient has significant hypotension with HOB elevated
         b) After thoracotomy, nonoperative ("good") lung down or supine with regular turning
   b. Maintain perfusion and adequate circulating volume.
      1) Fluids and/or blood transfusion may be necessary.
      2) Autotransfusion may be indicated if blood loss is greater than 400 ml.
   c. Control pain: narcotics given on a regular schedule
   d. Monitor for complications
      1) Atelectasis
      2) Shock

Rib Fracture, Sternal Fracture, and Flail Chest

1. Definition
   a. Rib fracture: break in the bony continuity of the ribs
   b. Sternal fracture: break in the bony continuity of the sternum
   c. Flail chest: instability of chest wall as a result of multiple rib or sternal fractures causing paradoxical movement of the chest wall during ventilation
      1) Two or more ribs broken in two or more places
      2) Fractured sternum
      3) Sternotomy that hasn't healed
2. Etiology
   a. Blunt trauma from motor vehicle collision, assault
   b. Relatively minor trauma in patients with the following:
      1) Osteoporosis
      2) Total sternectomy
      3) Multiple myeloma
3. Pathophysiology
   a. Rib fracture
      1) Fracture of the first and second rib is rare and requires extreme force so suspect underlying injury to great vessel, lungs, and spine
      2) If left lower rib fractures, suspect spleen injuries
      3) If right lower rib fractures, suspect hepatic injury
      4) Older adult patients are more likely to have complications because they are likely to have senile emphysema and concurrent cardiopulmonary disease.
   b. Sternal fracture
      1) Tremendous force (i.e., impact with steering wheel) required to cause sternal fracture
         a) This force may also cause myocardial contusion or cardiac tamponade.
      2) Most common location is the junction of the manubrium and body of the sternum.
   c. Flail chest (Fig. 4.41)
      1) Fractured segment is free of the bony thorax and moves independently in response to intrathoracic pressure.
         a) During inspiration, atmospheric pressure exceeds intrathoracic pressure on affected side, causing chest wall to move inward.
         b) On expiration, intrathoracic pressure exceeds atmospheric pressure, causing chest wall to move outward until the thorax contracts.
      2) The bellows effect of the thorax is lost; intrapleural pressure is less negative than normal.
      3) Ventilation is diminished; V_T is decreased, causing hypercapnia and resultant hypoxemia; atelectasis may occur.
      4) Increased work of breathing causes fatigue.
      5) Note related injuries: pulmonary contusion frequently accompanies flail chest; pneumothorax, pleural effusion may also be present
4. Clinical presentation
   a. Subjective
      1) Dyspnea
      2) Chest pain: related to inspiration, movement, coughing
      3) Chest tenderness to palpation
   b. Objective
      1) Tachycardia
      2) Tachypnea
      3) Diminished air movement at mouth and nose
      4) Ineffective cough
      5) Ecchymosis over thorax
      6) Paradoxical movement of flail segment
      7) Palpable detached segment, bony crepitation at fracture sites
      8) Subcutaneous emphysema with pneumothorax or laryngeal injury
      9) Breath sound changes: diminished breath sounds on affected side
      10) Clinical indications of hypoxia (Box 4.3)
   c. Diagnostic studies
      1) ABGs
         a) Decreased PaO_2
         b) Decreased SaO_2
         c) Increased $PaCO_2$
      2) Spirometry: decreased V_T and VC
      3) ECG: to assess for indications of myocardial contusion if sternal fracture
      4) Echocardiography: to assess for cardiac tamponade if sternal fracture
      5) CXR: rib and/or sternal fractures
      6) CT scan of chest: shows fractures
5. Collaborative management
   a. Establish and maintain airway, ventilation, and oxygenation.
      1) Oxygen per nasal cannula at 2 to 5 l/min to achieve a SpO_2 greater than 94% unless contraindicated; if patient has history of COPD, administer oxygen to achieve an oxygen saturation of ~90% by pulse oximetry
      2) Reestablishment of the thoracic bellows effect
         a) Stabilization of flail segment with hand or tape (temporary); avoid binding or constricting chest excursion
         b) Position on affected side if cervical spine fracture has been ruled out.
         c) Intubation and internal stabilization with mechanical ventilation may be necessary if patient cannot maintain adequate ventilation despite adequate analgesia.
            i) Indications: respiratory rate greater than 35, PaO_2 less than 60 mm Hg with supplemental oxygen; $PaCO_2$ greater than 50 mm Hg
            ii) Mechanical ventilation may need to be maintained for 3 weeks or longer
         d) Surgical internal fixation of rib and sternal fragments with plates and screws may be done for multiple rib fractures or flail chest, especially if thoracotomy is needed for another reason.
         e) Surgical reduction of displaced sternal fracture
      3) Chest physiotherapy
         a) Deep breathing and incentive spirometry
         b) Positioning for optimal ventilation: semi-Fowler or Fowler position

c) PD, percussion, vibration
      i) Do not percuss over fractured areas.
   d) Coughing; suctioning if coughing is ineffective and rhonchi are present
   e) Bronchoscopy may be necessary if airway clearance is inadequate.
 b. Provide adequate analgesia to encourage deep breathing (and coughing if indicated).
   1) Epidural analgesia
   2) IV narcotics
   3) Intercostal nerve blocks
   4) Intrapleural analgesia
 c. Assist in insertion of chest tube and establish water-seal drainage if pneumothorax is also present.
 d. Monitor for complications.
   1) Pain
   2) Nonunion
   3) Permanent chest wall deformity
   4) Atelectasis
   5) Pneumonia, abscess

Diaphragmatic Rupture

1. Definition: rupture of the diaphragm allowing the movement of abdominal contents into the thorax
2. Etiology: injury below nipple line, in flanks, or lateral chest wall
   a. Blunt trauma from motor vehicle collision, assault, or fall against an immobile object
   b. Penetrating injury such as from a gunshot or knife wound
   c. There may be a latent period after the injury.
3. Pathophysiology
   a. Opening in the diaphragm
      1) Blunt trauma
         a) More common on the left side because the left hemidiaphragm is weaker than the right, and the right hemidiaphragm is somewhat protected by the liver
         b) A sudden, dramatic increase in abdominal or thoracic pressure causes a tear in the diaphragm.
      2) Penetrating trauma causes a perforation in the diaphragm.
   b. The intrathoracic pressure is negative, and the intraabdominal pressure is positive.
   c. The size of the rupture determines the extent to which the organs migrate upward: the stomach and/or loops of intestine may enter the chest and compromise lung expansion.
   d. Ventilation problems are most evident if the left hemidiaphragm is affected because when the right hemidiaphragm is affected, the liver is fixed and cannot move upward into the thorax.
      1) Abdominal contents compress the lung on the affected side and may even cause mediastinal shift.
      2) The decrease in the effectiveness of the diaphragm causes ineffective ventilatory excursion.
4. Clinical presentation
   a. Subjective
      1) Dyspnea
      2) Dysphagia
      3) May have nausea, eructation
      4) Pain in shoulder, chest or abdomen
         a) Kehr sign: pain radiates to left shoulder (as a result of injury to the phrenic nerve)
         b) Exacerbated by supine position
   b. Objective
      1) Obvious injury to chest, abdomen
      2) Ecchymosis
      3) Tachypnea
      4) Tachycardia, hypotension
      5) Crepitus or deformity on palpation
      6) JVD if a mediastinal shift occurs
      7) Heart sounds may be shifted to opposite side of the injury.
      8) Diminished or absent breath sounds on the affected side
      9) Abdominal distention
      10) Bowel sounds audible over the affected side of the chest
      11) If chest tubes are placed for another condition, may see fecal matter or undigested food in the chest drainage system
   c. Diagnostic studies
      1) CXR
         a) Normal if no abdominal contents displaced in chest
         b) May have unilateral elevation of hemidiaphragm
         c) May have hollow or solid mass above the diaphragm (the stomach) may be visible
         d) May have mediastinal shift away from affected side
         e) May place NG tube before radiography, and tube will be seen in the chest
      2) CT of the chest and abdomen
         a) Confirms rupture of the diaphragm and any movement of abdominal contents into the thorax
         b) Focused assessment sonography trauma (FAST): indicates if intraabdominal fluid is present
5. Collaborative management
   a. Establish and maintain airway, ventilation, and oxygenation.
      1) Oxygen by nasal cannula at 2 to 6 l/min to maintain SpO$_2$ of 94% unless contraindicated; in patients with COPD, use pulse oximetry to guide oxygen administration to SpO$_2$ of 90%
      2) Elevation of HOB to 30 to 45 degrees; overbed table may be helpful for patient to lean on.
      3) Surgical intervention to pull the abdominal organs back into the abdomen and repair the diaphragm; prophylactic antibiotics will be prescribed
      4) Chest tube and drainage system as required for pneumothorax
      5) Deep breathing and incentive spirometry to prevent atelectasis
      6) NG tube placement to decompress the stomach

b. Maintain adequate circulation.
   1) IV access for fluid and medication administration
   2) Hydration
      a) IV fluids: usually 0.9% saline
      b) Avoidance of overhydration because the patient may have associated pulmonary contusion and be at risk for ARDS
c. Control pain, discomfort, and anxiety.
   1) NSAIDs and/or narcotic analgesics in doses that will allow patient to deep breathe and cough may be indicated.
   2) Anxiolytics may be indicated.
d. Monitor for complications.
   1) Atelectasis
   2) Pneumonia, abscess
   3) Bowel strangulation
   4) Tension viscerothorax: chest tube is indicated
   5) Sepsis
   6) Shock

Tracheobronchial Injury

1. Definition: disruption in the integrity of the tracheobronchial tree; usually occurs at the proximal trachea or near the carina
2. Predisposing factors
   a. Blunt trauma (e.g., motor vehicle collision [MVC], clothesline injury): most common cause resulting in a partial or complete tear of the tracheal or bronchial wall
   b. Deceleration injuries: can cause shearing forces between the fixed carina or proximal bronchus
   c. Rapid anteroposterior compression of the chest: can cause lateral traction on the lungs resulting in a tearing of the bronchus from the fixed carina
      1) Rupture can occur from an abrupt increase in pressure against a closed glottis.
   d. Compression of the trachea between the sternum and spinal column
   e. Penetrating trauma
3. Pathophysiology
   a. Injury causes a tear of the bronchial tree
   b. Ineffective ventilation as inspired air escapes into the thoracic cavity and does not reach the lungs
   c. Swelling can cause airway obstruction.
   d. Severity of symptoms related to the level of the injury, degree of injury, and airflow changes that occur
4. Clinical presentation
   a. Subjective
      1) History of trauma; injury may go unrecognized for 3 to 4 days
      2) Pain that increases with breathing and swallowing
      3) Dyspnea
   b. Objective
      1) Tachycardia
      2) Tachypnea
      3) Clinical indications of respiratory distress (Box 4.2)
         a) Sitting up and leaning forward
         b) Use of inspiratory accessory muscles in neck and shoulders
      4) Hoarse voice
      5) May have stridor
      6) Hemoptysis
      7) Chest contusion, ecchymosis, or wound
      8) Altered level of consciousness
      9) Subcutaneous emphysema palpated in the chest, face, neck, and/or suprasternal area
      10) Breath sound changes: decreased or absent on the affected side
      11) Hamman sign: mediastinal crunch associated with pneumomediastinum
      12) Persistent air leak from chest tube
   c. Diagnostic studies
      1) ABGs: may show hypoxemia
      2) Radiography
         a) Soft tissue lateral neck films
         b) Chest: pneumomediastinum below the carina
      3) Bronchoscopy: direct visualization of injury
5. Collaborative management
   a. Establish and maintain airway, ventilation, and oxygenation.
      1) After tracheobronchial injury is confirmed, prepare for RSI and intubation even if there is no evidence of respiratory compromise.
         a) Placement of ET below the level of injury
         b) Cricothyrotomy or emergent tracheostomy may be required.
      2) Oxygen by nasal cannula at 2 to 6 l/min to maintain SpO$_2$ of 94% unless contraindicated; in patients with COPD, use pulse oximetry to guide oxygen administration to SpO$_2$ of 90%
      3) Elevation of HOB to 30 to 45 degrees
      4) Open chest wounds should be covered; remove if clinical indications of tension pneumothorax occur.
      5) Thoracotomy for surgical repair
      6) Deep breathing and incentive spirometry to prevent atelectasis
      7) NG tube placement to decompress the stomach
   b. Maintain adequate circulation.
      1) IV access for fluid and medication administration
      2) Hydration
         a) IV fluids: usually 0.9% saline
         b) Warming of fluids, especially if patient is hypothermic
   c. Control pain, discomfort, and anxiety.
      1) NSAIDs and/or narcotic analgesics in doses that will allow patient to deep breathe and cough may be indicated.
      2) Anxiolytics may be indicated.
   d. Monitor for complications.
      1) Airway obstruction
      2) Acute respiratory failure
      3) Shock

Learning Activities

Chapter 4

1. Complete the following crossword puzzle to review pulmonary anatomy, physiology, and assessment.

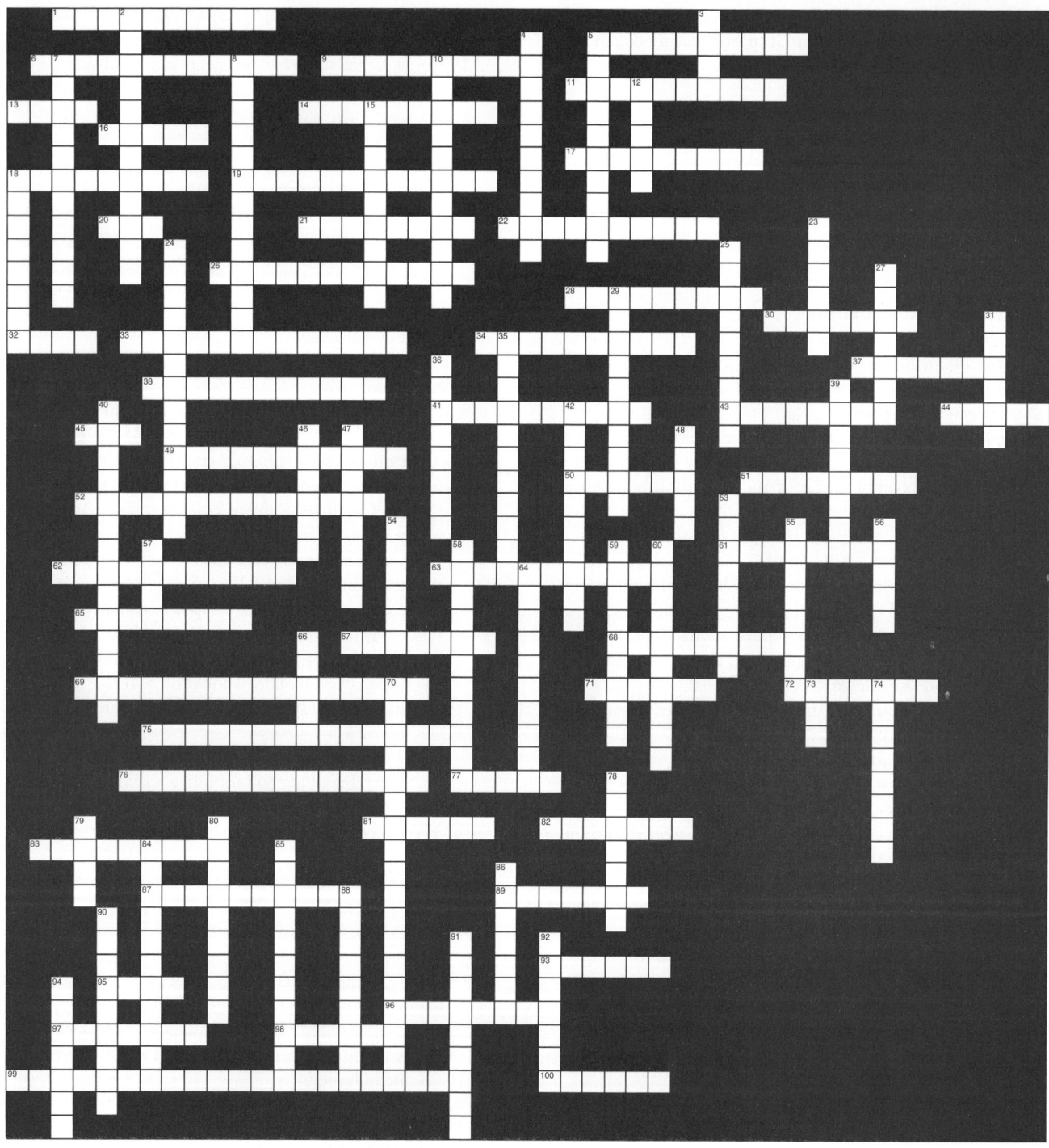

ACROSS

1. These structures increase the surface area in the nose
5. The flexible cartilage attached to the thyroid cartilage; closes to protect the larynx
6. The avascular membrane that can be punctured or opened with a scalpel to provide an emergency airway
9. The change in pressure for a given change in volume
11. Measurement of lung volumes
13. The type of cell that secretes histamine
14. This acid–base imbalance would cause the oxyhemoglobin dissociation curve to shift to the left
16. When deoxygenated blood comes in contact with nonventilated alveoli; V less than Q
17. Rapid breathing
18. A pulmonary embolism would decrease _____ relative to ventilation
19. These cellular organelles use oxygen and nutrients to make ATP
20. A decrease in surfactant would cause a decrease in compliance and an increase in _____ (abbrev.)
21. Alkalosis increases the _____ between hemoglobin and oxygen which impairs oxygen drop-off at the tissue
22. A phagocyte in the alveoli
26. In this type of acid–base imbalance, one system (i.e., respiratory or renal) changes as a result of an abnormality in the other system
28. These normal breath sounds are heard over peripheral lung
30. The passage through the vocal cords
32. A shift of the oxyhemoglobin dissociation curve to the _____ would improve pick-up at the lung but impair drop-off to the tissues
33. This gas is 20 × more diffusible than oxygen (2 words)
34. The area between the soft palate and the base of the tongue; the center for the gag reflex is located here
37. The area of the left lung that corresponds to the right middle lobe
38. The movement of air into and out of the lungs
41. Airway _____ affects the work of breathing
43. This nailbed change is associated with chronic hypoxia
44. Decreased compliance of the chest wall occurs in _____
45. This adventitious breath sound is associated with pleurisy
49. The eustachian tubes open into the _____
50. A dense concentration of lymphatic tissue which guards entryways into the GI or respiratory tracts
51. Noninvasive method of measuring arterial oxygen saturation
52. The lowest portion of the pharynx
61. The type of dead space which describes the air in the alveoli that are not perfused; V greater than Q
62. Measurement of expired carbon dioxide tension
63. This type of disorder is when expansion of the alveolus, lung, or chest wall is impaired, and compliance is decreased
65. An enzyme that breaks down elastic tissue
67. These chemoreceptors are primarily sensitive to blood carbon dioxide levels
68. A decrease in blood oxygen; manifested by a decrease in PaO_2 and SaO_2
69. These normal breath sounds are heard over the mainstem bronchi
71. The first portion of the trachea
72. Shift of this structure is seen with mediastinal shift
75. The cause of hypoxemia in myasthenia gravis would be alveolar _____
76. These receptors cause an increase in ventilation rate in response to body movement
77. In this type of acid–base imbalance, there are two disorders occurring concurrently
81. The area at the bifurcation of the trachea; rich in parasympathetic fibers
82. These sounds are heard when listening with a stethoscope to a patient with pneumonia or chronic bronchitis
83. The nutrient circulation of the lung is supplied by this artery
87. Surfactant is produced by the type II _____
89. A decrease in tissue oxygen; manifested by SNS innervation, cyanosis, restlessness or confusion
93. A cause of hypoxia even though the patient has a normal PaO_2
95. Percussion tone heard over pleural effusion
96. This acid–base imbalance causes vasodilation resulting in headache, flushed face, and hypotension
97. Shortness of breath
98. The terminal respiratory unit which has an alveolar-capillary membrane for the exchange of oxygen and carbon dioxide
99. This is caused most commonly by hypoxemia (2 words)
100. Respiratory pattern with normal rate and depth

DOWN

2. A procedure to view the bronchioles with a fiber-optic scope
3. This structure is primarily responsible for warming, humidifying, and filtering inspired air
4. These chemoreceptors are primarily sensitive to blood oxygen levels
5. The passive phase of ventilation
7. The first bronchial branch, which is part of the gas exchange unit is the _____ bronchiole
8. The _____ dissociation curve shows the relationship between PaO_2 and SaO_2
10. The active phase of ventilation
12. A shift of the oxyhemoglobin dissociation curve to the ___ would decrease the affinity between hemoglobin and oxygen
15. The main accessory muscles of expiration are the internal intercostal and _____ muscles
18. The pleural layer that is contiguous with the chest wall
23. _____ law is why the PaO_2 goes down if the $PaCO_2$ goes up (assuming room air)
24. Percussion tone heard over hyperinflated lung
25. Area of ventilation without perfusion (2 words)
27. This pressure is calculated by multiplying the FiO_2 (as a decimal) by the barometric pressure (760 mm Hg at sea level)
29. A lipoprotein that decreases surface tension and keeps the alveoli open at low distending pressure
31. The type of compliance which reflects the compliance of the lung and the chest wall

370 Chapter 4 The Pulmonary System

15. Match the ventilator mode, setting, or parameter with the correct description.

   ____ 1. Control
   ____ 2. Assist-control
   ____ 3. Synchronized intermittent mandatory ventilation
   ____ 4. Pressure support ventilation
   ____ 5. Pressure-controlled ventilation
   ____ 6. Independent lung ventilation
   ____ 7. High-frequency ventilation
   ____ 8. Pressure-regulated volume-controlled
   ____ 9. Bi-PAP
   ____ 10. Airway pressure release ventilation
   ____ 11. Tidal volume
   ____ 12. Positive end-expiratory pressure
   ____ 13. Sigh
   ____ 14. Peak inspiratory pressure
   ____ 15. FiO_2
   ____ 16. Plateau pressure
   ____ 17. Continuous positive airway pressure

   a. Augments a patient-initiated breath by using positive pressure to reduce the work of breathing
   b. Pressure measured at inflation hold, which is used to calculate static compliance
   c. Combines pressure support ventilation (PSV) and continuous positive airway pressure (CPAP)
   d. Useful for patients with unilateral lung disease, such as a pulmonary contusion
   e. Ventilator delivers a mandatory number of breaths per minute but allows the client to breathe spontaneously between set rate
   f. Varies the flow rate and flow waveform to deliver the desired volume at the desired pressure
   g. Provides short periods of lower pressure during CPAP to allow further expiration
   h. Uses small tidal volumes and rapid rates to keep airway pressures lower
   i. Maintains a closed circuit between control breaths so the patient cannot take additional breaths
   j. Ends inspiration when a preset pressure is reached; tidal volume is variable
   k. Occasional breaths with volume 1.5 to 2 times the tidal volume
   l. Positive pressure throughout the entire ventilatory process in a spontaneously breathing patient
   m. Volume of air given with each breath
   n. Percentage of oxygen expressed as a decimal
   o. Positive pressure maintained through the expiratory phase in a mechanically ventilated patient
   p. Pressure measured at the peak of inspiration which is used to calculate a dynamic compliance
   q. Allows the patient to trigger additional assisted breaths between control breaths

16. Identify four physiologic effects of PEEP and CPAP.
    a. _____
    b. _____
    c. _____
    d. _____

17. Identify if the following factors will cause a high-pressure or low exhaled volume alarm.

	High Pressure	Low Exhaled Volume
Cuff leak		
Bronchospasm		
Need for suctioning		
Disconnect		
Water condensation in tubing		
Pneumothorax		
ARDS		

18. Identify the values for the following parameters that indicate that the patient may be successfully weaned from mechanical ventilation.
    a. Spontaneous tidal volume_____
    b. Spontaneous vital capacity_____
    c. Maximal inspiratory pressure_____
    d. PaO_2 of at least _____ on an FiO_2 of no greater than _____ with no more than _____ cm H_2O PEEP.
    e. Rapid shallow breathing index _____

19. Complete the following table and determine if either of these patients is ready for weaning from mechanical ventilation.

	Patient A	**Patient B**
Age	38	64
Gender	F	M
Diagnosis	Asthma	ARDS
IBW	60 kg	75 kg
ABGs	FiO_2 of 0.28 pH 7.42 $PaCO_2$ 39 mm Hg HCO_3 25 mEq/l PaO_2 88 mm Hg SaO_2 98%	FiO_2 of 0.6 with 10 cm H_2O PEEP pH 7.32 $PaCO_2$ 50 mm Hg HCO_3 23 mEq/l PaO_2 55 mm Hg SaO_2 88%
Spontaneous V_T	350 ml	300 ml
Spontaneous vital capacity	650 ml	600 ml
Spontaneous minute ventilation		
NIF	−40 cm H_2O	−20 cm H_2O
Spontaneous respiratory rate	20/min	36/min
Rapid shallow breathing index (RSBI)		
Ready for weaning?		

20. Complete the following crossword puzzle regarding thoracic surgery and trauma.

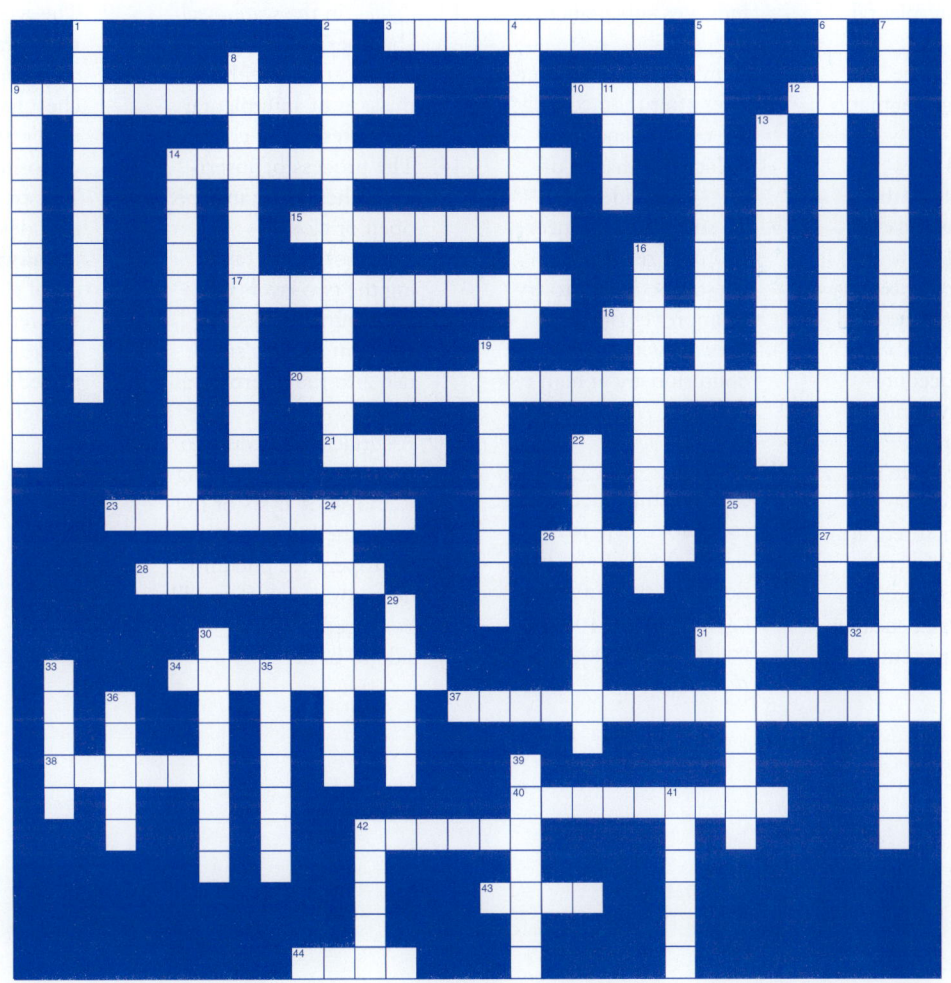

ACROSS

3. Rupture of this structure may cause bowel sounds to be heard over the thorax
9. A surgical procedure to remove an entire lung
10. This type of trauma can cause injury from acceleration/deceleration, direct impact, or compression
12. Patients with unilateral lung conditions (except pneumonectomy) should be placed on their _____ lung or their back
14. A surgical procedure to decrease the volume in a hemithorax after lung resection to prevent mediastinal shift
15. Edema and hemorrhage of the lung parenchyma caused by trauma is referred to as a pulmonary _____
17. The presence of lymph fluid in the interpleural space
18. _____ sign may be evident in diaphragmatic rupture
20. A connection between the bronchus and the pleura that causes a persistent air leak (2 words)
21. Another term for reduction pneumoplasty; used for emphysema (abbrev.)
23. A surgical procedure used in patients with myasthenia gravis
26. When two or more ribs are fractured or the sternum is fractured, a(n) _____ chest results
27. The type of pneumothorax that creates a sucking sound as the patient breathes
28. Patients with diaphragmatic rupture may have referred pain to the left _____
31. A type of sonography frequently used for trauma patients to quickly identify possible injuries (abbrev.)
32. A chest tube that is placed anterior and superior is intended to remove _____
34. A surgical procedure to remove a segment of the lung is referred to as a *segmental* _____
37. The presence of air and blood in the interpleural space; frequently surgically induced
38. This type of dysrhythmia is common after pneumonectomy
40. Crepitus around the chest tube insertion site indicates subcutaneous _____
42. Arm and shoulder exercises after thoracotomy are recommended to reduce the chance of _____ shoulder
43. To successively squeeze and then release the chest tube tubing to try to improve patency
44. Patients with pulmonary contusion are at high risk for _____ (abbrev.)

DOWN

1. A surgical procedure to remove hyperinflated areas of the lung done for patients with COPD; may also be called *lung volume reduction surgery*
2. Internal air leak indicates _____ fistula
4. The presence of blood in the interpleural space
5. This type of analgesia involves injection of a local anesthetic through a thoracostomy tube or catheter
6. A surgical procedure for cancer of the esophagus
7. This type of mechanical ventilation may be necessary in pulmonary contusion because one lung may be injured and the other not (3 words)
8. Pleural stripping for recurrent spontaneous pneumothorax
9. The presence of air in the interpleural space
11. Bubbling in the water-seal chamber indicates an air _____
13. _____ in the water-seal chamber indicates a patent chest tube with transmission of interpleural pressures to the chamber
14. The process of inserting a chest tube; may be open or closed
16. The process of fusing the two layers of the pleura by injecting an agent such as sterile talc into the interpleural space
19. A surgical procedure to remove a lobe of a lung
22. Removal of cysts or bullae in the lung
24. Postoperative pneumonectomy patients should be placed on their _____ side or back
25. A surgical procedure which opens the thorax
29. The type of pneumothorax that is caused by rupture of a congenital bleb or a fractured rib
30. A type of valve that may be used for pneumothorax with little or no liquid drainage
33. Epidural analgesia after thoracotomy should include a(n) _____ rate as well as patient-controlled analgesia
35. The presence of pus in the interpleural space
36. To hold the chest tube with thumb and forefinger of one hand and then slide the other thumb and forefinger down the tube and then release the first thumb and forefinger
39. The type of pneumothorax that results when pressure in the chest increases and the mediastinum shifts to the opposite side
41. This type of resection includes anastomosis of the airway proximal and distal to where the mass was removed
42. A chest tube that is placed lateral and inferior is intended to remove _____

21. List 10 possible causes of acute respiratory failure.

    a. _____
    b. _____
    c. _____
    d. _____
    e. _____
    f. _____
    g. _____
    h. _____
    i. _____
    j. _____

22. Match the cause of acute respiratory failure to the primary treatment.

    ____ 1. Upper airway obstruction   a. Antimicrobials
    ____ 2. Airway secretions   b. Deep breathing and incentive spirometry
    ____ 3. Overdosage of narcotics   c. Chest tube
    ____ 4. Bronchospasm   d. Positioning and airway placement
    ____ 5. Pneumothorax   e. Cholinergic drugs and mechanical ventilator
    ____ 6. Pneumonia   f. Encouragement of coughing; suctioning if cannot effectively cough
    ____ 7. Postoperative pain   g. PEEP
    ____ 8. ARDS   h. Bronchodilators
    ____ 9. Myasthenic crisis   i. Naloxone (Narcan)
    ____ 10. Atelectasis   j. Analgesics

23. Answer the following questions and explain your logic with a clinical example.
    a. If the PaO_2 is decreased, must the $PaCO_2$ be increased?
    _____
    b. If the $PaCO_2$ is increased, must the PaO_2 be decreased?
    _____

24. List five pulmonary and five nonpulmonary causes for acute respiratory distress syndrome (ARDS).

Pulmonary	Nonpulmonary
a.	f.
b.	g.
c.	h.
d.	i.
e.	j.

374 Chapter 4 The Pulmonary System

25. Match the treatment to the pathophysiology of ARDS. Choices may be used more than once.

____ 1. Pulmonary hypertension
____ 2. Intrapulmonary shunt
____ 3. Ventilation/perfusion mismatch
____ 4. Diffusion defect
____ 5. Pulmonary edema

a. PEEP
b. Nitric oxide
c. Fluid restriction and diuretics
d. High concentrations of oxygen
e. Prone positioning

26. Identify whether the following microorganisms are associated with community-acquired pneumonia (CAP) or health care-acquired pneumonia (HCAP). Choices may be used more than once.

Staphylococcus aureus	
Serratia marcescens	
Escherichia coli	
Legionella pneumophila	
Proteus mirabilis	
Bacteroides fragilis	
Hantavirus	

27. List three nursing interventions to prevent aspiration in a patient on enteral feedings.

a. _____

b. _____

c. _____

28. Complete the following table describing arterial blood gas changes in asthma using ↑ for increased, ↓ for decreased, or ↔ for no change.

Stage	PaO_2	$PaCO_2$	pH	Acid–Base Imbalance
I				
II				
III				
IV				

29. List four classifications of bronchodilators and an example of each.

Classification	Example
1.	
2.	
3.	
4.	

30. List three causes of pulmonary embolism in each of the following categories.

Hypercoagulability	Alteration in Blood Vessel	Venous Stasis

31. Match the treatment to the pathology in pulmonary embolism. Choices may be used more than once.

    ____ 1. Forward failure of left ventricle
    ____ 2. Pulmonary hypertension
    ____ 3. Occlusion of pulmonary blood supply
    ____ 4. Backward failure of right ventricle
    ____ 5. Low levels of antithrombin III
    ____ 6. V/Q mismatch

    a. Pulmonary embolectomy
    b. Dobutamine
    c. Heparin
    d. Tissue plasminogen activator (tPA)
    e. Fluids
    f. Oxygen

32. Identify whether the parameters in this case study are decreased, normal, or increased. Discuss implications and treatment goals.

    The patient is a 65-year-old woman admitted with a fractured hip. She had surgery 2 weeks ago. Earlier today she complained about chest pain, shortness of breath, and a feeling of doom. ABGs revealed respiratory alkalosis and hypoxemia. After she was transferred to the critical care unit, the physician inserted a pulmonary artery catheter to aid in diagnosis and evaluation of therapy. The patient's BSA is 1.6 m^2.

Parameter	↑, ↓, or Normal	Parameter	↑, ↓, or Normal
BP: 112/84 mm Hg		SV: 40 ml/beat	
MAP: 93 mm Hg		SI: 25 ml/m^2/beat	
HR 110 beats/min		SVR: 1364 dynes/sec/cm^{-5}	
RAP: 18 mm Hg		SVRI: 2182 dynes/sec/cm^{-5}	
PAP: 55/32 mm Hg		PVR: 618 dynes/sec/cm^{-5}	
PAm: 40 mm Hg		PVRI: 989 dynes/sec/cm^{-5}	
PAOP: 6 mm Hg		LVSWI: 30 g m/m^2	
CO: 4.4 l/min		RVSWI: 7 g m/m^2	
CI: 2.75 l/min/m^2		SvO$_2$: 58%	
SaO$_2$: 85% on 5 l/min by nasal cannula		DO$_2$I: 470 ml/min/m^2	

Implications and treatment goals: _____
_____
_____
_____
_____
_____

33. Match the clinical presentation to the type of chest trauma.

    ____ 1. Pulmonary contusion
    ____ 2. Flail chest
    ____ 3. Simple pneumothorax
    ____ 4. Hemothorax
    ____ 5. Tension pneumothorax
    ____ 6. Diaphragmatic rupture

    a. Chest pain, dyspnea, diminished breath sounds on affected side, hyperresonance to percussion, tracheal shift away from affected side
    b. Chest pain, dyspnea, diminished breath sounds on affected side, hyperresonance to percussion, tracheal shift toward affected side
    c. Ecchymosis at site of impact, chest tenderness, dyspnea, hemoptysis
    d. Epigastric pain, dyspnea, dysphagia, bowel sounds audible over affected side of chest
    e. Chest pain, dyspnea, diminished breath sounds on affected side, dullness to percussion
    f. Chest tenderness, dyspnea, paradoxical chest movement

376 Chapter 4 The Pulmonary System

34. Complete the following crossword puzzle to review pulmonary drugs and therapies.

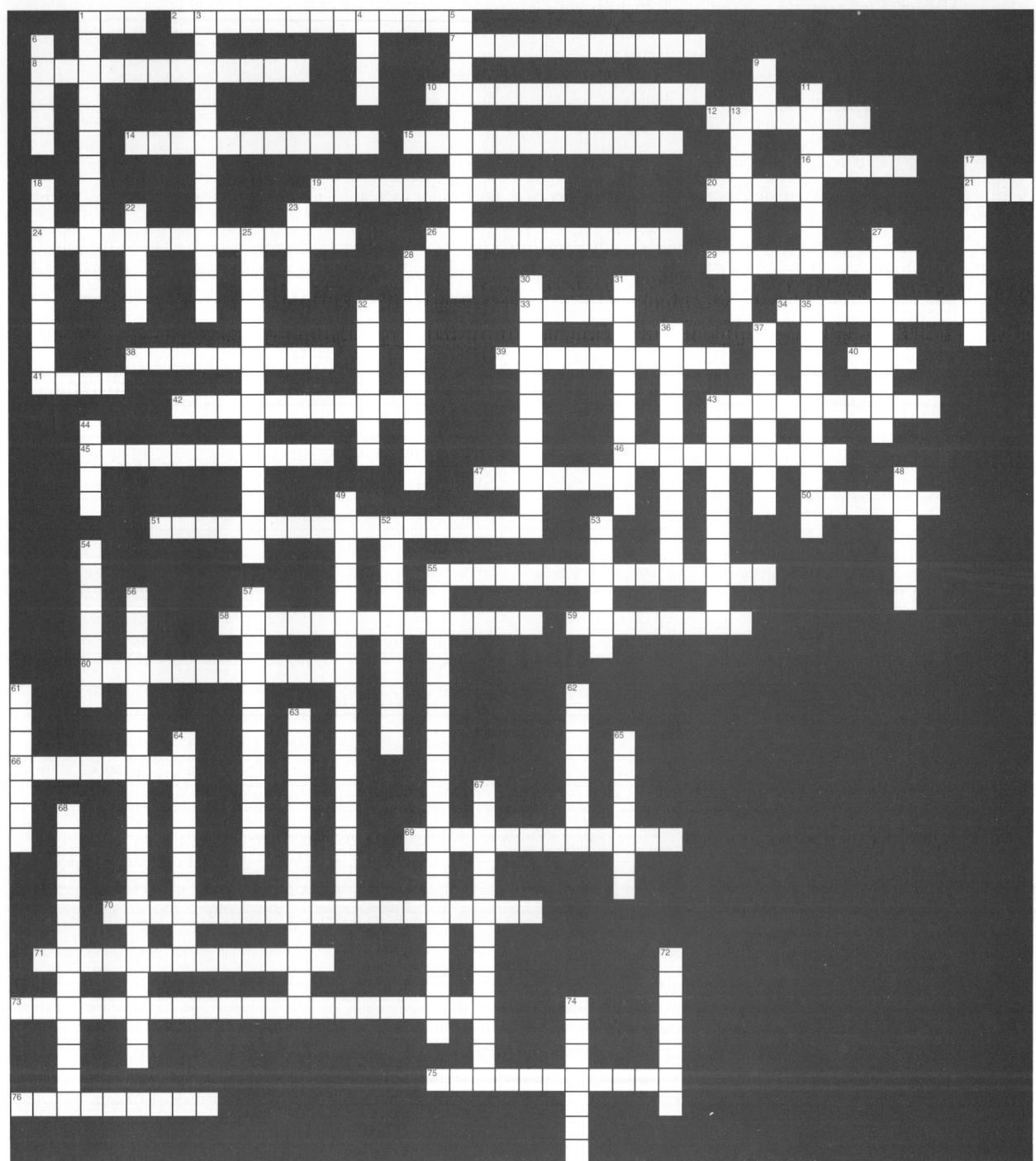

ACROSS

1. $PaCO_2$ of greater than 50 mm Hg and/or PaO_2 of less than 50-60 mm Hg (abbrev)
2. A drug that may be given in metabolic alkalosis; may cause metabolic acidosis
7. Inflammatory mediators including leukotrienes are released by _____ in ARDS
8. Pulmonary _____ is when the pulmonary vascular pressures are elevated
10. Results from release of erythropoietin in response to chronically low oxygen levels
12. A drug used to prevent extension or recurrence of a clot in patients with pulmonary embolism (generic)
14. Collapse of alveoli; frequently seen in postoperative patients
15. Pulmonary edema in ARDS is caused by increased capillary _____
16. The first treatment for asthma is the elimination of _____
19. This type of disorder is when expansion of the alveolus, lung, or chest wall is impaired and compliance is decreased
20. The most likely cause of ARDS
21. This may be caused by pulmonary hypertension (abbrev.)
24. A steroid that is frequently given by inhalation in patients with asthma (generic)

26. A beta₂ stimulant that may be given orally, subcutaneously, or by inhalation (generic)
29. Antibiotic _____ gram-positive bacterial strains have increased the mortality rate of health care-acquired pneumonia
33. Patient position recommended to optimize ventilation/perfusion matching in patients with ARDS
34. A pulmonary embolism would decrease _____ relative to ventilation
38. A drug used in patients with pulmonary embolism with acute right ventricular failure or refractory hypoxemia to break down the clot (generic)
39. Surfactant is produced by the type II _____
40. A decrease in surfactant would cause a decrease in compliance and an increase in _____ (abbrev)
41. Type of heparin that may be administered subcutaneously to prevent deep vein thrombosis and pulmonary embolism (abbrev)
42. Complication caused by hyperventilation in status asthmaticus
43. More likely to occur in the right lung
45. Treatment of pneumonia includes oxygen, bronchial hygiene, and _____
46. Drug used for stress ulcer prophylaxis that does not support gastric colonization (generic)
47. These sounds are heard when listening with a stethoscope to a patient with pneumonia or chronic bronchitis
50. Indicated when SaO₂ is less than 90%
51. This condition is characterized by an increase in the number and size of mucous and goblet cells
55. The cause of hypoxemia in myasthenia gravis would be alveolar _____
58. These receptors cause an increase in ventilation rate in response to body movement
59. A feeling of impending doom is a symptom of massive pulmonary _____
60. A prostanoid-type pulmonary vasodilator (generic)
66. Most community-acquired pneumonia caused by gram _____ bacteria
69. A procedure to view the bronchioles with a fiber-optic scope
70. This is caused by histamine
71. A diagnostic study to obtain fluid from the pleural space for analysis
73. This is caused by the decrease in PaO₂ in COPD, ARDS, and PE (2 words)
75. This type of disorder is when airway resistance is increased
76. This type of chest pain is sharp pain which occurs with deep inspiration

DOWN
1. IV antifungal (generic)
3. Fibrous exudate causes the _____ in pneumonia which is manifested by crackles, bronchial breath sounds, egophony, and whispered pectoriloquy
4. A form of noncardiac pulmonary edema caused by inflammatory mediators and surfactant deficiency (abbrev)
5. This type airway provides a relative seal to allow mechanical ventilation without the surgical risks of tracheostomy
6. When deoxygenated blood comes in contact with nonventilated alveoli; V less than Q
9. The most common pneumonia in AIDS patients (abbrev.)
11. These sounds are heard when listening with a stethoscope to a patient with atelectasis, pulmonary edema, and ARDS
13. This disorder is a chronic obstructive lung disease associated with the breakdown of elastic tissue, air trapping, and dyspnea
17. Chronic air _____ cause the shape of the thorax to change to be barrel-shaped
18. A beta₂ stimulant which is administered orally or by inhalation
22. Two common symptoms of pulmonary conditions are dyspnea and _____
23. The goal of oxygen therapy in this condition is to keep the SaO₂ at around 90% (abbrev.)
25. A drug that breaks down the disulfide bonds in mucus (generic)
27. Inflammation of the alveoli and bronchioles
28. A muscle paralytic that may be administered by IV infusion in patients on mechanical ventilation (generic)
30. This type of pneumothorax is most often associated with rupture of a congenital bleb
31. Bloody sputum; may be seen in lung cancer or tuberculosis
32. This habit is the No. 1 cause of COPD
35. Patients with obstructive disease have prolonged _____
36. Increased PaCO₂
37. A sedative frequently used in mechanically ventilated patients (generic)
43. Group of drugs that should be administered to allow a patient to breathe deeply after thoracotomy
44. The type of cell that secretes histamine
48. A gas which may be used in place of nitrogen in inspired air for patients with increased airway resistance
49. This diagnostic study is used to evaluate the adequacy of ventilation and oxygenation (3 words)
52. Another name for health care-acquired pneumonia
53. Also referred to as restrictive airway disease; mucosal swelling and smooth muscle spasm cause wheezing and increased airway resistance
54. These sounds are heard when listening with a stethoscope to a patient with asthma (plural)
55. Another term for type I acute respiratory failure (2 words)
56. Another term for type II acute respiratory failure (2 words)
57. An antibiotic which may be used to increase gastric motility (generic)
61. Shortness of breath
62. Placing a patient with an air embolism in a left lateral decubitus position with his or her head down is referred to as _____ maneuver (possessive)
63. This level increases in asthma, causing bronchospasm and increased mucus secretion
64. Airway _____ affects the work of breathing
65. Testing sputum for _____ is a common method to check for aspiration of enteral feeding
67. Impaired _____ is the risk factor most commonly associated with aspiration
68. A xanthine bronchodilator; also dilates pulmonary vasculature (generic)
72. Shift of this structure is seen with mediastinal shift
74. _____ triad are three things that predispose to clot formation: hypercoagulability, venous stasis, and vascular injury

The Neurologic System

CHAPTER 5

Selected Concepts in Anatomy and Physiology

General Information
1. Functions of the neurologic system
   a. Receiving stimuli from the internal and external environment over sensory pathways
   b. Communicating information between the body periphery and the central nervous system (CNS)
   c. Processing information received at reflex or conscious levels to determine appropriate responses
   d. Transmitting information over motor pathways to organs responsible for responding to the stimuli
2. Components of the neurologic system
   a. CNS
      1) Brain
      2) Spinal cord
   b. Peripheral nervous system
      1) Cranial nerves (CNs)
      2) Spinal nerves
      3) Peripheral nerves
   c. Autonomic nervous system (ANS)
      1) Sympathetic nervous system (SNS)
      2) Parasympathetic nervous system (PNS)

Microscopic Anatomy and Physiology
1. Nerve cells
   a. Neuroglia (also called *glial cells*)
      1) Neuroglia are more numerous than neurons (85% of the cells in the CNS are neuroglial).
      2) These cells provide support, nourishment, and protection to the neurons.
      3) Most tumors of the CNS are neuroglial because they are mitotic and can replicate themselves.
      4) Types
         a) Microglia
            i) Part of the reticuloendothelial system
            ii) Relatively rare in normal CNS tissue
            iii) Become mobile and travel to the area of damage when the neurons become damaged; microglia then enlarge and phagocytize tissue debris
         b) Oligodendroglia: responsible for myelin formation in the CNS
         c) Astrocytes
            i) May provide nutrients and regulate chemical environment for neurons
            ii) Wrap their foot processes around the epithelial cells of brain capillaries; this helps form the blood–brain barrier (BBB) (Sugarman, 2014).
            iii) Provide structure and support for nerve cells
            iv) May have indirect role in synaptic transmission
         d) Ependyma
            i) Line the ventricles of brain and central canal of spinal cord
            ii) Aid in secretion of cerebrospinal fluid (CSF)
   b. Neurons (Fig. 5.1)
      1) Transmit nerve impulses
      2) Ten billion in CNS; most are in the cerebral cortex
      3) Cannot regenerate in the CNS; can regenerate in peripheral nervous system by growing within the myelin if the cell body is intact
      4) Components
         a) Cell body (soma)
            i) Nucleus: controls metabolic processes of cell
            ii) Cytoplasm: contains organelles to carry out metabolic functions
         b) Axons
            i) Conduct impulses away from cell body to other neurons or to end organs
            ii) One axon per neuron
            iii) May be myelinated or unmyelinated
         c) Dendrites
            i) Conduct impulses toward cell body, which receives nerve impulses from the axons of other neurons
            ii) May be more than one dendrite
         d) Neurofibrils: thin, threadlike fibers forming a network in the cytoplasm

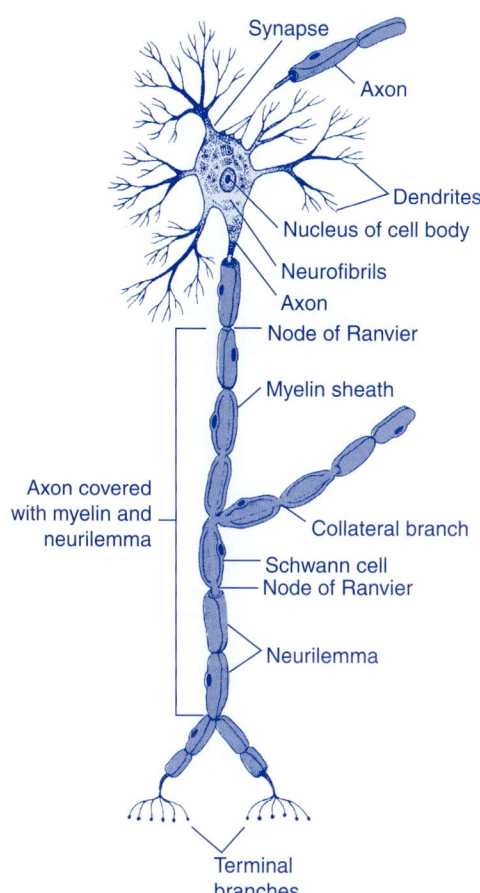

Fig. 5.1 The neuron. (From Black, J. M., & Hawks, J. A. [2009]. *Medical-surgical nursing: Clinical management for positive outcomes* [8th ed.]. Philadelphia: Saunders.)

- e) Nissl bodies
  - i) Specialize in protein synthesis with RNA
  - ii) Maintain and regenerate neuronal processes
- f) Myelin sheath
  - i) In some neurons, the axons covered with myelin, a white lipid substance, between the nodes of Ranvier
  - ii) Acts as insulation to speed conduction of impulses down the axon sheath
  - iii) Accounts for white color found in parts of brain and spinal cord
  - iv) Made by oligodendroglia in the CNS and by Schwann cells in the PNS
- g) Nodes of Ranvier
  - i) Constrictions occurring periodically along the axon where it is not covered by myelin
  - ii) Allows rapid conduction of impulses by saltatory conduction (node to node)
- h) Neurilemma
  - i) Outer coating of the neurons in the peripheral nervous system
  - ii) Provides for peripheral nerve regeneration
- i) Synaptic knobs: contain vesicles that store neurotransmitter substances

5) Categorization
  a) Direction of impulse formation
    i) Afferent sensory neurons transmit impulses to the spinal cord or brain.
    ii) Efferent motor neurons transmit impulses away from the brain or spinal cord.
    iii) Remember SA ME (sensory afferent, motor efferent).
    iv) Interneurons transmit impulses from sensory neurons to motor neurons.
  b) Number of processes
    i) Pseudounipolar (i.e., unipolar neurons) are sensory neurons (Mtui, Gruener, & Dockery, 2016).
      (1) One short process coming from the cell body
        (a) Bifurcates into a long peripheral branch and a long central branch
        (b) Peripheral branch sends sensory information from a somatic or visceral structure (i.e., skin, skeletal muscle, or intestinal wall)
          (i) Distal end of peripheral process ends in dendrite-like tendrils
          (ii) Receive information from certain receptors in skin, muscles, or joints
        (c) Central branch sends sensory information to the CNS.
          (i) In effect, the distal and central processes function together as a single axon (Naftel, Ard, & Fratkin, 2013).
        (d) True unipolar neurons found primarily in invertebrates.
        (e) Vertebrate neurons with a unipolar appearance are actually pseudounipolar.
          (i) Started as bipolar neurons
          (ii) During cell body development, a short part of the extensions fuse together, causing the stalk from which the peripheral and central processes project (Vanderah & Gould, 2016).
    ii) Bipolar neurons
      (1) Two distinct processes arising from the cell body
      (2) Commonly found in structures associated with the special senses (visual, auditory, and vestibular systems).
      (3) This type connects to rod and cone cells of the retina (Kierszenbaum & Tres, 2016; Naftel et al., 2013).
    iii) Multipolar neurons are the most common
      (1) Have multiple dendrites and a single axon

Table 5.1 Neurologic System Neurotransmitters

Name	Type	Region	Predominant Effect
Acetylcholine	Cholinergic	• Basal ganglia • Pyramidal cells • Parasympathetic branch of ANS	Excitatory
Norepinephrine	Amine	• Hypothalamus • Brainstem • Sympathetic branch of ANS	Inhibitory/excitatory
Dopamine	Amine	• Basal ganglia • Brainstem	Inhibitory
Serotonin	Amine	• Hypothalamus • Brainstem	Inhibitory
Gamma-aminobutyric acid (GABA)	Amino acid	• Basal ganglia • Cerebellum • Spinal cord	Inhibitory
Glycine	Amino acid	• Spinal cord	Inhibitory
Beta-endorphins	Peptide	• Spinal cord	Inhibitory
Substance P	Peptide	• Pain fibers in spinal cord	Excitatory

ANS, Autonomic nervous system.

        (2) Typical examples: pyramidal cells of the cerebral cortex and Purkinje cells and neurons of the cerebellar cortex (i.e., motor impulses or communication between neurons) (Kierszenbaum & Tres, 2016).
    c) Location
        i) Upper motor neurons (UMNs) originate above the brainstem.
        ii) Lower motor neurons (LMNs) originate below the brainstem.
2. Neurophysiology
   a. Impulse transmission
     1) Initiated by a stimulus: chemical, electrical, mechanical, thermal
     2) Change in permeability of the cell membrane to sodium
     3) Depolarization of the cell caused by sodium influx; initiation of an action potential
     4) Repolarization and return to normal resting polarized (ready) state occurs
     5) Synaptic transmission
        a) Unidirectional conduction of an impulse from one neuron to the next
        b) As the impulse nears the end of the axon, a release of neurotransmitter from the synaptic vesicles
        c) Diffusion of neurotransmitter across the synaptic gap changing the permeability of the cell membrane of the adjoining cell
        d) Continuation of the impulse to its end-organ or cell
        e) Types of synapses
           i) Axosomatic: the axon of one neuron synapses with the cell body of another neuron
           ii) Axodendritic: the axon of one neuron synapses with the dendrite of another neuron
           iii) Axoaxonic: the axon of one neuron synapses with the axon of another neuron
   b. Refractory periods
     1) Absolute: period of time when the nerve cannot be stimulated again
     2) Relative: period of time when the nerve can only be stimulated by a strong impulse
3. Cerebral neurotransmitters (Table 5.1)
   a. Function
     1) Neurotransmitters are released from the presynaptic vesicles and act as a chemical bridge for the transmission of impulses from one neuron to another.
     2) After synaptic transmission, the neurotransmitter is inactivated by an enzyme (e.g., cholinesterase deactivates acetylcholine).
   b. Types
     1) Excitatory neurotransmitters promote conduction of the impulse from one cell to the next.
     2) Inhibitory neurotransmitters increase resistance to depolarization.
4. Cerebral metabolism
   a. Oxygen requirements
     1) The brain weighs 2% of body weight but receives 20% of the cardiac output (CO) and uses 20% of oxygen delivered.
     2) The brain, especially the cerebral cortex, is very susceptible to change in oxygen delivery; the brainstem is the most resistant to hypoxic damage.
     3) Anoxia causes brain edema and neuron death.
   b. Nutrient requirements
     1) The brain has high metabolic energy needs.
     2) Glucose is the main source of cellular energy (adenosine triphosphate [ATP]).
        a) Triggered by the SNS, gluconeogenesis is a very important process because it causes the conversion of protein and fat to glucose; the brain does not require insulin to use glucose.

b) Hypoglycemia is associated with neurologic symptoms.
    i) Confusion usually occurs if blood glucose is less than 50 to 70 mg/dl.
    ii) Coma occurs if blood glucose is less than 20 mg/dl.
c) Although hyperglycemia does not cause direct neurologic effects, the osmotic effect may cause hyperosmolality and brain dehydration (e.g., hyperglycemic hyperosmolar state [HHS]).
3) Vitamins
   a) Thiamine (B_1) is important in the Krebs cycle; deficiency of B_1 causes Wernicke encephalopathy.
   b) Vitamin B_{12} is important in the spinal cord and peripheral nervous system; deficiency of vitamin B_{12} causes pernicious anemia and gradual deterioration of the CNS and peripheral nerves.
   c) Pyridoxine (B_6) is a coenzyme that participates in many enzymatic reactions in the CNS; deficiency of B_6 causes neuropathy and seizures.
   d) Niacin (nicotinic acid) is needed for the synthesis of coenzymes; deficiency of niacin causes pellagra.
5. BBB
   a. Not a true structure but a special permeability characteristic of the brain capillaries and choroid plexus
   b. Functions
      1) Acts to limit transfer of certain substances into extracellular fluid (ECF) or CSF of the brain
      2) Prevents toxic substances from readily entering the extracellular space of the nervous system; may hinder the effective use of certain drug therapies in the treatment of neurologic system problems
      3) May be altered by trauma, induction of some toxic elements, intracranial tumor, or brain irradiation

Macroscopic Anatomy and Physiology

1. Scalp: skin covering the cranium
   a. Made of five layers
      1) **S**kin: thicker than anywhere else in the body
      2) **C**utaneous tissue
      3) **A**dipose tissue
      4) **L**igament layer referred to as *galea aponeurotica*; moves freely over the skull
      5) **P**ericranium
   b. Blood vessels located in the subcutaneous tissue
      1) The scalp is very vascular.
      2) Blood vessels here do not contract well when injured.
      3) Scalp laceration can result in significant blood loss.
2. Skull (Fig. 5.2): bony structure of the head consisting of the cranium and the skeleton of the face
   a. The skull is composed of an inner table and outer table separated by cancellous (spongy) bone; this structure allows for maximum strength and minimal weight.
   b. The cranium is a bony vault that holds and protects the brain from external forces; volume capacity is approximately 1500 ml.
   c. The cranium consists of 8 bones
      1) Frontal: 1
      2) Parietal: 2
      3) Temporal: 2

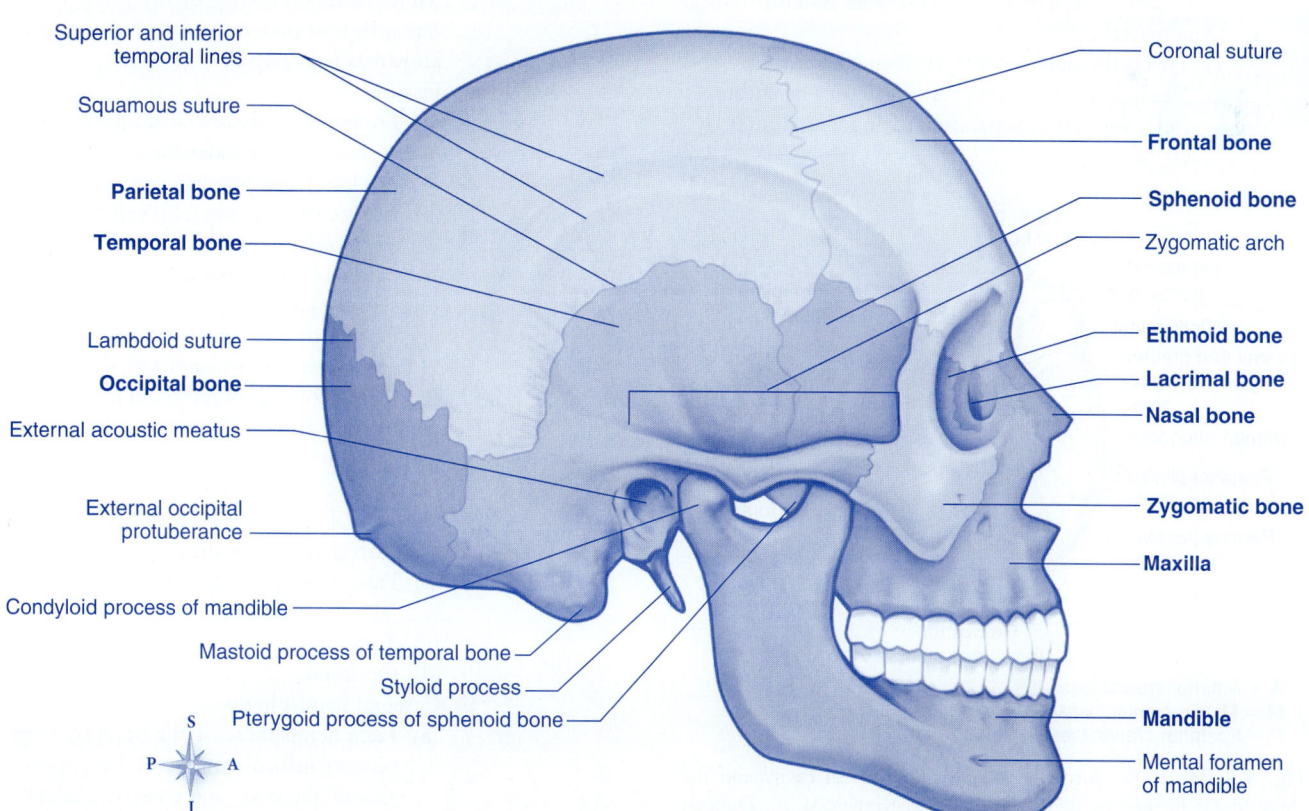

Fig. 5.2 Lateral view of skull. (From Patton, K. T., & Thibodeau, G. F. [2013]. *Anatomy & physiology* [8th ed.]. St. Louis: Mosby.)

4) Occipital: 1
5) Ethmoid: 1
6) Sphenoid: 1
d. The sphenoid bone divides interior of skull into 3 fossae (Fig. 5.3).
   1) Anterior fossa: contains the frontal lobes
   2) Middle fossa: contains the temporal, parietal, and occipital lobes
   3) Posterior fossa: contains the cerebellum
e. The foramen magnum is a large oval-shaped opening at the base of the skull; this is the location of the connection of the brain and spinal cord.
3. Meninges (Fig. 5.4): protective coverings of the brain and the spinal cord
   a. Pia mater
      1) This is the delicate layer that adheres to the surface of brain and spinal cord.
      2) This layer follows sulci and gyri of brain and carries branches of cerebral arteries with it.
         a) Sulci: shallow grooves or invaginations on the surface of the brain (deep sulci are referred to as *fissures*)
         b) Gyri: convolutions on the surface of the brain
      3) Blood vessels of pia form the choroid plexus.
   b. Arachnoid mater
      1) This is the middle layer of the meninges.
      2) The subarachnoid space is between the arachnoid mater and the pia mater.
         a) Contains larger blood vessels of brain
         b) Contains CSF
         c) Contains arachnoid villi (i.e., projections of arachnoid mater that serve as channels for absorption of CSF into venous system)
   c. Dura mater
      1) This is the outermost layer of meninges.
      2) Meningeal arteries and venous sinuses lie within clefts formed by separation of inner and outer layers of dura.
      3) The epidural space is between the skull and the dura mater.
         a) Only a potential space
         b) Site of epidural hemorrhage or hematoma
      4) The subdural space is between the dura mater and the arachnoid mater
         a) Only a potential space
         b) Site of subdural hemorrhage or hematoma
      5) There are several folds of the dura mater (Fig. 5.5).
         a) The falx cerebri separates the two cerebral hemispheres.
         b) The falx cerebelli separates the two cerebellar hemispheres.
         c) The tentorium cerebelli separates the cerebral hemispheres from the cerebellum.
         d) The diaphragma sellae canopies the sella turcica (where pituitary gland is located) and encloses the pituitary gland.
4. Brain
   a. General information
      1) Weighs approximately 1.5 kg
      2) Divided into cerebrum, brainstem, and cerebellum
   b. Telencephalon: two cerebral hemispheres connected by the corpus callosum
      1) Cerebrum (Fig. 5.6)
         a) Structure
            i) Outer layer of cerebral cortex is gray matter consisting of neuron cell bodies (six cell layers thick).
            ii) Deeper layers of each hemisphere are white matter consisting of myelinated axons with four paired masses of gray matter known as *basal ganglia*.
            iii) Fissures
               (a) Longitudinal fissure (also referred to as *falx cerebri*): divides the left and right cerebral hemispheres
               (b) Fissure of Rolando (also referred to as *central sulcus*): divides frontal lobe from parietal lobes; separates the motor and sensory strips
               (c) Fissure of Sylvius (also referred to as *lateral sulcus or Sylvian fissure*): divides frontal lobe from temporal lobes
         b) Cerebral cortical areas and functions (Table 5.2; Fig. 5.6)
            i) Lobes
               (a) Frontal: contains the precentral gyrus (also referred to as the *motor strip*)
               (b) Parietal: contains the postcentral gyrus (also referred to as the *sensory strip*)
               (c) Temporal
               (d) Occipital
            ii) Cerebral hemispheres
               (a) Each hemisphere of the brain receives sensory information from the opposite side of the body and controls skeletal muscles of the opposite side
               (b) Each hemisphere has specialization.

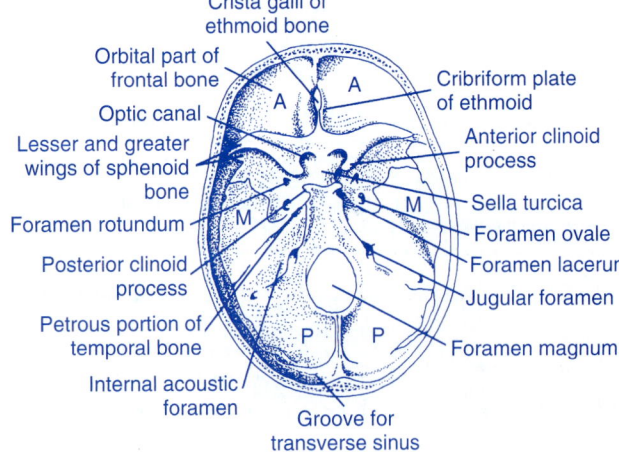

Fig. 5.3 Bones that form the floor of the cranial cavity and the three fossae formed by these bones. (From Kinney, M. R., Dunbar, S., Brooks-Brunn, J. A., Molter, N., & Vitello-Cicciu, J. [Eds.]. [1998]. *AACN's clinical reference for critical care nursing* [4th ed.]. St. Louis: Mosby.)

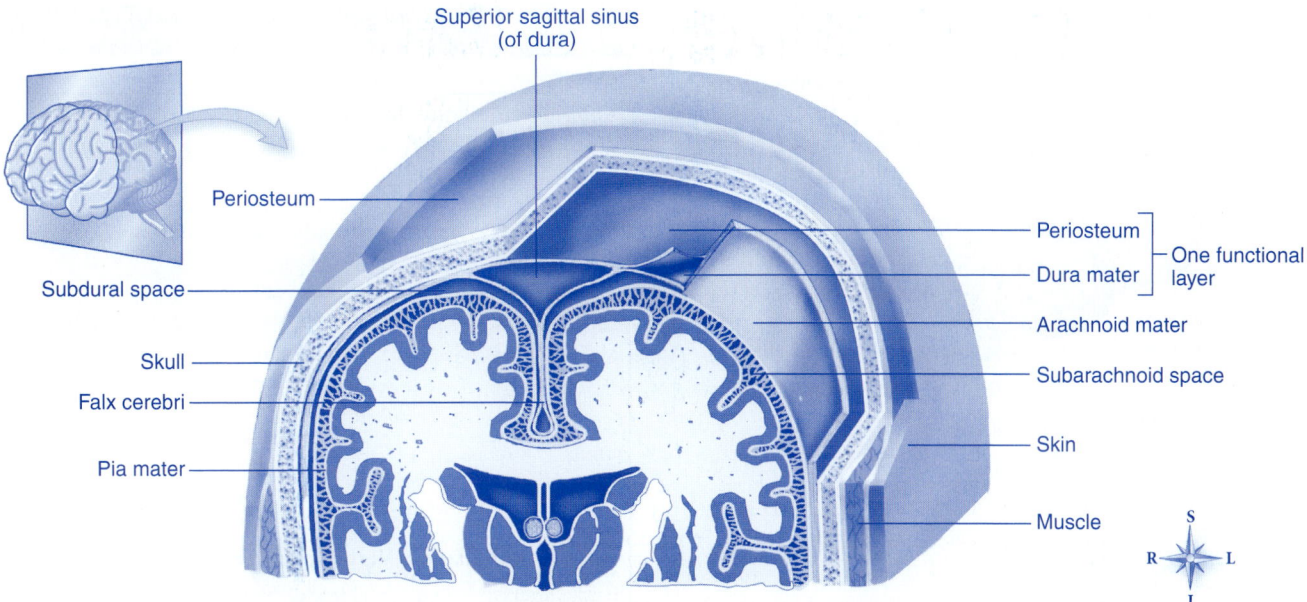

Fig. 5.4 Coverings of the brain. (From Patton, K. T., & Thibodeau, G. F. [2013]. *Anatomy & physiology* [8th ed.]. St. Louis: Mosby.)

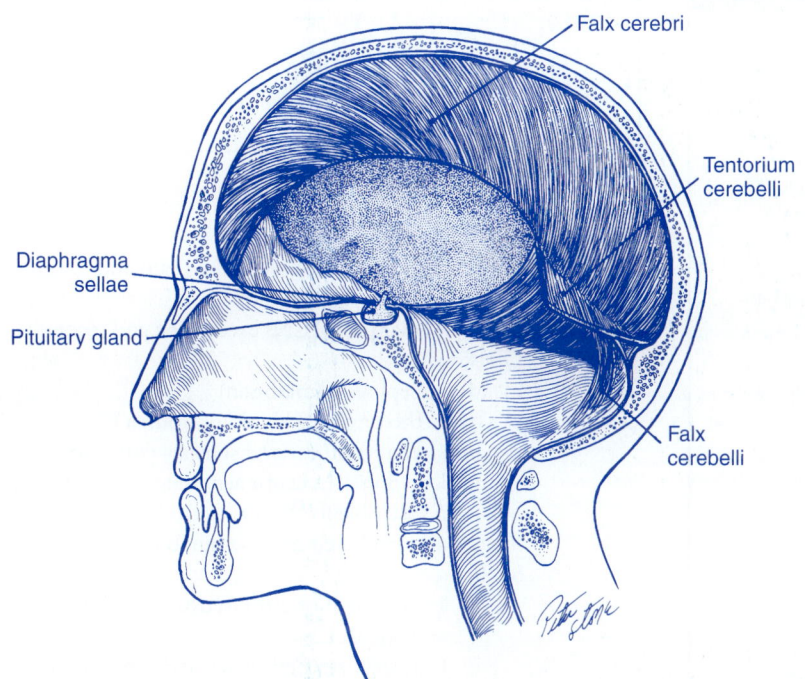

Fig. 5.5 Folds of the dura. (From Kinney, M. R., Dunbar, S., Brooks-Brunn, J. A., Molter, N., & Vitello-Cicciu, J. [Eds.]. [1998]. *AACN's clinical reference for critical care nursing* [4th ed.]. St. Louis: Mosby.)

(i) The left cerebral hemisphere is specialized for analysis, problem solving, language, mathematics, abstract reasoning, and interpretation of symbols.
(ii) The right cerebral hemisphere is specialized for visuospatial patterns, nonverbal communication, music, and artistic ability.
(c) Hemispheric dominance
   (i) Ninety percent of right-handed people are left hemisphere dominant.
   (ii) Sixty percent of left-handed people are right hemisphere dominant.
   (iii) Language centers are located in dominant hemisphere; lesions in dominant hemisphere frequently cause aphasia.
c) Corpus callosum: path for fibers to cross from one cerebral hemisphere to the other
d) Basal ganglia
   i) Major center of the extrapyramidal system
   ii) Functions
      (a) Regulates and controls motor integration
      (b) Influences posture
      (c) Allows fine voluntary movements
c. Diencephalon
   1) Thalamus: relay of incoming messages to appropriate areas of the brain

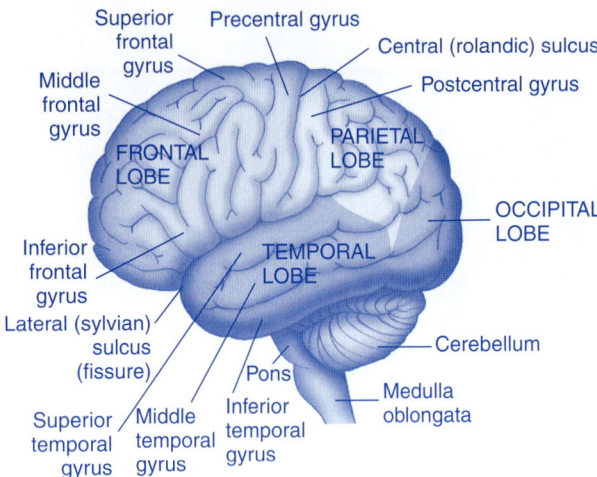

Fig. 5.6 Cerebral hemispheres. (From McCance, K. L., & Huether, S. E. [2014]. *Pathophysiology: The biologic basis for disease in adults and children* [7th ed.]. St. Louis: Mosby.)

Table 5.2	Cerebral Cortical Areas and Functions
Cerebral Cortical Area	**Functions**

Frontal lobe	• Personality
	• Behavior: ethical; moral; social
	• Intellectual functions
	  • Conscious thought
	  • Abstract thinking
	  • Judgment and foresight
	• Short-term memory
	• Voluntary motor function
	• Motor speech (Broca area in dominant hemisphere)

Parietal lobe	• Localization of sensory information to the body surface • Sensory integration and discrimination • Object recognition • Position sense • Body awareness • Body image
Temporal lobe	• Emotion • Long-term memory • Processing of olfactory, gustatory, auditory input • Sensory speech (Wernicke area in dominant hemisphere)
Occipital lobe	• Processing of visual input

Table 5.3	Cerebral Artery Distribution
Artery	**Areas**
Anterior Circulation: Internal Carotid System	
Anterior cerebral arteries	• Superior surface of the frontal and parietal lobes • Medial surface of cerebral hemispheres • Basal ganglia • Corpus callosum • Hypothalamus
Middle cerebral arteries	• Lateral surfaces of frontal, parietal, and temporal lobes • Superior surface of temporal lobe • Subcortical structures (e.g., thalamus, hypothalamus, basal ganglia) • Precentral (i.e., motor) gyri • Postcentral (i.e., sensory) gyri
Posterior Circulation: Vertebrobasilar System	
Basilar artery	• Most of brainstem • Cerebellum
Posterior cerebral arteries	• Thalamus • Medial portion of occipital lobe • Inferior portion of temporal lobe • Vestibular organs • Cochlear apparatus • Midbrain

2) Hypothalamus
   a) Temperature regulation
   b) Regulation of food and water intake
   c) Sleep patterns
   d) Autonomic responses
   e) Control of hormonal secretion of pituitary gland
3) Limbic system
   a) Self-preservation behaviors, including aggression
   b) Basic drives (e.g., food, sex)
   c) Affective aspect of emotional behavior
   d) Some aspects of memory

d. Brainstem
  1) Functions
    a) Relays messages between the brain and lower levels of the nervous system
    b) Is the origin of all CNs except first and second
  2) Divisions
    a) Mesencephalon (midbrain)
      i) Is the origin of third and fourth CNs
      ii) Contains motor and sensory pathways
      iii) Location of reticular activating system (RAS); responsible for arousal from sleep, wakefulness, and focusing of attention
    b) Pons
      i) Is the origin of fifth, sixth, seventh CNs and eighth CN
      ii) Connects cerebral cortex and cerebellum
      iii) Contains motor and sensory pathways
      iv) Contains respiratory centers
    c) Medulla oblongata
      i) Is the origin of 9th to 12th CNs
      ii) Connect motor and sensory tracts of spinal cord to medulla
      iii) Contains cardiac and respiratory centers
e. Cerebellum
  1) Coordinates muscle movement with sensory input
  2) Controls balance
  3) Influences muscle tone in relation to equilibrium
  4) Affects locomotion and posture
  5) Controls nonstereotyped movements
  6) Synchronizes muscle action
5. Cerebral circulation (Table 5.3)
  a. The brain receives 20% of CO.
  b. Arterial system (Fig. 5.7)

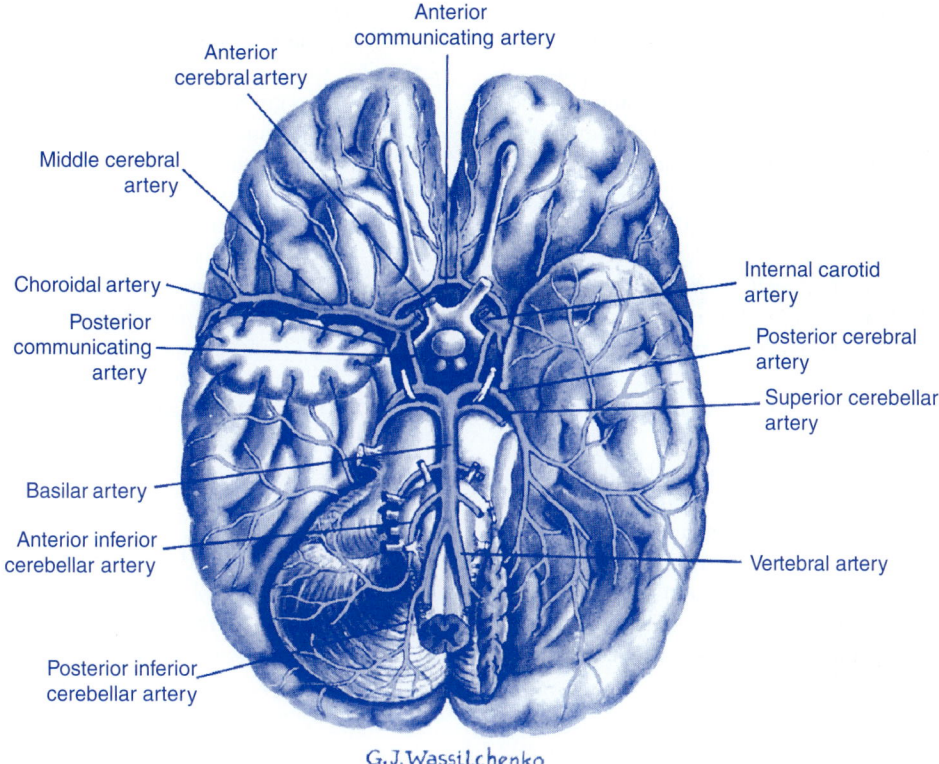

Fig. 5.7 Arterial system of the brain. (From Urden, L., Stacy, K., & Lough, M. [2010]. *Critical care nursing: Diagnosis and management* [6th ed.]. St. Louis: Mosby.)

1) External carotid system: arises from common carotid arteries
   a) Occipital arteries: supply the posterior fossa
   b) Temporal arteries: supply the temporal area
   c) Maxillary arteries: form the middle meningeal arteries
   d) Meningeal arteries: branches of external carotid arteries that supply dura mater (internal carotid and vertebral arteries supply pia and arachnoid mater)
      i) Anterior meningeal artery: supplies anterior portion of dura
      ii) Middle meningeal artery: supplies most of dura
      iii) Posterior meningeal artery: supplies occipital area of dura
2) Anterior circulation: internal carotid system
   a) Arises from common carotid arteries
   b) Accounts for 80% of cerebral perfusion
   c) Includes the following:
      i) Anterior cerebral arteries
      ii) Anterior communicating artery
         (a) Connects right and left anterior cerebral arteries
         (b) Forms anterior section of circle of Willis
      iii) Middle cerebral arteries
      iv) Posterior communicating arteries
         (a) Connect posterior cerebral arteries with the anterior circulation
         (b) Form posterior portion of circle of Willis
3) Posterior circulation: vertebrobasilar system
   a) Arises from subclavian arteries and joins at lower border of pons to form basilar artery
   b) Includes the following:
      i) Posterior cerebral arteries
      ii) Basilar artery
      iii) Anterior spinal artery: supplies anterior half of three quarters of spinal cord and medial aspect of brainstem
      iv) Posterior spinal arteries: traverse the cord along the dorsal roots
4) Circle of Willis
   a) Formed by internal carotids and vertebral arteries
   b) Permits collateral circulation if one of the carotid or vertebral arteries becomes occluded; unfortunately, many people have an incomplete circle of Willis, which prevents this collateral flow when injury or occlusion occurs
   c) Prone to aneurysmal formation because of multiple bifurcations
c. Cerebral blood flow (CBF)
   1) Brings oxygen and nutrients to the brain tissue for cellular energy production; waste products are removed from the blood
   2) CBF varies with changes in cerebral perfusion pressure (CPP) and diameter of the cerebrovascular bed.
      a) Normal CBF is approximately 50 ml/100 g/min.
      b) Normal cerebral oxygen extraction ratio is between 25% and 35%; an oxygen extraction ratio greater than 40% indicates an imbalance between oxygen supply and demand and impending cerebral ischemia.

i) Calculated by $SaO_2 - SjO_2 / SaO_2$ where SaO_2 is oxygen saturation of arterial blood by arterial blood gases (ABGs) or pulse oximetry and SjO_2 is the saturation of the venous blood from the jugular vein by a fiberoptic catheter placed in the jugular bulb

3) CPP = mean arterial pressure (MAP) − mean intracranial pressure (ICP)
   a) Changes in MAP or ICP affect CPP.
   b) Normal MAP is 70 to 105 mm Hg and normal ICP is 5.15 mm Hg; so normal CPP is 60 to 100 mm Hg.
   c) CPP less than 50 mm Hg is associated with impaired neuronal functioning.

4) Autoregulation is the ability of the brain to alter the diameter of the arterioles to maintain CBF at a constant level despite changes in CPP.
   a) When ICP approaches MAP, CPP decreases to the point where autoregulation is impaired, and CBF decreases.
   b) Limits of autoregulation are CPP between 50 and 150 mm Hg.
      i) CPP less than 50 mm Hg causes hypoperfusion (e.g., cardiopulmonary arrest, shock), causing anoxic encephalopathy.
      ii) CPP greater than 150 mm Hg causes hyperperfusion (e.g., hypertensive crisis), causing brain edema and hypertensive encephalopathy.

5) Factors affecting CBF
   a) Increase in CBF
      i) Hypercapnia
      ii) Hypoxemia
      iii) Decreased blood viscosity
      iv) Hyperthermia
      v) Drugs: vasodilators
   b) Decrease in CBF
      i) Hypocapnia
      ii) Hyperoxemia
      iii) Increased blood viscosity
      iv) Hypothermia
      v) Intracranial hypertension
      vi) Drugs: vasopressors
      vii) Cerebral vasospasm
   c) Drugs that are often used therapeutically to optimize CO, blood pressure (BP), and CPP and/or minimize oxygen consumption may result in decreased CO, BP, CPP, and CBF when used inappropriately or in excess.
      i) Negative inotropes (e.g., beta-blockers, barbiturates)
      ii) Vasodilators (e.g., nitroprusside, nitroglycerin)
      iii) Anesthetic agents
   d) Therapies used to manage intracranial hypertension, which are aimed at lowering $PaCO_2$ (i.e., hyperventilation), result in vasoconstriction, thereby reducing CBF and oxygenation.

d. Venous system
   1) The cerebrum has external veins that lie in the subarachnoid space on surfaces of hemispheres and internal veins that drain the central core of cerebrum and lie beneath corpus callosum.
   2) Both external and internal venous systems empty into venous sinuses that lie between dural layers.
      a) Superior sagittal sinus drains venous blood from the anterior portions of the brain.
      b) Cavernous sinus drains venous blood from the inferior portions of the brain.
      c) Transvenous sinus drains venous blood from the posterior portion of the brain.
   3) The internal jugular veins collect blood from dural venous sinuses.

6. CSF
   a. Characteristics
      1) Functions
         a) Cushions brain and spinal cord
         b) Allows for compensation for changes in ICP; displacement of CSF out of cranial cavity compensates for increases in intracranial volume to prevent increase in ICP
      2) Volume: 120 to 150 ml
         a) Distribution: 90 ml in lumbar subarachnoid space, 25 ml in ventricles, 35 ml in rest of subarachnoid space
         b) Daily synthesis: 500 ml
      3) Pressure: less than 200 mm H_2O, measured at lumbar level, with patient in side-lying position
   b. CSF production and reabsorption
      1) CSF is a transudate of plasma formed by choroid plexus in ventricles
         a) Choroid plexus: sheets of epithelial cells that project into the lumen of the ventricular spaces
         b) Majority (95%) of CSF produced in lateral ventricles
      2) CSF is absorbed via arachnoid villi, which return it to systemic circulation by the internal jugular veins; hydrostatic pressure gradient between CSF and venous sinus is one factor that determines CSF absorption.
   c. CSF communication system within brain (Fig. 5.8)
      1) Ventricles: hollow spaces that are lined with ependyma; contain specialized epithelium called *choroid plexus,* which produce CSF
         a) The lateral ventricles are the largest of the ventricles; one lies in each cerebral hemisphere.
         b) The third ventricle lies midline between the two lateral ventricles.
         c) The fourth ventricle lies in the posterior fossa.
      2) Pathway of CSF circulation (Fig. 5.9)

7. Spine and spinal cord
   a. Structure
      1) Vertebral column: composed of 7 cervical, 12 thoracic, 5 lumbar, 5 sacral, and 4 coccygeal vertebrae
      2) Spinal cord: 42 to 45 cm extending from superior border of atlas to upper border of second lumbar vertebrae (L2); continuous with the brainstem

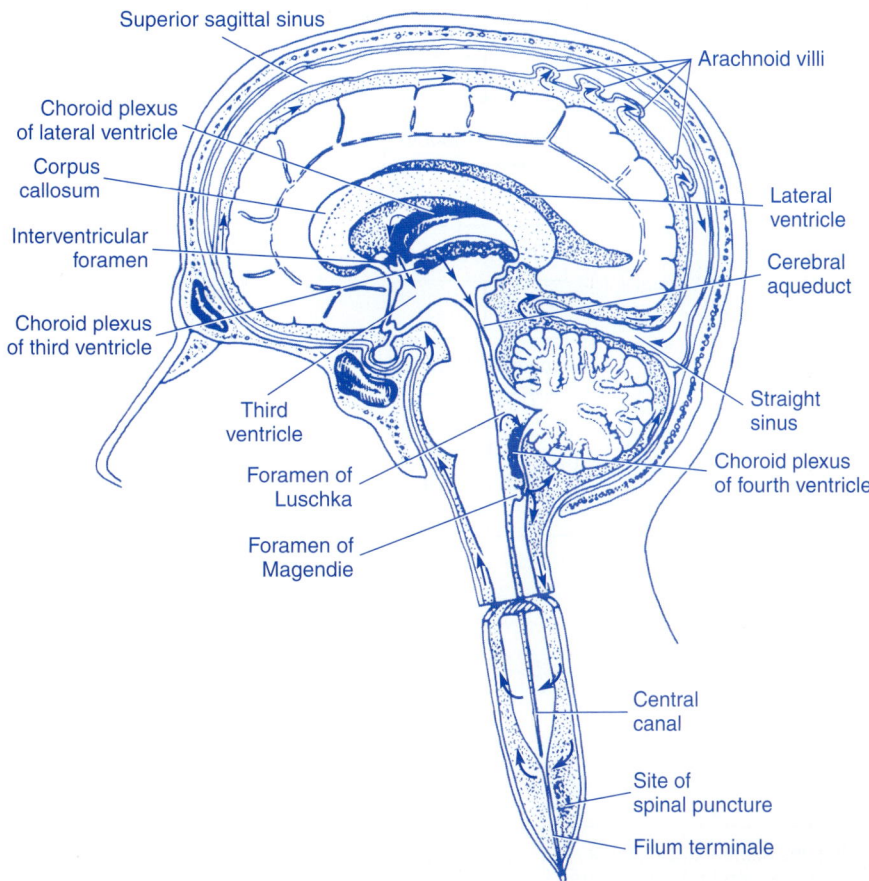

Fig. 5.8 Lateral view of the ventricular system. *Arrows* show the direction of cerebrospinal fluid circulation. (From Kinney, M. R., Dunbar, S., Brooks-Brunn, J. A., Molter, N., & Vitello-Cicciu, J. [Eds.]. [1998]. *AACN's clinical reference for critical care nursing* [4th ed.]. St. Louis: Mosby.)

- a) Meninges: pia mater, arachnoid mater, and dura mater
- b) Central canal: opening in the center of the spinal cord that contains CSF; communicates with the fourth ventricle
- c) Central gray horns that form an "H": contain mostly cell bodies (Fig. 5.10)
    - i) The anterior (or ventral) horn of gray matter contains cell bodies of efferent or motor fibers.
    - ii) The posterior (or dorsal) horn of gray matter contains cell bodies of afferent or sensory fibers.
    - iii) The lateral horns of gray matter contain preganglionic fibers of autonomic system.
- d) Columns of white matter that are fiber tracts surround the gray matter: contain mostly myelinated axons
    - i) Posterior tracts (dorsal columns) and the anterior and lateral spinothalamic tracts are ascending tracts that conduct sensory impulses from the spinal cord to the thalamus and cerebral cortex.
    - ii) Lateral tracts (the corticospinal and pyramidal) are descending tracts that conduct motor impulses from the brain to motor neurons in the anterior horn.
    - iii) Spinal tracts are named by column, origin, and termination (e.g., lateral corticospinal tract is located in the lateral column, originates in the cortex, and terminates in the spine; it is therefore a descending tract [cortex to spine]); Table 5.4 describes clinically significant tracts.
- 3) UMNs and LMNs
    - a) UMNs: located in the cerebral cortex and brainstem
        - i) Cell bodies lie in the motor area of the cerebral cortex.
        - ii) Axons pass through the spinal cord to synapse with the LMNs.
        - iii) Damage to UMN causes spastic paralysis and hyperactive reflexes.
    - b) LMNs: located in the spinal cord
        - i) Cell bodies lie in the anterior horn of gray matter in the spinal cord.
        - ii) Axons directly innervate striated muscle fibers.
        - iii) Damage to LMN causes flaccid paralysis and areflexia.
- b. Function
    - 1) Mediates the reflex arc (Fig. 5.11)
        - a) An involuntary response to a stimulus (e.g., touching hot stove causes reflex withdrawal of hand)

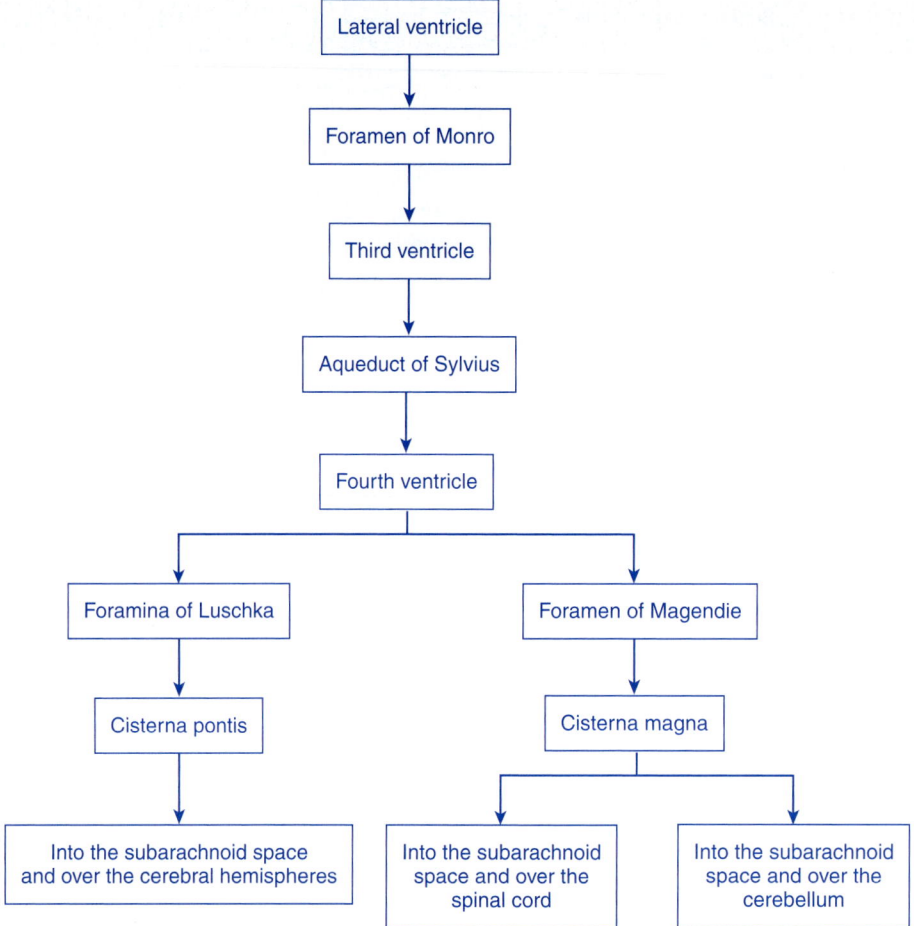

Fig. 5.9 Circulation of cerebrospinal fluid.

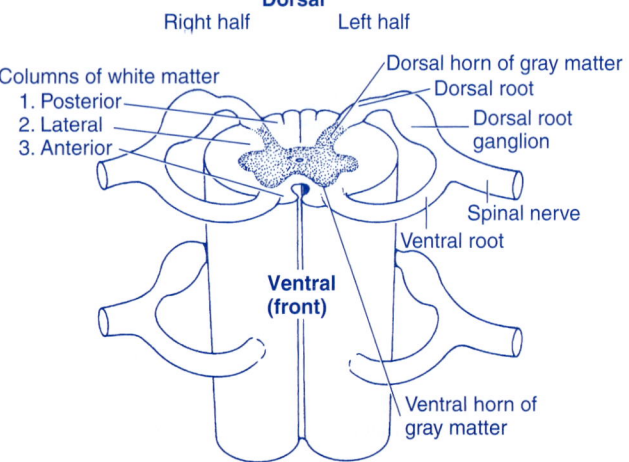

Fig. 5.10 Segment of the thoracic spinal cord in cross section. (From Kinney, M. R., Dunbar, S., Brooks-Brunn, J. A., Molter, N., & Vitello-Cicciu, J. [Eds.]. [1998]. *AACN's clinical reference for critical care nursing* [4th ed.]. St. Louis: Mosby.)

      b) Does not go beyond the spinal cord to the brain; does not require cerebral interpretation
      c) Components
         i) Receptor organ
         ii) Afferent neuron
         iii) Effector neuron
         iv) Effector organ

    2) Serves as the communicating pathway between the brain and the peripheral nervous system
8. Peripheral nervous system
   a. Spinal segments consist of 31 pairs of spinal nerves: 8 cervical (C1–C8), 12 thoracic (T1–T12), 5 lumbar (L1–L5), 5 sacral (S1–S5), and 1 coccygeal
     1) Fibers of spinal nerve
       a) Motor fibers
         i) Originate in anterior gray column of spinal cord
         ii) Form ventral root of spinal nerve and pass to skeletal muscles
       b) Sensory fibers
         i) Originate in spinal ganglia of dorsal roots
         ii) Peripheral branches distribute to visceral and somatic structures as mediators of sensory impulses to CNS.
     2) Dermatomes: each spinal nerve innervates a specific portion of the skin identified as the dermatome for that spinal nerve (Fig. 5.12 and Table 5.5).
     3) Spinal nerves form various nerve plexuses that innervate the skin and muscles throughout the body (Fig. 5.12).
       a) Cervical plexus: C1 to C4
       b) Brachial plexus: C5 to C8, T1
       c) Lumbar plexus: L1 to L4
       d) Sacral plexus: L4 to L5, S1 to S4
   b. CNs (Table 5.6) consist of 12 pairs of nerves that carry impulses to and from the brain.

Table 5.4 Spinal Cord Tracts and Functions

Tract	Column	Direction	Functions	Sidedness
Spinothalamic				
Lateral spinothalamic	Lateral	Ascending	• Pain • Temperature	Contralateral
Anterior spinothalamic	Anterior	Ascending	• Light touch • Pressure • Pain • Temperature	Contralateral
Spinotectal	Lateral	Ascending	• Tactile stimulation arousing consciousness	Contralateral
Spinocerebellar				
Dorsal spinocerebellar	Lateral	Ascending	• Reflex proprioception • Muscle tone and synergy	Ipsilateral
Ventral spinocerebellar	Lateral	Ascending	• Reflex proprioception • Muscle tone and synergy	Contralateral
Medial Lemniscal System				
Fasciculus gracilis	Posterior	Ascending	• Position sense • Vibratory sense • Pressure • Tactile localization • Two-point discrimination	Ipsilateral
Fasciculus cuneatus	Posterior	Ascending	• Position sense • Vibratory sense • Pressure • Tactile localization • Two-point discrimination	Ipsilateral
Pyramidal				
Lateral corticospinal	Lateral	Descending	• Voluntary movement	Contralateral
Ventral corticospinal	Lateral	Descending	• Voluntary movement	Ipsilateral
Corticobulbar		Descending	• Facial expression • Swallowing • Speech	Contralateral
Extrapyramidal				
Rubrospinal	Lateral	Descending	• Synergy and muscle tone	Contralateral
Lateral vestibulospinal	Anterior	Descending	• Posture and equilibrium	Ipsilateral
Medial vestibulospinal	Anterior	Descending	• Posture and equilibrium	Contralateral
Lateral reticulospinal	Lateral	Descending	• Muscle tone	Ipsilateral
Medial reticulospinal	Anterior	Descending	• Muscle tone	Ipsilateral
Tectospinal	Anterior	Descending	• Vision and hearing	Contralateral

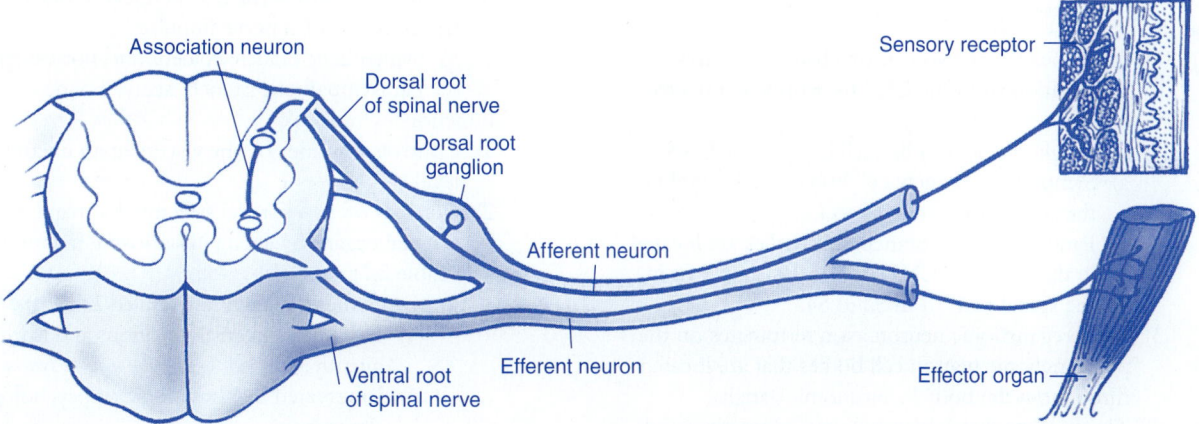

Fig. 5.11 Basic diagram of a reflex arc, including the sensory receptor, afferent neuron, association neuron, efferent neuron, and effector organ. (From Lewis, S. M., Heitkemper, M. M., & Dirksen, S. R. [2000]. *Medical-surgical nursing* [5th ed.]. St. Louis: Mosby.)

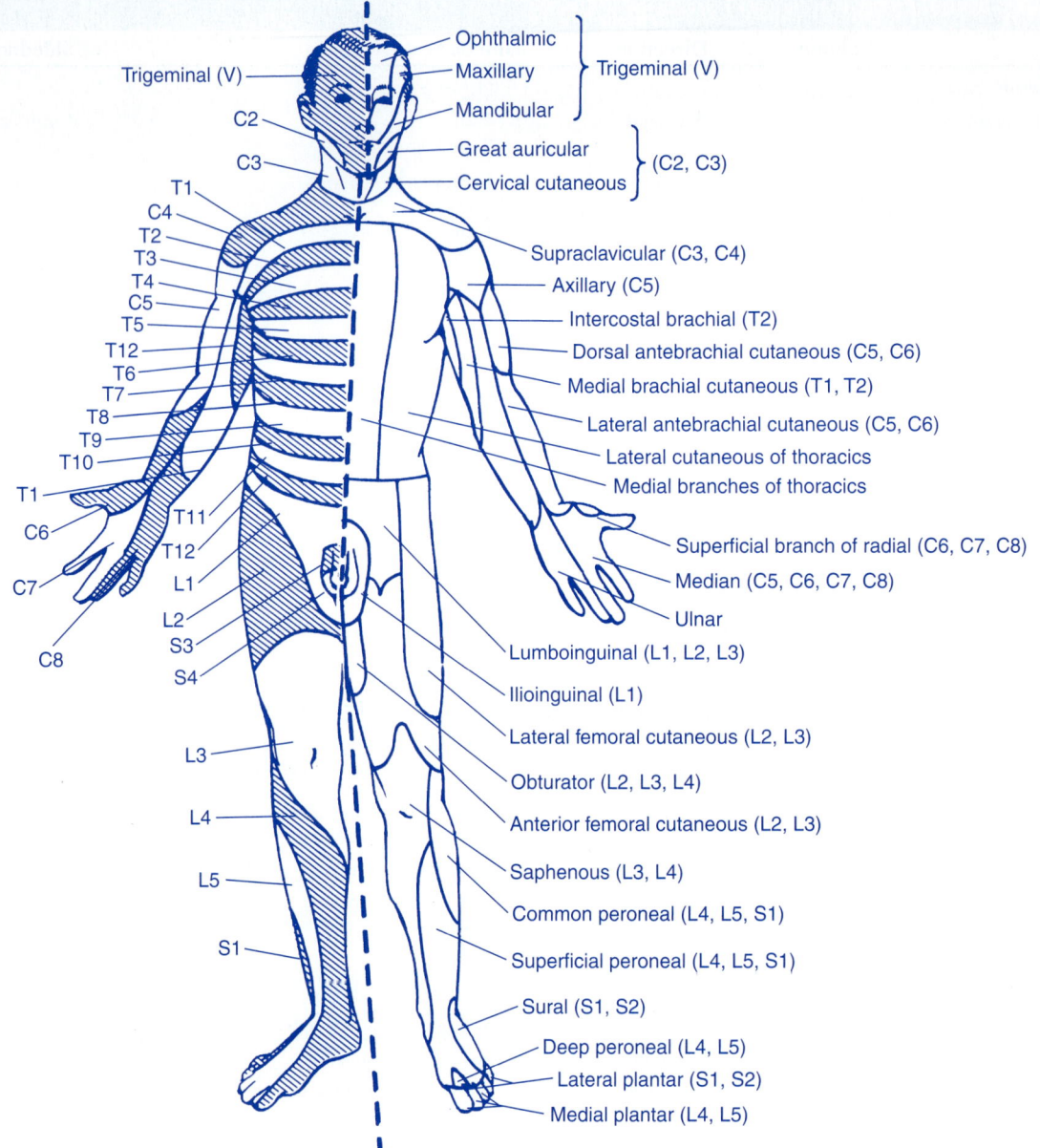

Fig. 5.12 *Left:* Dermatome distribution. *Right:* Peripheral distribution of cutaneous nerves. (From Long, B. C., Phipps, W. J., & Cassmeyer, V. L. [1993]. *Medical-surgical nursing: A nursing process approach* [3rd ed.]. St. Louis: Mosby.)

9. ANS
   a. Structure
      1) ANS consists of two neuron chains that carry information from the CNS to peripheral effector organs.
      2) Preganglionic neuron has cell body in the CNS.
         a) Sympathetic branch: cell bodies are located in the spinal cord from T1 to L2.
         b) Parasympathetic branch: cell bodies are located in the nuclei of CNs III, VII, IX, and X or in the spinal cord from S2 to S4.
      3) The preganglionic neuron axon terminates on the postganglionic neuron cell bodies that are located throughout the body in autonomic ganglia.
      4) The postganglionic neuron axon terminates and innervates the specific effector organs of the ANS.
      5) Neurotransmitters form a chemical bridge in transmission of a nerve impulse.
         a) Sympathetic branch: epinephrine; norepinephrine
         b) Parasympathetic branch: acetylcholine
   b. Function
      1) Controls activities of the viscera at an unconscious level
      2) Consists of two parallel systems that regulate visceral organs by acting in opposing manners (Table 5.7)
         a) Sympathetic branch (also called *adrenergic*)
            i) Dominates in crisis situations and is frequently referred to as *fight or flight system*
            ii) Innervated by physiologic or psychological stressors
            iii) Promotes activities that prepare the body for crisis situations

Table 5.5 Relationship of Spinal Cord Segments to Peripheral Nerves, Muscles, and Functional Ability

Spinal Cord Segment	Peripheral Nerves	Muscles	Functional Ability
C3–C5	• Phrenic nerve	• Diaphragm	• Diaphragmatic chest excursion
C5	• Spinal accessory nerve	• Trapezius	• Shoulder shrug
C5–C6	• Axillary nerve • Musculocutaneous nerve • Radial nerve	• Deltoid • Biceps • Brachioradialis	• Arm elevation • Forearm flexion
C6–C8	• Radial nerve	• Triceps • Extensor carpi radialis and ulnaris • Flexor carpi radialis and ulnaris	• Forearm extension • Wrist extension • Wrist flexion
C8, T1	• Median nerve • Ulnar nerve	• Adductor pollicis • Dorsal interossei	• Handgrip • Finger spreading
T1–T12	• Thoracic and lumbosacral branches	• Intercostals • Rectus abdominis and obliques	• Intercostal chest excursion • Rotation at waist
L1–L3	• Femoral nerve	• Iliopsoas • Quadriceps	• Hip flexion • Knee extension
L2–L4	• Deep peroneal nerve • Sciatic nerve	• Extensor hallucis and digitorum • Biceps femoris and hamstrings	• Foot dorsiflexion • Knee flexion
L5–S2	• Inferior gluteal nerve • Tibial nerve	• Gluteus maximus • Gastrocnemius	• Hip extension • Plantar flexion

Table 5.6 Cranial Nerve Summary

Number	Name	Memory Jogger: Name	Memory Jogger: Motor, Sensory, or Both	Functions
I	Olfactory	On	Some	Sensory • Smell
II	Optic	Old	Say	Sensory • Vision
III	Oculomotor	Olympus	Marry	Motor • Upward, lateral eye movement • Pupillary constriction • Eyelid elevation
IV	Trochlear	Towering	Money	Motor • Downward, medial eye movement
V	Trigeminal	Tops	But	Sensory • Sensation of scalp and face • Sensation of cornea of eye Motor • Temporal and masseter muscles
VI	Abducens	A	My	Motor • Lateral eye movement
VII	Facial	Fin	Brother	Sensory • Taste on anterior two thirds of tongue Motor • Muscles of facial expression • Eyelid closure • Lacrimal and salivary glands
VIII	Acoustic	And	Says	Sensory • Hearing • Equilibrium and balance
IX	Glossopharyngeal	German	Bad	Sensory • Taste on posterior one third of tongue • Pharynx Motor • Parotid gland

Continued

Table 5.6 Cranial Nerve Summary—cont'd

Number	Name	Memory Jogger: Name	Memory Jogger: Motor, Sensory, or Both	Functions
X	Vagus	Viewed	Business	Sensory • Pharynx, larynx, neck Motor • Palate, larynx, pharynx • Swallowing • Cardiac muscle • Secretory glands of pancreas and gastrointestinal tract
XI	Spinal accessory	Some	Marry	Motor • Shoulder and neck movement • Sternocleidomastoid and trapezius muscles
XII	Hypoglossal	Hops	Money	Motor • Tongue

Table 5.7 Autonomic Nervous System: Sympathetic and Parasympathetic Branch Function

	Sympathetic (Adrenergic)	Parasympathetic (Cholinergic)
Eyes	• Pupils dilate	• Pupils constrict
Heart	• Heart rate increases • Contractility increases • Coronary arteries dilate	• Heart rate decreases • Contractility decreases • No effect on coronary arteries
Lungs	• Bronchodilation	• Bronchoconstriction
Liver	• Glycogenolysis and lipolysis	• Glycogenesis
Gastrointestinal	• Salivary flow decreases • Gastric mobility and secretion decreases • Intestinal motility decreases	• Salivary flow increases • Gastric mobility and secretion increases • Intestinal motility increases
Urinary bladder	• Bladder relaxes • Sphincter closes	• Bladder contracts • Sphincter opens
Adrenal glands	• Secrete epinephrine, norepinephrine	• No effect
Skin	• Piloerection (goose pimples) • Increased perspiration	• No effect

   b) Parasympathetic branch (also called *cholinergic*)
      i) Dominant in moments of calm or "steady state"
      ii) Promotes activities that restore the body's energy sources

Neurologic Assessment

Interview

1. Chief complaint: why the patient is seeking help and duration of the problem
   a. Symptoms related to neurologic problems
      1) Head or spinal cord trauma
         a) Sequence of events
         b) Mechanism of injury
         c) Elapsed time
         d) Extent of injury
         e) Previous treatment
         f) Current status
      2) Change in consciousness (e.g., difficulty staying awake)
      3) Headache
         a) Focal or generalized
         b) Unilateral or bilateral
         c) With or without fever
            i) Headache with fever: infectious process (e.g., meningitis, encephalitis)
            ii) Headache without fever: intracerebral hemorrhage or tumor
         d) Time of day: early morning headache suggestive of tumor
      4) Seizures
         a) New onset
         b) Increased frequency if patient has history of epilepsy
      5) Visual changes
         a) Loss of a portion of the visual field
         b) Diplopia
         c) Photophobia: may be experienced with increased ICP or meningitis
         d) Nystagmus
      6) Impaired speech (e.g., dysarthria, aphasia)
      7) Change in mood (e.g., depression, euphoria, emotional lability)
      8) Change in thought processes (e.g., hallucinations, delusions, illusions, paranoia) and cognition
      9) Change in behavior (e.g., hygiene habits, inappropriate laughter, frequent crying)

10) Change in motor function
    a) Tremor
    b) Paresis
    c) Paralysis
11) Change in gait
12) Dizziness, syncope, vertigo
13) Change in sensory function
    a) Pain
    b) Paresthesia
    c) Anesthesia
14) Memory changes
15) Swallowing difficulties
16) Difficulties with activities of daily living (ADLs)
2. History of present illness: determine PQRST
   a. P
      1) Provocation: what provokes or worsens the pain?
      2) Palliation
         a) What relieves the pain?
         b) What was used but did not relieve pain?
   b. Q
      1) Quality: what does the pain feel like?
   c. R
      1) Region: where is the pain located?
      2) Radiation: if the pain radiates, where does the pain radiate?
   d. S
      1) Severity: how severe is the pain on a 0 to 10 scale with 0 being no pain and 10 being the most severe pain?
   e. T
      1) Timing
         a) Intermittent or continuous
         b) Relationship to other events or activities
         c) Time last seen normal: important in stroke assessment and determination of candidacy for fibrinolytic therapy
3. Past medical history
   a. Congenital disorders
      1) Spina bifida
      2) Cerebral palsy
      3) Down syndrome
   b. Childhood diseases: poliomyelitis
   c. Epilepsy
   d. Head trauma
   e. Infectious neurologic conditions
      1) Encephalitis
      2) Meningitis
   f. Neuromuscular disease
      1) Multiple sclerosis
      2) Myasthenia gravis
      3) Amyotrophic lateral sclerosis (ALS)
      4) Parkinson disease
   g. Spinal cord injury
   h. Alzheimer disease
   i. Cancer
   j. Cardiovascular disease
      1) Coronary artery disease: angina; myocardial infarction
      2) Valvular heart disease
      3) Hypertension
      4) Hyperlipidemia
      5) Dysrhythmia, especially atrial fibrillation
      6) Ventricular aneurysm
      7) Endocarditis
   k. Cerebrovascular disease
      1) Ischemic stroke
      2) Hemorrhagic stroke
      3) Carotid artery disease: bruit; prior carotid endarterectomy
   l. Diabetes mellitus
   m. Renal insufficiency or failure
   n. Pulmonary embolism (PE)
   o. Impairment of vision: use of eyeglasses, contact lenses, prosthesis
   p. Impairment of hearing: use of hearing aid
4. Family history
   a. Epilepsy
   b. Diabetes mellitus
   c. Cardiac disease
   d. Hypertension
   e. Cerebrovascular disease
      1) Ischemic stroke
      2) Hemorrhagic stroke
   f. Cancer
   g. Neurologic disorders
      1) ALS
      2) Huntington disease
      3) Muscular dystrophy
      4) Neurofibromatosis
      5) Tay-Sachs disease
      6) Myasthenia gravis
      7) Multiple sclerosis
      8) Alzheimer disease
      9) Tremor
      10) Dementia
   h. Psychiatric disorders
5. Social history
   a. Relationship with spouse or significant other; family structure
   b. Occupation: exposure to toxins (e.g., solvents, pesticides, arsenic, lead)
   c. Educational level
   d. Stress level and usual coping mechanisms
   e. Recreational habits
   f. Exercise habits
   g. Dietary habits
   h. Caffeine intake
   i. Tobacco use: record as pack-years (i.e., number of packs per day times the number of years the patient has been smoking).
   j. Alcohol use: record as alcoholic beverages consumed per month, week, or day.
   k. Drug use or abuse
   l. Toxin exposure
   m. Travel
   n. Handedness: left or right
6. Medication history
   a. Prescribed drug, dose, frequency, time of last dose
   b. Nonprescribed drugs
      1) Over-the-counter remedies
      2) Substance abuse
      3) Herbs
   c. Patient understanding of drug actions, side effects

d. Drugs frequently used for neurologic problems
   1) Tranquilizers
   2) Sedatives
   3) Aspirin
   4) Anticonvulsants
   5) Antihypertensives
   6) Platelet aggregation inhibitors
e. Drugs that may cause neurologic problems
   1) Tranquilizers
   2) Sedatives
   3) Aspirin
   4) Anticoagulants
   5) Alcohol

Vital Signs

1. Cushing triad: increased systolic BP with a decreased diastolic BP (widened pulse pressure), bradycardia, and abnormal respiratory pattern; late sign of increased ICP and impending herniation
2. BP
   a. Hypotension
      1) Hemorrhage
         a) Because the cranium is an inexpansible vault, intracranial hemorrhage cannot result in hypotension since herniation would result before significant hypotension.
         b) Consider other sources of bleeding (e.g., lacerated liver, ruptured spleen, thoracic trauma).
      2) General neurologic deterioration
      3) Of great concern because CPP = MAP − ICP
   b. Hypertension
      1) Systolic hypertension may be seen as a component of Cushing triad, a late sign of intracranial hypertension.
      2) May indicate a change in arterial resistance and associated with vessel occlusion (e.g., stroke)
   c. Pulse pressure: difference between systolic and diastolic
      1) Normal is 30 to 40 mm Hg.
      2) Increased pulse pressure is a component of Cushing triad, a late sign of intracranial hypertension.
3. Pulse
   a. Sinus bradycardia: a component of Cushing triad, a late sign of intracranial hypertension
   b. Sinus tachycardia
      1) Hypoxia
      2) Hemorrhage
      3) General neurologic deterioration
   c. Atrial dysrhythmias (e.g., premature atrial contractions, atrial fibrillation, atrial flutter) may be etiologic factors in ischemic stroke.
4. Ventilatory rate and rhythm (Fig. 5.13)
   a. Bradypnea
      1) Description: regular rhythm with rate less than 12 breaths/min
      2) Caused by CNS depression by injury, disease, or drugs
   b. Cheyne-Stokes respirations
      1) Increasing rate and depth of ventilation followed by decreasing rate and depth of ventilation and then apnea
      2) Causes
         a) Bilateral lesions of cerebral hemispheres
         b) Lesion of basal ganglia
         c) Cerebellar lesion
         d) Lesion of upper brainstem
         e) Metabolic condition
   c. CNS hyperventilation
      1) Sustained increased rate and depth of ventilation
      2) Causes
         a) Lesions of lower midbrain or upper pons
         b) May be secondary to transtentorial herniation
   d. Apneustic
      1) Apnea with inspiration followed by exhalation
      2) Cause: lesions of mid to lower pons
   e. Cluster
      1) 3 to 4 breaths of identical rate and depth followed by apnea, sequence repeated
      2) Cause: lesions of lower pons or upper medulla

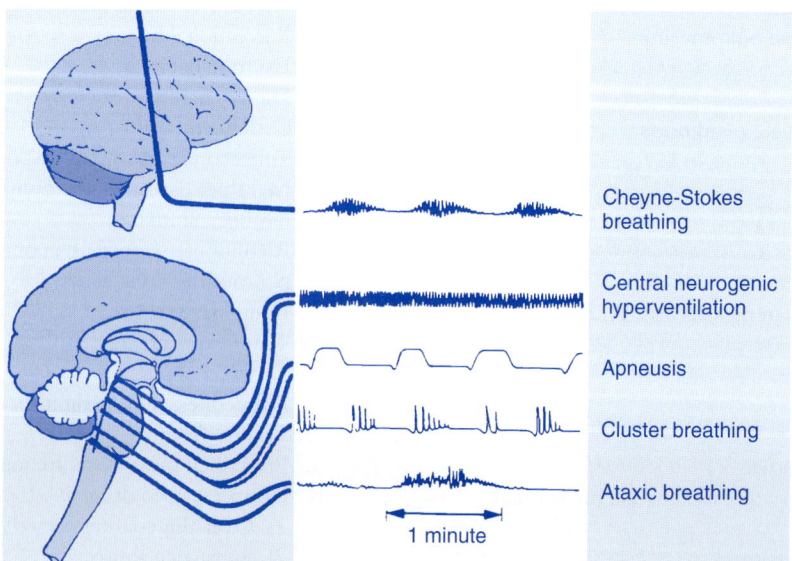

Fig. 5.13 Abnormal respiratory patterns with corresponding level of central nervous system activity. (From McCance, K. L., & Huether, S. E. [2014]. *Pathophysiology: The biologic basis for disease in adults and children* [7th ed.]. St. Louis: Mosby.)

f. Ataxic
1) No pattern to ventilation; completely irregular with mostly apnea
2) Cause: lesion of the medulla
5. Temperature
a. Decreased (subnormal)
1) Shock
2) Drug overdose
3) Metabolic coma (e.g., myxedema coma)
4) Terminal stages of neurologic disease
b. Increased
1) Infection
a) Systemic infection
b) CNS infection
2) Subarachnoid hemorrhage (SAH)
3) Seizures
4) Restlessness
5) Injury to hypothalamus: especially if inordinately elevated

General Appearance

1. Attire: appropriateness to age, environment
2. Grooming
   a. Hair
   b. Teeth
   c. Hygiene
   d. Nails
3. General behavior
   a. Demeanor
   b. Affect: facial expressions; body language
   c. Mood: euphoria, anger, depression, suicidal thoughts
4. Posture: gestures, fidgeting, restlessness, tremor, rigidity
5. Gait: ataxia is uncoordinated movements of the body.
6. Obvious physical defects
   a. Hemiparesis or hemiplegia
   b. Facial asymmetry
   c. Ptosis
   d. Tremor
   e. Amputations
   f. Mass response: decorticate or decerebrate posturing

Mental Status and Cognition

1. Level of consciousness (LOC): the most sensitive clinical indicator of a change in neurologic status
   a. Consciousness is a state of awareness: self; environment; responses to environment
      1) Arousal
         a) Measure of being awake
         b) Function of the RAS in the midbrain
      2) Awareness
         a) Involves interpreting sensory input and giving an appropriate response
         b) Requires both an intact RAS and cerebral hemispheres
   b. Evaluate the degree of stimulus to get a response
      1) Verbal stimuli
         a) Call the patient by name, speaking at normal voice volume.
         b) Ask the patient to make a fist with his or her hand; when performed, ask the patient to open the fist.
         c) Use increased volume (i.e., "yelling") if the patient does not respond to normal voice volume.
      2) Tactile stimuli: touch or shake the patient.
      3) Painful stimuli: use only if the other methods are unsuccessful; avoid trauma and bruising caused by pinching.
         a) Techniques to elicit a pain response
            i) Central: brain responds.
               (a) Pressure to trapezius muscle: squeeze large muscle mass between thumb and index finger; do not pinch skin.
               (b) Pressure to Achilles tendon: squeeze large muscle mass between thumb and index finger; do not pinch skin.
               (c) Supraorbital pressure
                  (i) Push up against the supraorbital ridge with thumb; exert gentle upward pressure.
                  (ii) Do not push into the eye socket; injury to the eye or vagal response may occur.
                  (iii) Do not use this technique in patients with facial fracture or cranial fracture.
               (d) Sternal rub: rub sternum gently with knuckle; if bruising results, discontinue using this technique.
            ii) Peripheral: spine responds.
               (a) Nailbed pressure: apply pressure to the nailbed using the flat surface of a pen or pencil.
                  (i) Useful in determining sensory and motor function but should not be used as the only method of evaluation of pain response
   c. LOC (Haymore, 2004)
      1) Normal: arouses easily, maintains wakefulness, speaks coherently, responds appropriately to stimuli
      2) Hypersomnia: prolonged sleeping time with normal sleep pattern
      3) Lethargy, obtundation, stupor
         a) These are confusing terms indicating diminishing LOC.
         b) It is recommended to describe the patient's response to stimuli and behavior rather than use these labels.
      4) Coma: absence of awareness and responsiveness caused by structural lesion or metabolic condition
      5) Persistent vegetative state: unaware of self and surroundings
         a) Sleep–wake patterns occur along with eye opening, but no response to stimuli occurs.
         b) Brainstem and hypothalamic function intact
      6) Locked-in syndrome: consciousness with near-complete paralysis
         a) Able to answer questions with eye blink
         b) Vision and hearing are preserved.
         c) Caused by lesion of midbrain or pons
      7) Brain death: absence of all cortical and brainstem function

d. Glasgow Coma Scale (GCS) (Table 5.8)
      1) Developed as a method to standardize observation of responsiveness in patients with traumatic brain injury
      2) Best or highest response is recorded; E (eye), M (motor), V (verbal) may be recorded separately along with a quantitative score.
      3) Note if certain responses cannot be evaluated because of any of the following:
         a) Endotracheal intubation or tracheostomy
         b) Aphasia
         c) Eyes swollen shut
      4) Parameters
         a) Minimum: 3
         b) Maximum (normal): 15
         c) Clinically significant: change of 2 points or more
   e. National Institutes of Health Stroke Scale (NIHSS) (Table 5.9)
      1) Used to assess the severity of presenting signs and symptoms
      2) Score over 22 indicates severe neurologic deficit
      3) Baseline assessment completed at admission; repeat assessments 2 hours after treatment, 24 hours after onset of symptoms, 7 to 10 after onset of symptoms, and 3 months after onset of symptoms
2. Cognitive function
   a. Orientation: patient may be alert but confused.
      1) Orientation to time
         a) Ability to give today's date (e.g., What is today's date?)
         b) Ability to state the year (e.g., What year is it?)
      2) Orientation to place
         a) Ability to identify surroundings (e.g., Where are you now?)
         b) Ability to state address (e.g., Where do you live?)
      3) Orientation to person
         a) Ability to identify self by name (e.g., Who are you? What is your name?)
         b) Recognition of friends, family
      4) Orientation to situation: ability to identify why they are in the hospital (e.g., Why are you here?)
   b. Memory
      1) How old are you?
      2) Remote memory: What is your birthday? Where were you born?
      3) Recent memory: What did you have for breakfast? What is your doctor's name?
   c. Short-term recall: Can the patient repeat three or four objects after 3 to 5 minutes?
   d. General knowledge: Ask a question about a current event.
   e. Attention span: Is the patient able to stay on a subject?
   f. Thought content: Note evidence of illusions, hallucinations, delusions, or paranoia.
   g. Calculation skills: Can you count backwards from 20 to 1?
   h. Judgment: Why are you here? What would you do if there were a fire in the wastebasket?
   i. Abstraction: Ask the patient to spell the word "world" backward.

Table 5.8 Glasgow Coma Scale

Parameter	Response	Score
Eye opening	Spontaneous	4
	To speech	3
	To pain	2
	None	1
	Untestable	U
Best motor response	Obeys commands	6
	Localizes pain	5
	Withdraws from pain	4
	Abnormal flexion (decorticate posturing)	3
	Abnormal extension (decerebrate posturing)	2
	None	1
	Untestable	U
Best verbal response	Oriented	5
	Confused	4
	Inappropriate	3
	Incomprehensible	2
	None	1
	Untestable	U

3. Speech and language
   a. Note punctuation, rhythm, stream of talk, sentence structure, appropriate use of words; speech should be fluent with expression of connected thoughts.
   b. If patient cannot use or understand verbal communication
      1) Can the patient understand or use gestures?
      2) Can the patient understand written language or write messages?
   c. Identify the presence of speech disorders.
      1) Dysphonia: difficulty producing sound
      2) Dysarthria: difficulty with articulation
      3) Dysprosody: lack of inflection while talking
      4) Aphasia: impaired understanding or expression of verbal or written language (or both)
         a) Receptive (sensory) aphasia: lesion in Wernicke area in temporal area
         b) Expressive (motor) aphasia: lesion in Broca's area in frontal area
         c) Global: both

Motor Function

1. Muscle size
   a. Symmetry
   b. Atrophy or hypertrophy
2. Symmetrical movement and strength of extremities
   a. Movement
      1) Spontaneous movement and symmetry of movement
      2) Assumption of a position of comfort
   b. Muscle strength (Table 5.10)
      1) Arm strength
         a) Test flexor and extensor muscle groups by evaluating strength against resistance.

Table 5.9 National Institutes of Health Stroke Scale

Item and Domain	Response	Score
1A Level of consciousness	• Alert, keenly responsive	0
	• Obeys, answers or responds to minor stimulation	1
	• Responds only to repeated stimulation or painful stimulation (excludes reflex response)	2
	• Responds only with reflex motor or totally unresponsive	3
1B Orientation	• Answers both correctly	0
Ask the month and patient age; must be exactly right.	• Answers one correctly or patient unable to speak because of any reason other than aphasia or coma	1
	• Answers neither correctly or too stuporous or aphasic	2
1C Response to commands	• Performs both tasks correctly	0
Ask patient to open and close eyes and then grip and release nonparetic hand.	• Performs 1 task correctly	1
	• Performs neither task correctly	2
2 Gaze	• Normal	0
Only horizontal movements tested	• Partial gaze palsy	1
	• Forced deviation or total gaze paresis not overcome by oculocephalic maneuver	2
3 Visual field	• No visual loss	0
Tested by confrontation	• Partial hemianopia	1
	• Complete hemianopia	2
	• Bilateral hemianopia (blind from any cause including cortical blindness)	3
4 Facial movement	• Normal symmetrical movement	0
Encourage patient to smile and close eyes or note symmetry of grimace in response to noxious stimuli if poorly responsive	• Minor paralysis (flattened nasolabial fold, asymmetry on smiling)	1
	• Partial paralysis (total or near-total lower face paralysis)	2
	• Complete paralysis (absence of facial movement upper/lower face)	3
5a Left arm motor function	• No drift—holds for full 10 seconds	0
Extend left arm palm down at 90 degrees (sitting) or 45 degrees (supine).	• Drifts down before 10 seconds but does not hit bed/support	1
	• Some effort against gravity, but cannot get up to 90 (or 45 if supine) degrees	2
	• No effort against gravity; limb falls	3
	• No movement	4
5b Right arm motor function	• No drift—holds for full 10 seconds	0
Extend right arm palm down at 90 degrees (sitting) or 45 degrees (supine).	• Drifts down before 10 seconds but does not hit bed/support	1
	• Some effort against gravity but cannot get up to 90 (or 45 if supine) degrees	2
	• No effort against gravity; limb falls	3
	• No movement	4
6a Left leg motor function	• No drift—holds for full 5 seconds	0
Extend left leg and flex at hip to 30 degrees.	• Drifts down before 5 seconds but does not hit bed or support	1
	• Some effort against gravity	2
	• No effort against gravity; limb falls	3
	• No movement	4
6b Right leg motor function	• No drift—holds for full 5 seconds	0
Extend right leg and flex at hip to 30 degrees.	• Drifts down before 5 seconds but does not hit bed or support	1
	• Some effort against gravity	2
	• No effort against gravity; limb falls	3
	• No movement	4
7 Limb ataxia	• Absent	0
Finger and nose and heel and shin done on both sides; not ataxia if hemiplegic or unable to comprehend; ataxia must be out of proportion to any weakness present	• Present in one limb	1
	• Present in two limbs	2
8 Sensory	• Normal	0
	• Pinprick less sharp or dull on affected side	1
	• Severe to total sensory loss; patient unaware of being touched	2

Continued

Table 5.9 National Institutes of Health Stroke Scale—cont'd

Item and Domain	Response	Score
9 Best language Name items; read short sentences.	• No aphasia	0
	• Some loss of fluency or comprehension	1
	• Severe aphasia—fragmentary communication; listener carries burden of communication	2
	• Mute, global aphasia. No usable speech or auditory comprehension	3
10 Dysarthria If not obviously present, have patient read.	• Normal	0
	• Slurs some words	1
	• So slurred as to be unintelligible, or mute	2
11 Extinction or inattention	• No abnormality	0
	• Inattention to any sensory modality or extinction to bilateral simultaneous stimulation in one sensory modality	1
	• Profound hemi-inattention or hemi-inattention to more than one modality; does not recognize own hand	2

From National Institutes of Health. (2008). NIH stroke scale. Retrieved August 2, 2011, from http://www.ninds.nih.gov/doctors/NIH_Stroke_Scale_Booklet.pdf

Table 5.10 Muscle Strength Grading Scale

Grade	Description
0/5	No movement or muscle contraction
1/5	Trace; no movement but evidence of muscle contraction
2/5	Not greater than gravity; movement with gravity eliminated
3/5	Greater than gravity; movement against gravity
4/5	Slight weakness; movement against some resistance
5/5	Normal; movement against full resistance

  b) Pronator drift
    i) Detection: have patient hold his or her arms out in front with palms up and eyes closed.
    ii) Normal: patient should be able to hold arms even for at least 20 seconds.
    iii) Abnormal: the weak arm begins to drift and pronate (turn palm downward).
  2) Leg strength
    a) Test flexor and extensor muscle groups by evaluating strength against resistance.
    b) Ask the patient to raise legs one at a time to 30 degrees off the bed from supine position and hold in place for a count to 5; observe for drift.
3. Muscle tone
  a. Flaccidity: no resistance to passive movement; flaccid paralysis is generally associated with LMN lesions but may also occur early in UMN lesions
  b. Hypotonia: little resistance to passive movement
  c. Hypertonia: increased muscle resistance to passive movement
  d. Rigidity: increased muscle resistance to passive movement of a rigid limb that is uniform through both flexion and extension (paratonic rigidity may occur in coma and is a sign of diffuse cerebral dysfunction)
  e. Spasticity: gradual increase in tone, causing increased resistance until tone is suddenly reduced
    1) Clonus, continued rhythmic contraction of a muscle after the stimulus has been applied, may be evident
    2) Spastic paralysis is associated with UMN lesions and emerges after resolution of the early flaccidity stage.
  f. UMN versus LMN (Table 5.11)
4. Coordination
  a. Point-to-point movements
    1) Finger-nose test: ask patient to touch his or her nose with the finger with eyes closed.
    2) Finger-finger test: ask patient to touch your finger with his or her finger.
    3) Heel-knee test: ask patient to run the heel of one foot down the opposite leg from the knee to the foot.
  b. Rapid, rhythmic alternating movements
    1) Pronation-supination test: ask patient to rapidly pronate and supinate his or her hand.
    2) Patting test: ask patient to rapidly pronate and supinate his or her hand against a leg.
  c. Figure-of-eight test: ask patient to draw a figure of eight in the air with his or her great toe.
5. Gait
  a. Tandem gait: patient asked to walk heel-to-toe in a straight line
    1) Normal: ability to walk heel-to-toe without difficulty
    2) Abnormal: loss of balance indicates cerebellar dysfunction
  b. Abnormal gaits
    1) Spastic: leg is held stiff and moved slowly; toes and lateral aspect of foot scrape the floor as the leg is moved; this indicates corticospinal tract lesion.
    2) Steppage: foot is lifted very high for each step with a distinctive slapping sound as it hits the floor; this indicates a peripheral nerve injury.
    3) Ataxic: feet are broad based, and steps are unsteady and staggering; this indicates cerebellar or dorsal column lesions.

Table 5.11　Locating Site of Motor Problems

	Lower Motor Neuron	Upper Motor Neuron	
		Pyramidal Tract	Extrapyramidal Tract
Effect	Flaccid paralysis Areflexia	• Spastic paralysis with hyperactive reflexes • Positive Babinski reflex	• No paralysis • Altered muscle tone and abnormal movements
Muscle appearance	Atrophy Small muscular contractions (fasciculation)	Mild atrophy from disuse	Tremor when at rest
Muscle tone	Decreased	Increased	Increased
Muscle strength	Decreased or absent	Decreased or absent	Normal
Coordination	Absent or poor	Absent or poor	Slowed
Examples	• Poliomyelitis • ALS • Guillain-Barré syndrome	• Stroke • Spinal cord injury • Multiple sclerosis • ALS	• Parkinson disease

ALS, Amyotrophic lateral sclerosis.

    4) Propulsive: body is bent forward, steps are short, momentum is increased, and falls are common; this indicates basal ganglia dysfunction (e.g., Parkinson disease).
    5) Waddling: pelvis opposite the weight-bearing hip drops and the trunk inclines, causing a waddle; this indicates proximal muscle weakness (e.g., muscular dystrophy).
    6) Scissors: thighs are held together, and each foot is alternately brought forward; this indicates a UMN lesion.
6. Station: tested by Romberg test
  a. Method: patient asked to stand with feet together and arms extended in front with eyes closed
  b. Normal: patient able to stand erect and steady; slight swaying may be seen
  c. Abnormal: patient loses balance; this indicates loss of position sense and/or cerebellar dysfunction
7. Involuntary movements
  a. Posturing may occur spontaneously or to pain in comatose patients; may also be considered a "mass response"
    1) Abnormal flexion (Fig. 5.14)
      a) Also called decorticate posturing
      b) Arms are flexed toward the body; legs are extended.
      c) Indicates a cerebral lesion
    2) Abnormal extension (Fig. 5.14)
      a) Also called decerebrate posturing
      b) Arms are extended, wrists are externally rotated, and legs are extended.
      c) Indicates a midbrain or brainstem lesion
    3) Opisthotonos
      a) Also referred to as arching
      b) Extension of arms and legs and arching of the back and neck
      c) May indicate a brainstem injury
    4) Flaccid posture: entire body is flaccid even with painful stimulation.

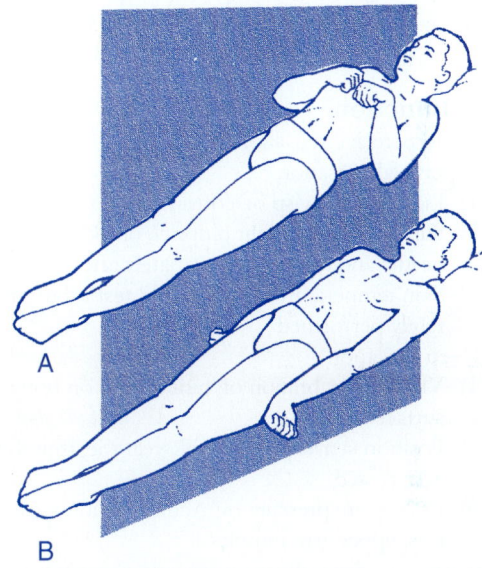

Fig. 5.14　**A,** Abnormal flexion (decorticate) posturing. **B,** Abnormal extension (decerebrate) posturing. (From Amidei, C. [2017]. Nervous system alterations. In M. L. Sole, D. Klein, & M. Moseley [Eds.], *Introduction to critical care nursing* [7th ed.]. St. Louis: Elsevier)

  b. Tremor
    1) Resting: Parkinson disease
    2) Intentional: cerebellar disease
    3) Flapping: metabolic encephalopathy (e.g., hepatic or renal failure)
    4) Physiologic: stress induced
    5) Senile: age induced
  c. Seizure: describe
    1) Preceding events: aura?
    2) Initial cry or sound
    3) Onset
      a) Initial body movements
      b) Deviation of head and eyes
      c) Chewing and salivation
      d) Posture of body
      e) Sensory changes

4) Tonic and clonic phases
    a) Progression of movements of body
    b) Skin color and airway
    c) Pupillary changes
    d) Incontinence
    e) Duration of each phase
5) LOC during seizure
6) Postictal phase
    a) Duration
    b) General behavior
    c) Memory of events
    d) Orientation
    e) Pupillary changes
    f) Headache
    g) Aphasia
    h) Injuries
7) Duration of entire seizure
8) Medications given and response
9) Findings on diagnostic studies
    a) Serum electrolytes
    b) Diagnostic imaging (e.g., computed tomography [CT], magnetic resonance imaging [MRI])
    c) Electroencephalography (EEG)

Sensory Function

1. Ability to perceive sensation
   a. Superficial sensation
      1) Light touch: wisp of cotton on skin
      2) Superficial pain: light pinprick on skin (use sterile needle and discard appropriately after testing)
      3) Skin temperature: hot and cold test tubes on skin; rarely performed
   b. Deep sensation
      1) Vibration: vibration of tuning fork on bony surface
      2) Position sense: position of great toe, thumb with eyes closed
      3) Deep pain: pressure on Achilles tendon, calf muscles, upper arm muscles
   c. Cortical or discriminatory sensation: requires cortical interpretation
      1) Two-point discrimination: ability to distinguish between one or two points; touch patient with two points at varying degrees of separation to see if the patient feels only one point or two points
      2) Stereognosis: ability to distinguish common objects placed in the hand with eyes closed
      3) Topognosis: ability to distinguish which finger is being touched with eyes closed
      4) Graphesthesia: ability to recognize numbers or letters traced on the skin with eyes closed
      5) Double simultaneous stimulation (tactile inattention testing): ability to differentiate between one point and two points when being touched by one or two points on opposite sides of the body in corresponding locations
   d. Ability to recognize objects through the special senses; inability referred to as *agnosia*
      1) Visual: occipital lobe
      2) Auditory: temporal lobe
      3) Tactile: parietal lobe
      4) Body parts and relationships: parietal lobe

Table 5.12 Dermatomal Levels for Bedside Assessment

Anatomical Location	Spinal Level
Front of neck	C3
Thumb	C6
Ring and little fingers	C8
Nipple line	T4
Umbilicus	T10
Groin crease	L1
Knee	L3
Anterior ankle and foot	L5
Lateral foot and heel	S1
Genitalia	S3, S4

   e. Distribution of sensory loss
      1) Entire side of body: parietal or thalamic lesion
      2) Dermatomal (Table 5.12; Fig. 5.12)
         a) Dermatome: skin area supplied by sensory fibers of a single spinal nerve
         b) Sensory loss below a dermatomal level: spinal cord lesion
         c) Sensory loss along a dermatome: spinal nerve lesion
      3) Peripheral nerve distribution (Fig. 5.12)
   f. Degrees of sensory loss
      1) Anesthesia: loss of sensation
      2) Dysesthesia: impaired sensation
      3) Hyperesthesia: increased sensation
      4) Hypesthesia: decreased sensation
      5) Paresthesia: burning, tingling sensation

Cranial Nerve Function Assessment

1. Olfactory (I)
   a. Test: patient's ability to identify familiar odors (e.g., coffee, cloves, tobacco, alcohol) tested; each nostril tested separately with eyes closed; rarely performed in acute care
   b. Normal: able to identify familiar odors
   c. Abnormal: unable to identify familiar odors; referred to as *anosmia*
2. Optic (II)
   a. Visual acuity: test by the following:
      1) Snellen chart
         a) Ask patient to read lines of the Snellen chart from a distance of 20 feet or use a pocket Snellen card for patients who are bed-bound.
         b) Record the number on the lowest line that the patient can read with 50% accuracy.
         c) Test with glasses or contact lenses.
      2) If patient cannot see well enough to read the Snellen chart, ask how many fingers you are holding up.
      3) If the patient cannot see well enough to tell you how many fingers you are holding up, assess whether he or she blinks to visual threat.
   b. Visual fields
      1) Test by confrontation: comparison of patient's visual field to examiner's visual field with eye on same side covered

2) Loss of vision or portion of visual field
   a) Unilateral blindness: lesion of eye, retina, or optic nerve
   b) Bitemporal hemianopsia: lesion of optic chiasm or lesion causing pressure on optic chiasm (e.g., pituitary tumor)
   c) Left homonymous hemianopsia: lesion of right optic tract
   d) Right homonymous hemianopsia: lesion of left optic tract
   e) Left homonymous hemianopsia with macular sparing: lesion of right geniculocalcarine tract
   f) Right homonymous hemianopsia with macular sparing: lesion of left geniculocalcarine tract
  c. Near vision
   1) Test: ask the patient to read newsprint at a distance of 12 inches or use pocket Snellen card.
   2) Normal: patient should be able to read newsprint at 1 foot.
  d. Funduscopic examination with ophthalmoscope to detect papilledema
   1) Optic disk is pushed forward.
   2) Disk margins are blurry.
   3) Indication of intracranial hypertension
    a) May be late in acute intracranial hypertension
    b) May be first sign in chronic intracranial hypertension (e.g., tumor)
3. Oculomotor (III), trochlear (IV), abducens (VI)
  a. Eyelids: elevation of the eyelid is controlled by CN III; ptosis may indicate CN III injury.
  b. Pupils
   1) Size
    a) Normal 2 to 6 mm
    b) Abnormal: clinically significant change is change of more than 1 mm.
     i) Pinpoint (and nonreactive)
      (a) Pontine lesion
      (b) Medication effect
       (i) Opiates (e.g., morphine)
       (ii) Miotics (e.g., pilocarpine)
     ii) Midsize (2 to 6 mm) but nonreactive: midbrain lesion
     iii) Unilateral large (>6 mm) and nonreactive (may be referred to as *blown or Hutchinsonian pupil*): pressure on oculomotor nerve on same side
     iv) Bilateral large (>6 mm) and nonreactive
      (a) Brainstem lesion
      (b) Medication effect
       (i) Parasympatholytics (e.g., atropine)
       (ii) Sympathomimetics (e.g., epinephrine)
   2) Equality
    a) Normal: equal
    b) Abnormal: unequal (referred to as *anisocoria*)
     i) Normal variation: 15% to 20% of the population has slightly unequal pupils (1 mm or less difference)
     ii) Abnormal: difference of more than 1 mm or change from baseline
     iii) Injury effects
      (a) Injury to parasympathetic fibers of the oculomotor nerve: ipsilateral (same side) pupil dilation
      (b) Injury to sympathetic fibers of the oculomotor nerves (e.g., Horner syndrome: ipsilateral pupil constriction)
   3) Shape
    a) Normal: round
    b) Abnormal
     i) Oval
      (a) May precede dilated pupil as a sign of pressure on the oculomotor nerve
      (b) Associated with ICP of 18 to 35 mm Hg
     ii) Irregular (e.g., keyhole shaped may be seen in patients after cataract removal due to concurrent iridectomy)
   4) Position
    a) Normal: midposition
    b) Abnormal
     i) Both eyes deviated toward one side
      (a) Unilateral pontine lesion
      (b) Fixed lesion such as tumor, stroke, or hemorrhage: toward the lesion and away from the hemiparesis
      (c) Seizure: away from the seizure focus and toward the hemiparesis
     ii) Downward deviation of both eyes (frequently with inward convergence): thalamic lesion
     iii) Downward deviation of one eye: CN III palsy
     iv) Medial deviation of one eye: CN IV palsy
   5) Reactivity to light
    a) Test
     i) Darken the room if pupils are small.
     ii) Use a small, bright penlight in front of each eye.
     iii) Note pupil constriction as the direct reaction.
     iv) Note pupil constriction of the opposite pupil as consensual reaction.
    b) Normal: brisk bilateral direct and consensual reaction to light
    c) Abnormal
     i) Sluggish or absent reaction; indicative of any of the following:
      (a) CN III pressure or injury
      (b) Hypothermia
      (c) Barbiturate intoxication
     ii) Hippus: pupil initially reacts briskly followed by an exaggerated rhythmic contraction and dilation of the pupil; may be normal but may be indicative of any of the following:
      (a) Early CN III pressure or injury
      (b) Midbrain injury
      (c) Barbiturate intoxication
   6) Accommodation
    a) Test: ask the patient to focus on a distant object and accommodate as the object moves closer.
    b) Pupils dilate when focusing on a far object.
    c) Pupils constrict when focusing on a near object.

7) Ciliospinal reflex
    a) Test: squeeze trapezius muscle and observe reaction of pupil on same side.
    b) Normal: ipsilateral pupil dilation with trapezius squeeze
    c) Abnormal: no response; indicative of interruption of sympathetic fibers of CN III
c. Extraocular movements (EOMs)
    1) Test: patient asked to keep head straight and follow your finger with eyes; move your finger in the direction of the six cardinal positions of gaze (Fig. 5.15)
    2) Normal: both eyes move conjugately in the direction of your finger.
    3) Abnormal: one or both eyes do not move to follow finger; indicative of CN injury or isolated muscular dysfunction
d. Abnormal eye movements
    1) Nystagmus: jerky eye movement that oscillates the eye back and forth quickly; may be seen in lesions of vestibular system or brainstem
    2) Dysconjugate eye movement: may indicate damage to the brainstem
    3) Conjugate eye movement: may indicate cerebral hemispheric damage
4. Trigeminal (V)
    a. Sensory branch
        1) Test
            a) Three branches (ophthalmic, maxillary, mandibular) tested on both sides with a wisp of cotton (light touch) and pinprick (superficial pain)
                i) Normal: detection of touch and pain
                ii) Abnormal: no detection of touch or pain
            b) Corneal blink reflex
                i) Detection: corneal touched with a wisp of cotton
                ii) Normal: bilateral blink; indicates intactness of CNs V and VII
                iii) Abnormal: decreased or absent blink; may indicate CN V injury (NOTE: Contact lens wearers have diminished corneal blink reflex.)
    b. Motor branch
        1) Test: face inspected for muscle atrophy, tremor; the masseter muscle palpated while the patient clenches teeth; the temporal muscles palpated as the patient squeezes eyes closed

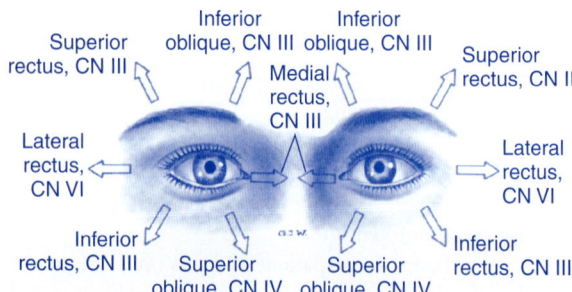

Fig. 5.15 The six cardinal positions of gaze. (From Seidel, H. M., Ball, J. W., Dains, J. E., & Benedict, G. W. [1991]. *Mosby's guide to physical examination* [2nd ed.]. St. Louis: Mosby.)

2) Normal: symmetry of muscle strength, no atrophy or tremor
3) Abnormal: asymmetry of muscle strength; may indicate CN V injury
5. Facial (VII)
    a. Motor branch
        1) Test: symmetry of facial expressions noted while patient raises eyebrows, frowns, smiles, and closes eyelids tightly
        2) Abnormal: asymmetry of facial expression; loss of nasolabial fold, eye remaining open; indicates CN VII injury (Bell palsy)
    b. Sensory branch
        1) Test: ability to taste sour and bitter on posterior tongue tested; rarely performed in acute care
        2) Normal: ability to taste
        3) Abnormal: inability to taste; indicates CN VII injury
6. Acoustic (VIII)
    a. Cochlear branch: hearing acuity
        1) Whisper test
            a) Test: face turned away and examiner whispers to see if patient can hear what is whispered
            b) Test each ear separately.
            c) This test differentiates between hearing and lip reading.
        2) Weber test
            a) Test: tuning fork placed at the midline vertex of skull
            b) Normal: patient hears equally on both sides.
            c) Abnormal: patient indicates difference between the two ears; hears the sound better with the "good" ear.
        3) Rinne test
            a) Test: tuning fork placed on the mastoid, when the patient can no longer hear the sound by bone, the tuning fork is moved to in front of the ear
            b) Normal: air conduction is usually better than bone conduction, so the patient should still be able to hear the sound when the tuning fork is moved in front of the ear after the patient reports not being able to hear the sound any longer by bone.
            c) Abnormal: inability to hear the sound by air after the cessation of the sound by bone; diminished air conduction is associated with middle ear infection or disease
    b. Vestibular branch
        1) Not tested directly; problems may be detected by symptoms such as nystagmus, vertigo, nausea, vomiting, pallor, sweating, and hypotension
        2) Reflexes: vestibular branch of CN VIII and connections with CNs III and VI provide information regarding integrity of the brainstem
            a) Oculocephalic reflex (also called *doll eyes reflex*) (Fig. 5.16)
                i) Prerequisites
                    (a) Cervical spine has been radiologically cleared.
                    (b) Patient must be unconscious.
                    (c) Eyes are held open so that eye movement can be observed.

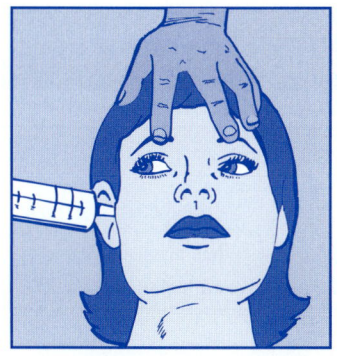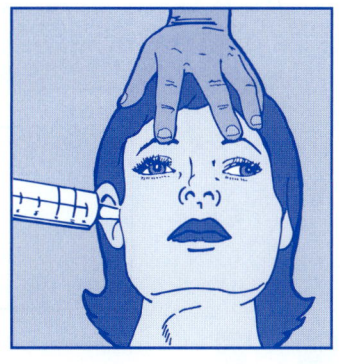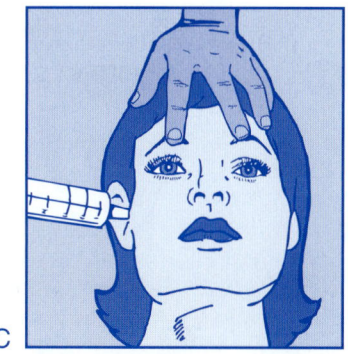

Fig. 5.16 Test for oculovestibular reflex (caloric ice-water test). **A,** Normal response—conjugate eye movements. **B,** Abnormal response—dysconjugate or asymmetric eye movements. **C,** Absent response—no eye movements. (From Boss, B., & Huether, S. [2014]. Alterations in cognitive systems, cerebral hemodynamics, and motor function. In K. McCance & S. Huether [Eds.], *Pathophysiology: The biologic basis for disease in adults and children* [7th ed.]. St. Louis: Elsevier.)

      ii) Test: head rotated side to side
      iii) Normal: eyes move in the opposite direction of the head (presence of doll eyes: like an expensive china doll); indicates supratentorial cause for the coma
      iv) Abnormal: eyes stay midline or turn to the same direction as the head (absence of doll eyes); indicates compression in the midbrain-pontine area
    b) Oculovestibular reflex (also called *caloric testing*) (Fig. 5.17)
      i) Prerequisites
        (a) Intact tympanic membrane
        (b) Absence of basal skull fracture
      ii) Test
        (a) Elevation of the head of bed (HOB) 30 degrees
        (b) Injection of 20 to 50 ml of iced water into the ear canal and against the tympanic membrane
      iii) Normal: nystagmus with deviation toward the irrigated ear
      iv) Abnormal
        (a) No eye movement
        (b) Dysconjugate eye movement
7. Glossopharyngeal (IX), vagus (X)
  a. Phonation
    1) Test: patient asked to say, "Ah"
    2) Normal: bilateral elevation of palate
    3) Abnormal: no elevation of palate on one side
  b. Speech
    1) Test: speech assessed; any hoarseness detected
    2) Normal: voice clear with ability to change volume and pitch
    3) Abnormal: hoarseness; indicates damage to the laryngeal branch of CN X
  c. Taste
    1) Test: ability to taste sour and bitter on posterior tongue tested; rarely performed in acute care
    2) Normal: ability to taste
    3) Abnormal: inability to taste sour or bitter
  d. Swallowing
    1) Test
      a) Hold tongue down with a tongue blade and touch each side of the pharynx with a cotton swab.
      b) Palpate elevation of larynx with swallow.
      c) If patient is conscious, give sip of water.
    2) Normal: involuntary swallow or gag when palate is stroked, elevation of larynx with swallow; effective swallow; indicates intactness of CNs IX and X
    3) Abnormal
      a) No swallow or gag; do not give fluids; position on side; have suction equipment available
      b) Cough on water swallow: request evaluation by speech and language pathologist.
  e. Gag
    1) Test: palate stroked with a tongue blade (NOTE: Do not perform this test within 2 hours after eating.)
    2) Normal: involuntary gag; indicates intactness of ninth and tenth CNs
    3) Abnormal: no gag (NOTE: Do not give fluids; do position on side and have suction equipment available.)
  f. Cough
    1) Test: touch hypopharynx with suction catheter.
    2) Normal: involuntary cough; indicates intactness of CNs IX and X
    3) Abnormal: no cough
8. Spinal accessory (XI)
  a. Test
    1) Sternocleidomastoid and trapezius muscles inspected for size and symmetry
    2) Patient asked to shrug shoulders as you push down with your hands on the shoulders
    3) Patient asked to turn head to each side against resistance
  b. Normal: symmetry; adequate muscle strength
  c. Abnormal: asymmetry; poor muscle strength
9. Hypoglossal (XII)
  a. Test
    1) Tongue inspected for atrophy, fasciculations, alignment
    2) Tongue strength tested with your index finger when the patient pushes his or her tongue against the cheek

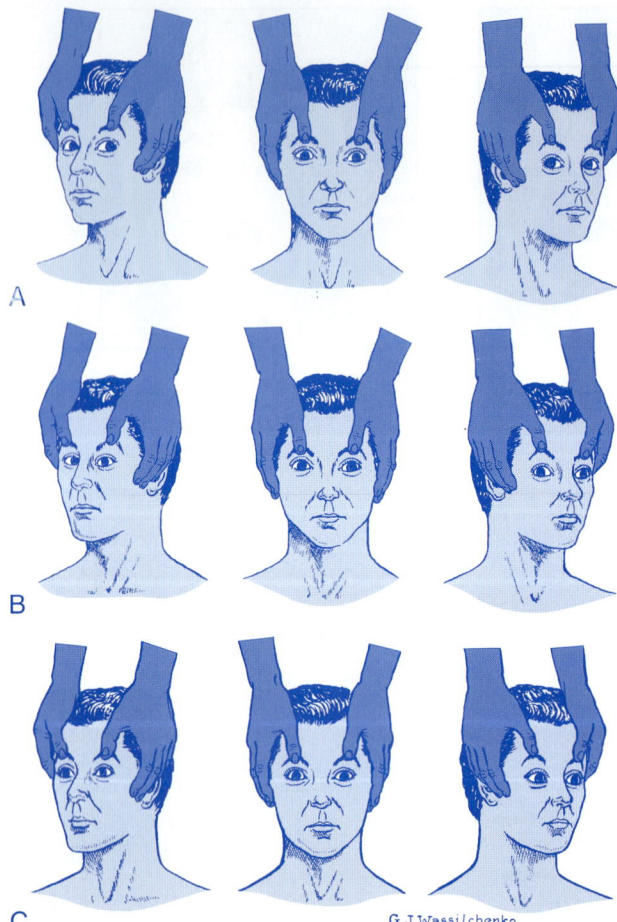

Table 5.13	Grading Scale for Deep Tendon Reflexes
Grade	Description
0	Absent
1+	Diminished
2+	Normal
3+	More brisk than average but may be normal
4+	Hyperactive with clonus

Fig. 5.17 Test for oculocephalic reflex response (doll eyes phenomenon). **A,** Normal response—eyes turn together to side opposite from turn of head. **B,** Abnormal response—eyes do not turn in conjugate manner. **C,** Absent response—eyes do not turn as head position changes. (From Boss, B., & Huether, S. [2014]. Alterations in cognitive systems, cerebral hemodynamics, and motor function. In K. McCance & S. Huether [Eds.], *Pathophysiology: The biologic basis for disease in adults and children* [7th ed.]. St. Louis: Elsevier.)

   b. Normal: no atrophy, fasciculations, midline alignment when protrudes, normal strength
   c. Abnormal: atrophy, fasciculations, or deviation from midline; decreased strength

Reflexes
1. Deep tendon (also called *muscle-stretch reflexes*)
   a. Test: tendon tapped with a reflex hammer
   b. Normal: contraction of the muscle and a jerk of affected limb
   c. Abnormal
      1) Hyporeflexia
         a) Less than normal contraction
         b) May be seen in hypocalcemia, hyperphosphatemia, hypomagnesemia, LMN lesion
      2) Hyperreflexia
         a) More than normal contraction; may be associated with clonus
         b) May be seen in hypercalcemia, hypophosphatemia, hypermagnesemia, and UMN lesion
   d. Grading scale (Table 5.13)
   e. Locations and spinal levels
      1) Jaw: CN V (trigeminal)
      2) Biceps: elbow flexion; C5 to C6
      3) Brachioradialis: wrist extension; C5 to C6
      4) Triceps: elbow extension; C7 to C8
      5) Patellar: knee extension; L2 to L4
      6) Achilles: foot extension; S1 to S2
2. Superficial reflexes
   a. Abdominal reflexes
      1) Test: abdomen stroked toward umbilicus with blunt end of cotton-tipped applicator
      2) Normal: umbilicus moves toward the quadrant that is stroked.
      3) Abnormal: no response; indicates lesion at T7 to T9 for upper abdomen; T11 to T12 for lower abdomen
   b. Cremasteric reflex
      1) Test: inner thigh stroked
      2) Normal: testis on stimulated side elevates.
      3) Abnormal: no response: indicates lesion at L1 to L2
   c. Plantar reflex
      1) Test: sole of the foot stroked with a blunt instrument (Fig. 5.18)
      2) Normal: toes curl downward.
      3) Abnormal (Babinski reflex): extension of great toe and fanning of other toes; indicates UMN lesion
3. Pathologic reflexes
   a. Babinski: described earlier
   b. Grasp
      1) Test: something (frequently finger) placed in the patient's hand
      2) Normal: releases grasp on command
      3) Abnormal: will not release grasp on command; infantile reflex: indicates diffuse cerebral dysfunction
   c. Sucking
      1) Test: corner of the patient's mouth touched
      2) Normal: no response
      3) Abnormal: patient purses lips and starts to suck; infantile reflex: indicates diffuse cerebral dysfunction
   d. Glabellar
      1) Test: patient's forehead tapped
      2) Normal: no response
      3) Abnormal: patient repeatedly blinks; indicates diffuse cerebral dysfunction

Miscellaneous
1. Clinical indications of neurologic trauma
   a. Scalp: tears or swelling
   b. Head and face

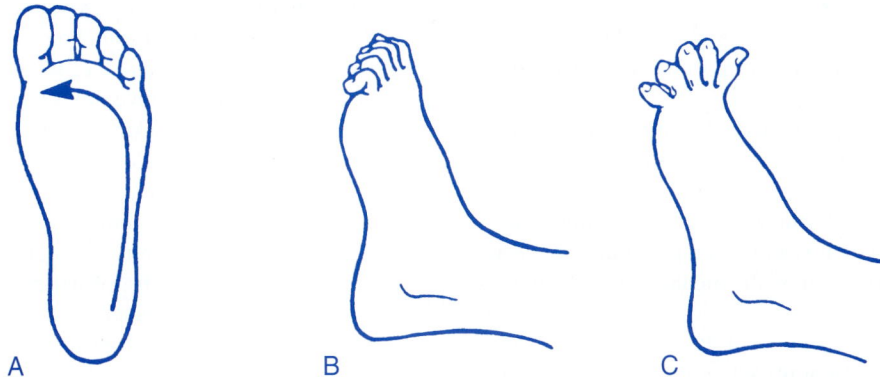

Fig. 5.18 Babinski reflex. **A,** Method of stroking sole of foot. **B,** Normal response (absence of Babinski reflex). **C,** Abnormal response (presence of Babinski reflex).

   1) Face, maxilla, and mandible should be palpated for fractures.
   2) Note Battle sign: bruising of mastoid (behind ear); indicative of basal (i.e., basilar) skull fracture (Fig. 5.19)
  c. Eyes
   1) Eye orbits should be palpated; note complaints of pain
   2) Visual acuity should be evaluated if corneal burn or trauma
   3) Note raccoon eyes: bruising around eyes indicative of basal skull fracture (Fig. 5.19)
  d. Nose
   1) Nose should be palpated; note complaints of pain.
   2) Note CSF leak: may be seen in basal skull fracture and may indicate a dural tear; referred to as *rhinorrhea*
      a) Differentiation of CSF from mucus by testing for significant glucose
         i) CSF glucose is normally 60% of serum glucose
         ii) Low levels of glucose may be seen with mucus
      b) CSF also leaves a "halo" on 4 × 4-inch gauze or linens; this refers to blood settling in the middle with a lighter-colored concentric ring around the blood (Fig. 5.19)
  e. Ears
   1) Note edema and trauma to external ear or ear canal.
   2) Note blood in external ear canal or blood behind ear drum: seen in basal skull fracture
   3) Note CSF leak from ear: seen in basal skull fracture and may indicate a dural tear; referred to as *otorrhea*
  f. Injury to teeth, tongue, gums, mucosa
  g. Alteration in consciousness
  h. Clinical indications of intracranial hypertension (see Intracranial Hypertension section)
 2. Clinical indications of meningeal irritation
  a. Nuchal rigidity: indicative of meningeal irritation (e.g., infection or hemorrhage)
  b. Brudzinski sign (Fig. 5.20)

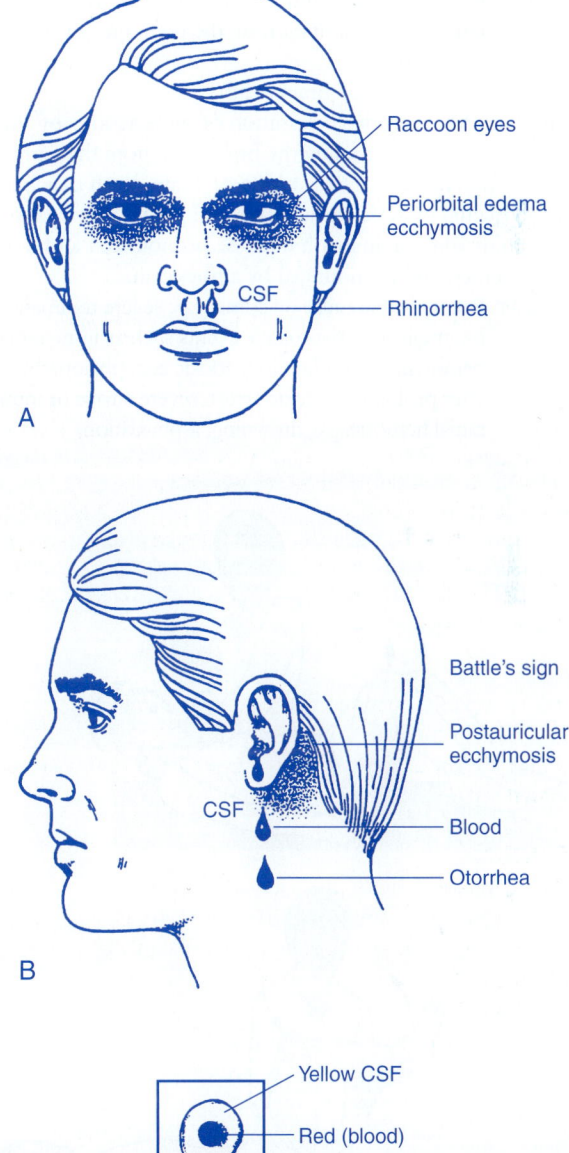

Fig. 5.19 A, Raccoon eyes and rhinorrhea. **B,** Battle sign with otorrhea. **C,** Halo sign. (From Barker, E. [2008]. *Neuroscience nursing: A spectrum of care* [3rd ed.]. St. Louis: Mosby.)

1) Prerequisite: cervical spine must be radiologically cleared.
2) Detection: chin brought toward chest and head moved forward
3) Normal: absence of neck pain and absence of involuntary adduction and flexion of knees toward body
4) Abnormal: neck pain and involuntary adduction and flexion of legs with attempts to flex the neck; indicates irritation of the meninges by infection or blood

c. Kernig sign (Fig. 5.20)
1) Detection: patient placed on his or her back and assisted to flex thigh toward chest until hip is at 90-degree angle; then leg extended at knee
2) Normal: ability to fully extend leg without pain
3) Abnormal: inability to fully extend leg when thigh is flexed toward abdomen; neck pain may also occur; indicates irritation of the meninges by infection or blood

3. Clinical indications of brain death
a. Criteria: irreversible cessation of all functions of the entire brain, including the brainstem; note that specific requirements for declaration of brain death may be affected by state law and hospital policy, however at minimum, brain death must be pronounced and documented and pronounced by a physician.
1) Recognizable cause of coma (e.g., severe traumatic brain injury or neurologic events such as intracranial hemorrhage or infarction, anoxic encephalopathy after prolonged cardiac arrest, severe stroke or intracranial hemorrhage, drowning, asphyxiation)

2) Exclude potentially reversible causes of coma and possible confounding factors, which could mimic brain death (e.g., fulminant Guillain-Barré syndrome, sedative drugs including alcohol, neuromuscular blocking agents, severe hypothermia, metabolic or endocrine disturbance, postcardiac arrest syndrome, severe overdose of CNS depressants or tricyclic antidepressants, and others)
  a) BP of 100 mm Hg or greater
    i) Correct hypotension with intravenous (IV) fluids, vasopressors, or inotropic medications
    ii) Neurologic examination is most reliable if systolic BP of 00 mm Hg or greater.
  b) Temperature greater than 32°C (90°F) (Establish normothermia; may need warming blankets) (Amidei, 2017; Dennison, 2013)
  c) Neurologic assessment (Arbour, 2013)
    i) Absence of brainstem function
      (1) Pupils fixed and dilated, no response to light (i.e., CN II [optic], III [oculomotor], and midbrain)
      (2) Absent ocular movements, which require functioning of CN III (i.e., oculomotor), CN IV (i.e., trochlear), CN VI (i.e., abducens), CN VIII (i.e., vestibulocochlear, pons, and midbrain)
      (3) No oculocephalic (i.e., doll's eyes) or oculovestibular reflexes
    ii) Negative CN assessment
      (1) No corneal reflex, which requires functioning of CN III (i.e., oculomotor), CN V (i.e., trigeminal), CN VII (i.e., facial), and pons
      (2) No gag or cough reflexes, which requires functioning of CN IX (i.e., glossopharyngeal), CN X (i.e., vagus), and medulla
    iii) Absence of responsiveness to noxious stimuli
    iv) Absence of movement
      (1) Including posturing, shivering, and seizures, either spontaneously or to central pain stimulation in the absence of sedation and neuromuscular blockade;
      2) Note: spinal reflexes and Babinski reflex may be present even in the presence of brain death
  d) Absence of spontaneous ventilation when tested for a sufficient time
    i) Can be 8 to 10 minutes if patient tolerates
    ii) $PaCO_2$ of greater than 60 mm Hg or 20 mm Hg or greater from baseline
    iii) Apnea testing (Arbour, 2013)
      (1) Stabilize body temperature of 36.5°C or greater (preferred)
        (a) Can be done at lower temperatures
        (b) Any additional time required for increase in CO_2 risks cardiovascular instability
      (2) Normalize $PaCO_2$ to range of 35–45 mm Hg

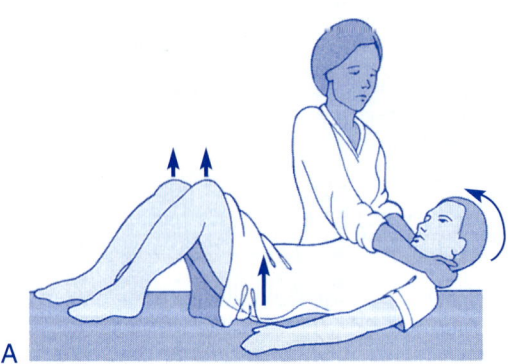
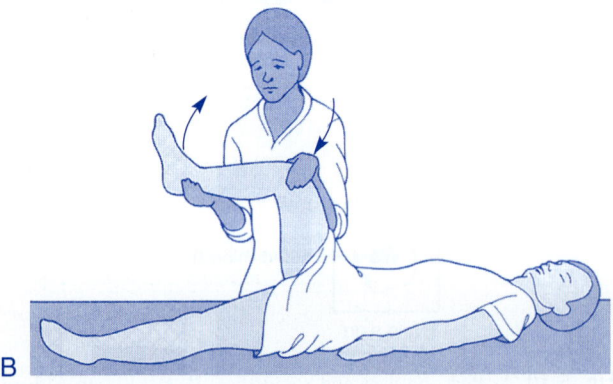

Fig. 5.20 A, Brudzinski sign. **B,** Kernig sign. (From Barker, E. [2008]. *Neuroscience nursing: A spectrum of care* [3rd ed.]. St. Louis: Mosby.)

(3) Maintain adequate circulating blood volume
(4) Administer 100% oxygen for 10 minutes or longer to PaO_2 of 200 mm Hg or greater; obtain ABG to confirm
(5) Disconnect the mechanical ventilator.
(6) Results of apnea testing consistent with brain death include
 (a) No movement of the chest and abdominal walls (consistent with no intrinsic respiratory drive)
 (b) Caution: must differentiate between movements associated with respiratory effort and movements produced in phase with the cardiac cycle.
(7) Measure ABGs to confirm $PaCO_2$ elevations 20 mm Hg or greater from baseline or reaching a threshold of 60 mm Hg $PaCO_2$
 iv) Reconnect ventilator.
 e) Indications for aborting apnea testing include (Arbour, 2013)
  i) Marked oxygen desaturation (i.e., <85% for >30 seconds) and/or
  ii) Unstable BP (i.e., <90 mm Hg systolic and unresponsive to drug therapy) and/or
  iii) Unstable cardiac rhythm (e.g., bradycardia, ventricular ectopy)
3) Clinical examination
 a) Absence of responsiveness to noxious stimuli
 b) Absence of movement, including posturing, shivering, and seizures, either spontaneously or to central pain stimulation in the absence of sedation and neuromuscular blockade; spinal reflexes and Babinski reflex may be present even in the presence of brain death
4) Optional confirmatory diagnostic and laboratory studies
 a) EEG: no electrical activity during a period of at least 30 minutes
 b) Cerebral angiography: no intracerebral filling in circle of Willis or at carotid bifurcation
 c) Cerebral blood flow scan: no uptake of radionuclide in brain parenchyma, indicating no CBF
 d) Transcranial Doppler: reverberating flow signals
b. One neurologic exam is now considered sufficient for diagnosing brain death in most states (Amidei, 2017)
 1) Brain death must be pronounced and documented by a physician.
 2) If two clinical examinations are completed, one is done by a neurologist or neurosurgeon.

Neurologic Monitoring

1. ICP
 a. Indications
  1) The need for ICP monitoring usually correlates with a GCS score of 8 or less.
  2) All of the following are potential diagnoses when ICP monitoring may be needed.
   a) Severe head trauma, especially if abnormal findings on admission CT scan
   b) Intracerebral masses
   c) SAH
   d) Intracerebral hemorrhage (e.g., massive stroke)
   e) Infectious processes (e.g., encephalitis, meningitis)
   f) Encephalopathy
    i) Anoxic encephalopathy (e.g., postcardiac arrest)
    ii) Reye syndrome
   g) Hydrocephalus
   h) Postcraniotomy
  3) ICP monitoring should be used if deep sedation, paralysis, or barbiturate coma is being used because LOC as an assessment parameter is eliminated.
 b. Purposes
  1) Diagnose intracranial hypertension.
  2) Allow drainage of CSF to maintain pressure.
  3) Observe effects of medical or nursing management.
  4) Predict outcomes: patients who sustain an ICP greater than 50 mm Hg for longer than 20 minutes have a very poor prognosis.
 c. General information
  1) CSF is considered the most accurate indication of ICP.
   a) The most accurate devices measure the pressure of CSF and are in contact with CSF.
   b) This contact with CSF creates an infection risk.
   c) Intraparenchymal devices: there is a linear relationship between intraventricular and intraparenchymal pressure measured with fiberoptic transducer-tipped probe.
  2) There are several types of ICP-measuring devices (Fig. 5.21 and Table 5.14)
   a) Insertion of all of these devices is either during craniotomy or through a small burr hole made with a twist drill using strict aseptic technique.
  3) There are three types of monitoring systems.
   a) Fluid-filled system
    i) Sensor: fluid-filled catheter or bolt that communicates the subarachnoid or interventricular space and the transducer
    ii) Closed fluid-filled system between the sensor and the transducer
     (a) Prime the system using preservative-free isotonic saline.
     (b) Do not add heparin; do not use a pressure bag or intermittent flush device.
     (c) Use Luer-Lok connections.
     (d) Do not routinely irrigate; subarachnoid bolts may be irrigated if specifically ordered with approximately 0.1 ml every 2 hours; dilute antibiotic solution may be prescribed as irrigation solution.
    iii) Transducer: converts the pressure signal to an electrical signal that can be recorded

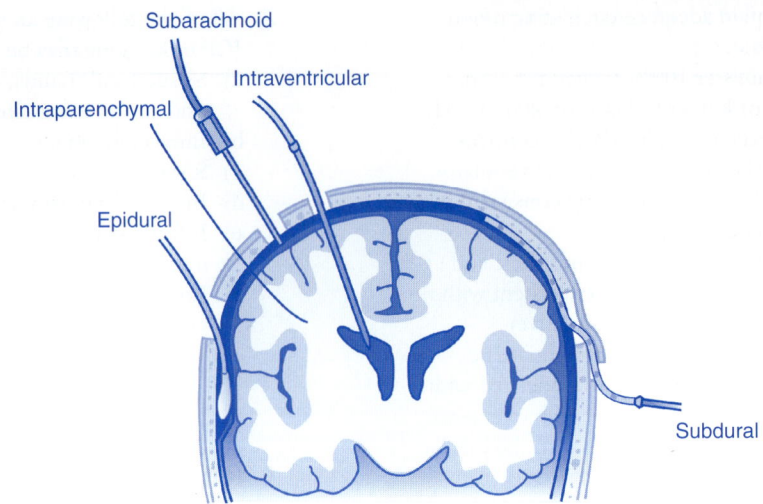

Fig. 5.21 Devices for the measurement of intracranial pressure. (From Carlson, K. K. [Ed.]. [2009]. *Advanced critical care nursing*. St. Louis: Saunders.)

Table 5.14	Intracranial Pressure Measuring Devices		
Device	**Location**	**Accuracy**	**Comments**
Intraventricular catheter	Lateral ventricle nondominant hemisphere is used if possible, but location of skull fracture and trauma may limit placement possibilities	Excellent; can test VPR	• Preferred because most accurate and reliable, low cost, and provides opportunity to drain CSF for specimen or treatment of intracranial hypertension • May be difficult to insert especially if ventricles are small or displaced • Therapeutic or diagnostic removal of CSF possible • Provides access for determination of volume-pressure relationship • May permit CSF leakage, but rapid CSF drainage may result in collapsed ventricle or subdural hematoma • May cause intracerebral bleeding or edema at cannula track • Infection rate, 2%–5% • Fluid-filled system used if intraventricular catheter is placed
Subarachnoid bolt or screw	Subarachnoid space	Fair; unreliable at high ICP	• Easy to insert; especially useful if ventricles are small • Inexpensive • Does not penetrate brain • Requires intact skull • Bolt can become occluded with clots or tissue causing a dampened waveform; may require irrigation, if ordered • Needs to be recalibrated frequently • Unable to drain CSF or to test VPR • Infection rate, 1%–2% • Fluid-filled system used
Epidural sensor or transducer	Between the skull and the dura	Variable; Increase in baseline drift over time may decrease accuracy (Arbour, 2004)	• Easy to insert • Does not penetrate brain or dura • Unable to drain CSF or to test VPR • Infection rate <1% • Head position has no effect on pressure reading • Cannot be rezeroed when in place • Epidural pressure is slightly higher than intraventricular pressure
Intraparenchymal transducer	1 cm into brain tissue	Excellent	• Easy to insert • Unable to drain CSF or to test VPR • Catheter relatively fragile; avoid sharp kinks or pulls • Head position has no effect on pressure reading • Cannot be rezeroed when in place • Risk of intracerebral bleeding and infection

CSF, Cerebrospinal fluid; *ICP*, intracranial pressure; *VPR*, volume-pressure response.

(a) Position the transducer at the level of the foramen of Monro; this correlates externally to the tragus of the ear.
(b) Connect the transducer cable to the pressure module of the bedside monitor.
  b) Continuous drainage system (Fig. 5.22)
    i) Place the drip chamber at the prescribed height above foramen of Monro; height is based on the desired upper limit for controlling the ICP.
    ii) Use commercial systems that have one-way flow valves and micropore filters on air vents.
  c) Fiberoptic transducer
    i) A fluid-filled system is not necessary.
    ii) The catheter is plugged directly into the monitor.
    iii) This system requires a special monitor module.
d. Measurement guidelines
  1) Explain procedure to the patient and family.
  2) Relevel and zero with each head position change if fluid-filled system.
  3) Do not stimulate patient before measures.
  4) Evaluate trends instead of one measurement.
  5) Assist with volume-pressure response (VPR) test (or *pressure-volume index*) as requested.
    a) Inject 1 ml of preservative-free isotonic saline in 1 second into an intraventricular catheter.
    b) Normal: increase in ICP of 2 mm Hg or less
    c) Low compliance: increase in ICP of 3 mm Hg or more
  6) If the ICP does not return to normal within 4 minutes after activity, compliance is poor.
e. ICP values (Amidei, 2017)
  1) Normal: 0 to 15 mm Hg

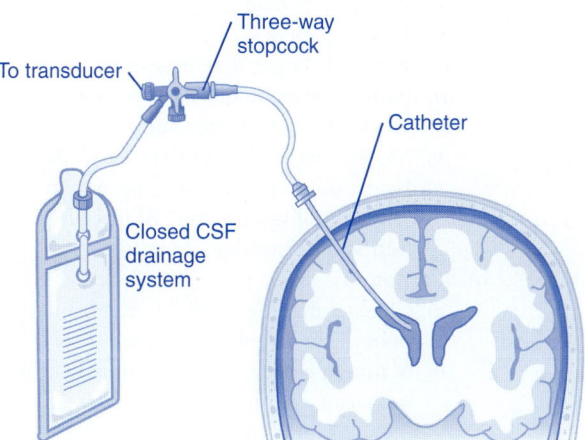

Fig. 5.22 Continuous drainage system. Continuous drainage involves placing the drip chamber of the drainage system at a specified level above the foramen of Monro (usually 15 cm). The system is left open to allow continuous drainage of cerebrospinal fluid into the chamber (which drains into a collection bag) against a pressure gradient that prevents excessive drainage and ventricular collapse. (From Carlson, K. K. [Ed.]. [2009]. *Advanced critical care nursing*. St. Louis: Saunders.)

  2) Increased ICP: greater than 20 mm Hg or greater persisting for 5 minutes or longer; this is a life-threatening event
    a) Sustained increases can lead in ICP to herniation (i.e., shifting of brain tissue for area of higher pressure to low pressure)
    b) Herniation syndromes
      i) Supratentorial (cingulate, central, and uncal herniation)
      ii) Infratentorial (cerebellar tonsil herniation)
f. ICP waveforms (Table 5.15)
  1) Normal actual time waveform (Fig. 5.23)
    a) P_1
      i) Percussion wave
      ii) Reflects ejection of blood from the heart transmitted through the choroid plexus
    b) P_2
      i) Tidal wave
      ii) Reflects elastic recoil during reduced systolic ejection phase of the cardiac cycle and arterial compliance within the brain
      iii) Normally, P_2 is approximately 60% of the height of P_1; when the amplitude of P_2 is greater than 60% of P_1 or becomes lost in the tracing, it is indicative of a decrease in compliance.
    c) P_3
      i) Dicrotic wave
      ii) Reflects closure of aortic valve
  2) Trend waveforms (Fig. 5.24)
    a) C waves (NOTE: Remember that C waves are cool.)
      i) Rapid, rhythmic oscillation of pressure without any relevance
      ii) Small spikes as high as 20 mm Hg at 6 per minute
      iii) Associated with changes in arterial BP and ventilation
    b) B waves (NOTE: Remember that B waves are bad.)
      i) Sharp, sawtooth-appearance waves
      ii) Pressures as high as 50 mm Hg lasting 30 seconds to 2 minutes
      iii) Related to changes in CBF
      iv) Although not significant alone, may precede A waves
    c) A waves (NOTE: Remember that A waves are awful.)
      i) Elevations on top of baseline elevation of ICP
      ii) Pressures reach 50 to 100 mm Hg and last 5 to 20 minutes
      iii) Pathologic waves produced by secondary changes in cerebral blood volume
      iv) Require immediate treatment
g. Prevent, detect, or treat complications of ICP monitoring.
  1) Infection (e.g., bacterial meningitis, bacterial ventriculitis)
    a) Risk factors associated with ICP monitoring-related infection

Table 5.15 Intracranial Pressure Waveforms

Waveforms	Description	Significance	Comments
Normal	• Low-amplitude fluctuations in ICP with pressure <15 mm Hg	• Normal	
C waves	• Rapid, rhythmic oscillation of pressure • Small spikes as high as 20 mm Hg at 6 per minute	• Not significant • Associated with changes in arterial BP, ventilation	
B waves	• Sharp, sawtooth appearance waves • Pressures as high as 50 mm Hg lasting 30 seconds to 2 minutes	• Probably not clinically significant but may precede A waves	• Do not perform any activities that may further increase ICP • Assess for reversible causes of increased ICP (e.g., jugular vein compression by cervical collar or tight tracheostomy ties, compromised airway, restlessness) • May indicate decreased brain compliance
A waves or plateau waves	• Elevations on top of baseline elevation of ICP • Pressures reach 50–100 mm Hg and last 5–20 minutes	• Most significant • Pathologic waves produced by secondary changes in cerebral blood volume • Ominous sign of decreasing cerebral compliance and rapidly progressing decompensation • Usually occur only in advanced stages of intracranial hypertension	• Requires treatment • Irreversible brain damage will occur if not resolved within 15 minutes
Terminal wave	• Flat wave with pressure of 50–100 mm Hg	• MAP = ICP, and CBF ceases • Indicative of brain death	
Dampened waveform	• Low-voltage wave with pressure notches	• May be caused by tubing kinks, blood in line, or stopcock positioned incorrectly	

BP, Blood pressure; *CBF*, cerebral blood flow; *ICP*, intracranial pressure; *MAP*, mean arterial pressure.

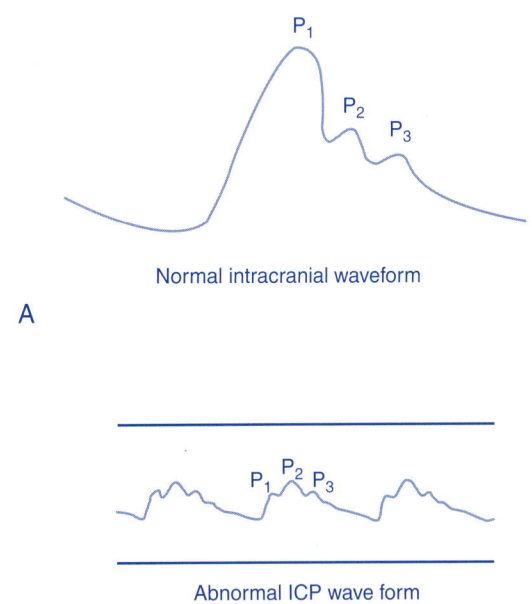

Fig. 5.23 Actual time intracranial pressure (ICP) waveforms. **A,** Normal ICP waveform. **B,** Abnormal waveform. Note that P_2 is more than 60% of P_1. (A from Barker, E. [2008]. *Neuroscience nursing: A spectrum of care.* [3rd ed.]. St. Louis: Mosby. B from Sole, M. L., Klein, D. G., & Moseley, M. J. [2009]. *Introduction to critical care nursing* [5th ed.]. Philadelphia: Saunders.)

      i) Intracerebral hemorrhage with intraventricular blood
     ii) Open head trauma
    iii) Postcraniotomy
    iv) ICP greater than 20 mm Hg
     v) Elderly patient
    vi) Burr hole larger than necessary
   vii) Nonsterile technique for insertion
  viii) Device that penetrates dura
    ix) Monitoring for longer than 3 to 5 days
     x) Irrigation of ICP monitoring system
    xi) Opening of system for CSF specimen collection, VPR testing, irrigation
b) Prevention
      i) Change dressing according to hospital policy using sterile technique.
     ii) Maintain closed system; limit irrigation; use strict aseptic technique if system must be interrupted (e.g., VPR test)
    iii) ICP monitoring is typically maintained for 3 to 7 days; the risk of infection increases the longer the catheter is in place.
c) Detection
      i) Monitor for clinical indications of infection.
        (a) Fever
        (b) Leukocytosis
        (c) Cloudy CSF

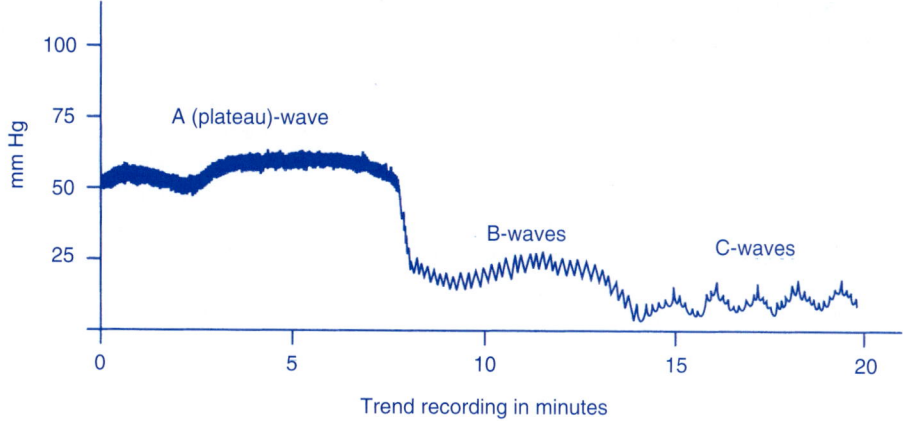

Fig. 5.24 Trend intracranial pressure waveforms. Remember that C waves are "cool," B waves are "bad," and A waves are "awful." (See text for more complete description). (From Barker, E. [2008]. *Neuroscience nursing: A spectrum of care* [3rd ed.]. St. Louis: Mosby.)

    ii) Monitor for laboratory findings indicating infection through routine CSF sampling.
       (a) Elevated CSF protein
       (b) Low CSF glucose (Normal CSF glucose is ~60% of serum glucose.)
       (c) Positive CSF bacterial culture
  d) Treatment: administer antibiotics as prescribed.
    i) IV antibiotic
    ii) Intrathecal antibiotic (usually aminoglycosides)
    iii) Irrigation of ICP catheter with very small volume (e.g., 0.1–0.2 ml) of antibiotic solution
2) Intercerebral hemorrhage, hematoma
  a) Monitor for change in color of CSF; change in neurologic status
  b) Maintain the air-fluid meniscus of the transducer at the level of the foramen of Monro; do not allow drainage bag to be lowered below the head.
3) CSF leak
  a) Use Luer-Lok connections.
  b) Maintain closed system.
4) CSF overdrainage
  a) Do not drain CSF below a pressure of 15 to 20 mm Hg unless specifically instructed.
  b) Ventricular collapse may cause hemorrhage.
5) Dislodgement or occlusion of catheter
6) CSF leakage around insertion site
7) Pneumoencephalopathy

2. CBF
  a. Techniques
    1) Diagnostic tests that provide a snapshot in time and provide excellent regional information about CBF
      a) Stable-xenon-enhanced computed tomography (XeCT)
      b) Perfusion computed tomography
      c) Perfusion MRI
      d) Single-photon emission computed tomography (SPECT)
      e) Positron emission tomography (PET)
    2) Continuous monitoring methods
      a) Laser flowmetry
        i) A laser light probe is placed over the brain area of interest either during craniotomy or by burr hole.
        ii) The light deflection is transformed into a CBF measurement.
        iii) Risks: infection, bleeding, displacement
        iv) Advantage: small size allows the probe to be placed in an ICP monitor.
      b) Thermal diffusion flowmetry
        i) A catheter with both a heat source and a thermistor is placed over the brain area of interest either during craniotomy or by burr hole.
        ii) CBF is determined by the difference between the temperature of the heat source and the thermistor; the greater the temperature difference, the lower the blood flow.
        iii) Risks: infection, bleeding, displacement
      c) Disadvantage: CBF is measured in a local area of the brain that may not reflect the global state of the brain or a specific region of interest.
    3) Intermittent measurement of CBF: transcranial Doppler ultrasound
      a) Doppler ultrasound probe placed over the skin on the cranium over the cranial windows where bone is very thin; different windows allow assessment of blood flow velocity through arteries (Harris, 2014).
        i) Temporal cranial window: middle, anterior, and posterior cerebral arteries; terminal internal carotid
        ii) Orbital cranial window: internal carotid artery siphon and ophthalmic artery
        iii) Occipital cranial window: vertebral and basilar arteries
      b) Normal flow velocity: less than 120 cm/sec
        i) Increase in flow velocity indicates that blood is flowing through a restricted area (e.g., vasospasm, stenosis) upstream from the probe.

ii) Decrease in flow velocity indicates obstruction downstream (e.g., carotid stenosis) from the probe.
iii) Mean flow velocity is average rate of blood flow through the artery.
iv) Peak flow velocity is much higher than the mean flow velocity and is subject to fluctuations in the patient's heart rate and BP and varies more widely than the mean flow velocity.
v) Mean flow velocity is considered more stable and thus a more reliable indicator of blood flow in the brain (Harris, 2014).
c) Disadvantage: need for technical expertise
b. CBF values (Berlin, 2017; Dennison, 2013)
1) Hyperemia: greater than 55 to 60 ml/100 g brain tissue/min
2) Average: 30 to 55 ml/100 g brain tissue/min
3) Altered LOC and EEG: 20 to 25 ml/100 g brain tissue/min
4) Isoelectric EEG and neurotransmitter failure: 15 to 20 ml/100 g brain tissue/min
5) Ion pump failure and cytotoxic brain edema: 10 to 15 ml/100 g brain tissue/min
6) Metabolic failure (i.e., calcium channels open, activation of intracellular enzymes): less than 10 ml/100 g brain tissue/min
3. Brain tissue oxygenation monitoring ($PbtO_2$)
a. Provides information about cerebral oxygen delivery to detect cerebral ischemia, a potential cause of secondary brain injury; secondary cerebral ischemia may occur even though ICP and CPP are normal
b. Indication: severe brain injury with risk of cerebral ischemia
c. Technique: a probe is placed into the white matter of the brain for global brain assessment or the penumbra of an injury for regional assessment.
d. Normal value: 20 to 50 mm Hg in uninjured tissue; less than 15 mm Hg is correlated with a poor outcome and increased chance of death
e. Risks: infection, hematoma
4. Jugular venous oxygen saturation (SjO_2) monitoring
a. Provides a global measure of oxygen reserve for the brain as a whole
b. Technique
1) Fiberoptic catheter placed into the jugular vein bulb to continuously monitor the oxygen saturation of the blood returning from the brain and intermittently sample venous blood gases
2) Comparison between arterial oxygen saturation and jugular venous oxygen saturation allows calculation of arteriovenous oxygen difference
c. Normal value: 55% to 75%; saturation less than 55% indicates brain ischemia
d. Limitations
1) May not be reliable if performed unilaterally because the oxygen content of each jugular bulb may differ
2) Normal values do not ensure adequate perfusion to all brain areas.
3) Prone to technical artifact and will not detect causes such as arteriovenous shunting

5. IN-Vivo Optical Spectroscopy (INVOS)
a. Technique
1) A sensor is placed on the forehead, either right or left of midline.
2) Low-intensity near-infrared light is passed into the patient's forehead, where it penetrates the skull and passes through the cerebral cortex.
3) The returned light at two distances from the light source allows determination of the regional oxygen saturation index (rSO_2), which is a measure of the oxygen saturation of the mixed arterial and venous blood in the brain cortex.
b. Interpretation: used for trending
1) Change in rSO_2 of 12 to 20 points or 20% to 30% correlates with changes in the neurologic status
2) rSO_2 index less than 50 is associated with poor outcome
6. Continuous EEG monitoring
a. Detects ischemia, severe metabolic and anoxic encephalopathy, drug intoxication, and seizures, including subclinical seizures
b. Technique: five electrodes are used to monitor two EEG leads
7. Bispectral Index (BIS): an EEG parameter developed to specifically measure patient's response to sedation and anesthesia
a. Electrodes are placed across the patient's forehead to detect electrical activity in the brain; changes reflect changes in the effects of sedative and anesthetic agents.
b. Values
1) Value of close to 100 corresponds to an awake state.
2) Value of 70 to 90 corresponds to light to moderate sedation.
3) Value of 40 to 70 corresponds to a moderate to deep level of sedation.
4) Value of 40 or less corresponds to a deep hypnotic state or barbiturate coma.
c. Advantage over traditional sedation scales (e.g., Ramsay, Riker): provides objective and reproducible data

Diagnostic Studies
1. Serum
a. Chemistries
1) Sodium: normal 136 to 145 mEq/l
2) Potassium: normal 3.5 to 5.0 mEq/l
3) Chloride: normal 96 to 106 mEq/l
4) Calcium: normal 8.5 to 10.5 mg/dl
5) Phosphorus: normal 3.0 to 4.5 mg/dl
6) Magnesium: normal 1.5 to 2.2 mEq/l or 1.8 to 2.4 mg/dl
7) Glucose: normal 70 to 110 mEq/l
8) Blood urea nitrogen (BUN): normal 5 to 20 mg/dl
9) Serum osmolality: normal 285 to 295 mmol/kg
10) Creatinine: normal 0.7 to 1.5 mg/dl
11) Lactate: normal <1 mmol/l
12) Enzymes
a) Total creatine kinase (CK): normal 55 to 170 units/l for males; 30 to 135 units/l for females
b) Lactate dehydrogenase: normal 90 to 200 IU/l

b. ABGs
1) pH: normal 7.35 to 7.45
2) PaCO₂: normal 35 to 45 mm Hg
3) HCO₃: normal 22 to 26 mEq/l
4) PaO₂: normal 80 to 100 mm Hg
5) SaO₂: normal greater than 95%
c. Hematology
1) Hematocrit: normal 40% to 52% for males; 35% to 47% for females
2) Hemoglobin: normal 13 to 18 g/dl for males; 12 to 16 g/dl for females
3) White blood cells (WBC): normal 3500 to 11,000 mm³
4) Erythrocyte sedimentation rate: normal up to 15 mm/hr for males; up to 20 mm/hr for females
d. Clotting profile
1) Prothrombin time (PT): normal 12 to 15 seconds; therapeutic 1.5 to 2.5 times normal
2) Partial thromboplastin time (PTT): normal 60–90 seconds; therapeutic 1.5 to 2.5 times normal
3) Activated partial thromboplastin time (aPTT): normal 25 to 38 seconds; therapeutic 1.5 to 2.5 times normal
4) Activated clotting time (ACT): normal 70 to 120 seconds; therapeutic 150 to 190 seconds
5) Thrombin time: normal 10 to 15 seconds
6) Bleeding time: normal 1 to 9.5 minutes
7) International normalized ratio (INR): normal less than 2.0
   a) Therapeutic range for atrial fibrillation: 1.5 to 2.5
   b) Therapeutic range for deep vein thrombosis (DVT) or PE: 2 to 3
   c) Therapeutic range for prosthetic valves: 2.5 to 3.5
8) Platelets: normal 150,000 to 400,000/mm³
e. Toxicology
1) Alcohol: normal 0 mg/dl
2) Dilantin: therapeutic 10 to 20 mcg/ml
2. Urine
a. Glucose: normal negative
b. Ketones: normal negative
c. Specific gravity: normal 1.005 to 1.030
d. Osmolality: normal 50 to 1200 mOsm/l
3. CSF analysis
a. Properties
1) Colorless, odorless; cloudy in bacterial meningitis
2) Specific gravity: normal 1.007
3) pH: normal 7.35
4) Chlorides: normal 120 to 130 mEq/l
5) Sodium: normal 140 to 142 mEq/l
6) Glucose: normal 60% of serum glucose value; decreased in bacterial meningitis
b. Protein: elevated in meningitis
1) By lumbar puncture (LP): normal 15 to 45 mg/dl
2) By cisternal puncture: normal 10 to 25 mg/dl
3) By ventricular puncture or catheter: normal 5 to 15 mg/dl
c. Cells
1) Leukocytes: normal 0 to 5/mm³
2) Erythrocytes: normal 0/mm³
   a) NOTE: Test tubes must be numbered to differentiate between traumatic puncture; if first test tube is bloody but others are clear, consider trauma; SAH would cause all test tubes to be equally bloody.
4. Other diagnostic studies (Table 5.16)

Intracranial Hypertension

Etiology
1. Mass lesion
   a. Hematoma
      1) Epidural
      2) Subdural
      3) Intracerebral
   b. Neoplasm
      1) Primary brain tumor
      2) Metastatic tumor
   c. Abscess
   d. Trauma: caused by local edema (e.g., contusion may act as a mass lesion)
2. Brain edema: most common cause of intracranial hypertension; may be localized or generalized
   a. Cytotoxic edema
      1) Intracellular swelling of neurons and glial cells
      2) Caused by any of the following:
         a) Hypoosmolality (e.g., low serum osmolality and sodium)
         b) Hypoxia (decreases ATP production, which impairs sodium-potassium pump)
         c) Cardiac arrest (cause of anoxic encephalopathy)
   b. Vasogenic edema
      1) Increase in ECF caused by breakdown of BBB; increased vascular permeability and leakage of plasma protein
      2) Begins locally; becomes generalized
      3) Caused by any of the following:
         a) Trauma (e.g., contusion)
         b) Tumors
         c) Hemorrhage
         d) Abscesses
         e) Surgical trauma (e.g., craniotomy)
3. Cerebrovascular alterations
   a. Arterial vascular occlusions with cytotoxic and vasogenic edema
   b. Venous outflow obstruction: caused by decreased venous return from head
      1) Neck rotation, hyperextension, hyperflexion
      2) Tracheostomy ties or cervical collar
      3) Increased intrathoracic pressure
         a) Valsalva maneuver (e.g., coughing, vomiting, straining at stool)
         b) Positive pressure mechanical ventilation
         c) Positive end-expiratory pressure
   c. Increase in CPP (caused by hypertensive crisis)
   d. Vasodilation (caused by hypercapnia, hypoxia, hyperthermia, vasoactive drugs)
4. Increase in CSF volume (i.e., hydrocephalus)
   a. Increase in production of CSF (e.g., choroid plexus disease)

Table 5.16 Neurologic Diagnostic Studies

Study	Purposes	Comments

Angiography	• Visualizes extracranial and intracranial vasculature
	• Identifies aneurysm, AVM, vasospasm, vascular tumors
	• Detects arterial occlusion and allows delivery of intraarterial therapy to restore blood flow
		• May cause local hematoma, vasospasm, vessel occlusion, allergic reaction to contrast media, transient or permanent neurologic dysfunction
		• Before test:
		  • Keep patient NPO for 4 hours and provide sedation before the study
		  • Check for allergy to iodine
		  • Evaluate renal function
		• After the test:
		  • Ensure hydration postprocedure (contrast medium used)
		  • Maintain bed rest for 8–12 hours
		  • Monitor arterial puncture point for hemorrhage or hematoma
		  • Monitor neurovascular status of affected limb
		  • Monitor for indications of systemic emboli
		  • Reevaluate renal function

Cisternography	• Views CSF flow • Identifies hydrocephalus • Evaluates CSF leakage through a dural tear • Evaluates abnormality of structures at the base of the brain and upper cervical cord region	• Contraindicated in intracranial hypertension
Computed tomography (CT) and computed axial tomography (CAT)	• Views intracranial structures: size, shape, location, shifts • Differentiates among tumors, hemorrhage, and infarction • Identifies hydrocephalus, brain edema, infectious processes, trauma, aneurysm, hematoma, AVM, brain atrophy, and subacute and old brain infarction • Evaluates arterial system if CTA studies performed	• Patient must be cooperative • Contrast media may be used; contrast media may be used after noncontrast CT • Check for allergy to iodine or seafood before study • Patient will be NPO for 4–8 hours before the study • Sedation may be given • Monitor for signs of allergic reaction • Encourage fluids • Evaluate renal function when contrast media used

Digital subtraction angiography (DSA): brain; spine	• Visualizes the vasculature, especially carotid and larger cerebral arteries
	• Evaluates occlusive vascular disease
	• Identifies tumors, aneurysms, AVM, and vascular abnormalities
		• May be done intravenously or intraarterially
		• If IV: less invasive with fewer complications than cerebral angiography
		• If intraarterial, care as for angiogram
		• Contrast media are used
		  • Check for allergy to iodine or seafood before study
		  • Patient will be NPO for 4–8 hours before the study
		  • Monitor for signs of allergic reaction
		  • Encourage fluids

Electroencephalography (EEG)	• Differentiates epilepsy from mass lesion • Detects focus of seizure activity • Evaluates drug intoxication • Evaluates electrical function of the brain which may be abnormal in the presence of cerebrovascular alterations • Localizes tumor, abscess, and other mass lesions • May be used in designation of brain death	• Stimulants, anticonvulsants, tranquilizers, and antidepressants may be withheld for 24–48 hours before the study • Hair shampooed before and after study
Electromyography (EMG); nerve conduction velocity studies	• Detects muscle disease • Identifies peripheral neuropathies, nerve compression • Identifies nerve regeneration and muscle recovery	• Patient must be cooperative • Contraindicated in patients taking anticoagulants, with bleeding disorders, or with skin infection • May be uncomfortable for patient
Electronystagmography (ENG)	• Detects nystagmus, which may aid in identification of cerebellar or vestibular problem	

Table 5.16 Neurologic Diagnostic Studies—cont'd

Study	Purposes	Comments
Evoked potential studies	• Evaluate brain's electrical potentials (i.e., responses) to external stimuli; evaluate sensory and somatosensory neurologic pathways • Identify neuromuscular disease, cerebrovascular disease, spinal cord injury, traumatic brain injury, peripheral nerve disease, and tumors • Determine prognosis in traumatic brain injury • Contribute to diagnosis of multiple sclerosis and brainstem injury	• Hair shampooed before and after study
Isotope ventriculography	• Visualizes CSF circulation system	• No CSF withdrawn • May cause meningeal irritation and aseptic meningitis
Lumbar puncture (LP) or cisternal puncture	• Obtains CSF for analysis • Measures CSF opening pressure (roughly equivalent to ICP for most patients if done recumbent and no blockage is present)	• Cisternal puncture is higher risk but may be used if scar tissue prevents lumbar puncture • Patient must be cooperative • Contraindicated in patients with intracranial hypertension because herniation may occur • Contraindicated in bleeding disorders and in patients receiving anticoagulants • Patient kept flat for 4–8 hours to prevent headache • May cause headache, low back pain, meningitis, abscess, CSF leak, or puncture of spinal cord
Magnetic resonance angiography (MRA) and magnetic resonance imaging (MRI)	• As for CT • Visualizes tissue state (diffusion and perfusion) so that early ischemic changes are apparent (CT cannot visualize most early changes) • Identifies vascular lesions, tissue abnormalities, hemorrhage, infarction, epileptic foci, and multiple sclerosis • Identifies patency of large veins and venous sinuses • Identifies brainstem abnormalities • Identifies type, location, and extent of brain injury	• Patient must be cooperative • Contraindicated in patients with any implanted metallic device, including pacemakers • Tends to overestimate degree of stenosis
Magnetic resonance spectroscopy (also known as nuclear magnetic resonance [NMR] spectroscopy)	• Measures biochemical changes in the brain tissue • Detects abnormal changes as in brain tumors, epilepsy, stroke, and traumatic brain injury	• Patient must be cooperative • Contraindicated in patients with any implanted metallic device, including pacemakers
Myelography	• Visualizes spinal subarachnoid space • Detects spinal cord lesions and cord or nerve root compression • Detects pressure on spinal nerve roots	• If done with oil-based iophendylate, patient must lie flat for 4–8 hours after study • May cause headache, nerve root irritation, allergic reaction, or adhesive arachnoiditis • If done with water-soluble metrizamide, patient should have head of bed elevated • May cause headache, nausea, vomiting, back and neck ache, chest pain, seizures, hallucinations, speech disorders, dysrhythmias, or allergic reaction • Encourage fluid intake with either type of dye
Nerve conduction velocity (NCV) studies	• Identifies peripheral neuropathies and nerve compression	• Needle electrodes are used
Oculoplethysmography (OPG)	• Indirectly measures ocular artery pressure • Reflects adequacy of cerebrovascular blood flow in the carotid artery	• Contraindicated in patients who have undergone eye surgery within the past 6 months, who have had lens implants or cataracts, or who have had retinal detachment • May cause conjunctival hemorrhage, corneal abrasions, or transient photophobia

Continued

Table 5.16 Neurologic Diagnostic Studies—cont'd

Study	Purposes	Comments
Pneumoencephalography	• Visualizes ventricular system and subarachnoid space • Identifies intracranial tumors • Identifies brain atrophy	• Care as for LP • Contraindicated in patients with intracranial hypertension • May cause headache, nausea, vomiting, autonomic dysfunction, herniation, subdural hematoma, air embolus, or seizures • Patient kept flat for 12–24 hours after the study
Positron emission tomography (PET) or single-photon emission-computed tomography (SPECT)	• Evaluates oxygen and glucose metabolism • Measures CBF, which may be altered by traumatic brain injury, seizure, ischemia, stroke, or neoplasm • Also used to evaluate dementia, depression, schizophrenia, and Alzheimer disease	• Patient must be cooperative • Contraindicated in pregnant and breastfeeding patients
Radioisotope brain scan	• Identifies tumors, cerebrovascular disease, infarction, trauma, infectious processes, seizures	• Generally replaced by CT scan • Reassure patient that amount of radioactive material is minimal • Patient must be cooperative • Contraindicated in pregnant and breastfeeding patients
Regional cerebral blood flow (xenon [^{133}Xe] inhalation)	• Evaluates blood flow to the cerebral cortex • Identifies cerebrovascular disease • Detects regions of increased or decreased perfusion • Determines presence of collateral blood flow • Evaluates the effect of vasospasm on tissue perfusion	• Assure patient that amount of radioactive material is minimal • Contraindicated in pregnant and breastfeeding patients
Skull radiography	• Detects skull fracture, facial fracture, tumor, bone erosion, cranial anomalies, air-fluid level in sinuses, abnormal intracranial calcification, and radiopaque foreign bodies	• Linear and basal fractures frequently missed by routine radiography • Contraindicated in pregnant patients
Somatosensory evoked potentials (SSEP)	• Evaluates neural pathways involving spinal cord, brainstem, thalamus, and cerebral cortex • Useful in diagnosis of multiple sclerosis, brain tumor, and spinal cord injury • Useful in determination of brain death	• Can be used on conscious or unconscious patients
Somnography	• Records EEG during sleep • Evaluates sleep and sleep disorders	
Spinal cord angiography	• Differentiates between spinal AVM, angioma, tumor, and ischemia	• As for angiography • May cause thrombosis of spinal vessels and allergy to contrast agent
Spine radiography	• Detects vertebral dislocation or fracture, degenerative disease, tumor, bone erosion, or calcification • Identifies structural spinal deficits and rules out associated cervical spine injuries	• Care must be taken to prevent fracture displacement and spinal cord injury • C1–C2 view best obtained via open mouth; C6–C7 best obtained with arms pulled down
Suboccipital puncture	• Obtains CSF for analysis • Measures CSF pressure • Rarely performed but may be useful when LP is contraindicated	• May cause trauma to the medulla
Transcranial Doppler	• Measures blood flow velocity through the cerebral arteries • Identifies vasospasm, emboli, vascular stenosis, and brain death	• Quality of findings and interpretation varies with user • Transtemporal window required (NOTE: lacking in 14% of general population)
Ventriculography	• Obtains CSF for analysis • Measures CSF pressure • Is used especially when intracranial hypertension contraindicates LP	• May cause meningeal irritation, seizures, herniation, intracerebral or intraventricular hemorrhage

AVM, Arteriovenous malformation; *CSF,* cerebrospinal fluid; *ICP,* intracranial pressure; *IV,* intravenous; *NPO,* nothing by mouth.

b. Decrease in reabsorption of CSF
   1) Communicating hydrocephalus (e.g., SAH, meningitis)
   2) Noncommunicating hydrocephalus (e.g., tumor, surgical, or traumatic edema, hemorrhage or infarction obstructing outflow of CSF)

Pathophysiology (Fig. 5.25)

1. Intracranial volumes
   a. Brain tissue: approximately 80% to 88%
      1) NOTE: Elderly patients and alcohol or drug abusers may have cerebral atrophy; traction on bridging vessels increases the risk of intracranial bleeding; hemorrhage or hematoma may be very large before symptomatic.
   b. Circulating blood: approximately 2% to 10%
   c. CSF: approximately 10%
2. ICP: the pressure exerted by brain tissue, blood, and CSF against the inside of the skull
   a. Measured as the pressure exerted by CSF within the ventricles of the brain
   b. Normal: 5 to 15 mm Hg
   c. Under normal circumstances, only slight fluctuation
3. Monro-Kellie hypothesis
   a. The cranium is an inexpansible vault.
   b. Inside the cranium is a closed system with three fluctuating volumes.
      1) Compensation is the ability of the cranium's contents to change or rearrange; compensation is more effective when volume increase is slower.
      2) If the volume of one of the constituents of the intracranial cavity increases, a reciprocal decrease in volume of one or both of the others will occur.
         a) Displacement of CSF from the cranium to the lumbar cistern
         b) Increased CSF reabsorption
         c) Compression of low-pressure venous system; blood is shunted to venous sinuses
   c. As successive units of any of the three volumes are added to the cranium, a critical point is reached where each additional unit of volume added increases ICP dramatically and herniation occurs.
      1) There is a volume-pressure relationship (Fig. 5.26).
      2) When the critical point is reached, herniation syndromes occur (Fig. 5.27 and Table 5.17).
         i) Increases in intracranial volume are compensated for by displacing CSF into the spinal subarachnoid space, displacing blood into the venous sinuses, or both; ICP remains normal despite increases in volume (i.e., flat part of curve) (Amidei, 2017).

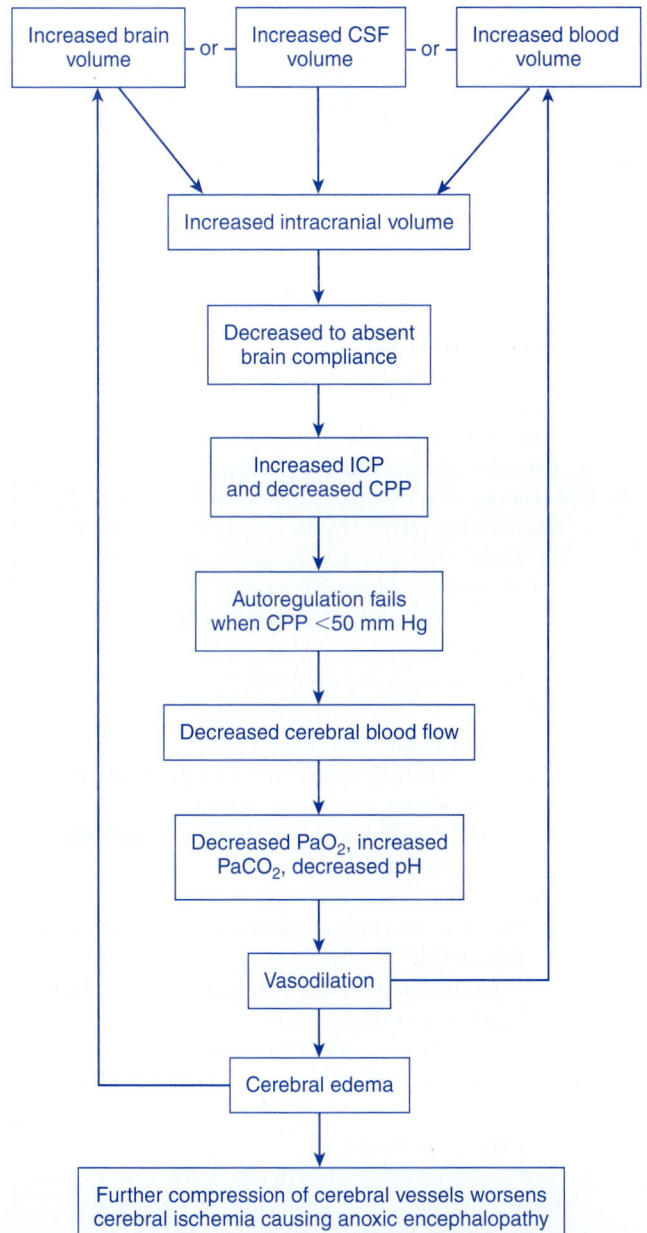

Fig. 5.25 Summary of pathophysiology of intracranial hypertension. *CPP,* Cerebral perfusion pressure; *CSF,* cerebrospinal fluid; *ICP,* intracranial pressure; *PaCO₂,* partial pressure of carbon dioxide in arterial blood; *PaO₂,* partial pressure of oxygen in arterial blood.

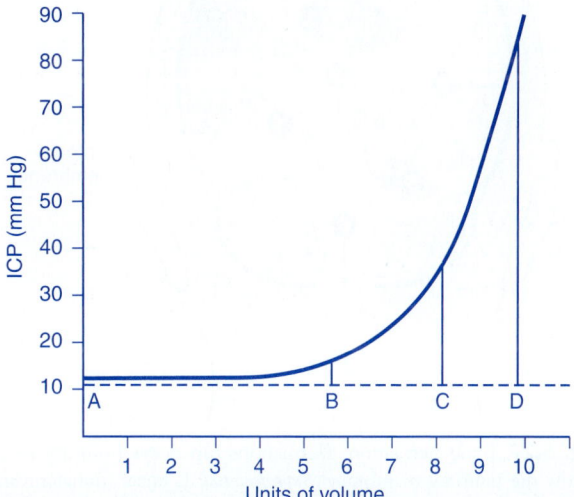

Fig. 5.26 Intracranial pressure–volume curve. Between points A and B, intracranial compliance is present (normal). With lost compliance, very small increases in volume can result in large and dangerous increases in ICP (points C and D). (From Amidei, C. [2017]. Nervous system alterations. In M. L. Sole, D. Klein, & M. Moseley [Eds.], *Introduction to critical care nursing* [7th ed.]. St. Louis: Elsevier.)

ii) Small increases in volume leads to a large increase in ICP (i.e., steep part of curve) when compensatory mechanisms fail. (Amidei, 2017).
4. Compliance
   a. The brain's ability to tolerate increases in volume without a corresponding increase in pressure.
   b. Compliance is poor if a small increase in volume causes a large increase in pressure.
5. CPP
   a. Pressure at which the brain tissue is perfused; used to estimate adequacy of CBF
   b. Calculated by subtracting ICP from MAP; MAP − ICP
   c. Normal CPP: 60 to 100 mm Hg; a CPP of greater than 60 mm Hg is considered a minimum desirable CPP in brain-injured patients
   d. Abnormal CPP
      1) CPP greater than 150 mm Hg disrupts the BBB and causes hyperperfusion and potentially brain edema.
      2) CPP less than 50 mm Hg causes hypoperfusion and brain ischemia (although CPP of 70 mm Hg is required in most brain-injured patients and some require an even higher CPP to perfuse the brain).
      3) CPP less than 40 mm Hg is associated with CBF that is 25% of normal.
      4) CPP less than 30 mm Hg causes irreversible ischemia.
      5) As ICP approaches MAP, CBF decreases; when they equalize, CBF ceases and brain death is inevitable.
6. Autoregulation: the intrinsic ability of the cerebral blood vessels to dilate or constrict in response to changes in the brain's environment
   a. Enables the cerebral blood vessels to maintain CBF in response to wide fluctuation in MAP
   b. Autoregulation fails if CPP is less than 50 or greater than 150 mm Hg
7. CBF
   a. Varies with changes in CPP and diameter of cerebrovascular bed
   b. Normal CBF: 50 ml/min/100 g of brain
   c. Increased ICP and decreased CPP decreases CBF; the brain receives less oxygen and nutrients eventually causing neuronal death
8. Decompensation: brain loses its ability to compensate
   a. Pressure on cerebral vessels slows blood flow to the brain.
   b. Diminished circulation produces ischemia and an accumulation of carbon dioxide and lactic acid.
   c. Hypoxia and hypercapnia trigger vasodilation, which increases blood volume and brain edema.
   d. Brain edema increases ICP further.
   e. Compression of cerebral vessels occurs and causes further ischemia.
   f. Eventually cerebral circulation stops, and brain death occurs.

Clinical Presentation
1. Stages of intracranial hypertension (Fig. 5.28)
2. Change in LOC
   a. Early: yawning, restlessness, confusion
   b. Late: diminishing LOC, posturing
3. CN changes
   a. Oculomotor (III)
      1) Early
         a) Ipsilateral pupil changes
            i) Change in size, shape (oval)
            ii) Sluggish reaction to light
         b) Conjugate eye deviation
      2) Late
         a) Ipsilateral pupil changes
            i) Dilated, nonreactive-to-light pupil or pupils
            ii) Ptosis
            iii) Dysconjugate eye movement with brainstem lesions
   b. Optic (II): visual changes
      1) Diplopia; blurring; decreased visual acuity; visual field deficit
      2) Papilledema: more likely to occur when ICP rises slowly rather than quickly
   c. Trigeminal (V): impaired corneal reflex
   d. Glossopharyngeal (IX) and vagus (X): impaired gag and swallowing
4. Motor changes: contralateral
   a. Due to compression or pressure on the corticospinal tracts
   b. Early: paresis, plegia
   c. Late: posturing
5. Vomiting: may occur especially with lesions below the tentorium
   a. Pressure on the vomiting center in the brainstem causes projectile vomiting without nausea.

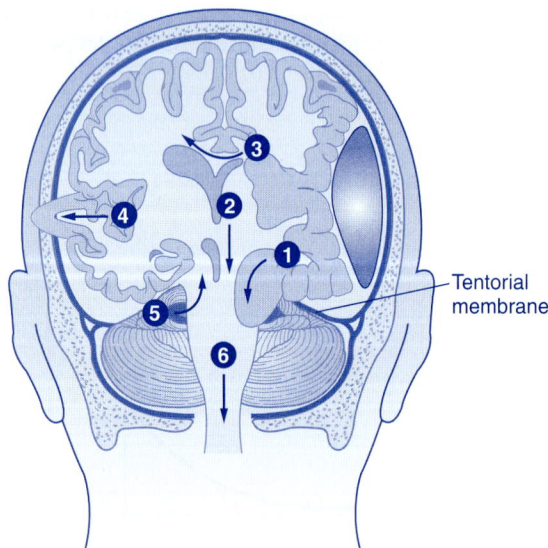

Fig. 5.27 Brain herniation. Herniations can occur both above and below the tentorial membrane. *Supratentorial:* 1, uncal (transtentorial); 2, central; 3, cingulate; 4, transcalvarial (external herniation through an opening in the skull). *Infratentorial:* 5, upward herniation of cerebellum; 6, cerebellar tonsillar moves down through foramen magnum. (From Boss, B., & Huether, S. [2014]. Alterations in cognitive systems, cerebral hemodynamics, and motor function. In K. McCance & S. Huether [Eds.], *Pathophysiology: The biologic basis for disease in adults and children* [7th ed.]. St. Louis: Elsevier.)

Table 5.17 Herniation Syndromes

Type of Herniation	Description	Symptomatology	Comments
Supratentorial			
Cingulate (or subfalcine) herniation	Expanding lesion of one hemisphere shifts laterally and forces the cingulate gyrus under the falx cerebri; compression of vessels causes brain edema, ischemia, and intracranial hypertension	• No specific clinical manifestations • May have altered LOC or plegia • Cheyne-Stokes ventilatory pattern may be seen	• Not life threatening but a sign of brain decompensation • If condition not controlled, uncal or central herniation will occur
Uncal herniation	Expanding lesion in middle fossa or temporal lobe causes a lateral displacement which pushes the uncus of the temporal lobe over the edge of the tentorium; uncus may be lacerated by sharp edge of tentorium	• First symptom is unilateral (ipsilateral) pupil dilation with sluggish reaction to light → fixed, dilated pupils • Decreased LOC • Ventilatory pattern change • Contralateral hemiplegia progressing to posturing	• Life-threatening when hemorrhage or brainstem compression occurs
Central (or transtentorial) herniation	Expanding lesions of the frontal, parietal, or occipital lobes or severe generalized edema cause downward displacement of the basal ganglia and diencephalon through the tentorial notch causing pressure on the midbrain	• First symptom is change in level of consciousness • Small, reactive pupils → fixed, dilated pupils • Ventilatory pattern changes → apnea • Decorticate posturing → flaccidity	• May be preceded by cingulate herniation • Life threatening
Transcalvarial herniation	Extrusion of brain tissue through the cranium	• No specific clinical manifestations	• May occur through an opening from a skull fracture, craniotomy site, or burr hole • Risk of infection
Infratentorial			
Upward transtentorial herniation	Expanding mass lesion of cerebellum, brainstem, or fourth ventricle causes protrusion of the central area of the cerebellum and the midbrain upward through the tentorial notch	• First symptom is unilateral (ipsilateral) pupil dilation • Obstructive hydrocephalus occurs with rapid deterioration of neurologic status	• May be life threatening
Downward cerebellar (or tonsillar) herniation	Expanding lesion of the cerebellum exerts downward pressure, sending cerebellar tonsils through the foramen magnum; compression and displacement of the medulla oblongata occurs	• Coma • Flaccid paralysis • Respiratory and cardiac arrest occur	• May be a complication of lumbar puncture when LP is performed in presence of high ICP • Causes death

CBF, Cerebral blood flow; *ICP*, intracranial pressure; *LOC*, level of consciousness; *LP*, lumbar puncture.

6. Headache: increasing severity but inconsistent symptom
7. Seizures may occur.
8. Reflexes: decrease in or absence of reflexes (e.g., cough, gag, corneal reflexes)
9. Vital sign changes
    a. Cushing triad
        1) Caused by pressure on or ischemia of vasomotor center in brainstem
        2) Components
            a) Increased systolic BP
            b) Widening pulse pressure due to diastolic BP being normal or decreased along with increased systolic BP
            c) Bradycardia
    b. Respiratory pattern changes dependent on location of injury
    c. Temperature: central hyperthermia may occur late in intracranial hypertension because of pressure on the thermoregulatory center in the hypothalamus.
10. ICP monitoring: elevated ICP
11. Diagnostic studies
    a. LP: contraindicated; may cause downward cerebellar herniation with medullary herniation and death
    b. CT scan: may show cause of intracranial hypertension or intracerebral shifts
    c. Cerebral angiography: may show cause of intracranial hypertension
    d. Skull radiography: may show cause of intracranial hypertension and/or shift of pineal gland or sella turcica; rarely performed
    e. EEG: evaluates brain wave activity
    f. Evoked potentials: assesses brainstem integrity

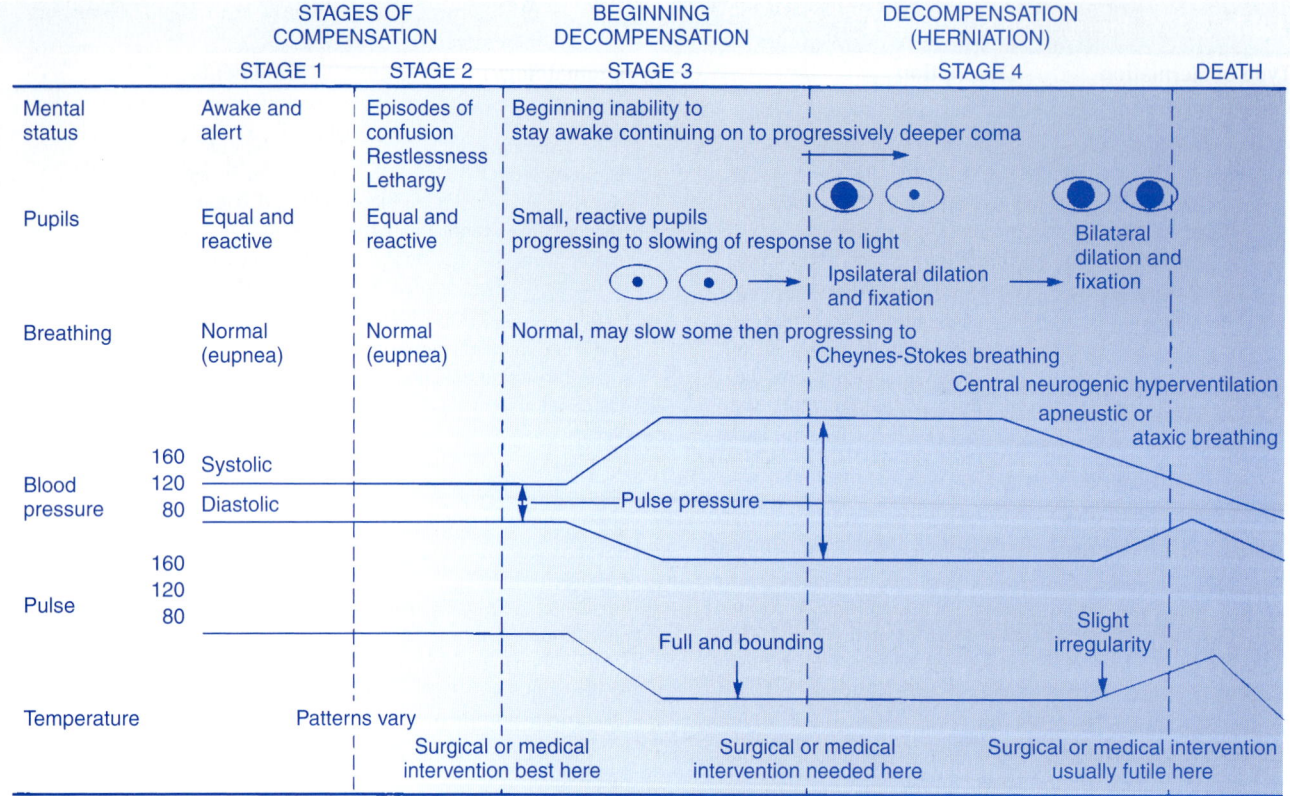

Fig. 5.28 Clinical correlates of compensated and decompensated phases of intracranial hypertension. (From Beare, P. G., & Myers, J. L. [1998]. *Principles and practice of adult health nursing*. [3rd ed.]. St. Louis: Mosby.)

g. Electrocardiography (ECG)
  1) May show prolonged QT interval
  2) Dysrhythmias: especially with SAH

Collaborative Management

1. Monitor closely for clinical indications of intracranial hypertension; assist with insertion of ICP monitoring device if patient requires continuous monitoring.
2. Recognize factors that increase ICP (Box 5.1); prevent as many of these factors that you can; space activities that increase ICP that cannot be eliminated.
3. Prevent intracranial hypertension.
   a. Assess neurologic status frequently.
   b. Maintain adequate venous drainage from head.
      1) Assess patient's response to HOB elevation by using ICP, CO, and BP and adjust accordingly; elevation of HOB to 30 degrees promotes venous drainage from the brain but may decrease CBF by decreasing BP.
      2) Maintain head and neck in straight alignment to prevent compression of jugular veins.
      3) Prevent compression of jugular veins by tracheostomy ties, cervical collar; loosen if necessary.
   c. Maintain patent airway and ventilation.
      1) Endotracheal intubation
         a) Necessary if protective reflexes are absent
         b) Indicated when GCS score is less than 8 even in the absence of typical signs of acute respiratory failure
      2) Mechanical ventilation may be necessary.
         a) Recognize that positive pressure mechanical ventilation will increase ICP; using lower tidal volumes may minimize this effect.
         b) Recognize that positive end-expiratory pressure will increase ICP; using only enough positive end-expiratory pressure (PEEP) to maintain adequate PaO_2 may minimize this effect.
   d. Prevent the increase in ICP caused by Valsalva maneuver.
      1) Instruct the patient to do the following:
         a) Exhale when turning in bed.
         b) Cough with mouth open if coughing is necessary.
         c) Avoid straining, bending, and sneezing.
         d) Avoid hip flexion greater than 90 degrees.
      2) Discourage isometric exercise.
         a) Do not use footboard to prevent footdrop.
         b) Use high-top tennis shoes, on for 2 hours and off for 2 hours.
      3) Administer stool softeners as indicated.
      4) Treat nausea with antiemetics to prevent vomiting.
      5) Administer analgesics and/or sedatives before activities that may increase ICP.
      6) Prevent increase in ICP associated with suctioning.
         a) Suction only if necessary.
         b) Limit suctioning to 10 seconds with no more than two passes. Hyperoxygenate between suction attempts and for 1 minute after the procedure (Amidei, 2017).
         c) Limit suction to less than 120 mm Hg.
         d) Ensure that the catheter occludes no more than half the diameter of the endotracheal tube.
         e) Hyperoxygenate with 100% oxygen before and after suctioning.

Box 5.1 Causes of Intracranial Pressure Elevations

Ventilation and/or Oxygenation Problems
- Airway obstruction
- Hypercapnia
- Hypoxia
- Suctioning without hyperoxygenation
- Deep breathing

Position Changes
- Prone position
- Trendelenburg position
- Extreme hip flexion (>90 degrees)

Decreased Venous Return from Head
- Neck flexion, hyperextension, or rotation
- Tight tracheostomy ties or cervical collar
- Increased intrathoracic pressure
- Positive-pressure mechanical ventilation
- Positive end-expiratory pressure
- Valsalva maneuver
- Straining at stool
- Vomiting
- Coughing
- Suctioning
- Isometric exercise

Increased Metabolic Rate
- Hyperthermia
- Seizure activity
- Rapid eye movement (REM) sleep

Stress
- Disturbing conversation
- Noise
- Bright lights
- Pain or noxious stimuli

---

        f) Lidocaine may be prescribed for IV use before suctioning to eliminate cough reflex.
        g) Do not suction via nose if there is evidence of head or facial trauma.
    e. Monitor ICP during nursing care activities (e.g., turning, suctioning, enteral feedings); space activities to allow ICP to return to normal before performing another activity that may increase ICP.
    f. Monitor ventilation and oxygenation; hypercapnia and/or hypoxemia may cause vasodilation and increase ICP.
      1) ABGs
      2) Pulse oximetry (SpO_2: oxygenation only)
      3) Capnography ($PaCO_2$: ventilation only)
    g. Maintain euvolemia.
      1) Hemodynamic monitoring may be necessary: Maintain pulmonary artery occlusion pressure (PAOP) at 10 to 15 mm Hg.
      2) Administer IV fluids as prescribed: Avoid hypotonic fluids (e.g., D_5W), which may contribute to brain edema.
    h. If CSF leakage is noted, do not pack nose or ears; apply mustache dressing under nose or 4 × 4-inch gauze over ear.
    i. Reduce anxiety.
      1) Reorient patient frequently to person, place, date, and time.
      2) Explain procedures thoroughly.
      3) Do not conduct or allow emotionally disturbing conversations at bedside.
      4) Encourage family members to touch and talk to patient; let them know that many patients report an awareness during altered LOC.
    j. Monitor ICP and calculate CPP; notify physician of significant changes or deteriorating trend.
4. Treat intracranial hypertension.
    a. Providing therapy aimed at reducing volume of one of the three components of ICP
      1) CSF: drainage of CSF if intraventricular catheter in place
        a) Drainage is usually initiated when the ICP is greater than 20 mm Hg.
        b) Do not drain to ICP less than 15 mm Hg unless specifically instructed; rapid CSF drainage may cause the brain to pull away from the dura, rupturing bridging veins and possibly causing subdural hematoma (SDH).
        c) Record volume of drainage.
        d) Maintain closed system and asepsis during fluid drainage; high risk for infection
      2) Circulating blood volume
        a) Hyperventilation (with a manual resuscitation bag or mechanical ventilator) decreases $PaCO_2$, which causes vasoconstriction of the cerebral arteries and a reduction of CBF.
          i) Should be performed only in the presence of acute neurologic deterioration suggesting herniation and only if other methods to reduce ICP have failed.
          ii) Hyperventilation may cause neurologic damage by decreasing cerebral perfusion.
          iii) SjO_2 or cerebral tissue monitoring is recommended to monitor oxygen delivery if $PaCO_2$ level is purposefully lowered to less than 35 mm Hg for an extended period.
          iv) Avoid hyperventilation when providing manual ventilation via bag-valve device (Amidei, 2017).
        b) Barbiturate-induced coma
          i) Actions
            (a) Decreases ICP by decreasing CBF and metabolism
            (b) Decreases metabolic rate and oxygen consumption of the brain
            (c) May shunt blood from healthy brain tissue to ischemic areas
          ii) Preferred agent: pentobarbital
            (a) Usually prescribed as 10 mg/kg IV over 30 minutes as a loading dose followed by 1 mg/kg/hr
            (b) Maintain barbiturate level of 2.5 to 4.0 mg/dl
          iii) Indications and expectations
            (a) Indicated when ICP is greater than 40 mm Hg despite aggressive therapy
            (b) Expect 10 mm Hg decrease in ICP within 10 minutes.

(c) Discontinued when the ICP has been normal for at least 24 to 72 hours; patient should be on anticonvulsants before discontinuance as seizures may occur
iv) Considerations
(a) Monitor hepatic and renal function.
(b) Monitor cardiac status and daily weight; may decrease cardiac contractility.
(c) Must be intubated and mechanically ventilated.
(d) Must have ICP monitor; systemic arterial and pulmonary arterial pressure monitoring are recommended.
(e) Protect the corneas by instilling artificial tears and taping the eyes shut or applying moisture chamber (i.e., plastic wrap taped in place over eyes).

3) Brain mass
a) Maintenance of euvolemia
i) Actions
(a) Maintains CO, MAP, and CPP
(b) Prevents hyperosmolality and increased blood viscosity which slows blood flow and may precipitate ischemia and occlusion
(c) Prevents brain edema caused by excess fluid administration
ii) Goals
(a) PAOP of 10 to 15 mm Hg or CVP of 5 to 10 mm Hg
(b) Serum osmolality less than 320 mmol/kg
(c) CPP greater than 60 mm Hg
iii) Considerations
(a) Isotonic crystalloids or colloids
(i) Colloids (e.g., dextran, albumin) frequently used but no evidence that they are superior to isotonic crystalloids and isotonic crystalloids are much more cost effective
(b) Hypertonic saline may be used.
(c) Blood and/or blood products may be needed if there has been significant blood loss.
(d) Hypotonic solutions (e.g., D_5W) should be avoided because they reduce serum osmolality and contribute to brain edema.
b) BP management (Amidei, 2017)
i) Usually maintain MAP between 70 and 90 mm Hg, but ICP and MAP must be monitored together to maintain a CPP of at least 70 mm Hg.
ii) Hypotension decreases CBF, which causes cerebral ischemia. Maintaining an adequate MAP and CPP may require manipulating SBP with vasopressors and fluids.
iii) Hypertension (>160 mm Hg systolic) can increase microvascular edema, which leads to worsening cerebral edema. However, an elevated BP may be required to provide adequate cerebral perfusion.
iv) Medications to decrease SBP
(1) Labetalol decreases sympathetic response and catecholamine release associated with neurologic injury.
(2) Nicardipine is a calcium channel blocker that does not affect cerebral vasculature and is more effective in providing rapid and tight control of BP than other antihypertensive.
v) Antihypertensives to avoid as they can cause cerebral vasodilation and can cause CBF and ICP. They should be avoided in patients with poor intracranial compliance.
(1) Vasodilators (e.g., nitroprusside, nitroglycerin)
(2) Calcium channel blockers (e.g., verapamil, nifedipine)
c) Administration of diuretics
i) Osmotic diuretics (e.g., mannitol)
(a) Actions
(i) Increases plasma osmolality which pulls fluid from brain tissue and decreases brain edema (this increase in intravascular volume is then eliminated by the kidney)
(ii) May decrease blood viscosity and increase CBF without raising ICP
(iii) May have a neuroprotective effect (under investigation)
(b) Dosage: usually prescribed as 0.25 to 1 g/kg IV; must be given with a 0.45-micron inline filter
(c) Onset and duration: starts to work within 15 minutes; lasts 2 to 6 hours; may be repeated every 1 to 4 hours
(d) Considerations
(i) Indwelling bladder catheter is recommended.
(ii) Monitor for clinical indications of fluid overload initially, especially in patients with history of cardiovascular disease.
(iii) Monitor for fluid deficit.
(iv) May mask diabetes insipidus (DI)
(v) Monitor for electrolyte imbalance.
(vi) Monitor serum osmolality; should be less than 320 mmol/kg
(vii) Rebound intracranial hypertension may be seen ~8 to 12 hours after mannitol; furosemide given with mannitol to reduce the incidence of rebound; because of this undesirable rebound effect, continuous hypertonic saline infusions are becoming standard of care for management of cerebral edema, with mannitol used for rescue dosing only

ii) Loop diuretics (e.g., furosemide)
    (a) Actions
        (i) Reduces intracranial volume by reducing overall body fluid
        (ii) Decreases CSF production (unknown mechanism)
    (b) Dosage: usually prescribed as 0.5 to 1 mg/kg IV
iii) Replacement of circulating volume must be ensured to prevent hyperviscosity and dehydration
d) Surgical removal of brain mass: cerebral lobectomy may be performed as last resort (usually nondominant temporal lobe)

b. Prepare patient for surgery if indicated.
   1) Débride open wounds and suture scalp laceration.
   2) Elevate depressed skull fracture and repair dural tears.
   3) Evacuate epidural or subdural hemorrhage or hematoma.
   4) Control intracranial hemorrhage or hematoma.

5. Decrease metabolic requirements of the brain.
   a. Administer prophylactic anticonvulsants as prescribed; usually no longer than 7 days
   b. Maintain normothermia (<38°C); hypothermia (~33°C), although experimental, may be ordered to further lower metabolic and oxygen requirements.
      1) Hyperthermia is aggressively treated as 1°C temperature elevation is associated with a 7% increase in metabolic rate and oxygen consumption.
      2) Central fever is directly attributed to brain injury and reflects hypothalamic dysfunction.
         a) Characterized by lack of sweating, absence of tachycardia, and may persist for days
         b) Controlled best by external cooling but avoid shivering; use hypothermia blanket
            i) Turn it off when the temperature reaches 38°C because the temperature of a neurologic patient will tend to drift downward after a hypothermia blanket is turned off.
            ii) Do not allow the patient to shiver; small doses of meperidine or promethazine HCl may be used to decrease shivering.
      3) Peripheral fever is associated with infection.
         a) Characterized by sweating and tachycardia
         b) Controlled best by antipyretics (e.g., acetaminophen)
      4) Large-bore central IV catheters may be placed for cooled solutions; less shivering is noted.
   c. Administer sedatives, muscle paralytics, and/or barbiturates as prescribed; preferred agents are short-acting and/or reversible.
      1) Analgesics and sedatives (e.g., morphine, propofol, midazolam)
         a) Actions: reduces restlessness or agitation to decrease metabolic rate and oxygen consumption
         b) Considerations
            i) Monitor ventilatory status.
            ii) May cause hypotension which will decrease CPP; fluid administration may be necessary to maintain preload
      2) Muscle paralysis (e.g., pancuronium, atracurium besylate, vecuronium)
         a) Actions
            i) Reduces skeletal muscle activity, metabolic rate, and oxygen consumption
            ii) Controls shivering and posturing, decreasing metabolic rate and oxygen consumption
         b) Considerations
            i) Must be mechanically ventilated
            ii) Protect the corneas by instilling artificial tears and taping eyes shut.
            iii) Always administer sedative with muscle paralytics.
      3) Barbiturate-induced coma
   d. Maintain a calm, quiet environment.
      1) Prevent loud noises and disturbing conversations.
      2) Encourage family to touch the patient and speak to them encouragingly; a high percentage of patients remember things that were said or read to them while they were "unconscious."

6. Maintain MAP and CPP.
   a. Assess for bleeding from chest, abdomen, pelvis, and extremities.
   b. Control scalp bleeding by applying pressure until sutured.
   c. Administer IV fluids as prescribed.
   d. Administer inotropes and/or vasopressors as prescribed to maintain MAP and CPP; maintain systolic BP ~140 mm Hg.
   e. Calcium channel blockers (e.g., nimodipine) may be used for vasospasm.

7. Monitor for complications.
   a. Permanent neurologic residual deficits
   b. Herniation
   c. Brain death

Encephalopathy

Definition
Global mental status dysfunction as a manifestation of a systemic or brain disorder

Etiology
1. Alterations in CPP such as anoxic or hypertensive encephalopathy (Fig. 5.29)
2. Buildup of toxins such as in uremic or hepatic encephalopathy
3. Cellular changes that alter neurologic function such as hypoglycemia and Wernicke encephalopathy
4. Metabolic imbalance such as hypothyroidism
5. Infection

Clinical Presentation: Varies with Etiology
1. Objective: varies
   a. Mild: memory loss, subtle personality changes
   b. Severe: dementia, loss of consciousness, seizures
2. Diagnostic studies: may clarify etiology

Collaborative Management
1. Maintain airway, oxygenation, and ventilation.
   a. Encourage deep breathing; if coughing is indicated (rhonchi are audible), instruct the patient to cough with mouth open.

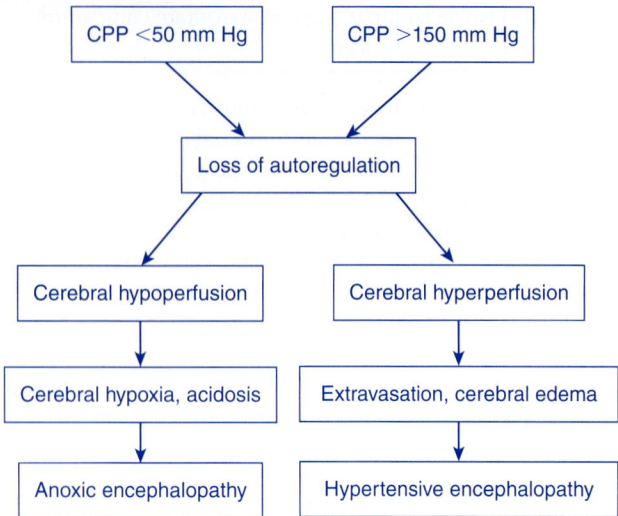

Fig. 5.29 Effects of significant alterations in cerebral perfusion pressure. *CPP*, Cerebral perfusion pressure.

   b. Administer oxygen to maintain SpO₂ of greater than or equal to 95% unless contraindicated.
   c. Assess swallow competency; have suction equipment available.
2. Resolve impairment in neurologic function if possible through treatment of cause.
3. Maintain adequate hydration and electrolyte balance.
   a. Administer isotonic fluids as prescribed.
   b. Monitor closely for indications of overhydration or dehydration; evaluate urine output and urine specific gravity hourly.
4. Maintain nutritional status: enteral nutritional support is preferred.
5. Prevent injury
   a. Administer prophylactic anticonvulsants as prescribed and use protective measures if seizure occurs
   b. Perform passive range of motion (ROM) and reposition the patient every 2 hours.
   c. Perform frequent skin assessment.
   d. Instill artificial tears every 2 hours to prevent corneal abrasions in patients who do not blink.
   e. Orient to time and place often; encourage family participation in reality orientation.

Craniotomy

Surgical Procedures
1. Craniotomy: opening of the cranium to allow access to the brain
   a. Supratentorial craniotomy is used to access the cerebral hemispheres and accomplish any of the following:
      1) Remove intracranial tumors, hematomas, abscesses, and epileptic foci.
      2) Clip or ligate aneurysm or arteriovenous malformations (AVMs) in the anterior circulation.
      3) Place ventriculovenous, ventriculopleural, or ventriculoperitoneal shunt.
      4) Débride fragments and necrotic tissue; elevate and realign bone fragments.
   b. Infratentorial craniotomy is used to access the brainstem and cerebellum to allow removal of cerebellar tumors and hemorrhages, acoustic neuromas, tumors of the brainstem or CNs, and abscesses.
   c. Transsphenoidal approach is frequently used to remove the pituitary gland; referred to as a *transsphenoidal hypophysectomy*
      1) A horizontal incision is made at the junction of the inner aspect of the upper lip and gingiva and extends laterally to the canine tooth on each side.
      2) The sella turcica is entered through the floor of the nose and the sphenoid sinus.
      3) Transsphenoidal hypophysectomy is indicated for pituitary tumor or to control pain associated with metastatic cancer.
2. Craniectomy: removal of a portion of the cranium
3. Cranioplasty: repair of the cranium usually with a synthetic material
4. Burr holes: small holes drilled through the cranium to allow access to underlying structures; frequently used for any of the following:
   a. Evacuation of epidural or SDH
   b. Insertion of intraventricular catheter for CSF drainage
   c. Insertion of another form of ICP monitoring device (e.g., subarachnoid bolt or fiberoptic catheter)

Preoperative Collaborative Management
1. Control pain and discomfort.
   a. Small doses of codeine or morphine may be prescribed.
   b. Care must be taken to avoid oversedation because it eliminates LOC, the most important assessment parameter.
2. Prepare patient for surgery.
   a. Anticonvulsants (e.g., phenytoin) may be initiated preoperatively.
   b. Hair is washed with an antimicrobial shampoo the night before surgery, the operative area is usually shaved in the operating room (OR) or the OR holding area.
   c. Baseline neurologic status should be carefully recorded.
      1) LOC
      2) GCS score
      3) Communication deficits
      4) Cognitive deficits
      5) Motor deficits
      6) Sensory deficits
      7) CN deficits
   d. Inform the patient and family what to expect after surgery.
      1) Equipment: IV catheter(s), oxygen therapy and possibly mechanical ventilation, indwelling bladder catheter, sequential compression stockings, possibly intraventricular catheter and ICP monitor
      2) Mild to moderate headache
      3) Photophobia
      4) Periorbital edema and bruising
      5) Head dressing and drain

Postoperative Collaborative Management
1. Prevent or monitor for clinical indications; treat intracranial hypertension.
   a. Perform frequent neurologic assessments.
      1) Compare results with preoperative status.
      2) Check vision in patients having hypophysectomy.

b. Monitor for clinical indications of intracranial hypertension (NOTE: This patient may have an intraventricular catheter in for monitoring ICP.)
c. Teach patient to avoid causes of intracranial hypertension (Box 5.1).
d. Prevent twisting of head or neck or flexion of neck to allow jugular vein drainage; support head, neck, and shoulders when turning patient in bed.
e. Control conditions that increase cerebral metabolic rate.
  1) Anticonvulsants for seizures
  2) Antipyretics, cooling blankets for hyperthermia
  3) Sedation as indicated for restlessness
  4) Muscle paralytics, barbiturates to decrease the oxygen requirements of the brain (ICP monitoring is required because the most important assessment parameter [LOC] is eliminated)
f. Administer treatments for intracranial hypertension as prescribed.
g. Prevent or treat hypertension and hypotension to maintain CPP of 60 to 100 mm Hg
h. Position patient appropriately.
  1) If supratentorial craniotomy
    a) Elevate HOB 30 degrees.
    b) If large mass is removed, do not allow the patient to lie on operative side.
  2) If infratentorial craniotomy
    a) Position flat on either side with small pillow under nape of neck.
    b) Do not allow on back for 48 hours because of impaired swallowing and decreased gag reflex.
  3) If transsphenoidal craniotomy (e.g., hypophysectomy): Elevate HOB 30 degrees.
  4) If insertion of interventricular shunt: position flat on nonoperative side.
  5) Other specific positioning may be prescribed by the surgeon.
2. Maintain airway, oxygenation, and ventilation
  a. Encourage deep breathing; if coughing is indicated (i.e., rhonchi are audible), instruct the patient to cough with mouth open.
  b. Administer oxygen to maintain SpO_2 of greater than or equal to 95% unless contraindicated.
  c. Assess swallow competency; have suction equipment available.
3. Maintain adequate hydration and electrolyte balance.
  a. Administer isotonic fluids as prescribed; avoid D_5W and other hypotonic solutions.
  b. Prevent overhydration, which can predispose to brain edema.
  c. Monitor closely for indications of overhydration or dehydration; evaluate urine output and urine specific gravity hourly.
  d. Assess head dressing hourly; notify surgeon if large amounts of drainage are noted.
4. Relieve headache.
  a. Inform patient to notify the nurse at the onset of headache; severe pain is not normal; notify physician.
  b. Administer small doses of morphine or codeine avoiding oversedation; when the patient can take oral medications, acetaminophen with codeine is usually used.
  c. Decrease environmental stimuli.
  d. Apply cool compresses to decrease periorbital edema; dressing may be clipped if too tight (clip on side opposite surgical site).
5. Prevent injury.
  a. Institute seizure precautions.
    1) Have suction equipment available.
    2) Have extra pillows available that can be placed between patient and side rails.
    3) Assess onset, progression, and postictal period if seizure occurs.
    4) Administer anticonvulsants as prescribed.
  b. Perform passive ROM and reposition the patient every 2 hours.
  c. Perform frequent skin assessment.
  d. Instill artificial tears every 2 hours to prevent corneal abrasions in patients who do not blink; a moisture chamber may be created using plastic wrap.
  e. Orient to time and place often; encourage family participation in reality orientation.
  f. Apply restraints only if indicated for self-protection.
6. Prevent or monitor for infection.
  a. Administer prophylactic and/or therapeutic antibiotics as prescribed.
  b. Monitor head dressing, drains for purulent drainage; assess wound during aseptic dressing changes for redness, swelling, induration, and drainage.
  c. Do not put tubes (e.g., suction catheter, nasogastric tube) into nose if patient has transsphenoidal approach; warn the patient not to blow or pick nose.
  d. Note drainage of CSF; CSF leak increases risk of intracranial infection.
    1) Assessment
      a) Rhinorrhea
      b) Otorrhea
      c) Excessive swallowing
    2) Management
      a) Mustache dressing for rhinorrhea
      b) 2 × 2-inch dressing over ear for otorrhea; sterile Uribag may also be used
  e. Monitor for and control hyperthermia: treat temperatures of greater than 38°C with hypothermia blanket and/or acetaminophen.
7. Monitor for complications.
  a. Intracranial hypertension: brain edema usually peaks in about 48 to 72 hours.
  b. Brain ischemia, infarction
  c. Cerebral hemorrhage
  d. CSF leak (NOTE: CSF leak is normal for up to 72 hours after transsphenoidal hypophysectomy.)
  e. CNS infection: encephalitis; meningitis
    1) Clinical indications of CNS infection: headache, photophobia, nuchal rigidity, positive Kernig and Brudzinski signs; fever
    2) Treatment: antibiotics
  f. Seizures
  g. Fluid and electrolyte imbalance

1) DI
   a) Pathophysiology
      i) Central or neurogenic DI (CNDI): decrease in production of antidiuretic hormone (ADH) or brain edema causes blockage in the pathway from the hypothalamus (where ADH is produced) to the posterior pituitary (where ADH is stored and released).
      ii) Nephrogenic DI: decrease in the responsiveness of the renal tubule to ADH
   b) Clinical indications: thirst; polydipsia; polyuria (4–20 l/day); specific gravity of urine 1.005 or less; increased serum sodium; hyperosmolality
      i) Usually occurs in three phases (John & Day, 2012)
         (a) First phase: polyuria caused by inhibition of ADH lasting a few hours to several days
         (b) Second phase (5–6 days): near normal urinary output caused by release of stored ADH.
         (c) Third phase: transient or permanent excessive urinary output caused by depletion of stored ADH or loss of functioning of cells producing ADH
         (d) If missing ADH is not corrected in TBI, CNDI causes severe dehydration and worsening electrolyte imbalance (John & Day, 2012).
   c) Treatment: fluid replacement, vasopressin (ADH) for central DI; drugs to increase the responsiveness of the renal tube to ADH (e.g., chlorpropamide) for nephrogenic DI
2) Syndrome of inappropriate antidiuretic hormone (SIADH)
   a) Pathophysiology
      i) Increase in production or release of ADH, ectopic (e.g., tumor) source of ADH, or increase in responsiveness of the renal tubule to ADH
      ii) Increase in renal retention of water causes hyponatremia by dilution
   b) Clinical indications: decreased urine output; weight gain; confusion and lethargy; specific gravity of urine 1.035 or greater; decreased serum sodium (high potential for seizures)
   c) Treatment: fluid restriction; diuretics; hypertonic (3%) saline may be necessary if sodium level very low
3) Cerebral salt wasting syndrome (CSW)
   a) Pathophysiology
      i) Poorly understood; hypotheses include the following:
         (a) Increased activity of the SNS causing exaggerated renal pressure-natriuresis
         (b) Presence of circulating natriuretic factors (e.g., atrial natriuretic peptide)
      ii) Ultimately, it is characterized by extracellular volume depletion caused by renal transport abnormalities in the presence of normal adrenal and thyroid function. (Peters [1950], as cited in Garimella & Springate [2017])
   b) Clinical indications: hyponatremia, hypovolemia, high or normal serum osmolality, high urine sodium, osmolality, and specific gravity, increased BUN
      i) Frequently confused with SIADH, which would cause hypervolemia, low serum osmolality, and dilutional hyponatremia
   c) Treatment: fluid and sodium replacement, possibly requiring hypertonic (3% or 5%) saline
      i) As opposed to SIADH, which requires primarily fluid restriction and possibly sodium replacement
   h. Hydrocephalus: frequently transient due to swelling
   i. DVT: prevention methods include the following:
      1) Use sequential compression devices rather than graduated elastic stockings because these patients are at high risk for DVT; they may be applied before surgery.
      2) Low-dose heparin may be prescribed; low-molecular-weight heparin (LMWH) may be used.
   j. Stress ulcer (frequently referred to as *Cushing ulcer*): prophylaxis with histamine$_2$ receptor antagonists or proton pump inhibitors is usually prescribed.

Traumatic Brain Injuries

Definitions
1. Concussion
   a. "Clinical syndrome characterized by immediate and transient alteration in brain function, including alteration of mental status and LOC, resulting from mechanical force or trauma" (American Association of Neurological Surgeons, 2017).
   b. Loss of consciousness or external signs of head trauma may be absent.
2. Contusions
   a. Blood leaking from an injured vessel; are most common in frontal lobes
   b. Severity depends on the amount of impact energy that is transmitted through the skull to the underlying brain tissue.
   c. The smaller the impact area, the greater the injury because of concentration of force (Boss & Huether, 2014).

Etiology
Blunt or penetrating trauma (risk is decreased by helmets, airbags, seatbelts, alcohol, drugs)
1. Motor vehicle collisions
2. Falls
3. Violence: assault; gunshot or knife wound
4. Sports-related injuries (e.g., boxing, football)
5. Industrial accidents

Pathophysiology
Fig. 5.30.

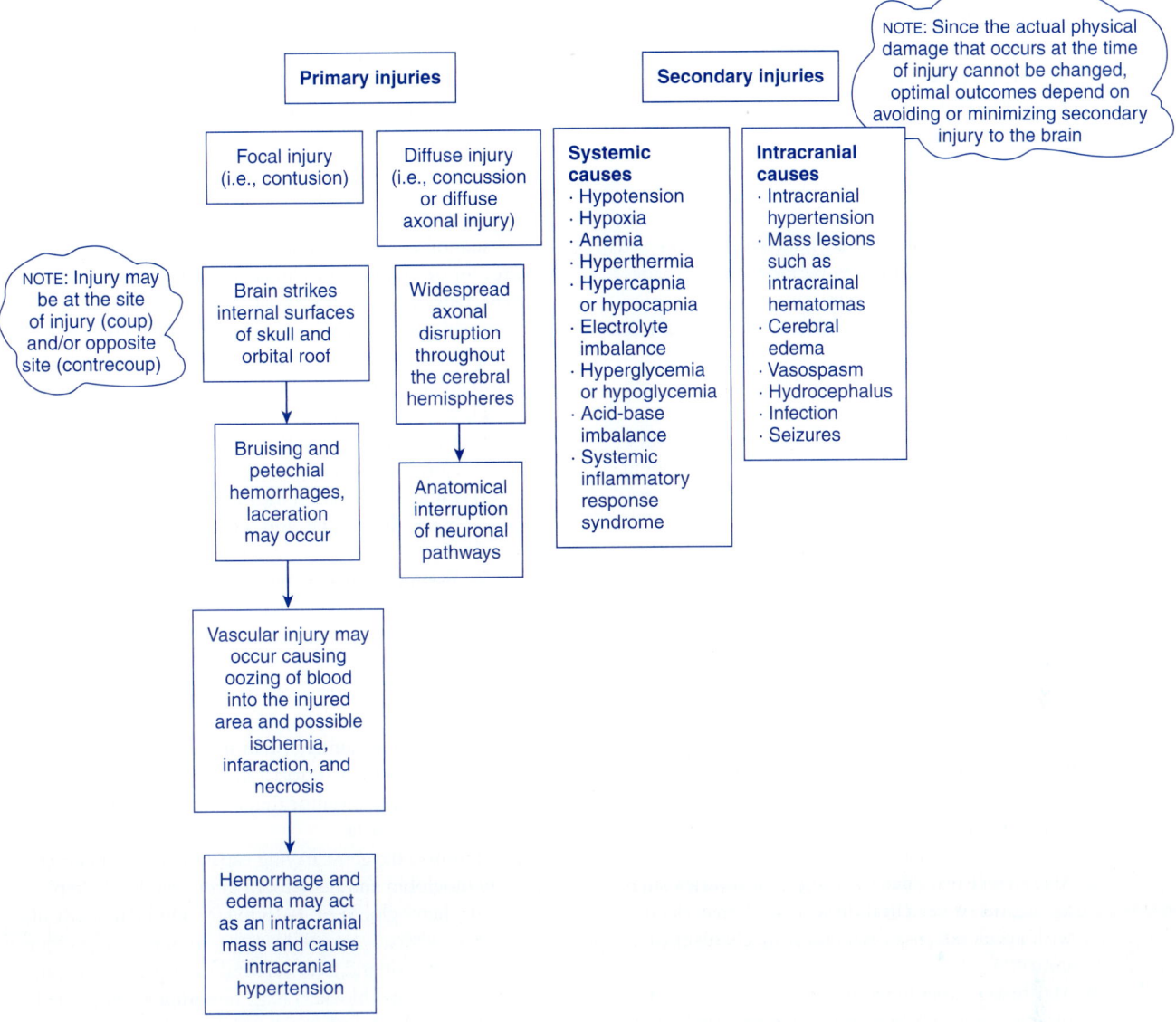

Fig. 5.30 Traumatic brain injuries: pathophysiology of primary injuries and possible causes of secondary injury.

Clinical Presentation
1. Classification of head injuries
   a. Mild: GCS score, 13 to 15
   b. Moderate: GCS score, 9 to 12
   c. Severe: GCS score, 3 to 8
2. Concussion
   a. Subjective (American Association of Neurological Surgeons, 2017; Dennison, 2013)
      1) Scalp tenderness or pain at injury site
      2) Prolonged headache
      3) Visual changes
      4) Dizziness
      5) Nausea
      6) Impaired balance
      7) Memory loss
      8) Ringing ears
      9) Difficulty concentrating
      10) Sensitivity to light
      11) Loss of smell or taste
   b. Objective
      1) Vomiting
      2) Restlessness
      3) Irritability
3. Contusion: signs vary depending on severity of trauma and area of brain involved; neurologic deficit persists less than 24 hours.
   a. Subjective
      1) History of precipitating event
      2) Memory loss
   b. Objective
      1) Possible change in LOC; usually no longer than 5 minutes
      2) Motor or sensory dysfunction
      3) CN dysfunction
      4) Focal neurologic signs (e.g., hemiparesis, hemiplegia may be seen)
      5) Loss of reflexes, which results in the individual falling to the ground

6) Seizures
7) Clinical indications of intracranial hypertension may be seen
8) Transient cessation of respiration (Boss & Huether, 2014)
4. Diffuse axonal injury
   a. Subjective
      1) History of precipitating event
   b. Objective
      1) Loss of consciousness may last days to weeks and is usually followed by long periods of retrograde and posttraumatic amnesia.
      2) May have purposeful movements, withdrawal from pain, and restlessness
      3) Posturing (i.e., decorticate or decerebrate) may be present.
      4) Permanent residual deficits in memory and cognitive and intellectual functioning occur; permanent residual psychological or personality changes are common.
      5) Death rates are high, and many of these patients may persist in a vegetative state; vegetative state is characterized by return of wakefulness (eyes open and sleep patterns observed) but without observable signs of cognition.
      6) Profound residual deficits
5. Diagnostic studies
   a. CT scan, MRI, magnetic resonance angiography (MRA), magnetic resonance spectroscopy (MRS)
      1) May show brain edema, areas of petechial hemorrhages with severe contusions, and hemispheric shift
      2) May detect presence of associated injuries such as carotid or vertebral dissection as may occur with acceleration–deceleration mechanism of injury
      3) May help predict functional recovery, degree of disability, and rehabilitation potential based upon measurement of chemicals in the brain
   b. EEG: may show brain wave abnormalities
   c. Somatosensory evoked potentials: may show prolongation of transmission of impulses through the brainstem to help predict whether there will be a return to consciousness

Collaborative Management

1. Perform a complete assessment for primary and secondary injuries.
   a. Remember that an adult with a head injury is not hypotensive because of blood loss from a closed head injury; therefore, look for other causes of hypotension.
   b. Remember that hypotension decreases CPP, increases the mortality rate dramatically, and contributes to secondary brain injury.
2. Maintain airway, ventilation, and oxygenation.
   a. Assume that the patient has a spinal injury until radiologic clearance of spine: do not tilt or hyperextend the head; use jaw-thrust technique to maintain open airway.
   b. Use oral or nasopharyngeal airway until lateral spine radiographs rule out fracture.
      1) Do not use nasopharyngeal airway or nasal suctioning if facial or skull fracture is present.
      2) Do not use oral airways in conscious patients because they stimulate the gag reflex.
   c. Assist with rapid sequence intubation if intubation is required.
   d. Administer oxygen as needed to maintain SpO_2 greater than or equal to 95% unless contraindicated.
   e. Prevent aspiration: position patient on side and have suction equipment available.
3. Prevent or monitor for clinical indications of intracranial hypertension (see Intracranial Hypertension section).
4. Maintain CPP of at least 60 mm Hg; MAP challenge with intraparenchymal PbO_2 monitoring to assess cerebral autoregulation and individualize MAP and CCP goals
   a. Therapies to increase MAP
      1) Identification and treatment of cause of hypotension if present
      2) Fluid resuscitation: isotonic crystalloids, colloids, hypertonic saline, and blood products as prescribed
      3) Vasopressors may be required in low systemic vascular resistance states (e.g., septic shock and neurogenic shock) or to raise MAP when ICP is elevated
   b. Therapies to decrease elevated ICP (see Intracranial Hypertension section)
5. Use therapies to maintain brain tissue oxygenation ($PbtO_2$) greater than 10 to 15 mm Hg using a specialized intraparenchymal monitor that accounts for all causes of brain tissue hypoxia.
   a. Optimize oxygen-carrying capacity by maintaining hemoglobin and hematocrit at desired levels (typically hemoglobin of 7–10 mg/dl and hematocrit of 25%–30%).
   b. Evaluate for and treat cerebral vasospasm with calcium channel blockers (e.g., nimodipine) as needed.
   c. Maintain body and brain euthermia to reduce oxygen consumption.
      1) Brain temperature probes are included in some intraparenchymal brain oxygen probe kits.
      2) Intravascular cooling may be used for maintenance of euthermia.
   d. Maintain PaO_2 greater than 90 mm Hg; evaluate for and treat acute lung injury, pneumothorax, or aspiration pneumonia as needed.
   e. Maintain upper-range normocapnia ($PaCO_2$ 40–45 mm Hg) if tolerated (i.e., may cause increased ICP); perform $PaCO_2$ challenge to assess CO_2 vasoreactivity and its effect on $PbtO_2$.
   f. Adjust ventilator settings as needed.
      1) Perform O_2 challenge to evaluate intraparenchymal $PbtO_2$ responsiveness.
      2) To decrease minute ventilation, allowing $PaCO_2$ to rise
         a) Decrease tidal volume.
         b) Decrease ventilation rate.
      3) To increase $PbtO_2$
         a) Increase FiO_2 considering guidelines to prevent oxygen toxicity.
         b) Increase PEEP.

i) Identify optimum PEEP by evaluating a pressure-volume curve.
ii) Avoid excessive PEEP since it may increase ICP.
c) Increase inspiratory time to increase mean airway pressure; the patient must be adequately sedated to prevent intolerance, agitation, and increased oxygen consumption.
d) Increase tidal volume (minimum, 4 ml/ kg ideal body weight for height).
e) Change ventilator modes to control pressure and volume (i.e., pressure-regulated, volume-controlled [PRVC]) but monitor closely for lung injury.
6. Prepare for surgery if indicated.
7. Prevent or monitor for complications.
   a. Vasogenic brain edema
   b. Neurogenic pulmonary edema
      1) Pathophysiology: thought to be caused by massive sympathetic discharge
      2) Clinical presentation: pulmonary edema with normal PAOP
      3) Treatment
         a) Elevate HOB 30 degrees, avoiding hip flexion.
         b) Administer codeine as prescribed for sedation.
         c) Administer osmotic diuretics (e.g., mannitol) and beta-blockers (e.g., propranolol) as prescribed.
         d) Use mechanical ventilation as necessary to maintain ventilation.
         e) Use oxygen and PEEP as necessary to maintain oxygenation.
         f) Weigh the benefits of PEEP (i.e., improves oxygenation by increasing the driving pressure of oxygen) against the risks (i.e., may increase ICP by reducing venous return).
   c. Sympathetic storm or dysautonomia
      1) Pathophysiology: an immediate sympathetic surge as an attempt to compensate for the effects of the injury
      2) Clinical presentation: hyperdynamic cardiac function with tachycardia, hypertension, hyperthermia, pupillary dilation, dysrhythmias, profuse sweating, hyperglycemia, agitation, muscle rigidity, and flexor or extensor posturing
      3) Treatment: sedatives, opiates (e.g., morphine), beta-blockers (e.g., propranolol or esmolol), dopaminergics (e.g., bromocriptine), alpha agonists (e.g., clonidine), GABA-B agonist (e.g., baclofen), and/or anticonvulsant (e.g., gabapentin)
   d. Cerebral vasospasm
   e. Seizures
   f. Fluid and electrolyte imbalance: DI, SIADH, CSW (see Craniotomy section)
   g. Stress ulcers (frequently referred to as *Cushing ulcers*)
   h. Postconcussion syndrome: persistent headache; inability to concentrate, memory problems, decreased problem-solving ability, irritability, emotional lability, depression, decreased libido, dizziness, tinnitus, diplopia, photophobia, decreased energy level, equilibrium disturbances
   i. Residual neurologic deficits
   j. Persistent coma

Skull Fractures

Etiology
1. Motor vehicle collisions
2. Falls
3. Violence: assault, gunshot wounds, knife wounds
4. Sports-related accidents (e.g., boxing or football)
5. Industrial injuries

Pathophysiology (Fig. 5.31)
1. Linear fractures (account for 80% of skull fractures)
   a. Fracture with no displacement of bone
   b. May interrupt major vascular channels
      1) Linear fractures of the temporal-parietal bones may tear the middle meningeal artery leading to epidural hematoma (EDH).
      2) Linear fractures of the occipital bone may tear the occipital artery leading to EDH.
2. Depressed
   a. Fracture that depresses outer table of skull
   b. May cause brain laceration
   c. May cause intracranial hematoma
3. Basal
   a. Fracture of base of skull
   b. May cause injury to one or more CNs or cause tearing of the dura with CSF leak

Clinical Presentation
1. Linear
   a. Subjective
      1) History of precipitating event or condition
      2) Scalp tenderness
   b. Objective
      1) Swollen, ecchymotic area on scalp
      2) May have scalp laceration (NOTE: Because of the mobility of the scalp, the fracture may not lie directly beneath laceration.)
2. Depressed
   a. Subjective
      1) History of precipitating event or condition
      2) Headache

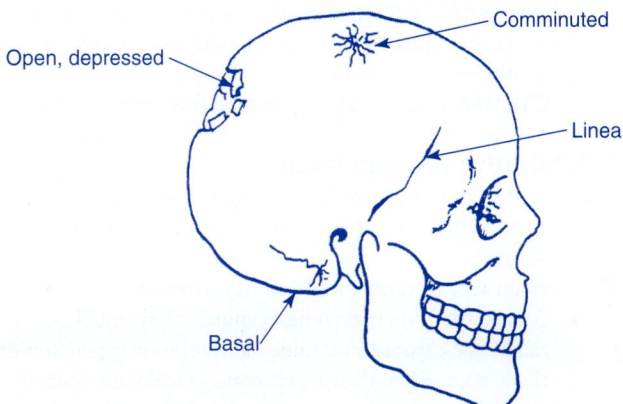

Fig. 5.31 Types of skull fractures. (From Barker, E. [2008]. *Neuroscience nursing: A spectrum of care* [3rd ed.]. St. Louis: Mosby.)

b. Objective
   1) May have altered LOC with focal neurologic deficits
   2) May have scalp laceration
      a) Open fracture: scalp laceration present
      b) Closed fracture: no scalp laceration present
   3) Hemiparesis, hemiplegia
   4) Seizures
   5) Depressed frontal fracture may cause CN I (olfactory) deficit (i.e., anosmia).
   6) Depressed temporal may cause CN VII (facial) or VIII (acoustic) deficits; may see ipsilateral facial paralysis (CN VII) or hearing or equilibrium problems (CN VIII).
3. Basal
   a. Subjective
      1) History of precipitating event or condition
   b. Anterior fossa
      1) May have rhinorrhea; usually lasts 2 to 3 days
      2) May have *raccoon eyes*; takes 3 to 4 hours after injury to develop
      3) May have injury to CNI (olfactory), causing anosmia
      4) May have facial fractures
   c. Middle fossa
      1) May have otorrhea or rhinorrhea
      2) May have CSF or blood behind the tympanic membrane if the tympanic membrane remains intact; may cause hearing deficit
      3) May have *Battle sign* (i.e., mastoid ecchymosis); takes 4 to 6 hours after injury to develop
      4) May have CN injuries
   d. Posterior fossa
      1) May have EDH, which may result in signs of intracranial hypertension
      2) May have cerebellar, brainstem, or CN signs
         a) Visual changes
         b) Tinnitus
         c) Facial paralysis
         d) Conjugate eye deviation
4. Diagnostic studies
   a. Skull radiography
      1) Linear or depressed skull fractures may be seen on plain films
      2) Basal skull fracture is difficult to confirm on radiography; pneumocephalus, opacity of the mastoid or sphenoid sinus, or an air-fluid level in one of the sinuses may be seen.
   b. CT, MRI: may visualize depressed fractures

Collaborative Management

1. Prevent or monitor for clinical indications or treat intracranial hypertension (see Intracranial Hypertension section).
2. Maintain airway, ventilation, and oxygenation.
   a. Assume that the patient has a spinal injury until radiologic clearance of spine: do not tilt or hyperextend the head; use jaw-thrust technique to maintain open airway.
   b. Use oral or nasopharyngeal airway until lateral spine radiographs rule out fracture; do not use nasopharyngeal airway or nasal suctioning if facial or skull fracture is present.
   c. Do not use oral airways in conscious patients because they stimulate the gag reflex.
   d. Assist with rapid sequence intubation if intubation is required.
   e. Administer oxygen as needed to maintain SpO_2 greater than or equal to 95% unless contraindicated.
   f. Prevent aspiration: position patient on side and have suction equipment available.
3. Linear
   a. Monitor for clinical indications of intracranial hypertension or neurologic deficit.
   b. No specific treatment required in the absence of neurologic symptoms
4. Depressed
   a. Monitor for clinical indications of intracranial hypertension or neurologic deficit.
   b. Protect brain under cranial defect from injury; position patient away from cranial defect.
   c. Prevent or monitor for intracranial infection from open fracture.
      1) Ensure meticulous cleansing and débridement of associated scalp laceration.
      2) Surgical intervention is indicated if the depression of the skull is greater than the thickness of the skull (5–7 mm) and should be done emergently if scalp laceration or brain laceration is present
      3) Note indications of infection: fever; leukocytosis; redness, swelling, or purulent drainage from wound
      4) Obtain culture if appropriate.
   d. Monitor for hemorrhage; removal of bone fragment from a venous sinus may result in hemorrhage; blood must be available
5. Basal
   a. Prevent CNS infection.
      1) Detect rhinorrhea of otorrhea; if present:
         a) Do not obstruct flow: use mustache dressing.
         b) Elevate HOB 30 degrees.
      2) Avert further tearing of dura by discouraging sneezing, blowing nose, and the Valsalva maneuver; instruct patient to cough with mouth open and to exhale when turning rather than holding the breath.
      3) Do not use nasal O_2, nasogastric tube, nasopharyngeal tube, or nasotracheal tube.
6. Monitor for complications.
   a. Linear: EDH
   b. Depressed
      1) Laceration of brain tissue by brain fragments
      2) Intracerebral hemorrhage or contusion
      3) CNS infection (e.g., meningitis, encephalitis)
   c. Basal
      1) Intracerebral hemorrhage
      2) CNS infection (e.g., meningitis, abscess)
      3) CN injury
      4) Carotid cavernous fistula
         a) Rare but serious complication
         b) Occurs when blood escapes from the carotid artery into the cavernous sinus

c) Clinical indications include bruit and pulsation of orbit over affected eye, exophthalmos, headache, and visual disturbances.

Intracranial Hemorrhage or Hematoma

Etiology: Usually Trauma
1. Intracranial hemorrhage: any bleeding occurring within the intracranial vault, including the parenchyma and surrounding meningeal spaces (Caceres & Goldstein, 2012)
2. SDH (15%–30% of patients with head trauma and 50%–70% of all hematomas)
   a. May occur spontaneously, particularly if patient has coagulation disorder or is taking anticoagulants
   b. Is prevalent in older patients with cerebral atrophy and alcoholics; may be bilateral
   c. May also be caused by purulent effusion
3. EDH (5%–8% of patients with head trauma and 20%–30% of all hematomas): often associated with linear skull fractures that cross major vascular channels
4. Intracerebral hematoma (ICH) (2%–20% of patients with head trauma)
   a. May occur as result of gunshot wound or stab wound, laceration of brain from a depressed skull fracture, severe acceleration–deceleration injury
   b. Intracerebral bleeding caused by aneurysm, AVM, vascular tumor, or rupture of a vessel caused by hypertension is described as a *hemorrhagic stroke* and is discussed in the Hemorrhagic Stroke section

Pathophysiology (Fig. 5.32)
1. SDH
   a. Usually venous bleeding; arterial origin is rare
   b. Accumulates below dura mater
   c. Classification
      1) Acute SDH: signs and symptoms occur within 48 hours after injury.
      2) Subacute SDH: signs and symptoms occur within 2 weeks after injury.
      3) Chronic SDH: signs and symptoms may occur weeks to months after injury.
         a) Fibroblasts accumulate around the hematoma and encapsulate it.
         b) Hemolysis of the clot liberates plasma proteins; this causes the encapsulated area to have a high osmotic pressure.
         c) This causes an influx of water and swelling of the mass.
2. EDH
   a. Usually arterial bleeding; associated with tearing of arteries from skull fractures
      1) Linear fractures of the temporal-parietal bones may tear the middle meningeal artery leading to EDH.
      2) Linear fractures of the occipital bone may tear the occipital artery, leading to EDH.
   b. May be caused by venous bleeding; associated with fractures that cross major vascular channels such as the superior sagittal or transverse sinus (posterior fossa EDHs are usually of venous origin)
   c. Accumulates above the dura mater
3. ICH: hematoma into brain mass itself: may be caused by bleeding from a missile injury (e.g., gunshot wound or knife) or severe acceleration–deceleration force that causes bleeding into deep cerebral tissues

Clinical Presentation
1. SDH
   a. Subjective
      1) History may include precipitating event or condition. (In chronic SDH, the patient may not be able to link to any particular event, either because she or he cannot remember or because there is no true precipitating event [spontaneous].)
      2) Headache
      3) Increasing irritability progressing to confusion progressing to decreased LOC
   b. Objective
      1) Decreased LOC
      2) Ipsilateral oculomotor paralysis
      3) Contralateral hemiparesis or hemiplegia
2. EDH
   a. Subjective
      1) History of precipitating event or condition
      2) History of short period of unconsciousness followed by lucid interval and then rapid deterioration; lucid interval may be absent if initial blow is significant
      3) Headache
   b. Objective
      1) Increasing irritability progressing to confusion progressing to decreased LOC
      2) Ipsilateral oculomotor paralysis
      3) Contralateral hemiparesis or hemiplegia
3. ICH
   a. Subjective
      1) History of precipitating event or condition

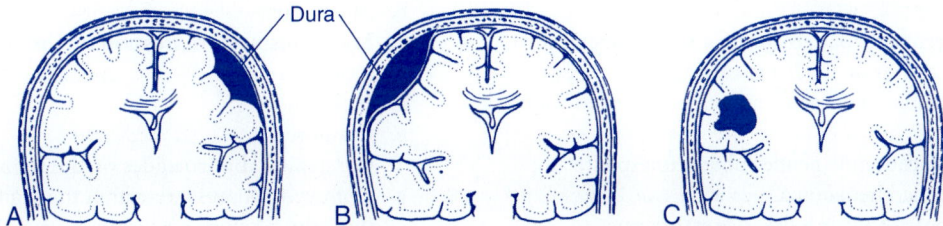

Fig. 5.32 Types of hematomas. **A,** Subdural. **B,** Epidural. **C,** Intracerebral. (From Carlson, K. K. [Ed.]. [2009]. *Advanced critical care nursing*. St. Louis: Saunders.)

b. Objective
1) Varies with area of brain involved, size of hematoma, and rate of blood accumulation
2) May or may not show clinical indications of intracranial hypertension
4. Diagnostic studies
   a. Skull and cervical spine radiographs: may reveal associated skull or spine fractures
   b. LP: contraindicated by intracranial hypertension
   c. CT scan: shows an area of increased density; may show midline shift
   d. MRI: shows hematoma
   e. Cerebral angiography (rarely performed): may reveal avascular area with displacement or stretching of vessels

Collaborative Management
1. Detect or treat cranial, intracranial, and extracranial injuries.
2. Maintain airway, ventilation, and oxygenation.
   a. Assume that the patient has a spinal injury until radiologic clearance of the spine: do not tilt or hyperextend the head; use jaw-thrust technique to maintain open airway.
   b. Use oral or nasopharyngeal airway until lateral spine radiographs rule out fracture; do not use nasopharyngeal airway or nasal suctioning if facial or skull fracture is present.
   c. Do not use oral airways in conscious patients because they stimulate the gag reflex.
   d. Assist with rapid sequence intubation if intubation is required.
   e. Administer oxygen as needed to maintain SpO$_2$ greater than or equal to 95% unless contraindicated.
   f. Prevent aspiration: position patient on side and have suction equipment available.
3. Prevent or monitor for clinical indications of intracranial hypertension (see Intracranial Hypertension section).
4. Prevent further bleeding; osmotic diuretics are generally not used since the tamponade effect of the hematoma helps to stop the bleeding.
5. Prepare patient for surgery.
   a. EDH and SDH
      1) Usually burr hole and clot evacuation, although small hematomas may be observed through serial CT scans to verify hematoma's gradual reabsorption
      2) Mortality rate increases dramatically if surgery is delayed.
   b. ICH
      1) Surgery is indicated if ICH is large or there is a deteriorating neurologic status.
      2) Alternative treatment to surgery: stereotactic aspiration
         a) Stereotactic placement of a small catheter into the center of the hematoma
         b) Urokinase is injected and catheter sealed for 6 hours
         c) Application of gentle suction to aspirate any liquefied hematoma
         d) Repeat of cycle 8 times over 2 days
      3) The FUNC (FUNCtion) score prediction tool (Rost et al., 2008) can be used following ICH to predict long-term functional independence to assist physicians, patients, and families in decision making regarding care and inclusion in clinical trials; variables include the following:
         a) ICH volume
         b) Patient age
         c) ICH location
         d) GCS score
         e) Pre-ICH cognitive impairment
6. Detect or treat postoperative rebleed and/or brain edema; monitor closely for clinical indications of intracranial hypertension or deterioration of neurologic status.
   a. HOB is usually elevated 20 to 30 degrees for acute and subacute SDH and EDH.
   b. Physician may request that HOB be flat on side after surgery for removal of chronic SDH.
7. Prevent seizure activity: administer anticonvulsants prophylactically or therapeutically as prescribed.
8. Monitor for complications.
   a. Intracranial hypertension
   b. Hydrocephalus
   c. CNS infection
   d. Fluid and electrolyte imbalance: DI, SIADH, CSW (see Craniotomy section)
   e. SIADH
   f. Seizures

Hydrocephalus

Definition
Excessive accumulation of CSF within the ventricular spaces of the brain
1. Noncommunicating or intraventricular hydrocephalus: caused by obstruction within the ventricular system
2. Communicating or extraventricular: caused by impaired reabsorption of CSF
   a. Hydrocephalus ex vacuo: associated with cerebral atrophy
   b. Normal-pressure hydrocephalus: associated with arachnoid obstruction caused by adhesions and thickening of the arachnoid

Etiology
1. Noncommunicating
   a. Congenital abnormalities in the ventricular system
   b. Mass lesions (e.g., tumor)
   c. Scarring
   d. SAH
2. Communicating
   a. SAH
   b. Meningitis
   c. Mass causing compression of the subarachnoid space
   d. Head injury
   e. Craniotomy
   f. Congenital abnormalities of the subarachnoid space
   g. High venous pressure within the sagittal sinus (e.g., thrombosis, sinus occlusion, heart failure)

Pathophysiology
Fig. 5.33.

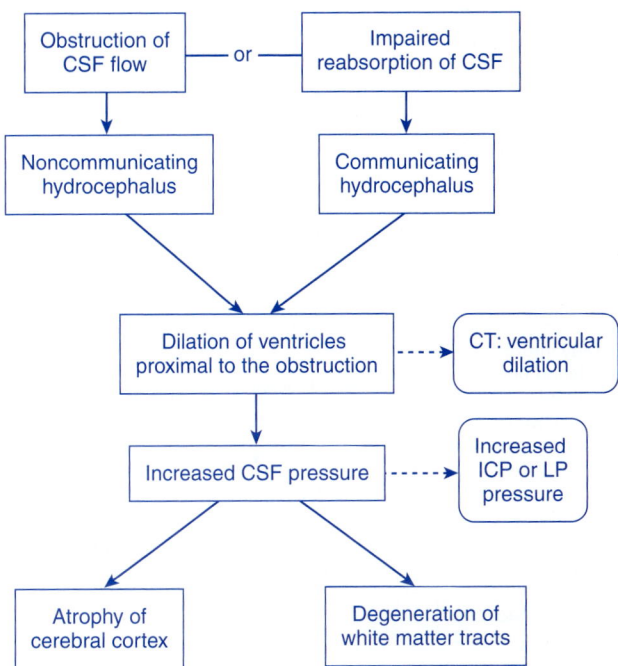

Fig. 5.33 Pathophysiology of hydrocephalus. *Dotted lines* connect pathology to clinical presentation. *CSF,* Cerebrospinal fluid; *CT,* computed tomography; *ICP,* intracranial pressure; *LP,* lumbar puncture.

Clinical Presentation
1. Subjective
   a. History of unsteady, broad-based gait with a history of falling and/or declining memory and cognitive function in normal-pressure hydrocephalus
   b. Headache
   c. Blurred vision, diplopia
   d. Nausea
2. Objective
   a. Change in LOC
   b. Inattentiveness
   c. Vomiting
   d. Ataxia
   e. Urinary incontinence
   f. May have clinical indications of intracranial hypertension
3. Diagnostic studies
   a. LP: shows increased pressure
   b. CT: shows increase in size of ventricles
   c. MRI: shows increase in size of ventricles
   d. Radioisotope cisternogram: useful in diagnosis of normal-pressure hydrocephalus

Collaborative Management
1. Maintain airway, ventilation, and oxygenation.
   a. Oropharyngeal or nasopharyngeal airway as needed to hold tongue away from hypopharynx in obtunded patient
   b. Endotracheal intubation as needed in patients without airway protective reflexes; sedation is recommended before intubation
   c. Oxygen as needed to maintain SpO_2 greater than or equal to 95% unless contraindicated
   d. Mechanical ventilation as needed for hypoventilation, hypercapnia, and respiratory acidosis
   e. Prevention of aspiration
      1) Position with HOB elevated 30 degrees.
      2) Assess swallow competency and have suction equipment available.
2. Prevent or treat intracranial hypertension.
   a. Treatment of cause
      1) Surgery for removal of mass lesion
      2) Ventricular bypass into the normal intracranial channel
   b. Measures to decrease CSF volume
      1) Ventriculostomy or lumbar drain
      2) Ventriculoperitoneal shunt
         a) Proximal tip in a lateral ventricle with distal tip placed in peritoneum
         b) Fluid from lateral ventricle is drained into the peritoneum
   c. Diuresis for normal-pressure hydrocephalus
3. Monitor for complications
   a. Intracranial hypertension
   b. Herniation

Hemorrhagic Stroke

Definition
Neurologic deficit caused by interruption of blood flow to the brain caused by vessel rupture

Etiology
1. Intraparenchymal brain hemorrhage (IPBH)
   a. Trauma: described in section on intracranial hematomas
   b. Hypertensive rupture of a cerebral vessel
   c. May also be caused by vascular intracerebral tumor, fibrinolytics, anticoagulants, bleeding disorders, and spontaneous hemorrhagic conversion of an ischemic infarct
2. Intraventricular hemorrhage: when ICH extends into ventricles (Caceres & Goldstein, 2012)
   a. It occurs more frequently in relatively large and deeply located (e.g., caudate nucleus and thalamus) hemorrhages.
   b. Generally associated with poor prognosis
3. SAH: hemorrhage into the subarachnoid space
   a. Cerebral aneurysm: weakened bulging area on an intracranial blood vessel; account for the majority of SAH
      1) Most cerebral aneurysms are small (2–6 mm), saccular, and occur at bifurcations in circle of Willis
         a) Saccular (i.e., berry) aneurysms: usually congenital defects
         b) Fusiform aneurysms: from atherosclerosis
         c) Mycotic aneurysms: from necrotic vasculitis and septic emboli (rare)
         d) Traumatic aneurysms: from skull fracture disrupting vessel (very rare)
   b. AVM
      1) A tangle of abnormal arteries and veins: arteries feed directly into veins without a capillary bed.
      2) Always congenital
      3) May occur in other circulatory systems including the spinal cord

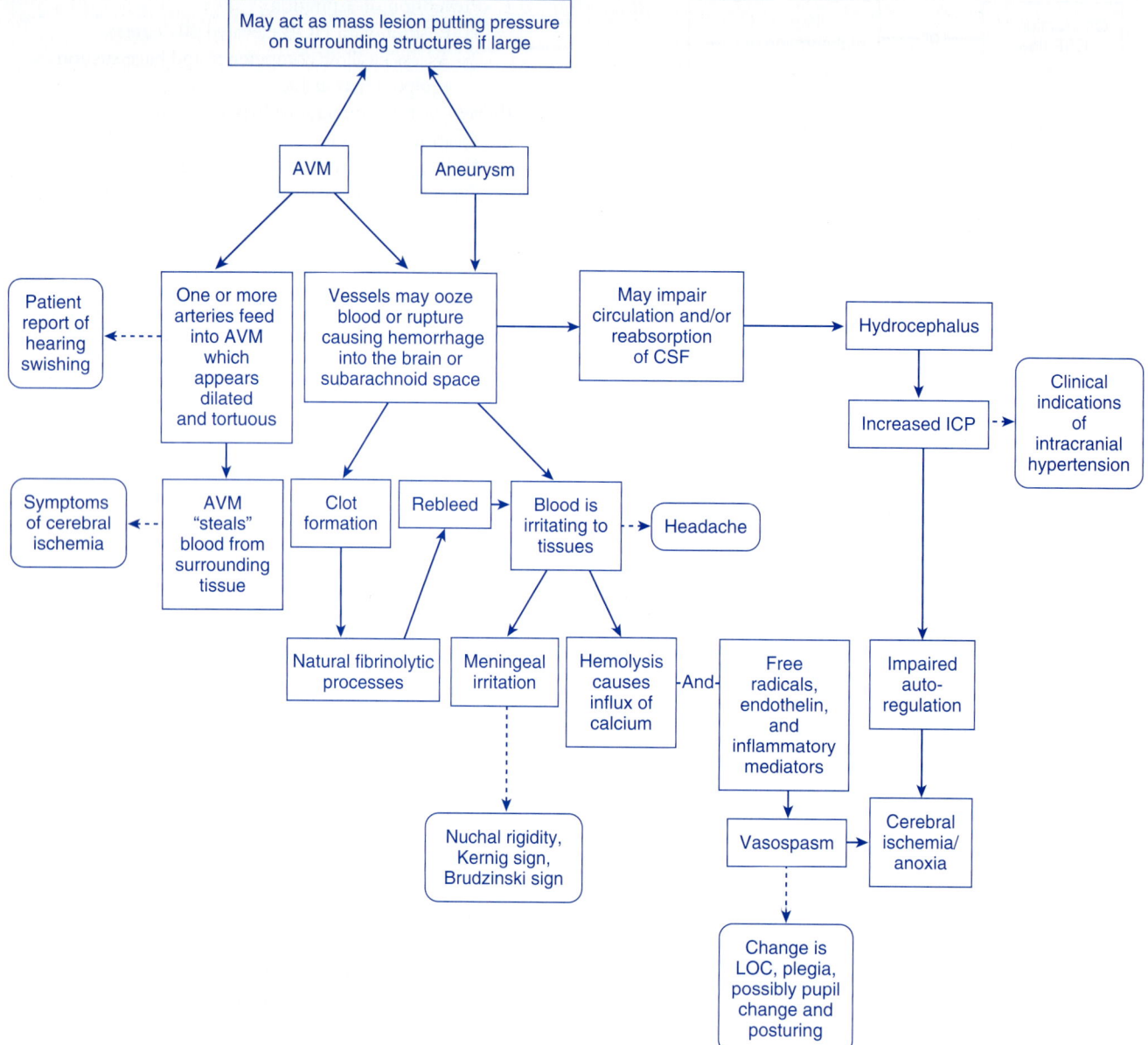

Fig. 5.34 Pathophysiology of hemorrhagic stroke. Dotted lines connect pathology to clinical presentation. *AVM,* Arteriovenous malformation; *CSF,* cerebrospinal fluid; *ICP,* intracranial pressure; *LOC,* level of consciousness.

Pathophysiology (Fig. 5.34)
1. Aneurysm
    a. Two contributing factors
        1) Congenital weakness
        2) Stress (e.g., hypertension)
    b. The aneurysm may act as mass lesion if intact and large.
    c. Weakness of an artery and high pressure (90% of ruptured aneurysm associated with hypertension) lead to hemorrhage; hemorrhage most likely when aneurysm is 8 to 10 mm in size
2. AVM: congenital tangle of arteries and veins

Clinical Presentation
1. Subjective
    a. History
        1) Hypertension present in 90% of cases of ruptured aneurysm
        2) Most patients have had a "warning leak" days or weeks before bleed
            a) Headache
            b) Generalized, transient weakness
            c) Fatigue
            d) Ptosis, diplopia, blurred vision
    b. Sudden, severe headache
        1) Frequently described as "the worst headache of my life"
        2) Sudden: described as a "thunder clap" or "like being hit in the head"
        3) Localized progressing to generalized
        4) May radiate to neck and back
    c. Nausea and vomiting may be present if severe bleed
2. Objective
    a. Restlessness progressing to altered LOC

1) Loss of consciousness is common in hemorrhage from aneurysm.
2) Loss of consciousness is uncommon in hemorrhage from AVM.
  b. If hemorrhage into ventricles
     1) Nuchal rigidity
     2) Photophobia
     3) Kernig sign, Brudzinski sign
     4) Hyperthermia
  c. Neurologic deficit
  d. Seizures
  e. Site and size determine specific clinical presentation
  f. Hunt and Hess aneurysm grading system (Table 5.18)
3. AVM specifically
  a. May have bruit and report a constant swishing sound in the head with each heartbeat
  b. Motor or sensory defects
  c. Aphasia
  d. Dizziness, syncope
4. Diagnostic studies
  a. Serum
     1) Hyponatremia may be present caused by SIADH or cerebral salt wasting
     2) PT and aPTT may be abnormal.
  b. ECG
     1) Changes that may occur with SAH
        a) Flattened, peaked, or inverted T wave
        b) Presence of U wave
        c) QT prolongation
     2) Dysrhythmias are common; torsade de pointes has been associated with SAH
  c. Echocardiography: may show decreased ejection fraction caused by "stunned" myocardium; mechanism unknown
  d. LP: performed only if CT is nondiagnostic and there are no clinical indications of intracranial hypertension
     1) Reveals bloody CSF, elevated protein in acute SAH; it is important to number the test tubes
        a) If only test tube #1 is bloody: traumatic tap
        b) If all test tubes are bloody: bloody tap
     2) Reveals xanthochromic (i.e., dark amber) CSF if hemorrhage occurred more than 5 days ago
  e. Transcranial Doppler: aids in diagnosing vasospasm
  f. CT: identifies extent of SAH or IPBH that may be suspicious of aneurysm; detects presence of hydrocephalus
  g. MRI or MRA
     1) May reveal small aneurysms that are not visualized with CT
     2) May reveal ICH and intraventricular blood
     3) May show vasospasm
  h. Cerebral angiogram: will illustrate size, shape, and location of aneurysm; allows direct evaluation for vasospasm

Collaborative Management

1. Maintain airway, ventilation, and oxygenation
   a. Maintain airway
      1) Oropharyngeal or nasopharyngeal airway may be needed to hold tongue away from hypopharynx in obtunded patient.
      2) Endotracheal intubation may be needed in patients without airway protective reflexes; sedation is recommended before intubation and administration of lidocaine may reduce the risk of increased ICP.
   b. Maintain oxygenation and ventilation.
      1) Administer oxygen as needed to maintain SpO_2 greater than or equal to 95% unless contraindicated.
      2) Initiate mechanical ventilation as needed for hypoventilation.
   c. Prevent aspiration.
      1) Position patient on side.
      2) Have suction equipment available.

Table 5.18 Aneurysm Grading Scales

Scale	Hunt and Hess Severity Scale	World Federation of Neurologic Surgeons	Fisher Scale
1	• Asymptomatic • Mild headache	• GCS score, 15 • No motor deficit	• CT shows no blood
2	• Moderate to severe headache • Nuchal rigidity • No focal deficit other than cranial nerve palsy	• GCS score, 13–14 • No motor deficit	• CT shows diffuse deposits of subarachnoid hemorrhage blood, no clots, no layers of blood >1 mm
3	• Mild mental status change (e.g., drowsy, confused) • Mild focal neurologic deficit	• GCS 13–14 • Motor deficit	• CT shows local clots or vertical layers of blood at ≥1 mm
4	• Stupor or moderate to severe hemiparesis	• GCS 7–12 • Motor deficit may be present or absent	• CT shows diffuse or no subarachnoid hemorrhage, but intracerebral or intraventricular clot
5	• Comatose or decerebrate posturing	• GCS 3–6 • Motor deficit may be present or absent	

CT, Computed tomography; *GCS*, Glasgow Coma Scale.
Adapted from EB Medicine, publisher of *Emergency Medicine Practice,* from: Aisiku I, Edlow JA, Goldstein J, Thomas LE. Emergency Medicine Practice. 2014;16(10):1–32. © 2014 EB Medicine. www.ebmedicine.net.

2. Minimize potential for rebleed and promote stabilization of patient: rebleed occurs most often within 10 days after hemorrhage.
   a. Maintain BP within 10% of prehemorrhage levels; hypotension is associated with hypoperfusion, and hypertension is associated with rebleeding
      1) Calcium channel blocker (e.g., nicardipine, alpha- and beta-blocker (e.g., labetalol or direct vasodilator (e.g., hydralazine) for hypertension
      2) Vasopressors (e.g., phenylephrine, norepinephrine) for hypotension
   b. Decrease environmental stimuli (these interventions may be referred to as *aneurysm precautions*).
      1) Provide a quiet, dimly lit private room.
      2) Enforce bed rest with HOB elevated 15 to 30 degrees.
      3) Instruct patient regarding how to avoid Valsalva maneuver (e.g., cough with mouth open, exhale when turning in bed, stool softeners).
      4) Instruct visitors that the patient should not be upset in any way; limit number of visitors and duration of visits.
      5) Do not perform any rectal procedures (e.g., rectal temperature, enemas).
      6) Provide sedation (usually phenobarbital) if patient is restless.
      7) Treat fever with acetaminophen.
   c. Administer analgesics for headache but avoid oversedation that would impair assessment.
      1) Use short-acting narcotics (e.g., morphine, fentanyl, codeine).
      2) Avoid benzodiazepines.
   d. Prepare patient for surgery or interventional neuroradiology procedures.
      1) Aneurysm
         a) Indications
            i) Surgery to secure the aneurysm is indicated within 72 hours
         b) Surgical
            i) Clipping: occlusion of the neck of the aneurysm with a ligature or metal clip; most common treatment especially if there is a well-defined neck
            ii) Wrapping or coating
               (a) Reinforcement of the sac with muscle, fibrin foam, or solidifying polymer
               (b) These procedures carry a higher risk of rebleeding, therefore complete obliteration is recommended.
            iii) Ligation: proximal ligation of a feeding vessel
            iv) Bypass grafts: redirect blood flow to prevent feeding an aneurysm.
         c) Endovascular procedures
            i) Detachable coils: made of soft platinum; the device molds itself into the inner diameter of the aneurysmal dilation to cause thrombosis; an average of five coils are needed to occlude the aneurysm; a clot forms and evidentially the base of the aneurysm endothelializes and is cut off
            ii) Intravascular balloon placement: silicone microballoon is placed into the aneurysm and detached.
      2) AVM
         a) Surgical excision
         b) Stereotactic radiosurgery if AVM may not be safely excised
         c) Glue embolization: injection of glue into the arterial pedicle to cause thrombosis and block blood flow into the malformation
         d) Embolization of the AVM with Silastic beads
         e) Preoperative embolization followed by surgical excision
      3) IPBH
         a) Surgical removal of the clot depends on the size and location of the clot, the patient's ICP, and neurologic status
            i) Massive hematoma (>3 cm diameter) with brainstem compression or intracranial hypertension
            ii) Hydrocephalus
            iii) Surgical-accessible lesions
      4) Provide postoperative management as described in the Craniotomy section; monitor for clinical indications of intracranial hypertension or rebleeding.
3. Prevent or monitor for clinical indications or treat intracranial hypertension (see Intracranial Hypertension section)
4. Prevent or monitor for ischemia related to vasospasm after SAH caused by aneurysm.
   a. Recognize risk factors that increase the risk of the occurrence and severity of vasospasm.
      1) Concomitant conditions
         a) Hyperglycemia: controlling serum glucose may reduce the risk of vasospasm after SAH.
      2) CT: diffuse, thick blood in the subarachnoid space on CT scan, especially if around the base of the brain
      3) Location: hemorrhage in one of the vessels of the circle of Willis
      4) Time frame: vasospasm occurs anytime from the third day postbleed to 2 to 3 weeks after the initial bleed (peak incidence 5–12 days)
      5) Significance: vasospasm is a leading cause of death after aneurysmal SAH.
   b. Monitor for clinical indications of vasospasm.
      1) Headache or worsening of headache
      2) Visual changes
      3) Change in LOC
      4) Confusion
      5) Pupil change
      6) Focal neurologic deficit (e.g., hemiparesis, aphasia)
      7) Seizures may occur
         a) Seizures, if occurring beyond 12 hours after hemorrhage, more likely caused by ischemic damage due to vasospasm Amidei, 2017
      8) Increase in ICP if being monitoring; blood may be visible in CSF if intraventricular catheter in place
      9) Transcranial Doppler
         a) Often performed daily after SAH or more often if indicated

b) Note trends in flow velocity; intracranial blood flow velocities greater than 100 to 120 cm/sec suggest vasospasm; greater than 200 cm/sec suggest severe vasospasm.
c) Correlate with clinical assessment.
10) Angiography
a) Definitive study for diagnosis of cerebral vasospasm
b) Narrowing of arterial vessels may be seen on angiography before clinical indications of vasospasm are noted.
c. Provide therapies for the prevention and treatment of cerebral vasospasm.
1) Early clipping with flushing of excess blood and clots from the basal cisterns
2) Calcium channel blockers to prevent and/or reduce vasospasm
a) Nimodipine is the preferred agent because it is lipid soluble and therefore able to cross the BBB.
  i) Dosage: 60 mg orally every 4 hours for 14 days posthemorrhage
  ii) Adverse effects: hypotension; dose may be reduced to 30 mg every 2 to 4 hours
b) Prolonged-release nicardipine implants may be placed parallel to the ruptured artery and adjacent to the clot.
c) Intrathecal nicardipine infusion may be administered via a lumbar drainage catheter.
3) Triple-H therapy (hypertension, hypervolemia, hemodilution)
a) Goals: to increase CPP and CBF and decrease risk of brain ischemia
b) No longer practiced; now it's more commonly referred to as hemodynamic augmentation and hemodilution is not included as outcomes were not found to be improved (Baggott & Aagaard-Kienitz, 2014)
c) Hypervolemia may increase CBF, but oxygen delivery is decreased.
d) Costs and complications increased with prophylactic hypervolemic and hypertensive therapy (Baggott & Aagaard-Kienitz, 2014).
e) Potential complications: pulmonary edema, myocardial ischemia, coagulopathy, electrolyte imbalance, rebleeding
4) Transluminal cerebral balloon angioplasty
a) Goal: widening of the stenotic segment with a balloon-tipped catheter
b) Limitation: can only be used with larger, accessible vessels
c) Complications
  i) Vessel rupture
  ii) Restenosis rarely occurs
5) Intraarterial injection of vasodilating agent (e.g., verapamil, nicardipine, nimodipine, milrinone, or papaverine)
a) Goal: relief of spasm of vessels too distal for the use of angioplasty; most beneficial when used during angioplasty
b) Complications: intracranial hypertension, brain ischemia

6) Magnesium: IV infusions may decrease cerebral ischemia and improve patient outcomes
7) Statins: may decrease vasospasm and the risk of mortality
5. Provide instruction and counseling regarding lifestyle modification and need for pharmacologic therapy.
a. Nonpharmacologic therapies
1) Weight normalization
2) Cessation of tobacco use
3) Limitation of alcohol consumption to 1 to 2 alcoholic beverages daily
4) Regular aerobic exercise in moderation
5) Complementary therapies: relaxation; imagery, biofeedback
6) Stress reduction
7) Yearly flu and pneumococcal vaccine
8) Recognition of symptoms of recurrence and when to call the physician
b. Pharmacologic agents
1) Control of hypertension, hyperlipidemia, and diabetes mellitus
6. Monitor for complications
a. Vasospasm (in aneurysms)
b. Rebleeding
c. Brain edema and intracranial hypertension
d. Hydrocephalus: may require temporary diversion with intraventricular catheter or lumbar drain and more long-term management through placement of a ventriculoperitoneal shunt
e. Fluid and electrolyte imbalance: DI, SIADH, CSW (see Craniotomy section)
f. Seizures: prophylactic anticonvulsants are frequently prescribed because the increase in BP, increase in metabolic rate and oxygen demand, and compromised ventilation and oxygenation during seizure activity could be devastating.
g. Dysrhythmias (e.g., prolonged QT interval and torsades de pointes)
h. DVT and PE: use sequential compression devices.

Ischemic Stroke

Definitions
1. Transient ischemic attack (TIA): episode of neurologic impairment attributed to focal cerebral ischemia
   a. Resolves within 24 hours (usually <1–2 hours)
   b. May be described as a zone of penumbra without central infarction
2. Ischemic stroke: sudden, severe disruption of the cerebral circulation with a subsequent loss of neurologic function caused by thrombus or embolus
3. Lacunar stroke: special subset of thrombotic stroke seen almost exclusively in hypertensive patients; small perforating vessel thrombosis

Etiology
1. Thrombosis
   a. Intracranial arteriosclerosis
   b. Extracranial (i.e., carotid) atherosclerosis
   c. Hypertension
   d. Hypercoagulability (e.g., polycythemia)

Box 5.2 Symptoms Occurring during Transient Ischemic Attacks

Anterior Circulation
- Ipsilateral monocular visual defect (amaurosis fugax) or homonymous hemianopsia
- Contralateral sensory or motor defects
- Aphasia (if dominant hemisphere affected)
- Ipsilateral headache
- Seizure activity

Posterior Circulation
- Bilateral visual defect; diplopia
- Bilateral sensory or motor defects
- Dysphagia
- Occipital headache
- Vertigo, syncope (drop attack), dizziness, ataxia

2. Embolism
    a. Mural thrombi
       1) Dysrhythmia (e.g., atrial fibrillation)
       2) Ventricular aneurysm
    b. Carotid artery atherosclerosis
    c. Bacterial endocarditis
    d. Valvular heart disease
    e. Prosthetic cardiac valves
    f. DVT with patent foramen ovale
    g. Air or fat embolism (see Chapter 4)

Pathophysiology (Fig. 5.35)
1. Risk factors include the following:
    a. Family history
    b. Hypertension
    c. Smoking

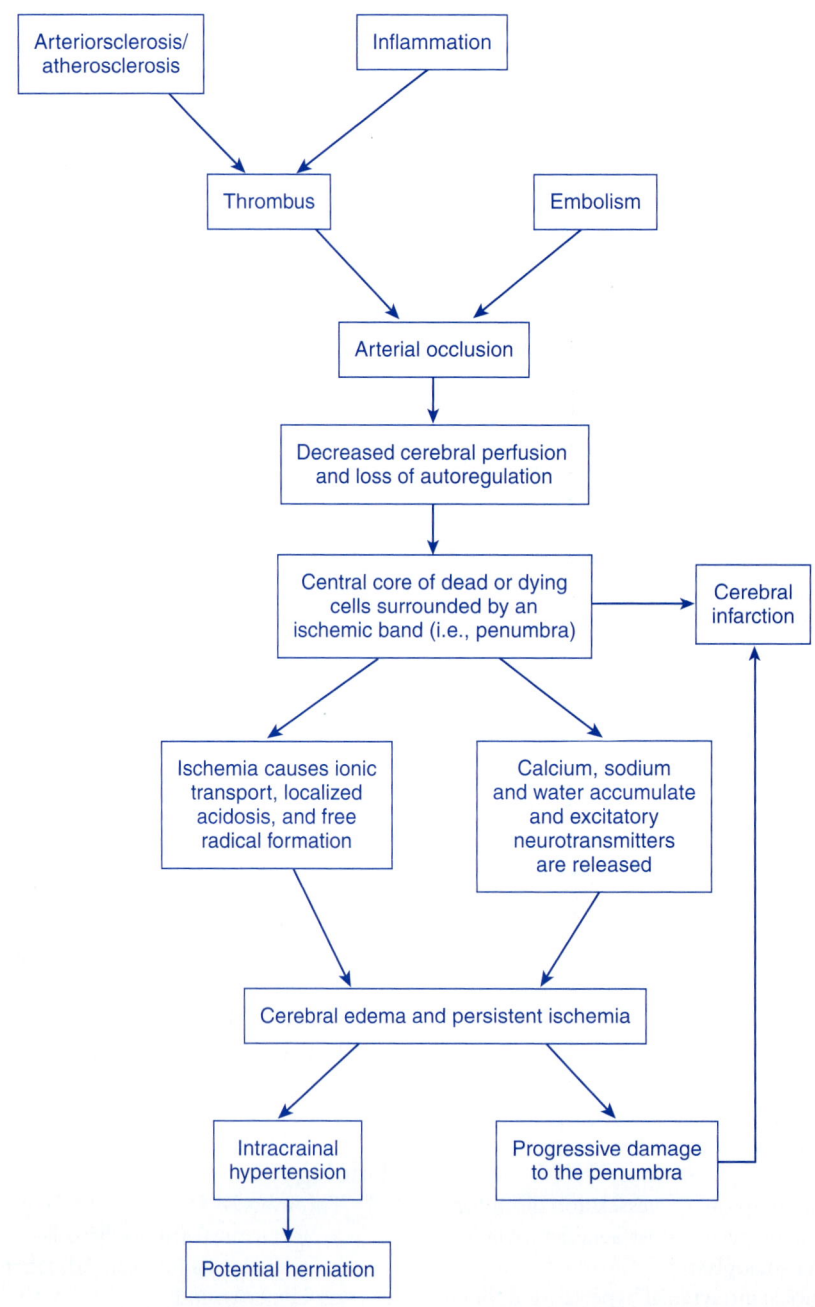

Fig. 5.35 Pathophysiology of ischemic stroke.

d. Diabetes mellitus
   e. Valvular heart disease
   f. Coronary artery disease
   g. Heart failure
   h. Hyperlipidemia
   i. Obesity
   j. Sedentary lifestyle
   k. Drugs
      1) Alcohol, especially heavy episodic consumption
      2) Stimulants (e.g., cocaine, phenylpropanolamine)
      3) Oral contraceptives
   l. Dysrhythmias, especially atrial fibrillation
   m. Hypercoagulability

Clinical Presentation
1. Subjective
   a. May have history of any of the following:
      1) TIA
      2) Hypertension
      3) Cardiovascular disease
      4) Arteriosclerosis
      5) Diabetes
   b. Sudden onset of signs and symptoms
      1) Thrombotic stroke usually occurs at night and is often discovered on awakening; likely caused by decrease in CO and BP with less flow through an area of critical stenosis
      2) Embolic stroke is more likely to occur when the patient is active.
2. Objective
   a. Varies depending on area of vessel involved and extent of injury (Box 5.3)
3. Diagnostic studies
   a. Serum
      1) Lipids: may be elevated
      2) Glucose
         a) Hypoglycemia may mimic stroke.
         b) Hyperglycemia frequently seen in stroke
      3) Clotting profile: baseline desirable before fibrinolytics
   b. ECG: may show dysrhythmias as a possible cause of cerebral emboli; Holter monitor may identify dysrhythmia
   c. Echocardiography: may show intracardiac source for cerebral emboli (e.g., ventricular aneurysm, bacterial endocarditis)
   d. Doppler carotid studies: may show carotid artery stenosis
   e. Transcranial Doppler: may be used to localize vessel occlusions and experimentally to assist with clot lysis
   f. CT
      1) Normal early in ischemic stroke
      2) Identifies the location and characteristics of subacute and old infarctions, the presence or absence of gross hemorrhage, and the presence or absence of a mass lesion
      3) May show distortion or shift of ventricles
      4) CT performed 24 hours postfibrinolytic therapy to rule out intracranial hemorrhage
   g. MRI
      1) Shows presence of early ischemic changes when CT scans still look normal
      2) Identifies changes in the cranial or spinal structures
   h. Cerebral angiography: identifies occlusion, stenosis, aneurysms, and hemorrhage in arterial system

Collaborative Management
1. Maintain airway, ventilation, and oxygenation.
   a. Maintain airway.
      1) Oropharyngeal or nasopharyngeal airway may be needed to hold tongue away from hypopharynx in obtunded patient.
      2) Endotracheal intubation may be needed in patients without airway protective reflexes.
   b. Maintain oxygenation and ventilation.
      1) Administer oxygen as needed to maintain SpO_2 greater than or equal to 95% unless contraindicated.
      2) Turn patient frequently; 60-degree lateral rotation therapeutic bed is helpful to prevent pneumonia in these patients.
      3) Initiate mechanical ventilation as needed for acute respiratory failure.
   c. Prevent aspiration.
      1) Position patient on side.
      2) Have suction equipment available.
2. Detect changes in neurologic status and restore or maintain CBF (Fig. 5.36).
   a. Use the NIHSS (Table 5.9) to assess changes in neurologic status.
   b. Correct possible causes and contributing factors.
      1) Assist in electrical or pharmacologic conversion of atrial fibrillation or administer anticoagulants to prevent mural thrombi.

Box 5.3 Clinical Indications Related to Vascular Occlusion

Anterior Cerebral Artery
- Impaired gait
- Contralateral paralysis of leg and foot
- Personality changes: flat affect; inappropriate emotional responses
- Mental impairment

Middle Cerebral Artery
- Hemiplegia of face and arm on contralateral side
- Contralateral sensory deficit
- Aphasia if dominant hemisphere affected
- Homonymous hemianopsia
- Apraxia, agnosia, neglect if nondominant hemisphere affected
- Dysarthria
- Dysphagia

Posterior Cerebral Artery
- Cortical blindness
- Perseveration (abnormal persistence of a response)
- Homonymous hemianopsia

Vertebral or Basilar Artery
- Weakness of tongue
- Ipsilateral facial numbness and weakness
- Dizziness
- Nystagmus
- Dysarthria
- Dysphagia
- Ataxia
- "Locked-in" syndrome (i.e., quadriplegia and mutism with intact consciousness)

2) Administer antihypertensives to control BP only if BP greater than 220/120 mm Hg, cardiac ischemia, heart failure, or aortic dissection exist, fibrinolytic therapy is planned, or intracerebral hemorrhage is identified on CT.
    a) Hypotension *must* be avoided since cerebral autoregulation is lost in the area of ischemia or infarction.
    b) Nicardipine, labetalol, or hydralazine may be used.
3) Control hyperglycemia with IV insulin infusion.
c. Administer fibrinolytics as prescribed.
    1) Goal: lysis of an occluding clot to restore blood flow to the compromised but potentially viable penumbra
    2) Seven Ds of stroke care (American Heart Association)

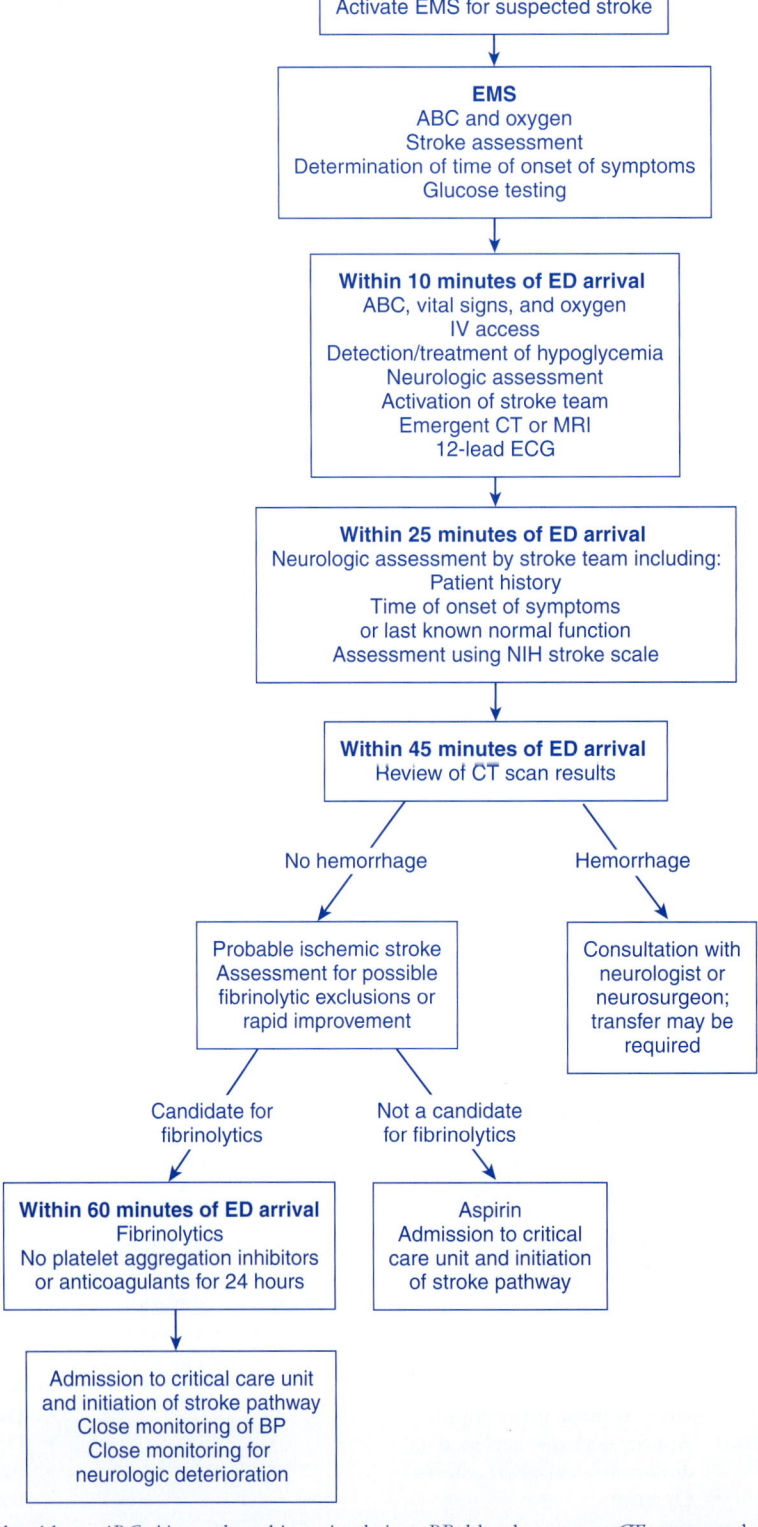

Fig. 5.36 Suspected stroke algorithm. *ABC*, Airway, breathing, circulation; *BP*, blood pressure; *CT*, computed tomography; *ECG*, electrocardiogram; *EMS*, emergency management system; *IV*, intravenous; *MRI*, magnetic resonance imaging; *NIH*, National Institutes of Health. (From Jauch, E. C., Saver, J. L., Adams, H. P., Bruno, A., Connors, J. J. B., Demaerschalk, B. M., . . . Yonas, H. (2013). Guidelines for the early management of patients with acute ischemic stroke. Stroke, 44(3), 870-947.)

a) Detection of early indications and determination of time of onset
   i) Time of onset is either witnessed or the time that last known normal neurologic function was noted.
b) Dispatch of emergency medical care
c) Delivery of the patient to the nearest facility capable of implementing the most current stroke guidelines
d) Door and rapid triage in the emergency department
e) Data collected to aid in decision making
   i) Baseline CT and/or MRI to exclude intracranial hemorrhage and other risk factors for intracranial hemorrhage
   ii) History, physical examination, laboratory
f) Decision made regarding whether the patient meets criteria for fibrinolytics and does not have contraindications (Box 5.4)
g) Drug within 3 to 4.5 hours of the onset of symptoms

Box 5.4 Inclusion and Exclusion Criteria for the Use of IV Recombinant Tissue Plasminogen Activator (rTPA) in Ischemic Stroke

Inclusion Criteria

Diagnosis of ischemic stroke causing measurable neurologic deficit
Onset of symptoms <3 hr before beginning treatment (either the witnessed onset of symptoms or the time last known normal if symptom onset was not witnessed)
Aged ≥18 yr

Exclusion Criteria

Significant head trauma or prior stroke in previous 3 mo
Symptoms suggest subarachnoid hemorrhage
Arterial puncture at noncompressible site in previous 7 days
History of previous intracranial hemorrhage
Intracranial neoplasm, arteriovenous malformation, or aneurysm
Recent intracranial or intraspinal surgery
Elevated blood pressure (systolic >185 mm Hg or diastolic >110 mm Hg)
Active internal bleeding
Acute bleeding diathesis, including but not limited to
Platelet count <100,000/mm^3
Heparin received within 48 hr, resulting in abnormally elevated aPTT greater than the upper limit of normal
Current use of anticoagulant with INR >1.7 or PT >15 sec
Current use of direct thrombin inhibitors or direct factor Xa inhibitors with elevated sensitive laboratory tests (e.g., aPTT, INR, platelet count, and ECT; TT; or appropriate factor Xa activity assays)
Blood glucose concentration <50 mg/dl (2.7 mmol/l)
CT demonstrates multilobar infarction (hypodensity greater than one third of the cerebral hemisphere)

Relative Exclusion Criteria

Recent experience suggests that under some circumstances—with careful consideration and weighting of risk to benefit—patients may receive fibrinolytic therapy despite one or more relative contraindications. Consider risk to benefit of IV rtPA administration carefully if any of these relative contraindications are present:
  Only minor or rapidly improving stroke symptoms (clearing spontaneously)
  Pregnancy
  Seizure at onset with postictal residual neurologic impairments
  Major surgery or serious trauma within previous 14 days
  Recent gastrointestinal or urinary tract hemorrhage (within previous 21 days)
  Recent AMI (within previous 3 months)

Inclusion and Exclusion Characteristics of Patients with Ischemic Stroke Who Could Be Treated with Intravenous Recombinant Tissue Plasminogen Activator Within 3 Hours from Symptom Onset

Additional Inclusion Criteria

Diagnosis of ischemic stroke causing measurable neurologic deficit
Onset of symptoms within 3–4.5 hr before beginning treatment

Additional Relative Exclusion Criteria

Age >80 yr
  Severe stroke (NIHSS score >25)
  Taking an oral anticoagulant regardless of INR
History of both diabetes and prior ischemic stroke

AMI, Acute myocardial infarction; *aPTT,* activated partial thromboplastin time; *CT,* computed tomography; *ECT,* electroconvulsive therapy *INR,* international normalized ratio; *IV,* intravenous; *NHISS,* National Institutes of Health Stroke Scale; *PT,* prothrombin time; *tPA,* recombinant tissue plasminogen activator; *TT,* thrombin time.
From Jauch, E. C., Saver, J. L., Adams, H. P., Bruno, A., Connors, J. J. B., Demaerschalk, B. M., . . . Yonas, H. (2013). Guidelines for the early management of patients with acute ischemic stroke. *Stroke,* 44(3), 870–947.

3) Dosage and routes
   a) IV alteplase
      i) Total dose: 0.9 mg/kg with maximum dose of less than or equal to 90 mg
      ii) Bolus: 10% of this total dose over 1 minute
      iii) Infusion: remaining 90% of this total dose administered over 60 minutes
      iv) Do not give aspirin, heparin, or warfarin for 24 hours (Gahart & Nazareno, 2017)
   b) Intraarterial
      i) Catheter is placed into the cerebral circulation under fluoroscopy
      ii) Dose of alteplase approximately half of IV dose
4) Management
   a) Monitor vital signs and neurologic status.
   b) Before fibrinolytic administration, maintain BP less than 185 mm Hg systolic and less than 110 mm Hg diastolic; labetalol, nicardipine, hydralazine, or enalaprilat are recommended.
   c) After fibrinolytic administration, maintain systolic BP less than 180 mm Hg and diastolic BP less than 105 mm Hg; postfibrinolytic therapy, BP should be managed with labetalol, nicardipine, or nitroprusside if necessary.
   d) Do not administer anticoagulants or platelet aggregation inhibitors for 24 hours after IV fibrinolytic.
   e) Repeat CT at 24 hours postfibrinolytic.
   f) Avoid punctures: arterial; IV, intramuscular, subcutaneous
      i) Apply pressure until hemostasis is achieved if punctures are required after fibrinolytics initiated
      ii) Insert multiple (usually two or three) IV catheters before initiation of fibrinolytic therapy; one of these catheters may be used for venous sampling
   g) Monitor stools, urine, emesis, sputum, saliva for blood
   h) Monitor for complications
      i) Hemorrhage
         (a) At site of vascular puncture: 80% incidence
         (b) Gastrointestinal or genitourinary bleeding: 15.20% incidence
         (c) Intracranial bleed: 1% incidence
d. Administer anticoagulants and platelet aggregation inhibitors as prescribed if fibrinolytics are contraindicated or after 24 hours after IV fibrinolytics.
   1) Anticoagulants (e.g., heparin) are especially important if emboli are of cardiac origin such as atrial fibrillation.
      a) LMWH subcutaneously may be used for DVT prophylaxis.
   2) Platelet aggregation inhibitors
      a) Oral agents (e.g., aspirin, Aggrenox, ticlopidine, clopidogrel) or IV agents abciximab, eptifibatide, tirofiban HCl as prescribed
         i) IV agents being studied for primary use within 24 hours of stroke symptoms
         b) Especially important in patients with carotid, intracranial, or vertebrobasilar artery stenosis
         c) Contraindicated for 24 hours after IV fibrinolytics
   e. Prepare patient for surgical procedures as requested.
      1) Endarterectomy or carotid artery angioplasty with or without stenting for patients with signs of cerebrovascular insufficiency who have not had completed stroke (see Vascular Disease section of Chapter 3).
      2) Intraarterial mechanical embolectomy with or without fibrinolytic administration
      3) Craniotomy with evacuation of clot depending on size, location, and neurologic status
      4) Decompressive hemicraniectomy where there are severe cerebral edema, hemispheric shifting, and potential herniation
3. Prevent or monitor for clinical indications or treat intracranial hypertension (see Intracranial Hypertension section) especially during the first 72 hours.
4. Maintain fluid and electrolyte balance and nutritional status.
   a. Administer IV fluids as prescribed.
   b. Assess gag and swallow reflexes before oral fluids; routine use of a bedside dysphagia screening tool is recommended.
   c. Initiate early enteral feedings within 24 to 48 hours if unable to take food by mouth
5. Decrease metabolic requirements.
   a. Enforce bed rest initially.
   b. Administer minor tranquilizers as prescribed but do not oversedate.
   c. Administer stool softeners as prescribed.
   d. Treat hyperthermia with antipyretics, passive cooling (i.e., fans), and cooling blankets; hypothermia therapy may be initiated.
6. Assess the patient's ability to communicate and establish means of communication; consult speech therapist as soon as possible in aphasic patients.
7. Protect patient from injury.
   a. Provide assistance during ambulation because patient may have postural imbalance related to hemiparesis or hemiplegia.
   b. Orient patient often and provide explanations of care because confusion and disorientation as well as memory deficits may occur concomitantly with aphasia.
   c. Administer prophylactic anticonvulsants as prescribed.
8. Prevent deformities, decubiti, and hazards of immobility.
   a. Reposition every 2 hours.
   b. Perform passive ROM exercises every 2 hours; assist with active ROM exercises when patient is able to assist.
9. Maximize independence in ADLs; allow the patient to do whatever he or she can.
10. Provide emotional support and encourage participation in support groups.
11. Provide instruction and counseling regarding lifestyle modification and need for pharmacologic therapy.
    a. Nonpharmacologic therapies
       1) Weight normalization
       2) Dietary modifications
          a) Low saturated fat
          b) Low (2–3 g) sodium
          c) American Diabetes Association diet for control of blood glucose for patients with diabetes

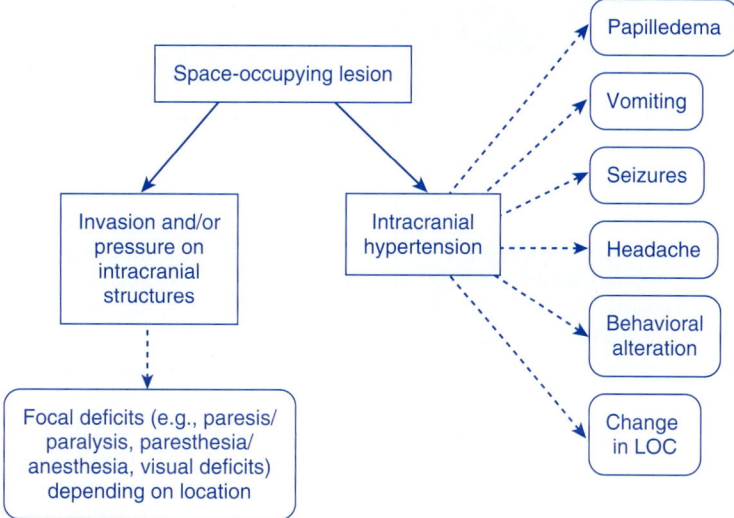

Fig. 5.37 Pathophysiology of brain tumors. *Dotted lines* connect pathology to clinical presentation. *LOC,* Level of consciousness.

  3) Cessation of tobacco use
  4) Limitation of alcohol consumption to 1 to 2 alcoholic beverages daily
  5) Regular aerobic exercise in moderation
  6) Complementary therapies: relaxation, imagery, biofeedback
  7) Stress reduction
  8) Yearly flu and pneumococcal vaccine
  9) Recognition of symptoms of TIA or stroke and when to call the physician
 b. Pharmacologic agents
  1) Control of hypertension, hyperlipidemia, and diabetes
  2) Platelet aggregation inhibitors and/or anticoagulants
  3) Discontinuance of oral contraceptive agents in premenopausal women and hormone replacement therapy in postmenopausal women
12. Monitor for complications.
 a. Persistent neurologic trauma
 b. Brain edema
 c. Seizures: prophylactic anticonvulsants
 d. Fluid and electrolyte imbalance: DI, SIADH, CSW (see Craniotomy section)
 e. Spastic paralysis may cause contractures.
  1) ROM
  2) Splints
 f. Pneumonia
 g. DVT, PE
  1) Subcutaneous LMWH or unfractionated heparin is usually used prophylactically.
  2) Sequential compression devices may also be used.
 h. Urinary tract infection, urosepsis
 i. Pressure ulcers

Brain Tumor

Etiology: Multifactorial or Unknown
1. Congenital
2. Hereditary factors

Pathophysiology (Fig. 5.37)
1. Primary brain tumors are categorized by their cell type; metastatic brain tumors are of the cell type of the primary tumor (Table 5.19).

Clinical Presentation
1. Subjective
 a. Headache
  1) Occurs at night after retiring
  2) Present and worse on awakening
  3) May be relieved by midmorning
 b. Visual changes
2. Objective
 a. Seizures: new onset
 b. Personality changes
 c. Vomiting without preceding nausea
  1) More common in morning
 d. Papilledema
 e. Change in LOC
 f. Hormonal changes if pituitary involved
 g. Specific to affected area of brain (Table 5.20)
3. Diagnostic studies
 a. Hormone levels: may be abnormal if pituitary tumor
 b. Chest radiography: may show primary tumor of lung
 c. Skull radiography: may show shift of pineal gland
 d. EEG: aids in identification of seizure activity
 e. Brain scan: identifies the tumor
 f. Bone scan: may show bone cancer
 g. CT: identifies the tumor
 h. MRI: identifies the tumor and effect on surrounding tissue
 i. Angiography: may show vascular shifts due to tumor or may show vascularity of tumor
 j. Biopsy: classifies tumor cell type

Collaborative Management
1. Prevent or monitor for clinical indications/treat intracranial hypertension (see Intracranial Hypertension section); glucocorticoids are frequently used to reduce brain edema
2. Maintain airway, oxygenation, and ventilation.

Table 5.19	Types of Brain Tumors
Type	**Comments**
Gliomas • Astrocytomas (initially benign but prone to become malignant) • Oligodendrogliomas (usually benign but may become malignant) • Ependymomas (usually benign but may become malignant) • Medulloblastomas (highly malignant) • Glioblastoma multiforme (highly malignant)	• Most in cerebrum, but medulloblastoma in cerebellum and ependymomas in ventricular system • Most grow rapidly, but medulloblastoma is rapidly invasive • Most nonencapsulated; cannot be incised completely
Meningioma	• Benign, slow growing • Usually encapsulated; surgical cure possible • Recurrence possible
Pituitary adenoma	• Usually benign • Surgical approach usually successful
Acoustic neuroma	• Benign or low-grade malignancy • Arise from sheath of Schwann cells found on eighth cranial nerve • Will regrow if not completely excised • Surgical resection often difficult because of location
Metastatic tumor	• Malignant • Cancer cells spread to the brain via the circulatory system, usually from lung, breast, or prostate cancer • Surgical resection difficult and prognosis poor

Table 5.20	Clinical Manifestations of Tumors Specific to Affected Area of Brain
Area	**Clinical Manifestations**
Frontal lobe	• Personality changes • Inappropriate behavior: loss of social behavior • Inappropriate affect: quiet, flat • Inattentiveness, inability to concentrate • Emotional lability • Recent memory loss • Decreased intellectual ability • Motor changes: hemiparesis, hemiplegia • Seizure activity possible • If dominant hemisphere: expressive aphasia
Parietal	• Sensory changes: hyperesthesia, paresthesia, loss of two-point discrimination • Constructional apraxia • Loss of right-left discrimination • Homonymous hemianopsia • Seizure activity possible
Temporal	• Poor judgment • Irritability • Regressive behavior • Auditory disturbances • Olfactory, visual, and gustatory hallucinations • Psychomotor seizures • If dominant hemisphere: receptive aphasia
Occipital lobe	• Visual disturbances: visual field defects • Visual hallucinations • Seizure activity possible: visual aura
Pituitary or hypothalamus	• Visual disturbances • Hormone imbalance: hypopituitarism or hyperpituitarism • Temperature regulation problems • Changes in sleep patterns
Brainstem	• Dysphagia • Vomiting • Ataxia • Nystagmus • Vomiting: with or without nausea • Decreased corneal reflex • Ventilatory pattern changes
Cerebellum	• Ataxia • Nystagmus • Unsteady gait • Decreased coordination • Vomiting: with or without nausea • Intentional tremors • Seizure activity possible

    a. Maintain airway.
        1) Oropharyngeal or nasopharyngeal airway may be needed to hold tongue away from hypopharynx in obtunded patient.
        2) Endotracheal intubation may be needed in patients without airway protective reflexes.
    b. Maintain oxygenation and ventilation.
        1) Administer oxygen as needed to maintain SpO_2 greater than or equal to 95% unless contraindicated.
        2) Initiate mechanical ventilation as needed for hypoventilation.
    c. Prevent aspiration.
        1) Position patient on side.
        2) Have suction equipment available.
3. Prepare patient for surgery, radiation, and/or chemotherapy.
    a. Surgery
        1) Purposes of craniotomy for brain tumor
            a) Debulk tumor to relieve pressure.
            b) Resect and remove tumor (usually followed by radiation).
            c) Insert shunt for hydrocephalus.
        2) Postcraniotomy care (see Craniotomy section)
    b. Radiation: after surgery for incompletely excised tumor or for nonsurgically accessible tumor
        1) Whole-brain radiation therapy in high doses or superfractionated therapy
        2) Brachytherapy or interstitial irradiation: placement of a radioactive source in contact with or implanted into the brain tumor
    c. Radiosurgery: closed-skull destruction of an intracranial target with ionizing beams of radiation; an intracranial guiding device aids in focusing the beams of radiation

1) Bragg peak proton beam
2) Linear accelerator radiosurgery
3) Gamma knife therapy
d. Chemotherapy
1) Used after debulking in combination with radiotherapy, after irradiation, or for tumor recurrence
2) Antineoplastic agent determined by tumor type; more than one agent may be used
4. Monitor for complications
a. Fluid and electrolyte imbalance: DI, SIADH, CSW (see Craniotomy section)
b. Brain ischemia
c. Hydrocephalus
d. Brain edema
e. Seizures
f. Herniation

Status Epilepticus

Definitions

1. Seizure: sudden, paroxysmal episode of exaggerated activity or abnormal behavior caused by excessive discharge of cerebral neurons; Table 5.21 describes types of seizures.
2. Status epilepticus: seizure activity of 30 minutes or more duration caused by a single seizure or a series of seizures in which there is no return of consciousness between seizures
    a. Note that a more current definition is seizure activity lasting at least 10 minutes because treatment is generally initiated within 10 minutes preventing the continuation of seizure activity for 30 minutes.

Etiology

1. Preexisting history of seizure disorder
    a. Withdrawal from anticonvulsant medications
    b. Acute alcohol withdrawal
    c. Acute withdrawal from chronically used drugs that have sedative or depressant effects (e.g., barbiturates)
    d. Acute condition which lowers the seizure threshold
2. No preexisting history of seizure disorder
    a. Brain trauma
    b. Stroke: ischemic or hemorrhagic
    c. CNS infection: meningitis, encephalitis, abscess
    d. Brain tumors
    e. Encephalopathy: anoxic (e.g., post–cardiac arrest), hypertensive, or metabolic
        1) Hypoglycemia
        2) Hepatic failure
        3) Uremia
        4) Hyperosmolality
    f. Electrolyte imbalance
        1) Hyponatremia
        2) Hypocalcemia
        3) Hypomagnesemia

Table 5.21 Types of Seizures

Type	Features	Duration
Generalized: Loss of Consciousness		
Absence (petit mal)	• Momentary loss of consciousness • Blank stare, cessation of activity • Eye blinking, lip smacking may occur • May lose muscle tone	Seconds
Tonic-clonic (grand mal)	• May be preceded by an aura and a cry from forced expiration • Loss of consciousness • Symmetrical tonic-clonic extremity movements • May experience apnea with cyanosis until tonic phase ends • May bite tongue, may be incontinent • Postictal fatigue, muscle soreness, confusion, lethargy, and/or headache	3–5 minutes
Myoclonic	• Short, abrupt muscle contractions of arms, legs, and torso • Contractions may be symmetrical or asymmetrical	Seconds
Clonic	• Muscle contraction and relaxation but slower than with myoclonic seizure	Several minutes
Tonic	• Abrupt increase in muscle tone of torso and face • Flexion of arms; extension of legs	Seconds
Atonic	• Abrupt loss of muscle tone • May cause falling and injuries related to fall	Seconds
Partial: Focal at Onset but May Evolve into a Generalized Seizure		
Simple partial	• Consciousness not impaired • Abnormal unilateral movement of arm, leg, or both • Patient may sense abnormal smell, sound, or sensation, such as numbness, tingling, or burning • Tachycardia or bradycardia, tachypnea, skin flushing, epigastric discomfort	Seconds to minutes
Complex partial	• Loss of consciousness but eyes may be open • Lip smacking, chewing, picking at clothing • Mumbling, speaking in repetitive phrases • Posturing or jerking movements • Postictal confusion, amnesia common	Minutes

g. Drug or alcohol withdrawal
h. Drug toxicity: lidocaine, meperidine, theophylline, salicylates, cyclic antidepressants, cocaine
i. Sepsis

Pathophysiology
Fig. 5.38.

Clinical Presentation
1. Subjective
   a. History may include precipitating event or condition
      1) History of epilepsy
      2) History of noncompliance in taking anticonvulsant drugs
      3) History of chronic drug or alcohol use
2. Objective
   a. Alteration in LOC
   b. Tonic and/or clonic body movements
   c. Incontinence of urine or stool
   d. Involuntary motor activities: lip smacking, swallowing, chewing
3. Diagnostic studies
   a. Evaluation of cause
      1) BUN: increased in uremia, hyperosmolality
      2) Liver function studies: increased in hepatic failure
      3) Drug and alcohol levels
      4) Anticonvulsant drug levels: subtherapeutic in noncompliance
   b. Serum
      1) Electrolytes: hyperkalemia
      2) Glucose: increased early; decreased late
      3) CK: increased
      4) Lactic acid: increased
      5) ABGs: may show hypercapnia, hypoxemia
   c. Urine: may show myoglobinuria
   d. Skull radiography: may show cause
   e. EEG: will show seizure activity
   f. CT, MRI, MRA: may indicate pathologic conditions (e.g., mass lesions)
   g. LP: may show meningitis as cause

Collaborative Management
1. Establish and maintain airway and adequate ventilation.
   a. Insert artificial airway if ventilation and oxygenation are inadequate.
      1) Use nasopharyngeal airway or nasotracheal intubation if mouth cannot be opened; do not try to force mouth open.
      2) Monitor ABGs and pulse oximetry.
   b. Maintain oxygenation and ventilation.
      1) Administer oxygen as needed to maintain SpO_2 greater than or equal to 95% unless contraindicated.
      2) Initiate mechanical ventilation as needed for hypoventilation.
   c. Prevent aspiration.
      1) Position on side: do not just turn head to side; turn body on side.
      2) Have suction equipment available; suction as indicated.
2. Protect patient from injury and prevent complications during seizure.
   a. Call for help.
   b. Do not leave patient.
   c. Loosen constrictive clothing.
   d. Remove pillow from under head.
   e. Turn patient to the side and maintain an open airway.

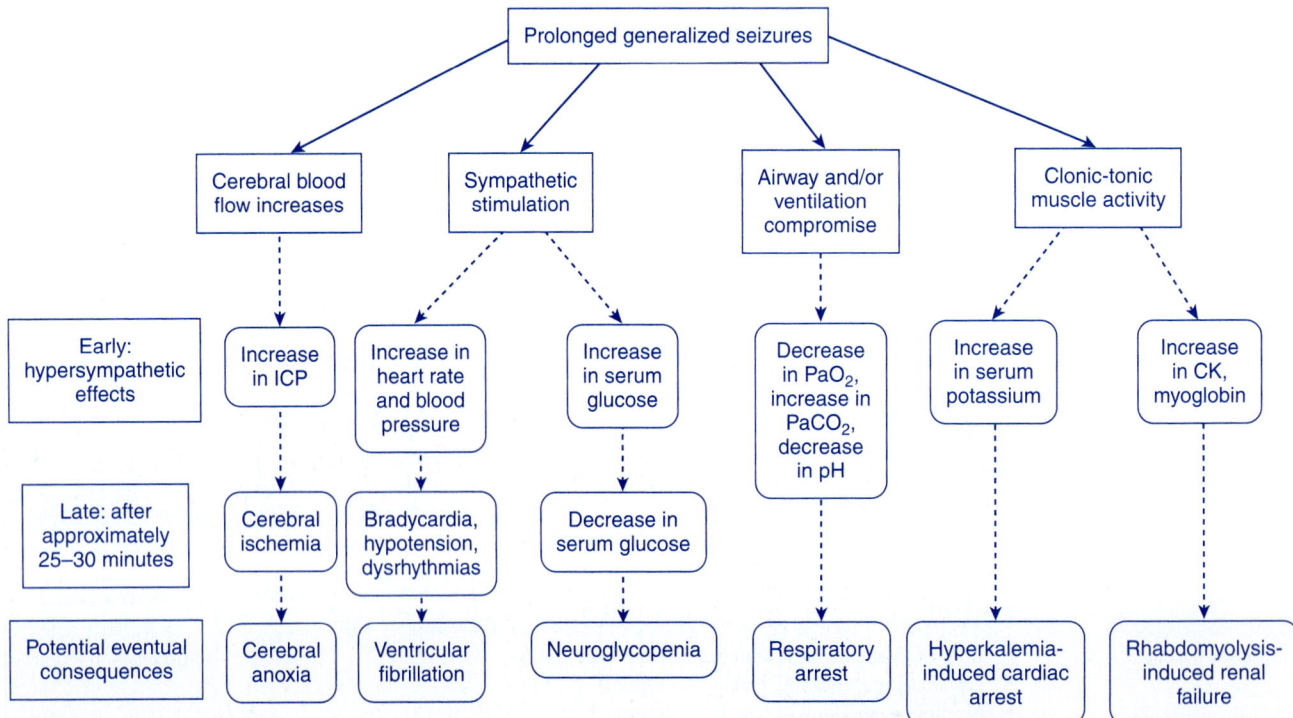

Fig. 5.38 Pathophysiology of status epilepticus. *Dotted lines* connect pathology to clinical presentation. *CK,* Creatine kinase; *ICP,* intracranial pressure; *PaCO₂,* partial pressure of carbon dioxide in arterial blood; *PaO₂,* partial pressure of oxygen in arterial blood.

f. Do not restrain but gentle guiding of extremities is acceptable.
g. Pad side rails with blankets or pillows.
h. Maintain privacy.
i. Assess for injury.
3. Assess for and eliminate causes or contributing factors.
   a. Analyze serum for glucose, sodium, potassium, calcium, phosphorus, magnesium, and BUN.
   b. Screen for drugs.
      1) Barbiturates
      2) Tricyclic antidepressants
      3) Alcohol
   c. Obtain anticonvulsant drug levels.
   d. Obtain blood cultures if patient is hyperthermic.
   e. Correct contributing factors that lower seizure threshold (e.g., hypoxemia, acid–base imbalance, electrolyte imbalance, hyperthermia, hypermetabolism).
4. Stop seizure activity.
   a. Initiate IV.
   b. Administer 100 mg of thiamine and 50 ml of $D_{50}W$ if alcohol ingestion or hypoglycemia is; Thiamine is given with the dextrose to prevent Wernicke encephalopathy, especially if patient has chronic malnutrition.
   c. Administer benzodiazepine or other drugs if seizures persist after dextrose and thiamine (Table 5.22).
      1) Benzodiazepine to stop the seizure
         a) First choice: lorazepam
         b) Second choice: diazepam
      2) Agents to prevent recurrence to be given after benzodiazepine
         a) Phenytoin
         b) Fosphenytoin
         c) Phenobarbital
      3) Other agents for refractory status epilepticus
         a) Pentobarbital
         b) Midazolam
         c) Propofol
         d) Levetiracetam
         e) Lacosamide
         f) Rarely used IV agents: thiopental, valproic acid, etomidate, paraldehyde, lidocaine
         g) Rarely used inhalation anesthetics: halothane, isoflurane, nitrous oxide
      4) Monitor closely for hypotension; administer fluids as prescribed.
      5) Monitor for respiratory depression; ventilation with manual resuscitation bag and mask may be required; endotracheal intubation may be required.
      6) Reduce the infusion rate as prescribed after at least 12 hours without seizures.
      7) Monitor serum drug concentrations and adjust drug dosages as prescribed to maintain optimal levels.
   d. Prepare patient for surgical procedures that may be required for removal of tumor, hematoma, or abscess.
5. Monitor and document duration of seizure activity, patient's LOC, and drugs.
   a. Aura: presence or absence; nature if present
   b. Cry: presence or absence
   c. Onset: site of initial body movements, deviation of head and eyes, chewing and salivation, posture of body, sensory changes
   d. Tonic and clonic phases: movement of body during progression; skin color and airway; pupillary changes; incontinence; duration of each phase
   e. Relaxation phase: duration and behavior
   f. Postictal phase: duration; ability to remember anything about the seizure; orientation; pupillary changes; headache; injuries
   g. Duration: from aura to relaxation
   h. Drugs administered
6. Monitor and assess condition closely to prevent complications.
   a. Insert nasogastric tube to prevent vomiting and aspiration.
   b. Monitor cardiac rate and rhythm and BP.
   c. Have cardiovascular drugs available.
   d. Assess neurologic status frequently.
7. Provide reassurance and comfort during postictal period.
   a. Elevate HOB 30 degrees.
   b. Reassure and reorient patient as he or she awakens.
   c. Provide privacy and calm environment.
   d. Discretely clean patient if he or she was incontinent.
   e. Allow the patient to sleep.
8. Maintain fluid and electrolyte balance.
   a. Assess electrolytes, calcium, magnesium, and renal and hepatic function.
   b. Monitor for indications of myoglobinuria (e.g., cola-colored urine); administer treatment for myoglobinuria as prescribed (fluids and osmotic diuretics [e.g., mannitol]).
9. Monitor for complications.
   a. Injury during seizure
   b. Acute respiratory failure
   c. Aspiration
   d. Acid–base imbalance, electrolyte imbalance
      1) Respiratory or metabolic acidosis
      2) Hyperkalemia
   e. Hypoglycemia: monitor serum glucose and administer parenteral dextrose as required.
   f. Hyperthermia: treat body temperature greater than 40°C with antipyretics and/or hypothermia blanket.
   g. Renal failure related to myoglobinuria
      1) Monitor serum CK to detect rhabdomyolysis and note change in urine color (i.e., cola colored) to detect myoglobinuria.
      2) Treat myoglobinuria with fluids, mannitol, and sodium bicarbonate as prescribed.
   h. Residual neurologic deficits

Central Nervous System Infections

Definitions
1. Meningitis: acute inflammation of the brain and spinal cord that may involve all meningeal membranes; may be bacterial, fungal, or viral
2. Encephalitis: acute inflammation of the parenchyma of the brain and meninges
3. Brain abscess: accumulation of pus within the brain tissue; surrounded by inflamed tissue

Table 5.22 Anticonvulsant Drugs

Medication	Actions or Use	Dose and Route	Time to Stop Seizure/ Duration of Anticonvulsant Effect	Side Effects	Nursing Implications
Phenytoin	Depresses seizure activity by altering ion transport in motor cortex	Status epilepticus: 10–20 mg/kg IV in 0.9% NS only Administer over 20–30 min Do not exceed a total dose of 1.5 g If seizure not terminated, consider other antiepileptic drugs, barbiturates, or anesthesia Follow with maintenance dose of 100 mg IV over 2 min every 6–8 hr	30 min/24 hr	• Bradycardia • Hypotension • Nystagmus or ataxia • Gingival hyperplasia • Agranulocytosis • Rash • Stevens-Johnson syndrome • Lymphadenopathy • Nausea • Cardiac arrest • Heart block	Slow rate if bradycardia, hypotension, or cardiac dysrhythmias occur Monitor ECG, BP, pulse, and respiratory function Dilute with 0.9% NS only Assess oral hygiene Assess for rash Monitor renal, hepatic, and hematologic status Interacts with many medications
Fosphenytoin	Depresses seizure activity by altering ion transport in motor cortex	Status epilepticus loading dose: 15–20 mg PE/kg IV Each 100–150 mg PE over a minimum of 1 min If full effect is not immediate, may be necessary to use with benzodiazepine Nonemergency loading dose: 10–20 mg PE/kg IV Maintenance dose: 4–6 mg PE/kg/24 hr	15 min/24 hr	• Transient ataxia • Dizziness • Headache • Nystagmus • Paresthesia • Pruritus • Somnolence Major or Overdose • Hypotension • Bradycardia • Heart block • Respiratory arrest • Ventricular fibrillation • Tonic seizures • Nausea or vomiting • Lethargy • Hypocalcemia • Metabolic acidosis • Rash	Slow infusion rate or temporarily stop infusion for bradycardia, hypotension, burning, itching, numbness, or pain along injection site Assess neurologic, respiratory, and cardiovascular status Assess seizure activity Monitor renal, hepatic, and hematologic status Catastrophic interactions possible with many medications
Levetiracetam	Mechanism of action unknown May inhibit intracellular sodium influx in motor cortex Depresses seizure activity	500 mg IV BID, titrate by 1000 mg/day every 2 wk for seizure control Maximum 3000 mg/day in divided doses	15–30 min/6–30 min	• Suicidal ideation • Muscle weakness • Dizziness • Psychosis • Decreased RBCs, hemoglobin, hematocrit	Adjust dose with acute kidney injury Monitor CBC Monitor for adverse changes in mental status

Drug	Action/Indication	Dose	Onset/Duration	Side Effects	Nursing Implications
Diazepam	Depresses subcortical areas of CNS Antiepileptic, sedative-hypnotic Antianxiety Adjunct medication to depress seizure activity	Status epilepticus: 5–10 mg IV Give 5 mg over 1 min May be repeated every 10–15 min for a total dose of 30 mg May repeat in 2–4 hr; or 0.2–0.5 mg/kg every 15–30 min for 2–3 doses Some specialists suggest 20 mg and titrate total dose over 10 min or until seizures stop Maximum dose in 24 hr is 100 mg	1–3 min/30 min	• Respiratory depression • Hypotension • Drowsiness • Lethargy • Bradycardia • Cardiac arrest • Hypoglycemia	• Monitor respiratory status, BP, HR • Assess IV site for phlebitis and venous thrombosis
Lorazepam	Depresses subcortical areas of CNS Antiepileptic Sedative-hypnotic Antianxiety	Status epilepticus: 4 mg IV over 1 min as initial dose May repeat once in 10–15 min if seizure continues; or 0.05 mg/kg to a total of 4 mg May repeat once in 10–15 min Do not exceed 8 mg in 12 hr	6–10 min/12–24 hr	• Airway obstruction • Apnea • Blurred vision • Confusion • Excessive drowsiness • Hypotension • Bradycardia • Respiratory depression • Somnolence	Same as diazepam
Phenobarbital	Barbiturate Sedative-hypnotic Anticonvulsant	Status epilepticus: Loading dose: 15–18 mg/kg as a single dose or in divided doses over 10–15 min May give an additional 5 mg/kg every 15–30 min up to a maximum total dose of 30 mg/kg. 20 mg/kg at a rate no faster than 50 mg/min (not actively seizing) or 100 mg/min (actively seizing)	20–30 min/6–10 hr	• Depression • Dermatitis • Angioedema • Fever • Headache • Hypotension • Nausea • Respiratory depression (hypoventilation) • Thrombocytopenic purpura • Vertigo • Thrombophlebitis	• Highly alkaline; use large veins, if possible • Assess IV site for phlebitis and venous thrombosis • Intraarterial injection will cause gangrene • Monitor hourly VS • Maintain patent airway • Monitor hematopoietic, renal, and hepatic systems in any extended therapy • Monitor serum levels as indicated; the therapeutic range in adults is 20–40 mcg/ml

BID, Twice a day; *BP*, blood pressure; *CBC*, complete blood count; *CNS*, central nervous system; *ECG*, electrocardiography; *HR*, heart rate; *IV*, intravenous; *NS*, normal saline; *PE*, phenytoin equivalence; *RBC*, red blood cell; *VS*, vital signs.

Etiology
1. Meningitis
   a. Bacterial
      1) Associated factors
         a) Otitis media
         b) Sinusitis, upper respiratory infection, or pneumonia
         c) Penetrating head injury
         d) Basal skull fracture
         e) Intracranial surgery
         f) ICP monitoring
         g) Septicemia, septic embolus
      2) Organisms
         a) *Haemophilus influenzae*
         b) *Neisseria meningitidis* (meningococcal)
         c) *Diplococcus pneumoniae* (pneumococcal)
         d) *Streptococcus pneumoniae*
         e) *Escherichia coli*
         f) *Enterobacter* spp.
         g) *Klebsiella* spp.
         h) *Pseudomonas* spp.
         i) *Serratia* spp.
         j) *Salmonella* spp.
         k) *Gonococcus* spp.
   b. Fungal
      1) Associated factors
         a) Immunosuppression
            i) AIDS
            ii) Histoplasmosis
            iii) After organ transplantation
            iv) Steroid therapy
            v) Cancer
         b) Contaminated needles or syringes from drug abuse
      2) Organisms
         a) Cryptococcosis
         b) Coccidioidomycosis
         c) Mucormycosis
         d) Candidiasis
         e) Aspergillosis
   c. Viral
      1) Associated factors
         a) Immunosuppression
      2) Organisms
         a) Coxsackievirus
         b) Echovirus
         c) Adenovirus
         d) Arbovirus
         e) Poliovirus
         f) Herpes simplex virus
         g) Myxovirus (e.g., influenza, mumps, measles)
         h) Western equine
   d. Parasitic
      1) *Plasmodium* spp. (i.e., malaria)
      2) *Toxoplasma gondii*
2. Encephalitis (almost always viral)
   a. Associated factors
      1) Mosquito or tick bite (i.e., arbovirus)
      2) Recent viral infection
      3) Recent vaccination: measles, mumps, rubella
      4) Immunocompromise
   b. Organisms
      1) Arbovirus (e.g., West Nile virus, eastern equine encephalitis)
      2) Herpes simplex
      3) Rubella
      4) Rubeola
      5) Mumps
      6) Mononucleosis
3. Brain abscess
   a. Associated factors
      1) Middle-ear and mastoid infection
      2) Sinus infection
      3) Penetrating head injuries, skull fractures
      4) Compound fractures
      5) Osteomyelitis of the skull
      6) Neurosurgical or oral surgical procedures
      7) Metastatic abscess
   b. Organisms
      1) Streptococci
      2) Staphylococci
      3) Pneumococci

Pathophysiology
Fig. 5.39.

Clinical Presentation
1. Meningitis
   a. Subjective
      1) History of precipitating event or condition
      2) Headache that gets progressively worse
      3) Chills
      4) Nausea, vomiting
      5) Photophobia, pain when moving eyes
   b. Objective
      1) Infectious signs
         a) Fever
         b) Tachycardia
         c) Chills
         d) Skin rash: most likely with meningococcal meningitis
      2) Meningeal irritation
         a) Nuchal rigidity
         b) Brudzinski sign
         c) Kernig sign
      3) Neurologic abnormalities
         a) Change in LOC
         b) Confusion, delirium
         c) CN involvement (e.g., pupil changes)
         d) Focal neurologic signs
         e) Seizures
   c. Diagnostic studies
      1) Serum
         a) Blood cultures: may be positive for causative organism
         b) WBC count: elevated
      2) LP
         a) Elevated CSF pressure (normal LP, 80–180 mm/H_2O, measured at lumbar level, with patient in side-lying position)
         b) Increased WBCs in CSF
         c) Elevated protein in CSF in most cases

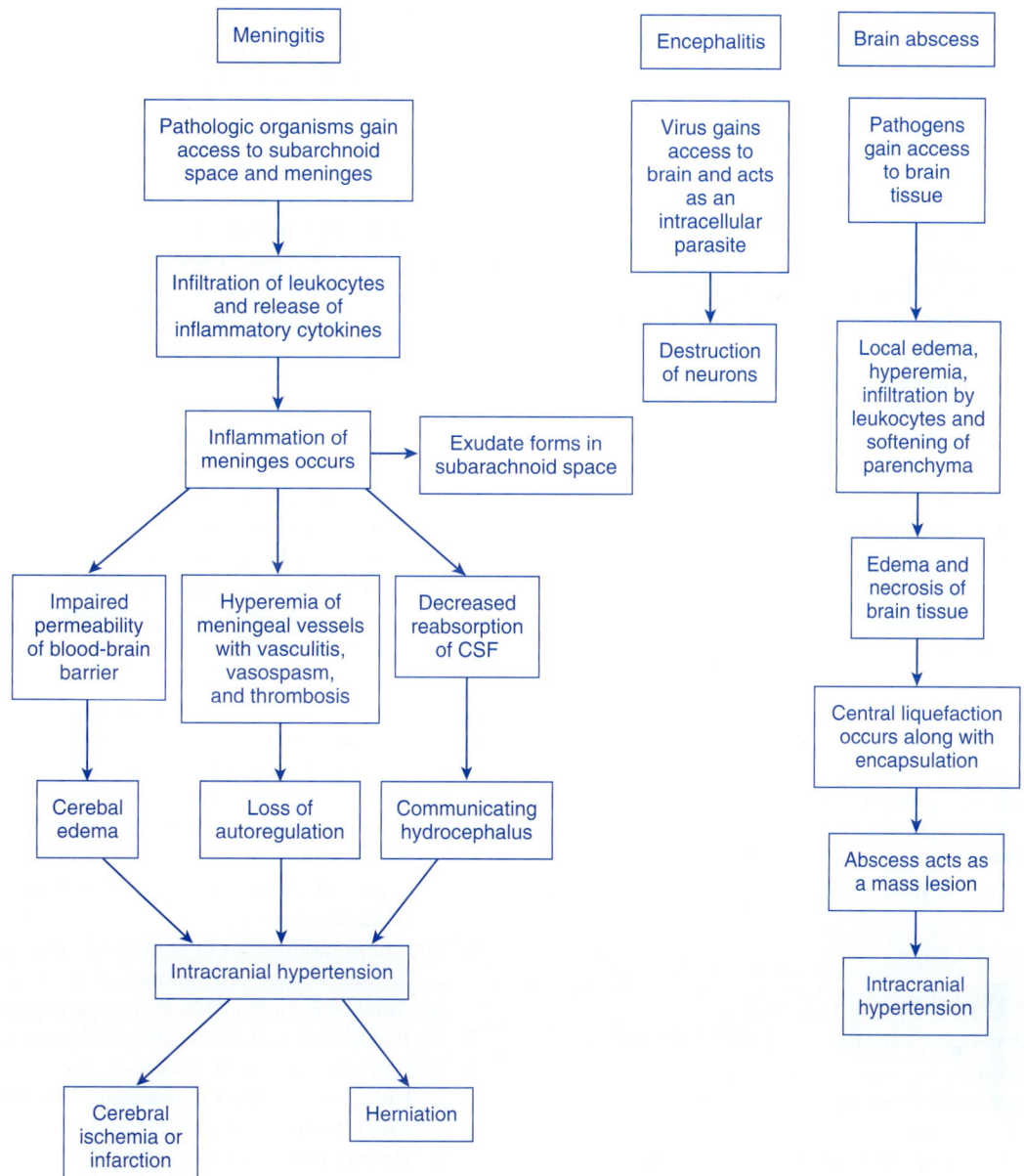

Fig. 5.39 Pathophysiology of brain central nervous system infections. *CSF,* Cerebrospinal fluid.

      d) Decreased glucose content in CSF in bacterial meningitis (NOTE: glucose in CSF is normally 60% of serum glucose)
      e) CSF is cloudy in bacterial meningitis
      f) Glucose content in CSF is normal and CSF is clear in viral meningitis.
      g) Culture: may identify organism
   3) CT: normal but CT scan of the head is frequently routinely obtained before the performance of an LP to identify occult intracranial abnormalities and avoid the risk of brainstem herniation secondary to the LP
2. Encephalitis
  a. Subjective
   1) History may include precipitating event or condition (e.g., mosquito or tick bite, contact with dead or sick bird).
   2) Headache
   3) Blurred vision, diplopia, photophobia
   4) Weakness
   5) Dysphagia
   6) Gastrointestinal symptoms may occur.
  b. Objective
   1) Change in LOC: lethargy, coma
   2) Fever
   3) Nuchal rigidity
   4) Dysphasia, aphasia
   5) Hemiparesis
   6) Nystagmus
   7) Facial muscle weakness
   8) Seizures
   9) Hallucinations
   10) Parkinsonian-like rigidity in tick-borne viral encephalitis

c. Diagnostic studies
  1) LP
    a) Elevated or normal pressure
    b) Elevated protein
    c) Increased WBC
    d) Normal or low glucose
    e) Culture: may identify organism
  2) Brain biopsy: required for diagnosis of herpes simplex encephalitis
  3) EEG: may show seizure activity
  4) CT: normal early in course; later low-density lesions may be seen
  5) MRI: may be more definitive than CT scan
  6) IgM antibody to West Nile virus for West Nile encephalitis in serum or CSF
3. Brain abscess
  a. Subjective
    1) History may include precipitating event or condition.
    2) Headache: constant and severe; increased with straining
    3) Malaise
    4) Irritability
    5) Chills
    6) Nausea, vomiting
    7) Muscle weakness
    8) Symptoms vary according to location in the brain
  b. Objective
    1) Change in LOC
    2) Confusion
    3) Hemiplegia
    4) Fever
    5) Nuchal rigidity may be present
    6) Dysphasia or aphasia
    7) Seizures
    8) Signs vary according to location of brain
  c. Diagnostic studies
    1) CT scan: may show localized changes in brain density
    2) EEG: may show electrical silence at abscess location
    3) LP
      a) Increased pressure
      b) Increased WBC count
      c) Elevated protein
      d) Normal glucose
    4) Brain biopsy: may identify organism
    5) Brain scan: locates abscess greater than 1 cm in size
    6) Angiogram: locate temporal lobe and cerebellar abscesses

Collaborative Management

1. Maintain airway, ventilation, and oxygenation.
  a. Maintain airway.
    1) Oropharyngeal or nasopharyngeal airway may be needed to hold tongue away from hypopharynx in obtunded patient.
    2) Endotracheal intubation may be needed in patients without airway protective reflexes.
  b. Maintain oxygenation and ventilation.
    1) Administer oxygen as needed to maintain SpO_2 greater than or equal to 95% unless contraindicated.
    2) Initiate mechanical ventilation as needed for hypoventilation.
  c. Prevent aspiration.
    1) Position patient on side.
    2) Have suction equipment available.
2. Treat infection.
  a. Administer antibiotics (need to be fat-soluble to cross BBB) to treat bacterial infection as prescribed.
  b. Administer antivirals to treat herpes simplex encephalitis as prescribed.
  c. Prepare patient for surgical excision and drainage of brain abscess.
3. Prevent or monitor for clinical indications/treat intracranial hypertension (see Intracranial Hypertension section)
  a. Steroids may be prescribed to decrease inflammation in bacterial meningitis: dexamethasone is usually prescribed either before or with the first dose of antibiotics.
4. Maintain fluid and electrolyte balance.
  a. Administer IV fluids as prescribed.
  b. Monitor for overhydration and DI.
5. Control body temperature to less than 38°C.
  a. Administer antipyretics.
  b. Use hypothermia blanket.
  c. Use meperidine as prescribed to control shivering (NOTE: Although chlorpromazine is sometimes used to prevent shivering, it lowers seizure threshold and should be avoided).
6. Prevent or monitor for or control seizures
  a. Institute seizure precautions.
  b. Administer anticonvulsant therapy as prescribed.
7. Treat headache with nonsedating analgesics (e.g., codeine).
8. Prevent transmission of disease.
  a. Universal precautions are adequate for most patients with CNS infections.
  b. Droplet precautions
    1) H. influenzae and N. meningitidis (i.e., meningococcal) may be transmitted by droplets generated during coughing, sneezing, talking, intubation, and bronchoscopy, so droplet precautions should be initiated if there is a clinical suspicion of one of these pathogens.
    2) These precautions should be continued for 24 hours after the start of effective antibiotic therapy until another organism is confirmed.
  c. Antibiotic prophylaxis for close contacts is indicated for H. influenzae and N. meningitidis (i.e., meningococcal).
  d. Vaccination
    1) Vaccination for H. influenzae is now incorporated into the routine immunization schedule for children.
    2) Vaccination for four serogroups of meningococcus (i.e., quadrivalent meningococcal vaccine) is recommended for high-risk populations, including military recruits, persons traveling to an area with high risk of meningococcal disease, college students living in dormitories, and patients postsplenectomy

3) Pneumococcal vaccine is thought to be about 50% effective in preventing pneumococcal meningitis.
9. Monitor for complications.
   a. Seizures: prophylactic anticonvulsant may be prescribed.
   b. Disseminated intravascular coagulation (DIC)
   c. Fluid and electrolyte imbalance: DI, SIADH, CSW (see Craniotomy section)
   d. Brain edema and intracranial hypertension
   e. Subdural effusions
   f. Hydrocephalus
   g. CN deficits
   h. Waterhouse-Friderichsen syndrome
      1) A major complication of meningococcal meningitis
      2) Overwhelming bacteremia with massive bilateral adrenal hemorrhage
      3) Causes acute adrenal crisis and potentially death
   i. Residual neurologic deficits (e.g., motor or cognitive deficits, memory loss, hearing or vision loss, seizure disorder)

Neuromuscular Disorders

Muscular Dystrophy
1. Definition: group of familial disorders that cause degeneration of skeletal muscle fibers; associated with progressive, symmetrical weakness and wasting of skeletal muscle groups
2. Etiology: genetic
3. Pathophysiology
   a. Degeneration of skeletal muscle fibers
   b. Replacement of muscle tissue with connective tissue and fat
   c. Number of muscle fibers is decreased and the remaining fibers are inflamed and may exhibit necrosis.
   d. Progressive weakness and muscle atrophy
4. Clinical presentation
   a. Subjective
      1) History of frequent falls
      2) Weakness
   b. Objective
      1) Muscle weakness and atrophy
      2) Lack of gross motor control
      3) Kyphoscoliosis is common
      4) Respiratory muscle weakness with tachypnea and decreased tidal volume
      5) Cardiac anomalies are common.
      6) Moderate developmental disability
      7) Smooth muscle dysfunction with megacolon, volvulus, and malabsorption syndromes
   c. Diagnostic studies: CK increased to approximately 10× normal

Multiple Sclerosis
1. Definition: a progressive demyelinating disorder of the white matter of the brain and spinal cord; the optic and oculomotor CNs and the spinal nerve tracts are most often affected; the peripheral nervous system is not affected
2. Etiology: genetic predisposition with environmental (e.g., viral) insult
3. Pathophysiology
   a. Possible precipitators include stress, fatigue, pregnancy, or respiratory tract infection
   b. Immune response results in recurrent inflammatory reaction leading to peripheral vasculitis
   c. Breakdown of BBB with migration of B lymphocytes into the CNS
   d. B lymphocytes secrete immunoglobulin G antibodies
   e. Macrophages remove degenerating myelin causing scattered demyelination of the white matter of the brain and spinal cord
   f. Proliferation of neuroglial tissue (i.e., gliosis) in the white matter of the CNS
   g. This proliferation causes hard yellow plaques of scar tissue, which damages the axon fiber.
   h. Nerve transmission is disrupted.
   i. Remission results from health of demyelinated areas but symptoms become irreversible as the disease progresses.
4. Clinical presentation
   a. Clinical course
      1) Exacerbations and remissions
      2) May progress rapidly causing death or disability, but most patients live productive lives with prolonged remissions
   b. Subjective
      1) Fatigue
      2) Sensory impairment (e.g., burning, pins and needles)
      3) Blurred vision, diplopia
      4) Urinary urgency
      5) Dysphagia
   c. Objectives
      1) Nystagmus
      2) Poor articulation
      3) Weakness
      4) Paralysis ranging from monoplegia to quadriplegia
      5) Spasticity and hyperreflexia
      6) Intentional tremor
      7) Ataxia
      8) Incontinence
   d. Diagnostic studies
      1) MRI: detects lesions and used to evaluate progression; most sensitive diagnostic test for multiple sclerosis
      2) CT: lesions within the brain's white matter
      3) CSF: elevated immunoglobulin G levels, normal WBC count, and normal protein levels
      4) EEG: frequently abnormal
      5) Evoked potential studies and somatosensory evoked potentials (SSEP): slowed conduction
   e. Specific syndromes
      1) Corticospinal syndrome: symmetrical muscle weakness, spastic paralysis, and bowel and bladder incontinence
      2) Brainstem syndrome: dysfunction of CNs III through XII with nystagmus, dysarthria, facial nerve weakness, and paresthesia
      3) Cerebellar syndrome: spastic gait, ataxia, intentional tremor, hypotonia
      4) Cerebral syndrome: optic neuritis, impaired vision, intellectual deterioration

Amyotrophic Lateral Sclerosis
1. Definition: chronic progressively debilitating disease that causes degeneration of the upper and LMNs and muscular atrophy
2. Etiology: unknown but the following may be factors:
    a. Genetic
    b. Virus
    c. Nutritional deficiency
    d. Metabolic interference
    e. Autoimmune process
3. Pathophysiology
    a. Glutamine may be a factor; accumulates to toxic levels at the synapses
    b. Reduction of the number of motor neurons in cortex, brainstem, and spinal cord and degeneration of remaining motor neurons
    c. Progressive degeneration of axons with loss of myelin
    d. Nonfunctional scar tissue replaces normal neuronal tissue in the corticospinal tract in lateral column of spinal cord.
4. Clinical presentation
    a. Subjective
        1) Generalized muscle weakness
        2) Dyspnea if brainstem involved
    b. Objectives
        1) Muscle atrophy, fasciculations, weakness
        2) Paralysis, especially forearms and hands
        3) Impaired speech, chewing, and swallowing with drooling and choking
    c. Diagnostic studies: primarily history and physical examination
        1) Electromyography (EMG): LMN denervation
        2) Muscle biopsy: lower motor degeneration

Guillain Barré Syndrome
1. Definition: acquired acute inflammatory demyelinating axonal polyneuropathy affecting motor more than sensory nerves; also referred to as acute inflammatory demyelinating polyradiculopathy or acute demyelinating polyneuropathy
2. Etiology: autoimmune disease triggered by a preceding bacterial or viral illness; associated infection usually *Campylobacter jejuni*
    a. Predisposing factors include the following:
        1) Surgery
        2) Vaccination
        3) Viral illness
        4) Rabies
        5) Hodgkin disease or other malignancy
        6) Lupus erythematosus
3. Pathophysiology
    a. Macrophages and lymphocytes destroy the myelin sheath of peripheral nerves
    b. Inflammation and swelling of axons
    c. Segmental demyelination of the peripheral nerves, both posterior (sensory) and anterior (motor) nerve roots
    d. Distance between nodes of Ranvier lengthens which impairs saltatory conduction along nerve roots
    e. Remyelination gradually transpires
    f. Autonomic nerve transmission may also be impaired
    g. Clinical course usually three phases
        1) Acute phase: from onset of symptoms to when no further deterioration develops; usually from 1 to 3 weeks
        2) Plateau phase: no change in symptoms; usually lasts up to 2 weeks
        3) Recovery phase: symptoms improve as remyelination occurs; usually lasts from months to years
4. Clinical presentation
    a. Subjective
        1) History of diarrhea or upper respiratory infection a few days or weeks before development of neurologic symptoms
        2) Numbness, pain, paresthesia, or paresis of the limbs
            a) Position and vibratory sensations are more affected than superficial sensation
            b) Paresthesias usually involving hands and feet
        3) Weakness and fatigue
    b. Objective
        1) Bilateral progressive paralysis beginning in legs and then progressing to arms, trunk, and face
            a) Loss of deep tendon reflexes
            b) Facial weakness caused by involvement of CN VII
            c) Bulbar (i.e., speech and swallowing) muscles may be involved, resulting in difficulty chewing, swallowing, dysarthria, and cough if bulbar weakness
            d) Usually plateaus or improves by fourth week
        2) Respiratory muscle weakness may cause tachypnea, decreased tidal volume, impaired cough, and acute respiratory failure
        3) Autonomic dysfunction may occur, manifested by tachycardia or bradycardia, hypotension or hypertension, ileus, urinary retention, and loss of or significant increase in perspiration
    c. Diagnostic studies
        1) CSF: high protein without cellular abnormality
        2) EMG and nerve conduction velocity studies show impairment of nerve transmission
        3) If acute respiratory failure: ABGs show decreased PaO_2, increased $PaCO_2$, decreased pH

Myasthenia Gravis
1. Definition: disorder of voluntary muscles caused by a defect in nerve impulse transmission at the neuromuscular junction
2. Etiology: acetylcholine receptor antibodies at the neuromuscular junction
    a. Genetic susceptibility
    b. Immunologic
    c. Lymphoid hyperplasia or tumor of thymus
3. Pathophysiology
4. Clinical presentation
    a. Clinical course: exacerbations and remissions
        1) Symptoms are milder on awakening and worsen as the day progresses.
        2) Short rest periods temporarily restore muscle function.

3) Symptoms may be more severe during menses, emotional stress, infection, and exposure to sunlight or cold.
   b. Subjective
      1) May have history of other autoimmune diseases such as systemic lupus erythematosus, rheumatoid arthritis, polymyositis, or Graves disease
      2) May have history of recurrent respiratory infection
      3) Exertional fatigue and weakness: worsens with activity and improves with rest
         a) Muscles of eyes, face, mouth, throat, and neck usually affected first: may complain of diplopia, choking, aspiration
   c. Objective
      1) Ptosis
      2) Impaired EOM
      3) Facial droop, expressionless face
      4) Extreme muscle weakness
      5) Difficulty chewing and swallowing
      6) Drooping jaw
      7) Bobbing head
      8) Weight loss related to nutritional impairment
      9) Nasal, low-volume but high-pitched monotonous speech pattern
      10) May have difficulty maintaining head in erect position
      11) If acute respiratory failure: ABGs show decreased PaO_2 and SaO_2, increased $PaCO_2$, decreased pH
   d. Diagnostic studies
      1) Edrophonium chloride test: strength increases significantly with administration of drug
      2) Repetitive single-fiber EMG: rapid fatigue of muscle fibers
      3) Nerve conduction studies: show slowed conduction
      4) Antibodies for acetylcholine receptor (AChR) and muscle-specific kinase (MuSK): positive
      5) CT and MRI of mediastinum to detect presence of thymoma

Collaborative Management of Neuromuscular Disorders

1. Maintain airway, ventilation, and oxygenation.
   a. Use oropharyngeal or nasopharyngeal airway as needed to hold tongue away from hypopharynx in obtunded patient.
   b. Assist with endotracheal intubation as needed in patients without airway protective reflexes; sedation is recommended before intubation.
   c. Encourage deep breathing.
   d. Administer oxygen as needed to maintain SpO_2 greater than or equal to 95% unless contraindicated.
   e. Initiate mechanical ventilation as needed for hypoventilation.
   f. Prevent aspiration.
      1) Position with HOB elevated 30 degrees.
      2) Assess swallow competency; have suction equipment available.
2. Promote comfort and treat pain.
   a. Gabapentin or amitriptyline is frequently used for neuropathic pain.
   b. Reposition frequently.
3. Maintain adequate hydration and electrolyte balance.
   a. Administer isotonic fluids as prescribed.
   b. Monitor closely for indications of overhydration or dehydration; evaluate urine output and urine specific gravity hourly.
4. Maintain nutritional status.
   a. Enteral nutritional support may be required if dysphagia precludes oral feeding.
5. Prevent injury.
   a. Perform passive ROM and reposition the patient every 2 hours.
   b. Obtain physical therapy consult.
   c. Perform frequent skin assessment.
   d. Instill artificial tears every 2 hours to prevent corneal abrasions in patients who do not blink; a moisture chamber may be created using plastic wrap.
   e. Orient to time and place often; encourage family participation in reality orientation.
6. Administer pharmacologic agents and therapies specific to diagnosis.
   a. Specific to muscular dystrophy: none
   b. Specific to multiple sclerosis
      1) Corticosteroids and adrenocorticotropin hormone (ACTH)
      2) Interferon and/or glatiramer, an immunomodulator
      3) Baclofen and tizanidine: muscle relaxants
      4) Monitor for the following complications
         a) Injuries from falls
         b) Constipation
         c) Urinary tract infection
         d) Pneumonia
   c. Specific to ALS
      1) Riluzole, an antiglutamate
      2) Dantrolene and baclofen: muscle relaxants
      3) Thyrotropin-releasing hormone
   d. Specific to Guillain-Barré syndrome
      1) Atropine for bradycardia or beta-blocker for tachycardia
      2) IV immune globulin
      3) Corticosteroids
      4) Plasmapheresis early: usually three to five plasma exchanges
      5) Anticoagulant (e.g., subcutaneous LMWH) for DVT prophylaxis
      6) Monitor for the following complications.
         a) Autonomic dysfunction
         b) SIADH
   e. Specific to myasthenic gravis
      1) Anticholinesterase drugs such as pyridostigmine
      2) Corticosteroids
      3) Immunosuppressants
      4) Azathioprine
      5) Cyclosporine
      6) Plasmapheresis
      7) Thymectomy

8) Monitor for the following complications, which may cause respiratory arrest:
    a) Myasthenic crisis: severe muscle weakness causes quadriparesis or quadriplegia, dyspnea, decreased tidal volume and vital capacity, pronounced dysphagia; occurs 3 to 4 hours after medication
    b) Cholinergic crisis: severe muscle weakness as in myasthenic crisis that occurs 30 to 60 minutes after anticholinesterase medication (especially if dose increase); other symptoms include diarrhea, cramping, fasciculation, bradycardia, pupillary constriction, increased salivation, increased perspiration

Learning Activities

CHAPTER 5

1. Complete the following crossword puzzle related to neurologic anatomy, physiology, and assessment.

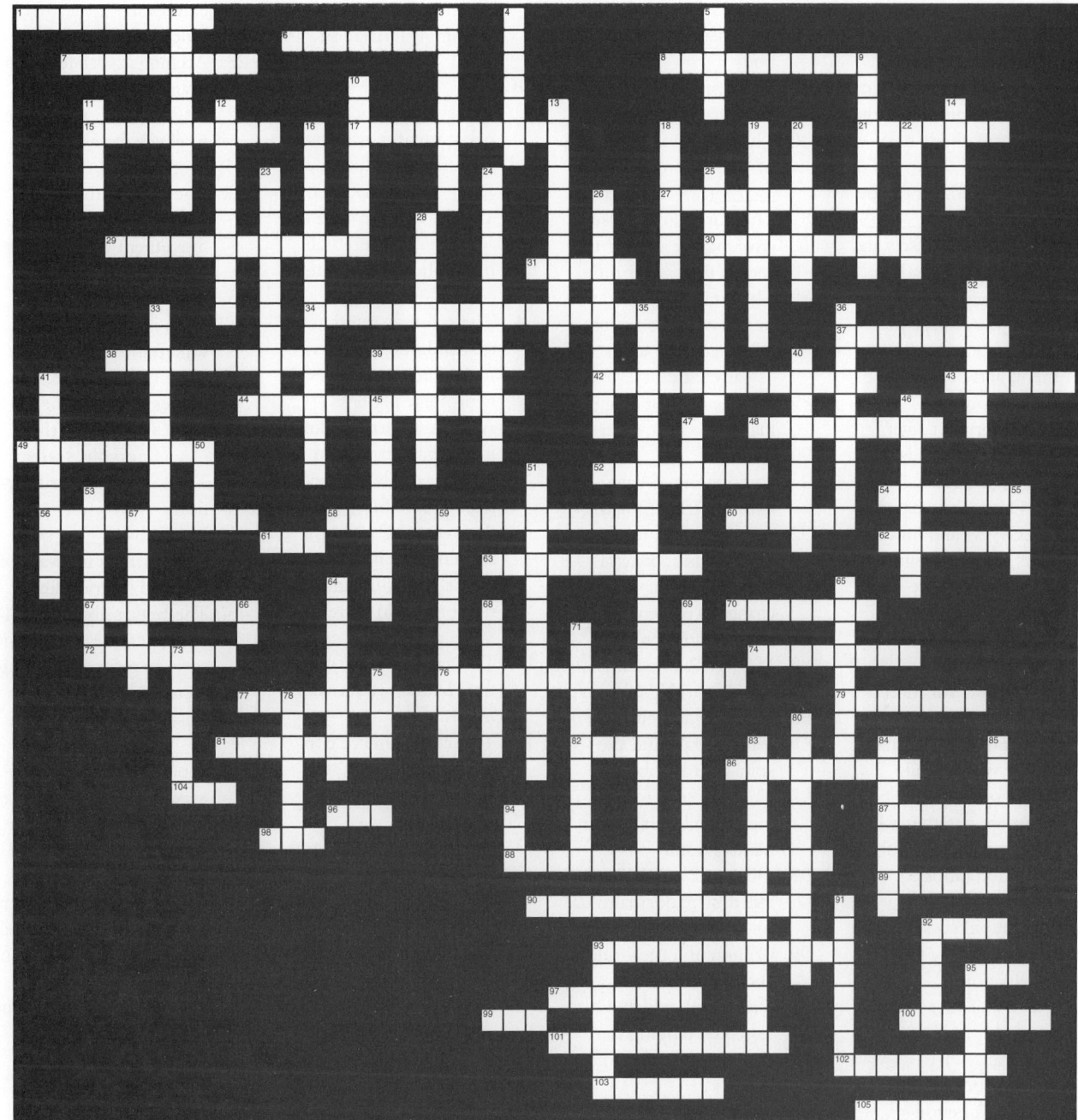

ACROSS

1. This lobe controls vision
6. During this refractory period, the nerve cannot be stimulated again
7. This type of aphasia is also referred to as sensory
8. CSF leak from the nose
15. This type of cell helps form the blood–brain barrier
17. A lack of inflection while talking
21. Unidirectional conduction of an impulse from one neuron to the next
27. A loss of sensation
29. This area of the diencephalon is responsible for temperature regulation
30. This type of aphasia is also referred to as motor
31. _____ test is conducted by placing tuning fork at midline vertex of skull
34. A chemical that acts as a bridge for transmission of impulses
37. These nerve cells line the ventricles of the brain and aid in secretion of CSF

457

38. Another term for *sympathetic*
39. The posterior portion of these lobes controls voluntary motor function
42. This spinal tract carries pain, temperature, light touch, pressure, and pain
43. These cells are responsible for the transmission of nerve impulses
44. This is the predominant neurotransmitter for the parasympathetic nervous system
48. The middle layer of the meninges is the _____ mater; blood vessels and cerebrospinal fluid are located here
49. These nerve cells provide support, nourishment, and protection of the neurons
52. The innermost layer of the meninges is the _____ (2 words)
54. This nerve originates at C3, C4, C5 and innervates the diaphragm
56. The cranial nerve that controls sensation on the face
58. These neurons are responsible for myelin formation in the CNS
60. The cranial nerve that allows you to smile
61. The most important assessment parameter in a patient with a neurologic condition (abbrev)
62. The nodes of _____ allow rapid conduction of impulses by saltatory conduction
63. The cranial nerve that controls pupillary constriction
67. These lobes control sensory function
70. Four paired masses of gray matter in the deeper layers of each hemisphere are called the basal _____
72. The inability to recognize objects through the special senses
74. CSF leak from the ears
76. The vascular structure which is invaluable for collateral circulation (3 words)
77. Loss of half of the visual field
79. The brain must have a continuous supply of oxygen and _____
81. The component of the neuron that conducts impulses toward the cell body
82. The respiratory centers are located in the _____
86. The outermost layer of the meninges is the _____ (2 words)
87. The normal response to stroking the sole of the foot is the _____ reflex
88. This branch of the autonomic nervous system may be described as "steady state"
89. An unsteady or staggering gait
90. Widened _____; component of the Cushing triad (2 words)
92. Another word for *body*
93. The intrinsic ability of cranium's contents to change to prevent increase in intracranial pressure
95. MAP ICP; normally 60 to 100 mm Hg (abbrev)
96. This acts as a cushion for the brain and the spinal cord (abbrev)
97. The type of paralysis seen with lower motor neuron lesion
98. (SBP + [2 × DBP]) divided by 3; normally 70 to 105 mm Hg (abbrev)
99. Contraction of a muscle and a jerk of the affected limb which is tested by tapping the tendon with a hammer (abbrev)
100. The type of paralysis seen with upper motor neuron lesion
101. A primary neurotransmitter for the sympathetic nervous system
102. This bone divides the interior of the skull into three fossae: anterior, middle, and posterior
103. The coating or sheath that speeds transmission along the axon; destroyed in multiple sclerosis
104. A diagnostic study to evaluate the brain's electrical activity (abbrev)
105. The _____ sign is pain in the neck when the leg is extended; indicates meningeal irritation

DOWN

2. The sympathetic and parasympathetic nervous systems constitute the _____ nervous system
3. The fold of the dura that separates the cerebral hemispheres from the cerebellum
4. The scoring system used to standardize observation of responsiveness in neurologic patients
5. A check for arm weakness if to ask the patient to hold her or his arms even and observe for _____
9. A synapse between the axon of one neuron and the cell body of another neuron would be referred to as _____
10. This cranial nerve controls lateral eye movement
11. This cranial nerve controls swallowing
12. Difficulty with articulation
13. This branch of the autonomic nervous system is frequently referred to as "fight or flight"
14. The cranial nerve that controls visual acuity
16. This type of hydrocephalus is most likely to occur from trauma, including surgical trauma
18. The inability to understand or express verbal communication
19. This type of neuron has one axon and more than one dendrite
20. Neurons that transmit impulses to the spinal cord or brain
22. Peripheral pain may be tested with pressure to the _____ (2 words)
23. Another term for *parasympathetic*
24. The opening at the base of the skull where the brain connects to the spinal cord (2 words)
25. This posturing is also referred to as abnormal extension
26. Unpleasant sensation
28. Arching associated with brain stem injury
32. This is a test of balance to check for cerebellar dysfunction
33. The part of the brain that coordinates muscle movement with sensory input
35. This area of the midbrain is responsible for wakefulness (3 words)
36. The cranial nerves, spinal nerves, and peripheral nerves constitute the _____ nervous system
40. The loss of motor function
41. In chronic _____ state the patient is unaware of self and surroundings
45. The brain's ability to tolerate increases in volume without a corresponding increase in pressure
46. C3–C5 innervates the _____
47. A pathologic reflex of grasping whatever is placed in the hand with failure to release on command
50. The component of the neuron that conducts impulses away from the cell body to other neurons or to end organs
51. This band of brain tissue connects the left and right cerebral hemispheres (2 words)
53. Double vision
55. The spinal _____ extends from the brain stem to L2
57. These neurons transmit impulses away from the spinal cord or brain
59. This posturing is also referred to as abnormal flexion
64. Difficulty with swallowing
65. This type of nerve cell is part of the

reticuloendothelial system and are responsible for phagocytosis
66. This test should never be performed if the patient has clinical indications of intracranial hypertension (abbrev)
68. Cerebrospinal fluid is produced in capillary networks called ___ plexuses
69. The enzyme that breaks down acetylcholine
71. An abnormal sensitivity to light
73. May be partial or generalized
75. _____ conduction is greater in the abnormal result of the Rinne test
78. This portion of the brainstem controls cardiac and respiratory centers
80. Slow movement
83. The intrinsic ability of the cerebral blood vessels to dilate or constrict to stable cerebral blood flow
84. This lobe controls long-term memory
85. Racoon eyes and Battle sign are indicative of _____ skull fracture
91. The protective coverings of the brain and spinal cord
92. The skin covering the cranium
93. This portion of the skull has eight bones
94. This pressure is the pressure exerted from the intracranial contents (abbrev)
95. The ____ triad is a late indication of intracranial hypertension

2. Match the area of the brain to the associated function.

___ 1. Anterior frontal lobe	a. Responsible for verbal expression
___ 2. Posterior frontal lobe	b. Regulates cardiac, vasomotor, and respiratory functions
___ 3. Parietal lobe	c. Receives visual stimuli
___ 4. Occipital lobe	d. Maintains equilibrium
___ 5. Temporal lobe	e. Regulates endocrine and autonomic functions
___ 6. Cerebellum	f. Receives auditory stimuli
___ 7. Medulla	g. Receives sensory stimuli
___ 8. Hypothalamus	h. Involved in emotional and sexual response
___ 9. Wernicke area	i. Responsible for language interpretation
___ 10. Thalamus	j. Contains the motor strip which controls voluntary motor functions
___ 11. Limbic system	k. Controls judgment, insight, and reasoning
___ 12. Broca area	l. Relays sensory and motor input to the cerebrum

3. Your patient has had a traumatic brain injury. His blood pressure is 80/50 mm Hg, and his intracranial pressure is 20 mm Hg. Calculate his cerebral perfusion pressure. Should you be concerned? Why? _____
_____

4. Identify the following physiologic alterations as being associated with either sympathetic or parasympathetic.

	Sympathetic	Parasympathetic
Bronchodilation		
Coronary artery dilation		
Hypersalivation		
Increased blood glucose		
Increased perspiration		
Increased intestinal motility		
Pupil constriction		
Tachycardia		

5. Think about the following ventilatory patterns and identify the site of lesion that would cause them.

Pattern	Site of Lesion
CNS hyperventilation	
Cheyne-Stokes respirations	
Cluster (or Biot)	
Ataxic	
Apneustic	

Chapter 5 The Neurologic System

6. Name and identify how to assess the cranial nerves.

Cranial Nerve	Name	Method of Assessment
I		
II		
III		
IV		
V		
VI		
VII		
VIII		
IX		
X		
XI		
XII		

7. List 10 factors that can increase intracranial pressure that can and should be eliminated.

a. _____
b. _____
c. _____
d. _____
e. _____
f. _____
g. _____
h. _____
i. _____
j. _____

8. Identify 6 interventions that can decrease intracranial pressure and identify if they decrease brain mass, CSF, or blood.

Intervention	What Is Decreased?
1.	
2.	
3.	
4.	
5.	
6.	

9. Match the following sign or symptom associated with the neurologic condition.

____	1. Brainstem lesion	a.	Kernig sign
____	2. Chronic subdural hematoma	b.	Fatigue and muscle weakness
____	3. Subarachnoid hemorrhage	c.	Ascending paralysis
____	4. Status epilepticus	d.	Change in LOC, pupillary changes, respiratory pattern changes, Cushing triad
____	5. Dural tear	e.	Periorbital edema
____	6. Postcraniotomy	f.	Increased LP pressure, vomiting
____	7. Upper motor neuron lesion	g.	Rhinorrhea
____	8. Meningeal irritation	h.	Personality change
____	9. Intracranial hypertension	i.	"Worst headache of my life"
____	10. Basal skull fracture	j.	Myoglobinuria
____	11. Guillain-Barré syndrome	k.	Absence of doll eyes (i.e., oculocephalic reflex)
____	12. Myasthenia gravis	l.	Babinski reflex
____	13. Hydrocephalus	m.	Battle sign

10. Your patient has had a hemorrhagic stroke. She has nuchal rigidity and decerebrate posturing. She does not vocalize at all and will not open her eyes even to pain. What is her Glasgow Coma Scale score? What grade severity is this on the Hunt and Hess aneurysm grading scale? _____

11. Identify the following factors as being associated with which complication of subarachnoid hemorrhage: vasospasm or rebleed.

	Vasospasm	Rebleed
Occurs either immediately after the bleed or between 7 and 10 days after the bleed		
Caused by calcium influx into the vessel		
Occurs any time after 3 days		
Treated with calcium channel blockers		
Caused by lysis of the protective clot		
Prevented by early clipping if the patient is stable enough		

12. List 5 ways that the use of fibrinolytics for ischemic stroke is different from fibrinolytics for myocardial infarction.
    a. _____
    b. _____
    c. _____
    d. _____
    e. _____

13. Describe CSF changes in the following conditions.

Bacterial meningitis	
Viral meningitis	
Subarachnoid hemorrhage	

14. List 5 observations to make and 5 interventions to perform during a seizure.

Observations to Make

Interventions

462 Chapter 5 The Neurologic System

15. Match the neuromuscular disorder to the pathophysiology of the disorder.

____ 1. Amyotrophic lateral sclerosis	a. Familial degeneration of skeletal muscle fibers
____ 2. Guillain-Barré syndrome	b. Acute inflammation and demyelination of motor more than sensory nerves
____ 3. Muscular dystrophy	c. Immune-mediated inflammation and destruction of myelin with replacement with glial scar tissue
____ 4. Multiple sclerosis	d. Autoimmune destruction of cholinergic receptors at the neuromuscular junction
____ 5. Myasthenia gravis	e. Degeneration of motor neurons in the brainstem and spinal cord

16. Complete the following crossword puzzle dealing with neurologic conditions and treatment.

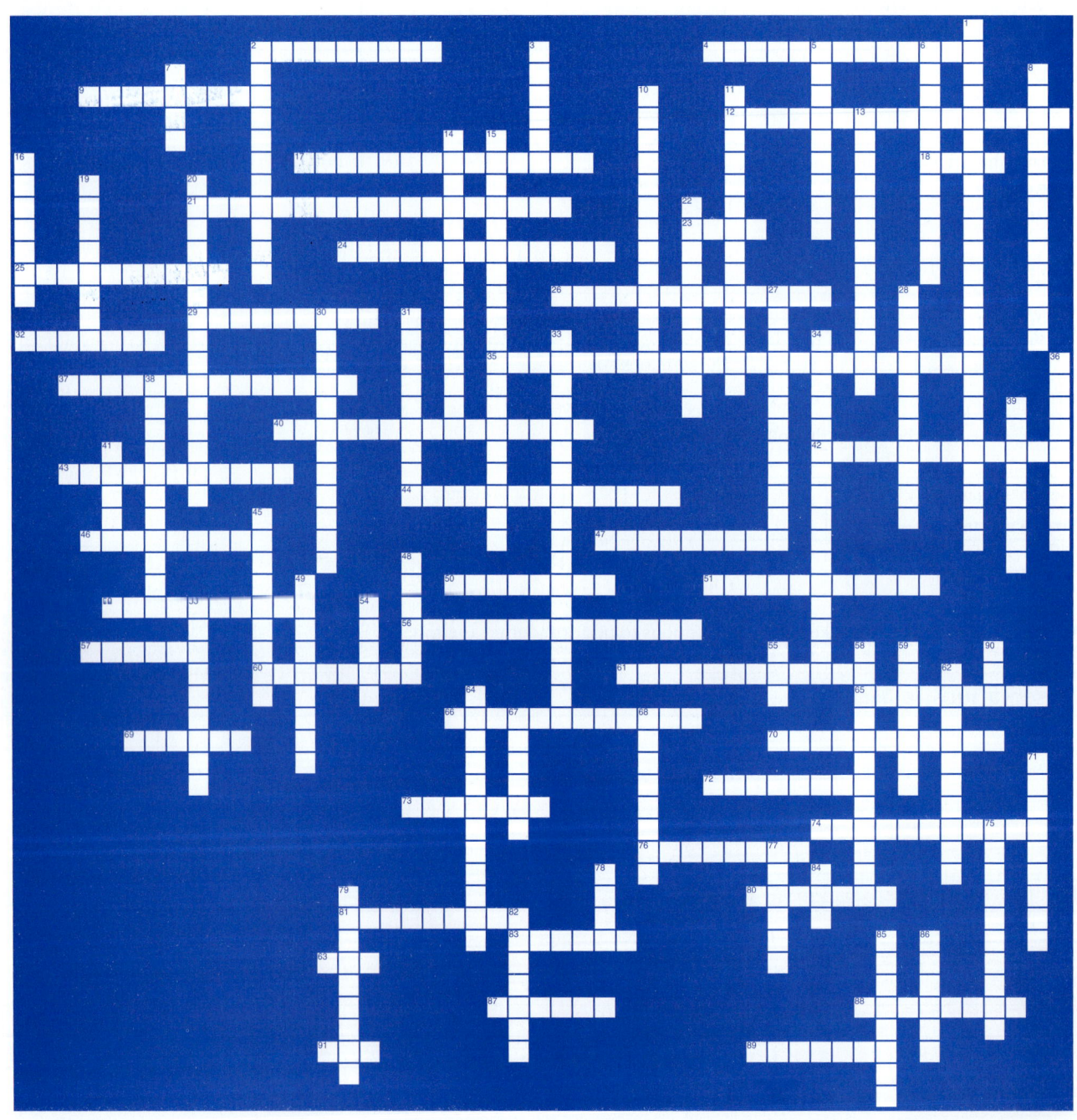

ACROSS

2. Herniation with a downward shift of the brain causing the brainstem to be pushed through the foramen magnum
4. Process that occurs in multiple sclerosis
9. Bruise on the brain
12. This type of hydrocephalus is most likely to occur from trauma, including surgical trauma
17. A treatment used in autoimmune disorders to remove antibodies
18. A subjective sensation that often precedes a seizure
21. Used to reduce central fever (2 words)
23. Early signs of multiple sclerosis primarily affect the _____ (plural)
24. This type of hydrocephalus may be caused by subarachnoid hemorrhage or meningitis
25. A common complication of chronic degenerative neuromuscular conditions
26. Used to reduce peripheral fever
27. Patients with status epilepticus may have _____ and require parenteral dextrose
29. This type of skull fracture may cause cranial nerve defects
32. A complication of cerebral aneurysm which frequently occurs about 7 to 10 days after the bleed
35. The primary risk and cause of death in neuromuscular disorders (3 words)
37. The head of the bed should be elevated after this type of craniotomy
40. This type of craniotomy is often used for removal of the pituitary gland
42. A major risk factor for stroke
43. This hypothesis states that the cranium is an inexpansible vault and if one of the three intracranial volumes goes up, one of the other two volumes must go down or a resultant increase in pressure will occur
44. Monitor patients with status epilepticus for this indication of rhabdomyolysis
46. Excessive _____ at synapses may be a factor in ALS
47. Speech impairment seen in myasthenia gravis
50. The most common type of cerebral aneurysm
51. This type of stroke is caused by aneurysm or arteriovenous malformation
52. Opening of the cranium
56. This type of drug is most likely to be used first to control seizures
57. Drooping of the eyelid; seen in myasthenia gravis
60. Skull fracture affecting this fossa may cause raccoon eyes and otorrhea
61. Repair of the cranium
63. The first sign of tentorial herniation is a change in _____ (abbrev)
65. _____ cerebral artery infarction, which usually does not manifest "typical" stroke symptoms
66. Brain stem lesions may cause this type of eye movement
69. Skull fractures affecting this fossa may cause rhinorrhea and Battle sign
70. This drug is frequently used to prevent or treat vasospasm (generic)
72. The primary symptom of hemorrhage from a cerebral aneurysm is sudden, severe _____
73. Elevation _____ in the CSF occurs in meningitis
74. Prolonged QT interval frequently seen in subarachnoid hemorrhage may cause this serious cardiac complication
76. This type of intracranial hematoma is caused by a venous bleed and causes symptoms that develop over several days
80. This type of partial seizure is associated with loss of consciousness
81. Guillain-Barré syndrome is characterized by _____ paralysis
83. This type of skull fracture of the temporal bone may tear the middle meningeal artery and cause epidural hematoma
87. This electrolyte is affected by diabetes insipidus, SIADH, and cerebral salt wasting syndrome
88. This type of stroke is caused by thrombus or embolism
89. A _____ lobe tumor tends to lead to personality changes
91. Focal cerebral ischemia that resolves within 24 hours (abbrev)

DOWN

1. Common cause of secondary brain injury (2 words)
2. Generalized seizures involve these phases (2 words)
3. This organ may be removed for myasthenia gravis
5. This drug may be used to reduce the increase in ICP associated with suctioning (generic)
6. Uncal herniation causes dilation of the _____ pupil
7. A _____ hole is drilled into the cranium to allow access for aspiration of a clot or to place an intracranial catheter for monitoring ICP
8. Stroke causes _____ paresis or plegia
10. This complication may occur after craniotomy, traumatic brain injury, hemorrhagic stroke, or meningitis
11. The head of the bed should be flat after this type of craniotomy
13. This type of meningitis is highly contagious
14. The enzyme that breaks down acetylcholine
15. This study is frequently used to evaluate patients after subarachnoid hemorrhage for vasospasm (2 words)
16. Tight cervical collar or trach ties may increase ICP by compressing these veins
19. An osmotic diuretic used for increased ICP
20. Cerebrospinal fluid is produced in capillary networks called _____ (2 words)
22. Shifting of the brain within or out of the cranium
28. This type of crisis occurs after an increase in anticholinesterase dose
30. Rupture of a cerebral aneurysm is sometimes referred to as a _____ hemorrhage because the blood vessels are located in this space
31. A complication of cerebral aneurysm that occurs most commonly about 3 to 5 days; treated with calcium channel blockers
33. This dysrhythmia is a common cause of ischemic stroke (2 words)
34. This disease is the result of decreased effect of acetylcholine at the neuromuscular junction (2 words)
36. Care after traumatic brain injury is primarily directed toward preventing this type of injury
38. This type of brain tumor is initially benign but is prone to become malignant
39. This type of hematoma is caused by an arterial bleed and causes rapid deterioration
41. A side-to-side herniation
45. This type of herniation occurs with bilateral processes such as cerebral edema; also called central herniation

48. When these muscles are affected in neuromuscular conditions, speech and swallowing difficulties result
49. This type of cerebral edema is caused by hyponatremia, ischemia, or hypoxia
53. Diabetes _____ is a complication of head trauma or craniotomy that causes polyuria
54. The first sign of uncal herniation is a dilated, sluggish or nonreactive _____
55. This degenerative neuromuscular disease selectively affects motor function (abbrev)
58. This type of encephalopathy is caused by severe elevation of BP
59. The _____ triad of vital sign changes is late signs of intracranial hypertension
62. Inflammation of the meninges
64. Central _____ is associated with injury to the hypothalamus and does not respond to antipyretics such as acetaminophen
67. Acute respiratory failure occurs in myasthenic _____
68. An abnormal weakness of an artery; most commonly occur in the circle of Willis
71. Patients with status epilepticus have elevated CK and _____
75. This type of crisis occurs in a patient with myasthenia gravis especially is infection or trauma
77. This type of encephalopathy is caused most often by out of hospital cardiac arrest
78. State of unconsciousness in which the patient cannot be awakened
79. This type of cerebral edema is caused by breakdown of the blood–brain barrier from trauma, tumor, abscess, hemorrhage
82. The ____ in the CSF is reduced in bacterial meningitis
84. Autoregulation fails if the ___ is less than 50 mm Hg or greater than 150 mm Hg (abbrev)
85. This test is used for myasthenia gravis; muscle weakness decreases when this drug is given
86. This type of rigidity occurs with meningeal irritation from infection or blood
90. A severe injury to the brain that causes prolonged unconsciousness, brainstem dysfunction, and profound residual deficits (abbrev)

The Endocrine System

CHAPTER 6

Selected Concepts in Anatomy and Physiology

Functions
The endocrine system regulates secretion of hormones that alter metabolic body functions, including all of the following:
1. Chemical reactions and transport of chemicals across cell membranes
2. Growth and development
3. Metabolism
4. Fluid and electrolyte balance
5. Acid–base balance
6. Adaptation
7. Reproduction

Components
1. Glands or glandular tissue that synthesize, store, and secrete hormones
    a. An endocrine gland is ductless but highly vascular.
    b. The location of endocrine glands is depicted in Fig. 6.1.
2. Hormones
    a. Definition: complex chemical substances produced in one part or organ of the body that initiate or regulate the activity of an organ or a group of cells in another part of the body
        1) The release of hormones occurs in response to a change in the cellular environment or to maintain regulated levels of certain substances.
            a) Chemical factors: blood glucose and calcium levels
            b) Endocrine factors: a hormone from one endocrine gland controlling another endocrine gland
            c) Neural control: stress causes release of catecholamines from the adrenal medulla
        2) Hormones are released directly into the bloodstream to be distributed throughout the body and to the target gland or target organ to initiate a response.
        3) Receptor cells are located on the target organ. Only organs with specific receptor cells can be affected by that specific hormone.
    b. Types include the following:
        1) Single amino acids (e.g., epinephrine, dopamine, thyroid hormones)
        2) Proteins (e.g., growth hormone, follicle-stimulating hormone)
        3) Steroids (e.g., androgens, aldosterone, cortisol)
    c. Endocrine glands and hormones significant in the care of critically ill patients are summarized in Table 6.1

Process of Hormone Synthesis, Secretion, Effect, and Suppression
Fig. 6.2.

Regulation of Hormones
1. The hypothalamus regulates the secretion of hormones through secretion of releasing factors.
2. The pituitary gland is stimulated by these releasing factors from the hypothalamus to secrete stimulating factors.
3. The target gland is then stimulated to secrete the hormone.
4. The hormone binds with receptors in the target cells.
5. Regulation
    a. Self-regulation based on the concentration of the hormone present in the circulation; may also be influenced by electrolyte levels, metabolites, osmolality, fluid status, and other hormones
    b. Negative feedback: most common
        1) High hormone levels inhibit the release of the releasing factor from the hypothalamus or stimulating factor from the pituitary gland or secretion of the hormone from the gland. (Fig. 6.2).
    c. Positive feedback: less common
        1) A hormone stimulates continued secretion until a specific level is reached.
    d. Neural regulation as a result of stimulation of sympathetic division of autonomic nervous system; when stress is removed, the sympathetic nervous system (SNS) is no longer stimulated, and epinephrine release is reduced

Endocrine Dysfunction
1. Classification
    a. Based on level of hormone activity

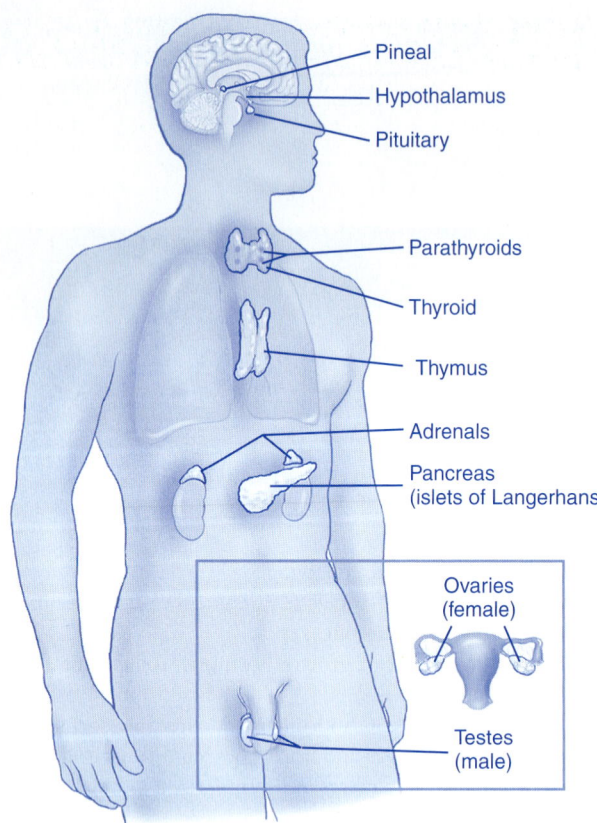

Fig. 6.1 Location of endocrine glands. (From Shiland, B. J. [2010]. *Mastering healthcare terminology* [3rd ed.]. St. Louis: Mosby.)

1) Hyperfunction: increased hormonal activity
2) Hypofunction: decreased hormonal activity
b. Based on location of dysfunctional gland or response
1) Primary disorders: disorder of the target gland (e.g., adrenal or thyroid gland)
2) Secondary disorder: disorder of the stimulating gland (e.g., pituitary)
3) Tertiary disorder: disorder of the hypothalamus
c. Based on acuity
1) Acute: beginning abruptly with marked intensity
2) Chronic: developing slowly and persisting for a long period of time, often for the remainder of the lifetime of the individual
2. Causes of endocrine dysfunction
a. Dysfunction of a particular gland
b. Altered secretion of the stimulating hormones for that gland
c. Altered response to the hormone itself at the target cell

Assessment of the Endocrine System

Interview
1. Chief complaint: Why is the patient seeking help and the duration of the problem? Because hormones affect every body tissue, numerous symptoms may indicate endocrine dysfunction.
   a. General
      1) Easy fatigability, lethargy
      2) Sleep disorders

Table 6.1 Endocrine Glands and Hormones Significant in the Care of Critically Ill Adults

Hormone	Actions	Releasing Factors	Target	Hypersecretion	Hyposecretion
Hypothalamus: Controls the Release of Pituitary Hormones					
Pituitary (Hypophysis)					
Anterior Pituitary (Adenohypophysis)					
Growth hormone (somatotropin)	• Stimulates protein anabolism • Mobilizes fatty acids • Conserves carbohydrates • Stimulates growth of bone, muscle, and cartilage	GHRH from hypothalamus in response to exercise, starvation, decreased amino acid levels, stress, hypoglycemia	All body cells capable of growth, especially muscle, bone, and cartilage cells	Giantism in children; acromegaly in adults	Dwarfism in children; possible decrease in organ weight in adults
Adrenocorticotropic hormone	• Stimulates growth and function of adrenal gland • Controls production and release of glucocorticoid hormones • Stimulates mineralocorticoid production • Stimulates androgen production	CRH from hypothalamus in response to hypoglycemia, decrease in cortisol levels, hypoxia, trauma, surgery, or physical or psychological stress	Cells of adrenal cortex	Cushing disease	Adrenal insufficiency (chronic) or adrenal crisis (acute)

Table 6.1	Endocrine Glands and Hormones Significant in the Care of Critically Ill Adults—cont'd				
Hormone	**Actions**	**Releasing Factors**	**Target**	**Hypersecretion**	**Hyposecretion**
Thyroid stimulating hormone (thyrotropin)	• Increases size and growth of thyroid cells • Increases synthesis of thyroid hormones • Releases stored thyroid hormones	TRH from the hypothalamus in response to cold temperature or a decrease in thyroid hormone levels	Cells of the thyroid gland	Hyperthyroidism	Hypothyroidism
Posterior Pituitary (Neurohypophysis)					
Antidiuretic hormone (vasopressin)	• Increases water reabsorption (inhibits diuresis) by kidney tubules and collecting ducts • Vasoconstriction of arterioles	Increase in serum osmolality; hypernatremia; hypovolemia; hypoxia; hypotension; pain; trauma; stress; nausea; pharmacologic agents	Distal renal tubules and collecting ducts; smooth muscle of arterioles and GI tract	SIADH	Diabetes insipidus
Thyroid Gland					
Triiodothyronine (T_3) and thyroxine (T_4) NOTE: T_3 is more biologically active.	• Stimulates metabolic rate • Increases protein synthesis • Increases carbohydrate and fat metabolism • Increases bone growth • Increases oxygen consumption • Increases metabolism and clearance of drugs	TSH from anterior pituitary; TRH from hypothalamus; cold temperature	Most body cells	Hyperthyroidism (chronic); thyroid storm or crisis (acute)	Hypothyroidism (chronic); myxedema coma (acute)
Thyrocalcitonin (calcitonin)	• Reduces plasma calcium levels by inhibiting bone lysis and decreasing calcium resorption by the kidney	Increase in serum calcium, magnesium, or glucagon	Bone cells, kidney cells	Not significant	Not significant
Parathyroid Gland					
Parathyroid hormone (parathormone)	• Increases serum calcium by accelerating bone breakdown with release of calcium into the blood, increasing calcium reabsorption from intestine, and decreasing kidney tubule reabsorption of calcium • Decreases blood phosphate levels by increasing phosphate loss in urine • Increases reabsorption of magnesium by the renal tubules	Low serum calcium or magnesium or high serum phosphate level; catecholamines; cortisol	Bone cells, cells of GI tract and kidney	Hypercalcemia and hypophosphatemia; osteoporosis and possibly renal calculi; decreased neuromuscular irritability and muscle weakness	Hypocalcemia and hyperphosphatemia; neuromuscular irritability and tetany

Continued

Table 6.1 Endocrine Glands and Hormones Significant in the Care of Critically Ill Adults—cont'd

Hormone	Actions	Releasing Factors	Target	Hypersecretion	Hyposecretion
Adrenal Cortex					
Glucocorticoids (i.e., cortisol)	• Increases blood glucose by stimulating gluconeogenesis and glycogenolysis in the liver • Inhibits glucose utilization by the cell • Inhibits protein anabolism • Promotes fatty acid mobilization • Inhibits inflammatory response	CRH from hypothalamus; ACTH from anterior pituitary	Most body cells	Cushing syndrome	Addison disease (chronic); adrenal crisis (acute)
Mineralocorticoids (i.e., aldosterone)	• Increases sodium and water reabsorption and potassium excretion	ACTH from anterior pituitary (minor effect); primary stimulus is renin-angiotensin system; decrease in serum sodium; increase in serum potassium	Distal and collecting tubules of kidney; sweat glands; salivary glands; intestines	Hyperaldosteronism	Addison disease (chronic); adrenal crisis (acute)
Adrenal Medulla					
Catecholamines (i.e., epinephrine, norepinephrine)	• Dilates pupils • Increases heart rate and contractility • Dilation of blood vessels to heart, brain, and skeletal muscle • Constriction of blood vessels to nonessential organs (i.e., skin, kidney, GI tract) • Bronchodilation • Increases in respiratory rate and depth • Increases in perspiration, peristalsis of esophagus and certain secretions in GI tract • Increases in blood sugar	SNS innervation: insulin; histamine; anxiety; fear; pain; trauma; exercise; temperature extremes; hypoxia; hypotension; hypovolemia; excess thyroid hormone	Most body cells, vascular beds, smooth muscle	Exaggeration or prolongation of normal effects; may be caused by adrenal medulla tumor called *pheochromocytoma*	May have decrease in stress response or no noticeable effect
Pancreas					
Glucagon (from alpha cells)	• Stimulates glycogenolysis and gluconeogenesis to increase blood glucose • Inhibits glycolysis • Increases lipolysis	Decrease in blood glucose; elevated blood amino acid; catecholamines; exercise; starvation	Most body cells, especially liver cells	Hyperglycemia	Hypoglycemia

Table 6.1	Endocrine Glands and Hormones Significant in the Care of Critically Ill Adults—cont'd				
Hormone	**Actions**	**Releasing Factors**	**Target**	**Hypersecretion**	**Hyposecretion**
Insulin (from beta cells)	• Enables glucose to move into the cell • Aids in muscle and tissue oxidation of glucose • Enhances storage of glycogen • Increases protein synthesis • Inhibits lipolysis	Increase in blood glucose; gastrin; increase in growth hormone; ACTH; glucagon	Most body cells, especially liver cells	Hypoglycemia	Hyperglycemia (diabetes mellitus)

ACTH, Adrenocorticotropin hormone; *CRH*, corticotropin-releasing hormone; *GHRH*, growth hormone-releasing hormone; *GI*, gastrointestinal; *SIADH*, syndrome of inappropriate antidiuretic hormone; *SNS*, sympathetic nervous system; *TRH*, thyrotropin-releasing hormone; *TSH*, thyroid-stimulating hormone

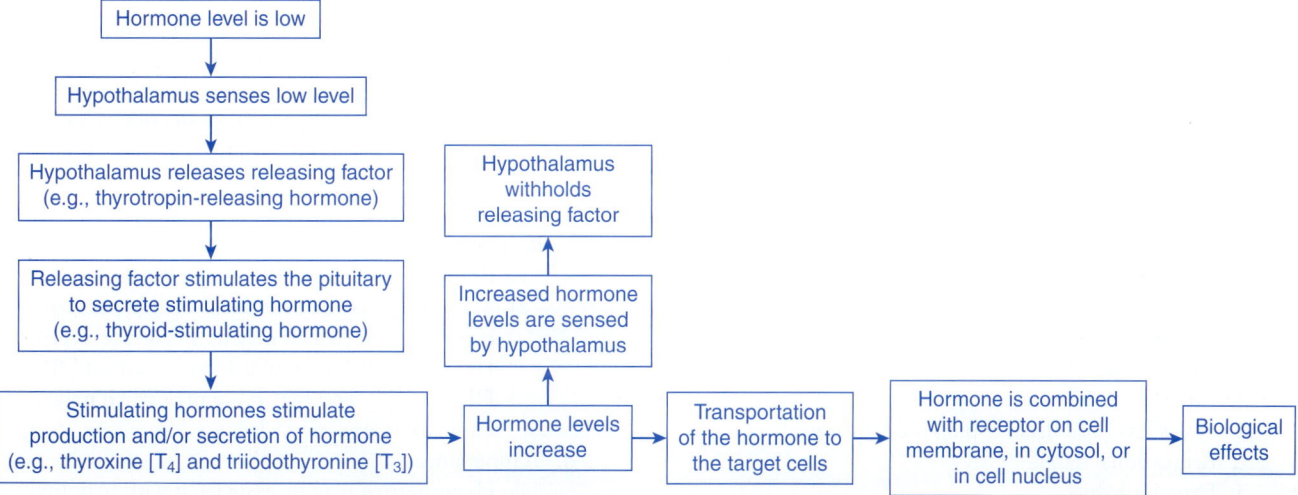

Fig. 6.2 Process of hormone secretion, effect, and suppression.

    3) Cold or heat intolerance
    4) Weight loss or gain, or rapid fluctuations in weight
    5) Increase in size of head, hands, or feet
  b. Dermatologic
    1) Pruritus
    2) Hair loss
    3) Changes in hair distribution
    4) Changes in quality of hair
    5) Changes in skin color or pigmentation
    6) Striae
    7) Changes in skin moisture
  c. Eyes: visual changes
  d. Neck
    1) Jugular neck vein distention
    2) Enlargement or nodules
  e. Cardiovascular
    1) Palpitations
    2) Syncope
  f. Pulmonary: dyspnea
  g. Neurologic
    1) Voice changes
    2) Tremors
    3) Nervousness
    4) Visual changes
    5) Loss of the sense of smell
    6) Headache
    7) Sensory changes
    8) Memory loss
    9) Personality changes
    10) Confusion, agitation
    11) Delusions, paranoia, depression
    12) Muscle twitching
    13) Seizures
  h. Gastrointestinal (GI)
    1) Change in appetite
    2) Nausea, vomiting
    3) Abdominal pain
    4) Constipation or diarrhea
    5) Incontinence
    6) Polyphagia
    7) Polydipsia
  i. Genitourinary
    1) Polyuria, oliguria, nocturia
    2) Incontinence
    3) Decreased libido
    4) Menstrual irregularities
  j. Musculoskeletal
    1) Muscle or joint pain or aching
    2) Muscle weakness

3) Muscle cramping
4) Muscle wasting
5) Twitching
6) Fractures
2. History of present illness: use PQRST format (provocation, palliation, quality, quantity, region, radiation, severity, timing).
3. Past medical history: past illnesses or pathologic conditions that may result in endocrine dysfunction
   a. Trauma
   b. Ischemia or infarction
   c. Neoplasm
   d. Inflammation, infection
   e. Autoimmune conditions
   f. Acquired immunodeficiency syndrome (AIDS)
   g. Irradiation, antineoplastic drugs
   h. Surgical removal of an endocrine gland
   i. Interruption of prescribed pharmaceutical agent for treatment of a preexisting chronic endocrine dysfunction
4. Family history
   a. Diabetes mellitus (DM)
   b. Cardiovascular disease
   c. Cerebrovascular disease
   d. Cancer
5. Social history
   a. Relationship with spouse or significant other; family structure
   b. Occupation
   c. Educational level
   d. Stress level and usual coping mechanisms
   e. Recreational habits
   f. Exercise habits
   g. Dietary habits
      1) Usual diet
      2) Compliance with prescribed limitations
   h. Fluid intake
   i. Caffeine intake
   j. Tobacco use: recorded as pack-years (number of packs per day times the number of years the patient has been smoking)
   k. Alcohol use: recorded as alcoholic beverages consumed per month, week, or day
   l. Toxin exposure
   m. Travel
6. Medication history
   a. Prescribed drug, dose, frequency, and time of last dose
   b. Nonprescribed drugs
      1) Over-the-counter drugs, supplements, and herbs
      2) Substance abuse
   c. Patient understanding of drug actions, side effects, and sick day management
   d. Pharmacologic agents used to treat chronic endocrine dysfunction
      1) Hormone replacement
      2) Hormone suppressive agents
      3) Agents that trigger release of hormone or potentiate the effect of the hormone
      4) Vitamins or minerals necessary for body synthesis of hormones
   e. Evaluation of patient's compliance with prescribed therapy
   f. Pharmacologic agents that may alter endocrine function by either stimulating or inhibiting hormone release or interfering with hormone action at the target tissue; pharmacologic agents that may cause endocrine dysfunction are listed under Etiology for each endocrine condition

Inspection and Palpation
1. Vital signs
   a. Blood pressure (BP): postural drop in BP (tilt positive): decrease of 15 mm Hg in systolic pressure when patient sits or stands caused by hypovolemia may be seen in diabetes insipidus (DI) or DM.
   b. Heart rate
      1) Bradycardia is frequently seen in hypothyroidism.
      2) Tachycardia may be associated with hyperthyroidism, infection (which may be a cause of diabetic ketoacidosis [DKA] or hyperglycemic hyperosmolar state [HHS]), hypovolemia (which may occur in DKA, HHS, or DI), and hypervolemia (which may occur in the syndrome of inappropriate antidiuretic hormone [SIADH]).
   c. Respiratory rate
      1) Bradypnea is frequently seen in hypothyroidism.
      2) Tachypnea may be associated with hyperthyroidism, infection (which may be a cause of DKA or HHS), hypovolemia (which may occur in DKA, HHS, or DI), and hypervolemia (which may occur in SIADH).
   d. Temperature
      1) Hypothermia may be associated with hypothyroidism.
      2) Hyperthermia may be associated with hyperthyroidism, with extreme hyperthermia during thyroid crisis.
      3) Hyperthermia may also indicate infection that may be a cause of DKA or HHS.
   e. Height and weight
      1) Weight increase may be associated with hypothyroidism or Cushing syndrome.
      2) Weight decrease may be associated with hyperthyroidism.
2. General survey
   a. Apparent health status
   b. Apparent age (consistency with chronologic age)
   c. Gross deformity or asymmetry
   d. Nutritional status
   e. Stature and posture
   f. Redistribution of body fat (e.g., Cushing syndrome [hyperadrenocortical function] causes redistribution of fat with "buffalo hump," "moon face," and thick trunk with thin arms and legs)
   g. Gynecomastia in men: may be related to hypogonadism, hyperthyroidism, or Cushing syndrome
   h. Mobility
   i. Level of consciousness: changes seen in cerebral function may occur.
   j. Presence of MedicAlert bracelet indicating chronic endocrine condition or steroid dependency

3. Head and neck
   a. Eyes
      1) Eyeballs
         a) Protruding eyeballs (exophthalmos): frequently seen in hyperthyroidism; eyelid lag frequently seen in patients with exophthalmos
         b) Sunken: may be seen in hypothyroidism or dehydration
      2) Strabismus: may be seen with hyperthyroidism
   b. Facial or periorbital edema: frequently seen in Cushing syndrome; may also be seen in hypothyroidism
   c. Changes in visual acuity and visual fields: may be related to pituitary tumor
   d. Facial bone structure: facial changes, including protruding forehead and prominent jaw, seen in acromegaly
   e. Thyroid gland (the only endocrine gland that can be palpated)
      1) Enlargement or palpable mass or nodule
      2) Tenderness
      3) Presence of thrill
4. Skin and appendages
   a. Skin color changes
      1) Addison disease causes characteristic "bronzing" of the skin.
      2) Gray-brown pigmentation around neck and axillae may be seen in Cushing syndrome.
      3) Yellowish skin discoloration may be seen in hypothyroidism.
   b. Skin temperature: changes frequently seen in thyroid conditions
   c. Skin moisture and turgor
      1) Warm, moist, paper-thin skin may be seen in hyperthyroidism.
      2) Dry, scaly skin may be seen in hypothyroidism.
      3) Decreased skin turgor may be seen in dehydration, which may be seen in DI, DKA, and HHS.
   d. Skin lesions: acne; spider angiomas
   e. Mucous membranes: note moisture.
   f. Scars (especially in neck area, which may indicate prior thyroid surgery)
   g. Bruising: increased bruising may be seen in Cushing syndrome.
   h. Striae: purplish striae on abdomen may be seen in Cushing syndrome.
   i. Hair changes
      1) Alopecia: may be seen in hyperthyroidism, hypothyroidism, and hypopituitarism
      2) Coarse hair: frequently seen in hypothyroidism
      3) Thin, silky hair: frequently seen in hyperthyroidism
      4) Increased body or facial hair: may be seen in acromegaly or Cushing disease.
   j. Brittle nails: frequently seen in hypothyroidism
   k. Enlargement and protrusion of tongue: may be seen in hypothyroidism or acromegaly
5. Cardiovascular
   a. Point of maximal impulse (PMI) displacement: may indicate cardiomegaly, which may be seen in hypothyroidism
   b. Heave: may be associated with heart failure, which may be seen in hyperthyroidism
   c. Peripheral pulses: increased or decreased quality
6. Pulmonary
   a. Odor of breath: acetone (fruity) breath noted in DKA
   b. Respiratory rate, depth, and rhythm
      1) Kussmaul pattern associated with metabolic acidosis such as DKA
7. Neurologic
   a. Level of consciousness or mental status changes: may be related to intracranial mass (e.g., pituitary tumor), cerebral edema, or dehydration (e.g., antidiuretic hormone [ADH] disorders)
   b. Pupil size, shape, and reactivity: changes may be related to intracranial mass (e.g., pituitary tumor) or cerebral edema.
   c. Motor tone and strength
   d. Sensation
   e. Tremors
8. GI: abdominal mass or organ enlargement
9. Genitourinary: suprarenal mass may indicate adrenal tumor (e.g., pheochromocytoma).

Percussion
1. Neurologic: changes in deep tendon reflexes (increased or decreased) may be related to serum sodium changes seen in DI or SIADH.

Auscultation
1. Head and neck: thyroid gland bruits
2. Cardiovascular: heart sound changes
   a. S_3: indicative of HF, which may be seen in patients with hyperthyroidism
   b. Systolic murmur: frequently heard in high cardiac output (CO) states (e.g., hyperthyroidism)
3. Pulmonary
   a. Crackles noted with fluid overload and pulmonary edema
   b. Stridor noted in hypocalcemia associated with hypoparathyroidism
4. GI: bowel sound changes (hyperactive or hypoactive)

Diagnostic Studies
1. Serum
   a. Sodium: normal 136 to 145 mEq/l
   b. Potassium: normal 3.5 to 5 mEq/l
   c. Chloride: normal 96 to 106 mEq/l
   d. Calcium: normal 8.5 to 10.5 mg/dl
   e. Ionized calcium: normal 4.5 to 5.6 mg/dl
   f. Phosphorus: normal 3 to 4.5 mg/dl
   g. Magnesium: normal 1.5 to 2.2 mEq/l
   h. Glucose: normal 70 to 110 mg/dl
   i. Glycosylated hemoglobin: normal 4% to 7%
   j. Osmolality: normal 280 to 295 mOsm/kg
   k. Blood urea nitrogen (BUN): normal 5 to 20 mg/dl
   l. Creatinine: normal 0.7 to 1.5 mg/dl
   m. Ketones: negative
   n. Thyroid-stimulating hormone (TSH): normal 2 to 10 mU/ml
   o. T_3: normal 0.2 to 0.3 mcg/dl
   p. T_4: normal 6 to 12 mcg/dl

Table 6.2 Forms of Antidiuretic Hormone Replacement

Drug	Route	Comments
Synthetic ADH		
Vasopressin (Pitressin synthetic)	• IV, IM, SC: 5–10 units two to four times/day	• Short duration (2–8 hr)
ADH Analogs		
Desmopressin (DDAVP [1,deamino-8-D-arginine vasopressin], Stimate, Minirin)	• Nasal: 10–60 mcg every 12 hr (one to four sprays when 0.1 mg/ml) • IV, IM, or SC: 2–5 mcg two times/day • Oral: 100–300 mcg two to three times/day	• Relatively long duration (8–24 hr) with few side effects • May cause nasal congestion if given intranasally • Administer IV DDAVP via central vein catheter
Lysine vasopressin (DIAPID)	• Nasal: one to two sprays two to four times/day	• Shorter duration (4–6 hours) than DDAVP

IM, Intramuscular; *IV*, intravenous; *SC*, subcutaneous.

---

q. Antithyroglobulin antibody: normal less than 1:100; used in differential diagnosis of thyroid disease
r. Radioactive iodine uptake test: normal 8% to 35%; increased in hyperthyroidism, iodine deficiency
s. Adrenocorticotropin hormone: normal 15 to 100 pg/ml in AM; less than 50 pg/ml in PM
t. Cortisol: normal 6 to 28 mcg/dl at 8 AM; 2 to 12 mcg/dl at 4 PM
u. ADH: normal 1 to 5 pg/ml
v. Provocation tests: assess the endocrine gland's ability to respond to stimulus
  1) Assess the endocrine gland's reserve capacity
  2) Confirm hypo- or hyperfunction of the endocrine gland
w. Arterial blood gases
  1) pH: normal 7.35 to 7.45
  2) $PaCO_2$: normal 35 to 45 mm Hg
  3) HCO_3: normal 22 to 26 mM
  4) PaO_2: normal 80 to 100 mm Hg
  5) SaO_2: normal 95% to 100%
x. Hematocrit: normal 40% to 52% for men; 35% to 47% for women
y. Hemoglobin: normal 13 to 18 g/dl for men, 12 to 16 g/dl for women
z. White blood cell (WBC) count: normal 3500 to 11,000/mm^3

2. Urine
  a. Glucose: normal negative
  b. Ketones: normal negative
  c. Specific gravity: normal 1.005 to 1.03
  d. Osmolality: normal 50 to 1200 mOsm/kg
  e. 17-hydroxycorticosteroids: normal 4.5 to 10 mg/24 hr for men, 2.5 to 10 mg/24 hr for women
  f. 17-ketosteroids: normal 8 to 15 mg/24 hr for men, 6 to 12 mg/24 hr for women
3. Radiologic studies
  a. Skull series
  b. Chest radiography
  c. Flat plate of abdomen (KUB)
  d. Computed tomography (CT) scan of head or abdomen
  e. Magnetic resonance imaging (MRI) of head or abdomen
  f. Pancreatic scan
  g. Thyroid scan
  h. Thyroid ultrasound
  i. Fine-needle aspiration biopsy of thyroid gland
  j. Adrenal angiography
  k. Brain scan
4. Other studies
  a. Electrocardiography (ECG)
  b. Electroencephalography

Endocrine Pharmacology

Antidiuretic Hormone
1. Actions
  a. Increases water reabsorption in the renal tubule
  b. Reduces portal venous pressure through vasoconstriction
  c. Causes contraction of coronary, splanchnic, GI, pancreatic, skin, and muscular vascular beds
2. Indications
  a. Cardiac arrest (see Chapter 3)
  b. GI hemorrhage (see Chapter 7)
  c. Vasogenic forms of shock (i.e., septic) (see Chapter 11)
  d. DI
3. Forms of ADH for DI (Table 6.2)
4. Side effects to monitor for: hypertension, chest pain, water intoxication, abdominal cramping

Insulin
1. Actions
  a. Facilitates uptake of glucose into cell
  b. Stimulates synthesis of proteins, carbohydrates, lipids, and nucleic acids
  c. Functions mostly in the liver, muscle, and adipose tissue
  d. Stimulates conversion of extra glucose to glycogen
2. Indication: hyperglycemia
3. Insulin preparations (Table 6.3)

Glucagon
1. Action: promotes the breakdown of glycogen, reduces glycogen synthesis, and stimulates biosynthesis of glucose to increase serum glucose level
2. Indication: hypoglycemia, beta-blocker intoxication with severe bradycardia

Table 6.3	Characteristics of Insulin Preparations		
Generic Name	Onset (min)	Peak (hr)	Duration (hr)
Short Duration, Rapid Acting			
Insulin lispro (SC)	15–30	0.5–2.5	3–6.5
Insulin aspart	10–20	1–3	3–5
Insulin glulisine	10–15	1–1.5	3–5
Short Duration, Slower Acting			
Human regular (IV)	Immediate	0.25–0.5	1–2
Human regular (SC)	30–60	1–5	6–10
Human regular (SC)	15–30	0.5–1.5	6.6
Intermediate Duration			
Human NPH (SC)	60–120	6–14	16–24
Insulin detemir	—	6–8	12–24*
Long Duration			
Insulin glargine	70	No discernible peak	24
Insulin degludec (SC)	—	30–90	>24

*Duration is dose dependent: At 0.2 unit/kg, duration is 12 hours, but at 2.5 units/kg, duration is 20 to 24 hours.
Adapted from Lehne, R. (2009). *Pharmacology for nursing care* (7th ed.). St. Louis: Saunders.
IV, Intravenous; *SC*, subcutaneous.

3. Administration: 0.5–1 mg intramuscular (IM), subcutaneous (SC), or intravenous (IV)
4. Comments
    a. IV glucose is preferred in patients with severe hypoglycemia.
    b. Adequate glycogen stores are required; therefore, ineffective if hypoglycemia is caused by starvation
    c. Consciousness is expected within 20 minutes if used in patients who are unconscious because of hypoglycemia; should be followed by oral carbohydrates and protein

Diabetes Insipidus

Definition
Clinical condition characterized by impaired renal conservation of water, resulting in polyuria, low urine specific gravity, dehydration, and hypernatremia; caused either by deficiency of ADH or decreased renal responsiveness to ADH

Etiology
1. Neurogenic (or central) DI: defect in synthesis or release of ADH caused by a defect in the hypothalamus, pituitary stalk, or posterior pituitary
    a. Primary: familiar, congenital, idiopathic
    b. Secondary
        1) Intracranial tumors: especially hypothalamic or pituitary; may be primary or metastatic tumor
        2) Extracranial neoplasm: leukemia; breast cancer
        3) Central nervous system (CNS) trauma: especially basal skull fracture
        4) Craniotomy
            a) Transient: edema postcraniotomy causes obstruction of the stalk between the hypothalamus and posterior pituitary.
            b) Permanent: hypophysectomy requires life-long replacement of ADH.
        5) Intracerebral aneurysm, hemorrhage
        6) CNS infections (e.g., meningitis, encephalitis)
        7) Radiation
        8) Cerebral hypoxia and/or anoxic brain syndrome
        9) Granulomatous diseases (e.g., sarcoidosis, tuberculosis)
        10) Drugs that inhibit the secretion of ADH (Box 6.1)
            a) Ethanol
            b) Phenytoin
            c) Chlorpromazine
            d) Reserpine
2. Nephrogenic DI: defect in renal tubular response to ADH; usually less severe than neurogenic DI
    a. Congenital
    b. Renal disease
        1) Renal insufficiency
        2) Pyelonephritis
        3) Renal transplant
        4) Polycystic kidneys
        5) Metabolic diseases affecting the kidneys
            a) Amyloidosis
            b) Sarcoidosis
            c) Multiple myeloma
    c. Drugs that block the effect of ADH on the renal tubules (Box 6.1)
        1) Lithium
        2) Demeclocycline (Declomycin), a tetracycline derivative
        3) Alpha-adrenergic agents (e.g., norepinephrine)
        4) Caffeine
        5) Amphotericin B
        6) Colchicine
        7) Vinblastine
    d. Result of electrolyte imbalance
        1) Severe hypokalemia
        2) Hypercalcemia

Box 6.1 Drugs Affecting the Action of Antidiuretic Hormone

Drugs that Decrease the Amount or Action of ADH (May Cause DI)
- Alpha-adrenergic agents (e.g., norepinephrine)
- Amphotericin B
- Caffeine
- Chlorpromazine
- Colchicine
- Demeclocycline, a tetracycline derivative
- Ethanol alcohol
- Lithium
- Phenytoin
- Reserpine
- Vinblastine

Drugs that Increase the Amount or Effect of ADH (May Cause SIADH)
- Amiodarone
- Analgesics and narcotics: fentanyl, morphine, acetaminophen, NSAIDs
- Anticonvulsants: carbamazepine
- Barbiturates
- Beta-adrenergic agents (e.g., isoproterenol)
- Ciprofloxacin
- Cytotoxic agents: vincristine; cyclophosphamide
- General anesthetics
- Haloperidol
- Nicotine
- Thiazide diuretics: hydrochlorothiazide
- TCAs: amitriptyline

ADH, Antidiuretic hormone; *DI*, diabetes insipidus; *NSAID*, nonsteroidal antiinflammatory drug; *SIADH*, syndrome of inappropriate antidiuretic hormone; *TCA*, tricyclic antidepressant.

---

  3. Psychogenic DI
     a. Caused by psychiatric disturbances with psychogenic polydipsia
     b. Also referred to as compulsive water drinking
  4. Dipsogenic DI: caused by an abnormality in the CNS thirst mechanism

Pathophysiology (Fig. 6.3)
1. Deficiency of ADH or inadequate renal tubule response to ADH, leading to inadequate antidiuresis
2. Diuresis of large volumes of hypotonic urine
3. Dehydration and hypernatremia
4. Potential shock or neurologic effects
5. Permanent versus temporary
   a. Permanent DI follows hypophysectomy (removal of pituitary gland).
   b. Temporary DI usually resolves within 3 to 5 days but may be up to 8 days.

Clinical Presentation
1. History of precipitating event: usually occurs within 24 hours of precipitating event, but clinical indications may not occur for 1 to 3 days because of utilization of stored ADH.
2. Subjective
   a. Thirst, especially for cold liquids
   b. Fatigue, weakness
3. Objective
   a. Polyuria: 5 to 15 l/24 hr; suspect DI if urine output is greater than 200 ml/hr for 2 consecutive hours
   b. Clinical indications of dehydration and volume depletion
      1) Weight loss
      2) Poor skin turgor
      3) Dry mucous membranes
      4) Sunken eyeballs
      5) Postural hypotension, tachycardia
      6) Decrease in central venous pressure (CVP) <2mm Hg, right atrial pressure (RAP) ,<2 mm Hg, and/or pulmonary artery occlusive pressure (PAOP) <8 mm Hg
   c. Neurologic signs resulting from hyperosmolality and hypernatremia
      1) Restlessness, confusion, irritability
      2) Seizures
      3) Lethargy, coma
4. Diagnostic
   a. Serum
      1) Sodium: elevated, greater than 145 mEq/l (hyperosmolar hypernatremia caused by water loss)
      2) BUN: elevated
      3) Serum osmolality: elevated, greater than 295 mOsm/kg
      4) Hematocrit: elevated
      5) Serum ADH level: decreased (less than 1 pg/ml)
   b. Urine
      1) Specific gravity: decreased; less than 1.005
      2) Osmolality: less than serum osmolality; less than 200 mOsm/kg
   c. Water deprivation test may be performed. (NOTE: Because of the risks of dehydration, this test usually is not performed in critically ill patients.)
      1) Prestudy weight, serum, urine osmolality, and urine specific gravity are measured.
      2) Fluid intake is withheld.
      3) Measurements are repeated hourly until one of the following occurs:
         a) Negative results: urine specific gravity exceeds 1.02; urine osmolality exceeds 800 mOsm/kg.
         b) Positive results: 5% of body weight is lost or urine specific gravity does not increase after 3 consecutive hours
      4) Discontinue if hypotension, tachycardia, or lethargy occurs.
      5) Inability to concentrate urine when fluid deprived suggests DI, and a vasopressin test should be performed
   d. Vasopressin test
      1) Exogenous ADH (usually 5 units of aqueous vasopressin) is administered subcutaneously; urine specimens are collected every 30 minutes for 2 hours and evaluated for quantity and osmolality.
         a) If neurogenic DI: urine output decreases and urine osmolality increases by more than 9%.
         b) If nephrogenic DI: no response to ADH will be seen.

Collaborative Management
1. Detect clinical indications of DI in high-risk patients.
   a. Monitor urine output hourly; measure urine specific gravity if indicated by an increase in urine output.

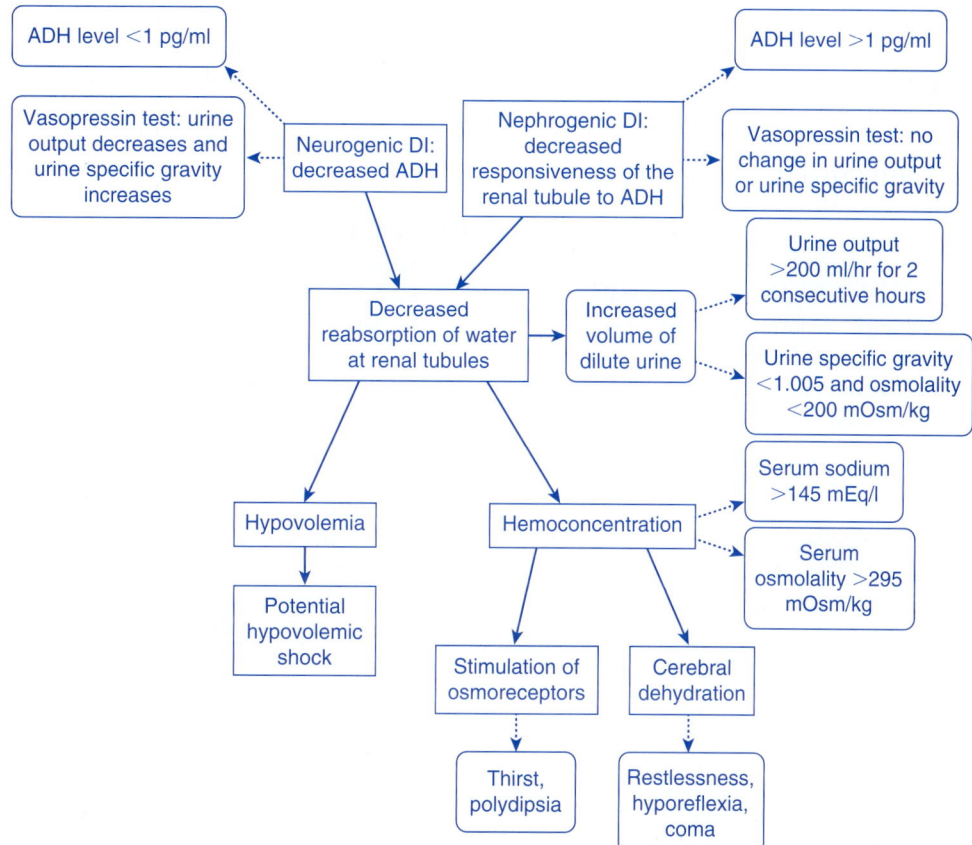

Fig. 6.3 Pathophysiology of diabetes insipidus (DI). *Dotted lines* connect pathology to clinical presentation. *ADH,* Antidiuretic hormone.

b. Monitor weight daily and estimate fluid loss (1 kg = 1 l).
c. Monitor serum sodium levels.
d. Note or calculate serum osmolality.
e. Monitor for clinical indications of hypovolemia and hypoperfusion.
f. Monitor closely for changes in neurologic status.
2. Correct fluid deficit.
   a. Type of volume replacement
      1) Normal saline until intravascular volume is replaced (even if the patient is hypernatremic) to avoid cerebral edema.
      2) Hypotonic solutions, such as 0.45% sodium chloride solution or D_5W to correct free water deficit, depending on degree of hyperosmolality when intravascular volume is restored
   b. Rate of volume replacement
      1) Half of free-water deficit is replaced over the first 24 hours, with the remaining deficit replaced over the next 48 hours.
      2) Hourly rate may initially be determined by volume of urine output and insensible losses (e.g., hourly urine output plus 50 ml/hr).
   c. Close monitoring for electrolyte losses and replace accordingly
3. Treat the cause.
   a. Administer exogenous ADH replacement as prescribed for neurogenic DI (Table 6.2).
   b. Assist in preoperative preparation and postoperative management after hypophysectomy if pituitary tumor is the cause; usually done by transsphenoidal approach
      1) Incision is made in the gingiva above the maxilla, and then the pituitary gland is removed through the sphenoid.
      2) Antibiotic-impregnated nasal packing is usually maintained for 48 to 72 hours.
      3) Cerebrospinal fluid (CSF) leak may be seen during first 72 hours; mustache dressing is used to collect CSF.
      4) Close monitoring of neurologic status, fluid and electrolyte balance, and urine output
   c. Administer ADH potentiator as prescribed for nephrogenic DI (Box 6.1).
      1) Thiazide diuretics (e.g., hydrochlorothiazide) and sodium restriction may be used.
         a) Causes mild sodium depletion that enhances water reabsorption
         b) May be combined with indomethacin or amiloride
   d. Administer pharmacologic agents as prescribed for obsessive-compulsive behavior (e.g., serotonin reuptake inhibitors, tricyclic antidepressants, or monoamine oxidase inhibitors) or psychogenic polydipsia.
4. Correct electrolyte imbalance.
   a. Potassium replacement usually required
   b. Frequent monitoring of serum sodium; serum sodium should be corrected no faster than 0.5 mEq/l per hour to reduce risk of seizure and cerebral edema.
5. Maintain patient safety.
   a. Safe environment: side rails up; call light within reach
   b. Seizure precautions
   c. Frequent reorientation

6. Monitor for complications.
   a. Coma
   b. Hypovolemic shock
   c. Thromboembolism

Syndrome of Inappropriate Antidiuretic Hormone

Definition
1. Clinical condition characterized by impaired renal excretion of water, resulting in oliguria, high urine specific gravity, water intoxication, and hyponatremia
2. Caused either by excess of ADH or an ADH-like substance or an increased renal responsiveness to ADH

Etiology
1. Neurogenic SIADH: increased production and/or release of ADH
   a. Pituitary tumor
   b. CNS trauma
   c. Stroke: thrombotic or hemorrhagic
   d. Intracranial hematoma
   e. CNS infection: encephalitis, meningitis
   f. CNS hemorrhage
   g. Guillain-Barré syndrome
   h. Cerebral infarction or atrophy
   i. Nonmalignant pulmonary disease
      1) Tuberculosis
      2) Pneumonia
      3) Lung abscess
      4) Chronic obstructive pulmonary disease
      5) Positive pressure ventilation
2. Ectopic SIADH: production of a substance indistinguishable from ADH by tissue
   a. Oat-cell (small cell) cancer of the lung
   b. Duodenal cancer
   c. Pancreatic cancer
   d. Prostatic cancer
   e. Leukemia
   f. Lymphoma: Hodgkin and non-Hodgkin
   g. Thymoma
   h. Lymphosarcoma
3. Nephrogenic SIADH: pharmacologic agents that increase ADH secretion or ADH effect (Box 6.1)
   a. General anesthetics
   b. Analgesics and narcotics: morphine, fentanyl, acetaminophen, nonsteroidal antiinflammatory drugs
   c. Barbiturates
   d. Thiazide diuretics: hydrochlorothiazide
   e. Tricyclic antidepressants: amitriptyline
   f. Haloperidol
   g. Amiodarone
   h. Cytotoxic agents: vincristine; cyclophosphamide
   i. Nicotine
   j. Anticonvulsants: carbamazepine
   k. Beta-adrenergic agents (e.g., isoproterenol)

Pathophysiology (Fig. 6.4)
1. Increased secretion of ADH or an ADH-like substance or increased renal responsiveness to ADH
2. Failure of negative feedback system: ADH secretion continues despite low serum osmolality.
3. Renal reabsorption of water increases.
4. Water intoxication
5. Hyponatremia, hypoosmolality
6. Potential cerebral edema and seizures

Clinical Presentation
1. Subjective
   a. Anorexia
   b. Nausea
   c. Dyspnea may be reported if pulmonary edema develops.
   d. Headache
   e. Inability to concentrate
   f. Muscle weakness and/or cramps
2. Objective
   a. Oliguria (less than 0.5 ml/kg/hr)
   b. Signs of fluid overload
      1) Tachypnea
      2) Hypertension
      3) Weight gain without edema
      4) Fever
      5) Jugular venous distention (JVD)
      6) Breath sound changes: crackles
      7) Increased CVP >6 mm Hg, pulmonary artery pressure (PAP) >25/15 mm Hg, PAOP >12 mm Hg
   c. GI
      1) Vomiting
      2) Diarrhea
      3) Diminished bowel sounds
   d. Neurologic
      1) Personality changes
      2) Altered level of consciousness: confusion, lethargy → coma
      3) Decreased deep tendon reflexes
      4) Seizures related to hyponatremia
3. Diagnostic studies
   a. Serum
      1) Sodium: decreased; frequently less than 120 mEq/l (hypoosmolar hyponatremia caused by water retention)
      2) Potassium: may be decreased
      3) Calcium: may be decreased
      4) BUN: decreased
      5) Osmolality: decreased; less than 280 mOsm/l
   b. Urine
      1) Specific gravity: elevated; greater than 1.03
      2) Osmolality: elevated; frequently greater than 1200 mOsm/l
      3) Urine sodium concentration >30 mmol
   c. Water load test: no longer recommended because 2014 *European Journal of Endocrinology* (EJE) guidelines indicate that this test is inaccurate and may be dangerous.

Collaborative Management
1. Detect clinical indications of SIADH in high-risk patients.
   a. Monitor urine output hourly; measure urine specific gravity if indicated by a decrease in urine output.

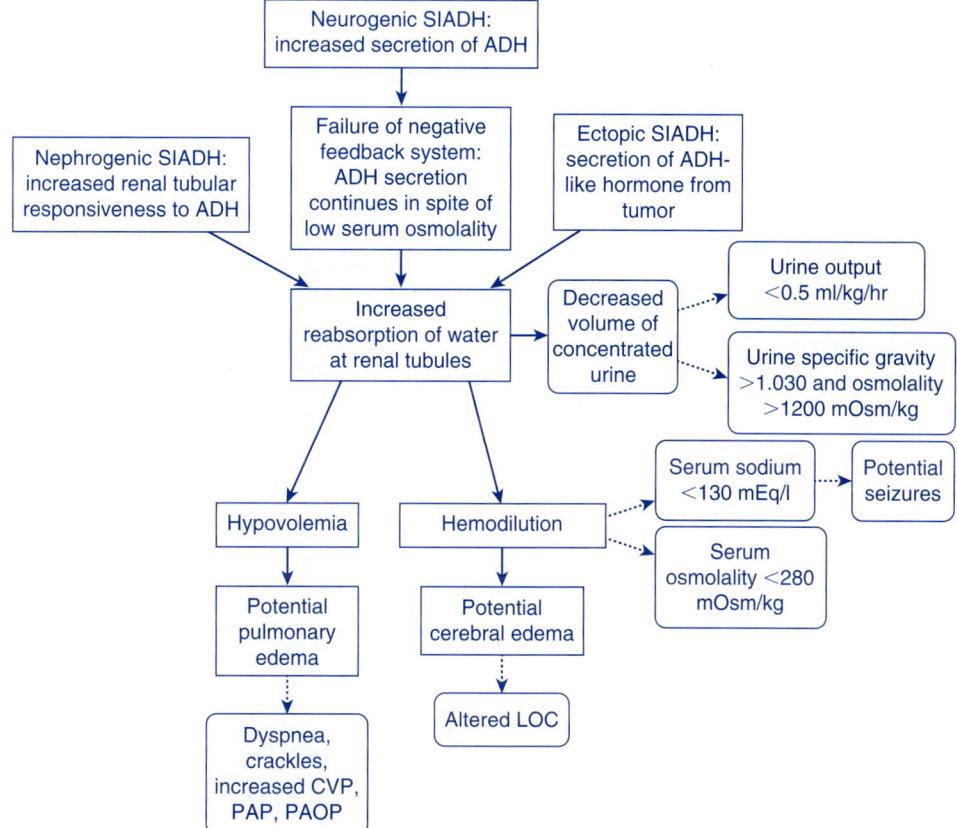

Fig. 6.4 Pathophysiology of syndrome of inappropriate antidiuretic hormone (*SIADH*). *Dotted lines* connect pathology to clinical presentation. *ADH,* Antidiuretic hormone; *CVP,* central venous pressure; *LOC,* level of consciousness; *PAOP,* pulmonary artery occlusive pressure; *PAP,* pulmonary artery pressure.

    b. Monitor weight daily (1 kg = 1 l).
    c. Monitor serum sodium levels.
    d. Note or calculate serum osmolality.
    e. Monitor for clinical indications of hypervolemia, pulmonary edema, and intracranial hypertension.
2. Treat the cause.
    a. Surgical intervention to remove malignant lesion if it is causative agent
    b. Phenytoin or lithium may be used to inhibit the action of ADH on the renal tubules, especially with ectopic ADH
    c. Discontinuance of causative drugs if possible
3. Correct fluid volume excess.
    a. Fluid restriction based on amounts lost in urine and insensible losses; usually restricted to 1000 ml/day
    b. Loop diuretics to promote water excretion
4. Correct electrolyte imbalance.
    a. Dietary sodium should be encouraged.
    b. Hypertonic (3%) saline is indicated in symptomatic patients.
        1) Generally IV infusion of a 50- to 150-ml bolus followed by a slow infusion of 150 to 200 ml of 3% saline over 4 to 6 hours.
        2) Treatment goal is to increase serum sodium by 1 to 2 mEq/l per hour until neurologic symptoms resolve.
        3) The rate of correction is then slowed to elevate the serum sodium no more than 8 to 10 mEq/l in a 24-hour period.
    c. Potassium replacement may be needed.

5. Provide for patient safety.
    a. Safe environment: side rails up; call light within reach
    b. Seizure precautions
    c. Frequent reorientation
6. Monitor for complications.
    a. Intracranial hypertension
    b. Seizures
    c. Coma

Diabetic Ketoacidosis

Definitions
1. DM: a group of metabolic diseases characterized by hyperglycemia (confirmed fasting serum glucose of greater than or equal to 126 mg/dl) that results from defects in insulin secretion, insulin action, or both
    a. Type 1 diabetes is characterized by beta cell destruction, usually leading to absolute insulin deficiency; previously known as juvenile-onset, type I, insulin-dependent DM (IDDM)
    b. Type 2 diabetes is characterized by insulin resistance and a relative (rather than absolute) insulin deficiency; previously known as age-onset, type II, non–insulin-dependent DM (NIDDM).
2. Hyperglycemic crises
    a. DKA: hyperglycemic crisis associated with cellular dehydration, volume depletion, metabolic acidosis, and elevated serum ketones; the most serious metabolic disturbance of type 1 DM. It can also occur in type II DM in severe stress states.

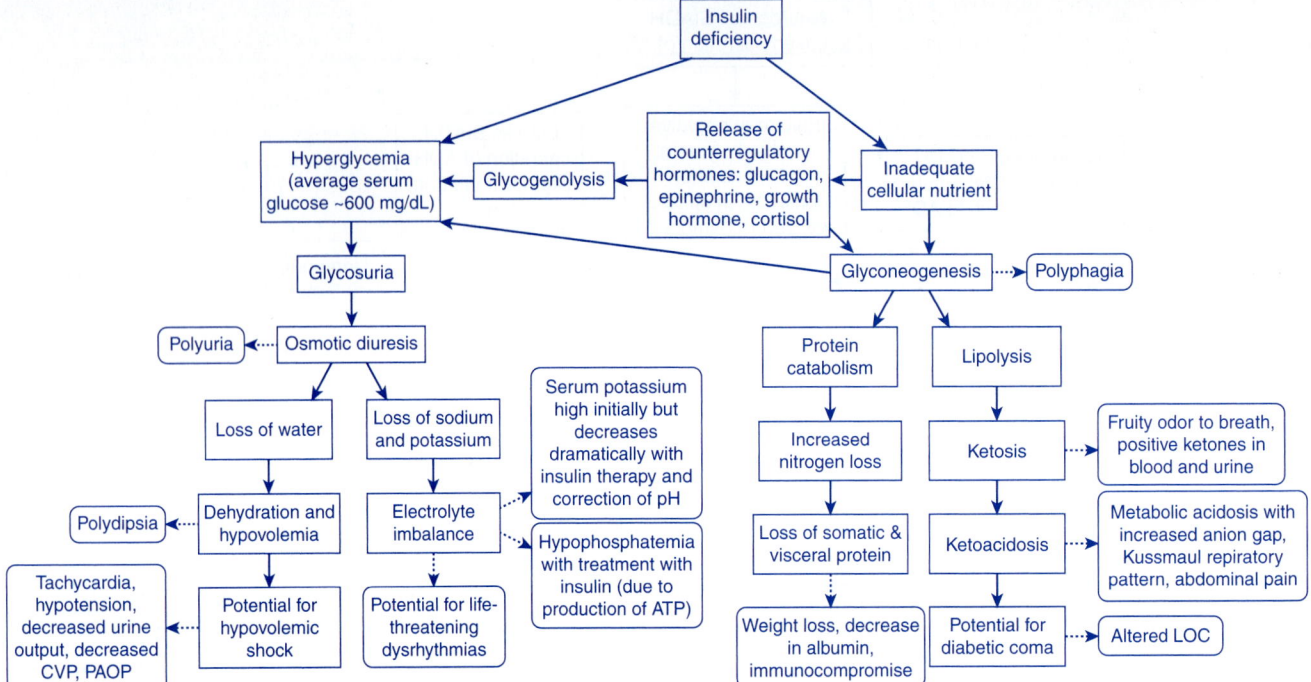

Fig. 6.5 Pathophysiology of diabetic ketoacidosis (DKA). *Dotted lines* connect pathology to clinical presentation. *ATP,* Adenosine triphosphate; *CVP,* central venous pressure; *LOC,* level of consciousness; *PAOP,* pulmonary artery occlusive pressure.

b. Hyperosmolar hyperglycemic state: hyperglycemic crisis associated with hyperglycemia and dehydration and the absence of ketone formation; most serious metabolic disturbance in type 2 DM

Etiology
1. Undiagnosed type 1 DM: 20% of patients with DKA
2. Causes in known type 1 DM
   a. Illness or infection
   b. Omission of exogenous insulin
   c. Trauma
   d. Surgery
   e. Noncompliance: too many calories
3. Causes in patients with or without diabetes
   a. Cushing syndrome
   b. Hyperthyroidism
   c. Pancreatitis
   d. Pregnancy
   e. Drugs
      1) Glucocorticoids (e.g., prednisone)
      2) Thiazide diuretics (e.g., hydrochlorothiazide)
      3) Phenytoin (Dilantin)
      4) Sympathomimetics (e.g., epinephrine)
      5) Diazoxide (Hyperstat)

Pathophysiology
Fig. 6.5.

Clinical Presentation
1. Subjective
   a. Nausea
   b. Abdominal pain
   c. Polyphagia initially; may progress to anorexia with acidosis
   d. Weakness, fatigue
   e. Polydipsia
   f. Weight loss
   g. Headache
   h. Visual disturbances
2. Objective
   a. General
      1) Flushed, warm, dry skin
      2) Poor skin turgor
      3) Sunken eyeballs
      4) Hypothermia or hyperthermia
      5) Dry mucous membranes
   b. Cardiovascular
      1) Tachycardia
      2) Pulse may have decreased quality: 1+/3+
      3) Hypotension
      4) Decreased CVP, PAP, PAOP, CO
   c. Pulmonary
      1) Kussmaul ventilatory pattern
      2) Acetone (fruity) odor to breath
   d. Neurologic
      1) Diminished deep tendon reflexes
      2) Lethargy progressing to coma
   e. Gastrointestinal
      1) Vomiting
      2) Hypoactive bowel sounds
   f. Renal
      1) Polyuria early
      2) Oliguria late
3. Diagnostic studies
   a. Laboratory
      1) Serum
         a) Glucose: elevated 300 to 800 mg/dl; average 600 mg/dl
         b) Sodium: normal, elevated, or decreased depending on hydration status

- c) Potassium
  - i) Elevated initially
  - ii) Decreased to normal or low as pH and dehydration are corrected
  - iii) Total body potassium is low.
- d) Anion gap: elevated; greater than 15
  - i) Formula: $(Na^+ + K^+) - (Cl^- + HCO_3^-)$
  - ii) Normal: 5–15
  - iii) Increase in anion gap indicates an increase in metabolic acid (e.g., ketoacids).
- e) Calcium: may be decreased
- f) Phosphorus: normal initially but decreases with treatment with insulin and fluids
- g) Magnesium: elevated initially and then decreased
- h) Ketones: elevated; greater than 3 mOsm/kg
- i) BUN and creatinine elevated with BUN:creatinine ratio greater than 10:1
- j) Serum osmolality: elevated; usually 295 to 330 mOsm/kg
- k) Lipids: may be elevated
- l) Arterial blood gases: metabolic acidosis frequently with some degree of respiratory compensation
  - i) pH less than 7.3
  - ii) HCO_3 less than 15
  - iii) $PaCO_2$ less than 35 mm Hg
- m) Hematocrit: elevated
- n) WBC count: elevated; unreliable indication of infection in DKA
2) Urine: positive for glucose and ketones
b. Electrocardiogram
1) May show changes associated with potassium levels
2) Sinus tachycardia is frequently seen.

Collaborative Management
1. Maintain oxygenation, ventilation, and circulation.
   a. Oxygen by nasal cannula to maintain SpO_2 at least 95% unless contraindicated
   b. Airway: intubation may be required if consciousness impaired
   c. Correction of fluid volume deficit
      1) Monitor for clinical and laboratory indications of dehydration, hypovolemia, and hypoperfusion.
      2) Establish IV access with at least one large-gauge catheter.
      3) Administer appropriate intravenous solution.
         a) Fluid loss averages approximately 6 to 9 l in DKA
            1) The goal is to replace the total volume loss within 24 to 36 hours with 50% of resuscitation fluid being administered during the first 8 to 12 hours.
            2) The optimal rate of initial fluid administration of isotonic fluid (0.9% saline) is a starting rate of 15 to 20 ml/kg/h (1–1.5 l/hr) for the first hour. After the initial hydration, fluids can be administered at a decreased rate of 4 to 14 ml/kg/hr.
            3) After initial restoration of volume loss evidenced by serum potassium greater than 3.3 mEq/l IV fluids can be changed to a 0.45% NaCl solution.
            4) Small amounts of potassium (20–30 mEq/l) are routinely added to IV fluids when serum potassium is between 3.3 and 5.3 mEq/l.
            5) When glucose levels fall below 200 to 250 mg/dl, IV fluids should be switched to dextrose-containing 0.45% NaCl solution at 150 to 250 ml/hr to prevent hypoglycemia, and/or insulin infusion rate should be decreased.
            6) Special considerations should be given to patients with heart failure and/or chronic kidney disease; these patients tend to retain fluids, so caution should be exercised during volume resuscitation in these patient groups.
            7) Urine output monitoring is crucial in patients with hyperglycemic crises.
2. Normalize serum glucose level gradually.
   a. Monitor serum glucose every hour initially.
      1) Goal of insulin therapy is to decrease serum glucose by 50 to 100 mg/dl each hour.
      2) Rapid correction of serum glucose is associated with hypoglycemia, hypokalemia, and cerebral edema
   b. When serum potassium is greater than 3.3 mEq/l, give initial bolus of regular insulin of 0.1 U/kg followed by continuous insulin infusion of 0.1 unit/kg/hr.
      1) If plasma glucose does not fall by at least 10% in the first hour of insulin infusion rate, 0.1 U/kg bolus of insulin can be given once more while continuing insulin infusion.
      2) Maintain blood glucose between 200 and 250 mg/dl by decreasing insulin or increasing dextrose concentration of IV fluids until serum bicarbonate is 15 mEq/l or greater and the anion gap is less than 10 to 12.
      3) At this point, stop IV fluid administration and IV insulin and start SC insulin at 0.5 to 0.8 U/kg.
3. Correct electrolyte imbalance.
   a. Monitor for clinical, laboratory, and ECG indications of hyperkalemia (initially) and hypokalemia, hypophosphatemia, and hypomagnesemia (with insulin therapy).
   b. Replace potassium as prescribed.
      1) Potassium levels are monitored every 1 to 2 hours initially.
      2) Insulin administration, correction of acidosis and hyperosmolality drive potassium intracellularly, resulting in hypokalemia that may lead to dysrhythmias and cardiac arrest.

3) If serum potassium decreases to less than 3.3 mEq/l during DKA treatment, insulin should be stopped and potassium administered intravenously.
4) Refractory hypokalemia suggests hypocalcemia and/or hypomagnesemia.
      c. Replace phosphorus as prescribed.
         1) Phosphorus is frequently low, especially with insulin therapy; replacement is indicated especially if patient is anemic or has heart failure, pneumonia, or any other cause of hypoxia (hypophosphatemia shifts the oxyhemoglobin curve to the left and impairs tissue oxygenation) or if the serum phosphate level is less than 1 mg/dl.
         2) Potassium replacement may result in hypocalcemia; therefore, close monitoring of both phosphorous and calcium levels is recommended.
      d. Replace magnesium as prescribed.
         1) Magnesium is frequently low.
         2) Usually replaced as 1 to 2 g of 10% solution if renal function is adequate
      e. Monitor sodium and replace as prescribed.
   4. Correct acid–base imbalance.
      a. Bicarbonate therapy is not indicated in mild and moderate forms of DKA because metabolic acidosis will correct with insulin therapy
      b. Administer sodium bicarbonate as prescribed. (NOTE: Sodium bicarbonate is only recommended for severe acidosis [pH 6.9 or less] and should be discontinued as soon as pH is 7.0.)
      c. Monitor for hyperchloremic acidosis caused by NaCl and KCl administration.
   5. Ensure patient safety.
      a. Prevent aspiration caused by paralytic ileus commonly seen in DKA.
         1) Keep head of bed elevated 30 degrees.
         2) Insert nasogastric tube as indicated.
      b. Maintain seizure precautions.
      c. Monitor serum glucose and electrolytes carefully.
   6. Identify and treat cause.
      a. Assess for source of infection: obtain cultures and administer antibiotics as prescribed.
      b. Assess knowledge level related to self-care; be alert to possible drug therapy errors, noncompliance with diet, and drug interactions.
   7. Monitor for complications.
      a. Cardiovascular
         1) Hypovolemic shock
         2) Dysrhythmias
         3) Thromboembolism
         4) Myocardial infarction
         5) Pulmonary edema
      b. Neurologic
         1) Cerebral edema
         2) Seizures
         3) Coma
      c. Pulmonary
         1) Acute respiratory distress syndrome (ARDS)
         2) Pulmonary embolism
      d. Endocrine: hypoglycemia
      e. Renal
         1) Acute renal failure
         2) Electrolyte imbalances: potassium, sodium, phosphorus, magnesium
      f. Sepsis
   8. Provide instruction and counseling regarding lifestyle modification and need for pharmacologic therapy.
      a. Nonpharmacologic therapies
         1) Monitoring and normalization of body weight
         2) Dietary modifications
            a) Low saturated fat
            b) American Diabetes Association diet for control of serum glucose
         3) Cessation of tobacco use
         4) Avoidance of alcohol
         5) Regular aerobic exercise in moderation
         6) Complementary therapies: relaxation; imagery, biofeedback
         7) Stress reduction
         8) Yearly flu and pneumococcal vaccine
         9) Recognition of symptoms of hyperglycemia and hypoglycemia and when to call the physician
         10) Measurement of body weight
      b. Pharmacologic agents
         1) Insulin therapy including sick day management
         2) Control of hypertension, hyperlipidemia, and thyroid disorders

Hyperglycemic Hyperosmolar State

Definition
Hyperglycemic crisis associated with the absence of ketone formation; most common severe metabolic disturbance in type 2 DM

Etiology
Usually seen in patients older than 50 years old with glucose intolerance or type 2 DM; frequently iatrogenic
   1. Noncompliance with diet or drug therapy in a patient with known type 2 DM
   2. Acute illness
   3. Trauma
   4. Surgery
   5. Infection
   6. Pancreatitis
   7. Burns
   8. Hepatitis
   9. Cushing syndrome
   10. Hyperthyroidism
   11. Renal disease
       a. Peritoneal dialysis
       b. Hemodialysis
   12. Hypertonic nutrition: enteral or parenteral
   13. Alcohol
   14. Drugs
       a. Glucocorticoids (e.g., prednisone)
       b. Thiazide diuretics (e.g., hydrochlorothiazide)
       c. Loop diuretics (e.g., furosemide)
       d. Phenytoin
       e. Diazoxide
       f. Immunosuppressive drugs
       g. Beta-blockers (e.g., propranolol)

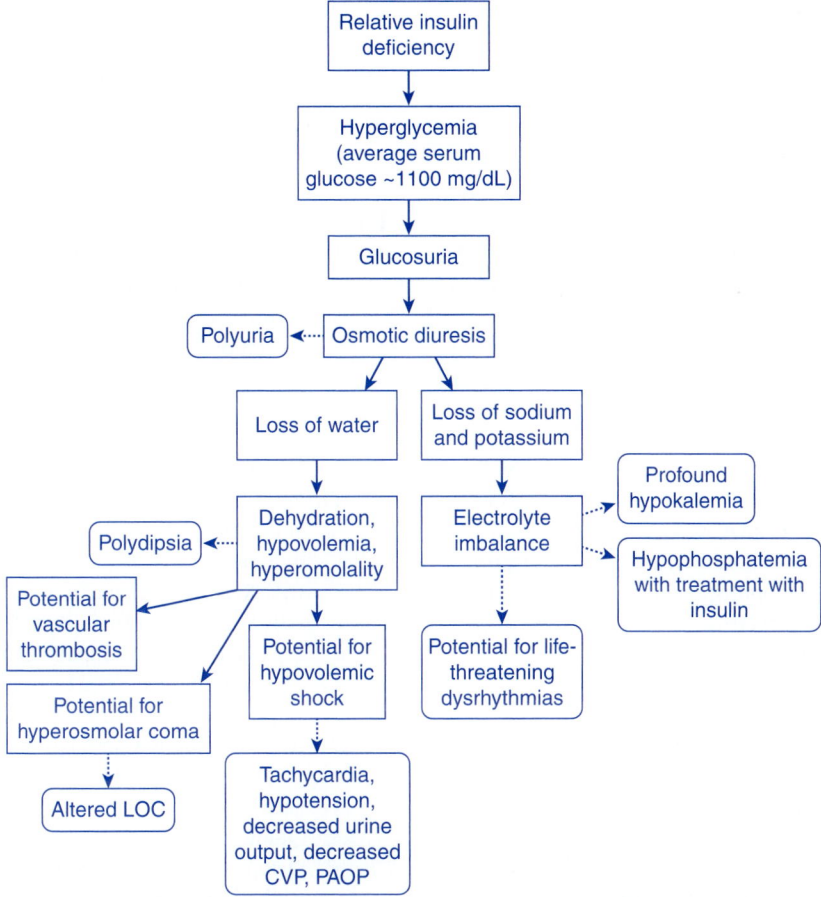

Fig. 6.6 Pathophysiology of hyperglycemic hyperosmolar state (HHS). *Dotted lines* connect pathology to clinical presentation. *CVP*, Central venous pressure; *LOC*, level of consciousness; *PAOP*, pulmonary artery occlusive pressure.

    h. Chlorpromazine
    i. Cimetidine
    j. Calcium channel blockers
    k. Mannitol
    l. Sympathomimetic drugs (e.g., epinephrine)
    m. Thyroid preparations

Pathophysiology
Fig. 6.6.

Clinical Presentation
1. Subjective: weakness, fatigue
2. Objective
    a. General
        1) Weight loss
        2) Flushed, warm, dry skin
        3) Poor skin turgor
        4) Polydipsia
        5) Fever common
    b. Cardiovascular
        1) Tachycardia
        2) Hypotension
        3) Decreased CVP, RAP, PAP, PAOP, CO, cardiac index (CI)
    c. Pulmonary: tachypnea
    d. Neurologic
        1) Sensory deficits: paresthesia
        2) Motor deficits: paresis, plegia
        3) Aphasia
        4) Decreased deep tendon reflexes
        5) Seizures
        6) Lethargy progressing to coma
    e. Renal
        1) Polyuria early
        2) Oliguria late
3. Diagnostic studies
    a. Serum
        1) Glucose, 600 to 2000 mg/dl; average, 1100 mg/dl
        2) Sodium: normal or elevated
        3) Potassium: decreased
        4) Calcium: may be decreased
        5) Phosphorus: decreased
        6) Magnesium: decreased
        7) Ketones: normal or only mildly elevated
        8) BUN and creatinine: elevated with BUN:creatinine ratio greater than 10:1
        9) Serum osmolality: elevated; usually greater than 330; may be as high as 450 mOsm/kg
        10) Arterial blood gases
            a) Normal pH or only mildly acidotic
                i) Acidosis, if present, is lactic acidosis related to hypoperfusion instead of ketoacidosis
        11) Hematocrit: elevated
        12) WBC count: elevated
    b. Urine
        1) Glucose: positive
        2) Ketones: negative or trace

c. Electrocardiogram
1) May show changes associated with potassium levels
2) May show sinus tachycardia

Collaborative Management
1. Maintain oxygenation, ventilation, and circulation (as for DKA).
    a. IV fluid replacement at appropriate rate: as for DKA except that total volume deficit is more significant (i.e., usually 8–15 l)
2. Normalize serum glucose level gradually (as for DKA).
    a. Even though HHS causes higher serum glucose levels, smaller amounts of insulin are needed to normalize serum glucose.
    b. IV insulin infusion usually discontinued when SC insulin is initiated
3. Correct electrolyte imbalance (as for DKA).
    a. Monitor for clinical, laboratory, and ECG indications of hypokalemia, hypophosphatemia, and hypomagnesemia (with insulin therapy).
4. Ensure patient safety (as for DKA).
5. Identify and treat cause.
    a. Assess for source of infection: obtain cultures and administer antibiotics as prescribed.
    b. Monitor serum glucose in patients on enteral and parenteral nutrition, glucocorticoids, dialysis, and diuretics.
    c. Assess knowledge level related to self-care; be alert to possible drug therapy errors, noncompliance with diet, and drug interactions.
6. Monitor for complications.
    a. Cardiovascular
        1) Hypovolemic shock
        2) Dysrhythmias
        3) Thromboembolism
        4) Myocardial infarction
        5) Pulmonary edema
    b. Neurologic
        1) Intracranial hypertension
        2) Cerebral edema
        3) Cerebral infarction
        4) Coma
    c. Pulmonary
        1) ARDS
        2) Pulmonary embolism
    d. Endocrine: hypoglycemia
    e. Renal
        1) Acute renal failure
        2) Electrolyte imbalances: potassium, sodium, phosphorus, and magnesium
    f. Sepsis
7. Provide instruction and counseling regarding lifestyle modification and need for pharmacologic therapy (as for DKA).

Hypoglycemia

Definition
Less than normal serum glucose level.

1. Any serum glucose level of less than 70 mg/dl is hypoglycemia.
2. Symptomatic hypoglycemia generally occurs at a serum glucose level of 50 mg/dl or less, but symptoms may occur if a sudden decrease in serum glucose occurs even though the level is not less than 50 mg/dl.

Etiology
1. Insufficient nutrient intake
    a. Missed or delayed meal
    b. Nausea, vomiting
    c. Interrupted tube feedings or parenteral nutrition
2. Excessive insulin dose
    a. Poor visual acuity causing dose inaccuracy
    b. Change from pork or beef insulin to human insulin
    c. Injection in area of improved absorption
3. Drugs
    a. Sulfonylurea (e.g., glyburide, glipizide, glimepiride) therapy
        1) Renal insufficiency potentiates effects.
        2) Hepatic insufficiency delays metabolism and excretion and impairs gluconeogenesis and glycogenolysis.
        3) Potentiated by salicylates, sulfonamides, phenylbutazone, alpha-glucosidase inhibitors (e.g., acarbose, miglitol)
    b. Ethanol
    c. Quinidine
    d. Disopyramide
    e. Alpha-blockers
    f. Salicylates
    g. Haloperidol
    h. Trimethoprim–sulfamethoxazole
4. Inadequate production of glucose
    a. Strenuous physical exercise or stress with inadequate adjustment of food intake and/or insulin dosage
    b. Excessive alcohol intake ingested without adequate food intake
    c. Glucagon deficiency
5. Postgastrectomy
6. Pancreatic islet cell necrosis: may occur with pentamidine therapy for *Pneumocystis carinii* infection; causes an acute increase in insulin release
7. Adrenal insufficiency
8. Severe liver disease
9. Pregnancy
10. Tumors
    a. Non–beta-cell tumors
        1) Malignant: sarcoma, mesothelioma, hepatomas, lymphoma, leukemia, adrenal carcinoma
        2) Benign: carcinoid and carcinoidlike tumors, pheochromocytoma
    b. Beta-cell tumors (i.e., insulinomas)

Pathophysiology
Fig. 6.7.

Clinical Presentation
1. Subjective
    a. Adrenergic (sympathetic) stimulation indicators

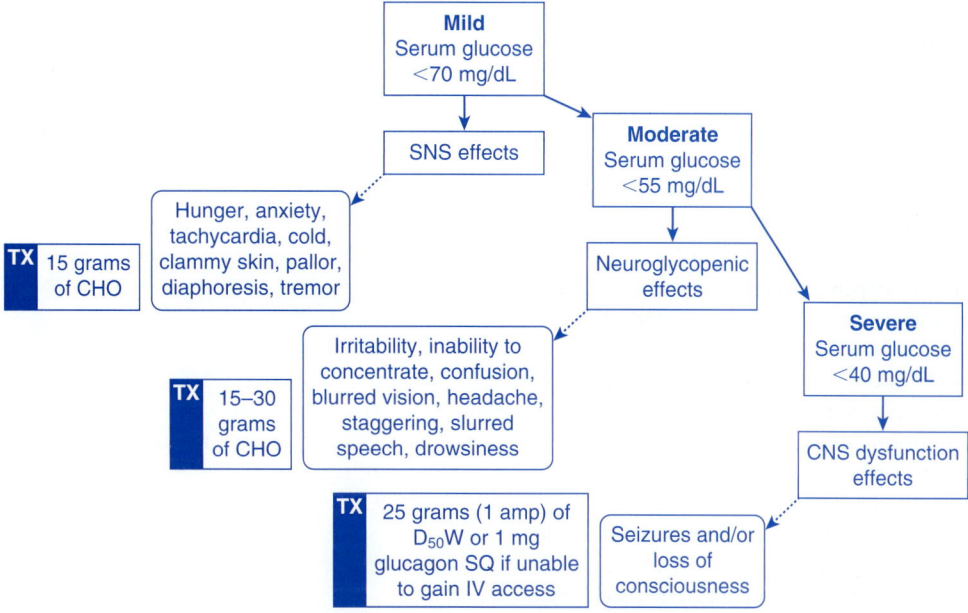

Fig. 6.7 Pathophysiology of hypoglycemia. *Dotted lines* connect pathology to clinical presentation. *CHO,* Carbohydrate; *CNS,* central nervous system; *SC,* subcutaneous; *IV,* intravenous; *SNS,* sympathetic nervous system; *Tx,* treatment.

      1) Palpitations
      2) Anxiety
      3) Nausea
      4) Weakness
   b. Neuroglycopenic indicators
      1) Hunger
      2) Anxiety
      3) Paresthesia
      4) Blurred vision, diplopia
      5) Headache
      6) Irritability, difficulty with concentration
      7) Fatigue
2. Objective
   a. Adrenergic (sympathetic) stimulation indicators
      1) Diaphoresis
      2) Pallor, cool skin
      3) Tremors
      4) Piloerection
      5) Tachycardia, tachypnea
   b. Neuroglycopenic indicators
      1) Vasomotor changes: hypotension
      2) Slurred speech
      3) Agitation
      4) Confusion
      5) Staggering gait
      6) Sensory changes: paresthesias
      7) Motor changes: paresis, hemiplegia, paraplegia
      8) Seizures
      9) Coma
   c. Nocturnal hypoglycemia
      1) Restless sleep
      2) Nightmares
      3) Early morning headache
3. Diagnostic
   a. Serum glucose: 70 mg/dl or less
      1) 20 to 40 mg/dl is associated with seizures.
      2) Less than 20 mg/dl is associated with coma.

> **Box 6.2** Foods Providing 15 g of Carbohydrates for Treatment of Hypoglycemia
>
> Three (5 g) glucose tablets
> 4 oz of apple or orange juice
> 4 oz of nondiet cola or other carbonated beverage
> 8 oz of skim or 1% milk
> 4 cubes or 2 packets of sugar

   b. Electrocardiogram: sinus tachycardia is seen.
   c. BUN, creatinine, liver function studies
   d. Drug screen for possible drug cause may be indicated.

Collaborative Management

1. Restore normal serum glucose level.
   a. Measure serum glucose level immediately when clinical indications of hypoglycemia occur.
   b. Administer 15 g (60 calories) of carbohydrates for conscious patients; for examples (Box 6.2).
      1) Glucose tablets or gel is **required** if the patient has been receiving an alpha-glucosidase inhibitor (e.g., acarbose, miglitol) because these agents block the conversion of carbohydrates to glucose.
   c. Administer parenteral glucose if patient is unconscious.
      1) $D_{50}W$ injection: usually 50 ml (25g) over 3 to 5 minutes
         a) Thiamine 100 mg IV recommended prior to dextrose administration, especially in alcoholics to prevent Wernicke encephalopathy
         b) $D_{10}W$ or D_5W infusion to follow as prescribed
      2) Glucagon 1 mg SC may be given to unconscious patients if unable to gain IV access

d. Provide longer acting carbohydrate source (milk, cheese, crackers) or regularly scheduled meal to avoid recurrence.
e. Reassess serum glucose 15 minutes after treatment and every 15 minutes until serum glucose is within normal range; an additional 50 ml of $D_{50}W$ may be required for refractory hypoglycemia.

2. Prevent injury.
   a. Maintain airway if patient is unconscious.
   b. Monitor closely for seizures; maintain seizure precautions.
3. Identify and treat cause of hypoglycemia.
   a. Assess serum glucose by laboratory or bedside glucose-monitoring device as indicated.
   b. Anticipate times when the patient is most likely to exhibit hypoglycemia.
      1) Be aware of peak times for administered insulin therapy (Table 6.3).
      2) Be aware of missed or late meals or snacks that predispose the patient to hypoglycemia.
      3) Be aware of excessive exertion that may predispose the patient to hypoglycemia.
      4) Note any drugs that the patient is receiving that may potentiate insulin.
      5) Be aware (and make patient and family aware) that beta-blockers block the SNS (early) symptoms of hypoglycemia; serum glucose testing should be done more frequently in patients on beta-blockers.
   c. Assess knowledge level related to self-care; be alert to possible drug therapy errors, noncompliance with diet, and drug interactions.
   d. Assist with additional diagnostic studies if hypoglycemia is experienced by a patient who is not known to have diabetes.
   e. Consider Somogyi phenomenon (insulin-induced posthypoglycemic hyperglycemia) as cause of early morning hyperglycemia (Fig. 6.8)
      1) The result of counterregulatory hormone secretion in response to hypoglycemia
      2) Results in early morning hyperglycemia after nighttime hypoglycemia; needs to be differentiated from dawn phenomenon (i.e., hyperglycemia caused by nocturnal elevations in growth hormone)
      3) Best documented by 3 AM serum glucose

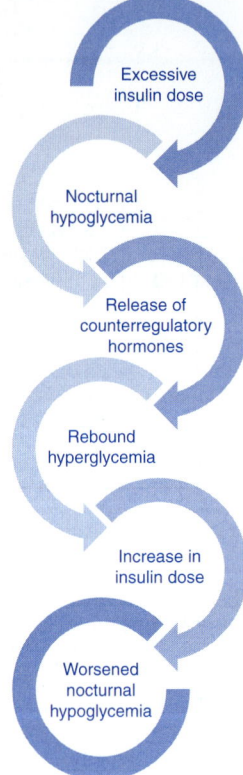

Fig. 6.8 Somogyi effect.

      4) Treated by a decrease in insulin dose and/or bedtime snack
   f. Administer hydrocortisone as prescribed if adrenal insufficiency is suspected.
4. Monitor for complications.
   a. Myocardial ischemia or infarction
   b. Seizures
   c. Coma
   d. Irreversible neurologic damage
5. Provide instruction and counseling regarding lifestyle modification and need for pharmacologic therapy.
   a. Importance of not skipping meals
   b. Recognition of symptoms of hyperglycemia and hypoglycemia and when to call the physician
   c. Insulin and/or oral hypoglycemic agents, including sick day management
   d. Control of hypertension, hyperlipidemia, and thyroid disorders

Learning Activities

CHAPTER 6

1. Complete the following crossword puzzle.

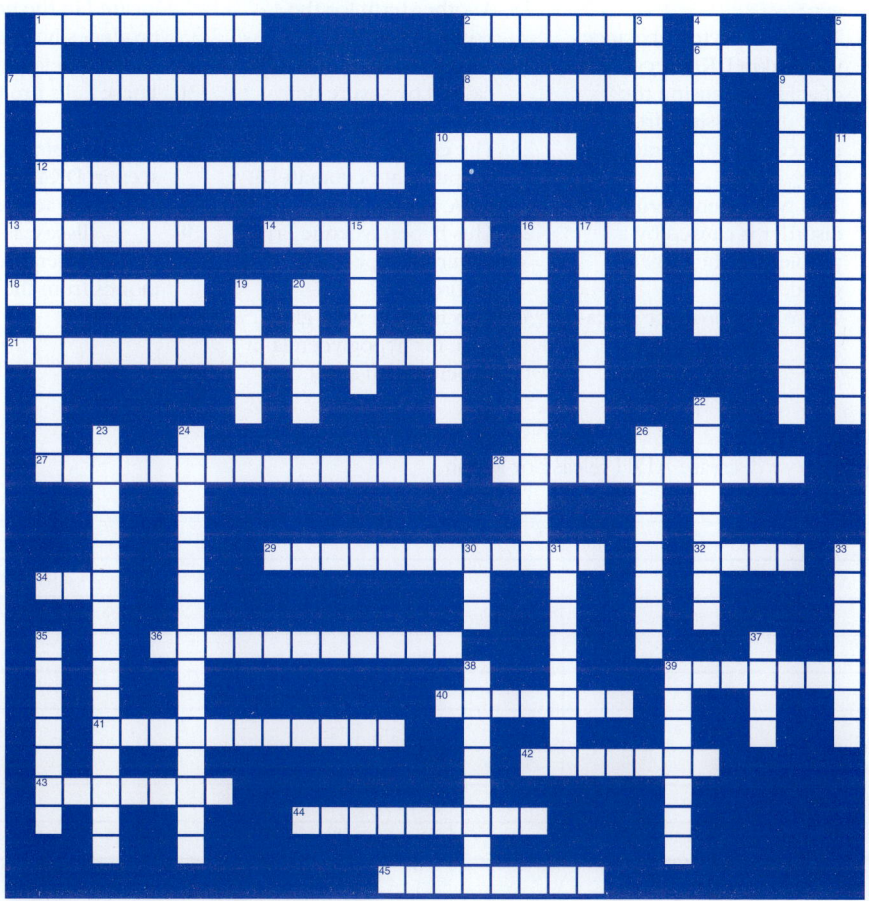

ACROSS

1. This organ produces glucagon and insulin
2. This area of the adrenal gland produces epinephrine and norepinephrine
6. This hormone is produced by the hypothalamus and stored in and released by the posterior pituitary (abbrev)
7. These hypoglycemic effects are caused by low brain glucose
8. This type of diabetes is caused by ADH deficiency
9. This hyperglycemic crisis occurs in type 2 DM or in patients with glucose intolerance (abbrev)
10. DKA causes an increase in this "gap"
12. This is most likely the result of insulin deficiency but also may be caused by stress, steroids, or insulin resistance
13. This hormone is considered a stress hormone and is produced by the adrenal cortex
14. This hormone triggers glycogenolysis and gluconeogenesis
16. In DI and HHS, the serum becomes _____
18. Hyperglycemia caused by counterregulatory hormones released in response to hypoglycemia
21. This electrolyte imbalance occurs with insulin therapy in DKA because glucose moves into the cell and increased amounts of ATP are produced
26. Another term for the anterior pituitary
27. This type of DI is caused by decreased responsiveness of the renal tubule to ADH
28. The treatment for hypoglycemia in a conscious patient is 15 g of ____
31. This hormone is produced by the anterior pituitary gland that causes the production and release of hormones from the adrenal cortex (abbrev)
33. This hormone is produced by the anterior pituitary that stimulates the thyroid gland (abbrev)
35. This type of drug blocks the early symptoms of hypoglycemia
38. This endocrine gland is located on top of the kidney
39. _____ syndrome is caused by an excess of hormones from the adrenal cortex
40. This electrolyte imbalance is noted in DKA as the acidosis is corrected and in HHS
41. This occurs in DKA but not in HHS
42. This hormone enables glucose to move into the cell
43. This type of endocrine disorder is caused by a problem with the pituitary gland
44. This type of diabetes is caused by insulin deficiency

485

DOWN

1. This benign tumor of the adrenal medulla causes labile hypertension
3. This hormone is secreted by the adrenal cortex and causes the retention of sodium and water
4. This is another name for ADH
5. The initial symptoms of hypoglycemia are caused by stimulation of the ___ (abbrev)
9. A serum glucose less than normal
10. This disorder is caused by excessive secretion of growth hormone in an adult
11. This type of DI results from a deficiency in the secretion of ADH from the posterior pituitary
15. The hormones from this area of the adrenal gland can be remembered as sugar (cortisol), salt (aldosterone), and sex (androgen)
16. This electrolyte imbalance is noted in DKA because of acidosis causing the shift of potassium from intracellular to extracellular
17. This type of endocrine disorder is caused by a problem in the target gland
19. These cells produce glucagon
20. This form of vasopressin replacement is used nasally in patients with permanent DI (abbrev)
22. This type of regulation controls the release or retention of hormones
23. Another term for the posterior pituitary
24. A complication in HHS caused by severe dehydration
25. The change in urine output that occurs in DI, DKA, and HHS
29. This hyperglycemic crisis occurs in type 1 DM (abbrev)
30. This is given with glucose for hypoglycemia in patients with substance abuse to prevent Wernicke encephalopathy
32. Regular insulin that has an immediate onset when administered IV (trade)
34. This endocrine gland is located in the neck and produces hormones that control metabolic rate
36. These cells produce insulin
37. _____ respirations are seen in DKA caused by metabolic acidosis
38. _____ disease is caused by a deficiency of hormones from the adrenal gland

2. Identify whether these factors increase or decrease ADH release or action.

Lithium	
Alcohol	
Positive-pressure ventilation	
Chlorpromazine	
Phenytoin	
Hydrochlorothiazide	
Anesthetic agents	
Demeclocycline	
Beta stimulants	
Morphine sulfate	

3. Identify whether these factors are increased or decreased in DI and SIADH.

	DI	SIADH
Serum ADH		
Urine output		
Urine specific gravity		
Urine osmolality		
Serum osmolality		
Serum sodium		
Right atrial/pulmonary artery occlusive pressures		

4. A 45-year-old man was admitted to the surgical intensive care unit yesterday after a craniotomy. Today his urine output has increased dramatically over the past couple of hours. His urine output has been 600 ml over the past 2 hours, and his urine is very dilute with a specific gravity of 1.004. Calculate his serum osmolality and identify the likely cause of the following laboratory values.

Serum sodium	158 mEq/l
Serum potassium	3.8 mEq/l
Serum glucose	110 mg/dl
BUN	32 mg/dl

Serum creatinine	1 mg/dl
Hematocrit	45%
Urine osmolality	195 mOsm/kg

_____
_____

5. Complete this table.

	DKA	**HHS**
Type of diabetes mellitus		
Onset		
Typical serum glucose range		
Presence of ketosis		
pH		
Anion gap		
Respiratory pattern		
Breath odor		
Serum osmolality		
Serum sodium		
Serum potassium		
BUN		
Average fluid deficit		

6. Identify the following clinical indications as DKA, HHS, or both.

Serum glucose >300 mg/dl	
Kussmaul respirations	
pH <7.3	
Positive serum and urine ketones	
Abdominal pain	
Dehydration	
Lethargy → coma	
Serum glucose >600 mg/dl	

7. Identify the following clinical indications as DKA, hypoglycemia, or both.

Headache	
Serum glucose >300 mg/dl	
Abdominal pain	
Cold, clammy skin	
Nervousness, tremors	
Polyuria	
Lethargy → coma	
Seizures → coma	
Glycosuria	
Tachycardia	
Agitation, difficulty with concentration	
Weakness, fatigue	
Fruity breath	
Serum glucose <70 mg/dl	

8. Match the following endocrine conditions with appropriate pharmacologic therapy. More than one therapy may be listed for each condition.

____ 1.	Neurogenic DI	a.	50% dextrose
____ 2.	Nephrogenic DI	b.	Parenteral fluids
____ 3.	DKA	c.	Insulin
____ 4.	HHS	d.	Thiazide diuretics
____ 5.	Hypoglycemia	e.	Vasopressin
____ 6.	SIADH	f.	Loop diuretics
		g.	Potassium
		h.	3% saline

The Gastrointestinal System

CHAPTER 7

Selected Concepts in Anatomy and Physiology

General Information About the Gastrointestinal System

1. Functions of the gastrointestinal (GI) system
   a. Digestion and absorption of nutrients
   b. Elimination of waste material
   c. Detoxification and elimination of bacteria, viruses, chemical toxins, and drugs
2. Processes of the GI system (Fig. 7.1)
   a. Ingestion
   b. Digestion
   c. Absorption
   d. Elimination
3. Structures of the GI system (Fig. 7.2)
   a. Alimentary canal: from the mouth to the anus
      1) Oropharynx
      2) Esophagus
      3) Stomach
      4) Small intestine: divided into duodenum, jejunum, and ileum
      5) Large intestine: divided into cecum, ascending colon, transverse colon, descending colon, sigmoid colon, and rectum
   b. Accessory organs of digestion
      1) Liver
      2) Gallbladder
      3) Pancreas
4. Cell layers
   a. All areas of the GI tract have the same cell layers (external to internal).
      1) Serosa: outermost layer that is frequently continuous with the peritoneum
      2) Muscularis
      3) Submucosa
      4) Mucosa: innermost layer that is exposed to dietary mucosa
5. Peritoneum
   a. The abdominal viscera are covered by the peritoneum.
      1) The parietal layer lines the abdominal cavity wall.
      2) The visceral layer covers the abdominal organs.
      3) The peritoneal cavity is a potential space between the parietal and visceral layers.
   b. There are two folds of the peritoneum.
      1) The mesentery contains blood and lymph vessels and attaches the small intestine and part of the large intestine to the posterior abdominal wall.
      2) The omentum contains fat and lymph nodes.
         a) Lesser omentum from lesser curvature of stomach and upper duodenum to the liver
         b) Greater omentum from stomach over the intestines

Alimentary Canal

1. Oropharynx
   a. Location: mouth to esophagus
   b. Description
      1) Oral cavity
         a) Lips
         b) Cheeks
         c) Palate
         d) Teeth
         e) Tongue
            i) Mucus glands
            ii) Serous glands
         f) Salivary glands
            i) Parotid glands (2)
            ii) Submandibular glands (2)
            iii) Sublingual glands (2)
      2) Muscles of mastication
      3) Pharynx
         a) Nasopharynx
         b) Oropharynx
         c) Laryngopharynx
   c. Secretions: saliva (Table 7.1)
      1) Stimulated by the thought, sight, smell, or taste of food
      2) Consists of:
         a) Ptyalin (amylase): begins the breakdown of polysaccharides (starches) to disaccharides
         b) Mucus: provides lubricant
         3) Volume: 1200 ml/day

489

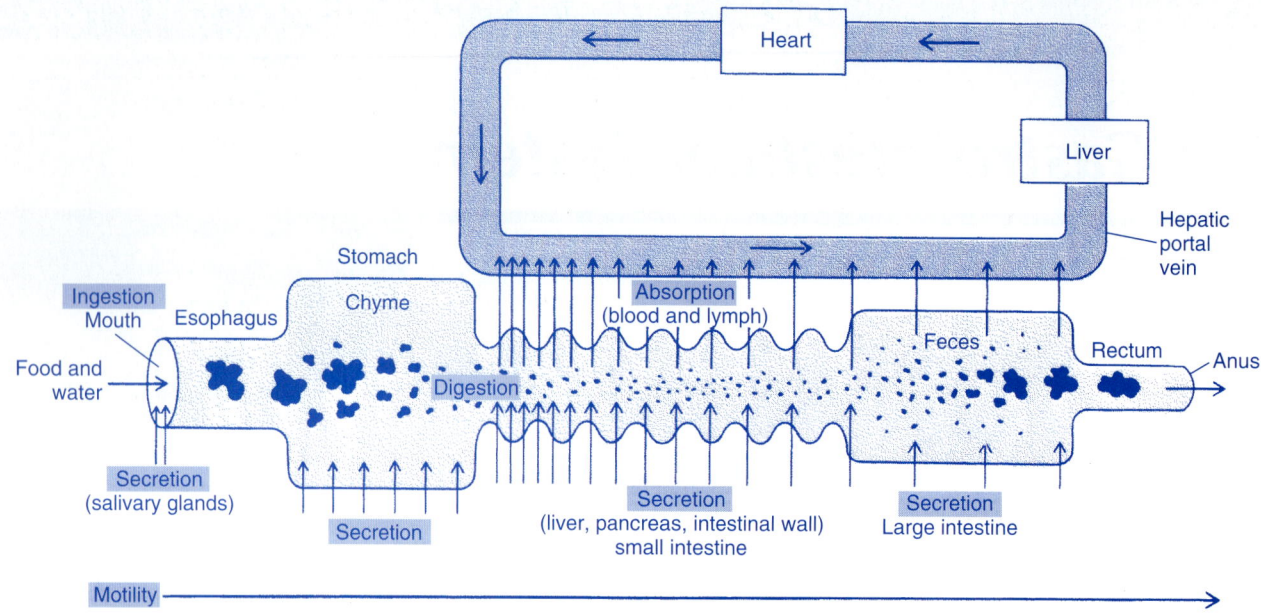

Fig. 7.1 Summary of processes of the gastrointestinal system. (From Kinney, M. R., et al. [1998]. *AACN's clinical reference for critical care nursing* [4th ed.]. St. Louis: Mosby.)

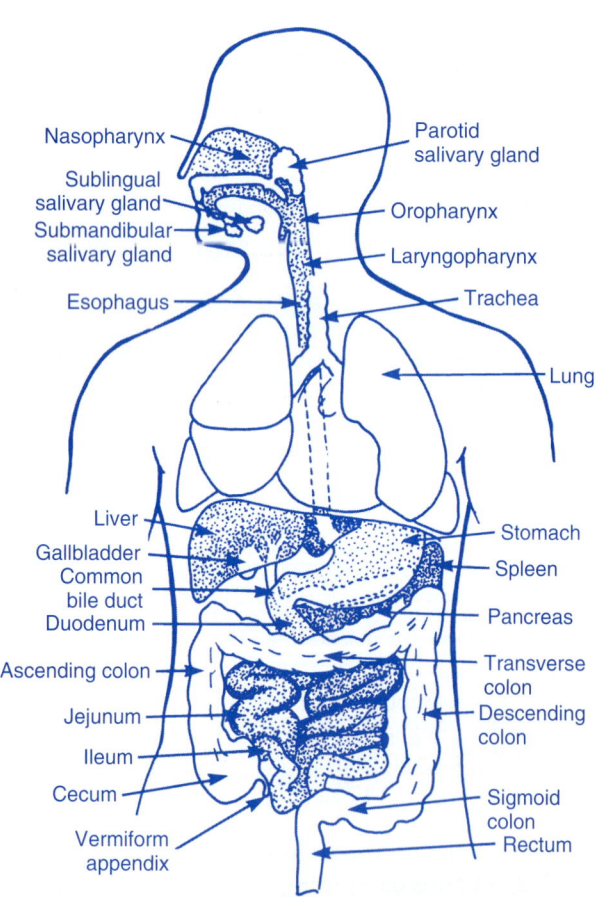

Fig. 7.2 Structures of the gastrointestinal system. (From Kinney, M. R., et al. [1998]. *AACN's clinical reference for critical care nursing* [4th ed.]. St. Louis: Mosby.)

    d. Process
       1) The teeth break up the food into smaller pieces to increase surface area for digestive enzymes to act (i.e., mastication).
       2) The masseter muscles are innervated by cranial nerve V (i.e., trigeminal).
       3) The tongue moves the food around in the mouth for better chewing and moves the food to the back of the throat to begin the process of swallowing.
       4) Swallowing (i.e., deglutition) consists of three stages; only stage one occurs in the mouth.
          a) Oral: The tongue forces the bolus of food into the pharynx; voluntary.
          b) Pharyngeal: The involuntary movement of the bolus of food from the pharynx to esophagus; the epiglottis closes to protect the larynx.
          c) Esophageal: The involuntary movement of the bolus of food from the esophagus to the gastroesophageal sphincter.
    e. Functions: Table 7.2
  2. Esophagus
    a. Location
       1) Lies behind the trachea
       2) Passes through the thoracic cavity and the diaphragm; passes through the diaphragm at the diaphragmatic hiatus
    b. Description: hollow tube from the pharynx to the stomach; approximately 25 cm in length and 2 cm in diameter
    c. Structure (Fig. 7.3)
       1) Cell layers (external to internal)
          a) Does not have a serosa layer

Table 7.1 Digestive Enzymes

Source	Enzyme	What It Acts On	What Is Produced
Salivary glands (saliva) (1200 ml/day)	• Ptyalin (amylase)	• Polysaccharides (starches)	• Disaccharides
Stomach (gastric juice) (2500 ml/day)	• Pepsin	• Proteins	• Polypeptides
	• Gastric lipase	• Emulsified fats	• Fatty acids • Glycerol
	• Renin	• Soluble milk protein	• Insoluble form
Liver (bile) (500–1000 ml/day)	• None	• Nonemulsified fats	• Emulsified fats
Pancreas (pancreatic juice) (1500 ml/day)	• Trypsin	• Denatured proteins • Polypeptides	• Peptides • Amino acids
	• Chymotrypsin	• Proteins • Polypeptides	• Peptides • Amino acids
	• Pancreatic lipase	• Emulsified fats	• Fatty acids • Glycerol
	• Pancreatic amylase	• Disaccharides	• Polysaccharides
	• Nucleases	• Nucleic acids	• Nucleotides
	• Carboxypeptidase	• Polypeptides	• Smaller polypeptides
Small intestine (2000 ml/day)	• Enterokinase	• Trypsinogen	• Trypsin
	• Aminopeptidase	• Polypeptides	• Smaller polypeptides
	• Dipeptidase	• Dipeptides	• Amino acids
	• Sucrase	• Sucrose	• Glucose • Fructose
	• Lactase	• Lactose	• Glucose • Galactose
	• Maltase	• Maltose	• Glucose
	• Nucleotidase	• Nucleotides	• Nucleosides • Phosphoric acid
	• Nucleosidase	• Nucleosides	• Purine • Pentose
	• Intestinal lipase	• Fat	• Glycerides • Fatty acids • Glycerol

Table 7.2 Functions of the Components of the Gastrointestinal System

Component	Function
Oropharynx	• Salivation • Ingestion • Mastication • Lubrication and moistening of food • First and seconds stage of swallowing
Esophagus	• Third stage of swallowing • Lubrication of food • Provision of vent for increased gastric pressures
Stomach	• Secretion of gastric enzymes • Mixing of food with gastric enzymes • Reduction of osmolality of food • Absorption of water • Movement of food through the pylorus
Small intestine	• Receipt of chyme from the stomach and move chyme forward to facilitate proper absorption of proteins, carbohydrates, fats, electrolytes, vitamins, minerals, drugs, and water • Receipt of bile and pancreatic fluid to aid in digestion • Movement of chyme via peristalsis and segmentation • Bacteria in the small intestine help break down and digest protein and, to some degree, fat

Continued

Table 7.2	Functions of the Components of the Gastrointestinal System—cont'd
Component	**Function**
Large intestine	• Secretion of mucus to lubricate and protect intestinal lining • Movement of chyme through colon to rectum and initiate urge to defecate • Storage of feces • Elimination of digestive wastes: defecation • Absorption of water and electrolytes • Synthesis of vitamins (folic acid, riboflavin, vitamin K, nicotinic acid) • Metabolism of blood urea to ammonia
Liver	• Secretion of bilirubin, bile salts, cholesterol, fatty acids, calcium, and other electrolytes into bile • Storage of amino acids, glucose, vitamins, minerals (copper, iron), and blood • Vitamins: riboflavin, nicotinic acid, pyridoxine, vitamins A, D, E, K, B_{12} • Conversion of complex sugars to simple sugars • Conversion of carbohydrates to fats • Conversion of stored glucose (glycogen) to glucose (process is called *glycogenolysis*) • Conversion of amino acids and fats to glucose (process is called *gluconeogenesis*) • Conversion of amino acids to fatty acids and triglycerides • Formation of phospholipids and cholesterol • Formation of lipoproteins from triglycerides and peptides • Conversion of amino acids to plasma proteins (e.g., albumin, fibrinogen, globulins) • Phagocytosis of old red blood cells • Formation of clotting factors and heparin • Conversion of ammonia to urea • Conversion of creatine to creatinine • Conversion of vitamin D_3 to 25-hydroxycholecalciferol • Detoxification of bacteria • Biotransformation of drugs to active and/or inactive metabolites • Deactivation of certain hormones
Gallbladder	• Collection, concentration, and storage of bile • Passageway for bile from liver to intestine • Regulation of bile flow • Release of bile

Pancreas	• Exocrine function
	  • Secretion of pancreatic juice for digestion of carbohydrates, proteins, and fats
	  • Secretion of bicarbonate to neutralize chyme
	• Endocrine function
	  • Secretion of insulin and glucagon

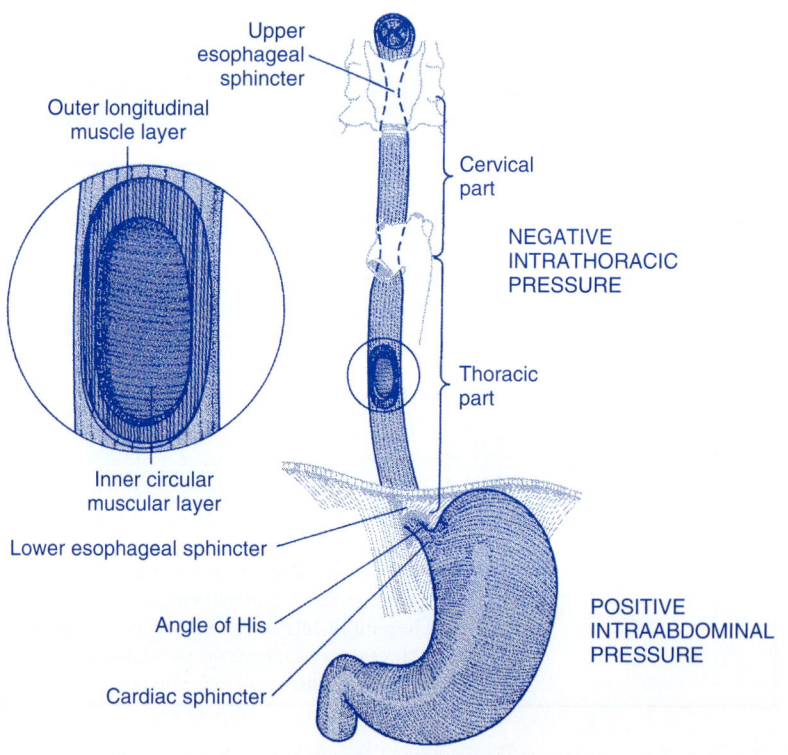

Fig. 7.3 Anatomy of the esophagus. (From Beare, P. G., & Myers, J. L. [1994] *Principles and practice of adult health nursing* [2nd ed.]. St Louis: Mosby.)

b) Muscularis
   i) Type of muscle
      (a) Upper one third: skeletal muscle
      (b) Lower two thirds: smooth muscle
   ii) Direction of muscle
      (a) Inner: circular
      (b) Outer: longitudinal
c) Submucosa
d) Mucosa: lined with mucous membrane, which secretes a protective mucoid substance
2) Sphincters
   a) Hypopharyngeal
      i) Also referred to as the *upper esophageal sphincter* (UES)
      ii) Made of cricopharyngeal muscle
   b) Gastroesophageal
      i) Also referred to as the *lower esophageal sphincter* (LES)
      ii) A physiologic rather than anatomic sphincter: consists of the last 2 to 4 cm of the esophagus
d. Secretions: mucus
e. Process: final phase of swallowing (involuntary)
   1) When a bolus of food enters the esophagus, the hypopharyngeal sphincter opens.
   2) Food is moved through the esophagus by gravity and peristaltic action; peristalsis is the alternating contraction and relaxation of muscle fibers that propels the substance in a wavelike motion through the esophagus, stomach, and intestines.
   3) The gastroesophageal sphincter opens and food enters the stomach.
   4) The process takes 5 to 10 seconds.
f. Functions: Table 7.2.

3. Stomach (Fig. 7.4)
   a. Location: inferior to the diaphragm with approximately 80% to 85% of the organ to the left of midline
   b. Description
      1) Largest dilation of the GI tract
      2) Approximately 25 to 30 cm in length and 10 to 15 cm at maximal diameter
      3) Relatively little muscle tone, which permits increased distention
   c. Structure
      1) Anatomical divisions
         a) Cardia: portion of stomach that immediately adjoins the esophagus
         b) Fundus: dome-shaped portion of stomach that extends left of the cardia
         c) Greater curvature: lateral, convex side
         d) Body: major area (belly) of stomach
         e) Lesser curvature: medial, concave side
         f) Antrum: lower portion close to pylorus
      2) Sphincters
         a) Cardiac: between esophagus and stomach
         b) Pyloric: between stomach and duodenum
      3) Layers of stomach wall (external to internal)
         a) Serosa: continuous with the peritoneum
         b) Muscularis
            i) Outer: longitudinal muscle fibers
            ii) Middle: circular muscle fibers
            iii) Inner: transverse muscle fibers
         c) Submucosa
            i) Blood vessels
            ii) Lymph vessels
            iii) Connective tissue
            iv) Fibrous tissues

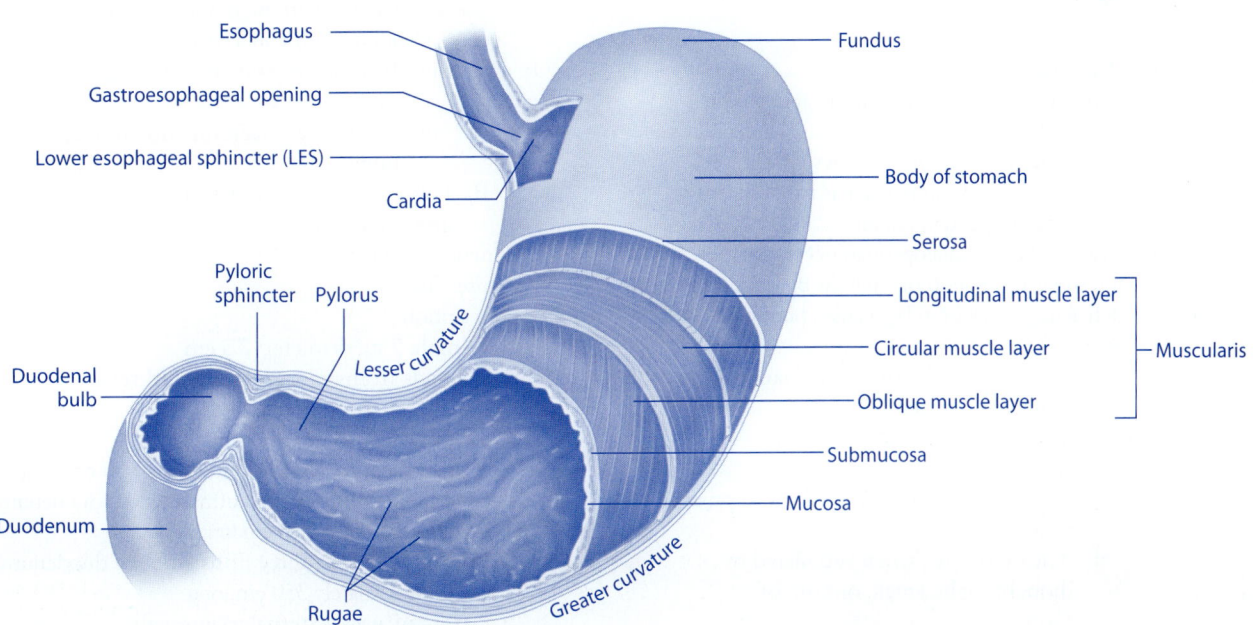

Fig. 7.4 Anatomy of the stomach. (From Patton, K. T. & Thibodeau, G. A. [2013]. *Anatomy & physiology* [8th ed.]. St Louis: Mosby.)

d) Mucosa: contains rugae, which are thick folds on the interior of the stomach; rugae do all of the following:
   i) Increase surface area for exposure
   ii) Allow for distention
   iii) Contain the openings of the gastric glands
e) Gastric glands
   i) Cardiac glands: just distal to the gastroesophageal junction; secrete pepsinogen and mucus
   ii) Oxyntic glands: fundic area
      (a) Mucous neck cells secrete mucus.
      (b) Chief cells secrete pepsinogen.
      (c) Oxyntic (also referred to as *parietal*) cells secrete:
         (i) Hydrochloric acid (HCl)
         (ii) Intrinsic factor
      (d) Enterochromaffin (endocrine) cells secrete serotonin.
   iii) Pyloric glands: antral area
      (a) Gastrin secreted by G-cells
      (b) Serotonin secreted by enterochromaffin cells
d. Secretions: Table 7.1.
   1) Description: Gastric secretions are clear and contain water, salts, enzymes, and HCl
   2) Gastric secretions are stimulated when a bolus of food enters the upper portion of the stomach.
   3) Gastric secretions contain the following
      a) Hydrochloric acid
         i) Stimulated by histamine, acetylcholine, and gastrin
         ii) Functions
            (a) Denature protein and break intermolecular bonds
            (b) Activate a number of enzymes secreted by stomach
            (c) Kill bacteria
      b) Pepsinogen
         i) Activated by hydrochloric acid to form pepsin
         ii) Function: Pepsin catalyzes splitting of bonds between particular types of amino acids in protein chains.
      c) Intrinsic factor: mucoprotein necessary for intestinal absorption of vitamin B_{12} in the ileum; deficiency of vitamin B_{12} causes pernicious anemia
      d) Mucus: contributes to the maintenance of the gastric mucosal barrier
   4) Control of gastric secretion
      a) Cephalic phase
         i) Mediated by the parasympathetic nervous system (PNS)
         ii) Release of HCl when stimulated by thought, sight, smell, or taste of food
      b) Gastric phase
         i) Enhances acid secretion
         ii) Stimulated by distention of stomach and digestion products of food
      c) Intestinal phase
         i) Continuation of gastric acid secretion but in lesser amounts
         ii) Stimulated by distention, hypertonic solution, acid, and fat within duodenum
e. Process
   1) As food moves toward the pyloric sphincter at the distal end of the stomach, peristaltic waves increase in force and intensity.
   2) The food bolus becomes a substance known as *chyme*.
   3) Gastric motility is affected and controlled by various factors.
      a) Affected by the following:
         i) Quantity and pH of contents
         ii) Degree of mixing
         iii) Peristalsis
         iv) Ability of the duodenum to accept the chyme
      b) Controlled by the following:
         i) Sympathetic nervous system (SNS) and PNS
         ii) Reflexes
         iii) Gastric hormones
   4) Chyme is pumped through the pyloric sphincter into the duodenum.
   5) The stomach empties as chyme moves through the pyloric channel.
      a) Rate of gastric emptying proportional to the volume of the stomach's contents
      b) Regulation of gastric emptying affected by the following:
         i) Consistency of the fluid chyme; liquids selectively move through the pylorus before solids
         ii) Receptiveness of the duodenum
      c) Factors inhibiting gastric emptying
         i) Chyme with high lipid content
         ii) High acidity in antrum
         iii) Emotions: pain, anxiety, sadness, hostility
         iv) Hormones: secretin and cholecystokinin
      d) Food usually stays in the stomach 2–6 hours after ingestion.
f. Function: Table 7.2.
4. Small intestine
   a. Description
      1) Length: 7 m; diameter: 2.5 cm
      2) Extends from pylorus to ileocecal valve
   b. Structure
      1) Divisions
         a) Duodenum: short segment only 30 cm long
         b) Jejunum: the next two fifths after the duodenum; approximately 250 cm long
         c) Ileum: the last three fifths after the duodenum; approximately 350 cm long
      2) Layers of wall (external to internal)
         a) Serosa: continuous with the peritoneum
         b) Muscular
         c) Submucosal
         d) Mucosal

3) Sphincters
   a) Pylorus: from stomach to duodenum
   b) Ileocecal: controls flow of contents into large intestine and prevents reflux from the large intestine back into the ileum
4) Villi
   a) Fingerlike projections of mucosa and submucosa prominent in duodenum and jejunum increase surface area.
   b) Contain a single lymph vessel called a *lacteal* and a dense capillary bed to aid in absorption
   c) Contain many different types of cells to absorb fat, carbohydrate (CHO), or protein and secrete enzymes and mucus
      i) Brunner glands: cells that secrete mucus; primarily in duodenum
      ii) Goblet cells: cells that secrete mucus
      iii) Crypts of Lieberkühn: cells that produce watery mucus called *succus entericus*, a carrier substance for absorption of nutrients when the villi come in contact with the chyme
      iv) Paneth cells: uncertain function but may regulate intestinal flora
      v) Peyer patches
         (a) Cells in mucosa and submucosa
         (b) Lymphoid follicles that carry out antibody synthesis
c. Secretions (Table 7.1)
   1) Stimulated by the presence of chyme in the duodenum and release of gastric hormones
d. Process
   1) Movement of chyme
      a) During fasting and sleeping states: Muscle contraction moves from antrum to ileum to sweep the gut of contents.
      b) During eating state
         i) Concentric, segmenting contractions take place in the jejunum; help to mix secretions of the small intestines with the chyme particles
         ii) Slow, propulsive contractions (peristalsis) slowly push the chyme in the direction of the large intestine.
         iii) Continuous shortening and lengthening of the villi constantly stir the intestinal contents.
      c) The movement of chyme from the small intestine to the large intestine regulated by gastroileal reflex; increased contractions in the ileum as the chyme nears the large intestine
      d) Movement of chyme through small intestine approximately 3 to 10 hours
e. Function: Table 7.2.
5. Large intestine
   a. Description: length, 90 to 150 cm; diameter, 4 to 6 cm extending from the ileum to the anus
   b. Structure
      1) Divisions (Fig. 7.5)
         a) Cecum

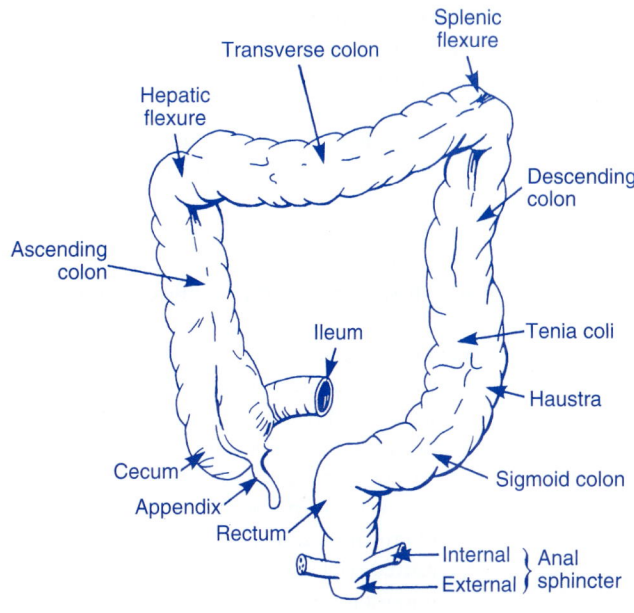

Fig. 7.5 Anatomy of the large intestine. (From Kinney, M. R., et al. [1998]. *AACN's clinical reference for critical care nursing* [4th ed.]. St. Louis: Mosby.)

         b) Colon
            i) Ascending colon
            ii) Transverse colon
            iii) Descending colon
            iv) Sigmoid colon
         c) Rectum
      2) Flexures
         a) Hepatic: bend at the liver; in the right upper quadrant (RUQ)
         b) Splenic: bend at the spleen; in the left upper quadrant (LUQ)
      3) Sphincters
         a) Ileocecal: from small intestine to cecum
         b) Anal: internal and external anal sphincters
      4) Layers of large intestinal wall
         a) Serosa: continuous with the peritoneum
         b) Muscularis
         c) Submucosa
         d) Mucosa
   c. Process
      1) Movement of intestinal contents
         a) Haustral shuttling
            i) Periodic uncoordinated tonic contractions or segmentations of both the longitudinal and circular muscles
            ii) Contents displaced short distances
            iii) Weak peristaltic contractions that move the chyme through the large intestine
         b) Phasic, random, nonpropulsive contractions
            i) Last 30 seconds to 2 minutes
            ii) Contents displaced short distances in both directions
            iii) Mixes the stool material and helps in the absorption of liquid contents without advancement toward the anus

c) Spontaneous mass movements
　i) Fecal contents are pushed forward by mass movements that typically occur only a few times each day.
　ii) Mass movements are stimulated by gastrocolic reflexes initiated when food enters the duodenum from the stomach, especially after the first meal of the day.
　iii) These movements move feces into the rectum.
　iv) The defecation reflex occurs when feces enters the rectum; peristaltic waves in the rectum and relaxation of the internal and external anal sphincter occur.
　v) Afferent impulses are transmitted to the sacral segment of the spinal cord, from which reflex impulses are transmitted back to the colon and rectum, initiating relaxation of the internal anal sphincter.
　vi) Evacuation of the colon may be facilitated by Valsalva maneuver.
2) Factors that enhance colonic motility
　a) High-residue diet
　b) Hyperosmolality
　c) Fluids
　d) Irritation of colon (e.g., spicy foods)
　e) Irritant laxatives
3) Factors that inhibit colonic motility
　a) Low-residue diet
　b) Anticholinergic drugs
　c) Opiates
4) Movement of fecal contents through small intestine approximately 12 hours
d. Function: Table 7.2.

Accessory Organs of Digestion (Fig. 7.6)
1. Liver
　a. Location: in RUQ, fitting snugly against right inferior diaphragm
　b. Description
　　1) Largest organ in the body: 1.5 kg
　　2) Attached to the abdominal wall by the falciform ligament, which also divides the left and right lobes
　　3) Four main lobes
　　　a) Right: larger than left
　　　b) Left
　　　c) Caudate
　　　d) Quadrate
　　4) Covered by a thick capsule of connective tissue (called *Glisson capsule*); contains blood vessels and lymphatics
　　5) Capsule covered by a layer of serosa continuous with the peritoneum
　c. Structure
　　1) Lobes are divided into lobules.

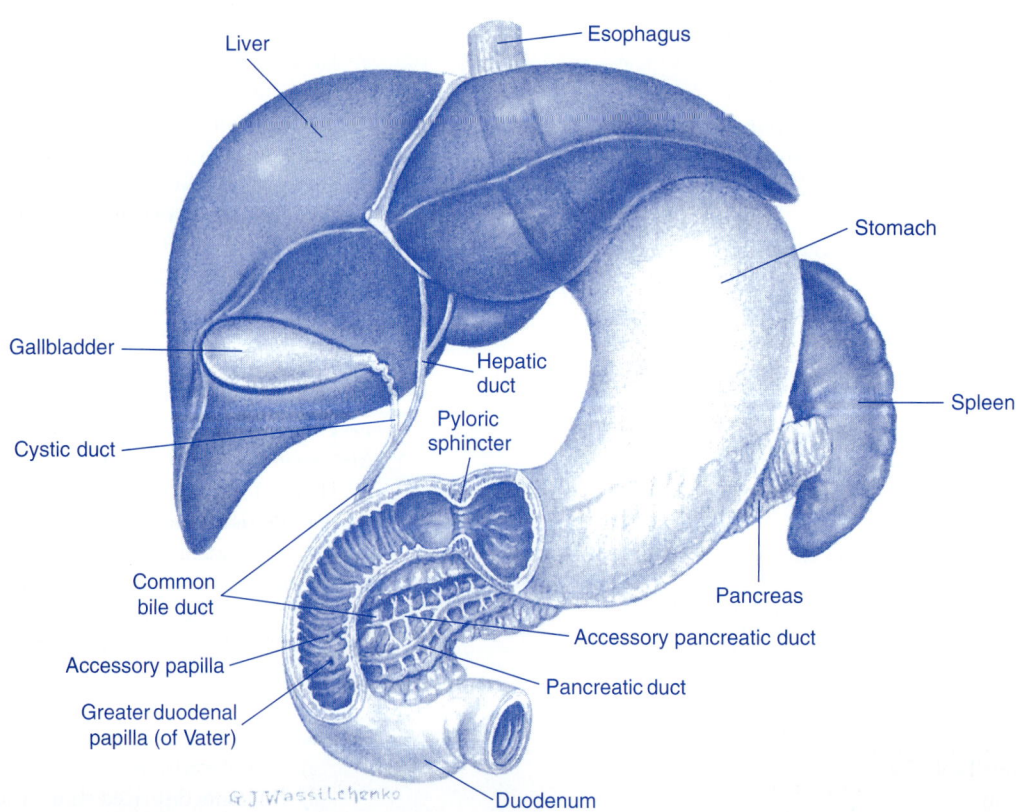

Fig. 7.6 Accessory organs of the gastrointestinal system. (From Doughty, D. B., & Jackson, D. B. [1993]. *Gastrointestinal disorders: Mosby's clinical nursing series.* St Louis: Mosby.)

2) Lobules are the functioning unit of the liver; there are more than 1 million lobules.
   a) Hepatic cells (hepatocytes) are arranged in chains around a central vein.
   b) Blood flows through sinusoids, which separate the hepatic chains.
   c) The sinusoids receive oxygenated blood from branches of the hepatic artery and nutrient-rich blood from branches of the hepatic portal vein; the hepatic cells remove oxygen, nutrients, and toxins from the blood.
   d) Each lobule has its own hepatic artery, portal vein, and bile duct, collectively called the *portal triad*.
   e) The lobule is composed of branching plates of liver cells radiating from center to periphery.
   f) Kupffer cells, which are responsible for phagocytosis, line the sinusoids; Kupffer cells are a part of the reticuloendothelium system; they destroy old or defective red blood cells and remove bacteria and foreign particles from the blood.
   g) Ducts
      i) Bile canaliculi are located between the hepatic cells and empty bile into the small bile ducts.
      ii) Small bile ducts join to form the right and left hepatic ducts.
      iii) Left and right hepatic ducts merge to form the common hepatic duct.
      iv) Cystic duct from the gallbladder joins the common hepatic duct to form the common bile duct (Fig. 7.7).
      v) The pancreatic duct joins the common bile duct and together they empty into the duodenum through the ampulla of Vater.
      vi) The sphincter of Oddi is a valve in the common bile duct, which regulates the passage of bile from the common bile duct into the duodenum.
   d. Secretions: bile (described under Gallbladder)
   e. Function: Table 7.2.
2. Gallbladder
   a. Location
      1) Attached to undersurface of liver
      2) Connected to the upper portion of the duodenum by the common bile duct
   b. Description
      1) Saclike organ about 7 to 10 cm in length and 3 cm in diameter
      2) Storage capacity of 50 to 70 ml
      3) Layers (exterior to interior)
         a) Serous layer: continuous with the peritoneum
         b) Smooth muscle layer
         c) Mucous membrane layer has rugae which allow an increase in gallbladder size
   c. Structure
      1) There are four anatomical divisions of the gallbladder.
         a) Fundus: distal portion of the body that forms a blind sac
         b) Body: connects the fundus to the infundibulum
         c) Infundibulum: connects the body to the neck
         d) Neck: narrows into the cystic duct
      2) The cystic duct merges with the common hepatic duct to form the common bile duct, which joins with the pancreatic duct to form ampulla of Vater.
      3) The sphincter of Oddi is at the terminal end of the common bile duct, located at the entrance into the duodenum.
         a) Regulates the flow of bile and pancreatic juices into the intestine
         b) Inhibits the entry of bile into the pancreatic duct
         c) Prevents reflux of intestinal contents into the duct
   d. Secretions (Table 7.1)
      1) Bile
         a) Bile is produced by the liver and stored in the gallbladder.
         b) The gallbladder contracts in response to the hormone cholecystokinin when food is present in the small intestine; release is stimulated when fatty food is present in the small intestine.
         c) The action of bile is to assist in the absorption of fats by emulsifying the fat and breaking down large fat droplets into small droplets.
         d) Bile is composed of the following:
            i) Water
            ii) Bile pigments
            iii) Bile salts
            iv) High concentration of cholesterol
            v) Some neutral fat, phospholipid, and inorganic salts

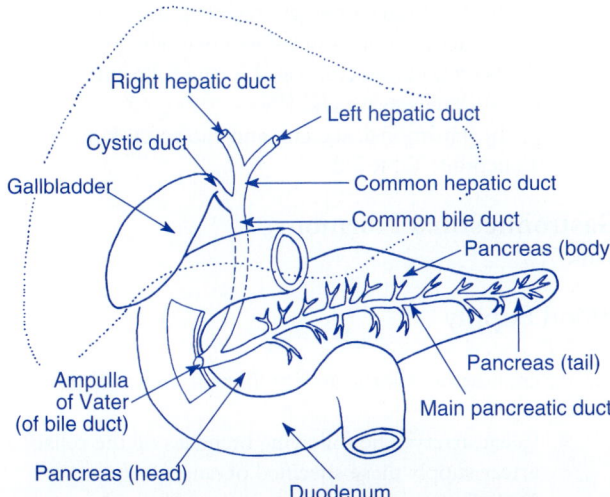

Fig. 7.7 Ductal systems of the gastrointestinal tract. (From Kinney, M. R., et al. [1998]. *AACN's clinical reference for critical care nursing* [4th ed.]. St. Louis: Mosby.)

e) The major bile pigment is bilirubin, a breakdown product of hemoglobin (Hgb).
   i) Metabolism (Fig. 7.8)
      (a) The heme portion of the Hgb molecule is converted to bilirubin by reticuloendothelial cells, released into the bloodstream, and binds to albumin as fat-soluble, unconjugated bilirubin (indirect).
      (b) In the liver, indirect bilirubin is bound to glucuronic acid to form water-soluble conjugated (direct) bilirubin, which is excreted into the hepatic ducts.
   e. Process
      1) Contraction of the gallbladder is stimulated by the hormone cholecystokinin.
   f. Function: Table 7.2.
3. Pancreas
   a. Location: lies in the posterior curvature of the stomach; lies behind duodenum and spleen (Fig. 7.6)

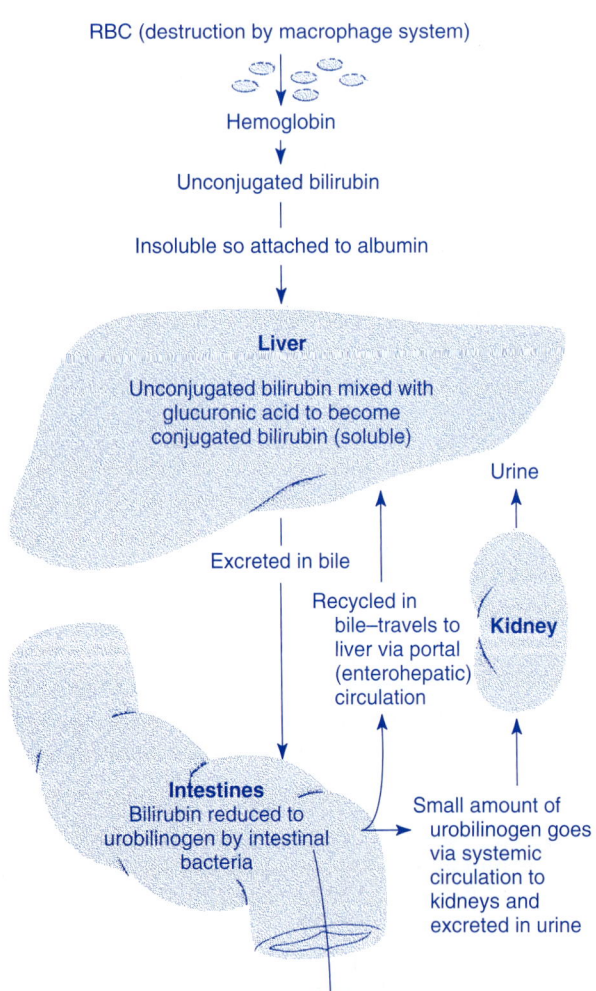

Fig. 7.8 Bilirubin metabolism. *RBC,* Red blood cell. (From Lewis, S. M., Heitkemper, M. M., & Dirksen, S. R. [2000]. *Medical-surgical nursing: Assessment and management of clinical problems* [5th ed.]. St. Louis: Mosby.)

   b. Description
      1) Length: 15 to 20 cm; diameter: 5 cm
      2) Anatomical divisions
         a) Head: over the vena cava in the C-shaped curve of the duodenum
         b) Body: lies behind the duodenum and extends across the abdomen behind stomach
         c) Tail: under the spleen
      3) Not surrounded by a capsule
   c. Structure
      1) Connected lobes are formed by lobules.
      2) Lobules are clustered cells.
      3) The acini are arranged around a small central lumen; they secrete their enzymes into the central lumen.
      4) These central lumina are drained into ductules.
      5) Ductules drain into intralobular ducts, which drain into interlobular ducts, which empty into the pancreatic duct (also called the *duct of Wirsung*).
      6) The pancreatic duct runs from the tail to the head of the pancreas and unites with the common bile duct to form the ampulla of Vater, which empties into the duodenum.
      7) Cells have exocrine and endocrine functions.
         a) Acinar cells have exocrine (through a duct) functions.
         b) Alpha and beta cells of the islets of Langerhans have endocrine (ductless) functions.
            i) Alpha cells secrete glucagon.
            ii) Beta cells secrete insulin.
            iii) Delta cells secrete somatostatin.
   d. Secretions: Table 7.1.
      1) Pancreatic secretions are triggered by the presence of undigested food in the small intestine.
      2) Acinar cells secrete a high concentration of sodium bicarbonate, water, sodium, potassium, and digestive enzymes (lipase, amylase, trypsin, ribonuclease, deoxyribonuclease).
         a) Trypsinogen: secreted in inactive form; activated in contact with bile salts
         b) Chymotrypsinogen: secreted in inactive form; activated in contact with bile salts
      3) Secretions are controlled by the following:
         a) Vagus nerve and PNS
         b) Hormonal: secretin and cholecystokinin
   e. Functions: Table 7.2

Gastrointestinal Hormones
Table 7.3.

Blood Supply
Fig. 7.9.
1. Arterial: aorta → aortic arch → thoracic arch → abdominal aorta →
   a. Celiac artery: The following branches of the celiac artery supply these specified organs:
      1) Left gastric: supplies stomach and esophagus
      2) Hepatic to right gastric: supplies stomach
      3) Gastroduodenal: supplies stomach and duodenum
      4) Cystic: supplies gallbladder
      5) Splenic: supplies stomach, pancreas, and spleen

Table 7.3	Gastrointestinal Hormones		
Hormone	**Source**	**Stimulus for Release**	**Action**
Gastrin	Gastric mucosa of the antrum of the stomach and the pylorus	Partially digested proteins in pylorus	• Stimulates release of gastric juices
Secretin	Duodenal mucosa	Partially digested proteins, fats, and acids in intestine	• Inhibits gastric motility and acid secretions • Pancreatic bicarbonate secretion
Cholecystokinin	Duodenal mucosa	Fats in duodenum	• Increases gallbladder contraction • Decreases stomach tone
Gastric inhibitory peptide	Small intestine mucosa	Fat and carbohydrate in duodenum	• Stimulates secretion of insulin • Decreases motor activity of the stomach • Slows emptying of gastric contents into the small intestine
Vasoactive intestinal peptide	Small intestine mucosa	Acid in the duodenum	• Stimulates intestinal juice • Inhibits gastric secretion
Enterogastrone	Small intestine mucosa	Partially digested proteins, fats, and acids in intestine	• Inhibits gastric secretion and motility • Relaxation of sphincter of Oddi and contraction of gallbladder
Villikinin	Small intestine mucosa	Chyme in intestine	• Stimulates movement of intestinal villi
Pancreozymin	Duodenal mucosa	Partially digested proteins, fats, and acids in duodenum	• Stimulates pancreatic juice

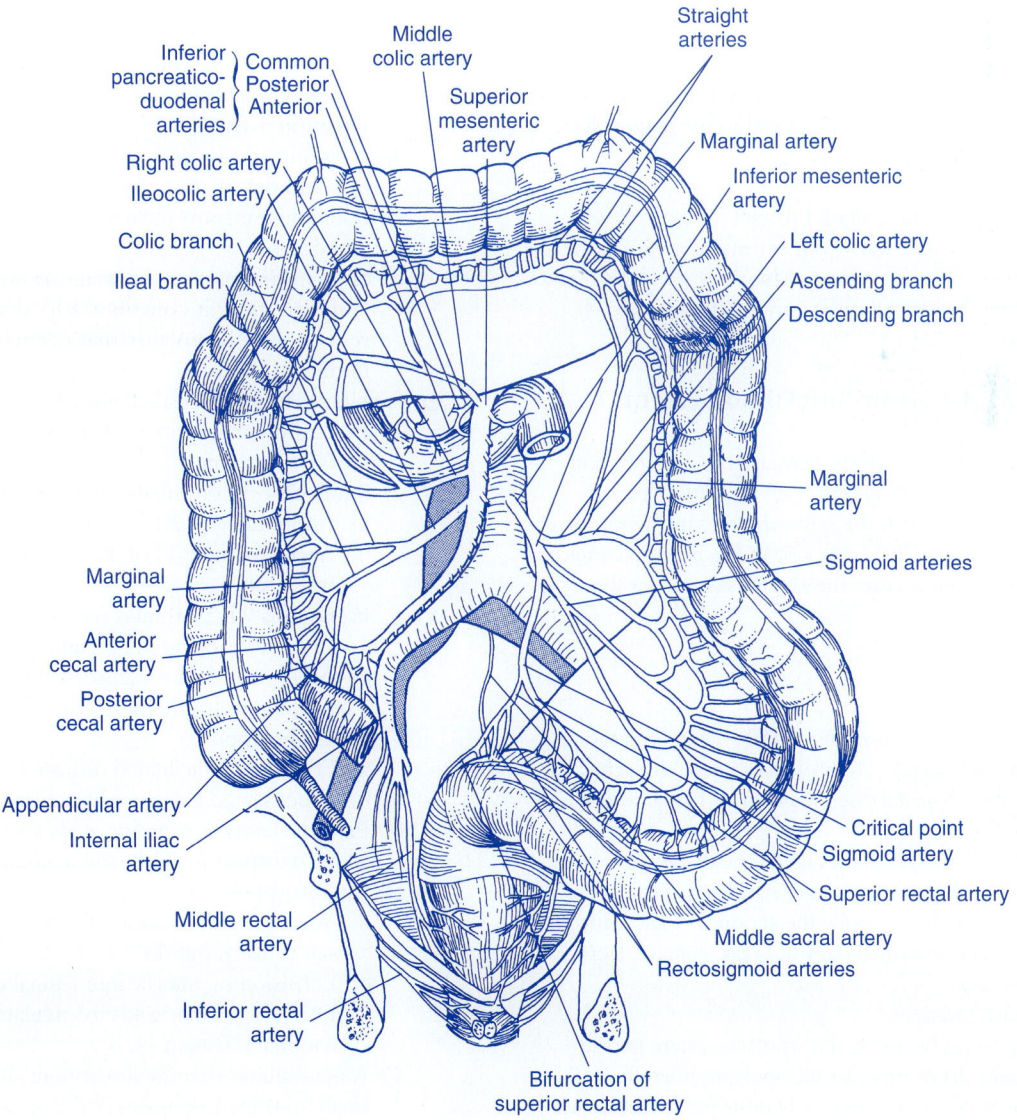

Fig. 7.9 Arterial blood supply of the gastrointestinal system. (From Society of Gastroenterology Nurses and Associates SGNA [1993]. *Gastroenterology nursing: A core curriculum.* St Louis: Mosby.)

b. Superior mesenteric arteries supply the following:
   1) Jejunum
   2) Ileum
   3) Cecum
   4) Ascending colon
   5) Part of transverse colon
c. Inferior mesenteric arteries supply the following:
   1) Transverse, descending, and sigmoid colon
   2) Rectum
d. Hepatic artery and vein supply the liver.
2. Venous
   a. Portal vein collects and delivers blood from entire venous drainage of GI tract to liver; branches: gastric; splenic; superior mesenteric; inferior mesenteric
   b. Portal vein subdivides into liver sinusoids, which then unite with branches from hepatic artery to form hepatic vein, which empties into inferior vena cava
   c. Partially metabolized digestive products are brought to liver sinusoids, where hepatocytes complete the next stage of metabolism.

Nervous Innervation

1. Extrinsic
   a. PNS: increases the activity of the GI tract; innervated via the vagus nerve
   b. SNS: decreases the activity of the GI tract; innervated via SNS fibers, which run parallel to the major blood vessels of the GI tract
2. Intrinsic
   a. Located inside the wall of GI tract
   b. Consists of extensions from extrinsic nerves of the autonomic nervous system (ANS)
   c. Form two major and three minor networks of plexuses

Functions of the Gastrointestinal System

1. Ingestion
   a. Ingestion begins with the sensation of hunger, controlled by the feeding center of the hypothalamus.
   b. Ingestion ends with the sensation of satisfaction provided by the satiety center also in the hypothalamus.
   c. Food and liquids enter the alimentary tract at the mouth.
2. Secretion: Table 7.1.
3. Digestion
   a. CHO: 4 kcal/g
      1) Digestion begins in the mouth, where polysaccharides (starch) are broken down to disaccharides (e.g., sucrose, lactose, maltose) by the action of ptyalin (amylase).
      2) The process continues when the disaccharides are broken down to monosaccharides (e.g., glucose, galactose, fructose) by the action of pancreatic amylase and intestinal enzymes (e.g., sucrase, lactase, maltase).
   b. Proteins: 4 kcal/g
      1) Digestion begins in the stomach, where pepsin breaks down proteins into polypeptides.
      2) The process continues when the polypeptides are broken down into peptides and amino acids in the small intestine by the action of trypsin, chymotrypsin, carboxypeptides from the pancreas, and aminopeptidases and dipeptidase from the intestinal villi.
   c. Fats: 9 kcal/g
      1) Digestion of fats that are already emulsified (e.g., cream and butter) begins in the stomach by lipase.
      2) Digestion of nonemulsified fat occurs in the small intestine with emulsification of the fat by bile and pancreatic lipase.
      3) Fat is broken down into glycerol and fatty acids.
4. Absorption
   a. Basic absorption mechanisms
      1) Active transport requires an energy source (e.g., adenosine triphosphate) to move substances into and out of the cell; substances absorbed by active transport include proteins, glucose, sodium, and potassium.
      2) Passive diffusion is passive movement from an area of high solute concentration to an area of low solute concentration; substances absorbed by passive diffusion include free fatty acids and water.
      3) Facilitated diffusion is movement that requires a carrier that moves into the cell, but energy is not required; a substance absorbed by facilitated diffusion is fructose.
      4) Nonionic transport is movement of solutes freely into and out of the cell; substances absorbed by nonionic transport include unconjugated bile salts and drugs.
      5) Solvent drag is flow of water to higher osmotic concentration; it contributes to absorption and reduction in osmolality that occurs in the jejunum.
   b. Specific absorption in small intestine
      1) Electrolyte absorption: active transport from all areas of intestine
      2) Water absorption: small and large intestine
         a) Approximately 2 l of fluid is ingested daily.
         b) Approximately 7 l of fluid is secreted by the GI tract daily.
         c) Of this 9 l, 7500 ml is reabsorbed with only 1500 ml reaching the cecum.
         d) Additional fluid is reabsorbed in the large intestine, but only 200 ml is lost in the stool.
      3) CHO absorption
         a) Fructose by facilitated diffusion
         b) Glucose and galactose by active transport
      4) Protein absorption: amino acids absorbed by active transport in ileum and jejunum
      5) Fat absorption
         a) Micellar solubilization of fatty acid with bile salt to form micelle
         b) Diffusion of micelle into jejunal cell
         c) Delivery of fatty acids to circulation via lymphatic system
      6) Water-soluble vitamin absorption: all areas of small intestine by passive diffusion (absorption of vitamin B_{12} requires intrinsic factor)

7) Fat-soluble vitamin absorbed in jejunum; bile salts required
8) Calcium absorption mainly in duodenum; vitamin D required
9) Iron absorption by active transport all areas of the intestine but especially in duodenum; stored as protein-bound iron
5. Synthesis
   a. Bacteria in the large intestine produce vitamin K.
   b. Peyer patches in the small intestine play a role in antibody synthesis.
6. Effect on fluid and electrolyte balance
   a. Gastric losses are acidic; increased gastric losses (e.g., nasogastric [NG] suction, vomiting) cause metabolic alkalosis, hypokalemia, hyponatremia, and hypovolemia.
   b. Intestinal losses are alkaline: Increased intestinal losses (e.g., biliary losses, pancreatic fistula, intestinal suction, diarrhea) cause metabolic acidosis, hypokalemia, hyponatremia, and hypovolemia.

Assessment of the Gastrointestinal System

Interview

1. Chief complaint: why the patient is seeking help and duration of the problem
   a. Nonspecific problems or complaints
      1) Change in appetite
      2) Fatigue or weakness
      3) Unintentional weight loss or weight gain
      4) Fever and chills
   b. Abdominal pain: describe PQRST (Table 7.4)
      1) Provocation: relationship to food, drugs, activity, position, bowel movements, breathing, and stress
      2) Palliation
         a) Ineffective or effective treatments
         b) Alleviating factors (e.g., position)
      3) Quality: sharp, dull, tearing, cramping, burning, gnawing, stabbing, aching, colicky
         a) Visceral pain
            i) Dull, poorly localized
            ii) May be caused by organic lesions or functional disturbance within the GI tract
         b) Somatic pain
            i) Sharp, well localized
            ii) May be caused by inflammation of abdominal organs which causes peritoneal irritation
         c) Referred pain
            i) Pain experienced at a distance from the disease process
            ii) May be explained by the embryologic origins of the structures involved
      4) Region: location
         a) May be poorly localized
         b) May be referred pain
            i) Pain may be felt in a remote area that is supplied by the same nerve as the diseased or damaged organ.
            ii) The pain is usually sharp and localized but not over area of injury.
      5) Radiation
      6) Severity: 0 to 10 scale
      7) Timing: constant, intermittent; duration
   c. Abdominal distention
      1) Bloating (i.e., subjective feeling of abdominal fullness) versus distention (i.e., objective increase in abdominal girth)
      2) Abdominal volume must be increased by at least 1 l for physical enlargement to occur.
   d. Change in bowel elimination
      1) Change in color of stools
         a) Clay-colored stools indicate biliary obstruction.
         b) Tarry stools (melena) indicate upper GI bleeding.
         c) Bloody stools (hematochezia) indicate lower GI bleeding.
      2) Change in consistency or shape of stools
         a) Flattened on one side may indicate partial obstruction.
      3) Change in frequency of stools
      4) Excessive flatus
      5) Use of laxative or enemas
      6) Relationship to food, drugs, and alcohol
   e. Nausea or vomiting
      1) Onset and duration
      2) Frequency
      3) Character and color; presence of blood in vomitus (hematemesis)
      4) Palliation
         a) Ineffective or effective treatment
         b) Alleviating factors
      5) Timing
         a) Time of day
         b) Relationship to food, odors, drugs, alcohol, activity, bowel movements
      6) Aggravating factors
      7) Associated pain
   f. Abdominal trauma
      1) Gunshot entrance and exit wound
      2) Knife wounds
      3) Burns or abrasions
      4) Ecchymotic areas associated with blunt trauma
   g. Dentition problems
      1) Caries
      2) Gingivitis
      3) Poor-fitting dentures
   h. Odynophagia (i.e., painful swallowing)
   i. Dysphagia (i.e., difficulty swallowing)
   j. Dyspepsia (i.e., impaired digestion): may be manifested by indigestion, nausea, abdominal pain, bloating, belching, or early satiety
   k. Eructation (i.e., belching)
   l. Flatulence
   m. Edema
   n. Abnormal bruising or bleeding
   o. Jaundice
   p. Change in color of urine: dark brown or orange urine may indicate biliary obstruction
   q. Pruritus
   r. Fecal incontinence
   s. Rectal bleeding
   t. Anal discomfort or pressure

Table 7.4 Differentiation of Abdominal Pain

Condition	Description of Pain	Associated Signs and Symptoms
Abdominal aortic aneurysm	• Abdominal • Ripping or tearing • May radiate to back	• Pulsatile mass in abdomen • If ruptured, clinical indications of hypoperfusion and shock
Appendicitis	• Epigastric or periumbilical pain; later localizes to RLQ • Dull to sharp • May be referred to right shoulder • McBurney sign: pain with palpation at McBurney's point (i.e., point at ⅓ the distance between the right anterior iliac crest and the umbilicus) • Rovsing's sign: pain in RLQ with palpation of LLQ indicates peritoneal irritation • Iliopsoas sign: abdominal pain caused by hyperextension of right hip	• Anorexia, nausea, vomiting • Fever • Diarrhea • Leukocytosis • Clinical indications of peritoneal irritation if ruptured
Cholecystitis	• Epigastric or RUQ • Cramping • May be referred to below right scapula • Murphy sign: pain with deep breath while the nurse palpates under the right costal margin	• Nausea and vomiting especially after fatty foods • Abdominal tenderness in RUQ • Leukocytosis
Diverticulitis	• LUQ • Cramping • Tenderness over descending colon	• Vomiting, diarrhea • Fever, chills • Bloating
Gastritis	• Epigastric or slightly left of midline • May be described as indigestion	• Nausea and vomiting • May have hematemesis • Abdominal tenderness
Intestinal obstruction	• Epigastric or periumbilical • Sharp if small intestine; dull if large intestine	• Change in bowel habits • Melena or hematochezia • Hyperactive to hypoactive bowel sounds
Mesenteric ischemia	• Diffuse midabdominal • Severe	• Nausea and vomiting may occur • Diarrhea or constipation
Pancreatitis	• Epigastric or periumbilical LUQ • Boring; worsened by lying down • May be referred to back, left flank, or left shoulder	• Nausea and vomiting • Mild fever • Abdominal tenderness • May have Cullen sign (i.e., bluish discoloration at umbilicus) indicating intraperitoneal bleeding or Grey Turner sign (i.e., bluish discoloration at flanks) indicating retroperitoneal bleeding • May be jaundiced
Peptic ulcer	• Epigastric or RUQ • Gnawing or burning • May be referred to back	• Abdominal tenderness • Hematemesis (gastric) or melena (duodenal) • Clinical indications of peritoneal irritation if perforated
Strangulated hernia	• Localized • Severe • Generalized if bowel obstruction	• Distention if bowel obstruction

LLQ, Left lower quadrant; *LUQ*, left upper quadrant; *RLQ*, right lower quadrant; *RUQ*, right upper quadrant.

2. History of present illness: Use PQRST format.
3. Past medical history
   a. Past illnesses
      1) Gastroesophageal reflux disease (GERD)
      2) Jaundice
      3) Anemia
      4) Obesity: use of liquid diets, GI bypass, gastric balloon, and so on
      5) Eating disorders (e.g., bulimia, anorexia nervosa)
      6) Substance abuse
         a) Alcohol
         b) Drug abuse
         c) Chronic drug use of potentially hepatotoxic agents such as acetaminophen
      7) Peptic ulcer disease
      8) GI hemorrhage
      9) Cholelithiasis
      10) Hepatic disease
         a) Cirrhosis
         b) Hepatitis
         c) History of blood transfusion
      11) Pancreatitis
      12) Cancer
      13) Irritable bowel syndrome

14) Inflammatory bowel disease (e.g., ulcerative colitis, Crohn disease, antibiotic-associated colitis, *Clostridium difficile* colitis)
15) Diverticulitis
16) Polyps
17) Hemorrhoids
18) Renal disease
19) Cardiovascular disease
20) Diabetes mellitus
21) Chronic obstructive pulmonary disease (COPD) (high incidence of peptic ulcer disease)
   b. Past injury: abdominal trauma
   c. Past surgical procedures
   d. Past diagnostic studies (e.g., endoscopy, radiography, stool examination for occult blood)
   e. Food intolerances or allergies; type of reaction if allergy
4. Family history
   a. Eating disorders (e.g., obesity, anorexia nervosa, bulimia)
   b. Anemia
   c. Peptic ulcer disease
   d. Pancreatic disease (e.g., pancreatitis, pancreatic cancer)
   e. Diabetes mellitus
   f. Liver disease (e.g., cirrhosis, hepatitis)
   g. Malabsorption syndrome
   h. Inflammatory bowel disease (e.g., ulcerative colitis, Crohn disease)
   i. Irritable bowel syndrome
   j. Alcoholism
   k. Cancer
5. Social history
   a. Relationship with spouse or significant other; family structure
   b. Occupation
   c. Educational level
   d. Stress level and usual coping mechanisms
   e. Recreational habits
   f. Exercise habits
   g. Dietary habits
      1) Appetite
      2) Usual foods
      3) Number and time of meals and snacks
      4) Fluid intake
      5) Food restrictions
         a) Intolerances
         b) Prescribed restrictions
         c) Religious restrictions
      6) Change in eating habits
   h. Usual bowel habits
   i. Caffeine intake
   j. Tobacco use: Record as pack-years (number of packs per day times the number of years of smoking).
   k. Alcohol use: Record as alcoholic beverages consumed per month, week, or day.
   l. Exposure to toxins or infectious disease
   m. Travel
6. Medication history
   a. Prescribed drugs, dose, frequency, time of last dose
   b. Nonprescribed drugs
      1) Over-the-counter drugs, including herbal drugs and remedies
      2) Substance abuse
   c. Patient understanding of drug actions and side effects
   d. Drugs causing potential problems for patients with GI problems
      1) Antibiotics
      2) Aspirin
      3) Nonsteroidal antiinflammatory drugs (NSAIDs) (e.g., ketorolac [Toradol], ibuprofen [Motrin])
      4) Corticosteroids
      5) Acetaminophen (Tylenol)
      6) Many drugs have anorexia, nausea, or vomiting as side effects
      7) Many drugs are hepatotoxic (Box 7.1).
   e. Drugs frequently used for GI problems
      1) Antacids, H_2 receptor antagonists, proton pump inhibitors
      2) Stool softeners
      3) Laxatives
      4) Cathartics
      5) Anticholinergics
      6) Corticosteroids
      7) Antidiarrheals
      8) Antiemetics
      9) Tranquilizers
      10) Sedatives
      11) Barbiturates

Vital Signs
1. Blood pressure (BP):
   a. sitting, lying, standing, especially in hemorrhaging patient;
   b. systolic BP less than 100 mm Hg and heart rate (HR) greater than 100 beats/min indicates at least a 20% reduction in blood volume
2. HR
3. Respiratory rate
4. Temperature
5. Height
6. Weight
7. Body mass index (BMI): takes into account not just weight but also height to indicate body fat; goal for most people is a BMI of 18 to 25

Inspection
1. Landmarks (Fig. 7.10)
   a. Xiphoid
   b. Costal margin
   c. Midline
   d. Umbilicus
   e. Anterior superior iliac crest
   f. Symphysis pubis
   g. The abdomen may be divided into:
      1) Four quadrants (Fig. 7.11): Horizontal and vertical lines intersect at the umbilicus.
      2) Nine regions (Fig. 7.12)
2. General survey
   a. Apparent health status
   b. Apparent age relative to chronological age
   c. Level of consciousness
   d. Gross deformity
   e. Nutritional status
   f. Stature or posture
      1) Patient flexing his or her knees to relieve abdominal tension is frequently seen in peritonitis.

Box 7.1 Hepatotoxic Agents

6-Mercaptopurine
Acetaminophen
Acetylsalicylic acid (ASA)
Allopurinol
Amiodarone
Amitriptyline
Ampicillin
Carbamazepine
Carbon tetrachloride
Chlorambucil
Chloramphenicol
Chlordiazepoxide
Chlorpromazine
Chlorpropamide
Cimetidine
Clindamycin
Cyclosporine
Dantrolene
Diazepam
Doxepin
Erythromycin estolate
Ethanol
Ethrane
Ferrous sulfate
Fluothane
Haloperidol
Halothane
Hydrochlorothiazide
Imipramine
Indomethacin
Isoniazid
Ketoconazole
Meprobamate
Methotrexate
Methyldopa
Monoamine oxidase (MAO) inhibitors
Nicotinic acid
Oral contraceptives
Oxacillin
Penicillin
Penthrane
Phenazopyridine
Phenobarbital
Phenylbutazone
Phenytoin
Probenecid
Prochlorperazine
Promethazine
Propoxyphene
Propylthiouracil (PTU)
Quinidine
Rifampin
Sulfonamides
Tetracyclines
Tolbutamide
Trimethobenzamide
Tripelennamine

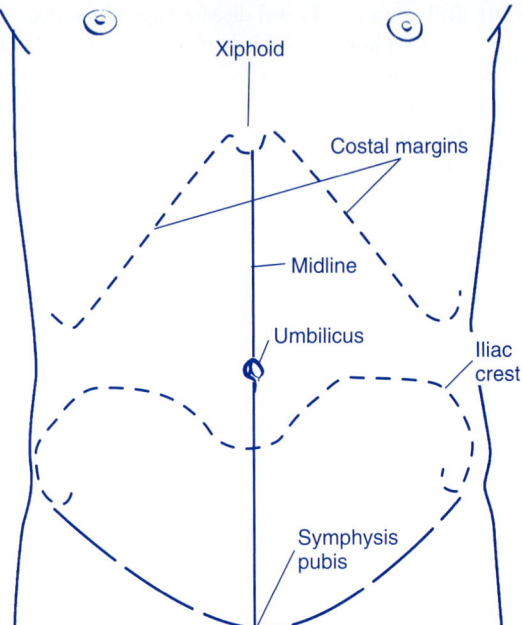

Fig. 7.10 Landmarks of the abdomen.

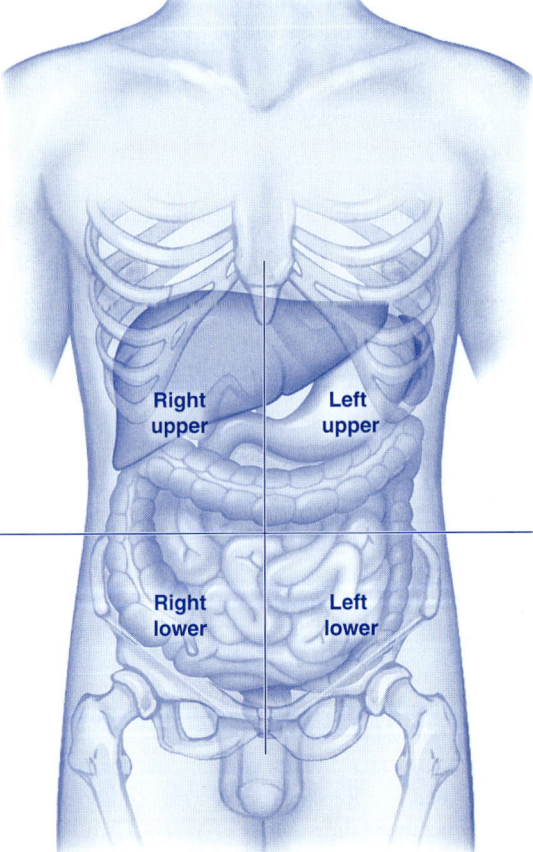

Fig. 7.11 The abdomen divided into four quadrants: right upper quadrant (RUQ), left upper quadrant (LUQ), right lower quadrant (RLQ), and left lower quadrant (LLQ). (From Patton, K. T., & Thibodeau, G. A. [2013]. *Anatomy & physiology* [8th ed.]. St Louis: Mosby.)

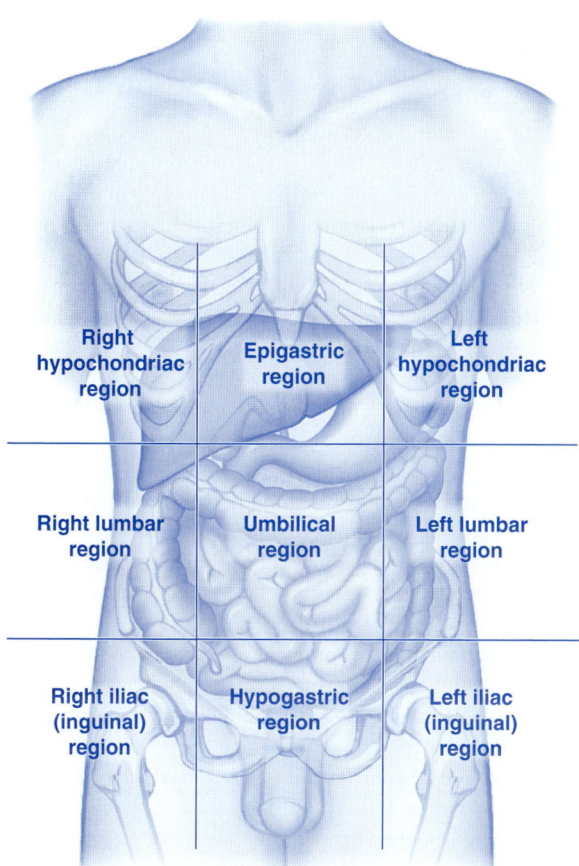

Fig. 7.12 The abdomen divided into nine regions: epigastric, umbilical, hypogastric, right and left hypochondriac, right and left lumbar, and right and left iliac (inguinal). (From Patton, K. T., & Thibodeau, G. A. [2013]. *Anatomy & physiology* [8th ed.]. St Louis: Mosby.)

2) Patient leaning forward to relieve abdominal pain is frequently seen in pancreatitis.
   g. Gait
3. Mouth
   a. Lips: color; texture; lesions; swelling; symmetry
   b. Gums: inflammation; retraction; hypertrophy; bleeding; lesions
   c. Teeth: caries; state of repair; occlusion; dentures: fit; gum ulceration caused by ill-fitting dentures
   d. Tongue: swelling; laceration; lesions; coating
   e. Mucosa: moisture; lesions; color
   f. Odor
      1) Fetor hepaticus: sweet fecal odor caused by hepatic failure
      2) Feculent breath: foul fecal odor caused by severe bowel obstruction
      3) Severe halitosis: foul odor may be caused by poor dental hygiene or neoplasms of esophagus or stomach
4. Skin
   a. Color: should be homogeneous over the entire abdomen
      1) Pallor: anemia
      2) Jaundice: occurs when bilirubin is greater than 3 mg/dl; associated with any of the following:
         a) Liver disease
         b) Biliary obstruction
         c) Excessive hemolysis
      3) Bluish: due to infiltration of the abdominal wall with blood
         a) Location
            i) Grey Turner sign: ecchymosis to flanks indicative of retroperitoneal bleeding (e.g., from pancreas, duodenum, kidneys, vena cava, aorta)
            ii) Cullen sign: ecchymosis around umbilicus indicative of intraperitoneal bleeding (e.g., liver or spleen)
         b) Causes
            i) Hemorrhagic pancreatitis
            ii) Infarcted bowel
            iii) Ruptured ectopic pregnancy
   b. Lesions or discoloration
      1) Scars: trauma or surgical procedures
      2) Striae
         a) Usually vertical
         b) Initially pinkish or bluish, become silvery with time
         c) May be caused by pregnancy, obesity, or ascites
         d) Purplish striae may be caused by Cushing syndrome
      3) Rash
      4) Ecchymosis
      5) Abrasions
      6) Spider angioma: may be associated with
         a) Vitamin B_{12} deficiency
         b) Liver disease
         c) Pregnancy
      7) Palmar erythema: seen in cirrhosis and hepatic failure
   c. Shiny, edematous abdomen
      1) Ascites: intraperitoneal fluid frequently associated with cirrhosis, intraabdominal malignancy (e.g., liver, ovarian), or right ventricular failure
      2) Anasarca: entire body edema, which may be seen in end-stage heart failure or renal failure
   d. Superficial vascularity
      1) May be caused by obstruction of inferior vena cava or portal vein
      2) Caput medusae: pronounced dilation of the periumbilical veins radiating from the umbilicus; seen in severe portal venous hypertension
   e. Stoma: location; color; drainage; condition of peristomal skin
   f. Draining wounds: location; drainage; condition of surrounding skin
   g. Fistula: location; drainage; condition of surrounding skin
5. Contour of abdomen
   a. Profile
      1) Normal: flat from xiphoid process to pubic symphysis

2) Scaffold: concave abdomen seen in malnutrition
3) Distention or protuberance
   a) Diffuse and symmetrical
      i) Fat
      ii) Flatus
      iii) Fetus (i.e., pregnancy)
      iv) Feces (i.e., obstruction)
      v) Fluid (i.e., ascites)
      vi) Fatal growths (i.e., malignancy)
      vii) Fibroids
   b) Distention in upper quadrants: gastric dilation; pancreatic cyst, malignancy
   c) Distention in lower quadrants: pregnancy; uterine fibroid; distended bladder; ovarian tumor
   d) Distention in one quadrant: hernia; tumor; cyst; obstruction; organomegaly
6. Abdominal girth
   a. Measure abdominal girth at largest area.
   b. Mark on either side of tape measure so that measurements are consistently at same location.
   c. One-inch increase is equal to an increase in intraabdominal volume of 500 to 1000 ml.
7. Weakness of abdominal wall
   a. Diastasis recti abdominis: abnormal separation of the two abdominal rectus muscles when the patient tenses abdominal muscles by raising his or her head from the bed
   b. Hernia: abdominal, umbilical, or inguinal
8. Movement of abdomen
   a. Breathing: normal
      1) Women generally breathe thoracically when upright.
      2) Both men and women generally breathe abdominally when supine.
   b. Peristalsis: abnormal to see waves of peristalsis across the abdomen: generally associated with intestinal obstruction
   c. Aortic pulsation: normally visible at the end of expiration in a supine patient especially if patient is thin; pulsatile swelling in the epigastrium suggests an abdominal aortic aneurysm or an epigastric solid tumor overlying the aorta
9. Umbilicus
   a. Color
      1) Bluish (Cullen sign): caused by infiltration of the abdominal wall with blood
      2) Inflammation: may be seen with poor hygiene
   b. Contour
      1) Deeply inverted: obesity
      2) Everted: pregnancy or ascites
      3) Nodular (Sister Mary Joseph nodule): may indicate intraabdominal carcinoma (especially stomach) with metastasis to the navel

Auscultation
1. Auscultation is done before percussion or palpation to prevent "stirring up" the abdomen; therefore, order for physical assessment of the abdomen is inspection, auscultation, percussion, and palpation.
2. Preparation: may be helpful to put pillow under knees to relax abdominal muscles
3. Bowel sounds
   a. Method
      1) Use diaphragm with light pressure for 1 minute in each of the four abdominal quadrants.
      2) Disconnect NG suction.
      3) If bowel sounds are hypoactive, 5 minutes of auscultation without audible bowel sounds is required before documenting the absence of bowel sounds.
   b. Normal bowel sounds: bubbling or soft gurgling noises heard every 5 to 20 seconds in an irregular pattern; heard in all quadrants
      1) Return of bowel motility after surgery
         a) Small intestine: 4 to 24 hours
         b) Stomach: 2 to 4 days
         c) Colon: 3 to 7 days
      2) Feeding before return of bowel sounds after surgery is now considered safe.
      3) Bowel sounds are not considered an indication of feeding tolerance.
   c. Abnormal bowel sounds
      1) Very infrequent or absent bowel sounds
         a) Functional obstruction: paralytic ileus
         b) Advanced mechanical intestinal obstruction
      2) Loud, hyperactive (but normal pitched) bowel sounds: hyperperistalsis (e.g., diarrhea, catharsis caused by GI bleeding)
      3) High-pitched "rushing" bowel sounds: early mechanical small intestinal obstruction
      4) Low-pitched "rushing" bowel sounds: early mechanical large intestinal obstruction
4. Succussion splash: roll patient side to side while listening over left upper quadrant; indicative of pyloric obstruction
5. Vascular sounds
   a. Method. Use bell over specified areas.
   b. Bruits
      1) Listen over midline and renal and femoral arteries.
      2) If bruit is noted, check circulation to extremities; if decreased blood flow is noted, aneurysm should be suspected.
         a) Notify physician.
         b) Keep patient quiet.
         c) Do not palpate abdomen.
   c. Venous hum: hum of medium tone created by blood flow in a large, engorged vascular organ such as liver or spleen
6. Peritoneal friction rub: scratchy sound heard over inflamed spleen or neoplastic liver

Percussion
1. Percussion tones normally heard over abdomen
   a. Dull: liver, full sigmoid colon, full bladder
   b. Flat: bone
   c. Tympany: gastric bubble, bowel
2. Tests for ascites
   a. Fluid wave: Tap one side of the abdomen and feel for the wave to hit the hand on other side of abdomen; have a colleague or the patient place the ulnar surface of his or her hand at the abdomen's midline to stop skin transmission.

b. Shifting dullness: Percuss dullness indicating fluid at flanks while patient is supine, mark fluid level, turn patient on one side, and note shift of dullness line.
  c. Midline dullness: Dullness at midline with the patient is leaning forward in a standing position indicates intraabdominal fluid.
3. Organ borders
  a. Liver
    1) Dullness between right lung resonance and bowel tympany
    2) Normal span, 6 to 12 cm in the right midclavicular line
    3) Enlarged and tender in right ventricular failure (RVF), hepatitis, and mononucleosis
    4) May be large or small in cirrhosis
    5) Absence of liver dullness: may indicate free air in peritoneum from bowel perforation
  b. Spleen
    1) Dullness under left diaphragm
    2) If percussible, should be less than 7 cm at the left midaxillary line
  c. Stomach: tympany under left costal margin
  d. Bladder
    1) Dullness above symphysis pubis
    2) Percussible only if enlarged
  e. Intestine
    1) Tympany over abdomen
    2) May percuss dullness over left lower quadrant (LLQ) if sigmoid colon is full

Palpation

1. Method
  a. Warm hands.
  b. Examine each quadrant.
  c. Always palpate tender areas last.
  d. Carry on conversation with patient to keep him or her (and the abdominal muscles) relaxed and place a pillow under the knees and a pillow under the head.
2. Light palpation: use fingertips to depress 1 to 2 cm; note the following:
  a. Temperature
  b. Moisture
  c. Superficial skin reflexes: movement of the umbilicus toward the quadrant that is stroked
  d. Voluntary guarding
    1) Patient may voluntarily splint abdominal muscles, especially when sensitive spot is touched; watch for nonverbal indicators of pain during palpation.
  e. Involuntary guarding or rigidity
    1) Diffuse rigidity suggests an infectious, neoplastic, or inflammatory process in the peritoneal cavity.
    2) Rigid, boardlike abdomen is associated with acute perforation of a viscus with spillage of air or GI contents into the peritoneal cavity.
  f. Tender areas
  g. Large masses
    1) If mass is pulsatile, refrain from additional abdominal palpation because it may be an abdominal aortic aneurysm.
    2) If mass is not pulsatile, describe the following:
      a) Size
      b) Location
      c) Consistency
      d) Contour
      e) Tenderness
      f) Mobility
3. Deep palpation: Use one hand on top of the other to depress 4 to 5 cm.
  a. Do not use deep palpation in the following situations:
    1) Polycystic kidneys
    2) After renal transplant
    3) Malignant tumor: may cause seeding
    4) Recent surgery
  b. Note the following:
    1) Direct tenderness
      a) Associated with local inflammation of the abdominal wall, the peritoneum, or a viscus
    2) Rebound (or indirect) tenderness (also referred to as *Blumberg sign*)
      a) Performed by pressing into the tender area and then letting go
      b) If the pain is exacerbated when pressure is released, rebound tenderness is present, and peritoneal inflammation is suspected.
      c) Rebound tenderness is especially significant when it occurs at a site away from the area of direct tenderness.
    3) Organ size
      a) Liver edge: may be palpable
        i) Ask patient to take a deep breath; move hand in and up to check for tenderness, smoothness of edge.
          (a) Tenderness is frequently caused by hepatitis or engorgement caused by right ventricular failure.
          (b) A hard, lumpy liver is associated with cancer or cirrhosis.
        ii) A normal sized liver may be palpable especially in patients with COPD caused by hyperinflation of lungs; hepatomegaly exists only if liver span by percussion is greater than 12 cm.
      b) Gallbladder: palpable only if enlarged with stones; if palpable, located under liver edge in right upper quadrant
    4) Splenic tenderness
      a) Palpate left side of abdomen with patient in lateral decubitus position.
      b) Note any tenderness.
      c) Spleen is palpable only if significantly enlarged (e.g., injury, leukemia, mononucleosis, portal hypertension).
    5) Aortic pulsation: Check for lateral expansion, which may indicate an aneurysm.
4. Ballottement
  a. Gentle repetitive bouncing of tissues against the hand
  b. May be used to evaluate organ enlargement

Intraabdominal Pressure

1. Definitions
   a. Intraabdominal pressure (IAP): the pressure within the abdominal cavity
      1) Normal IAP is ~5 to 7 mm Hg
      2) Variations in IAP
         a) Position changes
         b) Obesity
         c) Breathing, mechanical ventilation, positive end-expiratory pressure
   b. Abdominal perfusion pressure: difference between the mean arterial pressure (MAP) and the IAP; greater than 60 mm Hg is desirable
   c. Intraabdominal hypertension (IAH): sustained or repeated elevation of IAP greater than or equal to 12 mm Hg
      1) Grade I: 12 to 15 mm Hg
      2) Grade II: 16 to 20 mm Hg
      3) Grade III: 21 to 25 mm Hg
      4) Grade IV: greater than 25 mm Hg
   d. Abdominal compartment syndrome (ACS): sustained intracranial pressure (ICP) greater than 20 mm Hg that is associated with new organ dysfunction or failure
      1) Primary: condition associated with injury or disease in the abdominal-pelvic region
      2) Secondary: condition that does not originate from the abdominal-pelvic region
      3) Recurrent: condition in which ACS redevelops after previous surgical or medical treatment of primary or secondary ACS
2. Methods of measurement
   a. Assist with placement of an access for measuring IAP
      1) Via a catheter (e.g., peritoneal dialysis catheter) inserted into peritoneal cavity and attached to a transducer
      2) Via a catheter inserted into the sample port of an indwelling urinary catheter and attached to a transducer (Fig. 7.13)
         a) Accuracy of this method is affected by neurogenic bladder, abdominal packing, elevation of the head of the bed, pelvic fracture or hematoma, and intraperitoneal adhesions.
   b. Attach a pressure monitoring system with the air-fluid interface of the transducer leveled to the midaxillary line at the iliac crest (Gallagher, 2010).
   c. Place the patient in supine position.
   d. After drainage of the bladder, remove air from the system and then instill 25 ml of isotonic sterile saline into the bladder.
   e. Allow 30 to 60 seconds equilibration time after instillation of saline before measurement of pressure.
   f. Measure the pressure at end-expiration.
3. Conditions associated with risk for intraabdominal hypertension and abdominal compartment syndrome include the following:
   a. Conditions that cause an increase in intraabdominal volume
      1) Intraabdominal or retroperitoneal masses
      2) Ascites or hemoperitoneum
      3) Pneumoperitoneum (e.g., laparoscopic procedures)
      4) GI tract dilation (e.g., gastroparesis, ileus, volvulus, intestinal obstruction)
      5) Abdominal or pelvic trauma
         a) Pelvic fractures
         b) Intraperitoneal or retroperitoneal hemorrhage or hematoma
         c) Visceral edema due to ischemia and/or massive fluid resuscitation
      6) Use of military antishock trousers or pneumatic antishock garments

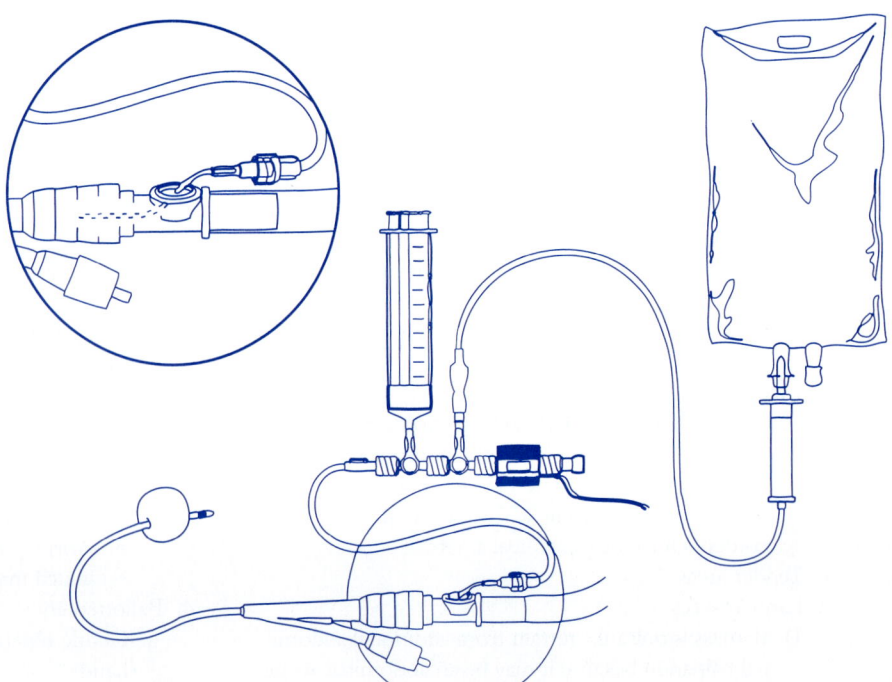

Fig. 7.13 Measurement of intraabdominal pressure using an intravenous catheter into the specimen port of the urinary drainage tubing. (From Cheatham, M. L. [1999]. Intra-abdominal hypertension and abdominal compartment syndrome. *New Horizons, 7*[1], 96-115.)

b. Conditions that decrease abdominal wall compliance
   1) Abdominal surgery
   2) Abdominal wall bleeding
c. Conditions that affect both intraabdominal volume and abdominal wall compliance
   1) Obesity
   2) Sepsis, severe sepsis, septic shock
   3) Acute pancreatitis
   4) Massive fluid resuscitation
   5) Major burns
   6) Liver or kidney transplantation
4. Clinical implications
   a. A critical level of IAH has not been established; an IAP of 25 mm Hg has been traditionally considered a critical value, although levels as low as 10 mm Hg may cause organ dysfunction.
   b. There is a volume-pressure curve. The abdominal wall can compensate for increases in intraabdominal volume up to a point; then any additional increase in intraabdominal volume results in a rapid increase in IAP and compromised organ perfusion.
   c. Pathophysiologic consequences of intraabdominal hypertension
      1) Cardiovascular
         a) Increased HR
         b) Increased central venous pressure (CVP), PAP, PAOP
         c) Increased systemic vascular resistance (SVR)
         d) Decreased cardiac output or cardiac index
         e) Decreased venous return from extremities
      2) Pulmonary
         a) Increased respiratory rate
         b) Decreased tidal volume, increased $PaCO_2$, decreased PaO_2, SaO_2
         c) Decreased compliance: increased intrathoracic pressure; increased peak inspiratory pressure
         d) Increased intraalveolar fluid
         e) Increased risk of compression atelectasis
      3) Neurologic
         a) Increased ICP
         b) Decreased cerebral perfusion pressure (CPP)
      4) Renal
         a) Decreased glomerular filtration rate and urine output
         b) Urethral compression
      5) GI
         a) Decreased portal, celiac, and mesenteric blood flow
            i) Severe mesenteric ischemia may occur and lead to multiple organ dysfunction syndrome (MODS).
         b) Increased intestinal permeability and bacterial translocation that increase risk of sepsis
         c) Increased risk of peptic ulcer
      6) Immunology: release of proinflammatory cytokines that may lead to systemic inflammatory response syndrome (SIRS) and MODS
      7) Elevated serum lactate, metabolic acidosis
5. Treatment of intraabdominal hypertension and abdominal compartment syndrome
   a. Measure IAP at least every 2 to 4 hours in patients at risk for IAH; continuous monitoring is indicated for high-risk patients; titrate therapy to maintain IAP less than 15 mm Hg.
   b. Optimize hydration status and avoid excessive fluids.
      1) Hypertonic crystalloids, colloids, or both to allow expansion of vascular volume without excessive fluid volume
      2) Diuresis, dialysis, and/or ultrafiltration as indicated
      3) Hemodynamic monitoring is recommended to guide fluid administration.
   c. Improve abdominal wall compliance.
      1) Head-of-bed (HOB) elevation at 20 degrees between pressure readings
         a) Avoid prone positioning.
         b) Consider reverse Trendelenburg position.
      2) Encouragement to take deep breaths to prevent atelectasis and facilitate venous return to the heart
      3) Sedation and analgesia; neuromuscular blockade may be considered
      4) Removal of constrictive dressing, binders, eschar
   d. Decompress the GI tract as prescribed
      1) Gastric and/or rectal tube
      2) Prokinetic agents (e.g., metoclopramide, erythromycin)
      3) Slowing or discontinuance of enteral nutrition
      4) Enemas
      5) Colonoscopic decompression
   e. Evaluate and eliminate intraabdominal space-occupying lesions
      1) Abdominal ultrasonography or computed tomography (CT) scan
      2) Paracentesis if free fluid is cause
      3) Surgical evacuation of hematoma, mass lesion, and so on
   f. Optimize perfusion
      1) Goal-directed fluid resuscitation
      2) Maintenance of abdominal perfusion pressure greater than or equal to 60 mm Hg; fluids, inotropic agents, and/or vasopressors may be necessary
   g. Prepare the patient for decompression laparotomy as requested in symptomatic patients with IAP of greater than or equal to 25 mm Hg or greater than 15 mm Hg with evidence of organ ischemia.
      1) Surgical approach is most commonly a full midline laparotomy from xiphoid to pubis.
         a) Less invasive procedures such as a subcutaneous linea alba fasciotomy may be used.
      2) Excess fluid, blood, and blood clots are removed.
      3) Recognize that reperfusion washes anaerobic metabolic byproducts from the viscera, which may cause hypotension; fluids, mannitol, and sodium bicarbonate may be used before and during decompression surgery.
      4) The abdomen is left open after surgery for repair after swelling has subsided (usually within 5–7 days).
         a) Vacuum-assisted closure may be used after surgery to continue to reduce edema.

Diagnostic Studies

1. Serum chemistries
   a. Sodium: normal 136 to 145 mEq/l; elevated in dehydration from severe diarrhea or intestinal obstruction
   b. Potassium: normal 3.5 to 5.0 mEq/l; decreased in GI losses from upper or lower GI tract
   c. Chloride: normal 96 to 106 mEq/l
      1) Elevated in dehydration
      2) Decreased in vomiting, diarrhea, or intestinal obstruction
   d. Calcium: normal 8.5 to 10.5 mg/dl; decreased in acute pancreatitis
   e. Phosphorus: normal 3 to 4.5 mg/dl
      1) Elevated in intestinal obstruction
      2) Decreased in malnutrition or malabsorption syndromes
   f. Magnesium: normal 1.5 to 2.2 mEq/l; decreased in chronic diarrhea
   g. Glucose: normal 70 to 110 mEq/l; elevated in diabetes mellitus, pancreatitis
   h. Blood urea nitrogen (BUN): normal 5 to 20 mg/dl
   i. Creatinine: normal 0.7 to 1.5 mg/dl
   j. Gastrin: normal, less than 200 nn/l; elevated in Zollinger-Ellison syndrome (gastrin-producing pancreatic tumor) or G-cell hyperplasia that may cause peptic ulcer disease
   k. Ammonia: byproduct of protein metabolism
      1) Normal 15 to 110 mOsm/dl
      2) Elevated in hepatic failure, renal failure, heart failure
   l. Iron: normal 50 to 150 mcg/dl
   m. Iron-binding capacity: normal 250 to 410 mcg/dl
   n. Lactate: negative
   o. Carcinoembryonic antigen (CEA): normal less than 2 ng/ml; elevated in cancer of the colon, lung, pancreas, stomach, breast, head, neck, prostate
   p. Bilirubin
      1) Total: normal 0.3 to 1.3 mg/dl; elevated in hepatic disease, biliary obstruction, and excessive hemolysis
      2) Direct (i.e., conjugated): normal 0.1 to 0.3 mg/dl; elevated in biliary obstruction
      3) Indirect (i.e., unconjugated): normal 0.1 to 1.0 mg/dl; elevated in hepatic disease or excessive hemolysis
   q. Serum proteins
      1) Total protein: normal 6 to 8 g/dl
      2) Albumin: normal 3.5 to 5 g/dl; half-life is 19 to 20 days, so poor indicator of acute changes in nutritional status
      3) Prealbumin: normal 15 to 35 mg/dl; half-life is only 2 to 3 days, so indicates changes in nutritional status better than albumin
      4) Transferrin: normal 250 to 300 mg/dl; half-life is only 8 to 10 days, so indicates changes in nutritional status better than albumin
      5) Globulin: normal 1.5 to 3 g/dl
      6) Albumin/globulin ratio (A/G): normal 1.5/1 to 2.5/1; reverse in chronic hepatitis, chronic liver disease
      7) Fibrinogen: normal 0.1 to 0.4 g/dl
   r. Serum lipids
      1) Cholesterol: normal 150 to 200 mg/dl
      2) Triglycerides: normal 40 to 150 mg/dl
   s. Pepsinogen: normal 200 to 425 units/ml
      1) Elevated in hemoconcentration
      2) Decreased in malnutrition or hemorrhage
   t. Enzymes
      1) Alkaline phosphatase (ALP): normal 30 to 85 IU/l; elevated in cirrhosis, rheumatoid arthritis, biliary obstruction, liver tumor, hyperparathyroidism
      2) Amylase: normal 56 to 190 IU/l; elevated in acute pancreatitis, pancreatic cancer, pancreatic pseudocysts, perforated peptic ulcer, mesenteric thrombosis, ectopic pregnancy, renal failure, mumps
      3) Lipase: normal up to 150 units/l; elevated in acute or chronic pancreatitis, duodenal ulcer, biliary obstruction, cirrhosis, hepatitis; stays elevated longer than amylase in pancreatitis
      4) Alanine aminotransferase (ALT): normal 5 to 36 units/ml
         a) Formerly called *SGPT*
         b) Elevated in hepatitis, cirrhosis, liver tumor, hepatotoxic drugs, cholestasis, infectious mononucleosis
      5) Aspartate aminotransferase (AST): normal 15 to 45 units/ml
         a) Formerly called *SGOT*
         b) Elevated in hepatitis, cirrhosis, acute pancreatitis, skeletal muscle disease or trauma, liver tumor
      6) Gamma-glutamyl transferase (GGT): normal 5 to 38 IU/l; elevated in hepatitis, cirrhosis, liver tumor, cholestasis, alcohol ingestion, myocardial infarction (MI)
      7) Lactate dehydrogenase (LDH): normal 90 to 200 IU/l; elevated in hepatitis, hemolytic anemia, pancreatitis, muscular dystrophy, pulmonary infarction, MI, pernicious anemia, renal disease
   u. Serology for viral hepatitis
2. Hematology
   a. Hematocrit (Hct): normal 40% to 52% for males; 35% to 47% for females
   b. Hgb: normal 13 to 18 g/dl for males; 12 to 16 g/dl for females
   c. White blood cell (WBC) count: normal 3500 to 11,000 mm^3
      1) Differential: shift to left (increase in bands) indicates acute infection
   d. Erythrocyte sedimentation rate: normal up to 15 mm/hr for males; up to 20 mm/hr for females
3. Clotting profile: may be abnormal in liver disease
   a. Prothrombin time (PT): normal 12 to 15 seconds; therapeutic 1.5 to 2.5 times normal
   b. Activated partial thromboplastin time (aPTT): normal 25 to 38 seconds; therapeutic 1.5 to 2.5 times normal
   c. Activated clotting time (ACT): normal 70 to 120 seconds; therapeutic 150 to 190 seconds
   d. Thrombin time: normal 10 to 15 seconds
   e. Bleeding time: normal 1 to 9.5 minutes

    f. International normalized ratio (INR): normal less than 2
    g. Platelets: normal 150,000 to 400,000/mm^3
4. Urine
    a. Glucose: normal negative
    b. Ketones: normal negative
    c. Amylase: normal negative
    d. Bilirubin: normal negative
    e. Urobilinogen: normal 0.3 to 3.5 mg/dl
        1) Elevated in hepatocellular disease
        2) Decreased in complete biliary obstruction
    f. Specific gravity: normal 1.005 to 1.030
    g. Osmolality: normal 50 to 1200 mOsm/l
5. Gastric contents
    a. Gastric analysis with a NG tube
        1) Histamine or insulin is administered before collection of a sample of gastric contents.
        2) Gastric contents are analyzed for the presence of hydrochloric acid.
        3) Have antihistamine (e.g., diphenhydramine) and 50% dextrose available.
    b. pH determination
        1) Method
            a) Flush NG tube with 20 ml of tap water and then clear tube with air before aspirating.
            b) Do not use the same syringe used to give antacids or H$_2$ receptor antagonist to obtain the sample for pH testing.
        2) Used for the following:
            a) To determine tube placement: stomach pH 1 to 3; intestine pH 6.5 or greater
            b) To determine effectiveness of H$_2$ receptor antagonist and/or antacid therapy: pH of 3.5 to 5 is desirable
6. Stool
    a. Fecal occult blood test: normal negative
    b. Ova, parasites, blood (OPB): normal negative; specimen must be warm
    c. Fecal fat: normal 5 g/24 hr
        1) Elevated in cystic fibrosis, Crohn disease, biliary tract obstruction, pancreatic duct obstruction
        2) Specimen must be sent to laboratory in a wax-free container.
    d. Pus: normal, none
    e. Urobilinogen: normal 0 to 4 mg/day
        1) Decreased in biliary obstruction
        2) Specimen must be sent to laboratory in a light-resistant container.
    f. Culture: normal intestinal flora
    g. Assay for clostridium difficile toxin A or B: positive is diarrhea is caused *C. difficile*, an opportunistic infection caused primarily by suppression of normal flora by antibiotic therapy
7. Other diagnostic studies (Table 7.5)

Gastrointestinal Drugs (Table 7.6)

Decrease Gastric Acidity or Protect the Gastric Mucosa

1. Indications: prevention or treatment of peptic ulcer
2. Types of agents and specific actions
    a. Antacids
        1) Examples
            a) Aluminum-magnesium complex
            b) Magnesium hydroxide and aluminum hydroxide
            c) Calcium carbonate

Table 7.5 Gastrointestinal Diagnostic Studies

Study	Evaluates	Comments

Angiography: celiac or mesenteric	• Evaluates portal vasculature
	• Diagnoses source of GI bleeding
	• Evaluates cirrhosis, portal hypertension, vascular damage resulting from trauma, intestinal ischemia, tumors
	• May be used to treat GI bleeding using vasopressin
		• Bowel preparation (e.g., cathartics) as prescribed
		• NPO for 8 hr before the study
		• Sedative is usually prescribed before the procedure
		• Contrast media used
		  • Check for allergy to iodine before the study
		  • Monitor for allergic reaction after procedure
		  • Ensure hydration after procedure
		• Keep extremity in which catheter was placed immobilized in a straight position for 6–12 hr
		• Monitor arterial puncture point for hemorrhage or hematoma
		• Monitor neurovascular status of affected limb
		• Monitor for indications of systemic emboli

Barium enema (also called lower GI series) NOTE: Meglumine diatrizoate may be used, especially if bowel perforation is suspected.	• Visualizes the movement, position, and filling of various segments of the colon after instillation of barium by enema • Diagnoses colorectal lesions, diverticulitis, inflammatory bowel disease, strictures, fistulas • Evaluates colon size, length, and patency	• Low-fiber diet for 1–3 days before the study • Bowel preparation with bowel irrigation (e.g., GoLYTELY) and cathartics • NPO for 8–12 hr before study • Cathartics must be given after study • Contraindicated if bowel perforation or obstruction exists

Continued

Table 7.5 Gastrointestinal Diagnostic Studies—cont'd

Study	Evaluates	Comments
Barium swallow, upper GI series, and small bowel follow-through NOTE: Ordered according to which area or areas need to be evaluated (e.g., upper GI with small bowel follow-through means stomach, pylorus, duodenum; barium swallow with upper GI means esophagus, stomach, pylorus) NOTE: Meglumine diatrizoate may be used, especially if bowel perforation is suspected.	• Visualize the position, shape, and activity of the esophagus, stomach, duodenum, and jejunum • Diagnose esophageal lesions, varices, or esophageal motility disorders, hiatal hernia, gastric ulcers and tumors, small bowel obstruction, small bowel lesions, Crohn disease • Evaluate gastric and small bowel motility	• Bowel preparation with bowel irrigation (e.g., GoLYTELY) and cathartics • NPO for 8–12 hr before study • Cathartics must be given after study • Contraindicated if bowel perforation or obstruction exists

Cholecystography (oral, intravenous, percutaneous transhepatic, or common bile duct)	• Assesses gallbladder function, patency of the biliary system, and presence of gallstones
	• Diagnoses extrahepatic or intrahepatic jaundice, biliary calculi, biliary obstruction, common bile duct injury
		• Percutaneous transhepatic cholangiography is contraindicated in patients with bleeding disorders
		• Fatty meal the day before the study, but the evening meal is fat free
		• Enema may be given the evening before the study
		• NPO 8–12 hr before the study
		• Contrast medium is administered orally the evening before the study, administered intravenously immediately before the study, injected percutaneously into the bile duct, or injected directly into the common bile duct during surgery
		  • Check for allergy to iodine before the study
		  • Monitor for allergic reaction after procedure
		  • Ensure hydration after procedure
		• Monitor for clinical indications of bile leakage, hemorrhage, or peritonitis after percutaneous transhepatic cholangiography

CT scan of abdomen	• Diagnoses tumors, pancreatic cancer or cysts, pancreatitis, biliary tract disorders, obstruction versus nonobstructive jaundice, cirrhosis, liver metastases, ascites, lymph node metastases, aneurysm
	• Evaluates vasculature and focal points found on nuclear scans
	• Used to direct biopsy of tumors or aspiration of abscess
		• No special preparation required
		• If contrast medium is used:
		  • Check for allergy to iodine before the study
		  • Monitor for allergic reaction postprocedure
		  • Ensure hydration postprocedure

ERCP	• Diagnoses biliary stones, ductal stricture, ductal compression, neoplasms of the pancreas and biliary system • Evaluates patency of biliary and pancreatic ducts, jaundice, pancreatitis, cholecystitis, hepatitis	• Same as for esophagogastroduodenoscopy • Contraindicated if patient is uncooperative or if bilirubin is greater than 3.5 mg/dl • Monitor for clinical indications of pancreatitis (most common complication) after study • Monitor for clinical indications of sepsis

Table 7.5	Gastrointestinal Diagnostic Studies—cont'd	
Study	**Evaluates**	**Comments**
Endoscopy • Esophagogastroduodenoscopy • Colonoscopy • Proctosigmoidoscopy	• Directly visualize mucosa of areas of the GI tract • Esophagogastroduodenoscopy can be extended to visualize the pancreas and gallbladder • Esophagogastroduodenoscopy is used to diagnose esophagitis, esophageal ulcers, esophageal strictures, esophageal varices, hiatal hernia, gastritis, gastric ulcers, pyloric obstruction, pernicious anemia, foreign bodies, duodenal inflammation or ulcers and to evaluate esophageal or gastric motility, bleeding, lesions, status of surgical anastomoses • Esophagoscopy, gastroscopy may also be used therapeutically for sclerosis of varices • Proctosigmoidoscopy diagnoses rectosigmoid cancer, strictures, polyps, inflammatory processes, hemorrhoids and evaluates bleeding from rectosigmoid, surgical anastomoses • Colonoscopy diagnoses diverticular disease, obstruction, strictures, radiation injury, polyps, neoplasms, bleeding, ischemia • Colonoscopy or sigmoidoscopy may be used therapeutically for removal of polyps • Biopsies may be taken during any endoscopy	• Sedation may be prescribed, especially for colonoscopy • Bowel preparation with gastric irrigation (e.g., GoLYTELY) and cathartics required before lower GI endoscopy • NPO 4–8 hr before study • Keep NPO until gag reflex returns if sedation used • Monitor closely after procedure for clinical indications of perforation or hemorrhage
Flat plate of abdomen (may also be referred to as *KUB*)	• Diagnoses perforated viscus, paralytic ileus, mechanical obstruction, intraabdominal mass • Evaluates the distribution of visceral gas (and identifies free air in the peritoneum indicative of bowel perforation) • Evaluates organ size	• No preparation required

Liver biopsy	• Obtains tissue specimen for microscopic evaluation
	• Diagnoses liver disease or malignancy
		• May be performed open or closed
		  • Open is done in surgery
		  • Closed biopsy may be done at bedside
		• Clotting profile is evaluated preprocedure
		  • Closed biopsy is contraindicated if platelet count is less than 100,000/mm^3
		• Patient must be cooperative because he or she must take a deep breath and hold for closed biopsy
		• Type and crossmatch for 2 units of blood preprocedure
		NPO for 4–8 hr before study
		Postprocedure
		• Position patient on right side for 2 hr
		• Pressure dressing is applied, and the patient is on bed rest for 24 hr
		• Observe for:
		  • Hemorrhage (e.g., subphrenic hematoma): hypotension or dyspnea
		  • Pneumothorax: dyspnea; chest pain; diminished breath sounds on right; hypoxemia
		  • Sepsis: fever; leukocytosis; rebound tenderness

Liver scan	• Diagnoses cirrhosis, hepatitis, tumors, abscesses, cysts, tuberculosis	• No preparation required

Continued

Table 7.5 Gastrointestinal Diagnostic Studies—cont'd

Study	Evaluates	Comments
MRI	• Evaluates liver, biliary tree, pancreas, spleen • Differentiation between cyst and solid mass • Diagnoses hepatic metastasis • Evaluates abscesses, fistulas, source of GI bleeding • Used for staging of colorectal cancer	• Cannot be used in patients with any implanted metallic device, including pacemakers • No special preparation required • Cannot be done on a patient being mechanically ventilated • Must be able to lie flat and still for ~30–60 minutes during the scan; sedation may be necessary
Paracentesis	• Analysis of fluid removed during peritoneal tap • Diagnoses intraperitoneal bleeding with diagnostic peritoneal lavage	• Monitor for peritoneal leakage after tap • Monitor for clinical indications of infection or peritonitis after tap
Percutaneous transhepatic cholangiography	• Diagnoses extrahepatic or intrahepatic jaundice, biliary calculi, bile duct obstruction, bile duct injury • Evaluates the patency of the biliary ductal system	• Contraindicated in uncorrected coagulopathy, allergy to iodine, severe ascites, cholangitis • Monitor closely for clinical indications of bleeding or peritonitis
Percutaneous transhepatic portography	• Diagnoses esophageal varices and visualizes portal venous circulation	• As for angiography
Radionuclide imaging (hepatobiliary scintigraphy) • HIDA scan • PIPIDA scan	• Diagnoses hepatocellular disease, hepatic metastasis, biliary disease, lower GI bleeding, gastric reflux	• NPO 2 hr before study • Must be able to lie flat and still for 60 minutes during the scan
Schilling test	• Evaluates ileal absorption of vitamin B_{12} • Diagnoses pernicious anemia caused by intrinsic factor and inadequate ileal absorption of intrinsic factor–vitamin B_{12} complex	• IM vitamin B_{12} and oral radioactive B_{12} are given and 24-hour urine specimen is collected
Ultrasonography of abdomen	• Evaluates the pancreas, biliary ducts, gallbladder, liver • Identifies tumor, abdominal abscesses, hepatocellular disease, splenomegaly, pancreatic or splenic cysts • Differentiates obstructive from nonobstructive jaundice	• All barium must have been cleared from the GI tract before ultrasonography • NPO for 8 hr before study • If for evaluation of gallbladder: fat-free meal the evening before study • Must be able to lie flat and still for 30 minutes during the procedure

CT, Computed tomography; *ERCP*, endoscopic retrograde cholangiopancreatography; *GI*, gastrointestinal; *HIDA*, hepatobiliary; *IM*, intramuscular; *MRI*, magnetic resonance imaging; *NPO*, nothing by mouth; *PIPIDA*, paraisopropyliminodiacetic acid.

Table 7.6 Selected Gastrointestinal Drugs

Drug	Administration	Adverse Effects	Nursing Implications
Octreotide acetate	• For GI hemorrhage • SC: 50–150 mcg bid or tid • IV injection (for GI bleeding): 25–50 mcg followed by IV infusion • IV infusion (for GI bleeding): 25–50 mcg/hr for 48 hr	• Orthostatic hypotension • Anorexia, nausea, vomiting, abdominal pain • Diarrhea, constipation, steatorrhea • Abdominal bloating, flatulence • Increase in liver enzymes • Anxiety • Dizziness • Drowsiness • Heartburn • Hypoglycemia or hyperglycemia • Rectal spasm	• Monitor HR and BP • Monitor for GI complaints and bleeding and serum glucose • Note contraindication: known hypersensitivity • Note that this drug is tolerated better than vasopressin for GI bleeding, especially in patients with CAD • Note pain or burning at injection site • Do not administer if precipitation or discoloration occurs
Prototype PPI: pantoprazole sodium	• IV injection: 40 or 80 mg over 2 min; may also be diluted in 100 ml and infused over 15 min; followed by infusion • IV infusion: 8 mg/hr • PO: 40 mg twice daily	• Headache • Diarrhea, abdominal pain, flatulence • Rash • Hyperglycemia	• Monitor for GI complaints and bleeding and serum glucose • Note contraindications: known hypersensitivity

Table 7.6 Selected Gastrointestinal Drugs—cont'd

Drug	Administration	Adverse Effects	Nursing Implications
Prototype H₂ receptor antagonist: ranitidine	• PO: 150 mg once or twice daily or 300 mg at bedtime • IM: 50 mg every 6–8 hr • IV injection: 50 mg in 20 ml slowly every 6–8 hr or 50 mg in 100 ml over 15–20 min • IV infusion: mix 300 mg in 250 ml (1.2 mg/ml); usual dose 6.25–12.5 mg/hr	• Dizziness • Elevated liver enzymes, hepatotoxicity • Headache • Malaise	• Monitor HR, BP, liver enzymes, gastric pH • pH is maintained at 3.5 or greater • Note contraindications: known hypersensitivity • Use cautiously in liver disease, renal disease
Vasopressin	For GI hemorrhage • IV infusion: mix 100 units/100 ml (1 IU/ml) and administer at 0.1–0.8 IU/min (concurrent nitroglycerin is recommended with doses higher than 0.4 IU/min) • Administer through CVC	• Bradycardia • Hypertension • Fever • Water intoxication (SIADH), hyponatremia • Nausea, abdominal cramps • Tremor • Headache • Seizures • Coma • Constriction of cardiac arteries, resulting in chest pain and myocardial ischemia	• Monitor HR, BP, daily weight, serum sodium • Note contraindications: known hypersensitivity, nephritis • Use cautiously in coronary artery disease • Administer NTG as prescribed concurrently with IV vasopressin infusion to prevent potential complications related to cardiac ischemia • Prevent extravasation because necrosis may occur; treat with phentolamine (Regitine)

bid, Twice a day; *CAD*, coronary artery disease; *CVC*, central venous catheter; *GI*, gastrointestinal; *IV*, intravenous; *NTG*, nitroglycerin; *SC*, subcutaneous; *SIADH*, syndrome of inappropriate antidiuretic hormone secretion; *tid*, three times a day.

---

    2) Actions
        a) Buffers gastric acid
        b) Increases pH to decrease the activity of pepsin
  b. Histamine (H₂) receptor antagonists
    1) Examples
        a) Cimetidine
        b) Ranitidine
        c) Famotidine
        d) Nizatidine
    2) Action: blocks the action of histamine on parietal cells to inhibit volume and concentration of gastric secretions
  c. Proton pump inhibitors
    1) Examples
        a) Omeprazole
        b) Lansoprazole
        c) Pantoprazole sodium
    2) Action: inactivate hydrogen pump causing prevention of the formation of HCl by parietal cells
  d. Mucosal protectant (prostaglandin E₁-analog)
    1) Example: misoprostol
    2) Actions
        a) Enhances the body's normal gastric mucosal protective mechanisms
        b) Increases mucosal blood flow
        c) Decreases gastric acid secretion
  e. Mucosal protectant
    1) Example: sucralfate
    2) Actions
        a) Combines with gastric acid and forms an adhesive protective coating over an ulcer crater
        b) Adsorbs pepsin

3. Controversies of prophylaxis
  a. Costs of prophylaxis are considerable, and the number needed to treat to prevent even one case of GI bleeding is significant.
  b. Risks of changing the pH of the gastric secretions
    1) May impair digestion
    2) May impair absorption of drugs normally absorbed in the acid environment of the stomach
    3) May increase the risk of pneumonia: Bacteria that are normally killed in the acid medium of the stomach live, proliferate, and ascend the esophagus and are silently aspirated into the lungs.
  c. Who should probably definitely receive prophylaxis?
    1) Patients already exhibiting GI bleeding (although not technically prophylaxis at this point)
    2) Patients with a history of GI bleeding
    3) Patients with head injury
    4) Patients with burns

Gastrointestinal Hemorrhage

1. Octreotide acetate
  a. GI indications
    1) Severe diarrhea associated with carcinoid tumors or vasoactive intestinal peptide tumors
    2) GI bleeding (off-label use)
    3) GI or pancreatic fistula (off-label use)
    4) After partial pancreatectomy (Whipple procedure) (off-label use)
  b. Actions
    1) Inhibits release of vasodilatory hormones to cause vasoconstriction of the viscera and decrease portal vein flow and portal hypertension

2) Suppresses secretion of serotonin, gastroenteropancreatic peptides, and growth hormones
3) Stimulates fluid and electrolyte absorption from GI tract and prolongs GI transmit time
2. Vasopressin
   a. GI indication: GI hemorrhage
   b. Actions: constricts mesenteric arterioles and decreases portal circulation and pressure

Malnutrition

Definitions
1. Malnutrition: Dietary intake of essential nutrients is insufficient to meet the metabolic demands of the body.
   a. Macronutrients: CHO, protein, fat
   b. Micronutrients: vitamins, minerals, water
2. Types of malnutrition
   a. Marasmus: gradual wasting of body fat and somatic muscle with preservation of visceral proteins as seen in prolonged starvation and chronic illness
   b. Kwashiorkor: visceral protein wasting with preservation of fat and somatic muscle as seen in poverty; the patient may appear well-nourished, overweight, or obese, and edema may be present
   c. Mixed marasmus and kwashiorkor: type most commonly seen in hospitalized patients and associated with the highest mortality and morbidity rates

Etiology
1. Decreased nutrient intake
   a. Recent weight loss
   b. Recent change in diet; fad or limited diet
   c. Eating disorder (e.g., obesity, bulimia, anorexia nervosa). NOTE. Obesity is not the same as overnourished, and many obese patients are protein malnourished.
   d. Anorexia
   e. Nausea
   f. Difficulty chewing or swallowing (e.g., stomatitis, dysphagia)
   g. Depression
   h. Alcoholism or drug addiction
   i. Social history of poverty, disability, living alone
   j. Loss of the sense of taste or smell
   k. Use of drugs known to alter dietary intake or food utilization (e.g., antacids, antibiotics, laxatives, antineoplastics)
2. Decreased absorption
   a. Diseases of the GI tract
   b. Malabsorptions (e.g., diarrhea, steatorrhea)
   c. Parasites
   d. Pernicious anemia
   e. Intestinal bypass or resection
   f. Drugs (e.g., antacids, cholestyramine, neomycin, alcohol)
3. Increased nutrient losses
   a. Recurrent vomiting, diarrhea
   b. GI disease such as peritonitis, inflammatory bowel disease
   c. Diabetes mellitus
   d. Hemorrhage
   e. Peritoneal dialysis or hemodialysis
4. Increased nutrient requirements
   a. Recent surgery or trauma
   b. Chronic illnesses such as malignancy or renal, liver, lung, or heart disease or diabetes mellitus
   c. Prolonged hypercatabolic state (e.g., multiple trauma, major surgery, sepsis, burns)
   d. Hyperthyroidism
   e. Hypoxia
5. Nosocomial malnutrition: related to mismanagement or inattention to nutritional requirements of hospitalized patients
   a. NPO (nothing by mouth) status for diagnostic studies or postoperatively
   b. Feedings not advanced
   c. Wait and see
      1) If appetite improves
      2) If nausea, vomiting resolves
      3) If ileus resolves

Pathophysiology
1. Atrophy of mucosal cells in the small bowel can occur in as little as 72 hours without nutrient intake in individuals with even minor acute illness or injury; this cell atrophy is a major facilitator for bacterial translocation, a common cause of sepsis and MODS in critically ill patients.
2. Inadequate calories cause glycogenolysis and gluconeogenesis.
3. Stress of critical illness; stress hormones cortisol and glucagon have catabolic functions
   a. Hypermetabolism
   b. Glycogenolysis with increased glucose utilization
   c. Gluconeogenesis with increased protein and fatty acid utilization
   d. Insulin resistance
   e. Depletion of lean body tissue
4. Glycogenolysis, gluconeogenesis, and stress hormones all lead to hyperglycemia.
   a. Level of serum glucose is related to the degree of illness or injury.
   b. Hyperglycemia requires treatment with insulin to keep serum glucose within normal levels because hyperglycemia interferes with immune function.
   c. Recommended goal for glucose in critically ill patients is 80 to 120 mg/dl (Urden, Stacey, Lough, 2017).
5. Malnutrition causes immunodeficiency, poor wound healing, and eventually organ failure.

Clinical Presentation
1. Subjective
   a. Anorexia
   b. Diarrhea
   c. Weakness, fatigue, apathy
   d. Irritability
   e. Headache
2. Objective
   a. Dull, brittle, dry hair; hair loss

- b. Integumentary changes
    1) Pale, dry, flaky skin
    2) Poor skin turgor
    3) Poor wound healing
    4) Peripheral edema
    5) Transverse ridging of fingernails
- c. Oral changes
    1) Fissures at angles of lips (cheilosis)
    2) Hyperemic tongue; papillae may be hypertrophic or atrophic
    3) Gum and teeth problems: loss of teeth; dental caries; bleeding or receding gums
- d. Muscle wasting
- e. Ascites
- f. Hepatomegaly, splenomegaly
- g. Neurologic changes
    1) Altered mental status
    2) Loss of balance and coordination
- h. Weight loss
    1) Degrees of loss: 10% loss is significant; 20% loss indicates malnutrition
    2) Loss of more than 1 kg/week associated with primarily protein loss
    3) Body mass index (BMI)
        a) Formula: Weight (kg)/Ht (m) × Ht (m)
        b) Optimal: 20 to 25
        c) Obesity: greater than 25
        d) Underweight: less than 20
- i. Diminished skinfold and arm circumference measurement (rarely used in critical care)
    1) Triceps skinfold
        a) Measurement of skinfold thickness with calipers
        b) Reflects measurement of the subcutaneous fat reserves of the body; normal 7.5 to 16.5 mm; less than 3 mm indicates severely depleted fat stores
    2) Midarm muscle circumference
        a) Measurement of middle of upper nondominant arm
        b) Reflects measurement of body's muscle stores
3. Diagnostic studies
    a. Visceral protein measurements
        1) Albumin: decreased
            a) Reflects changes in nutritional status slowly because half-life is 10 to 20 days
                i) Normal: 3.5-5 g/dl
                ii) Mild depletion: 2.8 to 3.4 g/dl
                iii) Moderate depletion: 2.1 to 2.7 g/dl
                iv) Severe depletion: less than 2.1 g/dl
            b) May be secondary to liver disease, nephrotic syndrome, or hypercatabolism
            c) May reflect overhydration
        2) Prealbumin: decreased
            a) More reliable than albumin for monitoring overall protein status in acute care setting; half-life, 24 hours
        3) Transferrin: decreased; half-life, 8 to 10 days
        4) Retinol-binding protein: decreased; half-life, 10 hours; decreases with even minor stress; significance not fully understood
        5) Hgb or Hct: may be decreased
        6) Tests for immunocompetence
            a) Total lymphocyte count (TLC): decreased
                i) Formula: TLC = WBC (in mm^3) × % of lymphocytes
                    (a) Normal: 1500 to 2500/mm^3
                    (b) Mild depletion: less than 1500/mm^3
                    (c) Moderate depletion: less than 1200/mm^3
                    (d) Severe depletion: less than 800/mm^3
                ii) May be decreased by stress, steroids, renal failure
                iii) May be increased by infection, leukemia, myeloma
            b) Cell-mediated immunity: skin tests for the following:
                i) *Candida albicans*
                ii) Mumps
                iii) Purified protein derivative (PPD) of tuberculin
    b. Somatic (skeletal) protein measurements
        1) Midarm muscle circumference
        2) 24-hour urine specimen for creatinine
    c. Nitrogen balance study may show negative nitrogen balance.
        1) Requires 24-hour dietary record to evaluate nitrogen intake and 24-hour urine collection to measure urine urea nitrogen and evaluate nitrogen loss
        2) Reliable only when renal function is normal

Collaborative Management

1. Prevent or detect negative nitrogen balance and malnutrition.
    a. Weigh daily at same time and on same scale.
    b. Monitor diagnostic studies reflective of visceral protein stores (e.g., albumin, transferrin, prealbumin).
2. Ensure delivery of adequate and appropriate nutrients.
    a. Indication for nutritional support: when the patient is required to be NPO for more than 5 days or if patient is unable to meet nutritional needs with oral feedings
        1) Note that 1 l of 5% dextrose provides only 170 kcal; although this provides fluids and delays gluconeogenesis for a short period of time, catabolism occurs after approximately 5 days at basal metabolic rate and earlier in a hypermetabolic patient.
    b. Nutritional support within 48 hours of injury or critical illness may lessen the hypercatabolic state; nutritional support does the following:
        1) Promotes anabolism to prevent negative nitrogen balance and loss of visceral and somatic protein stores
        2) Provides needed nutrients for cellular energy
        3) Supports healing and the immune system
        4) Enhances feeling of well-being
    c. Calculation of nutritional requirements
        1) Protein
            a) Basal protein requirement is 0.8 g/kg/day.
            b) Most critically ill patients require approximately 1.5 g/kg/day.

c) Patients with direct protein loss (e.g., crush injuries, burns, hemorrhage) require 2 to 3 g/kg/day.
d) Note that too much protein is associated with azotemia.
2) Calories: 25 to 80 kcal/kg/day; varies according to age, activity level, metabolic rate, nutritional status, severity of illness, and other factors
   a) Basal or minimal illness: 25 kcal/kg/day
   b) Moderate illness: 35 kcal/kg/day
   c) Sepsis or extensive trauma: 45 kcal/kg/day
   d) Burns: 80 kcal/kg/day
   e) Note that overfeeding is associated with electrolyte imbalance, especially hypophosphatemia.
3) Fluids: 25 to 35 ml/kg/day with an additional 150 ml/day for each degree of body temperature above 37°C

d. Distribution of nutrients to ensure adequate nonprotein calories to prevent protein catabolism
   1) Protein: 15% to 20%
   2) CHO: 50% to 60%
   3) Fats: 20% to 30%
      a) Note that propofol (Diprivan) is delivered in a 10% lipid emulsion vehicle, and these fat calories need to be included in total calorie allotments; consult with the dietitian regarding the amount of propofol that the patient is receiving in a 24-hour period so that these fat calories are included in the nutritional support plan.

e. Specialty supplements and effects
   1) Glutamine
      a) Nonessential neutral amino acid that plays an important role in maintaining normal intestinal structure and function; essential acid at times of stress and hypercatabolism, specifically burns, trauma, wound healing
      b) Provision of glutamine to stressed patients is thought to support the integrity of the gut and decrease the rate of protein catabolism.
         i) Glutamine deficiency causes gut mucosal atrophy and eventually intestinal necrosis, leading to bacterial translocation and sepsis.
         ii) Glutamine supplementation provides enterocytes their preferred energy source and prevents gut-induced SIRS.
      c) Use of glutamine in patients with intracranial pathology is questionable, especially if seizures are occurring, because glutamine is a predominant stimulatory neurotransmitter.
   2) Arginine
      a) Semiessential amino acid
      b) Provision of arginine is thought to do the following:
         i) Promote nitrogen retention.
         ii) Improve protein turnover.
         iii) Improve wound healing.
         iv) Enhance immune function by increasing T-helper cells and decreasing T-suppressor cells.
         v) Aid in production of nitric oxide, a potent regulator of vascular tone and cardiac contractility.
      c) Arginine supplementation reduces the risk of infection and sepsis and promotes wound healing.
   3) Nucleotides
      a) Have a role in energy transfer
      b) Provision of nucleotides enhances natural killer (NK) cell activity and supports growth and function of metabolically active cells, such as lymphocytes and macrophages.
   4) Branched-chain amino acids: leucine, isoleucine, valine
      a) Have beneficial effects on nitrogen balance in patients under stress
      b) These are especially helpful in patients with hepatic failure or encephalopathy, but temporary lowering of daily protein intake is likely to produce the same effect.
   5) Medium-chain triglycerides (MCTs)
      a) These are less irritating and more easily absorbed by the small bowel mucosa.
      b) They may be better than long-chain triglycerides (LCTs) for patients with compromised GI function, SIRS, or sepsis.
   6) Essential polyunsaturated fatty acids (PUFAs): omega-6 (e.g., linoleic acid) and omega-3 (e.g., α-linolenic acid) fatty acids: aid in efficient functioning of the immune system
   7) Dipeptide/tripeptide formulas: may be used for patients with malabsorption (e.g., severe Crohn disease, bowel edema, inflammation, or ischemia)

f. Administer nutritional support either enterally or parenterally (Fig. 7.14).
g. Administer enteral nutritional support (Table 7.7) to patients with a functioning GI tract requiring nutritional support; remember "if the gut works, use it."
h. Administer parenteral nutritional support (Table 7.8) to patients without a functioning GI tract requiring nutritional support; may also be used with oral or enteral nutrition to increase the amount of nutrients provided in hypermetabolic patients
i. Ensure a smooth transition from enteral or parenteral feedings to oral nutrition.
   1) Consult with the dietitian and the physician regarding plans for this transition.
      a) Parenteral to enteral feeding: The total parenteral nutrition (TPN) rate is cut in half when half to one third of the patient's total caloric requirements are met by enteral feeding and discontinued when total caloric requirements are met by enteral feedings.
      b) Parenteral to oral diet
         i) Start with clear liquids and advance to full liquids while observing for aspiration.

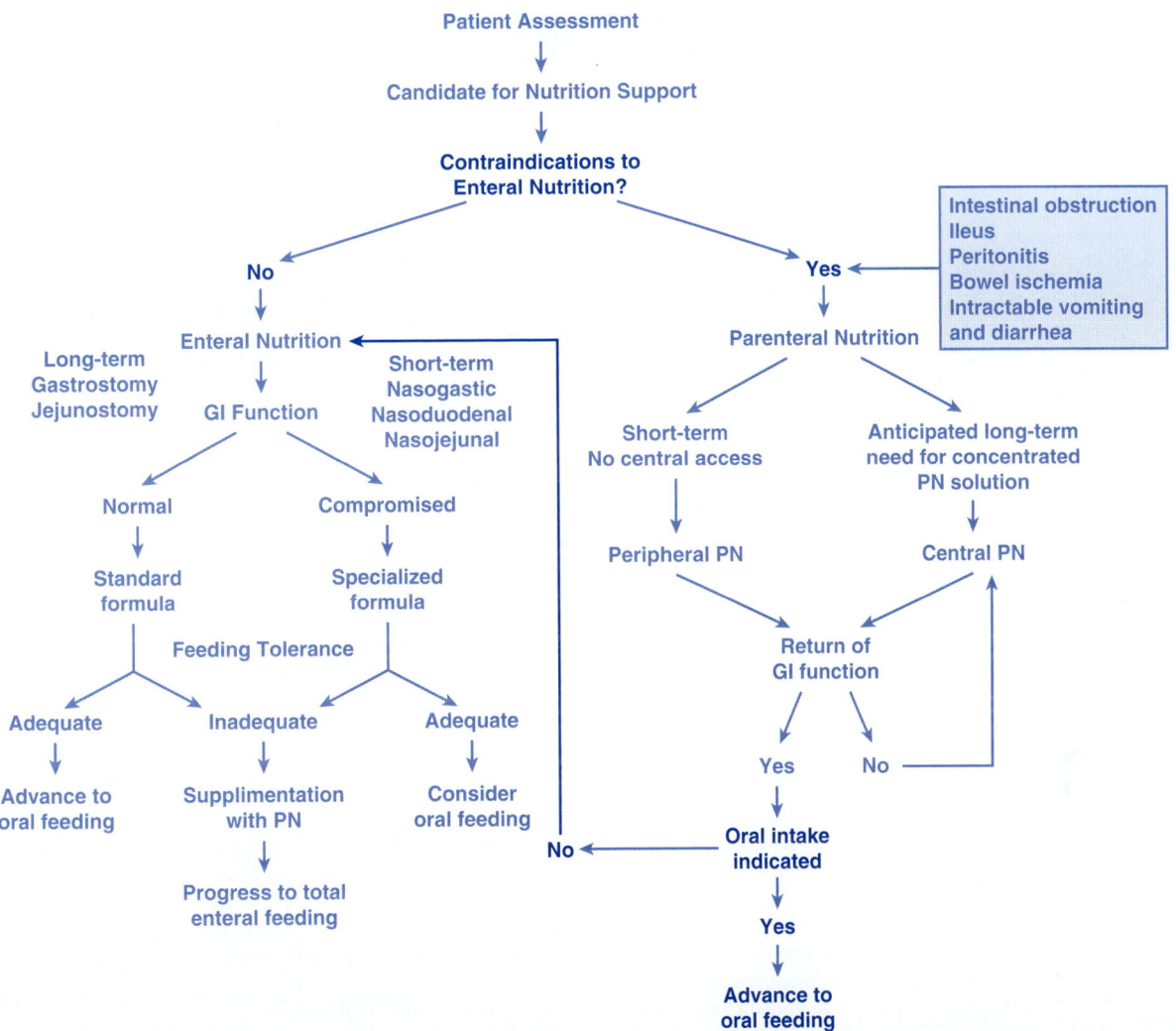

Fig. 7.14 Route of administration of specialized nutrition support. *GI*, Gastrointestinal; *PN*, parenteral nutrition. (Redrawn from Ukleja A, et al. Standards for nutrition support. *Nutr Clin Pract*, 25[4]:403, 2010.)

Table 7.7	Enteral Nutritional Support
Consideration	**Comments**
Indication	Patient has functioning GI tract but unable to consume adequate nutrients

Advantages	• Preferred route for patients with functional GI tract
	  • Maintenance of gut structure and absorptive ability
	  • Reduced incidence of sepsis by prevention of translocation of GI bacteria into blood or lymph
	  • Fewer complications than parenteral route
	  • Lower cost than parenteral route
	  • Early enteral

Disadvantages	• Decreased gastric and intestinal motility often accompanies critical illness and may lead to an inability to achieve adequate caloric intake as well as increase the risk of gastroesophageal reflux with resultant aspiration

Contraindications	• Absolute contraindications
	  • Diffuse peritonitis
	  • Intestinal obstruction
	    • Functional obstruction (e.g., paralytic ileus)
	    • Structural obstruction (e.g., tumor, volvulus, adhesion)
	  • Intestinal perforation
	• Relative contraindications
	  • Gastrointestinal ischemia
	  • Enterocutaneous fistula
	  • Severe acute pancreatitis, especially if hemorrhagic
	  • Severe malabsorption

Continued

Table 7.7	Enteral Nutritional Support—cont'd
Consideration	**Comments**

Routes and choice of tubes	Routes
	• Gastric
	  • Advantages
	    • Maintains natural bactericidal quality of acid environment
	    • Provides some protection from stress ulceration
	  • Disadvantage: increases risk of aspiration especially in patients with gastric atony, which is common in critically ill patients
	    • PEG may decrease this risk since the tube does not cause gastroesophageal sphincter incompetence
	• Intestinal
	  • Advantage: reduces risk of gastroesophageal regurgitation and microaspiration of gastric contents
	  • Disadvantage: placing tube is frequently difficult because critically ill patients frequently have delayed gastric motility; placement methods may include the following:
	    • Blind insertion
	      • Turn patient to right side and twist tube during advancement after gastric confirmation
	      • Air insufflation technique: instillation of 350–500 ml of air into the stomach
	      • Use of metoclopramide
	    • Fluoroscopic or endoscopic placement (e.g., PEJ)
	    • Surgical (needle jejunostomy tube)
	Choice
	• Small-gauge tube that is placed below the gastroesophageal sphincter (e.g., PEG tube or jejunostomy tube [including needle jejunostomy, which may be done at the conclusion of a laparotomy] is preferred, especially in patients with potential for impaired gastric motility and high risk of aspiration (Bourgault et al., 2007)
	• Short term (less than 6 weeks)
	  • Nasogastric or orogastric tube
	  • Nasointestinal or orointestinal tube (this may be advanced to the duodenum or jejunum)
	  • Needle jejunostomy
	• Long term (greater than 6 weeks)
	  • Gastrostomy
	  • Jejunostomy

Types of formulas	• Monomeric (also referred to as *elemental*) diets (e.g., Vivonex, Vivonex HN, Criticare HN, Vital HN, Travasorb NH, Impact, Stresstein) contain predigested nutrients: required when feeding is delivered distal to presence of digestive enzymes (distal jejunum); hyperosmolar
	• Polymeric formulas contain intact protein and require a functional GI system
	  • Intact protein and lactose-free enteral diets (e.g., Sustacal, Ensure, Enrich, Osmolite)
	  • Intact protein, lactose-free, high-density enteral diets (e.g., Magnacal, Isocal HCN, Sustacal HC, Ensure Plus, Ensure Plus HN)
	  • Blenderized meat-based enteral diets (e.g., Vitaneed, Compleat B)
	  • Specialized enteral diets
	    • Immune-boosting formulas (e.g., Immune-Aid, Impact, Perative, Replete): contain glutamine, arginine, and/or nucleotides
	    • Trauma (e.g., TraumaCal, Traum-Aid HBC, Vivonex TEN)
	    • Hepatic (e.g., Travasorb Hepatic, Hepatic-Aid): increased branched-chain amino acids
	    • Pulmonary (e.g., Pulmocare): higher proportion of fats, less CHO to reduce CO_2 production
	    • Renal (e.g., Travasorb Renal, Amin-Aid): essential amino acids
	    • Diabetic (e.g., Glucerna, Suplena)
	    • Fiber-containing formulas (e.g., Ensure with fiber, Jevity, Sustacal with fiber)
	• Modular
	  • CHO (e.g., Polycose, Nutrisource Modular System [carbohydrate])
	  • Protein (e.g., ProMod, Nutrisource Modular System [protein])
	  • Lipid-Medium Chain Triglycerides (e.g., MCT oil, Nutrisource Modular System [lipid])
	  • Lipid-Long Chain Triglycerides (e.g., Nutrisource Modular System [lipid LCT])
	• Note calorie concentration (most 1 kcal/ml, but some critical care solutions have 2 kcal/ml and Pulmocare, which is higher in fat, has 1.5 kcal/ml)
	• Note osmolality (isotonic is 250–350 mOsm/l; hypertonicity contributes to dehydration and diarrhea)

Pattern of delivery	• Intermittent (cannot be used below the pylorus) • Continuous; provides more protection from stress ulcers • Cyclic: feeding may be discontinued for periods of time during the 24-hr period; infusion frequently initiated during nighttime hours

Table 7.7	Enteral Nutritional Support—cont'd
Consideration	**Comments**

Monitor	• Position of the feeding tube
	  • Radiography is the only reliable method for confirming placement of enteral tubes; radiography should be obtained to confirm desired placement before administering formula or medication by the tube for the first time
	  • Other nondefinitive methods include:
	    • pH of aspirate may be helpful but not definitive: pH of 1–3 in stomach without pH-altering drugs, 3–5 in stomach with pH-altering drugs, greater than 7 in small intestine
	    • Color of aspirate may be helpful but not definitive
	      • Stomach: green, cloudy, or colorless
	      • Intestine: yellow or brown
	      • Tracheobronchial: tan, white, pale yellow, or clear
	    • Auscultation over stomach when air is injected through the tube (air insufflation) is NOT recommended because of poor sensitivity
	• GI tolerance of enteral feeding
	  • Abdominal distention or complaints of discomfort or fullness
	  • Vomiting
	  • Excessive residual volumes
	• Intake and output totaled every 8–12 hr
	• Weight daily
	• Bedside glucose testing by fingerstick q 6 hr; serum glucose by laboratory daily
	• Electrolytes daily
	• BUN daily
	• Proteins, trace elements, liver function studies weekly

General guidelines	• Start feedings within 24–48 hr of admission or when fully resuscitated and hemodynamically stable
	• Use an infusion pump for continuous infusion
	• Do not add blue food coloring (or methylene blue) to the enteral feeding; it is no longer recommended to add blue food coloring to enteral feedings for the following reasons:
	  • May result in generalized absorption of the dye from the GI tract; more likely in patients with multiple organ failure
	    • Discoloration of body fluids and tissues
	    • May cause fatal liver toxicity
	  • Causes questionable specificity because discoloration of tracheal secretions may have occurred by systemic route
	  • May result in infection because of contamination of the food coloring
	  • Interferes with occult blood testing
	  • Causes allergic reactions in some people because of the presence of FD&C yellow No. 5
	  • Has relatively low sensitivity as an indication of aspiration
	• Keep HOB elevated 30 to 45 degrees during and 30–60 min after intermittent feeding and continuously for continuous feeding
	• Give formula full strength but start at 25 ml/hr; increase rate by 25 ml/hr every 4 hr if tolerated until desired rate achieved
	• Check for residual volume every 4–6 hr or before next intermittent feeding; checking residuals is not recommended with small-lumen tubes because they tend to collapse and aspiration of gastric contents can cause clogging (Kenny & Goodman, 2010)
	  • If the residual is greater than 200 ml (Kenny & Goodman, 2010)
	    • The aspirate should be reinstilled in the absence of abdominal pain or distention; flush with water after reinstallation of aspirate
	    • The feeding should be continued and rechecked in 1 hr
	      • If the residual is still greater than 200 ml, the infusion should be stopped for 4 hr and then rechecked
	        • If the residual is still greater than 200 ml, notify physician
	        • If the residual is less than 200 ml, restart feeding at 50% the original rate and monitor
	    • Note that frequent interruptions may compromise adequacy of nutritional support
	  • If large residual volumes continue to limit feeding and impair nutritional support, consider the following interventions:
	    • Place the patient on the right side for 20 min before recheck
	    • Consult with the physician regarding the use of a drug to increase gastric motility (e.g., metoclopramide [Reglan], erythromycin); erythromycin has the potential risk of bacterial resistance
	    • Advance the tube to below the pylorus (intestinal motility usually not affected by same factors as gastric motility)
	    • Consult with the dietitian regarding a more calorie-dense formula in order to reduce required volume
	    • Monitor and treat hyperglycemia to avoid gastroparesis
	• Use strict aseptic technique in administration of enteral feedings; discard feeding system after 24 hr if an open system or after 48 hr if a closed system
	• Administer free water in volume of 1 ml/kcal to prevent hyperosmolality

Continued

Table 7.7 Enteral Nutritional Support—cont'd

Consideration	Comments

Complications of enteral alimentation	• Clogged feeding tube
	  • Recognize factors that increase risk of clogging the tube
	    • Calorie-dense formula
	    • Protein formulas
	    • Instillation of crushed medications
	    • Small-bore feeding tube
	    • Gravity drip
	  • Prevent clogging
	    • Use an infusion pump for continuous feedings and by flushing with water when indicated
	      • Flush with 30 ml of water before and after medication administration via tube
	      • Flush with 30 ml of water before and after intermittent feedings or every 4 hr with continuous feedings
	      • Flush with 30 ml of water after checking for residuals
	      • Flush with 30 ml of water every 4 hr
	    • Use liquid-form medications when possible
	  • Attempt to reestablish patency of a clogged tube by flushing with warm water (note that cranberry juice or cola has not been shown to be more effective than water); if warm water is not successful in unclogging the tube, a physician's order for pancreatic enzymes or pancreatic enzyme–sodium bicarbonate suspension may be requested (note that proper tube placement confirmation is crucial before using pancreatic enzymes); tube replacement may be required
	• Tube displacement
	• Tape tube securely and monitor for a change in external length
	• Prevent vomiting with antiemetics
	• Nausea or vomiting
	  • Slow feeding
	  • Allow feeding to come to room temperature before infusion
	  • Reduce osmolality of the feeding by diluting with water
	  • Decrease amount of fat in feeding
	  • Administer lactose-free formula
	  • Consider the use of drugs to increase gastric motility (e.g., metoclopramide [Reglan], erythromycin)
	  • Consider the need to move the tube from the stomach into the duodenum
	• Endotracheal aspiration of tube feeding
	  • Elevate HOB 30–45 degrees at all times if feeding is continuous; during and for 30–60 min after intermittent feeding
	  • Keep cuff inflated during feeding if patient is intubated or has tracheostomy
	  • Check for residual volumes every 4–6 hr if administering gastric feedings through a large-bore tube
	• Diarrhea
	  • Caused by decreased plasma COP because of low serum proteins
	    • Maintain adequate nutritional support; diarrhea will resolve when plasma proteins are more normal
	    • Administer IV albumin as prescribed
	  • Bacterial contamination
	    • Wash hands before manipulation of equipment and use clean technique; wipe top of formula cans with an alcohol wipe
	    • Utilize a closed system if possible
	    • Change administration system daily or according to policy
	    • Do not allow solutions to hang at room temperature for more than 4 hr if an open system or 24 hr if a closed system
	    • Avoid antidiarrheals, which slow peristalsis and increase the risk of sepsis
	  • Hypertonicity
	    • Initiate enteral feedings at a slow rate and/or half strength; gradually increase rate and/or strength
	    • Use isotonic solutions if possible; dilute hyperosmolar feeding with free water
	  • Alteration in normal flora from antibiotics and proliferation of *Clostridium difficile*
	    • Administer metronidazole (Flagyl) or vancomycin
	    • Encourage yogurt (with active cultures) or *lactobacillus acidophilus* to restore normal flora
	  • Also:
	    • Consider the addition of fiber (e.g., Jevity)
	    • Use only lactose-free formulas
	    • Consider discontinuance of causative medications (e.g., elixirs containing sorbitol or antacids)
	    • Administer pancreatic enzymes for pancreatic insufficiency

Table 7.7 Enteral Nutritional Support—cont'd

Consideration	Comments

	• Constipation
	  • Add fiber
	  • Increase free water
	  • Increase activity if possible
	  • Administer laxative as prescribed
	• Dehydration
	  • Monitor daily weight and intake and output
	  • Administer free water as indicated
	• Electrolyte imbalance
	  • Treat cause (e.g., diarrhea)
	  • Monitor serum electrolytes
	  • Replace electrolytes as prescribed
	  • Consult with the physician and dietician regarding modification of formula
	• Hyperglycemia
	  • Monitor serum glucose every 6 hr
	  • Consult with physician and dietician regarding modification of formula
	  • Administer insulin as prescribed
	• Overfeeding
	  • Monitor renal and liver function studies
	  • Monitor for fluid overload, hyperglycemia, hyperlipidemia, electrolyte imbalance
	  • Consult with the physician and dietician regarding caloric and protein prescriptions

	• Refeeding syndrome
	• Start feedings slowly, especially in high-risk patients (e.g., NPO for several days, existing malnutrition, alcoholism, sepsis); may take 24–48 hr to get intake to recommended level of nutrition
	  • Monitor glucose, potassium, phosphorus; insulin, electrolyte replacement may be required
	• Inadequate feeding (Bourgault et al., 2007)
	  • Minimize interruptions
	  • Stop feedings immediately before minor procedures and then restart within 1 hr after procedures
	  • Stop feedings no more than 4 hr before major procedures

BUN, Blood urea nitrogen; *CHO*, carbohydrate; *COP*, colloidal oncotic pressure; *GI*, gastrointestinal; *HOB*, head of bed; *IV*, intravenous; *PEG*, percutaneous endoscopic gastrostomy; *PEJ*, percutaneous endoscopic jejunostomy.

Table 7.8 Parenteral Nutritional Support

Considerations	Comments
Indications	• When the enteral route is contraindicated (Table 7.7) • When the enteral route is ineffective (high caloric needs or shock)

Routes	• Central vein: referred to as *total parenteral nutrition* (TPN)
	  • Allows the administration of hypertonic glucose solutions because of rapid dilution by blood as the solution enters the great vessel
	  • Subclavian or internal jugular usually used; PICC may also be used
	• Peripheral vein: referred to as *peripheral parenteral nutrition* (PPN)
	  • Used for patients who cannot take in sufficient nutrition enterally for 5–7 days but are not hypermetabolic
	  • Not usually adequate to provide sufficient calories for critically ill patients because of osmolality (and therefore calorie) limitations

Type of catheter	• Short term: peripheral or central venous catheter; multilumen catheter usually used to provide lumen for parenteral nutrition, lumen for blood or fluids, lumen for parenteral drugs • Long term: Hickman, Broviac, or Groshong catheter; Infuse-a-Port; Port-A-Cath

Solution: 1 l of standard TPN formula (25% dextrose and 8.5% amino acids) provides ~1000 kcal (1 kcal/ml)	• CHO: hypertonic dextrose
	  • Concentrations
	    • TPN: usually 25% but may be as high as 35% dextrose
	    • PPN: no more than 10% dextrose
	  • CHO and fats provide enough calories for maximal protein sparing effect
	  • Dextrose provides 3.4 cal/g

Continued

Table 7.8 Parenteral Nutritional Support—cont'd

Considerations	Comments

	• Protein: crystalline amino acids 2.5%–8.5%; includes essential and nonessential (note that no more than 5% amino acid solution via parenteral line [i.e., PPN]) amino acids and provides 4.3 cal/g
	  • Specialized formulas are available for specific diseases
	    • Hepatic failure (e.g., HepatAmine, Branch Amin): branched-chain amino acids
	    • Renal failure (e.g., RenAmin, NephrAmine): essential amino acids
	• Fats: oil-in-water emulsions composed of soybean oil or a combination of soybean oil and safflower oil that provide fatty acids as long-chain triglycerides
	  • 30%–50% of nonprotein calories should be supplied by lipids not exceeding 2.5 g/kg/day
	    • Linoleic acid, the only essential fatty acid, should provide at least 4% of the total calorie intake to prevent deficiency of essential fatty acid
	    • Excessive amounts of lipids may have a detrimental effect on pulmonary function and the reticuloendothelial system
	  • Concentrations
	    • 10% lipids provide 1.1 kcal/ml
	    • 20% lipids provide 2 kcal/ml
	    • 30% lipids provide 3 kcal/ml
	• Medium-chain triglycerides are immediately oxidized for fuel and may be preferred in SIRS and sepsis
	• Electrolytes: sodium chloride; potassium; calcium; magnesium; phosphate
	• Buffer: acetate or bicarbonate
	• Minerals: iron; zinc; copper; manganese; cobalt; iodine; chromium; selenium
	• Vitamins: multivitamins 1 ampule daily
	  • Vitamin K (10–20 mg) should be administered every week; may be given IM or SC or added to TPN solution as phytonadione
	  • Thiamine replacement should be considered, especially when chronic alcohol ingestion is known or suspected, to prevent Wernicke's encephalopathy
	• 3-in-1 admixture has everything in one infusion rather than lipid piggybacked in separately
	  • Advantages: lower cost with less equipment, waste, and nursing time
	  • Disadvantage: risk of solution instability; monitor closely for a cream-colored layer (also referred to as *creaming*) or a complete emulsion crack with a separation of the oil and water and return to pharmacy if separation noted

Possible additives	• Regular insulin (note that sliding scale insulin still must be administered as needed) • Heparin • H_2 receptor antagonists • Metoclopramide • NOTE: All additives should be added under laminar hood (in pharmacy department) rather than on nursing unit.
Monitor	• Vital signs and infusion rate at least every 4 hr (depending on the acuity of the patient) • Intake and output totaled every 8–12 hr • Weight daily • Bedside glucose testing by fingerstick q 6 hr; serum glucose by laboratory daily • Electrolytes daily • BUN daily • CBC, proteins, trace elements, liver function studies, triglycerides, cholesterol, platelet count, prothrombin time weekly • Catheter site

General guidelines	• Use strict sterile technique during catheter insertion and management
	• Assess patient for central venous catheter insertion complications (pneumothorax, hemothorax, chylothorax, arterial puncture); request chest radiography after insertion of central venous catheter; do not initiate fluids at a rate faster than KVO until chest radiography confirms placement
	• Ensure a dedicated catheter or lumen of a multilumen catheter for TPN infusion
	  • Do not use a catheter or lumen that has been previously used for CVP measurements or for the prolonged administration of crystalloid solution or blood products
	  • Do not use the catheter (or lumen) for drawing blood samples or infusing any other fluids
	• Assess the solution before infusion
	  • Examine expiration date and discard any expired solutions
	  • Do not hang cloudy solutions
	  • Monitor closely for emulsion crack if hanging 3-in-1 solution (also called *total nutrient admixture* [TNA]); do not hang solution if a layer of fat is seen separated at top of bag
	• Initiate at 1200–2400 cal/day and increase to desired caloric intake as prescribed
	• Remove from refrigerator 30 min before infusing
	• Keep rate constant (volumetric pump required)

Table 7.8 Parenteral Nutritional Support—cont'd

Considerations	Comments
	• Use an inline filter; 0.22 micron if lipids are piggybacked in distal to filter; 1.2 micron if TNA used because smaller filter will not allow lipids to flow through • Change dressing every 48 hr or according to hospital policy or anytime that the dressing becomes soiled • Gauze and tape or semipermeable transparent dressing (e.g., Op-Site, Tegaderm); note that semipermeable transparent dressing has been associated with a higher rate of catheter-related infection and sepsis than standard gauze and tape probably because of inadequate permeability and infrequency of dressing change; they should not be used in patients with oily skin or acne near catheter insertion site • Change tubing every 24–72 hr or according to hospital policy; lipid tubing (including TNA tubing) should be changed every 24 hr • Do not allow a bag to hang more than 24 hr

Complications	• Allergic reaction (especially to lipids)
	  • Note fever, chills, shivering, chest or back pain
	  • Stop infusion
	• Infection and sepsis
	  • Use meticulous aseptic technique with all aspects of catheter care; change dressing every 48 hr or whenever soiled; change tubing every 24–72 hr; minimize number of entries into the system
	  • Monitor for clinical indications of catheter-related sepsis: fever, leukocytosis, glucose intolerance, redness, swelling, tenderness, and purulent drainage at insertion site
	  • Obtain blood cultures (not through this catheter), remove catheter and culture tip
	• Hyperglycemia
	  • Monitor serum glucose levels
	  • Administer insulin therapy; usually administered as insulin drip if serum glucose greater than 500 mg/dl
	• Hyperosmolar nonketotic dehydration
	  • Monitor serum glucose levels
	  • Administer insulin therapy; usually administered as insulin drip if serum glucose greater than 500 mg/dl
	  • Administer 5% dextrose and hypotonic saline (¼ or ½) or D_5W (depending on patient's serum osmolality) to correct free water deficit
	  • Discontinue TPN until patient is stable as prescribed
	• Hypoglycemia
	  • Prevent interruption of TPN infusion (e.g., catheter occlusion or accidental removal)
	  • Use infusion pump (required)
	  • Never discontinue TPN abruptly unless for HHS
	• Electrolyte imbalances: hyperchloremic metabolic acidosis; hyponatremia; hypokalemia; hypocalcemia; hypomagnesemia; hypophosphatemia
	  • Adjust TPN solution concentration and/or alteration of infusion rate as prescribed
	• Refeeding syndrome: fluid imbalance; hypokalemia; hypophosphatemia; hypoglycemia or hyperglycemia
	  • Monitor fluid, electrolyte, glucose levels especially during the first 24–48 hr after TPN initiated
	  • Adjust TPN solution concentration and/or alteration of infusion rate as prescribed
	• Increased CO_2 production
	  • Monitor closely for clinical indications of hypercapnia; request ABGs as indicated
	  • Decrease the percentage of calories supplied by CHO and increase percentage of calories supplied by fats if hypercapnia occurs or during weaning
	• Air embolism
	  • Prevent air embolus by the following:
	  • Ask the patient to hold his or her breath or perform Valsalva maneuver during catheter insertion, tubing changes, and catheter removal
	  • Purge all air from tubing before attachment to catheter
	  • Use air-eliminating filters on central line tubing
	  • Use Luer-Lok connections
	  • Note dyspnea, hypotension, churning murmur over precordium, confusion
	  • If clinical indications of air embolism do occur:
	  • Place patient in Trendelenburg position on left side
	  • Aspirate air with a syringe attached to the central venous catheter
	  • Administer oxygen
	• Subclavian thrombosis (rare)
	  • Monitor for swelling of involved arm, face, neck, erythema, fever
	  • Remove catheter
	  • Administer fibrinolytic or anticoagulation therapy as prescribed

ABG, Arterial blood gas; *BUN*, blood urea nitrogen; *CBC*, complete blood count; *CHO*, carbohydrate; *CVP*, central venous pressure; D_5W, 5% dextrose in water; *HHS*, hyperglycemic hyperosmolar state; *IM*, intramuscular; *KVO*, keep vein open ; *PICC*, percutaneously inserted central catheter; *SC*, subcutaneous; *SIRS*, systemic inflammatory response syndrome; *TNA*, total nutrient admixture.

ii) Advance to solid food after 2 to 3 days of liquids and decrease TPN by half if at least 500 kcal is consumed.
iii) Discontinue nutritional support when the patient is able to tolerate sufficient oral nutrition for 2 to 3 days.
iv) High-protein and high-calorie drinks, shakes, and puddings may be used as nutritional supplements to augment small, frequent meals.
c) Enteral to oral diet
i) Monitor oral intake and use nutritional supplements to boost caloric intake if needed.
ii) Cyclic enteral feeding may be considered if calorie intake is consistently inadequate; usually administered at night
2) Continue to monitor daily weight and food intake during transition times.
3. Provide frequent oral hygiene; teeth should be brushed before meals to avoid aspiration of harmful bacteria.
4. Prevent skin breakdown.
a. Monitor for changes in edema.
b. Keep skin clean and dry.
c. Turn every 2 hours and use special mattresses as indicated.

Gastroesophageal Reflux Disease and Esophagitis

Definitions
1. GERD: persistent reflux of stomach content that occurs more than twice a week
2. Esophagitis: inflammation of the lining of the esophagus

Etiology
1. GERD
    a. Increased intraabdominal pressure (e.g., obesity, pregnancy)
    b. Hiatal hernia
    c. Decreased LES pressure
    d. Smoking, alcohol
    e. Dietary factors
        1) Caffeine
        2) Fried or fatty foods
        3) Onions, garlic, spices
        4) Tomato-based sauces
        5) Citrus fruits
        6) Chocolate
        7) Mint flavoring
2. Esophagitis
    a. GERD
    b. Achalasia (i.e., neurogenic impairment of esophageal motility that affects the lower two thirds of the esophagus)
    c. Medications (e.g., NSAIDs, potassium supplements)

Pathophysiology
1. Malfunction of the LES leads to reflux of acidic contents back up into the esophagus.
2. When reflux occurs, food or fluid can be tasted in the back of the mouth, and a burning sensation occurs when stomach acid refluxes back into the esophagus.
3. Exposure to pepsin and trypsin enzymes along with bile salts causes a chemical irritation and initiation of the inflammatory process (i.e., esophagitis).

Clinical Presentation
1. Subjective
    a. Burning or discomfort up and down epigastric area
        1) Increases when bending over
        2) May radiate to the back, chest, and neck
        3) Worse about 30 minutes after eating
        4) May feel like something is stuck in the upper chest area
    b. May complain of dyspnea
    c. May complain of excessive salivation
2. Objective
    a. Cough
    b. Belching
    c. Lesions in mouth; frequently herpes
    d. Halitosis
    e. Tenderness in epigastric area with palpation
    f. Wheezing, especially if pulmonary aspiration
    g. Hoarseness
3. Diagnostic studies
    a. Upper GI and barium swallow: to evaluate motility and identify reflux
    b. Endoscopy: to evaluate the condition of the esophageal and gastric mucosa
    c. Esophageal manometry: to measure the function of the LES

Collaborative Management
1. Maintain airway, oxygenation, and ventilation.
    a. Elevation of the head of the bed to 30 to 45 degrees, especially after meals
2. Prevent further damage to the gastric mucosa caused by gastric irritants, hyperacidity, or an impaired mucosal barrier.
    a. Discontinuance of any gastric irritants
    b. Pharmacologic agents that decrease gastric acidity and/or protect gastric mucosa
        1) Antacids (e.g., magnesium hydroxide and aluminum hydroxide)
        2) Histamine (H2) receptor antagonist (e.g., ranitidine, famotidine)
        3) Proton-pump inhibitors (e.g., omeprazole, pantoprazole, esomeprazole)
        4) Prokinetic agents (e.g., bethanechol, metoclopramide)
3. Evaluate for and treatment of H. pylori
4. Provide patient and family teaching.
    a. Nutrition consultation to provide instruction regarding dietary modifications
    b. Abdominal breathing exercises to strength the antireflux barrier of the LES
5. Monitor for complications.
    a. Gastric ulceration
    b. Perforation

c. GI hemorrhage
   d. Shock
   e. Barrett esophagus: condition in which the color and composition of the cells lining the lower esophagus change because of repeated exposure to stomach acid; may lead to esophageal cancer

Upper Gastrointestinal Hemorrhage

Definitions
1. Peptic ulcer: a sharply defined erosion in mucosa, which may involve the submucosa and muscular layers of the esophagus (~5%), stomach (~15%), or duodenum (~80%)
2. Esophageal varices: dilation of the submucosal esophageal veins
3. Mallory-Weiss tear: acute longitudinal tear of the esophagus caused by forceful retching
4. Gastritis: a generalized inflammation of the gastric mucosa

Etiology
1. Peptic ulcer
   a. *Helicobacter pylori:* a bacterial infection that has been identified as a common cause of recurrent ulcer disease
   b. Other predisposing factors
      1) Genetic predisposition
      2) Smoking
      3) Diet
         a) Coffee or tea
         b) Carbonated beverages
         c) Beer
      4) Drugs and therapies
         a) Antineoplastics
         b) Radiation therapy
         c) Drugs that alter the mucosal barrier
            i) Alcohol
            ii) NSAIDs (e.g., acetylsalicylic acid, ibuprofen, indomethacin)
         d) Drugs that decrease gastric mucosal renewal: corticosteroid, phenylbutazone
         e) Drugs that increase acid stimulation
            i) Coffee (because of peptides, not caffeine)
            ii) Nicotine
            iii) Reserpine
         f) Hormones (e.g., estrogen)
      5) High physiologic stress situation
         a) COPD
         b) Multiple traumas
         c) Major surgery
         d) MI
         e) Hepatic failure
         f) Renal failure
         g) Burns: referred to as Curling ulcer
         h) Neurologic trauma: referred to as *Cushing ulcer*
            i) Cerebral trauma
            ii) Spinal cord injury
            iii) Neurosurgery
         i) Acute respiratory distress syndrome (ARDS)
         j) Mechanical ventilation for more than 5 days
         k) Coagulopathy
         l) Sepsis
         m) Shock
         n) Multiple organ dysfunction syndrome
2. Cirrhosis: portal hypertension
   a. Cirrhosis
      1) Alcoholic cirrhosis: most likely
      2) Viral or toxic hepatitis
      3) Chronic biliary obstruction
      4) Chronic right ventricular failure
   b. Portal vein thrombosis
   c. Hepatic venous outflow obstruction
   d. Congenital hepatic fibrosis
   e. Schistosomiasis: a parasitic infection
3. Mallory-Weiss tear: forceful retching and vomiting (e.g., alcoholism, particularly binge drinking, or bulimia)
4. Gastritis
   a. Dietary intolerances, especially milk intolerance
   b. Alcohol
   c. Drugs such as aspirin, steroids, NSAID
   d. Uremia
   e. Certain systemic diseases such as hepatitis
   f. Ingestion of strong acids or alkalis (referred to as corrosive gastritis)

Pathophysiology
Fig. 7.15.

Clinical Presentation
1. Peptic ulcer
   a. Subjective
      1) History: epigastric pain, previous ulcer, previous GI bleeding, alcoholism, liver disease
      2) Epigastric pain
      3) Fatigue, weakness
      4) Thirst
      5) Anxiety
   b. Objective
      1) Bleeding
         a) Blood or coffee-grounds material appears in vomitus if gastric ulcer
         b) Black stools if duodenal
         c) If bleeding is gradual, faintness, fatigue, and pallor may be the only indications.
      2) Hyperactive bowel sounds
      3) Patient may have signs of acute abdomen if ulcer perforates (Box 7.2); other terms for an acute abdomen include *surgical abdomen* and *hot belly*
   c. Diagnostic studies
      1) Serum
         a) Gastrin level: may be elevated in gastric ulcer
         b) Amylase: elevated if perforation causes penetration into the pancreas and causes acute pancreatitis
         c) Total proteins, albumin, and transferrin may be decreased because many of these patients are malnourished.
         d) CBC: anemia
         e) Hgb, Hct: decreased but changes may take 4 to 6 hours after acute bleed

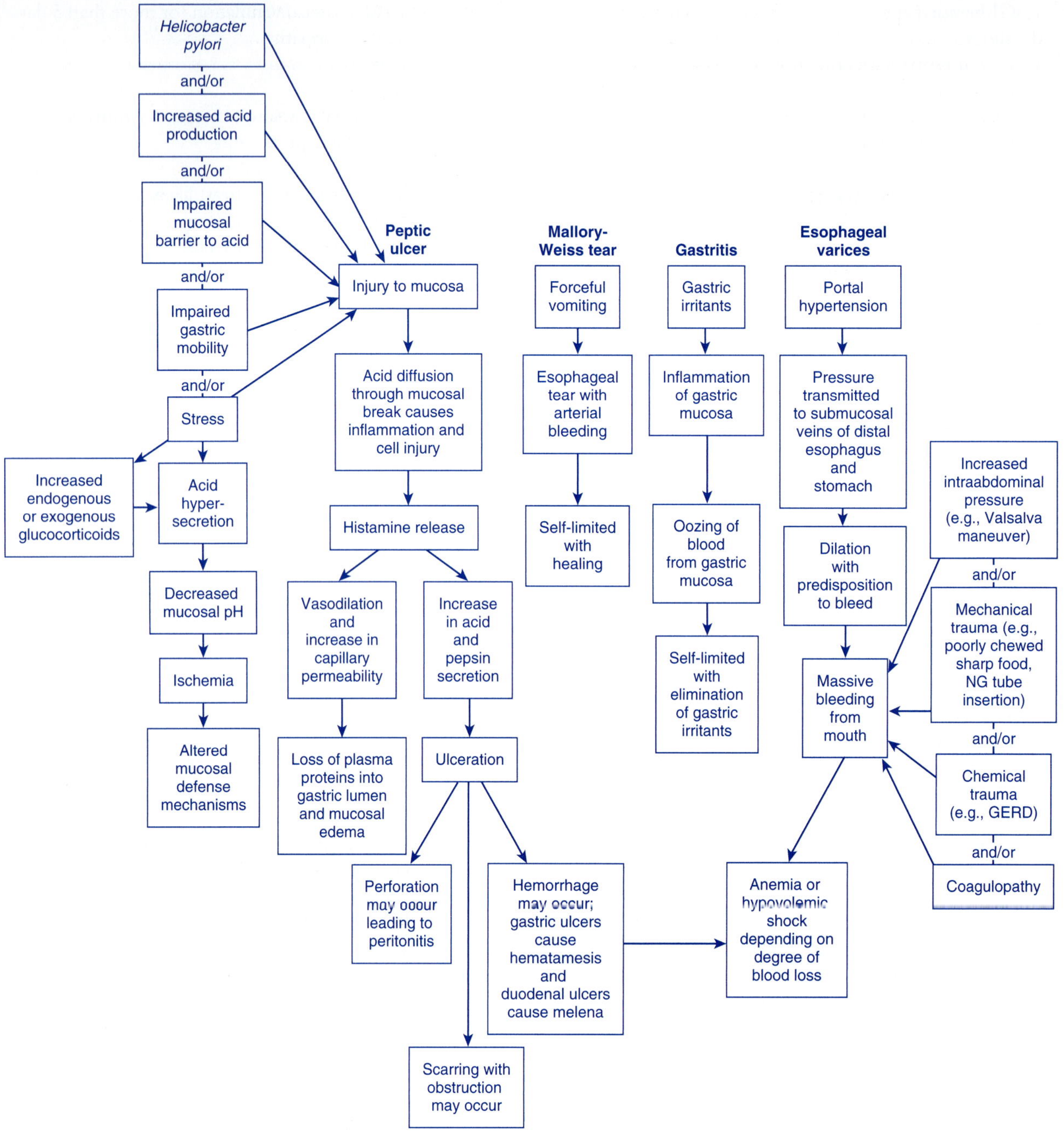

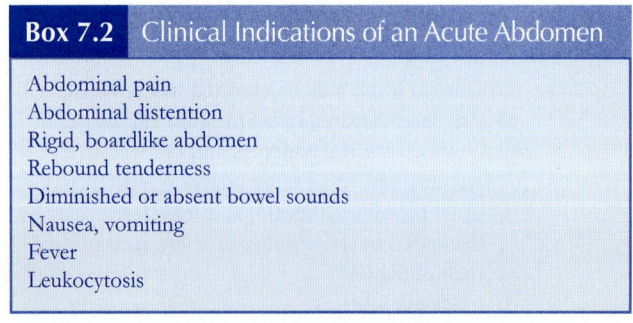

Fig. 7.15 Pathophysiology of upper gastrointestinal hemorrhage. *GERD,* Gastroesophageal reflux disease; *NG,* nasogastric.

Box 7.2	Clinical Indications of an Acute Abdomen

Abdominal pain
Abdominal distention
Rigid, boardlike abdomen
Rebound tenderness
Diminished or absent bowel sounds
Nausea, vomiting
Fever
Leukocytosis

    f) Clotting studies: PT, aPTT prolonged if liver is affected
2) Gastric analysis: may show hyperacidity or blood in the gastric secretions
3) Stools for occult blood: positive
4) Electrocardiogram (ECG): may show indications of ischemia (e.g., ST-T wave changes)
5) Flat plate of abdomen: may show free air under diaphragm indicating perforation
6) Gastroscopy: important in differentiating cause of upper GI bleeding; can determine ulcer presence, location, and stage of healing

7) Upper GI series: may show anatomic deformity created by ulcer crater; may show delayed gastric emptying if edema or scarring is present
8) Biopsy: may be done to rule out gastric cancer or malignant gastric ulcer
9) Angiography
   a) Rarely performed
   b) May reveal bleeding site or sites
   c) May include the placement of a catheter for intraarterial administration of vasopressors (e.g., vasopressin)
2. Esophageal varices
   a. Subjective
      1) History of precipitating causes (e.g., excessive, chronic alcohol intake)
      2) Report of sudden, painless hemorrhage orally
   b. Objective
      1) Bright red blood gushing from mouth (average blood loss is 10 units)
      2) Jaundice
      3) Abdominal distention
      4) Hyperactive bowel sounds
      5) Melena
      6) Hepatomegaly
      7) Splenomegaly
      8) Clinical indications of hypoperfusion: tachycardia; tachypnea; hypotension; cool, clammy skin; decreased urine output; agitation; confusion
   c. Diagnostic studies
      1) Serum
         a) BUN: elevated
         b) Bilirubin: may be elevated
         c) Albumin: decreased because of liver disease
         d) AST, ALT, LDH: elevated because of liver disease
         e) Hematology: Hgb, Hct decreased
         f) Clotting studies: PT, aPTT prolonged because of liver disease
         g) Arterial blood gases: may reveal metabolic acidosis related to shock and hypoperfusion
      2) Stool: positive for occult blood
      3) ECG: may show indications of ischemia (e.g., ST-T wave changes)
      4) Barium swallow: reveals the presence of esophageal varices
      5) Esophagogastroduodenoscopy: reveals the presence of esophageal varices
      6) Percutaneous transhepatic portography: reveals esophageal varices and measures pressure in the portal circulation
      7) Angiography
         a) Rarely performed
         b) May reveal bleeding site or sites
         c) May include the placement of a catheter for intraarterial administration of vasopressors (e.g., vasopressin)
3. Mallory-Weiss tear: hematemesis after forceful vomiting
4. Gastritis: coffee-grounds hematemesis

Collaborative Management

1. Ensure airway, oxygenation, and ventilation.
   a. Position for optimal ventilation and to prevent aspiration.
      1) Elevate HOB 30 to 45 degrees.
      2) Turn to left side.
   b. Administer oxygen as necessary to maintain SpO$_2$ at 94% unless contraindicated; in patients with COPD, administer oxygen to achieve a SpO$_2$ of ~90%.
   c. Ensure availability of oropharyngeal suctioning equipment at bedside.
   d. Assist with endotracheal intubation as requested to reduce risk of aspiration.
      1) Before balloon tamponade for esophageal varices: recommended to prevent obstruction of airway in case of accidental dislodgement of the esophageal balloon
      2) Before endoscopy if indicated
2. Maintain hemodynamic stability.
   a. Monitor blood loss and hemodynamic stability.
      1) Insert large-bore orogastric or NG tube and perform gastric lavage.
         a) Note that gastric lavage does not truly aid in clotting as previously believed and may actually dislodge clots; purposes of gastric lavage include the following:
            i) Monitor bleeding.
            ii) Remove nitrogenous materials (i.e., blood) out of the gut so that they will not be converted to ammonia nitrogenous materials from the GI tract.
            iii) Allow visualization during endoscopy.
         b) Use room temperature saline for lavage; problems with the use of iced lavage.
            i) Less effective in cessation of bleeding
            ii) Prolongation of clotting times
            iii) Hypothermia
               (a) Causing a shift of the oxyhemoglobin dissociation curve to the left, decreasing tissue delivery of oxygen
               (b) Causing the patient to shiver, increasing oxygen consumption
      2) Insert indwelling urinary catheter to evaluate hourly urine output.
      3) Assist with insertion of arterial catheter and pulmonary artery catheter in patients with severe hemorrhage.
   b. Replace circulating blood volume.
      1) Insert at least two short (1¼-inch) large-gauge (16 or 18) peripheral intravenous (IV) catheters; blood is drawn for laboratory analysis and for type and crossmatch for two units of blood during the catheter insertion.
      2) Administer crystalloids initially as prescribed; colloids may also be prescribed.
         a) Maintain urine output of 0.5 to 1 ml/kg/hr.
         b) Maintain PAOP of ~12 to 15 mm Hg.
         c) Avoid lactated Ringer solution (LRS) in patients with liver disease.

3) Administer blood and blood products as prescribed.
   a) Red packed cells should be given early if significant blood loss is suspected to prevent tissue hypoxia; indications include the following:
      i) Persistent hemodynamic instability after 2 l of crystalloid
      ii) Hct less than 25%
      iii) Clinical indications of hypoperfusion (Table 2.2)
   b) Fresh blood is preferred, especially in patients with liver disease, because it is lower in ammonia than banked blood.
   c) After multiple transfusions, consideration should be given to replacement of clotting factors, platelets, and calcium.
c. Control bleeding
   1) Administer octreotide acetate (Sandostatin) as prescribed (Table 7.6).
   2) Administer vasopressin intravenously as prescribed (Table 7.6).
   3) Assist with diagnostic or therapeutic endoscopy.
      a) Diagnostic: to identify the specific cause of the bleeding
      b) Therapeutic for peptic ulcer or Mallory-Weiss tear
         i) Endoscopic thermal therapy uses heat to cauterize the bleeding vessel.
         ii) Endoscopic injection therapy uses hypertonic saline, epinephrine, or dehydrated alcohol to cause localized vasoconstriction of the bleeding vessel.
      c) Therapeutic for esophageal varices
         i) Endoscopic injection therapy (i.e., sclerotherapy)
            (a) A sclerosing agent (ethanolamine oleate, morrhuate sodium, sodium tetradecyl) is injected into the varix and surrounding tissue; the sclerosing agent causes variceal inflammation, venous thrombosis, and eventually scar tissue; repeated injections may be necessary to completely decompress the bleeding varix and decrease the risk of recurrent hemorrhage.
            (b) Varices are categorized as I to IV by their size; class III and IV are at high risk to bleed if not already bleeding.
            (c) Monitor for complications of sclerotherapy.
               (i) Retrosternal pain
               (ii) Transient fever
               (iii) Transient dysphagia
               (iv) Local ulceration
               (v) Pulmonary symptoms, including diminished breath sounds
               (vi) Bleeding
               (vii) Stricture
               (viii) Perforation
               (ix) Sepsis
            (d) Sclerosing is repeated in 4 to 7 days and every 6 to 8 months thereafter.
         ii) Esophageal variceal ligation: Rubber bands or O-rings are placed on the target vessels at gastroesophageal junction.
   4) Stop bleeding in esophageal varices through measures that lower venous pressure.
      a) Administer beta-blockers (e.g., propranolol) as prescribed.
      b) Assist in placement of a multiple-lumen tube for balloon tamponade (Fig. 7.16 and Table 7.9) if bleeding cannot be controlled pharmacologically, endoscopically, or through use of transjugular intrahepatic portosystemic shunt (TIPS) (Fig. 7.17).
d. Correct coagulopathy; frequently significant in patients with esophageal varices and liver disease
   1) Administer vitamin K as prescribed; recombinant clotting factors (e.g., rFVIIa) may be prescribed.
   2) Monitor closely for bleeding.
   3) Monitor clotting studies.
   4) Avoid invasive procedures and injections.
3. Prepare patient for surgery if necessary to control bleeding.
   a. Peptic ulcer
      1) Indications for surgery
         a) Continuation of bleeding despite treatment
         b) Administration of greater than eight units of blood over 24 hours
         c) Hemorrhage to the point of hypotension or shock
         d) Rebleeding after homeostasis achieved
         e) Perforation with evidence of pneumoperitoneum
      2) Surgical interventions
         a) Oversewing of bleeding point
         b) Vagotomy: dividing the vagus nerve along the esophagus
            i) Decreases acid secretion in the stomach
            ii) If ulcer is prepyloric, vagotomy should be performed to prevent obstruction.
         c) Vagotomy and pyloroplasty
            i) Pyloroplasty: surgical procedure in which the pylorus is cut and resutured to relax the muscle and widen the opening into the duodenum
         d) Vagotomy and antrectomy
            i) Antrectomy: surgical removal of the antrum to decrease acidity
               (a) With gastroduodenal reconstruction (i.e., Billroth I) (Fig. 7.18, *A*)
               (b) With gastrojejunal reconstruction (i.e., Billroth II) (Fig. 7.18, *B*)

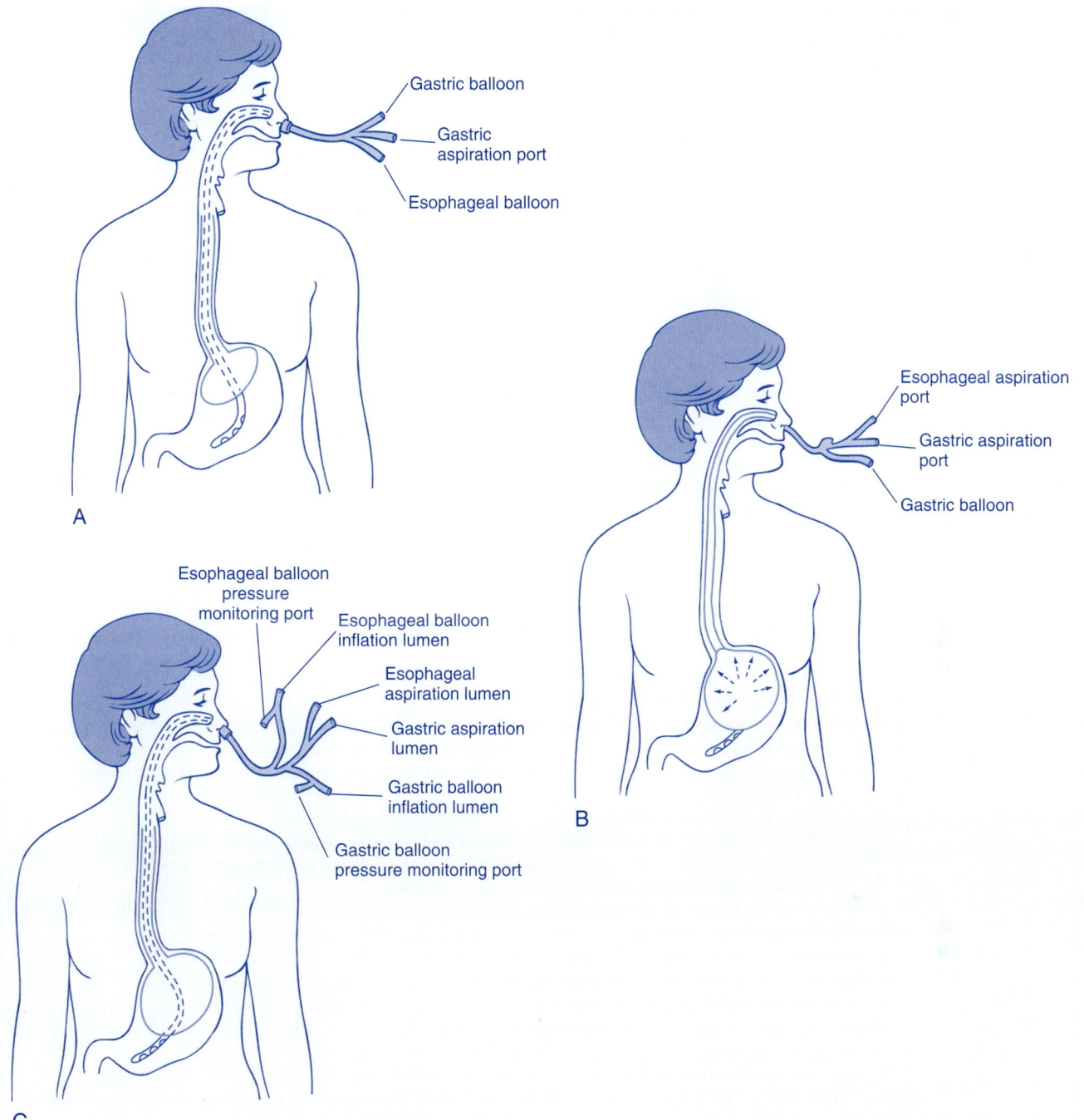

Fig. 7.16 Esophageal tamponade tubes. **A,** Sengstaken-Blakemore tube. **B,** Linton tube. **C,** Minnesota tube. (From Urden, L., Stacy, K., & Lough, M. [2009]. *Critical care nursing: Diagnosis and management* [6th ed.]. St. Louis: Mosby.)

    e) Total gastrectomy: gastrectomy with anastomosis of esophagus to the duodenum or jejunum (Fig. 7.18, *C*)
        i) Monitor for:
            (a) Early dumping syndrome (hyperosmolality effect related to a hyperosmolar bolus of food being "dumped" into the duodenum because of absence of pyloric valve and normal, more gradual gastric emptying): occurs within 30 minutes after eating; dizziness, weakness; tachycardia; cool, clammy skin
            (b) Late dumping syndrome (hyperinsulinism effect related to an increase in insulin production by the pancreas in response to a large bolus of food causing an increase in blood glucose): occurs 2 hours after meal; complaints of dizziness, weakness, restlessness; tachycardia; cool, clammy skin; malabsorption

Table 7.9 Balloon Tamponade for Esophageal Varices

Action	• Applies pressure to esophageal and intragastric varices
Tubes	• Linton (L): gastric balloon; esophageal suction; gastric suction • Minnesota (M) tube: esophageal balloon; gastric balloon; esophageal suction; gastric suction
Lumens	• Gastric balloon: 200–500 ml for SB tube; 450–500 ml for M tube; 700–800 for L tube • Esophageal balloon: usually 20 mm Hg (25 cm H_2O) but may be as high as 30–40 mm Hg to control bleeding • Gastric suction: nonvented • Esophageal suction: nonvented

Insertion	Generally done by physician but may be done by specifically trained nurse
	• Check balloon for leaks before insertion by inflating with air and putting in a basin of saline
	• Use viscous lidocaine or Cetacaine to anesthetize the nose and posterior pharynx
	• The catheter is advanced to ~50-cm mark
	• The gastric balloon is inflated to ~200–300 ml; the lumen is double clamped to prevent leakage
	• The catheter is pulled back until resistance is met and then a nasal sponge is placed at the nose to keep the gastric balloon up against the gastroesophageal junction
	  • A football helmet with face mask may also be used. If a helmet is used, check fit closely; skin breakdown is frequently caused by an ill-fitting helmet
	  • 0.5–1.0 kg weight may be hung over the end of the bed
	• The esophageal balloon is inflated to a pressure of 20–40 mm Hg until bleeding is controlled; the lumen is double clamped to prevent leakage
	• The suction lumens are connected to intermittent low suction (these are nonvented)
	• Label all lumens
	• Obtain chest radiography to check placement

Management	• Monitor and maintain airway
	  • Elevate HOB to 45 degrees unless patient is unconscious; if patient is unconscious, elevate HOB 15 degrees on left side
	  • Have suction equipment available
	  • Intubation is desirable but not absolutely required
	    • Suction the oropharynx and nasopharynx often because the patient cannot swallow with the tube in
	    • Not as much of an issue with Minnesota tube because there is suction above the esophageal balloon
	  • A small nasogastric tube may be inserted into the nostril opposite the SB tube to drain secretions that collect above the esophageal balloon
	• Maintain pressures at prescribed levels
	  • Periodic deflation at specific intervals (e.g., every 4 hours) may be prescribed because the pressures required to control bleeding exceed the pressure of capillary filling, and ischemia or necrosis may occur
	    • Monitor closely for bleeding during any time of deflation
	• Have scissors at bedside to release pressure from esophageal balloon if it accidentally moves into the pharynx and acute respiratory distress occurs
	• Keep second tube in the room for replacement if necessary
	• Maintain traction on tube to keep gastric balloon pulled up against the gastroesophageal junction
	• Note amount of pressure and volume in each part of tube; maintain inflation of balloons
	• Ensure patency of the gastric suction lumen and keep connected to low intermittent suction to prevent aspiration or retention of blood in the gut which is likely to increase ammonia levels
	• Monitor closely for skin breakdown at mouth or nose; lubricate every 8 hr with water-soluble lubricant
	• Deflation of the esophageal balloon is usually done at 24 hr; deflation of the gastric balloon is usually done at 48 hr; monitor closely for recurrent bleeding when balloons are deflated

Complications	• Airway obstruction • Aspiration • Perforation of esophagus: sudden epigastric or substernal pain, respiratory distress, increased bleeding, shock • Dysrhythmias • Chest pain • Bronchopneumonia • Laceration, ulceration of stomach • Pressure necrosis of hypopharynx, esophagus, or upper stomach • Hiccoughs

HOB, Head of bed.

    (c) Pernicious anemia: related to removal of parietal cells that make intrinsic factor necessary for the absorption of vitamin B_{12} in the ileum

  b. Esophageal varices
    1) Indications for surgery
      a) Continuation of bleeding despite treatment
      b) Administration of greater than 8 units of blood over 24 hours

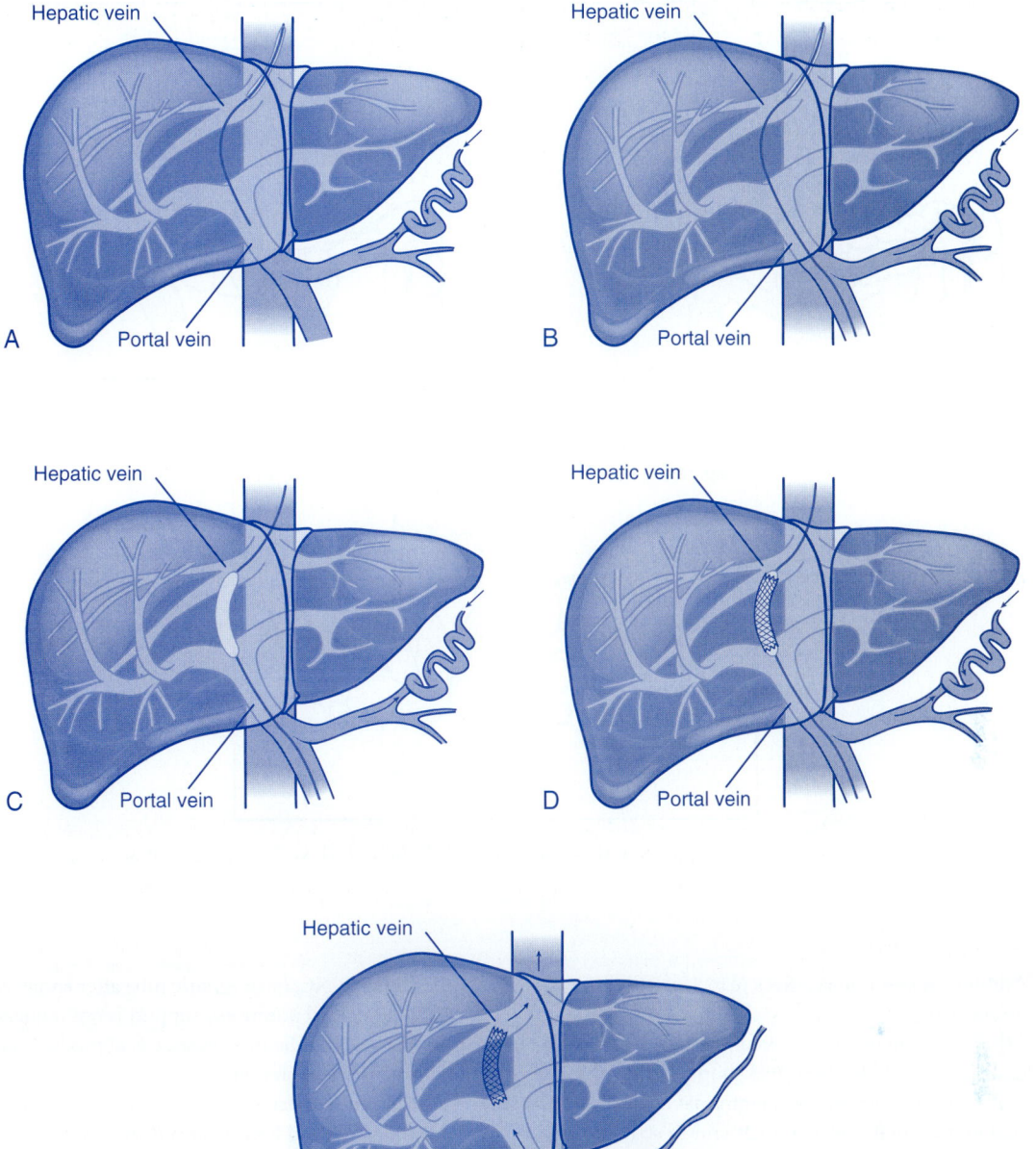

Fig. 7.17 Transjugular intrahepatic portosystemic shunt. **A,** Needle directed though the liver parenchyma to the portal vein. **B,** Needle and guidewire passed down to the midportal vein. **C,** Balloon dilation. **D,** Deployment of the stent. **E,** Intrahepatic shunt from the portal to the hepatic vein. (From Urden, L., Stacy, K., & Lough, M. [2013]. *Critical care nursing: Diagnosis and management* [7th ed.]. St. Louis: Mosby.)

       c) Hemorrhage to the point of hypotension or shock
       d) Rebleeding after homeostasis achieved
    2) Portal-systemic shunt: portacaval, mesocaval, or splenorenal
       a) Lowers portal pressure by diverting blood flow
       b) Associated with a higher incidence of hepatic encephalopathy and avoided if possible
    3) TIPS
       a) Invasive angiographic method; less invasive than surgical shunt
       b) Shunts blood between the portal and systemic venous systems entirely within the liver; connection is made between the hepatic and portal veins and a stent is placed in the tract
       c) Complications: hemorrhage; renal failure; septic shock; shunt stenosis; hepatic encephalopathy
  4. Prevent encephalopathy.
    a. Remove nitrogenous materials from the GI tract.
      1) Perform gastric lavage with room-temperature saline so that bacteria in GI tract cannot digest the globin (i.e., protein).

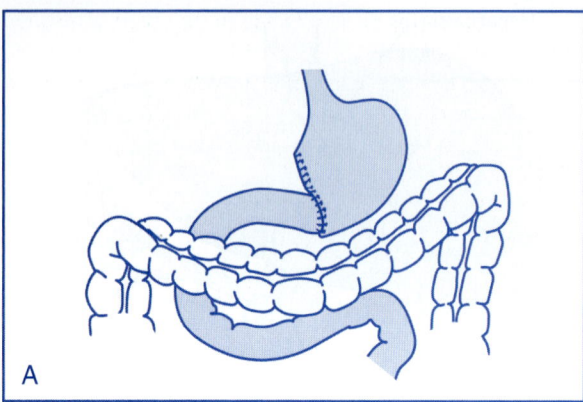
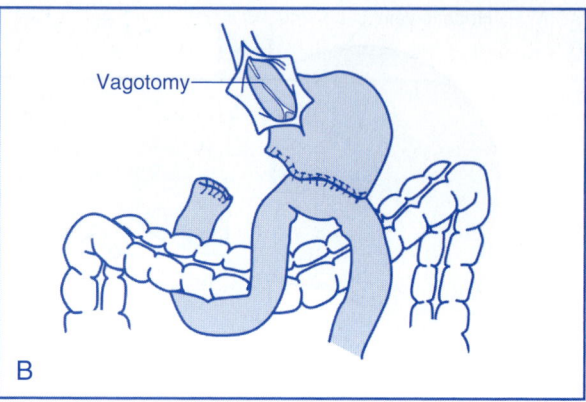
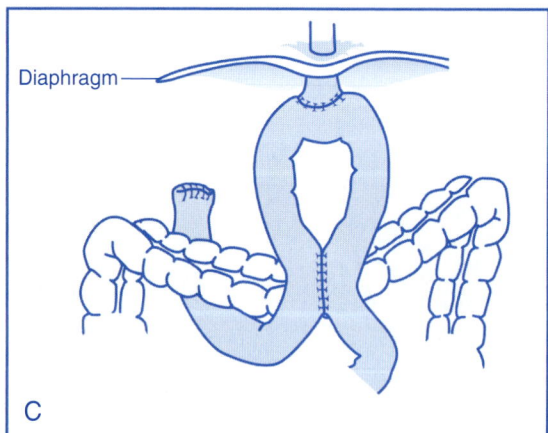

Fig. 7.18 Gastric resection procedures. **A,** Billroth I. **B,** Billroth II. **C,** Total gastrectomy.

   2) Administer osmotic laxatives (e.g., lactulose) as prescribed.
   3) Administer enemas as ordered.
  b. Monitor patients with portacaval shunts closely for clinical indications of elevated ammonia levels (e.g., confusion, irritability, decreased attention span, apathy, slurring of speech).
5. Prevent further damage to the gastric mucosa caused by gastric irritants, hyperacidity, or an impaired mucosal barrier.
  a. Discontinue any gastric irritants.
  b. Administer pharmacologic agents that decrease gastric acidity and/or protect gastric mucosa (Table 7.6).
   1) Decrease gastric pH to 3.5–5 (normal pH of gastric secretions, 1–3).
     a) Antacids (e.g., aluminum-magnesium complex, magnesium hydroxide and aluminum hydroxide, calcium carbonate
     b) Histamine (H_2) receptor antagonist (e.g., ranitidine, famotidine, nizatidine)
     c) Proton pump inhibitors (e.g., omeprazole, lansoprazole, esomeprazole)
   2) Provide agents to improve the mucosal barrier to acid.
     a) Prostaglandin E_1-analog (e.g., misoprostol)
     b) Mucosal protectant (aluminum hydroxide, sulfated sucrose): (e.g., sucralfate)
  c. Provide required nutritional support by enteral route if possible.
  d. Remove NG or orogastric tube after lavage is completed (and enteral nutritional support is not required) because the gastric tube may increase acid production by stimulating gastric secretion.
  e. Administer drug therapy for *Helicobacter pylori;* any of the following combinations may be prescribed:
   1) Bismuth subsalicylate + metronidazole + tetracycline + H_2 receptor antagonist
   2) Omeprazole + clarithromycin
   3) Ranitidine bismuth citrate + clarithromycin
   4) Lansoprazole + amoxicillin + clarithromycin
   5) Lansoprazole + amoxicillin
6. Decrease anxiety.
  a. Maintain a calm and reassuring approach.
  b. Administer anxiolytics as prescribed and indicated; avoid hepatotoxic agents if the patient has liver disease.
  c. Keep the patient and family informed regarding patient status.
  d. Encourage discussion of fears and concerns.
  e. Assess for alcohol withdrawal syndrome (Box 7.3); if present:
   1) Administer central nervous system depressants (e.g., diazepam [Valium], chlordiazepoxide [Librium]) as prescribed.
     a) Most drugs used for this purpose, including diazepam and chlordiazepoxide, have potential for liver toxicity; dosage is adjusted and liver function studies are monitored.

> **Box 7.3 Alcohol Withdrawal Syndrome**
>
> | Early | Late |
> |---|---|
> | Mild tachycardia | Marked tachycardia |
> | Mild hypertension | Marked hypertension |
> | Nausea, vomiting | Hyperthermia |
> | Diaphoresis | Dehydration |
> | Pruritus | Delirium |
> | Visual disturbances | Delusions |
> | Time disorientation | Hallucinations |
> | Tremors | Tonic-clonic seizures |
> | Anxiety, agitation | |
> | Sleep disturbances | |

2) Reorient frequently.
3) Encourage family attendance.
7. Maintain fluid and electrolyte balance: Evaluate sodium, potassium, calcium, and magnesium and replace as prescribed.
8. Maintain nutritional status by administering appropriate nutrients when appropriate.
   a. Recommendations for patients with peptic ulcer
      1) Provide bland proteins and fats in small, frequent meals.
      2) Avoid stimulants of gastric secretions (e.g., coffee, tea, cola, spicy foods, alcohol).
      3) Progress to full diet as soon as possible.
   b. Recommendations for patients with esophageal varices
      1) Give clear liquids initially; progress diet as indicated.
      2) Avoid alcohol-containing mouthwash and drugs.
      3) Encourage thorough chewing of foods, especially hard, sharp foods such as crackers because they may mechanically injure varices, causing recurrence of bleeding.
9. Monitor for complications.
   a. Aspiration pneumonitis
   b. Recurrent bleeding, hemorrhage
   c. Perforation
   d. Peritonitis
   e. Penetration into surrounding tissues (e.g., acute pancreatitis)
   f. Gastric outlet syndrome related to ulcer inflammation and mucosal edema
   g. Obstruction caused by ulcer scarring at the pylorus
   h. MI
   i. Cerebral infarction
   j. Disseminated intravascular coagulation (DIC)
   k. Sepsis
   l. Shock: hypovolemia or septic

Hepatic Failure and Encephalopathy

Definitions
1. Hepatic failure: inability of the liver to perform organ functions
   a. Acute liver failure (ALF) (previously referred to as *fulminant hepatic failure*): onset of coagulopathy (INR greater than or equal to 1.5) and any degree of encephalopathy within 25 weeks of the appearance of symptoms of liver failure in the absence of underlying liver disease (Larson, 2010)
2. Hepatic encephalopathy: neurologic failure as a result of hepatic failure

Etiology
1. Acute liver failure
   a. Hepatotoxic drugs (Box 7.1) (e.g., acetaminophen, halothane, methyldopa, isoniazid [INH], 3,4-methylenedioxy methamphetamine [Ecstasy]) or toxins (*Amanita* mushrooms, carbon tetrachloride, sea anemone sting)
   b. Viruses
      1) Fulminant viral hepatitis (Table 7.10)
      2) Herpes simplex
      3) Herpes zoster
      4) Epstein-Barr
      5) Adenovirus
      6) Cytomegalovirus
   c. Ischemia (e.g., shock and multiple organ dysfunction syndrome [MODS])
   d. Trauma
   e. Reye syndrome
   f. Budd-Chiari syndrome (i.e., hepatic vein obstruction)
   g. Acute fatty liver of pregnancy
   h. Acute hepatic vein occlusion
2. Chronic liver failure with an acute situation (e.g., peritonitis, GI hemorrhage, catabolism)
   a. Cirrhosis
   b. Wilson disease
   c. Primary or metastatic tumors of the liver

Pathophysiology (Fig. 7.19)
1. Cirrhosis
   a. Liver parenchymal cells are progressively destroyed and replaced with fibrotic tissue, resulting in impaired hepatic function; three quarters of the liver can be destroyed before symptoms appear.
   b. Distortion, twisting, and constriction of central sections cause impedance of portal blood flow and portal hypertension.
2. Fulminant hepatitis: Liver cells fail to regenerate, and necrosis occurs.

Clinical Presentation
1. Subjective
   a. History of precipitating event
   b. Irritability
   c. Personality change
   d. Disorientation
   e. Weakness, fatigue
   f. Anorexia, nausea, vomiting
   g. Right upper quadrant dull abdominal pain
   h. Abdominal fullness
   i. Change in bowel habits
   j. Weight loss
2. Objective
   a. General: emaciation, cachectic appearance
   b. Cardiovascular
      1) Tachycardia, dysrhythmias
      2) Bounding pulses
      3) Hypertension or hypotension
      4) Flushed skin

Table 7.10	Types of Viral Hepatitis			
Type	Route	Incubation Period (weeks)	Onset/Chronicity	Comments
A (HAV; infectious hepatitis, enteric hepatitis)	Fecal–oral	2–6	Acute onset Chronicity does not develop	• 99% resolves but 1% becomes fulminant • Treatment is supportive
B (HBV; serum hepatitis)	Parenteral Sexual Perinatal	4–24	Insidious onset Chronicity develops in less than 5%	• 1% becomes fulminant • 15%–25% develop liver cancer • Treatment includes interferon alfa-2b (Intron A); antivirals such as lamivudine (Epivir) or famciclovir (Famvir) may also be prescribed
C (HCV; non-A, non-B hepatitis; posttransfusion hepatitis)	Parenteral Sexual Perinatal	2–20	Insidious onset Chronicity develops in 50%–60%	• 20%–50% develop cirrhosis • 20% develop liver cancer • 20% develop liver failure • Treatment includes interferon alfa-2b (Intron A) or peginterferon alpha-2b (Peg-Intron) and ribavirin (Virazole); may also include corticosteroids
D (HDV; delta virus)	Superinfection or coinfection in patient with chronic hepatitis B	4–24	Acute onset Chronicity common with superinfection	• Up to 30% become fulminant • Most have worsening active hepatitis • Treatment is as for hepatitis B
E (HEV; enteric non-A, non-B hepatitis)	Fecal–oral Perinatal	2–8	Acute onset Chronicity does not develop	• Generally benign and self-limiting; however, 10%–20% mortality rate when it occurs during pregnancy
F (HFV)	Parenteral Sexual Perinatal			• Now considered a variant of hepatitis B
G (HGV)				• Very little known

        5) Spider angioma on upper trunk, face, neck, arms
        6) Jugular venous distention
        7) Distended superficial vessels on abdomen (caput medusae)
    c. Pulmonary
        1) Tachypnea or hyperpnea
        2) Decreased respiratory excursion
    d. Neurologic
        1) Peripheral neuropathy
        2) Slow, slurred speech
        3) Asterixis
        4) Hyperactive reflexes
        5) Seizures
        6) Positive Babinski reflex in encephalopathy
        7) Extreme lethargy or coma in encephalopathy
    e. GI
        1) Fetor hepaticus
        2) Ascites
        3) Hematemesis
        4) Hepatomegaly early; liver atrophy occurs later
        5) Splenomegaly
        6) Ascites
        7) Bowel sounds: diminished
        8) Clay-colored (pale) stools if biliary obstruction
        9) Steatorrhea (i.e., excessive fat in stool)
       10) Esophageal varices or hemorrhoids
    f. Renal
        1) Oliguria
        2) Dark amber urine
    g. Hematologic or immunologic
        1) Abnormal bruising, bleeding
        2) Susceptibility to infection
        3) Poor wound healing
    h. Integumentary
        1) Jaundice; usually noted in the sclera first
        2) Palmar erythema
        3) Petechiae
        4) Bruises
        5) Edema
        6) Pruritus
        7) Spider angioma
    i. Endocrine changes
        1) Hypogonadism: testicular atrophy and reduced testosterone levels in men
        2) Gynecomastia in men
        3) Altered hair distribution
3. Diagnostic studies
    a. Serum
        1) Sodium: may be decreased or normal
        2) Potassium: may be decreased
        3) Calcium: may be decreased
        4) Magnesium: may be decreased

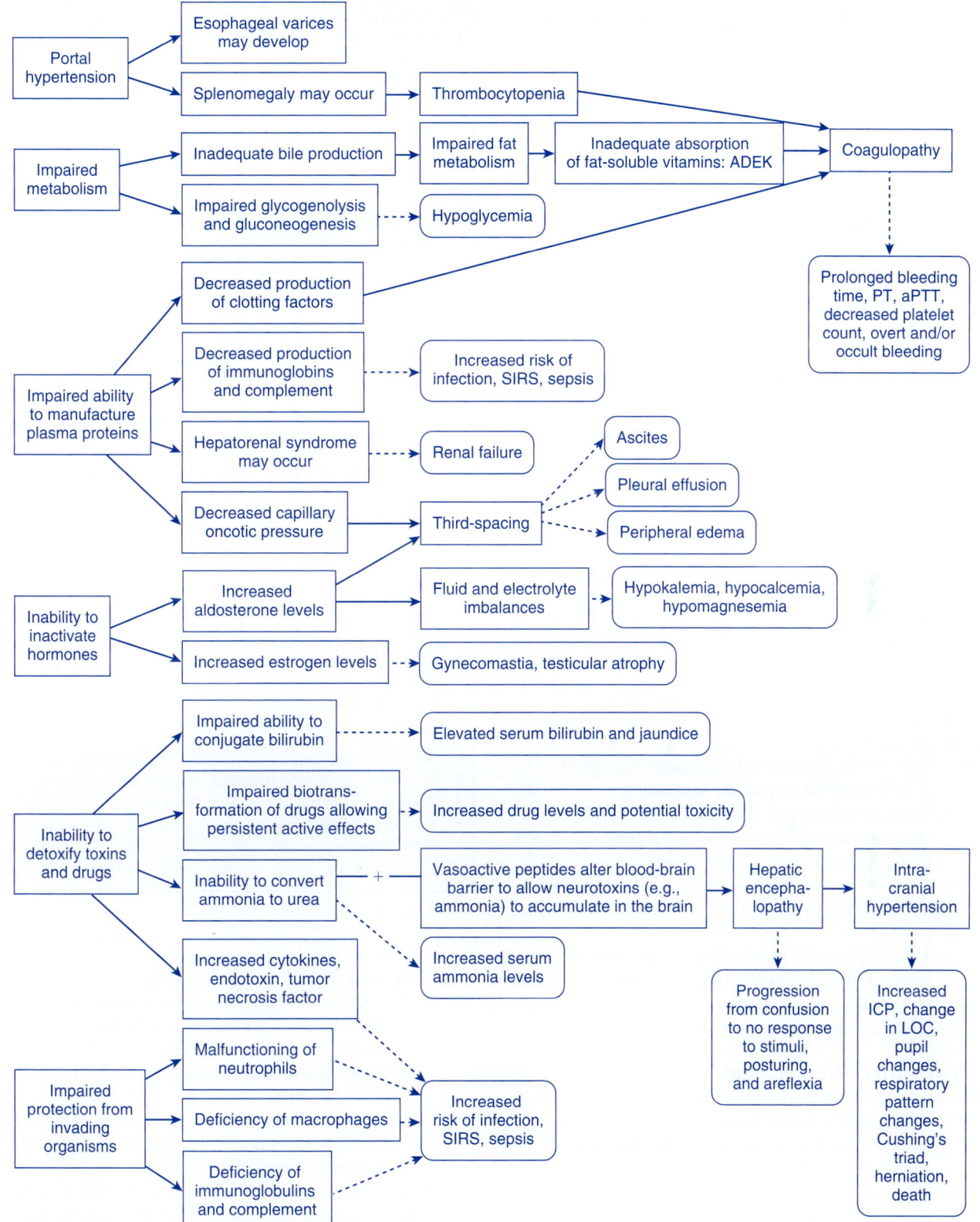

Fig. 7.19 Pathophysiology of hepatic failure. *Dotted lines* connect pathology to clinical presentation. *aPTT,* activated partial thromboplastin time; *ICP,* intracranial pressure; *LOC,* level of consciousness; *PT,* prothrombin time; *SIRS,* systemic inflammatory response syndrome.

5) BUN: may be elevated because of dehydration, hepatorenal syndrome, or GI bleeding
6) Glucose: may be elevated or decreased
7) Creatinine: may be elevated due to hepatorenal syndrome
8) Cholesterol: elevated
9) ALT, AST, LDH: elevated
   a) AST/ALT ratio greater than 1 suggests chronic liver failure or tumor.
   b) AST/ALT ratio less than 1 suggests hepatitis.

10) ALP: elevated
11) Bilirubin: elevated
12) Ammonia: elevated in encephalopathy
13) Total protein, serum albumin, fibrinogen: decreased
14) Hgb, Hct: may be decreased if hemorrhage or hypersplenism
15) WBC count: decreased; if normal or elevated, infection may be present
16) Platelets: decreased in splenomegaly
17) Arterial blood gases
    a) Respiratory alkalosis
    b) Hypoxemia may be seen
  b. Urine
    1) Sodium: decreased
    2) Bilirubin: elevated in biliary obstruction
    3) Urobilinogen
        a) Elevated in hepatocellular disease
        b) Decreased in complete biliary obstruction
  c. Chest radiography: may show pleural effusion or atelectasis
  d. Flat plate of abdomen: may reveal hepatosplenomegaly; abdominal haziness may be seen if ascites is present
  e. Abdominal ultrasonography: may reveal intraabdominal fluid if ascites is present
  f. Barium swallow or esophagogastroduodenoscopy may be done to identify presence of esophageal varices.
  g. Liver scan: may show diffuse changes of cirrhosis
  h. Liver biopsy: may show fatty infiltration (early) or severe degeneration and scarring (advanced)
  i. Endoscopic retrograde cholangiopancreatography (ERCP): may identify biliary obstruction
  j. Paracentesis: Cytologic examination may be done to rule out malignancy; ascites fluid has low specific gravity, low protein concentration, and cell counts.
  k. Electroencephalography (EEG): shows abnormal and generalized slowing in patients with encephalopathy
  l. Lumbar puncture: may be done to rule out neurologic cause of altered consciousness; CSF shows increase in glutamine
4. Stages of encephalopathy (Box 7.4)

Collaborative Management
1. Identify and treat cause of hepatic failure.
   a. Administer N-acetylcysteine for acetaminophen toxicity; must be administered within 24 hours of acetaminophen ingestion
   b. Administer antivirals (e.g., acyclovir, ganciclovir) as prescribed for viral causes; interferon may also be prescribed.
   c. Prevent further injury to the liver.
      1) Avoid hepatotoxic drugs.
      2) Avoid alcohol-containing mouthwash or medications.
   d. Monitor liver function studies.
2. Maintain airway, oxygenation, and ventilation.
   a. Elevate HOB 30 to 45 degrees, especially if ascites restricts diaphragmatic excursion.

Box 7.4 Stages of Encephalopathy

Stage I
- Mild confusion
- Decreased attention span
- Difficulty performing simple arithmetic computations (e.g., count backward from 100 by 7s)
- Decreased response time
- Forgetfulness
- Mood changes
- Slurred speech
- Personality changes
- Irritability
- Disruption in sleep–wake patterns
- EEG normal

Stage II
- Lethargy
- Confusion
- Apathy
- Aberrant behavior
- Tremor and asterixis (also referred to as *liver flap*)
- Inability to reproduce simple designs (constructional apraxia)
- Slowing of normal EEG

Stage III
- Somnolent with diminished responsiveness to verbal stimuli
- Severe confusion and incoherence after arousal
- Speech incomprehensible
- Tremor and asterixis
- Hyperactive deep tendon reflexes
- Hyperventilation
- EEG abnormal

Stage IV
- No response to stimuli or abnormal (e.g., decorticate or decerebrate) posturing to stimuli
- Areflexia except for pathologic reflexes
- Positive Babinski reflex
- Fetor hepaticus
- EEG abnormal

EEG, Electroencephalography.

   b. Monitor for and prevent aspiration.
      1) Use artificial airways as necessary in patients with altered consciousness and airway protective mechanisms (e.g., gag reflex).
      2) Intubation is usually required at stage III hepatic encephalopathy.
   c. Administer oxygen as necessary to maintain SpO_2 at 94% unless contraindicated; in patients with COPD, administer oxygen to achieve a SpO_2 of ~90%.
   d. Assist in management of ascites that cause decreased diaphragmatic excursion and ventilation difficulties.
      1) Monitor closely for clinical indications of atelectasis.
      2) Assist with paracentesis as necessary; patient may need paracentesis if extremely dyspneic.
      3) Administer aldosterone antagonists (also referred to as *potassium-sparing diuretics*) (e.g., spironolactone [Aldactone]) as prescribed; loop diuretics may also be required as aldosterone antagonists tend to lose their effectiveness over time.

4) Restrict sodium to 500 mg/day and restrict fluids to 1500 ml/day as prescribed; be alert to clinical indications of hypovolemia.
5) LeVeen or Denver shunt may be performed when patient is stable.
   a) Surgical procedures that shunt ascites fluid into the superior vena cava
   b) LeVeen shunt uses positive abdominal pressure caused by descent of the diaphragm during inspiration to open an intraperitoneal valve and shunt fluid from the peritoneum to the superior vena cava.
   c) Denver shunt adds a subcutaneous pump that can be compressed manually to irrigate the intraperitoneal tubing.
  e. Control respiratory alkalosis associated with hyperammonemia.
     1) Avoid assist-control mode because it will perpetuate the problem.
     2) Use synchronized intermittent mandatory ventilation (SIMV); muscle paralysis and sedation may be required to control $PaCO_2$ levels.
  f. Monitor closely for ARDS.
     1) Monitor for clinical indications of respiratory distress and SpO_2.
     2) Use mechanical ventilation strategies to prevent ventilator-induced lung injury: VT ~6 ml/kg.
3. Maintain adequate circulating volume and fluid and electrolyte balance.
  a. Monitor closely for indications of fluid and electrolyte imbalances.
     1) Monitor vital signs and hemodynamic parameters; invasive hemodynamic monitoring is usually indicated in stage III and IV hepatic encephalopathy.
     2) Weigh daily at same time on same scale.
     3) Measure abdominal girth daily for patients with ascites.
     4) Monitor serum osmolality, sodium, potassium, calcium, and magnesium.
  b. Maintain circulating blood volume.
     1) Administer colloids as prescribed to improve capillary oncotic pressure and reduce third spacing; avoid protein-containing colloids (e.g., albumin) in hepatic encephalopathy.
     2) Administer crystalloids as prescribed; avoid LRS because the liver is responsible for converting lactate to bicarbonate.
  c. Maintain vascular tone: Vasopressors may be necessary, especially in stage III or IV hepatic encephalopathy.
  d. Administer electrolyte replacement as prescribed.
  e. Monitor for hepatorenal syndrome.
     1) Observe urine output closely; note clinical indications of hepatorenal syndrome.
        a) Oliguria (i.e., less than 0.5 ml/kg/hr)
        b) Low urinary sodium
        c) Elevated BUN, serum creatinine
        d) Low serum sodium (i.e., dilutional hyponatremia)
        e) Moderately reduced GFR (less than 50 ml/min) as evaluated by 24-hour urine
     f) Monitor for hepatopulmonary syndrome (i.e., intrapulmonary vascular dilations)
        1) Hypoxia caused by ventilation-perfusion mismatch
     2) Administer diuretics as prescribed while monitoring closely for clinical indications of intravascular depletion and azotemia.
        a) Avoid thiazide diuretics.
        b) Use aldosterone antagonists (also frequently referred to as potassium-sparing diuretics) (e.g., spironolactone) as prescribed.
        c) Use loop diuretics as prescribed; sometimes administered after albumin
           i) Albumin pulls fluid back into the intravascular space.
           ii) Furosemide (Lasix) then eliminates fluids by preventing reabsorption of sodium and water in the renal tubules.
     3) Prepare patient for hemodialysis or continuous renal replacement therapy (CRRT) as prescribed; unfortunately, frequently unresponsive to treatment
        a) CRRT preferred because less likely to precipitate rapid osmolar shifts that can cause intracranial hypertension
  f. Administer H_2 receptor antagonists and/or antacids as prescribed to maintain a pH of 3.5 to 5 to reduce the risk of stress ulcer and GI hemorrhage.
4. Prevent and reduce elevated levels of toxins including ammonia.
  a. Stop nitrogen-containing drugs: ammonium chloride, urea
  b. Administer lactulose (combination of galactose and fructose) orally or via NG tube as prescribed.
     1) Acts as a chelating (bonds with) agent of ammonia by changing gut pH, which results in ammonia excretion
     2) Changes gut flora to foster growth of non–ammonia-forming bacteria
     3) Acts as an osmotic laxative; dose is usually adjusted for two semiformed stools per day
  c. Administer antibiotic to kill the bacteria that convert nitrogenous wastes to ammonia as prescribed.
     1) Rifaximin (Xifaxan) is a nonabsorbable antibiotic that is now preferred over neomycin.
     2) Neomycin has been traditionally used and may be prescribed by oral or NG tube; if used, monitor for auditory or renal toxicity.
  d. Administer magnesium citrate orally and/or tap water enemas as prescribed to remove nitrogenous wastes from the GI tract.
  e. Prevent constipation with fiber, stool softeners, or enemas.
  f. Assist with the use of liver support systems.
     1) Hemodialysis: blood circulated through a porous filter for rapid removal of fluid and solutes
     2) CRRT: blood circulated through a porous filter for slow removal of fluid and solutes

3) Hemoperfusion: hemodialysis or CRRT with a charcoal or resin exchange filter added
4) Therapeutic plasma exchange: plasma removed and replaced by donor plasma
5) Bioartificial liver support: Blood flows through a hollow fiber cartridge loaded with either cultured human or porcine hepatocytes.
6) Extracorporeal liver perfusion: blood circulated through a human or animal liver in vitro

5. Prevent, assess for, or treat intracranial hypertension and progression of hepatic encephalopathy.
    a. Perform frequent neurologic checks; invasive ICP monitoring may be used, especially in grade III and IV hepatic encephalopathy.
    b. Avoid hepatotoxic agents (Box 7.1).
    c. Avoid sedatives and analgesics and/or reduce dosage if necessary; diphenhydramine (Benadryl) or oxazepam (Serax) may be used for restlessness because they can safely be eliminated.
    d. Provide adequate rest; maintain bed rest in hepatic encephalopathy.
    e. Avoid activities that increase ICP (Intracranial Hypertension section of Chapter 5).
        1) Teach the patient to avoid Valsalva maneuver and other activities that increase intraabdominal or intrathoracic pressure.
        2) Maintain normal PaCO$_2$ and hypoxemia, which increase ICP.
    f. Institute seizure precautions.
    g. Administer hypertonic saline or mannitol (Osmitrol) and/or drainage of cerebrospinal fluid (if ICP catheter in place) as prescribed for cerebral edema.

6. Decrease portal hypertension.
    a. Administer beta-blockers as prescribed.
    b. Prepare the patient for a shunt as requested
        1) Interventional radiologic procedure: TIPS (described in the GI Hemorrhage section)
        2) Surgical procedure (e.g., portacaval shunt): associated with higher incidence of hepatic encephalopathy than TIPS

7. Maintain normal serum glucose and nutritional status.
    a. Monitor serum glucose every 4 to 6 hours.
    b. Administer IV dextrose solution continuously; D10 may be required to prevent hypoglycemia.
    c. Increase dietary protein (0.6–1 g/kg/day) for patients with cirrhosis and hepatic failure but restrict dietary protein (to less than 0.5 g/kg/day) in hepatic encephalopathy.
        1) Ensure that adequate CHO is provided to prevent muscle (protein) catabolism and muscle wasting (caloric requirements, 35–40 kcal/kg/day).
        2) Add protein in 20-g increments during recovery from encephalopathy.
    d. Use appropriate route for nutritional support.
        1) Oral: Administer antiemetics as prescribed before each meal and whenever indicated to prevent nausea (nausea is a significant impairment to oral nutritional intake in these patients).
        2) Enteral
            a) Necessary in patients with altered consciousness
            b) Elemental formulas (e.g., Vivonex) frequently used while maintaining protein restrictions if indicated (i.e., hepatic encephalopathy)
        3) Parenteral
            a) Branched-chain amino acid formulas may be used in encephalopathy; dextrose and lipids are needed to prevent the metabolism of parenteral amino acids or somatic protein (i.e., catabolism) for energy requirements.
    e. Administer vitamins and minerals.
        1) Fat-soluble (i.e., A, D, E, K) vitamins
        2) Thiamine and other B vitamins

8. Prevent and monitor for injury and infection.
    a. Prevent and monitor for skin breakdown.
        1) Alleviate pruritus.
            a) Cornstarch baths
            b) Skin lubricating lotions
        2) Place hands in cotton gloves at night to prevent scratching during sleep.
        3) Administer cholestyramine as prescribed to reduce bile pigment accumulation in skin.
    b. Prevent and monitor for bleeding.
        1) Avoid aspirin and NSAIDs
        2) Avoid invasive procedures, including injections, if possible.
        3) Administer vitamin K, fresh-frozen plasma, and platelets as prescribed.
        4) Administer aminocaproic acid as prescribed.
    c. Monitor closely for clinical indications of infection and sepsis.
        1) Administer microbials as prescribed: antibiotics and antifungals.

9. Assess for clinical indications of alcohol withdrawal syndrome (Box 7.3).
    a. Administer sedatives as prescribed; most of these agents, including chlordiazepoxide and diazepam, are hepatotoxic, so doses are adjusted and liver enzymes are monitored.
    b. Avoid alcohol-containing mouthwash or medications.

10. Participate in consideration of long-term treatment of hepatic failure.
    a. Early evaluation of candidacy for liver transplantation

11. Monitor for complications.
    a. Malnutrition resulting in immunosuppression, poor wound healing, and edema
    b. Coagulopathy
    c. Hemorrhage may be caused by:
        1) Esophageal varices
        2) Coagulopathy
        3) DIC
    d. Hypoglycemia
    e. Electrolyte imbalance
    f. Acute respiratory failure related to intrapulmonary shunt or noncardiac pulmonary edema
    g. Pancreatitis
    h. Infection, sepsis
    i. Acute renal failure related to hepatorenal syndrome, acute tubular necrosis, or hypovolemia

j. Seizures
k. Cerebral edema

Acute Pancreatitis

Definition
Acute inflammation of the pancreas; forms include the following:
1. Mild acute pancreatitis (previously referred to as interstitial pancreatitis)
   a. Edematous pancreas with little necrosis damage
   b. Hypovolemia may occur as a result of fluid leak into the peritoneal cavity
   c. Usually resolves within approximately 7 days
2. Severe acute pancreatitis (also referred to as *edematous interstitial pancreatitis*) (previously referred to as *necrotizing pancreatitis*)
   a. Extensive necrosis of pancreas and peripancreatic tissue and fat
   b. Erosion into blood vessels with hemorrhage
   c. SIRS frequently occurs.
   d. High incidence of complications and death

Etiology
1. Obstruction of common bile duct
   a. Cholelithiasis
   b. Post-ERCP
   c. Gallstone migration
   d. Alcoholism
2. Alcoholism
   a. Chronic alcohol intake leads to secretory and structural changes in the pancreas, contributing to duct obstruction.
   b. Alcohol increases the amount of trypsinogen.
3. Hypertriglyceridemia
4. Drugs
   a. Thiazide diuretics
   b. Furosemide
   c. Estrogen
   d. Procainamide
   e. Tetracycline
   f. Sulfonamides
   g. Corticosteroids
   h. Azathioprine
   i. Opiates
5. Peptic ulcer with perforation
6. Cancer, especially tumors of pancreas or lung
7. Injury to pancreas
   a. Trauma
   b. Surgical
      1) Gastric
      2) Biliary
      3) Duodenal
   c. Iatrogenic
8. Radiation injury
9. Pregnancy: third trimester; ectopic pregnancy
10. Ovarian cyst
11. Hyperparathyroidism or other causes of hypercalcemia
12. Lupus erythematosus
13. Infections
    a. Mumps
    b. Coxsackievirus B
    c. Mycoplasma
    d. Infectious mononucleosis
    e. Viral hepatitis
    f. Human immunodeficiency virus (HIV)
    g. Intestinal parasites (e.g., *Ascaris*)
14. Ischemia (e.g., shock and multiple organ dysfunction syndrome)
15. Postcardiopulmonary bypass
16. Infection, sepsis
17. Hereditary factors
18. Idiopathic (20% of cases)

Pathophysiology
Fig. 7.20.

Clinical Presentation
1. Subjective
   a. Abdominal pain
      1) Precipitation: may occur after a heavy, especially if fatty, meal or a drinking binge
      2) Palliation: may be eased by leaning forward or by assuming a fetal position
      3) Quality: "boring"
      4) Region: diffuse in epigastrium but may be left upper quadrant
      5) Radiation: to back or flanks
      6) Severity: moderate to very severe
      7) Timing: sudden onset; constant
   b. Associated symptoms
      1) Abdominal tenderness, guarding
      2) Nausea, vomiting, retching
      3) Dyspepsia
      4) Flatulence, diarrhea
      5) Weight loss
      6) Weakness
2. Objective
   a. Tachycardia
   b. Hypotension may be seen because of decreased circulating volume due to effusion or hemorrhagic; may be decreased because of septic shock
   c. Fever: usually low grade (e.g., 37.8–39°C)
   d. Jaundice if biliary obstruction
   e. Vomiting
   f. Hematemesis
   g. Grey Turner sign or Cullen sign may be seen with hemorrhage
   h. Abdominal distention
   i. Bowel sounds: decreased or absent
   j. Indications of peritoneal irritation: involuntary guarding during palpation of the abdomen, rebound tenderness
   k. Epigastric mass may be palpable, especially if pseudocyst
   l. Ascites may be present.
   m. Steatorrhea (bulky, pale, foul-smelling, floating)
   n. Breath sounds changes: may be diminished because of atelectasis, pleural effusion, or ARDS; crackles may also be heard
   o. Chvostek or Trousseau signs may be positive in hypocalcemia.

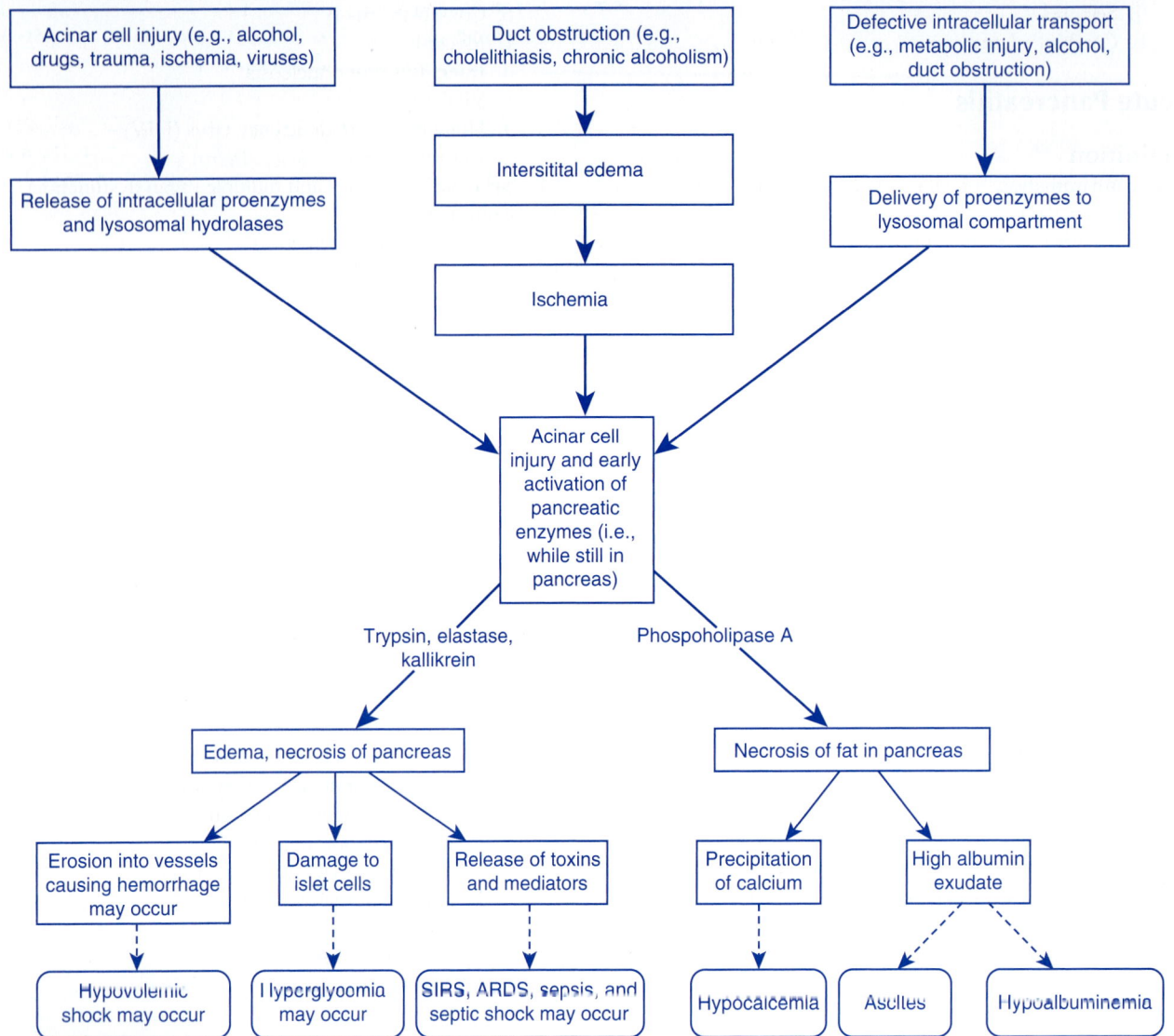

Fig. 7.20 Pathophysiology of pancreatitis. *Dotted lines* connect pathology to clinical presentation. *ARDS*, Acute respiratory distress syndrome; *SIRS*, systemic inflammatory response syndrome.

3. Diagnostic studies
   a. Serum
      1) Potassium: decreased
      2) Calcium: decreased
      3) Magnesium: decreased
      4) Glucose: elevated if endocrine function of the pancreas is compromised
      5) Triglycerides: may be elevated
      6) Amylase: usually elevated to greater than three times normal
         a) Peaks at 4 to 24 hours after onset of symptoms; usually returns to normal within 4 days
         b) May not be elevated when pancreatitis is caused by hypertriglyceridemia
      7) Lipase: elevated
         a) Stays elevated longer than amylase
         b) More specific than amylase
      8) Albumin: decreased
      9) BUN: may be elevated because of hypovolemia
      10) AST, ALT, LDH, ALP, bilirubin: elevated in liver or biliary disease
      11) Hct: decreased with hemorrhage; elevated with hemoconcentration because of third spacing
      12) WBC count: usually elevated with shift to the left
      13) Arterial blood gases
         a) Metabolic acidosis
         b) Respiratory complications may cause respiratory acidosis and hypoxemia.
   b. Urine: amylase usually elevated
   c. Stool: increase in fecal fat
   d. ECG: may suggest MI (e.g., ST-T wave elevations)
   e. Chest radiography
      1) May show bilateral or only left pleural effusion, elevated left hemidiaphragm, left atelectasis
      2) May show pulmonary complications of pancreatitis (e.g., atelectasis, pneumonia, ARDS, pleural effusion)
   f. Flat plate of abdomen
      1) May show cause (e.g., cholelithiasis)
      2) May show ileus and bowel dilation
      3) May show calcified pancreatic stones

g. Upper GI
   1) May show delayed gastric emptying
   2) May show enlargement of duodenum
   3) May show presence of dilated loop of smooth bowel adjacent to the pancreas
h. Abdominal ultrasonography: may show pancreatic swelling, edema, gallstones, pseudocyst, or peripancreatic fluid collections
i. CT scan with contrast
   1) May show enlargement, edema, or necrosis of the pancreas
   2) May show complications of pancreatitis (e.g., pancreatic pseudocyst or abscess)
   3) Balthazar and Ranson's system for grading pancreatitis by CT findings
      a) Grade A: normal pancreas
      b) Grade B: focal or diffuse enlargement of pancreas
      c) Grade C: mild peripancreatic inflammatory changes
      d) Grade D: fluid collection in a single location
      e) Grade E: multiple fluid collections or gas within the pancreas or peripancreatic inflammation
j. MRI: shows inflammatory changes within the pancreas
k. ERCP
   1) Contraindicated in acute pancreatitis; used more often in chronic pancreatitis
   2) Identifies ductal changes or calculi
l. Hepatobiliary (HIDA) scan: may identify hepatocellular disease from biliary obstruction as cause of pancreatitis
m. Peritoneal lavage: positive for blood in hemorrhagic pancreatitis
4. Ranson's prognostic criteria
   a. Scoring
      1) Each of the following criteria increases the severity (and mortality) in pancreatitis.
         a) Only one or two criteria: mild pancreatitis; mortality rate, approximately 1%
         b) More than six criteria: severe pancreatitis; predicted mortality rate, greater than 60%
   b. Criteria
      1) At the time of admission or diagnosis
         a) Age over 55 years
         b) WBC count over 16,000/mm^3
         c) Serum glucose greater than 200 mg/dl
         d) Serum LDH greater than 350 units/l
         e) Serum AST greater than 250 units/l
      2) After 48 hours
         a) Hct drop greater than 10%
         b) Increase in BUN greater than 5 mg/dl
         c) Calcium less than 8 mg/dl
         d) Base deficit greater than 4 mEq/l
         e) Estimated fluid sequestration greater than 6 l
         f) PaO$_2$ less than 60 mm Hg

Collaborative Management

1. Maintain airway, oxygenation, and ventilation.
   a. Elevate HOB 30 to 45 degrees, especially if ascites restricts diaphragmatic excursion.
   b. Administer oxygen as necessary to maintain SpO$_2$ at 94% unless contraindicated; in patients with COPD, administer oxygen to achieve a SpO$_2$ of ~90%.
   c. Monitor SpO$_2$ closely and evaluate work of breathing in detection of development of atelectasis and/or ARDS.
2. Maintain adequate circulating volume and fluid and electrolyte balance.
   a. Administer crystalloids and colloids as prescribed to restore circulating blood volume.
   b. Monitor sodium, calcium, potassium, magnesium, and phosphate.
      1) Administer calcium replacement orally or intravenously as prescribed.
      2) Administer potassium replacement as prescribed.
      3) Restrict sodium to 500 mg/day for patients with ascites.
   c. Measure abdominal girth daily in patients with ascites.
   d. Measure intraabdominal pressure if intraabdominal hypertension is suspected.
   e. Weigh daily at same time on same scale.
3. Decrease release of and destruction by pancreatic enzymes.
   a. Assist with treatment of cause.
      1) Alcohol cessation if alcohol related
      2) Cholecystectomy after resolution of pancreatitis if caused by cholelithiasis
      3) Discontinuance of offending drug if drug induced
      4) Statins, niacin, fibrates, or omega-3 fatty acids if related to hypertriglyceridemia
   b. Provide appropriate nutritional support
      1) Severe acute pancreatitis
         a) Maintain NPO status during acute phase and with any recurrence of pain.
         b) Enteral nutrition via nasojejunal tube prevents atrophy of the gut lymphoid tissue and prevents the overgrowth of bacteria in the intestine, thereby maintaining its permeability and improving outcomes.
      2) Mild acute pancreatitis
         a) Oral feeding can be restarted when abdominal pain is decreasing and inflammatory markers are improving.
   c. Insert NG tube to decompress the stomach and decrease risk of vomiting until ileus is resolved.
   d. Administer drugs as prescribed to decrease secretion of pancreatic enzymes (Table 7.6).
      1) Octreotide acetate IV or subcutaneously
      2) Histamine$_2$ receptor antagonists IV
   e. Keep environment free of food odors.
   f. Perform mouth care with water or normal saline only; do not use alcohol-containing or flavored mouthwash or toothpaste.
4. Prevent and treat pain and discomfort.
   a. Maintain bed rest; encourage knee flexing while in supine position to relax abdominal muscles.
   b. Maintain quiet environment, comfortable temperature, and dim lighting.

c. Administer analgesics.
  1) Opiates (e.g., morphine, hydromorphone) preferably administered via patient-controlled analgesia (PCA)
     a) NOTE: Although meperidine for years has been considered the analgesic of choice in acute pancreatitis, recent studies show no significant difference between morphine and meperidine in the degree of spasm of the sphincter of Oddi.
  2) Neurolytic block of the celiac plexus for severe persistent pain
d. Use nonpharmacologic pain relief methods (e.g., imagery, distraction).
e. Treat nausea with prescribed antiemetics.
f. Ensure adequate sleep and rest.
5. Administer appropriate nutritional support considering restrictions.
  a. Administer nutritional support during acute phase of illness.
    1) Parenteral nutrition initially
    2) Enteral nutrition below the duodenum after ileus is resolved
       a) Although enteral feeding has traditionally been thought to be contraindicated in acute pancreatitis, recent studies indicate that enteral feeding may be safely administered if the tube is below the ligament of Treitz (e.g., jejunostomy tube).
       b) Advantages over parenteral nutrition include the following:
          i) Maintains immune responsiveness and gut integrity
          ii) Reduces risk of bacterial translocation
          iii) Fewer complications
  b. Clear liquids or elemental diet (e.g., Vivonex) may be used after inflammation subsides (pain subsides, serum amylase normal), progressing to low-fat, full liquids and eventually progressing to a regular diet.
  c. Avoid alcohol and food high in fat.
  d. Administer fat-soluble vitamins, thiamine, and folic acid as prescribed.
  e. Monitor serum glucose levels closely and administer glucose or insulin as indicated.
6. Prevent and monitor for infection.
  a. Prophylactic antibiotics as prescribed
    1) Antibiotics are prescribed that effectively penetrate the pancreatic tissue and provide good coverage against gram-negative enteric and anaerobic organisms (e.g., imipenem–cilastatin, ofloxacin, metronidazole).
    2) If no improvement after 1 week, CT-guided aspiration may be performed; bacteria in aspirate suggest infected pancreatic necrosis and indicate the need for surgery.
  b. Monitor for clinical indications of abscess formation (e.g., increase in abdominal pain, vomiting, fever, leukocytosis).
7. Prepare patient for surgical measures for relief of pancreatitis if necessary (during acute phase, surgery is performed only if absolutely necessary).
  a. Cholecystectomy if bile reflux is the cause of pancreatitis
  b. Drainage and removal of abscess or pseudocysts
  c. Pancreatic resection or total pancreatectomy
    1) Used if pancreas and/or other organs are necrotic
    2) After surgical debridement of necrotic tissue, the abdomen may be left open and packed or closed with drains in place.
    3) Total pancreatectomy results in diabetes and other metabolic difficulties.
       a) Islet cell autotransplantation is sometimes performed.
       b) Segmental pancreatic autotransplantation is sometimes performed: part of viable pancreatic tissue reimplanted following total pancreatectomy
8. Maintain normal serum glucose levels.
  a. Monitor serum glucose levels closely.
  b. Administer insulin as indicated and prescribed.
  c. Maintain constant infusion of TPN solution or enteral feedings.
9. Assess for clinical indications of alcohol withdrawal syndrome (Box 7.3).
  a. If present, administer sedatives as prescribed; most of these agents, including chlordiazepoxide and diazepam, are hepatotoxic; doses are adjusted, and liver enzymes are monitored.
  b. Avoid alcohol-containing mouthwash or medications.
10. Monitor for complications.
  a. Hypoglycemia or hyperglycemia
  b. Hypocalcemia
  c. Pseudocysts
    1) Caused by collection of inflammatory debris, pancreatic secretions, and necrotic tissue in the pancreatic tissue; may cause compression of portal vein or bile duct or rupture and peritonitis and sepsis
    2) Clinical presentation includes pain or ache in the abdomen, a feeling of bloating, or poor digestion of food.
    3) Complications related to the pseudocyst include infection of the pseudocyst with a pancreatic abscess, bleeding into the pseudocyst, or intestinal obstruction of the intestine by the pseudocyst.
    4) Collaborative management includes nothing for small cysts or drainage by surgical, endoscopic, or percutaneous approach for larger cysts.
  d. Pancreatic abscess
    1) Caused by accumulation of pus in or near the pancreas
    2) Clinical presentation includes fever, palpable mass, abdominal tenderness, nausea, vomiting, and leukocytosis.
    3) Collaborative management includes surgery for drainage.
  e. Pancreatic fistula
    1) Caused by a communication between the pancreas and the skin
    2) Clinical presentation includes drainage of extremely alkaline pancreatic secretions onto the skin and severe excoriation.
    3) Collaborative management includes fluid and electrolyte replacement; octreotide acetate (Sandostatin) may be used.

f. Hypovolemic shock
  1) Caused by exudate of protein-rich fluid into retroperitoneal space or by erosion into the vascular bed and hemorrhage
  2) Clinical presentation includes tachycardia, hypotension, oliguria, and other indications of hypoperfusion.
  3) Collaborative management includes volume resuscitation, including crystalloids, colloids, blood administration for hemorrhagic pancreatitis
g. SIRS
h. Pleural effusion
i. ARDS
j. GI bleeding
k. DIC
l. Sepsis
m. Acute renal failure
n. Perforation

Intestinal Infarction, Obstruction, and Perforation

Definitions
1. Intestinal infarction: necrosis of the intestinal wall resulting from ischemia
2. Intestinal obstruction: failure of the intestinal contents to progress forward through the lumen of the bowel; may be partial or complete
   a. Mechanism
     1) Functional obstruction: caused by loss of peristalsis; usually referred to as paralytic ileus
     2) Structural (i.e., mechanical) obstruction: caused by factors that occlude the bowel lumen
   b. Severity
     1) Simple: luminal obstruction without compromise of blood supply
     2) Strangulated: luminal obstruction with compromise of blood supply
   c. Extent: partial versus complete
   d. Location: proximal versus distal
3. Intestinal perforation: penetration of the lumen of the intestine with resultant spillage of intestinal contents into the peritoneal cavity

Etiology
1. Infarction
   a. Arteriosclerosis
   b. Vasculitis
   c. Mural thrombus, emboli: post-MI; atrial fibrillation; ventricular aneurysm; endocarditis
   d. Hypercoagulability (e.g., polycythemia, postsplenectomy)
   e. Surgical procedures involving aortic clamping (e.g., abdominal aortic aneurysm repair)
   f. Vasopressors
     1) Endogenous caused by sympathetic nervous system stimulation (e.g., shock)
     2) Exogenous (e.g., norepinephrine, high-dose dopamine)
   g. Strangulated intestinal obstruction
   h. Intraabdominal infection
   i. Cirrhosis
2. Obstruction
   a. Functional (i.e., paralytic ileus): most common type of intestinal obstruction
     1) Abdominal surgery
     2) Hypokalemia
     3) Intestinal distention
     4) Peritonitis
     5) Intestinal ischemia
     6) Severe trauma
     7) Spinal cord injury
     8) Ureteral distention
     9) Pneumonia
     10) Pleuritis
     11) Subphrenic abscess
     12) Pancreatitis
     13) Acute cholecystitis
     14) Pelvic abscess
     15) Narcotics (e.g., morphine)
     16) Sepsis
   b. Structural (i.e., mechanical)
     1) Small bowel: Most obstructions occur in the small bowel, especially at the ileum.
       a) Postoperative adhesions: most common
       b) Incarcerated hernia
       c) Volvulus
       d) Foreign body
       e) Neoplasm
       f) Crohn disease
     2) Large bowel: most often the sigmoid colon
       a) Neoplasm: most common
       b) Stricture
       c) Intussusception
       d) Diverticulitis
       e) Fecal or barium impaction
3. Perforation
   a. Peptic ulcer
   b. Bowel obstruction
   c. Appendicitis, diverticulitis
   d. Penetrating wound

Pathophysiology
Fig. 7.21.

Clinical Presentation
1. Infarction
   a. Subjective
     1) May have history of precipitating event
     2) Anorexia
     3) Pallor
     4) Abdominal pain
       a) Severe cramping, periumbilical or nonspecific diffuse
       b) Abdominal pain related to mesenteric ischemia may be referred to as *abdominal angina.*
     5) Abdominal tenderness
     6) Urgency to have a bowel movement
   b. Objective
     1) Tachycardia
     2) Hypotension
     3) Tachypnea
     4) Fever

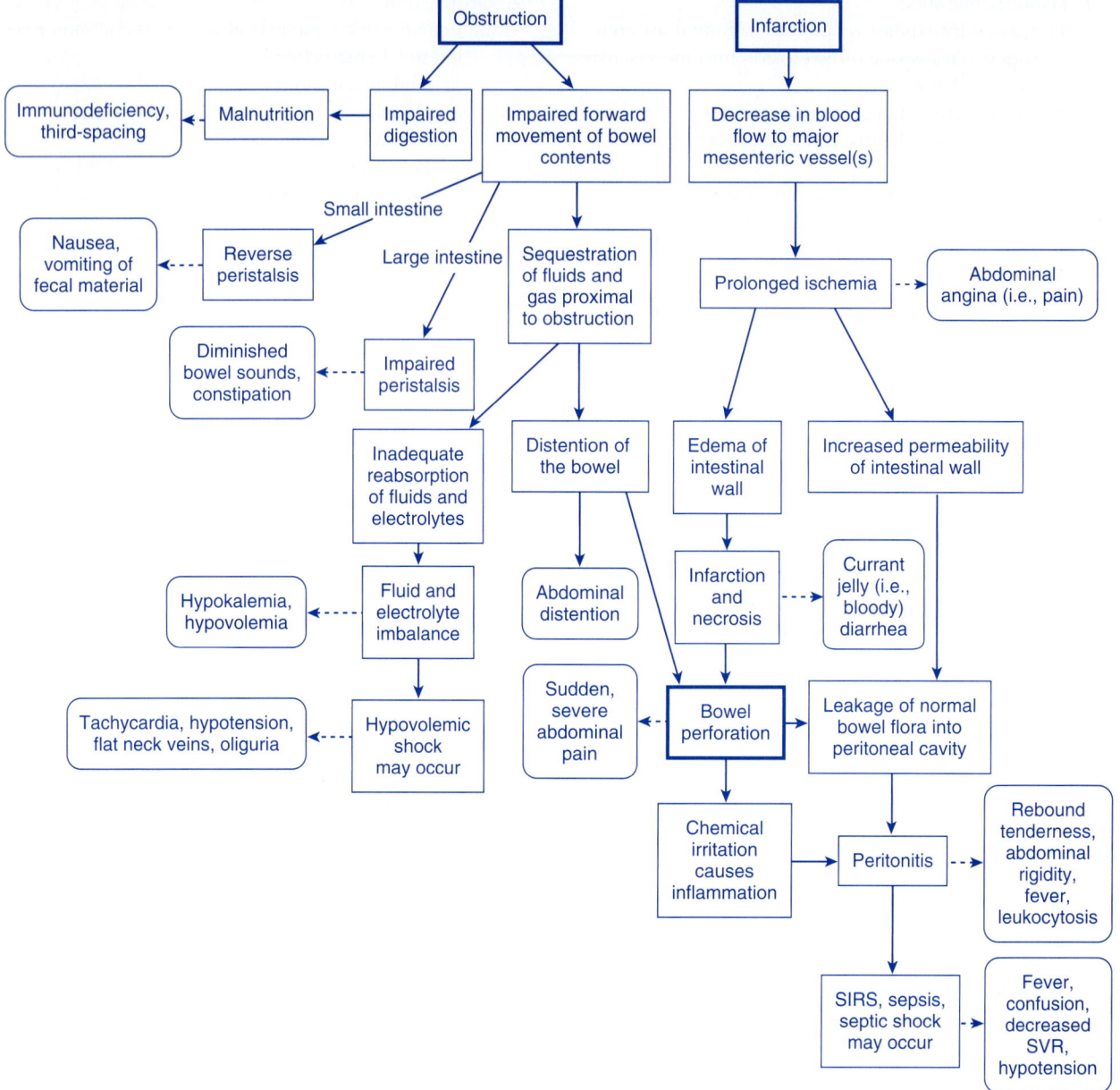

Fig. 7.21 Pathophysiology of intestinal obstruction, infarction, and perforation. *Dotted lines* connect pathology to clinical presentation. *SIRS,* Systemic inflammatory response syndrome; *SVR,* systemic vascular resistance.

      5) Clinical indications of dehydration
      6) Vomiting: persistent, may be bloody
      7) Abdominal distention
      8) Abdominal guarding and rigidity
      9) Urgent and bloody diarrhea
     10) Hypoactive or absent bowel sounds
     11) Weight loss
  c. Diagnostic studies
    1) Serum
      a) BUN: elevated because of dehydration
      b) ALP: elevated
      c) Amylase: elevated
      d) Hct: elevated
      e) WBC count: elevated
      f) Arterial blood gases: metabolic acidosis
    2) Stool: guaiac positive
    3) Angiography: shows occlusion of the arterial supply
    4) Sigmoidoscopy: shows dusky, ischemic bowel

2. Obstruction
  a. Small bowel
    1) Subjective
      a) May have history of precipitating event
      b) Abdominal pain
        i) Pain that is colicky and of shorter duration with bilious vomiting may be more proximal; pain that is progressive and lasting for several days with abdominal distention may be more distal.
        ii) Steady, severe, localized pain may indicate strangulation.
      c) Changes in bowel habits
        i) Early or partial bowel obstruction: normal stools or diarrhea
        ii) Late or complete obstruction: constipation or absence of stools

2) Objective
    a) Vomiting early: may be projectile and/or fecal
        i) Clear gastric fluid: obstruction at the pylorus
        ii) Gastric contents and bile
            (a) Obstruction in the proximal small intestine
            (b) Paralytic ileus
        iii) Brown fecal: obstruction in the distal small intestine
    b) Abdominal distention
    c) Clinical indications of dehydration
    d) Bowel sounds: high-pitched
        i) Increased early
        ii) Decreased late
3) Diagnostic studies
    a) Serum
        i) Sodium: may be decreased, increased, or normal depending on hydration level and serum osmolality
        ii) Potassium: decreased
        iii) Chloride: decreased
        iv) BUN: elevated due to dehydration
        v) Hct: elevated
        vi) WBC count: elevated
        vii) Arterial blood gases: usually metabolic acidosis, but metabolic alkalosis may be seen with proximal obstruction and gastric losses
    b) Upper GI: may show point of obstruction
    c) Flat plate of abdomen: shows dilated loops of gas-filled bowel
    d) CT: aids in differentiation of cause and location of obstruction
    e) MRI: aids in differentiation of cause and location of obstruction
b. Large bowel
    1) Subjective
        a) May have history of precipitating event
        b) Dull pain
        c) Change in bowel habits: thin, ribbonlike stools progressing to constipation to absence of stools with watery discharge
        d) Decrease in flatus
    2) Objective
        a) Vomiting late
        b) Abdominal distention
        c) Bowel sounds: low-pitched
            i) Increased early
            ii) Decreased late
        d) Melena may occur if large bowel obstruction is caused by ulcerative colitis, cancer, or diverticulitis.
    3) Diagnostic studies
        a) Serum
            i) Sodium: may be decreased, increased, or normal depending on hydration level and serum osmolality
            ii) Potassium: decreased
            iii) Chloride: decreased
            iv) BUN: elevated because of dehydration
            v) CEA: elevated if caused by cancer
            vi) Hct: may be elevated because of dehydration or decreased because of hemorrhage; large intestinal tumor frequently causes slow bleeding
            vii) WBC count: elevated
            viii) Arterial blood gases: metabolic acidosis
        b) Stools: may be positive for occult blood in large bowel obstruction because of ulcerative colitis, cancer, or diverticulitis
        c) Flat plate of abdomen: shows dilated loops of gas-filled bowel
        d) Barium enema: may show point of obstruction
        e) Endoscopy: obstruction may be visible on sigmoidoscopy or colonoscopy
3. Perforation
    a. Subjective
        1) Abdominal pain
        2) Abdominal tenderness
        3) Anorexia
        4) Nausea
    b. Objective
        1) Tachycardia
        2) Tachypnea
        3) Fever
        4) Vomiting
        5) Rigid, "boardlike" abdomen
        6) Rebound tenderness
        7) Absence of liver dullness due to free air in peritoneum
        8) Bowel sounds: diminished or absent
    c. Diagnostic studies
        1) Serum: WBC count elevated
        2) Flat plate of abdomen: free air in peritoneum may be seen
        3) Upper GI: contraindicated

Collaborative Management

1. Maintain airway, oxygenation, and ventilation.
    a. Elevate HOB 30 to 45 degrees.
    b. Administer oxygen as necessary to maintain SpO_2 at 94% unless contraindicated; in patients with COPD, administer oxygen to achieve a SpO_2 of ~90%.
2. Maintain adequate circulating volume and fluid and electrolyte balance.
    a. Assess fluid status.
        1) Weigh daily at the same time on the same scale.
        2) Hemodynamic monitoring may be necessary during fluid resuscitation.
    b. Administer crystalloids and colloids as prescribed to restore circulating blood volume.
    c. Administer blood and blood products as needed; whole blood or packed cells should be given early if significant bleeding is suspected; after multiple transfusions, consideration should be given to replacement of clotting factors, platelets, and calcium.
    d. Monitor sodium, calcium, potassium, and phosphate; administer electrolyte replacement as indicated.
    e. Discontinue vasopressors if cause of ischemia.
3. Prevent and treat pain and discomfort.
    a. Maintain bed rest.
    b. Maintain quiet environment, comfortable temperature, and dim lighting.

c. Administer analgesics (e.g., morphine) (Note: Analgesics are sometimes withheld until the diagnosis is made).
   d. Encourage knee flexing while in supine position to relax abdominal muscles.
   e. Use nonpharmacologic pain relief methods (e.g., imagery, distraction, music).
   f. Treat nausea with prescribed antiemetics.
   g. Perform mouth care after emesis.
4. Prevent perforation of bowel if obstruction is present.
   a. Discontinue all oral intake.
   b. Insert a NG tube or orogastric tube as prescribed to decompress the stomach, prevent vomiting, and reduce the risk of aspiration.
   c. Administer drugs as prescribed to enhance GI motility in partial intestinal obstruction.
      1) Erythromycin
      2) Metoclopramide HCl
      3) Octreotide
   d. Insert a rectal tube as prescribed to reduce trapped air in complete large bowel obstruction.
   e. Prepare patient for therapeutic colonoscopy as requested.
      1) Air insufflation for intussusception
      2) Cecal dilation or endoscopic balloon duodenal dilation for small bowel obstruction
   f. Assist with palliative procedures to enhance quality of life in patients with terminal disease associated with bowel obstruction.
      1) Insertion of distal gastric or jejunal tubes
      2) Colonic dilation
      3) Insertion of intestinal stents
5. Prepare the patient for surgery as requested: Surgery is indicated for vascular obstruction, complete bowel obstruction, and bowel perforation; a strangulated obstruction is a surgical emergency.
   a. Bowel preparation with cathartics, enemas, and sterilization prior to surgery
      1) Nonabsorbable aminoglycoside (e.g., neomycin) usually is used for bowel sterilization.
      2) Do not give cathartics or enemas for patients who are completely obstructed.
   b. Procedures
      1) Infarction
         a) Exploratory laparotomy and embolectomy and/or arterial reconstruction with resection of irreparably damaged bowel
      2) Obstruction
         a) Correction of cause
            i) Laparoscopic adhesiolysis: for obstruction caused by adhesion
            ii) Herniorrhaphy: for reduction of hernia
            iii) Reduction of volvulus or intussusception
         b) Bowel resection: may require temporary or permanent bowel diversion with colostomy
            i) Right hemicolectomy: for tumors in the cecum and ascending colon
            ii) Left hemicolectomy: for tumors of the descending and sigmoid colon; prepare patient for the possibility of colostomy (temporary or permanent) in cases of left-sided obstruction
            iii) Transverse colectomy: for tumors of the middle or left transverse colon
            iv) Low anterior resection: for proximal and midrectal tumors
            v) Abdominoperineal resection: for malignant lesions of the lower sigmoid colon, rectum, and anus; requires permanent colostomy
      3) Perforation
         a) Repair of perforation may require bowel resection; a temporary bowel diversion may be performed to allow the anastomosis to heal.
         b) Antibiotic lavage may be done during surgery.
   c. Answer the patient's questions about the planned procedures.
   d. Prepare the patient for adjuvant therapy if required for colon cancer.
      1) Chemoembolization: the infusion of a concentrated dose of an antineoplastic agent into the hepatic artery to embolize the agent
      2) Radiation therapy
      3) Brachytherapy: the placement of radioactive seeds in the area where the tumor was removed
      4) Chemotherapy: the administration of an antineoplastic agent before, during, or after surgery
      5) Cryosurgery: the freezing of liver metastasis
6. Prevent or monitor for infection.
   a. Administer antibiotics as prescribed.
   b. Reduce leakage of intestinal bacteria and risk of peritonitis and sepsis if perforation has occurred.
      1) Keep the patient immobilized to reduce the chemical irritation to the peritoneum.
      2) Antibiotics are given preoperatively.
      3) Antibiotic lavage may be done during surgery.
      4) Antibiotics are given postoperatively.
   c. Monitor closely for clinical indications of infection and sepsis.
      1) Measure temperature every 4 hours.
      2) Assess HR and BP hourly.
      3) Note changes in mental status.
      4) Note changes in color and character of wound drainage.
      5) Monitor changes in WBC count.
   d. Clean around drains aseptically and protect skin around drains postoperatively.
7. Administer appropriate nutritional support considering restrictions.
   a. Administer nutritional support parenterally in the acute phase.
   b. Provide oral feedings and advance diet when condition and postoperative paralytic ileus have resolved.
   c. Administer vitamin and mineral supplements as prescribed.
8. Monitor for complications.
   a. Fluid and electrolyte imbalance
   b. Hemorrhage
   c. Sepsis
   d. Peritonitis

e. Respiratory distress secondary to abdominal distention
f. Shock: hypovolemic or septic
g. Abscess
h. Perforation

Abdominal Trauma

Definition
Trauma that occurs between the nipple line to midthigh

Etiology
1. Penetrating trauma (e.g., motor vehicle collision, assault, sharp instruments [e.g., knife, gunshot wound, impalement])
2. Blunt trauma (e.g., motor vehicle collision, assault, fall, sport injury)
3. Iatrogenic trauma
   a. Peritoneal tap
   b. Endoscopy
   c. Biopsy
   d. Cardiopulmonary resuscitation

Pathophysiology
1. Seldom a single-organ injury
2. High-velocity penetrating trauma
   a. Extensive destruction of contact tissue
   b. Severe associated blast effect on the surrounding tissues
   c. Liver most often affected by penetrating trauma
3. Blunt trauma
   a. Caused by direct injury, crushing force between two objects, acceleration/deceleration, shearing, or twisting
   b. Pressure injury
   c. Spleen most often affected by blunt trauma; pancreas is frequently injured with spleen

Clinical Presentation
1. Subjective
   a. Abdominal pain: may be poorly localized or referred
      1) Kehr sign: left shoulder pain indicative of splenic rupture caused by blood below diaphragm that irritates the phrenic nerve
      2) Rovsing sign: pain in right lower quadrant with palpation of left lower quadrant indicates peritoneal irritation
   b. Abdominal tenderness
2. Objective
   a. Seat belt sign: ecchymosis across the lower abdomen caused by seat belt
   b. Hematoma: Note location.
      1) Hematoma in flank area may be seen in renal injury.
   c. Entrance and exit wounds
   d. Grey Turner or Cullen sign: may be seen
   e. Coopernail sign (ecchymosis of scrotum or labia): indicative of fractured pelvis
   f. Rigid abdomen: may indicate intraabdominal bleeding
   g. Ballance sign (i.e., resonance over right flank with patient on left side): indicative of ruptured spleen
   h. Diminished femoral pulses: may be seen in vascular injury
   i. Loss of liver dullness: indicates perforation with free air in peritoneum
   j. Clinical indications of hypoperfusion or shock (Table 3.2)
   k. Clinical indications of perforation (e.g., severe abdominal pain, fever, nausea, vomiting)
   l. Clinical indications of peritonitis (e.g., involuntary guarding, abdominal rigidity, rebound tenderness)
   m. Specifics related to organ injured (Table 7.11)
3. Diagnostic studies
   a. Serum
      1) Glucose: elevated because of stress
      2) Amylase: may be elevated if injury to pancreas or bowel
      3) ALT, AST, and LDH: may be elevated if liver injury
      4) Hgb, Hct: decreased with hemorrhage
      5) WBC: may be elevated if infection is present or if spleen is ruptured
      6) Platelets: elevated if spleen is injured
      7) PT, aPTT: may be prolonged
      8) Drug and alcohol screens: results may be positive

Table 7.11 Clinical Indications of Organ Injury

Organ	Suspect Injury to This Organ if	Clinical Indications of Injury	Complications
Liver	• Seat belt sign • Local sign of injury (RUQ) • Lower right rib fracture • Blunt or penetrating trauma • Acceleration/deceleration MVC • Presence of other abdominal injuries	• RUQ pain, tenderness, and guarding • Referred pain to right shoulder • Increase in abdominal girth and rigidity • Increased pain on inspiration • Clinical indications of shock • Leukocytosis • Elevated ALT, AST, LDH • Decreased Hgb and Hct • Abnormal clotting studies • Chest radiography: elevated diaphragm on right side • Injury evident on FAST • Positive peritoneal lavage if performed	• Shock • Infection, sepsis • Subdiaphragmatic abscess • Clotting abnormalities • Atelectasis, pneumonia, ARDS • Hepatic failure

Continued

Table 7.11 Clinical Indications of Organ Injury—cont'd

Organ	Suspect Injury to This Organ if	Clinical Indications of Injury	Complications
Spleen	• Seat belt sign • Local sign of injury (LUQ) • Lower left rib fractures • Left pneumothorax • Blunt or penetrating trauma to abdomen • Acceleration/deceleration MVC • Presence of other abdominal injuries	• LUQ pain, tenderness, and guarding • Increased abdominal girth and rigidity • Kehr sign • Ballance sign • Increased pain on inspiration • Clinical indications of shock • Decreased Hgb and Hct • Injury evident on FAST • Positive peritoneal lavage • Shock	• Shock • Atelectasis, pneumonia, ARDS • Infection, sepsis especially if splenectomy performed • Subdiaphragmatic abscess
Pancreas	• Seat belt sign • Presence of other abdominal injuries • MVC • Blunt or penetrating trauma to abdomen	• Epigastric, back, or shoulder pain • Abdominal tenderness and guarding • Increased abdominal girth • Diminished bowel sounds • Clinical indications of shock • Hyperglycemia or hypoglycemia • Elevated serum lipase • Leukocytosis • Positive peritoneal lavage for amylase but unreliable because the pancreas is located retroperitoneally	• Shock • Diabetes • Pancreatitis • Pancreatic abscess or pseudocyst • Pancreatic fistula • Atelectasis, pneumonia, ARDS
Stomach	• Penetrating trauma to abdomen • Presence of other abdominal injuries	• Epigastric or LUQ pain and tenderness • Hematemesis or bloody aspirate from NG tube • Rebound tenderness • Clinical indications of shock • Leukocytosis • Positive peritoneal lavage • Free air on flat plate of abdomen	• Atelectasis, pneumonia, ARDS • Gastric fistula
Intestine	• Seat belt sign • Presence of other abdominal injuries • Blunt trauma with deceleration • Penetrating injury	• Local sign of injury (e.g., ecchymosis, abrasion) • Nausea, vomiting • Abdominal pain: may be referred or rebound • Absent bowel sounds • Leukocytosis • Positive peritoneal lavage for blood and fecal matter • Free air on flat plate of abdomen • Positive fecal occult blood test	• Ileus • Peritonitis, sepsis • Abscess • Intestinal ischemia, infarction, obstruction, perforation • Fistula
Abdominal vessels	• Other abdominal injuries • Blunt or penetrating abdominal injury • Sudden deceleration in MVC or fall	• Clinical indications of shock • Abdominal distention and guarding • Increased abdominal girth and rigidity • Abdominal bruit • Diminished femoral pulses if aorta or iliac injury • Mottled lower extremities • Cullen sign • Decreased Hgb and Hct • Shock	• Shock • Mesenteric ischemia or infarction • Infection, sepsis

ALT, Alanine aminotransferase; *ARDS*, acute respiratory distress syndrome; *AST*, aspartate aminotransferase; *FAST*, focused abdominal sonography for trauma; *Hb*, hemoglobin; *Hct*, hematocrit; *LDH*, lactate dehydrogenase; *LUQ*, left upper quadrant; *MCV*, mean corpuscular volume; *NG*, nasogastric; *RUQ*, right upper quadrant.

    b. Urine
        1) May show hematuria if renal trauma
        2) May show myoglobinuria if crush injury has occurred
    c. Stool: may be positive for occult blood
    d. Chest radiography: used to rule out concurrent thoracic injury; identify free air under diaphragm
    e. Flat plate of abdomen: may show free air in peritoneum if stomach or bowel is perforated
    f. IV pyelogram: if hematuria is present to look for renal trauma
    g. Angiography: may show vascular injury
    h. CT scan or MRI: to identify areas of injury

i. Focused abdominal sonography for trauma (FAST)
   1) Use: detects fluid or blood in the pericardium, abdomen, or pelvis and allows visualization of the spleen and liver
      a) Although it cannot reliably identify injury to intraabdominal organs (requires CT), it can accurately predict the need for laparotomy in trauma patients; very good sensitivity and excellent specificity
   2) Advantages over diagnostic peritoneal lavage (DPL)
      a) More rapid: generally completed in less than 5 minutes
      b) Requires no preparation
      c) Noninvasive
      d) No contraindications
j. DPL: may be done to assess for intraabdominal bleeding, although FAST is usually the preferred screening study
   1) Assist with placement of peritoneal catheter; if gross blood is obtained with catheter insertion, immediate exploratory laparotomy is indicated.
   2) Instill 1 l of normal saline over 15 to 20 minutes.
   3) Move the patient side to side after fluid instillation to distribute the lavage fluid.
   4) Drain.
   5) Send for analysis.
      a) Considered positive if lavage fluid is grossly bloody or contains the following:
         i) RBC greater than $100,000/mm^3$
         ii) WBC greater than $500/mm^3$
         iii) Amylase greater than 175 units/dl
         iv) Bile, bacteria, intestinal content
      b) Considered positive if newsprint cannot be read through the lavage fluid (i.e., newsprint sign)
      c) Major limitation of peritoneal lavage is that it does not detect diaphragmatic or retroperitoneal injuries
k. Specifics related to organ injured (Table 7.11)

Collaborative Management

1. Maintain airway, oxygenation, and ventilation.
   a. Stabilize the cervical spine.
   b. Elevate HOB 30 to 45 degrees to allow for optimal diaphragmatic excursion.
   c. Administer oxygen as necessary to maintain SpO_2 at 94% unless contraindicated; in patients with COPD, administer oxygen to achieve a SpO_2 of 90% by pulse oximetry.
   d. Place oropharyngeal or nasopharyngeal airway in patients with altered consciousness; assist with endotracheal intubation if required.
2. Detect bleeding and maintain adequate circulating volume.
   a. Detect bleeding by performing head-to-toe assessment and assisting with peritoneal lavage; peritoneal lavage is especially important in an unconscious patient because subjective report of tenderness or pain is absent.
   b. Insert indwelling urinary catheter to evaluate hourly urine output unless contraindicated; contraindications include the following:
      1) Blood around the urinary meatus
      2) Perineal or scrotal hematoma
      3) Displacement of the prostate gland noted during rectal exam by physician
   c. Assist with insertion of arterial catheter and pulmonary artery catheter in patient with hemodynamic instability.
   d. Insert two short (1¼-inch) large-gauge (16- or 18-gauge) peripheral IV catheters; draw blood samples for laboratory analysis and type and crossmatch for blood.
   e. Administer intravenous fluids to restore circulating blood volume.
      1) Crystalloids
      2) Colloids
      3) Blood and blood products
         a) Whole blood or packed cells should be given early if significant bleeding is suspected.
         b) Consideration should be given to replacement of clotting factors, platelets, and calcium after multiple transfusions.
   f. Control bleeding.
      1) Pressure can be applied to overt bleeding site.
      2) Prepare patient for exploratory laparotomy as indicated.
         a) Penetrating injury invading the peritoneum
         b) Clinical indications of perforation (e.g., acute abdomen)
         c) Free air in peritoneum on radiograph
         d) Shock
         e) GI hemorrhage
         f) Massive hematuria
         g) Evisceration
         h) Positive peritoneal lavage
         i) Surgical indications on CT scan or angiography
3. Prevent and treat pain and discomfort.
   a. Maintain bed rest.
   b. Maintain quiet environment, comfortable temperature, and dim lighting.
   c. Administer analgesics (e.g., morphine); may be contraindicated until diagnoses are made
   d. Encourage knee flexing while in supine position to relax abdominal muscles in patients with peritoneal irritation.
   e. Use nonpharmacologic pain relief methods (e.g., imagery, distraction, music).
4. Maintain fluid and electrolyte balance.
   a. Monitor sodium, calcium, potassium, magnesium, and phosphate.
   b. Administer electrolyte replacement as indicated.
5. Decompress GI tract.
   a. Insert NG tube; use orogastric tube in patients with midface fractures.
   b. Monitor NG output for color, amount, and odor of drainage.
   c. Cover any eviscerated organs with saline-soaked pads.

6. Administer appropriate nutritional support considering restrictions.
    a. Administer nutritional support parenterally acutely.
    b. Provide oral feeding and advance diet when condition is surgically resolved.
    c. Administer vitamin and mineral supplements.
7. Prevent or monitor for infection.
    a. Observe for signs of peritonitis (e.g., fever, peritonitis, leukocytosis).
    b. Monitor abdominal girth.
    c. Administer antibiotics as prescribed; antibiotic lavage may be performed during exploratory laparotomy if bowel perforation has occurred.
    d. Maintain asepsis of wounds and drains.
    e. Monitor bowel sounds.
    f. Evaluate tetanus immunization status and administer tetanus toxoid if indicated for penetrating trauma, abrasion, cuts, and so on.
8. Monitor for complications.
    a. Obstruction
    b. Perforation
    c. Peritonitis
    d. Pancreatitis
    e. Infection, abscess, sepsis
    f. Hemorrhage
        1) Retroperitoneal
        2) Intraperitoneal
    g. Shock: hypovolemic or septic
    h. DIC
    i. Atelectasis, pneumonia, ARDS
    j. Organ failure
    k. Abdominal compartment syndrome

Gastrointestinal Surgery

Procedures Frequently Requiring Critical Care
Table 7.12 and Figs. 7.22 through 7.26.

Postoperative Management for Gastrointestinal Surgeries
1. Maintain airway, oxygenation, and ventilation.
    a. Monitor airway patency and use artificial airways as indicated; many of these patients will still be intubated and receiving mechanical ventilation.

Table 7.12 Gastrointestinal Surgical Procedures Frequently Requiring Critical Care

Surgical Procedure	Description	Indications
Billroth I (also referred to as *gastroduodenostomy*) (Fig. 7.18)	• Resection of the antrum of the stomach and anastomosis of the remainder of the stomach to the duodenum	• Ulcer or malignancy
Billroth II (also referred to as *gastrojejunostomy*) (Fig. 7.18)	• Resection of the antrum of the stomach and anastomosis of the remainder of the stomach to the jejunum, leaving the duodenal stump and accompanied by a vagotomy	• Ulcer or malignancy
Complete gastrectomy (Fig. 7.18)	• Removal of the stomach with anastomosis of the esophagus to the jejunum, leaving the duodenal stump	• Ulcer or malignancy
Whipple procedure (also referred to as *radical pancreaticoduodenectomy*) (Fig. 7.22)	• Removal of the lower stomach and duodenum with anastomosis of the remaining stomach to the jejunum with partial or total pancreatectomy and a possible splenectomy	• Cancer of the pancreas • May also be performed for resection of necrotic tissue as a result of pancreatitis
Esophagogastrectomy (Fig. 7.23)	• Removal of all or a portion of the esophagus, possibly with a portion of the stomach, with anastomosis to the remaining portion of the stomach	• Cancer of the lower and middle third of the thoracic esophagus • Corrosive esophagitis
Esophagoenterostomy (may also be referred to as *esophagogastrectomy with a colon interposition*) (Fig. 7.24)	• Removal of all or a portion of the esophagus along with replacement with a segment of the colon	• Cancer of the esophagus • Corrosive esophagitis
Colon resection with end-to-end anastomosis; may include colostomy	• Removal of a portion of the colon; may include formation of a colostomy • Temporary colostomy may be developed to temporarily divert bowel contents to allow for healing of the anastomosis • May be performed laparoscopically	• Tumor, bleeding, inflammation, necrosis, or trauma of the large intestine
Total colectomy and ileostomy	• Removal of the entire large intestine and the formation of a stoma from the end of the ileum • May also include surgical formation of a continent ileostomy (i.e., Kock pouch) or ileoanal reservoir	• Ulcerative colitis

Table 7.12 Gastrointestinal Surgical Procedures Frequently Requiring Critical Care—cont'd

Surgical Procedure	Description	Indications
Abdominoperineal resection	• Removal of the anus, rectum, and sigmoid colon with creation of a permanent colostomy	• Malignancy of the rectum
Restrictive Procedures for Morbid Obesity		
Vertical banded gastroplasty (VBG)	• Partitioning of the stomach near the gastroesophageal junction to create a small gastric pouch and outlet • Less commonly performed today because of lack of sustained weight loss	• Morbid obesity (e.g., BMI greater than $40 kg/m^2$ or BMI of greater than $35 kg/m^2$ with serious medical problems)
Gastric banding (Fig. 7.25)	• Placement of a prosthetic device around the gastric cardia to limit oral intake • May be done laparoscopically	• Morbid obesity (e.g., BMI greater than $40 kg/m^2$ or BMI of greater than $35 kg/m^2$ with serious medical problems)
Malabsorptive Procedures for Morbid Obesity		
Intestinal bypass	• Formation of an anastomosis between the upper small intestine and the lower small intestine or large intestine • Less commonly performed today because of high complication rate	• Morbid obesity (e.g., BMI greater than $40 kg/m^2$ or BMI of greater than $35 kg/m^2$ with serious medical problems)
Roux-Y gastric bypass (RYGB) (Fig. 7.26)	• Combines gastric restriction and malabsorption; in addition to creating a gastric pouch, the small bowel is resected so that the upper jejunum is connected to the pouch and the lower jejunum is anastomosed to the biliopancreatic limb; digestive juices do not come into the small bowel until the lower jejunum, so absorption is decreased • Usually performed via laparoscopic technique	• Morbid obesity (e.g., BMI greater than $40 kg/m^2$ or BMI of greater than $35 kg/m^2$ with serious medical problems)

BMI, Body mass index.

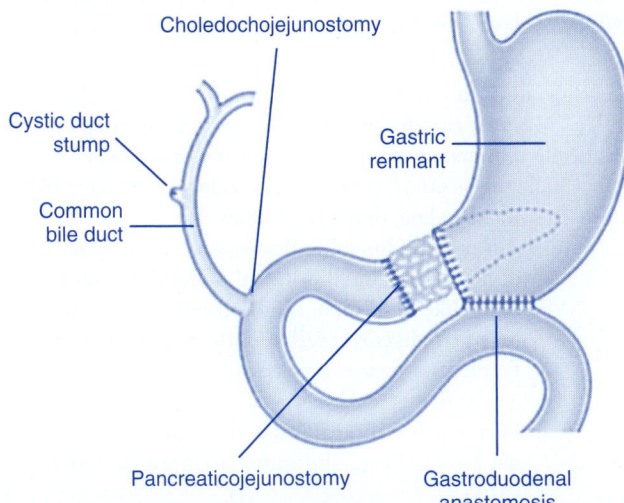

Fig. 7.22 Whipple procedure (also referred to as *radical pancreaticoduodenectomy*). (From Lewis, S. M., et al. [2011]. *Medical-surgical nursing: Assessment and management of clinical problems* [8th ed.]. St. Louis: Mosby.)

    b. Monitor SpO_2 and administer oxygen to maintain SpO_2 at 94% until contraindicated.
    c. Position the patient with HOB elevated to 30 to 40 degrees unless contraindicated; a side-lying position is frequently more comfortable for patients who have had rectal or perineal procedures.
    d. Use short-term breathing trials to evaluate the patient's ability to maintain spontaneous breathing so that weaning and extubation can be accomplished as soon as possible.
    e. Encourage deep breathing and incentive spirometry.
    f. Maintain hydration, encourage leg exercises, and ambulate as soon as possible to prevent deep vein thrombosis (DVT) and pulmonary embolism.
2. Prevent or monitor for fluid volume deficit and/or electrolyte imbalance.
    a. Monitor vital signs, hemodynamics, urine output, daily weights, and laboratory values.
        1) Use CVP or pulmonary artery catheter when in place to evaluate fluid status.
        2) Evaluate electrolyte values as indicated.
        3) Monitor Hgb and Hct as indicated.
        4) Weigh daily.
    b. Administer fluids as prescribed: crystalloids and colloids.
    c. Monitor drains if in place for change in amount or character of drainage.

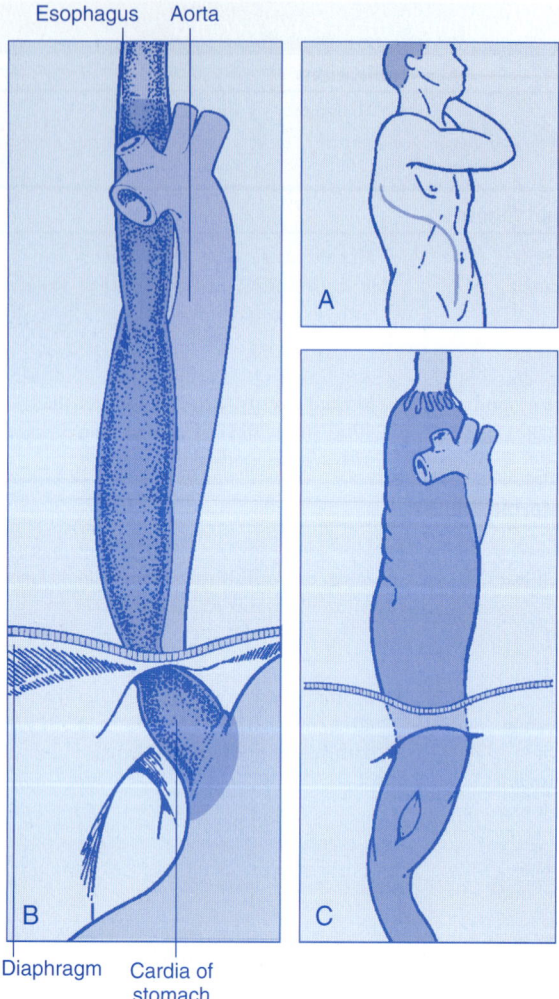

Fig. 7.23 Esophagogastrectomy. **A,** Incision. **B,** *Shaded portion* to be resected. **C,** Completed reconstruction. (From Beare, P. G., & Myers, J. L. [1998]. *Adult health nursing* [3rd ed.]. St. Louis: Mosby.)

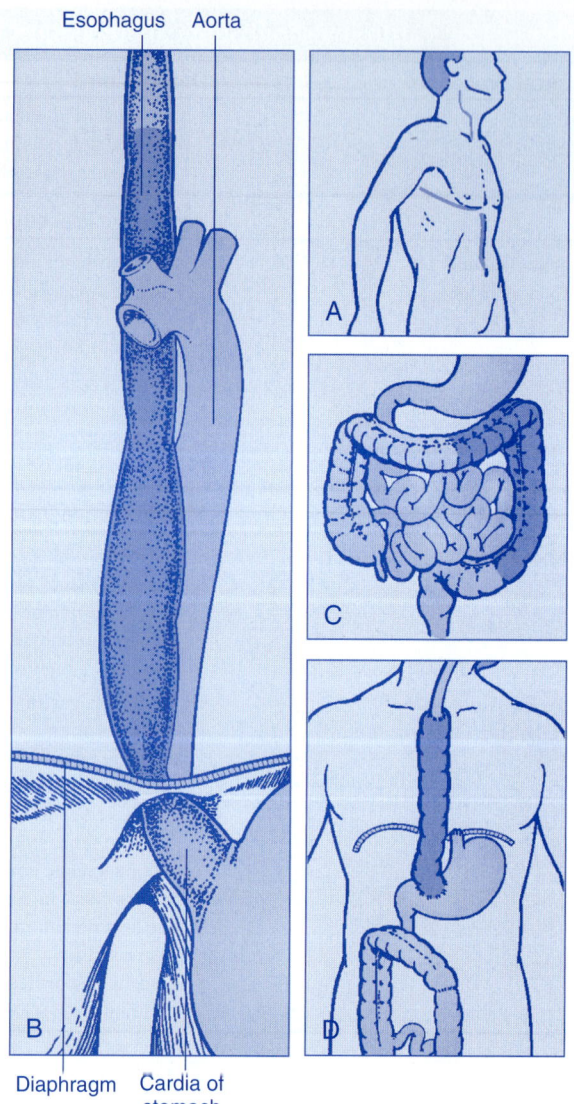

Fig. 7.24 Esophagoenterostomy. **A,** Incision. **B,** *Shaded portion* to be resected. **C,** Portion of colon to be used. **D,** Completed reconstruction. (From Beare, P. G., & Myers, J. L. [1998]. *Adult health nursing* [3rd ed.]. St. Louis: Mosby.)

  d. Expect mobilization of third-spaced fluids and increase in urine output on second or third postoperative day; monitor for changes in electrolyte levels.
  e. Monitor for petechiae, ecchymosis, changes in clotting profile, and frank bleeding that may indicate a coagulopathy, such as DIC.
3. Prevent or treat pain.
  a. Administer narcotics (e.g., morphine, hydromorphone, fentanyl) by PCA as prescribed; epidural analgesia may be used.
  b. Administer NSAIDs as prescribed to augment the analgesic effect of narcotics by acting as antiprostaglandins.
    1) Initially ketorolac
    2) Oral agents (e.g., ibuprofen, naproxen) when able to take drugs by mouth
  c. Use noninvasive pain control measures.
  d. Teach the patient how to splint the incision during coughing; teach the family how to assist.
  e. Administer antiemetics for nausea; provide mouth care after each episode of vomiting and assess positioning of NG tube if still in place.

4. Prevent or monitor for infection.
  a. Monitor closely for clinical indications of infection.
    1) Evaluate temperature at least every 4 hours.
    2) Assess color, character, and odor of drainage from incision line, drains, and tubes.
    3) Assess for clinical indications of peritonitis (e.g., abdominal pain, abdominal distention, rigid, boardlike abdomen, rebound tenderness, diminished or absent bowel sounds, nausea, vomiting, fever, leukocytosis) caused by anastomosis leak.
    4) Monitor for clinical indications of intraabdominal abscess (e.g., abdominal pain, fever, leukocytosis).
  b. Administer antibiotics prophylactically and therapeutically as prescribed.
  c. Provide incision and drain care aseptically.
    1) Protect the skin from excoriation by changing incisional dressing and dressings around drains as indicated.

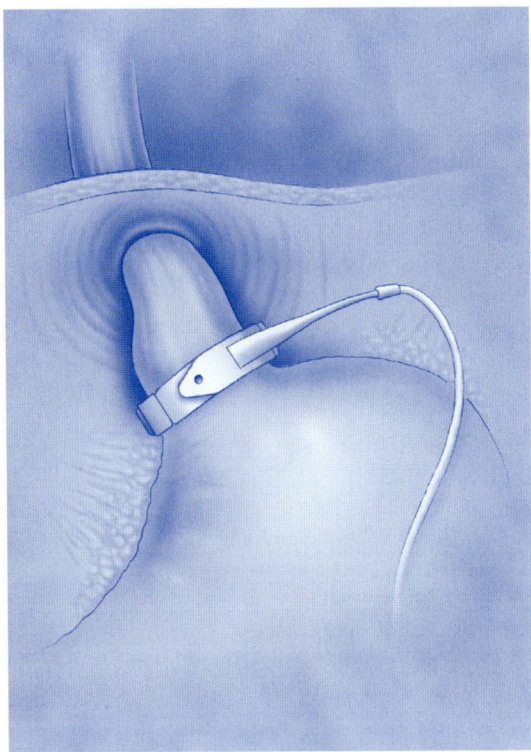

Fig. 7.25 Example of gastric banding. (From American Association of Operating Room Nurses. [2004]. AORN bariatric surgery guideline. *AORN J, 79*[5], 1026-1052.)

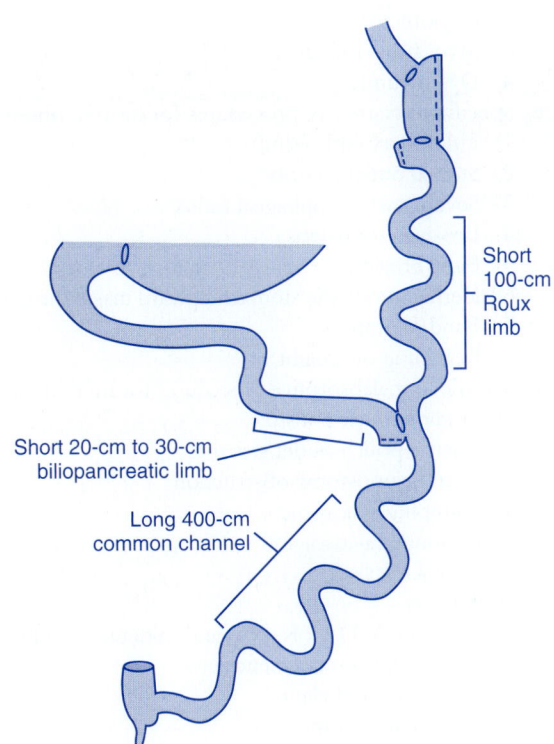

Fig. 7.26 Example of gastric bypass: Roux-en-Y proximal gastric bypass. (From American Association of Operating Room Nurses. [2004]. AORN bariatric surgery guideline. *AORN J, 79*[5], 1026-1052.)

2) Change packing as prescribed.
   a) Some patients may have wounds that are left open and packed with saline-soaked dressings.
      i) Do not use packing soaked with Betadine (iodine); known effects of Betadine on open wounds include the following:
         (a) Toxic to fibroblasts
         (b) Decreases epithelialization
         (c) Increases susceptibility to infection
         (d) Iodine may be absorbed and cause nephrotoxicity.
   b) Do not allow dressings to become dry (i.e., wet to dry); the dressings should be still moist (i.e., wet to moist) at the time of removal and replacement to prevent disruption of granulating tissue.
3) Irrigate the wound with saline as prescribed.
   a) Do not use hydrogen peroxide because it is damaging to new epithelium.
4) Monitor closely for a fistula tract.
   a) Look for small openings along or near the incision or drain site; output is usually green or yellow.
   b) Protect the skin from potentially excoriating drainage by placing a wound drainage bag over the fistula; also allows measurement of fluid loss and collection of sample for electrolyte analysis to guide fluid and electrolyte replacement.
   d. Monitor serum glucose and administer insulin to keep serum glucose within normal limits.
   e. Assess approximation of wound edges for indications of possible dehiscence or evisceration.
5. Reduce acidity of gastric secretions.
   a. Maintain NPO status while gastric suction is required.
   b. Administer antacids, H_2 receptor antagonists, and/or proton pump inhibitors as prescribed.
   c. Administer octreotide acetate (Sandostatin) as prescribed to suppress secretion of pancreatic peptides post-Whipple.
6. Maintain GI integrity.
   a. Monitor and maintain NG tube until return of bowel sounds.
      1) Ensure proper tube placement; do not manipulate a tube placed during surgery without consulting surgeon.
   b. Monitor closely for indications of anastomosis leak.
   c. Monitor for return of bowel sounds, flatus, and bowel movements.
   d. Assess and provide bowel diversion care as indicated (bowel resection with formation of a temporary or permanent bowel diversion).
      1) Maintain intactness of bowel diversion appliance.
      2) Keep peristomal skin clean and dry.
      3) Report any change in the drainage from the ileostomy or colostomy.
         a) Ileostomy: watery, excoriating, and continuous
         b) Ascending colostomy: watery or semisolid, excoriating, and continuous

c) Transverse colostomy: pastelike or semisolid and occurs at unpredictable intervals; may be 3 to 5 days postoperative before any drainage
d) Descending or sigmoid colostomy: formed stools that may be at predictable intervals (e.g., after breakfast) especially with irrigation routine; may be 3 to 5 days postoperative before any drainage
  4) Assess color of stoma and report any indications of ischemia.
   a) Stomal color should be the same color as the oral mucosa, and it should be moist; report darkening such as burgundy or black.
  5) Report any stomal prolapse or retraction.
7. Maintain or improve nutritional status.
 a. Assess nutritional status: weight, BUN, serum albumin, total protein, Hgb and Hct
 b. Administer TPN initially as prescribed and progress diet as prescribed: usually small, frequent meals are indicated.
 c. Administer enteral feedings as prescribed; a jejunostomy tube may be placed for nutritional support.
 d. Monitor for diarrhea.
 e. Administer oral pancreatic enzymes with each meal as prescribed post-Whipple.
8. Provide size-sensitive care for patients with obesity.
 a. Ensure that appropriate bariatric equipment is available.
  1) Avoid derogatory terms such as "big boy bed."
 b. Recognize and discuss prejudice based on size and weight.
 c. Provide privacy and dignity.
  1) Weigh the patient in private.
  2) Close doors and curtains when examining the patient.
  3) Maintain confidentiality.
9. Assist with adjustment to diagnosis of cancer if malignancy present.
 a. Provide accurate information and clarification about the diagnosis, prognosis, and treatment plan when information is requested.
 b. Be realistic but do not eliminate hope.
 c. Give patient and family members time to discuss their feelings and concerns; encourage expression of goals for treatment.
 d. Refer patient and family to support groups or for counseling as indicated.
 e. Prepare the patient and family for additional treatments for malignancy if indicated such as the following:
  1) Radiation therapy
  2) Antineoplastic drug therapy
10. Monitor for complications.
 a. General
  1) Anastomosis leak
  2) Atelectasis, pneumonia, ARDS
  3) DVT, pulmonary embolism
  4) Infection, sepsis
  5) Prolonged ileus
  6) GI bleeding
  7) Stenosis or stricture
  8) Fistula
  9) Organ failure
   a) Cardiac
   b) Hepatic
   c) Pulmonary
   d) Renal
 b. Specific to gastric resections
  1) Dumping syndromes
   a) Early: hyperosmolality causing hypovolemic effect
   b) Late: hypoglycemia caused by hyperinsulinemic response
  2) Pernicious anemia
  3) Diarrhea
  4) Chronic gastritis
 c. Specific to Whipple procedure
  1) Delayed gastric emptying
  2) Pancreatic fistula
  3) Intraabdominal abscess
  4) Hemorrhage: usually caused by injury to portal vein or vena cava
  5) Wound infection
  6) Diabetes
  7) Pancreatic exocrine insufficiency
  8) Pancreatitis
  9) Marginal ulceration
 d. Specific to esophagogastrectomy
  1) Esophageal stenosis or anastomotic stricture
  2) Chylothorax
  3) Myocardial ischemia
  4) Dysrhythmias
 e. Specific to restrictive procedures for morbid obesity
  1) Pulmonary embolism
  2) Stomal outlet stenosis
  3) Severe gastroesophageal reflux
  4) Erosive esophagitis
  5) Band erosion
  6) Herniation of the stomach upward inside the band
  7) Band migration
  8) Regaining of weight
 f. Specific to malabsorptive procedures for morbid obesity
  1) Pulmonary embolism
  2) Gastric pouch outlet stricture
  3) Jejunojejunostomy obstruction
  4) Dumping syndrome
  5) Prolonged nausea and vomiting
  6) Cholelithiasis
  7) Anemia
  8) Vitamin (A, D, E, K, B_{12}) and mineral (calcium, folic acid, iron) deficiencies
  9) Electrolyte imbalance
  10) Lactose intolerance
  11) Anemia
  12) Offensive, foul-smelling soft bowel movements and flatus
11. Provide instruction to the patient and family regarding wound care, pharmacologic agents prescribed for home use, and signs/symptoms to report to the physician.

LEARNING ACTIVITIES

CHAPTER 7

1. Complete the following crossword puzzle related to gastrointestinal anatomy, physiology, and assessment.

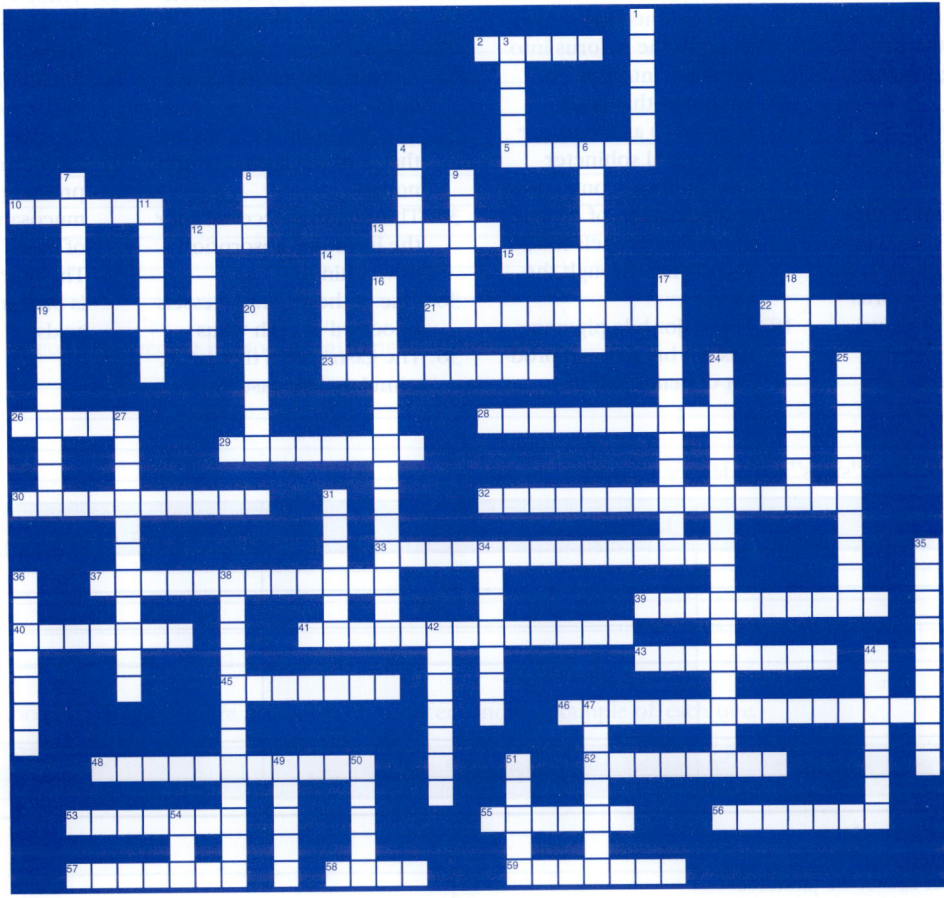

ACROSS

2. GI secretions are controlled by this nerve and the parasympathetic nervous system
5. Gastric losses are ___ so excess losses cause metabolic alkalosis
10. Dome-shaped portion of the stomach that extends left of the cardia
12. The branch of the autonomic nervous system that speeds gastric emptying (abbrev)
13. Fingerlike projections of mucosa and submucosa in the duodenum and jejunum that increase surface area
15. Fluid produced by the liver and store in the gallbladder
19. Enzyme in saliva that begins the breakdown of polysaccharides to disaccharides
21. Absorption of this type of vitamins requires the presence of bile salts; examples are ADEK (two words)
22. The accessory organ responsible for the conversion of ammonia to urea
23. The hollow tube that passes from the pharynx, through the diaphragm, and to the stomach
26. The last section of the small intestine
28. This structure protects the airway by closing during swallowing
29. The accessory organ with both endocrine and exocrine functions
30. The membrane that covers the abdominal viscera
32. The hormone that stimulates contraction of the gallbladder
33. The process of breaking down stored carbohydrate
37. The nutrient source that is broken down into glucose, fructose, and galactose
39. The first portion of the alimentary canal
40. Absorption of this mineral requires vitamin D
41. Another term for *swallowing*
43. The vitamin that plays a chief role in the metabolic breakdown of glucose to yield energy in body tissue
45. These glands are also referred to as parietal cells; they secrete hydrochloric acid and intrinsic factor
46. The process of converting fat and protein to glucose
48. The accessory organ responsible for the storage and release of bile
52. The phase of gastric secretion that is stimulated by the thought, sight, smell, or taste of food
53. The cells that line the sinusoids of the liver and are responsible for phagocytosis
55. These cells are in the pancreas and responsible for exocrine function
56. The nutrient source that is broken down into amino acids
57. The flexure of the large intestine that is in the RUQ

557

Chapter 7 The Gastrointestinal System

12. List five common causes of paralytic ileus.

    a. _____

    b. _____

    c. _____

    d. _____

    e. _____

13. List five classic indications of an "acute abdomen" seen in intestinal perforation.

    a. _____

    b. _____

    c. _____

    d. _____

    e. _____

14. Complete the following table. You may include more than one condition for each but include only conditions discussed in this chapter.

Clinical Finding	Condition
Elevated lipase, amylase	
Sudden, painless hematemesis	
Decreased protein	
Rebound tenderness	
Jaundice	
Hypocalcemia	
Bleeding tendencies	
Elevated ammonia	
Bloody diarrhea	
Hyperbilirubinemia	
Fetor hepaticus	
High-pitched rushing bowel sounds	
Succussion splash	
Asthma, chronic cough, laryngitis	
Management	**Condition**
Irrigate NG tube until clear	
Neomycin and lactulose	
Sclerosis during endoscopy	
Aldosterone antagonist diuretics	
NPO status	
Sengstaken-Blakemore tube	
Volume and blood replacement	
Billroth I or II	
Proton pump inhibitors	

Chapter 7 The Gastrointestinal System   561

15. Complete the following crossword puzzle related to gastrointestinal conditions.

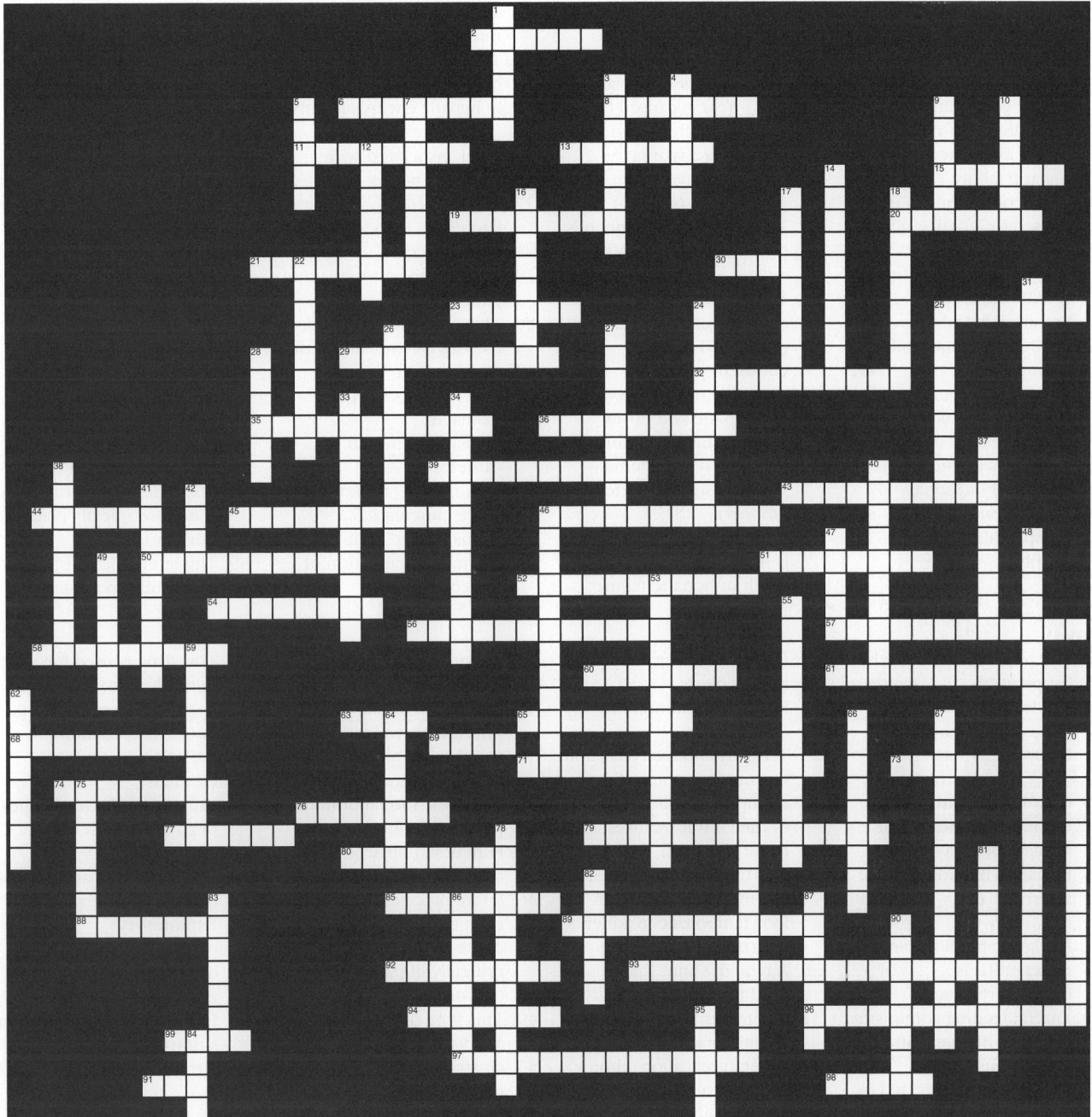

ACROSS

2. This type of ulcer causes an erosion in the mucosa of the esophagus, stomach, or duodenum
6. This antibiotic is used in hepatic encephalopathy to kill intestinal bacteria that convert nitrogenous wastes to ammonia (generic)
8. Along with fibrinogen and globulins, responsible for the conversion of amino acids to plasma proteins
11. This type of pain is experiences at a distance from the disease process
13. _____ procedure is also called a pancreatoduodenectomy
15. Most specific laboratory test for pancreatitis
19. A deficiency of this vitamin commonly seen in alcoholism
20. An abnormal accumulation of fluid in the peritoneal cavity
21. Conditionally essential amino acid that enhances the immune system and promotes wound healing
30. Screening echo used in abdominal trauma (abbrev)
23. Abdominal pain experienced with mesenteric ischemia is frequently described as abdominal _____
25. This syndrome may occur after gastric resection; may be classified as early or late
29. _____ sign is a bluish tint to the flanks that is indicative of retroperitoneal bleeding (2 words)
32. A drug used in GI hemorrhage to suppress gastrin (generic)
35. The location of pain in acute pancreatitis
36. A flapping tremor seen in hepatic encephalopathy
39. Term for belching
43. A drug that acts as mucosal barrier used to protect the gastric mucosa (generic)

Chapter 7   The Gastrointestinal System

44. Type of enteral feeding with supplemental fiber
45. This condition may be caused by ulcer, appendicitis, diverticulitis, or intestinal obstruction; causes peritonitis
46. A syndrome of renal failure associated with hepatic failure
50. This type of anemia is caused by a deficiency of intrinsic factor
51. _____ sign is indicative of splenic rupture
52. Vomiting blood
54. IV proton pump inhibitor (brand name)
56. The gentle repetitive bouncing of tissues again the hand; used to evaluate organ enlargement
57. A luminal intestinal obstruction with compromise of blood supply
58. This condition is manifested by coffee-ground gastric aspirate
60. An obstruction here is manifested by vomiting and a succussion splash
61. _____ tear is caused by forceful retching and vomiting (2 words)
63. This test may cause pancreatitis (abbrev)
65. The type of drug frequently prescribed for patients with ascites
68. This treatment for esophageal varices is performed during endoscopy
69. A stent is placed between the hepatic and portal veins in this procedure performed in patients with esophageal varices (abbrev)
71. Hepatic _____ is neurologic failure as a result of hepatic failure
73. Intestinal perforation causes an _____ abdomen and requires surgical intervention
74. This osmotic diuretic may be used for cerebral edema in hepatic encephalopathy
76. _____ ulcer is a stress ulcer associated with cerebral trauma
77. *Helicobacter* _____ is a bacterium associated with peptic ulcer
79. A common cause of acute pancreatitis
80. This procedure divides the vagus nerve along the esophagus to decrease acid secretion in the stomach
85. Type of parenteral catheter
88. Serum _____ is elevated in acute pancreatitis
92. A "maneuver" that facilitates evacuation of the colon
93. This tube has three lumens and may be used for balloon tamponade in patients with esophageal varices (2 words)
94. This macronutrient is restricted in hepatic encephalopathy
96. A drug commonly used for suicide gesture that is a major cause of hepatic failure in adolescents (generic)
99. A serious pulmonary complication of acute pancreatitis (abbrev)
97. This diuretic is frequently used for fluid retention in hepatic failure; blocks aldosterone (generic)
98. Small bowel obstruction causes reverse peristalsis and vomiting that is ___
91. A gastric feeding tube that is endoscopically placed (abbrev)
89. This antibiotic may be used to stimulate peristalsis

Down

1. The term for tarry stools
3. Esophageal _____ causes sudden, painless hemorrhage by mouth; caused by portal hypertension
4. _____ sign is a bluish discoloration around the umbilicus; indicative of intraabdominal bleeding
5. Hepatitis B is sometimes referred to as _____ hepatitis
7. Analgesic of choice in pancreatitis is _____ or hydromorphone
9. Enteral feeding administration may be intermittent, continuous, or _____
10. Serum _____ is elevated in acute pancreatitis and is more specific than serum amylase
12. Hepatitis A and E are sometimes referred to as _____ hepatitis
14. Collection of inflammatory debris, pancreatic secretions, and necrotic tissue in the pancreas
16. May be caused by biliary obstruction, liver disease, or excessive hemolysis
17. An amino acid that is considered essential at times of hypercatabolism
18. An osmotic laxative frequently used in hepatic encephalopathy (generic)
22. Causes coffee-ground hematemesis
24. H2 receptor antagonist (generic)
25. Term for impaired digestion
26. Occurs as a result of a disruption in the integrity of the GI tract; causes an acute abdomen
27. This tube has four lumens and may be used for balloon tamponade in patients with esophageal varices
28. A type of shunt that is used for ascites
31. A complication of vasopressin therapy that causes water intoxication (abbrev)
33. May be used for GI hemorrhage but may cause myocardial or mesenteric ischemia (generic)
34. A common description of the appearance of the stool seen with mesenteric infarction (2 words)
37. This type of enteral formula is required is feeding is delivered distal to the jejunum
38. One controversy regarding the use of drugs that alter the pH of the gastric secretions is the increased incidence of _____
40. The route of nutritional support used in functional or structural obstruction
41. Term for difficulty swallowing
42. _____ sign is caused by phrenic nerve irritation by subphrenic blood
46. Intraabdominal _____ is when the intraabdominal pressure is above normal
47. Functional obstruction of the bowel
48. Spore-producing bacterium that is a common cause of diarrhea in critically ill patients (2 words)
49. This type of pain is sharp and well localized
53. clostridium difficile infection is usually initially treated with _____ (generic)
55. Another term for bright red blood per rectum
59. Bowel diversion that is most likely to cause skin erosion if excellent containment is not achieved
62. This type of pain is dull and poorly localized
64. _____ is a stress ulcer associated with burns
66. Inflammation of the liver
67. Conversion of fat or protein to glucose
70. A complication of hernia that may cause bowel ischemia or infarction
72. This drug is used for acetaminophen toxicity; must be administered within 24 hours of acetaminophen ingestion (generic)
75. Elevated _____ levels cause neurologic changes in patients with hepatic encephalopathy
78. Electrolyte imbalance seen in acute pancreatitis
81. Exploratory _____ may be necessary to localize organ injury or hemorrhage in trauma patients
82. Hypertension of this circulation system is seen in cirrhosis
83. _____ tenderness indicates that pain is more severe on release than with pressure
84. Procedure now preferred over intestinal bypass for weight reduction for patients with morbid obesity (abbrev)
86. These must be kept at the bedside for a patient with balloon tamponade
87. The preferred method of nutritional support; should be used unless contraindications exist
90. Generalized, massive edema
95. The form of fluid replacement that is indicated for acute hemorrhage

16. Read the case study and answer the question.
    A patient is in the intensive care unit after undergoing a gastric resection for stomach cancer and has been started on a regular diet before transfer out of the unit. Within minutes of eating, the patient becomes diaphoretic and weak; he complains of abdominal cramping and palpitations. His blood pressure is 102/70 mm Hg, heart rate is 96 bets/min, and respirations are 22 breaths/min. What condition explains these clinical findings?

17. Read the case study and answer the question.
    A postoperative abdominal surgery patient weighing 700 lb (318 kg) develops acute onset of dyspnea and chest pain. Arterial blood gas values are pH is 7.35, paO_2 is 74 mm Hg, $PaCo_2$ is 30 mm Hg, and O_2 saturation is 90%. Chest radiography shows an enlarged cardiac silhouette, a prominent pulmonary artery, and mild right pleural effusion. The 12-lead electrocardiogram demonstrates T-wave inversions in the anterior leads. These findings suggest that this patient most likely developed what postoperative complication?

18. Read the case study and answer the question.
    A patient admitted with severe abdominal discomfort and fatigue notes that the patient tested positive for *Helicobacter pylori* and has a history of cigarette smoking. The patient develops nausea and abdominal tenderness. His vital signs are blood pressure of (BP) 123/80 mm Hg, pulse of 89 beats/min, and respirations of 15 breaths/min. Within 15 minutes, the patient vomits, and his emesis contains coffee grounds. His vital signs now are BP of 100/68 mm Hg, pulse of 120 beats/min, and respirations of 24 breaths/min. What medical orders would you expect for this patient?

19. Read the case study and answer the questions.
    Mrs. G is a 54-year-old woman with a history of rheumatoid arthritis. She has taken nonsteroidal antiinflammatory drugs for several years. She was recently treated with warfarin for a deep vein thrombosis. Mrs. G is admitted to the intensive care unit with an upper gastrointestinal bleed because she is vomiting bright red blood. She is pale and diaphoretic and complains of epigastric pain. Her vital signs are:
    BP 70/40; HR 130 bpm, sinus in origin; RR 30 breaths/min; temperature is 101.3°F tympanic. Mrs. G's urine output is 15 ml/h. Her hemoglobin is 9 g/dl.
    a. What would you expect Mrs. G's ABG results to be upon admission to the ICU?

    b. The physician orders an IV infusion of Pitressin for Mrs. G. What adverse effects should you monitor for?

    c. An upper GI study is performed on Mrs. G, and she is diagnosed with a bleeding ulcer. What other complications would you need to monitor Mrs. G for?

20. Match the following terms with the condition (answers will be used more than once).

____ 1. Acute GI hemorrhage	a. Metabolic acidosis
____ 2. Acute pancreatitis	b. Metabolic alkalosis
____ 3. Acute liver failure	
____ 4. Antacid overuse	
____ 5. Hypoglycemia	

The Renal System

CHAPTER 8

Selected Concepts in Anatomy and Physiology

General Information
1. Functions of the renal system
   a. Regulation of homeostasis and the body's internal environment
      1) Regulation of extracellular fluid volume
      2) Regulation of extracellular fluid osmolality
      3) Regulation of electrolyte balance
      4) Excretion of metabolic wastes
      5) Regulation of acid–base balance (in conjunction with the pulmonary system)
   b. Production and release of hormones
      1) Regulation of blood pressure (BP) influenced by aldosterone and antidiuretic hormone (ADH)
      2) Stimulation of red blood cell (RBC) production via erythropoietin
      3) Synthesis and release of prostaglandins
   c. Participation in activation of vitamin D
2. Components of the renal system (Fig. 8.1)
   a. Two kidneys
   b. Two ureters
   c. Urinary bladder
   d. Urethra

Functional Anatomy
1. General characteristics of the kidney
   a. Location of kidney
      1) Posterior abdominal wall behind peritoneum
      2) Opposite last thoracic and first three lumbar vertebrae on each side of spine
      3) Right kidney slightly lower than left as a result of liver location
   b. Size, shape, weight of the kidney
      1) Size: approximately 10 × 5 × 2.5 cm or approximately fist sized
      2) Shape: beanlike with convex lateral border, convex and concave medial border; long axis approximately vertical
      3) Weight: 120 to 170 g per kidney
2. Extrarenal structures
   a. Renal capsule
      1) Thin, smooth layer of fibrous membrane that surrounds each kidney
      2) Acts as a protective layer
      3) Prevents kidney swelling
      4) Contains pain receptors
   b. Perirenal fat and renal fascia
      1) Support and protect the kidney
      2) Hold kidney in place
   c. Adrenal gland (also referred to as the *suprarenal gland*): rests on top of each kidney
   d. Hilum
      1) Concave notch of medial aspect of kidney
      2) Entry site for renal artery and nerves
      3) Exit site for renal vein and ureter
   e. Ureters
      1) Fibromuscular tubes located behind peritoneum; extend from kidney to posterior part of bladder floor
      2) Ureter walls composed of smooth muscle with mucosa lining and fibrous outer coat
      3) Collect urine from the renal pelvis and propel it to the bladder by peristaltic waves
      4) Ureters enter the superior, posterior bladder at an oblique angle; this angle and the peristaltic action of the ureters prevent reflux of urine.
   f. Bladder
      1) Located behind symphysis pubis, below the peritoneum
      2) Collapsible bag of smooth muscle
      3) Acts as a reservoir for urine until sufficient amount accumulates for elimination; expels urine from body by way of urethra
         a) Adults void approximately 5 to 9 times/day
         b) Volume of each voiding usually 100 to 300 ml but may be as much as 1 l
   g. Urethra
      1) Located behind symphysis pubis, anterior to the vagina in females; extends through the prostate gland and penis in males

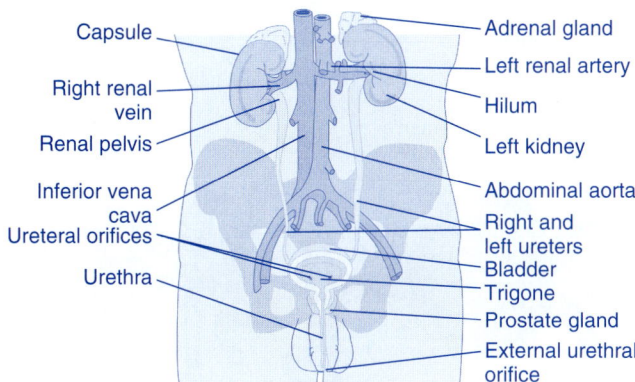

Fig. 8.1 The kidneys and other structures of the urinary tract. (From Montague, S. E., Watson, R., & Herbert, R. [2005]. *Physiology for nursing practice* [3rd ed.]. Oxford: Baillière Tindall.)

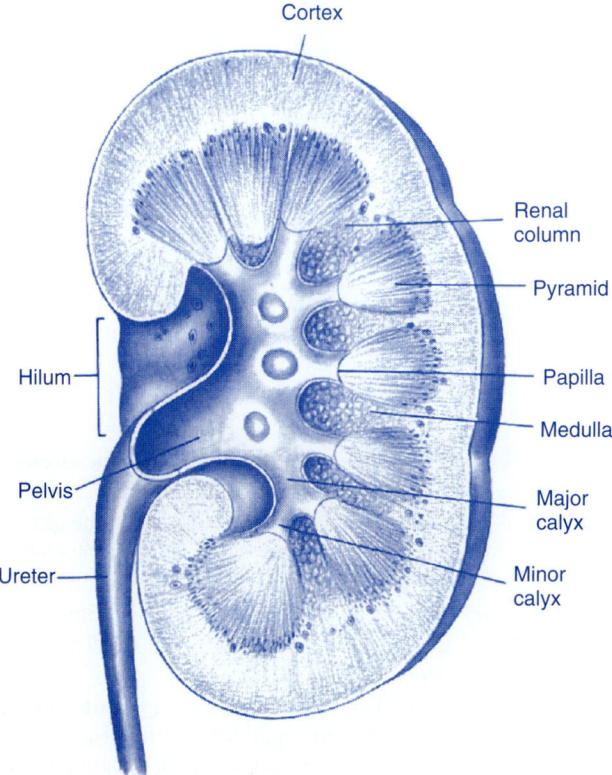

Fig. 8.2 Cross-section of the kidney. (From Thompson, J. M., McFarland, G. K., Hirsch, J. E., & Tucker, S. M. [2002]. *Mosby's clinical nursing* [5th ed.]. St Louis: Mosby.)

    2) Acts as passageway for expulsion of urine from the urinary bladder to the urinary meatus, where it is expelled from the body
3. Renal structures (Fig. 8.2)
  a. Renal parenchyma
    1) Cortex
      a) Approximately 1 cm wide, reddish-brown, and granular appearance
      b) Metabolically active portion of kidney where aerobic metabolism occurs and ammonia and glucose are formed
      c) Site of glomerulus, proximal and distal tubules

    2) Medulla
      a) Approximately 5 cm wide, darker than cortex and striated
      b) Composed of 6 to 10 pyramids formed by collecting tubules and ducts
        i) Pyramids are triangular wedges of medullary tissue and are composed of collecting tubules.
        ii) Columns are inward extensions of cortical tissue between the pyramids; much of the kidney's blood vessels and nerves are in these columns.
        iii) Renal lobe is composed of a pyramid and surrounding cortical tissue.
      c) Site of deepest part of Henle loop
  b. Renal sinus: spacious cavity filled with adipose tissue, the renal pelvis, minor and major calyces, and the origin of the ureter
    1) Calyces
      a) Calyces are cuplike structures that drain the papillae.
      b) Eight to 12 minor calyces open into two to three major calyces that form the renal pelvis.
    2) Renal pelvis
      a) Papillae are at the apices of the renal pyramids; collecting tubules drain into minor calyces at papillae.
      b) Renal pelvis is like a small funnel tapering into the ureter; formed by the union of several calyces
      c) Urine flows from collecting duct to renal pelvis and into the ureter.
  c. Nephron: microscopic functional unit of kidney (Fig. 8.3)
    1) Approximately 1 million in each kidney
    2) Able to compensate for significant degree of nephron destruction by:
      a) Filtering a greater solute (dissolved substances) load
      b) Hypertrophy of remaining functional nephrons
    3) Types of nephrons
      a) Cortical (85% of nephrons are cortical nephrons)
        i) The glomerulus is located in outer cortex.
        ii) Cortical nephrons contain short loops of Henle that dip into the outer edge of the medulla.
      b) Juxtamedullary (15% of nephrons are juxtamedullary nephrons)
        i) The glomerulus is located in inner cortex.
        ii) Juxtamedullary nephrons contain long loops of Henle that penetrate deep into medulla.
        iii) These nephrons are important in the kidney's ability to concentrate urine.

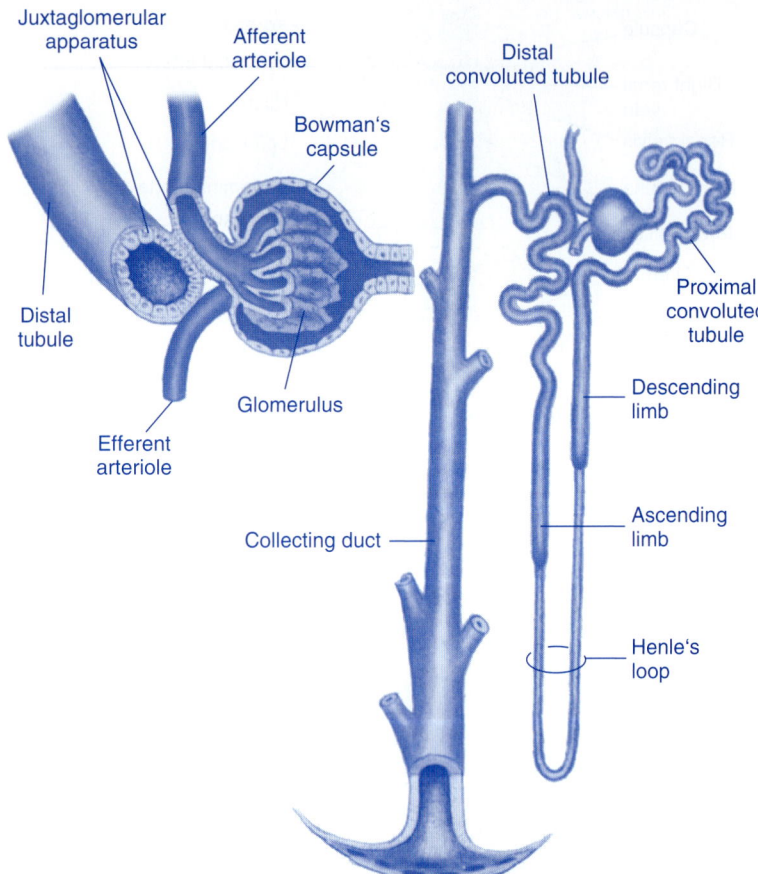

Fig. 8.3 Components of the nephron. (From Urden, L. D., Stacy, K. M., & Lough, M. E. [2010]. *Critical care nursing: Diagnosis and management* [6th ed.]. St. Louis: Mosby.)

  4) Functional segments
    a) Renal corpuscle: consists of Bowman capsule and glomerulus
      i) The glomerulus is a cluster of tightly coiled capillaries that produces an ultrafiltrate; a portion of this ultrafiltrate eventually becomes urine.
      ii) Bowman capsule is the funnel-shaped upper end of the proximal tubule.
    b) Renal tubules
      i) Segmentally divided into proximal convoluted tubule, loop of Henle, distal convoluted tubule
      ii) Responsible for reabsorption and secretion, which alter the volume and composition of the ultrafiltration to form the final urine volume and composition
    c) Collecting duct
      i) Several nephrons converge into a collecting duct.
      ii) The collecting duct relays the urine from the tubules to the minor calyx.
  d. Renal vasculature
    1) Pathway of blood supply
      a) Renal arteries branch from the aorta.
      b) The renal arteries branch into interlobar arteries → arcuate arteries → interlobular arteries
      c) The interlobular arteries become the afferent arteriole that forms the glomerulus.
      d) The efferent arteriole leads out of the glomerulus and forms the peritubular capillary network.
      e) The efferent arteriole from the juxtamedullary nephron forms a different capillary network called the *vasa recta*.
        i) The vasa recta is a complex of long straight capillary loops that run parallel to the ascending and descending loop of Henle.
        ii) The vasa recta plays an important role in concentrating interstitial fluid found in the medulla.
        iii) Blood flow through the vasa recta is sluggish.
      f) The peritubular capillary network leads to the interlobular vein that leads to the arcuate vein.
      g) The arcuate vein leads to the interlobar vein that leads to the renal vein.
      h) The renal vein empties into the inferior vena cava.
    2) Renal blood flow
      a) The kidneys receive 20% to 25% of the cardiac output (CO), or approximately 1200 ml/min (600 ml/min for each kidney).

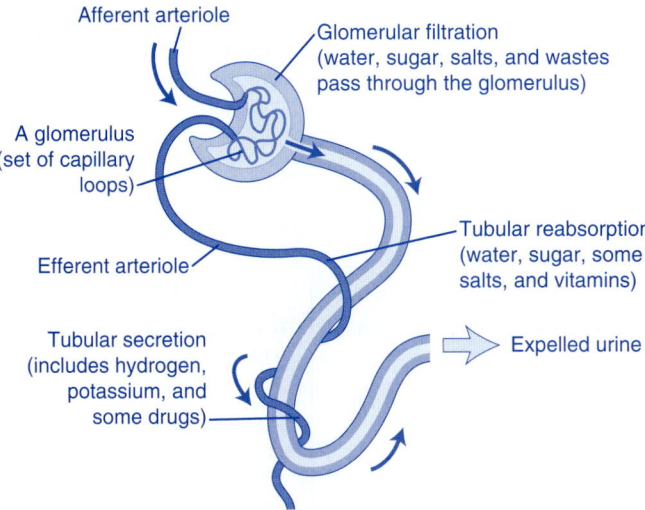

Fig. 8.4 Processes of filtration, secretion, and reabsorption in the formation of urine. (From Leonard, P.C. [2005]. *Building a medical vocabulary with Spanish translations* [6th ed.]. St. Louis: Saunders.)

      b) Autoregulation maintains constancy in glomerular filtration rate (GFR).
         i) Systemic arterial pressure between 80 and 180 mm Hg prevents large changes in GFR because of the ability of the afferent arteriole to constrict or dilate.
           (a) Increases in mean arterial pressure (MAP) cause constriction of the afferent arteriole that prevents the increased arterial pressure from raising the pressure in the glomerulus.
           (b) Decreases in MAP cause dilation of the afferent arteriole, so more blood is allowed to flow into the glomerulus.
         ii) Autoregulation fails at MAP of 60 mm Hg or less.
     3) Juxtaglomerular apparatus consists of the macula densa and the juxtaglomerular cells.
        a) The macula densa is a part of the distal tubule that lies close to the afferent and efferent arterioles.
        b) Juxtaglomerular cells produce and store the enzyme renin that is secreted in response to hypotension.
   e. Lymphatics
     1) There is an abundant supply of lymphatics to the kidney.
     2) Lymphatics from the kidney drain into thoracic duct.
   f. Nervous innervation
     1) The autonomic nervous system (ANS) supplies the primary innervation of the kidney and the urinary tract.
     2) The renal plexus is formed by the superior splanchnic and inferior splanchnic nerves and enters the kidney at the hilum; the bladder, ureters, and urethra are supplied by the inferior mesenteric plexus, the hypogastric plexus, and the pubic nerve from the sacral region.
     3) Both the sympathetic nervous system (SNS) and the parasympathetic nervous system (PNS) innervate the kidney, but the SNS has the prominent effect on the kidney; SNS fiber endings are found in the afferent and efferent arterioles and in all sections of the tubule; effects on the kidney include the following:
        a) Low level: increased sodium reabsorption within the proximal tubule
        b) Moderate level: constriction of afferent and efferent arterioles decreases renal blood flow and GFR
        c) High level: predominant effect of afferent arteriole constriction; extreme reduction in renal blood flow and potential cessation of GFR

Physiology

1. Formation of urine involves three processes: filtration, reabsorption, and secretion (Fig. 8.4); major functions of each portion of the nephron (Fig. 8.5)
   a. Glomerular filtration: The pressure of the blood within the glomerular capillaries causes blood to be filtered into Bowman capsule, where it begins to pass down to the tubule.
     1) Filtration is the transfer of water and dissolved substances through a permeable membrane from a region of high pressure to low pressure.
     2) Filtration depends on hydrostatic pressure, which may be affected by the following:
        a) Diminished renal perfusion from hypovolemia
        b) Occlusion of the glomeruli from diabetic neuropathy
        c) Alteration in the plasma protein concentration from hypoproteinemia
        d) Alterations in the basement membrane from an autoimmune disorder
        e) Arteriolar constriction from SNS stimulation or vasopressors
     3) GFR
        a) Dependent on the following:
           i) Permeability of the capillary walls
           ii) Vascular pressure
           iii) Filtration pressure

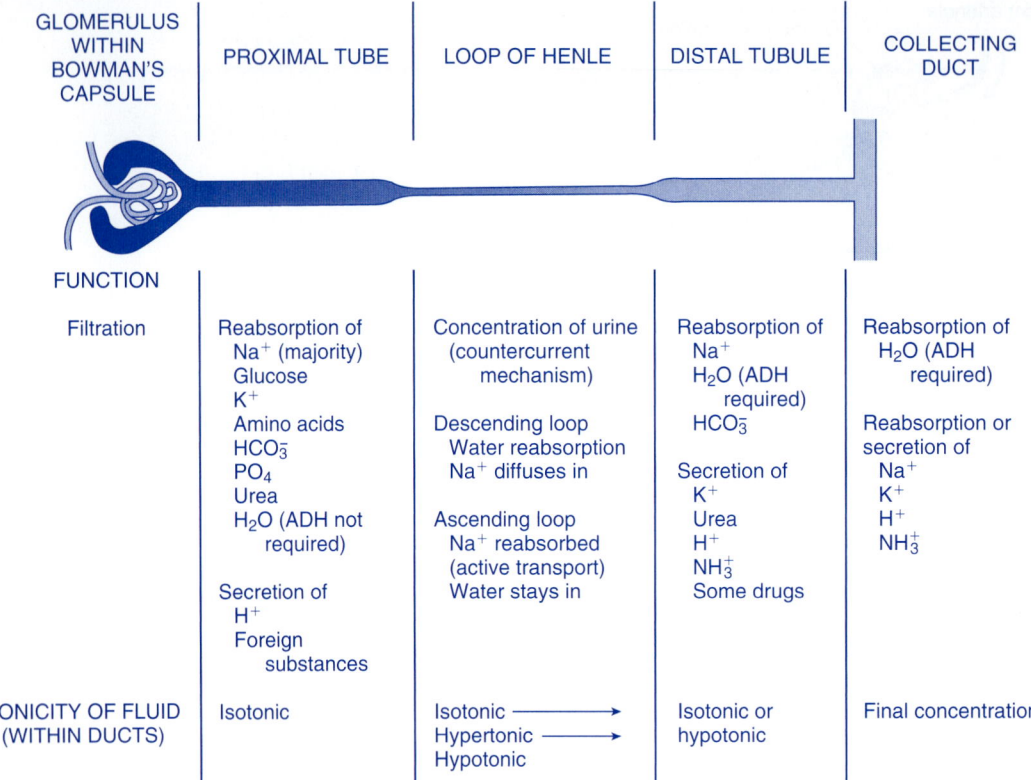

Fig. 8.5 Major functions of each portion of the nephron. *ADH,* Antidiuretic hormone. (From Sole, M. L., Klein, D. G., & Moseley, M. J. [2005]. *Introduction to critical care nursing* [4th ed.]. Philadelphia: Saunders.)

    b) Clearance: complete removal of a substance from the blood
        i) Clearance of a substance equals GFR if the tubules neither reabsorb nor secrete the substance.
        ii) Clearance of a substance is less than GFR if the tubules secrete the substance.
        iii) Clearance of a substance is greater than GFR if the tubules secrete the substance.
    c) Clinically measured by creatinine clearance because creatinine is filtered by the glomeruli and not reabsorbed by the tubules
        i) Formula for GFR =

$$\frac{U_x \times v}{P_x}$$

where: x = substance freely filtered through the glomerulus and not secreted or absorbed by tubules (e.g., creatinine); P = plasma concentration of x (e.g., creatinine); v = urine flow rate/min; and U = urine concentration of x (e.g., creatinine).
        ii) Creatinine clearance is a calculation of GFR by comparing serum creatinine with the amount of creatinine excreted in the urine over a 24-hour period.
        iii) GFR must be maintained at a constant rate, and autoregulation ensures this constant rate; systemic MAP must be maintained between 80 and 180 mm Hg to maintain regulation.

    4) The glomerular membrane is a porous but semipermeable membrane.
        a) Glomerular filtrate (also called *ultrafiltrate*) is similar in composition to blood except that it lacks blood cells, platelets, and large plasma proteins; water, sodium, glucose, potassium, chloride, phosphate, urea, uric acid, creatinine, ammonia, phenol, calcium, and magnesium pass through the glomerular membrane.
        b) Glomerular filtrate volume is usually 120 ml/min, but 99% of this is reabsorbed in the renal tubule.
    b. Reabsorption: passage of a substance that the body needs from the lumen of the tubules through the tubular cells and into the capillaries
      1) Processes
        a) Active transport
            i) The force used when the cell membranes must move molecules "uphill" against a concentration gradient
            ii) Requires the use of energy and a carrier substance; the substance combines with a "carrier" and diffuses through the tubular membrane, where they reenter the bloodstream
            iii) Substances moved by active transport include glucose, protein, amino acids, and phosphate.

b) Passive transport: processes of osmosis and diffusion
   i) Diffusion: the passive movement of solute from an area of higher concentration to an area of lower concentration; urea and electrolytes are moved by diffusion
   ii) Osmosis: the passive movement of water from an area of lower solute concentration to an area of higher solute concentration
2) Maximal tubular transport capacity: maximum amount of a substance that can be completely reabsorbed in 1 minute and reflects the renal threshold of a substance; if this threshold is exceeded, the substance appears in the urine (e.g., glucosuria)
c. Tubular secretion: passage of a substance not needed by the body from the capillaries through the tubular cells into the lumen of the tubule
d. Countercurrent mechanism uses the juxtamedullary nephrons with their long loops of Henle and occurs within the renal medullary interstitium.
   1) Countercurrent multiplication is the mechanism that enables the body to excrete urine with an osmolality higher than the osmolality of serum.
      a) Sodium chloride is transported out of the filtrate as it moves up the ascending limb of the loop of Henle, but water is not able to follow because this limb is impermeable to water.
      b) Some of sodium chloride enters the peritubular capillaries and is removed from the kidney, but some reenters the descending limb of the loop of Henle, making the filtrate more concentrated than the blood from which it was derived.
      c) This process increases the osmotic pressure in the capillaries and tubules of the papillary region of the kidney until it is four times stronger than that of the blood in the afferent arteriole.
   2) Countercurrent exchange is the maintenance component of the countercurrent mechanism.
      a) The vasa recta minimize the loss of solute from the interstitium by passive diffusion, maintaining the osmotic gradient necessary for the countercurrent multiplication process.
e. A total of 99% of the glomerular filtrate is reabsorbed from the tubules (especially the proximal limb); the remaining 1% is excreted as urine output.
   1) Normal urine output is approximately 1500 ml/day.
   2) Urine composition
      a) Water
      b) Nitrogenous wastes: urea, uric acid, creatinine, ammonia
      c) Ions: potassium, sodium, calcium, chloride, bicarbonate, hydrogen, phosphate, sulfate
      d) Hormones and their breakdown products
      e) Vitamins: particularly water-soluble B vitamins and vitamin C
      f) Toxins
      g) Drugs
   3) Abnormal constituents: glucose, albumin, RBCs, calculi, casts, pigments
2. Excretion of metabolic waste products
   a. Urea
      1) Protein (either ingested or borrowed from protein stores) is broken down into amino acids and nitrogenous wastes.
      2) Urea nitrogen is the endproduct of protein metabolism; it circulates in the bloodstream and is excreted in the urine.
      3) Blood urea nitrogen (BUN) varies with protein intake and hydration status, so BUN provides an unreliable evaluation of renal function.
   b. Creatinine
      1) Creatinine is a waste product of muscle metabolism.
      2) A normal kidney excretes creatinine at a rate equal to the kidney's blood flow or GFR.
      3) Serum creatinine is a better test for evaluation of renal function than BUN; urine creatinine clearance, which provides a comparison of serum creatinine and 24-hour urine creatinine, is an even better evaluation of renal function.
3. Renal regulation of acid–base balance (for more on acid–base balance, Chapter 4)
   a. Tubular excretion of H^+ ions in exchange for sodium reabsorption
   b. Bicarbonate reabsorption into the circulation or excretion into the urine
   c. Excretion of H^+ ions in the urine as NH_4Cl, H_2PO_4, H_2O
   d. Renal response to acidosis
      1) Increased hydrogen ion secretion
      2) Increased bicarbonate reabsorption
      3) Production of ammonia to accommodate hydrogen ion excretion
   e. Renal response to alkalosis
      1) Decreased hydrogen ion secretion
      2) Increased bicarbonate excretion
      3) Decreased production of ammonia
4. Fluid balance
   a. Body fluids are dilute solutions of water and solutes.
   b. Measurement methods
      1) Milliliter (ml): the unit of measure for fluid volume
      2) Milliequivalent (mEq): the unit of measure for chemical combining activity of an electrolyte
      3) Milliosmoles (mOsm): the unit of measure for osmotic pressure based on the number of dissolved particles in solution
         a) Osmolality and osmolarity: frequently used interchangeably, although most calculations of body fluids are based on osmolality
            i) Osmolality: number of osmoles per kilogram of solution; expressed as mOsm/kg
               (a) Blood
                  (i) Normal 280 to 295 mOsm/kg
                  (ii) Main constituent: sodium

(b) Urine
(i) Normal 50 to 1200 mOsm/kg H_2O
(ii) Main constituents: urea and sodium
ii) Osmolarity: number of osmoles per liter of solution
(a) Isotonic: the tonicity of body fluids; osmolarity of 280 to 295 mOsm/l
(b) Hypotonic: lower tonicity than body fluids
(c) Hypertonic: higher tonicity than body fluids
c. The human body is mostly water.
1) Volume
a) Men: 60% of total body weight in adult males is water.
b) Women: slightly less water at 55% of total body weight because of a higher percentage of body fat
c) Older adults: less water at 45% to 55% of total body weight
d) Obesity: body water decreases with increasing body fat
2) Distribution (Fig. 8.6, A)
a) Intracellular
i) Fluid contained within the cells
ii) Accounts for 40% of total body weight
b) Extracellular
i) Fluid outside the cells
ii) Accounts for 20% of total body weight
iii) Distribution
(a) Interstitial
(i) Fluid surrounding the cells
(ii) Accounts for 15% of total body weight
(b) Intravascular
(i) Fluid contained within the blood vessels
(ii) Accounts for approximately 4% of total body weight
(c) Transcellular
(i) Fluid contained within specialized cavities of the body (e.g., cerebrospinal, pericardial, pleural, synovial, intraocular, digestive fluids)
(ii) Accounts for approximately 1% of total body weight
d. Homeostasis is the state of internal equilibrium within the body; fluid, electrolyte, and acid–base are in balance.
1) Water and solutes are in constant movement and are exchanged continuously.
a) Most of the membranes of the body are semipermeable, allowing free movement of water and many nonelectrolytes and selective movement of electrolytes according to concentration gradients.
b) Movement of fluids, electrolytes, and other solutes occurs by the following processes:
i) Diffusion: Solutes move from an area of higher solute concentration to an area of lower solute concentration.
ii) Osmosis: Solutions move from an area of lower solute concentration to an area of higher solute concentration.

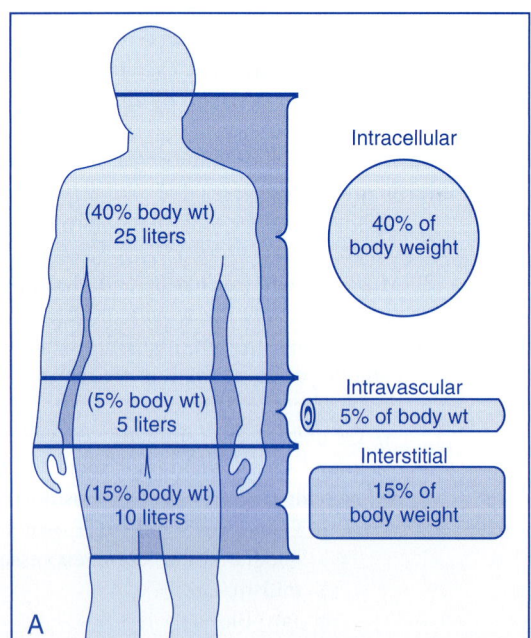
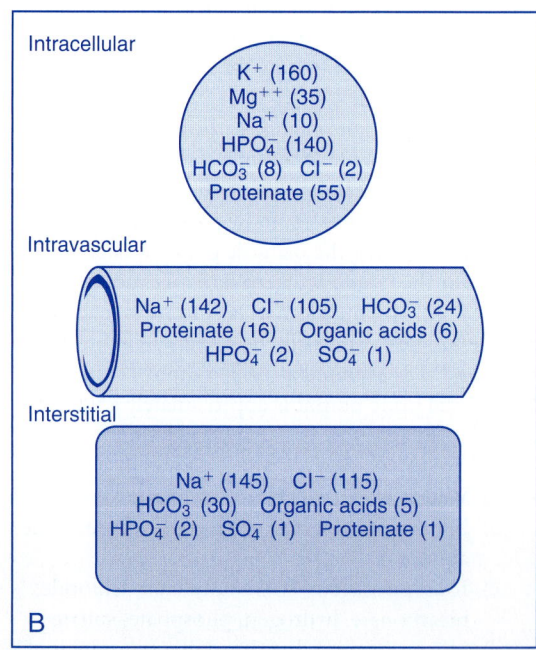

Fig. 8.6 A, Distribution of body fluids. **B,** Electrolytes by fluid compartment. (From Urden, L. D., Stacy, K. M., & Lough, M. E. [2010]. *Critical care nursing: Diagnosis and management* [6th ed.]. St. Louis: Mosby.)

iii) Active transport: use of an energy source to move solutes from an area of lower solute concentration to an area of higher solution concentration
iv) Filtration: use of the pushing pressure of hydrostatic pressure to move water and selective solutes through a semipermeable membrane

c) Movement into and out of the cell occurs by diffusion, osmosis, and active transport.
   i) Hydrostatic pressures push.
      (a) Capillary hydrostatic pressure pushes fluid out of capillary and into interstitium.
      (b) Interstitial hydrostatic pressure pushes fluid out of interstitium and into the capillary.
   ii) Colloidal oncotic pressures pull.
      (a) Capillary colloidal oncotic pressure pulls and holds fluid in the capillary.
      (b) Interstitial colloidal oncotic pressure pulls and holds fluid in the interstitium.
   iii) Starling's law of the capillaries describes the movement of fluid into and out of the capillaries (for more on capillary dynamics, Chapter 3)
      (a) Pressure differences at the venous and arterial ends of the capillaries influence the direction and rate of water and solute movement.
      (b) Pressures pushing fluid out of the capillary dominate at the arterial end; pressures pushing fluid back into the capillary dominate at the venous end.

d) Pathology
   i) Third spacing: fluid accumulation in any space that is not intravascular or intracellular (e.g., interstitial edema, ascites, pleural effusion, pericardial effusion)
      (a) Heart failure (HF): Peripheral edema is caused by venous congestion and excessive hydrostatic pressure at the venous end.
      (b) Malnutrition: Decrease in plasma proteins decrease capillary colloidal oncotic pressure and allow excessive fluid to leak out of the capillary.
      (c) Fluid resuscitation with hypotonic solutions (e.g., D_5W): Fluids with osmolality less than serum cause movement of fluid out of the vascular bed into the interstitium.

2) Normal functioning of cells requires constancy of the body's compartments; imbalances disrupt homeostasis.

e. Water exchanges occur continuously.
   1) Loss of water: total ~2400 ml/24 hr
      a) Lungs (400 ml)
      b) Skin (400 ml)
      c) Kidneys (1500 ml)
      d) Intestines (100 ml)
      e) Losses are increased by any of the following:
         i) Increased respiratory rate
         ii) Fever
         iii) Hot, dry environment
         iv) Injury to the skin (e.g., burns)
   2) Gains of water: total ~2400 ml/24 hr
      a) Liquids (1500 ml)
      b) Food (500 ml)
      c) Oxidation of food and body tissues (400 ml)

f. Body fluid is regulated by the following mechanisms:
   1) Thirst
      a) Thirst mechanism is located in the anterior hypothalamus; osmoreceptor cells sense changes in serum osmolality and initiate impulses to produce the thirst sensation and the release of ADH.
      b) The mechanism is stimulated by any of the following:
         i) Intracellular dehydration
         ii) Hypertonic body fluids
         iii) Extracellular fluid loss
         iv) Hypotension or decreased CO
         v) Angiotensin
         vi) Dry mouth
      c) The effect of thirst is the conscious desire to drink fluids (NOTE: Thirst is unreliable in older adults and confused individuals.)
   2) ADH
      a) ADH is produced by the hypothalamus, stored in and released by the posterior pituitary gland; release may be altered by intracranial processes (e.g., head injury, tumors, craniotomy) and extracranial processes (e.g., mechanical ventilation, tuberculosis).
      b) ADH is stimulated by any of the following:
         i) Hyperosmolality of extracellular fluid
         ii) Decrease in extracellular fluid volume
         iii) Hyperthermia
      c) Effects of ADH include the following:
         i) Acts on distal and collecting tubules, causing more water to be pulled from the tubule back into the blood
         ii) Increases total volume of body fluid by decreasing urine volume
   3) Renin-angiotensin-aldosterone (RAA) system (Fig. 3.22)
      a) RAA system is stimulated by any of the following:
         i) Decreased BP stimulating stretch receptors in juxtaglomerular cells
         ii) SNS stimulation
         iii) Hyponatremia, hyperkalemia
         iv) Increased adrenocorticotropin hormone (ACTH) levels

b) Effects of the RAA system include the following:
   i) Angiotensin II causes vasoconstriction and secretion of aldosterone, a mineralocorticoid produced by the adrenal cortex.
   ii) Aldosterone stimulates the renal tubules to reabsorb more sodium and water, which causes sodium retention, water retention, and decreased urine volume.
   iii) Vasoconstriction and sodium and water retention increase BP, which decreases renin secretion.
4) Atrial natriuretic peptide (ANP)
   a) ANP is a hormonelike substance that is synthesized and stored by specialized atrial muscle cells.
   b) ANP secretion is stimulated by the following:
      i) Volume expansion
      ii) Elevated cardiac filling pressures
   c) Effects of ANP include the following:
      i) Increased excretion of sodium and water by the kidney
      ii) Decreased synthesis of renin and decreased release of aldosterone
5) Countercurrent mechanism of kidney: mechanism for concentration and dilution of urine

5. Electrolyte balance
   a. Solutes are substances dissolved in a solution and may be electrolytes or nonelectrolytes.
      1) Nonelectrolytes (e.g., glucose, proteins, lipids, oxygen, carbon dioxide, urea, creatinine, bilirubin) are solutes without an electrical charge; they stay intact in solution.
      2) Electrolytes are solutes that dissociate into positive or negative ions when in solution and will generate an electrical charge when in solution.
         a) Electrical charge
            i) Cations are positively charged ions
               (a) Major intracellular cation is potassium (K^+)
               (b) Major extracellular cation is sodium (Na^+)
               (c) Other cations: Ca^{++}; Mg^{++}; H^+
            ii) Anions are negatively charged electrolytes.
               (a) Major intracellular anion is chloride (Cl^-)
               (b) Major extracellular anion is phosphate (PO_4^{3-})
               (c) Other anions: HCO_3^-
            iii) In each fluid compartment, the various cations and anions balance each other to achieve electrical neutrality; there is no net charge within a fluid compartment (Fig. 8.6, *B*).
   b. Renal regulation of electrolytes
      1) Excretion and/or retention of electrolytes
      2) Filter and reabsorb about half of unbound serum calcium and activate vitamin D_3, a compound that promotes intestinal calcium absorption
      3) Regulates phosphorus excretion
   c. Summary of electrolyte normal values, roles, regulation, and food sources (Table 8.1)
6. Renal role in regulation of BP
   a. Juxtaglomerular apparatus is a combination of specialized cells located near the glomerulus at the junction of the afferent and efferent arterioles; juxtaglomerular cells contain granules of inactive renin.
   b. RAA system as depicted in Fig. 3.22
7. RBC synthesis and maturation
   a. Erythropoietin secretion
      1) Stimulates production of RBCs in bone marrow
      2) Prolongs life of RBC
   b. Postulated methods of erythropoietin synthesis and stimulus for secretion
      1) Normal kidneys either produce erythropoietin or synthesize an enzyme that catalyzes its formation.
      2) Stimulation for formation is believed to be decreased PaO_2 in renal blood.
   c. Interference in this process causes anemia in patients with chronic renal failure.
8. Prostaglandin synthesis
   a. Process occurs primarily in the medulla.
   b. Types of prostaglandins are as follows:
      1) Vasodilators: PGE_2, PGD_2, PGI_2
      2) Vasoconstrictor: PGA_2

Table 8.1 Electrolyte Summary

Electrolyte	Functions	Regulation and Factors Affecting Serum Level
Sodium: normal 136–145 mEq/l	• Maintains extracellular osmolality and volume • Maintains active transport mechanism in conjunction with potassium • Influences the kidney's regulation of the body's water and electrolyte status • Promotes the irritability of nerve tissue and the conduction of nerve impulses • Facilitates muscle contraction • Aids in some enzyme activities • Combines with bicarbonate and chloride to help regulate acid–base balance	• Aldosterone: causes sodium and water retention • GFR: sodium excretion is increased when GFR is high; decreased when GFR is low • "Third factor": promotes sodium excretion by inhibiting sodium reabsorption; suppression of this factor ensures sodium reabsorption • Increase in sodium concentration stimulates water retention by ADH release diluting sodium back to normal level • Some excretion through skin in perspiration

Table 8.1	Electrolyte Summary—cont'd	
Electrolyte	**Functions**	**Regulation and Factors Affecting Serum Level**
Potassium: normal 3.5–5.0 mEq/l	• Promotes transmission of nerve impulses • Maintains intracellular osmolality • Activates several enzymatic reactions • Helps regulate acid–base balance • Influences kidney function and structure • Promotes myocardial, skeletal, and smooth muscle contractility	• Aldosterone: increase in intracellular potassium or decrease in serum sodium causes aldosterone release and potassium excretion • GFR: potassium excretion is directly related to GFR in a normal kidney • Obligatory loss: the kidneys are unable to conserve potassium; it may be flushed out by diuresis even in the presence of a body deficit; 40–50 mEq lost each day • Renal failure: if kidneys fail to excrete potassium normally from the body (e.g., renal failure), toxic levels can occur • pH: potassium shifts into the cell in alkalosis (causing hypokalemia) and out of the cell in acidosis (causing hyperkalemia)
Calcium: normal 8.5–10.5 mg/dl or 4.5–5.8 mEq/l (NOTE: Calcium is affected by albumin levels; to correct calcium, add 0.8 mg/dl for each 1-g/dl decrease in albumin.)	• Hardens and strengthens bones and teeth • Aids in blood coagulation • Transmits neuromuscular impulses • Maintains cellular permeability • Serves essential role in cardiac contractility	• PTH: stimulated by a decrease in serum calcium; promotes calcium transfer from bone to plasma and aids in renal and intestinal absorption • Phosphorus: inhibits calcium absorption; calcium and phosphorus have an inverse relationship; if calcium goes up, phosphorus goes down and vice versa • Vitamin D: necessary for GI absorption; promotes calcium absorption • Calcitonin: aids transfer of calcium from plasma to bone which directly lowers serum calcium • Albumin: 50% of serum calcium is bound to serum albumin; therefore, a decrease in serum albumin will lower the total calcium level but not the ionized calcium level and the patient will not have symptoms of hypocalcemia • pH: alkalosis increases binding between albumin and calcium so that the patient will exhibit symptoms of hypocalcemia, although total body calcium is normal; acidosis decreases binding between albumin and calcium so that the patient may exhibit symptoms of hypercalcemia • Corticosteroids: contribute to demineralization of the bone and calcium loss; large doses decrease calcium absorption in GI tract • Diuretic effect: calcium is lost, along with potassium and magnesium, in patients on diuretics
Phosphorus: normal 3.0–4.5 mg/dl	• Aids in structure of cellular membrane • Essential for glucose metabolism in RBCs; produces 2,3-DPG as an endproduct • Regulates the delivery of oxygen to the tissues; 2,3-DPG encourages unloading between hemoglobin and oxygen • Essential for ATP or high-energy phosphate formation • May be connected to DNA, RNA, genetic coding • Helps maintain bone hardness • Aids in enzyme regulation (ATPase) • Used by kidney to buffer hydrogen ions (PO_4)	• PTH: inhibits renal reabsorption of phosphates; calcium and phosphorus have an inverse relationship; if calcium goes up, phosphorus goes down and vice versa • Alterations in GFR affect phosphate excretion; increased GFR decreases reabsorption of phosphorus; decreased GFR increases reabsorption of phosphorus

Continued

Table 8.1 Electrolyte Summary—cont'd

Electrolyte	Functions	Regulation and Factors Affecting Serum Level
Magnesium: normal 1.5–2.5 mEq/l	• Aids in neuromuscular transmission • Aids in cardiac contractility • Activates enzymes for cellular metabolism of CHO and proteins • Aids in maintaining the active transport mechanism at the cellular level • Aids in the transmission of hereditary information to offspring	• Not completely understood • Factors that influence calcium and potassium balance also affect magnesium • Deficiencies of these electrolytes usually occur together (e.g., diuretics cause the loss of all three) • Availability of sodium: sodium is necessary for the absorption of magnesium • Diuretics: cause the loss of excessive magnesium • PTH: affects magnesium reabsorption as it does calcium
Chloride: normal 96–106 mEq/l	• Maintains serum osmolality (along with sodium) • Combines with major cations to form important compounds (e.g., NaCl, HCl, KCl, CaCl) • Helps maintain acid–base balance through HCl production	• Indirectly affected by aldosterone • Changes almost always linked to sodium • pH: acidosis causes bicarbonate to be reabsorbed while chloride is excreted; alkalosis causes bicarbonate to be excreted while chloride is reabsorbed

ADH, Antidiuretic hormone; *ATP,* adenosine triphosphate; *CHO,* carbohydrate; *GFR,* glomerular filtration rate; *GI,* gastrointestinal; *PTH,* parathyroid hormone; *RBC,* red blood cell; *2,3-DPG,* 2,3-diphosphoglyceric acid.

    c. Release is stimulated by vasoactive substances (e.g., angiotensin, norepinephrine, bradykinins).
    d. Effects of prostaglandins include the following:
       1) Modulate the vasoconstrictive effects of angiotensin and norepinephrine; interference with this process may be one factor contributing to hypertension in patients with renal failure
       2) Increase renal blood flow, which results in arterial vasodilation, inhibition of the distal tubule's response to ADH, and promotion of sodium and water excretion
9. Renal role in bone mineralization
    a. Vitamin D is metabolized by the kidney from an inactive form to an active metabolite called *1,25-dihydroxycholecalciferol,* necessary for the absorption of calcium and phosphorus from the intestine.
    b. Interference in this process causes osteodystrophy in patients with chronic renal failure.

Assessment of Fluid, Electrolyte, and Renal Status

Interview

1. Chief complaint: common symptoms of fluid, electrolyte, or renal conditions
    a. Flank or costovertebral angle (CVA) pain
       1) Unilateral or bilateral
       2) Constant or intermittent
       3) Aggravated by CVA percussion
       4) Dull ache to stabbing or throbbing pain
       5) Relieved only by analgesics or treatment of underlying disease
       6) Accompanying findings: hematuria; pyuria; change in urine volume
       7) Possible causes: renal calculi, bladder cancer, bacterial cystitis, acute glomerulonephritis, obstructive uropathy, perirenal abscess, polycystic kidney disease, acute pyelonephritis, renal infarction, renal cancer, renal trauma, renal vein thrombosis, acute pancreatitis
    b. Changes in pattern of urination
       1) Frequency: frequent voiding
       2) Nocturia: getting up at night to void (more than twice)
       3) Dysuria: painful urination
       4) Urgency: a feeling of the need to void immediately
       5) Hesitancy: difficulty starting the flow of urine
       6) Change in stream
       7) Retention: incomplete emptying of the bladder
       8) Incontinence: inability to control urination
       9) Enuresis: incontinence of urine in bed at night
    c. Change in urine output: increased or decreased amount
    d. Change in appearance of urine
       1) Dilute: clear to light yellow
       2) Concentrated: dark, amber
       3) Pyuria: cloudy
       4) Hematuria: pink to red
       5) Bilirubinemia: orange to brown
       6) Myoglobinuria: tea or cola colored
       7) Hemoglobinuria: wine colored
    e. Neurologic
       1) Visual changes: may be associated with uremia or fluid or electrolyte imbalance
       2) Paresthesias: may be associated with hypocalcemia
       3) Headaches: may be associated with fluid imbalance or uremia
       4) Seizures: may be associated with uremia or fluid or electrolyte imbalances
       5) Decreased ability to concentrate: may be associated with uremia or fluid or electrolyte imbalances
       6) Apathy: may be associated with uremia

f. Cardiovascular
   1) Palpitations: may be seen with dysrhythmias in electrolyte imbalance
   2) Chest pain: may be seen with uremia or electrolyte imbalance
   3) Edema: may be associated with uremia, fluid overload, or hypoproteinemia
g. Pulmonary
   1) Dyspnea: may be seen in patients with renal failure as the result of left ventricular failure or pleural effusion
   2) Hemoptysis: seen in Goodpasture syndrome
h. Gastrointestinal (GI)
   1) Halitosis: foul odor to breath; urinelike odor to breath may be associated with uremia; metallic taste in mouth
   2) Anorexia: may be associated with uremia
   3) Nausea or vomiting: may be associated with uremia, electrolyte imbalance, or fluid overload
   4) Constipation or diarrhea: may be related to fluid imbalance
i. Musculoskeletal
   1) Joint pain: may be associated with uremia, fluid imbalance, or electrolyte imbalance
   2) Muscle weakness: may be associated with electrolyte imbalance
   3) Muscle pain or cramps: may be associated with uremia or electrolyte imbalance
j. Dermatologic
   1) Pruritus: may be associated with uremia
   2) Bruising: may be associated with uremia
   3) Delayed healing: may be associated with uremia
k. Sexual
   1) Impotence: may be related to uremia
   2) Diminished libido: may be related to uremia
   3) Infertility: may be related to uremia
l. Other general symptoms
   1) Fatigue: may be associated with uremia
   2) Fever: may be associated with infection or dehydration
   3) Thirst: may be associated with fluid imbalance
   4) Change in body weight: may be associated with uremia or fluid imbalance
2. History of present illness
   a. PQRST
   b. Accompanying symptoms
3. Past medical history
   a. Renal and urinary tract
      1) Urinary tract infection (UTI)
      2) Calculi
      3) Renal insufficiency or failure
         a) Dialysis
         b) Renal transplantation
      4) Surgical procedures
   b. Cardiovascular
      1) Hypertension
      2) Arteriosclerosis or atherosclerosis
      3) Heart failure (HF)
      4) Bacterial endocarditis
   c. Pulmonary: tuberculosis
   d. Endocrine and metabolic
      1) Diabetes mellitus
      2) Gout
   e. Immunologic and hematologic
      1) Connective tissue disorders
         a) Lupus erythematosus
         b) Scleroderma
      2) Goodpasture syndrome: hemoptysis with glomerulonephritis
      3) Hemophilia
      4) Disseminated intravascular coagulation
      5) Sickle cell disease
      6) Malignancy
      7) Blood transfusion
   f. Gynecologic: toxemia of pregnancy
   g. Infection
      1) Recent beta-hemolytic streptococcal infection
      2) UTI
4. Family history
   a. Renal
      1) Inherited glomerulonephritis
      2) Polycystic disease
      3) Inherited nephritis (Alport syndrome)
      4) Amyloidosis
      5) Malignancy
   b. Cardiovascular
      1) Hypertension
      2) Coronary artery disease
   c. Immunologic and hematologic
      1) Hemophilia
      2) Sickle cell disease
   d. Endocrine: diabetes mellitus
5. Social history
   a. Occupational exposure to toxins: lead, mercury, pesticides, methanol, radiation, carbon tetrachloride, phenol
   b. Exercise habits: strenuous exercise in an unconditioned person may cause rhabdomyolysis
   c. Fluid intake: type of fluids
   d. Smoking: increased incidence of bladder cancer
   e. Use of saccharin: increased incidence of bladder cancer
6. Medication history
   a. Potentially nephrotoxic agents
      1) Antimicrobials
         a) Aminoglycosides
         b) Cephalosporins
         c) Sulfonamides
         d) Amphotericin B
         e) Bacitracin
         f) Rifampin
      2) Nonsteroidal antiinflammatory agents (e.g., ibuprofen, indomethacin, aspirin)
      3) Angiotensin-converting enzyme (ACE) inhibitors (e.g., captopril, enalapril)
      4) Antineoplastics (e.g., cisplatin, methotrexate)
      5) Analgesics containing phenacetin
      6) Cyclosporin A
      7) Methanol, ethylene glycol
      8) Carbon tetrachloride
      9) Contrast media
      10) Heavy metals (e.g., lead, arsenic, mercury, uranium)
      11) Insecticides and fungicides
      12) Phencyclidine (PCP) and other street drugs
   b. Diuretics
   c. Antihypertensives

b) Not as accurate an indicator of renal failure as is creatinine because BUN levels fluctuate greatly with protein intake, but creatinine levels are relatively unchanged by protein intake and hydration level
2) Abnormal values
  a) Increased with decreased renal blood flow or urine production, dehydration, some neoplasms, and certain antibiotics; increased BUN is also referred to as *uremia*
  b) Decreased in pregnancy, overhydration, severe liver disease, malnutrition
3) BUN: creatinine ratio: normally ~10:1
  a) When BUN is elevated disproportionately to the creatinine (e.g., BUN:creatinine ratio, 20:1), consider an extrarenal cause such as one of the following:
    i) Volume depletion (i.e., prerenal)
      (a) Insufficient fluid intake
      (b) Excessive fluid loss
        (i) Diuresis
        (ii) Vomiting
    ii) Poor renal perfusion
      (a) Shock
      (b) Sepsis
      (c) Decreased CO
      (d) Renovascular disease
    iii) Protein catabolism
      (a) Starvation
      (b) Blood in the GI tract
      (c) Corticosteroids
  b) When BUN and creatinine are both elevated while maintaining the normal 10:1 ratio, consider a renal cause such as acute or chronic renal failure.
  c) When BUN:creatinine is lower than normal
    i) Decreased protein intake
    ii) Liver dysfunction
c. Creatinine: normal 0.7 to 1.5 mg/dl
1) Nonprotein endproduct of muscle metabolism
  a) More accurate than BUN in evaluating renal function because creatinine is normally filtered by the glomerulus and not reabsorbed by the tubule
  b) Unaffected by diet and fluid intake
2) Abnormal values
  a) Increased
    i) A twice-normal (~3 mg/dl) creatinine level suggests 50% nephron loss.
    ii) Greater than 10 mg/dl indicates end-stage renal disease with less than 10% of nephrons still functioning.
  b) Decreased: muscular dystrophy
d. Electrolytes
1) Sodium: normal 136 to 145 mEq/l
2) Potassium: normal 3.5 to 5.0 mEq/l
3) Chloride: normal 96 to 106 mEq/l
4) Calcium: normal 8.5 to 10.5 mg/dl
5) Phosphorus: normal 3.0 to 4.5 mg/dl
6) Magnesium: normal 1.5 to 2.2 mEq/l

e. Anion gap: a calculated parameter (Table 8.2)
1) Calculated by subtracting the anions from the cations
  a) (Sodium + Potassium) − (Chloride + Carbon dioxide content or Bicarbonate)
  b) Normal 5 to 15
2) Helpful in determination of cause of metabolic acidosis
  a) A normal anion gap indicates that the reason for the metabolic acidosis is bicarbonate loss.
  b) An elevated anion gap indicates that the reason for the metabolic acidosis is an acid gain (e.g., lactic acid, ketoacid, toxins).
f. Glucose: normal 70 to 110 mEq/l

Table 8.2 Anion Gap

Considerations	Comments
Calculation of anion gap	$(Na + K) - (Cl + [HCO_3$ or CO_2 content$])$
Normal value	5-15
Causes of metabolic acidosis with normal anion gap: bicarbonate loss	Intestinal loss of bicarbonate • Diarrhea • Pancreatic fistula • Ureterosigmoidostomy Renal loss of bicarbonate • Carbonic anhydrase inhibitors (e.g., acetazolamide [Diamox]) • Aldosterone antagonists (also referred to as *potassium-sparing diuretics*) (e.g., triamterene, spironolactone) • Renal tubular acidosis • Adrenal insufficiency • Primary hypoaldosteronism Excessive gain of chloride • Large quantities of normal saline • Ammonium chloride • Arginine hydrochloride
Causes of metabolic acidosis with increased anion gap: metabolic acid gain	Renal failure Lactic acidosis • Shock • Hypoxemia or hypoxia • Severe anemia • Status epilepticus • Cyanide poisoning Ketoacidosis • Diabetic ketoacidosis • Starvation • Alcohol Drugs and toxins • Salicylates • Methanol • Ethylene glycol • Paraldehyde • High-dose carbenicillin • Rhabdomyolysis

g. Arterial blood gases
  1) pH: normal 7.35 to 7.45
  2) PaCO$_2$: normal 35 to 45 mm Hg
  3) HCO$_3$: normal 22 to 26 mEq/l
  4) PaO$_2$: normal 80 to 100 mm Hg
h. Hematology
  1) Hematocrit: normal 40% to 52% for males; 35% to 47% for females
     a) Measures portion of blood volume occupied by RBCs
     b) Increased in dehydration or polycythemia
     c) Decreased with low RBCs or with normal hemoglobin and water overload
  2) Hemoglobin: normal 13 to 18 g/dl for males; 12 to 16 g/dl for females
  3) White blood cell (WBC) count: normal 3500 to 11,000/mm^3
i. Clotting profile
  1) Prothrombin time (PT): normal 12 to 15 seconds
  2) Activated partial thromboplastin time (aPTT): normal 25 to 38 seconds
  3) Thrombin time: normal 10 to 15 seconds
  4) Bleeding time: normal 1 to 9.5 minutes
  5) Platelets: normal 150,000 to 400,000/mm^3
j. Serum proteins
  1) Total protein: normal 6 to 8 g/dl
  2) Albumin: normal 3.5 to 4.5 g/dl
k. Serum lipids
  1) Cholesterol: normal 150 to 200 mg/dl
  2) Triglycerides: normal 40 to 150 mg/dl

2. Urine
  a. Visual examination: clear, yellow
  b. Glucose: normal negative; glycosuria occurs when renal threshold for glucose is exceeded; renal threshold is variable and patient specific, so there is no accurate method to predict serum glucose
  c. Ketones: normal negative; ketonuria is seen in catabolism (e.g., starvation or diabetic ketoacidosis [DKA])
  d. Protein: normal 0 to 8 mg/dl
     1) Proteinuria may occur after ingestion of a high-protein meal or can accompany renal changes of pregnancy.
     2) Consistent proteinuria suggests compromise of the glomerular membrane (e.g., nephrotic syndrome, glomerulonephritis).
  e. Myoglobin: normal negative or less than 20 ng/ml; myoglobinuria indicates muscle breakdown
  f. Hemoglobin: normal negative; hemoglobinuria indicates free hemoglobin in the urine such as occurs in hemolytic blood transfusion reaction, hemolytic or sickle cell anemia, fresh-water drowning, burns, disseminated intravascular coagulation (DIC)
  g. Bilirubin: normal negative; urobilinogen indicates biliary obstruction or liver disease
  h. Specific gravity: normal 1.005 to 1.030
     1) Increased with any condition causing hypoperfusion of kidneys leading to oliguria (e.g., shock, severe dehydration, proteinuria, glycosuria, contrast media)
     2) Decreased in diabetes insipidus (DI), overhydration, and when renal tubules lose their ability to reabsorb water and concentrate urine as in early pyelonephritis
  i. Osmolality: normal 50 to 1200 mOsm/kg
     1) Measures number of particles per unit of water in urine
     2) Depends on the circulating titer of ADH and the rate of urinary solute excretion; should be 1.5 times that of serum osmolality
     3) Increased in fluid volume deficit caused by retention of fluid by the body
     4) Decreased in fluid volume excess caused by fluid being excreted by the kidney
  j. Creatinine clearance
     1) Estimate of GFR
     2) Urine specimen for 24-hour period and a serum creatinine required
     3) Normal 85 to 135 ml/min
  k. Culture and sensitivity: normal no bacteria present; if bacteria are present, appropriate antibiotic therapy is identified
  l. pH: normal 4 to 8 with an average of 6
     1) Increased urinary acidity indicates that the body is retaining bicarbonate.
     2) Decreased urinary acidity (more alkaline) indicates that the kidney is retaining sodium and acids.
        a) Alkaline urine may be associated with UTI.
        b) Alkaline urine and serum acidosis are associated with renal tubular acidosis.
  m. Spot urine electrolytes
     1) Evaluates the kidney's ability to conserve sodium and concentrate urine
     2) Measures sodium, potassium, and chloride concentrations in the urine
        a) Sodium: normal 40 to 220 mEq/l
        b) Potassium: normal 25 to 120 mEq/l
        c) Chloride: normal 110 to 250 mEq/l
  n. Sediment
     1) Casts: precipitation from the kidney that takes the shape of the tubule where it was formed; normally none or occasional hyaline casts
        a) Hyaline casts: small amounts normal, but large amounts indicative of significant proteinuria
        b) Erythrocyte casts: indicative of glomerulonephritis or vasculitis
        c) Leukocyte casts: indicative of infectious process
        d) Granular casts: indicative of acute tubular necrosis, interstitial nephritis, acute or chronic glomerulonephritis, chronic renal failure
        e) Fatty casts: indicative of lipoid nephrosis or nephrotic syndrome
        f) Renal tubular casts: indicative of acute kidney injury (AKI)
     2) Bacteria: abnormal in catheterized specimen
     3) Erythrocytes: small numbers normal; large numbers indicative of glomerulonephritis, interstitial nephritis, malignancy, infection, calculi, cystitis, or trauma

4) Leukocytes: small numbers normal; large numbers indicative of infection, interstitial nephritis
5) Renal epithelial cells: indicative of acute tubular necrosis, glomerulonephritis, interstitial nephritis
6) Crystals: indicative of stone formation
7) Eosinophils: indicative of allergic reaction in kidney
3. Other diagnostic studies (Table 8.3)

Drugs Affecting the Renal System

Diuretics
1. Action: excretion of fluid and sodium
2. Indications
    a. Hypertension
    b. HF
    c. Edema
        1) Pulmonary (usually a loop diuretic)
        2) Cerebral (usually mannitol)

Table 8.3 Renal Diagnostic Studies

Study	Purposes	Comments
Computed tomography (CT)	• Provides a view of kidneys, retroperitoneal space, bladder, and prostate • Evaluates kidney size • Evaluates the kidney for tumors, abscesses, and obstruction	• No special preparation required • Can be safely used in patients with renal failure • Contrast medium may be used
Cystometrography	• Evaluates the pressure exerted against the wall of the bladder to evaluate bladder tone	• No special preparation required • Urinary catheter inserted and saline instilled into bladder Postprocedure • Monitor for clinical indications of urinary tract infection
Cystoscopy	• Visualizes bladder and urethra for identification of pathology	Preprocedure • NPO after midnight if general anesthesia is to be used • Administer sedative if prescribed • No special preparation required Postprocedure • Pink-tinged urine is normal, but gross hematuria is abnormal; monitor urine output • Encourage fluids
Intravenous pyelography (IVP)	• Evaluates position, size, shape, and location of kidneys • Provides visualization of internal kidney (parenchyma, calyces, pelvis) • Evaluates filling of renal pelvis • Outlines ureters and bladder • Identifies presence of cysts and tumors • Identifies obstruction, congenital abnormality	• Also called excretory urogram • Contraindicated in renal insufficiency, multiple myeloma, pregnancy, congestive HF, sickle cell disease • Bowel preparation (e.g., cathartics as prescribed) • NPO for 8 hours before the test • Contrast media used 　• Check for allergy to iodine before the study 　• Monitor for allergic reaction postprocedure 　• Ensure hydration postprocedure
Kidneys, ureters, and bladder (KUB) radiography	• Outlines kidneys, ureters, and bladder • Evaluates size, shape, and position of kidneys • Identifies location of calculi	• Also called *flat plate of abdomen* • Bowel preparation (e.g., cathartics may be prescribed if to be followed by IVP)
Magnetic resonance imaging (MRI)	• Differentiation between cyst and solid mass • Identifies infarction, trauma, obstruction	• More specific than renal ultrasonography or CT scan because it shows subtle density changes • Cannot be used in patients with any implanted metallic device, including pacemakers • No special preparation required
Nephrotomography	• Evaluates segments of the kidney at different levels • Differentiates cysts from solid masses	• Bowel preparation (e.g., cathartics as prescribed) • NPO for 8 hours before the test • Contrast media used 　• Check for allergy to iodine before the study 　• Monitor for allergic reaction postprocedure 　• Ensure hydration postprocedure

Table 8.3 Renal Diagnostic Studies—cont'd

Study	Purposes	Comments

Renal angiography	• Evaluates renal vasculature
	• Identifies renal artery stenosis
	• Identifies cysts, tumors, infarction, trauma
		• Bowel preparation (e.g., cathartics) as prescribed
		• NPO for 8 hr before the test
		• Sedative is usually prescribed before the procedure
		• Contrast media used
		  • Check for allergy to iodine before the study
		  • Monitor for allergic reaction postprocedure
		  • Ensure hydration postprocedure
		Postprocedure
		• Keep extremity in which catheter was placed immobilized in a straight position for 6–12 hr
		• Monitor arterial puncture point for hemorrhage or hematoma
		• Monitor neurovascular status of affected limb
		• Monitor for indications of systemic emboli

Renal biopsy	• Obtains tissue specimen for microscopic evaluation	• May be performed open or closed • Clotting profile is evaluated preprocedure • Type and crossmatch for 2 units of blood preprocedure • Usually not performed if patient has only one functioning kidney (unless being done to evaluate possible transplant rejection) • Closed biopsy contraindicated in bleeding abnormalities, polycystic disease, hydronephrosis, neoplasm, UTI, and uncooperative patient Postprocedure • Pressure dressing is applied, and the patient is on bed rest for 24 hr • Observe for hematuria, flank pain, or hypotension
Renal radionuclide scan (renogram)	• Evaluates position, size, shape, and location of kidneys • Identifies obstruction, abscesses, cysts, tumors • Evaluates renal perfusion • Evaluates glomerular filtration, tubular function, and excretion • Assesses status of renal transplant	• Assure patient that the amount of radioactive material is minimal • Do not schedule within 24 hours after IVP • Ask patient to void before scan • Encourage fluids after the procedure

Retrograde pyelography	• Evaluates position, size, shape, and location of kidneys
	• Outlines ureters and bladder
	• Identifies presence of cysts and tumors
	• Identifies obstruction
		• Does not require the kidney to excrete dye so may be used in patients with renal insufficiency
		• Bowel preparation (e.g., cathartics as prescribed)
		• NPO for 8 hours before the test
		• Contrast media used
		  • Check for allergy to iodine before the study
		  • Monitor for allergic reaction postprocedure
		  • Ensure hydration postprocedure
		• Monitor patient for clinical indications of urinary tract infection or sepsis

Ultrasonography	• Evaluates fluid versus solid mass • Identifies obstructions • Identifies cysts, abscesses, tumors, polycystic kidney disease • Identifies hemorrhage • Identifies urinary tract obstruction and leaks	• No special preparation required • Can be safely used in patients with renal failure • Contrast media may be used
Voiding cystourethrography	• Identifies abnormalities of lower urinary tract to determine presence of reflux and residual urine	• No special preparation required • Encourage fluids postprocedure

HF, Heart failure; *NPO*, nothing by mouth; *UTI*, urinary tract infection.

3) Peripheral
d. Drug toxicity (forced diuresis) (usually mannitol)
e. Renal pigments (e.g., hemoglobinuria, myoglobinuria) (usually mannitol)
3. Types of diuretics and specific actions
   a. Thiazide diuretics
      1) Examples
         a) Hydrochlorothiazide
         b) Chlorthalidone
         c) Chlorothiazide
         d) Polythiazide
         e) Indapamide
         f) Metolazone
      2) Actions
         a) Inhibit sodium reabsorption in the ascending loop of Henle and the early distal tubule
         b) Decrease water reabsorption
      3) Potential adverse effects
         a) Hyponatremia
         b) Hypokalemia
         c) Hypercalcemia
         d) Hypomagnesemia
         e) Hypovolemia
         f) Hyperglycemia
         g) Hyperuricemia
         h) Increased BUN
         i) Hepatitis
         j) Anemia, thrombocytopenia, neutropenia
   b. Loop diuretics: used most often in critical care because of their potency
      1) Examples
         a) Furosemide
         b) Ethacrynic acid
         c) Bumetanide
         d) Torsemide
      2) Actions
         a) Inhibit sodium reabsorption in the ascending loop of Henle
         b) Decrease water reabsorption
      3) Potential adverse effects
         a) Hyponatremia
         b) Hypokalemia
         c) Hypocalcemia
         d) Hypomagnesemia
         e) Hypochloremic alkalosis
         f) Hypovolemia
         g) Hyperglycemia
         h) Hyperuricemia
         i) Increased BUN
         j) Hearing loss
         k) Thrombocytopenia, agranulocytosis, leukopenia, anemia
   c. Osmotic diuretics
      1) Example: mannitol
      2) Actions
         a) Expand intravascular volume and increase GFR
         b) Increase osmolality of the tubular fluid leading to decreased absorption of sodium and water
      3) Potential adverse effects
         a) Hyponatremia
         b) Hypokalemia
         c) Hypocalcemia
         d) Hypomagnesemia
         e) Initial intravascular hypervolemia followed by hypovolemia
         f) Increased intravascular volume may cause pulmonary edema in patients with poor cardiac function.
         g) Hyperglycemia
         h) Hyperuricemia
         i) Increased BUN
         j) Confusion
      4) Aldosterone antagonists (frequently referred to as *potassium-sparing diuretics*)
         a) Examples
            i) Spironolactone
            ii) Triamterene
            iii) Amiloride
         b) Actions
            i) Act as an aldosterone antagonist
            ii) Block sodium and potassium exchange mechanism in the distal tubule, causing loss of sodium and water and retention of potassium
         c) Potential adverse effects
            i) Hyponatremia
            ii) Hyperkalemia
            iii) Hypocalcemia
            iv) Hypomagnesemia
            v) Hypovolemia
            vi) Hyperchloremic metabolic acidosis
      5) Carbonic anhydrase inhibitors
         a) Examples: acetazolamide
         b) Actions
            i) Block the action of carbonic anhydrase in the proximal tubule, preventing bicarbonate and sodium reabsorption
            ii) Cause increased water loss and a decrease in serum pH; may be used to treat metabolic alkalosis
         c) Potential adverse effects
            i) Hyponatremia
            ii) Hypokalemia
            iii) Hypocalcemia
            iv) Hypomagnesemia
            v) Hypovolemia
            vi) Hyperchloremic metabolic acidosis
            vii) Thrombocytopenia, agranulocytosis, leukopenia, anemia
   d. Selected diuretics (Table 8.4)

Dopaminergic Stimulators

1. Dopamine infused at low doses is (i.e., 1-2 mcg/kg/min) has been thought to be specific to dopaminergic receptors.
   a. Results are often unpredictable, and dopamine can cause several alpha- and beta-induced side effects (Abay, Reyes, Everts, & Wisser, 2007).
   b. Diuretic effect is thought to be caused primarily by the inotropic effect of beta$_1$ stimulation.
2. Fenoldopam mesylate
   a. Actions
      1) Dilates arterial system, decreasing afterload

Chapter 8   The Renal System   583

Table 8.4	Selected Diuretics		
Drug	**Administration**	**Adverse Effects**	**Nursing Implications**
Furosemide	• PO: 20–80 mg/day • IV injection: 20–120 mg; administer at rate not to exceed 10 mg/min; if initial dose is ineffective, the next dose is usually double the original dose • IV infusion: mix 250 mg in 250 ml (1 mg/ml); usual dose is 0.1–0.75 mg/kg/hr; not to exceed 4 mg/min • Maximum: 1 g/day • Do not mix with acidic solutions Other loop diuretics • Torsemide: 5–20 mg/day PO or IV (over 2 min); may be titrated to desired effect but single dose should not exceed 200 mg • Bumetanide: 0.5–1.0 mg IV; may be repeated at 2- to 3-hr intervals	• Hypotension • Hypovolemia • Nausea, vomiting, abdominal pain • Rash • Electrolyte imbalance: hypocalcemia, hypokalemia, hypomagnesemia, hyponatremia • Acid–base imbalance: hypochloremic alkalosis • Increased uric acid and BUN • Renal failure • Hyperglycemia • Photosensitivity • Thrombocytopenia, agranulocytosis, leukopenia, neutropenia, anemia • Transient deafness (with rapid IV injection)	• Monitor HR, BP, urine output, serum electrolytes, BUN, creatinine, uric acid, CBC, daily weights • Monitor patients also on digitalis for clinical indications of digitalis toxicity • Monitor serum glucose in patients with diabetes mellitus • Monitor for clinical indications of gout • Note contraindications: known hypersensitivity to sulfonamides, anuria, hypovolemia, electrolyte depletion • Sulfonamide-sensitive patients may have allergic reaction to these drugs (furosemide, bumetanide, torsemide) because they are all sulfa derivatives • Use cautiously in diabetes mellitus, dehydration, severe renal disease, gout, hepatic disease • Do not administer if solution is yellow or if precipitate is present • Teach patient about potassium-rich foods
Mannitol	• IV infusion: 1–2 g/kg over 30–60 min; average dose 50–100 g • Use inline filter when administering mannitol	• Tachycardia • Nausea, vomiting • Fluid and electrolyte imbalance • Pulmonary edema • Thirst • Phlebitis • Seizures • Rebound cerebral edema 8–12 hr after diuresis	• Monitor BP, HR, urine output, serum osmolality, serum electrolytes, BUN, uric acid, daily weights • Note contraindications: known hypersensitivity, active intracranial bleeding, anuria, severe dehydration • Use cautiously in severe renal failure, HF, dehydration • Check bottle or ampule for crystallization: discard and replace • Monitor closely for rebound effect: return of clinical indications of intracranial hypertension 8–12 hr after mannitol

BP, Blood pressure; *BUN*, blood urea nitrogen; *CBC*, complete blood count; *HF*, heart failure; *HR*, heart rate; *IV*, intravenous; *PO*, oral.

   2) Stimulates dopamine D1 receptors in the kidneys, causing diuresis
  b. Indications
   1) Hypertension

Fluid and Electrolyte Imbalances

Hypovolemia
1. Etiology
  a. Insufficient intake
  b. Inadequate replacement following excess fluid loss
  c. Excessive fluid losses
   1) Hemorrhage
   2) GI losses
      a) Nasogastric or intestinal suction
      b) Vomiting
      c) Diarrhea
      d) Fistula
   3) Renal losses
      a) Diuretics
      b) Aldosterone insufficiency (i.e., Addison disease)
      c) Diuretic phase of AKI
      d) Osmotic diuresis caused by hyperglycemia
   4) Increased insensible losses
      a) Diaphoresis
      b) Tachypnea
   5) Draining wounds
  d. Intravascular to extravascular shift (also called third spacing)
   1) Ascites
   2) Intestinal obstruction
   3) Peritonitis
   4) Burns
2. Clinical presentation
  a. Subjective
   1) Weakness
   2) Anorexia, nausea, vomiting, constipation
   3) Thirst
   4) Syncope
  b. Objective
   1) Tachycardia
   2) Orthostatic hypotension

3) Low-grade fever
4) Flushed skin (fluid loss) or cool, clammy skin (blood loss)
5) Flat jugular veins even when patient in flat position
6) Dry, sticky tongue and mucous membranes
7) Poor skin turgor
8) Lethargy, disorientation, coma
9) Oliguria
10) Weight loss greater than 5% of body weight
11) Hemodynamic changes: decreased CVP, PAOP, CO; increased systemic vascular resistance (SVR)
   c. Diagnostic studies
      1) Hematocrit and serum osmolality increased if fluid lost; hematocrit decreased if blood lost
      2) Urine specific gravity greater than 1.03 if ADH osmoreceptor mechanism is intact
      3) BUN increased with normal creatinine (i.e., prerenal)
3. Collaborative management
   a. Monitor urine output, input and output (I & O), daily weight, and laboratory studies.
   b. Treat the cause.
      1) Antiemetics for vomiting
      2) Antidiarrheals for diarrhea
      3) Control of hemorrhage: local pressure, prepare patient for surgery
      4) Antibiotics for infection
   c. Replace fluids carefully to prevent hypervolemia.
      1) Oral fluids for mild deficits
      2) Parenteral fluids for moderate or severe deficits; replace fluids lost with similar fluids (e.g., blood for hemorrhage, normal saline [NS] with electrolytes for excessive diuresis)
      3) Close monitoring for clinical indications of fluid overload (e.g., S_3, crackles)
   d. Provide frequent oral and skin care.

Water Loss Syndromes

Serum osmolality greater than 295 mOsm/kg (may be referred to as hyperosmolar [or hypovolemic] hypernatremia)
1. Etiology: water loss in excess of sodium loss
   a. Inadequate water intake
   b. Hypertonic fluids or enteral feedings
   c. DI
   d. Diabetes mellitus
   e. Excess total parenteral nutrition (TPN)
   f. Watery diarrhea
2. Clinical presentation
   a. Subjective
      1) Weakness
      2) Thirst
      3) Syncope
   b. Objective
      1) Tachycardia
      2) Hypotension
      3) Low-grade fever
      4) Flushed skin
      5) Dry, sticky tongue and mucous membranes
      6) Poor skin turgor
      7) Thirst
      8) Mental irritability, confusion
      9) Oliguria to anuria (except DI)
   c. Diagnostic studies
      1) Hematocrit and serum osmolality increased
      2) Serum sodium increased (concentration effect)
3. Collaborative management
   a. Monitor urine output, I & O, daily weight, and laboratory studies.
   b. Treat the cause.
      1) Vasopressin for central DI; chlorpropamide for nephrogenic DI
      2) Insulin for diabetes mellitus and hyperglycemia
      3) Antidiarrheals for diarrhea
      4) Antiemetics for nausea and vomiting
   c. Provide appropriate volume replacement and normalize serum osmolality: administer water in excess of sodium (e.g., D_5W or ½ NS).
   d. Maintain adequate urine output with adequate volume replacement.
   e. Provide frequent oral and skin care.

Hypervolemia

1. Etiology
   a. Excessive intake of fluid
      1) Excess oral or parenteral fluids
      2) Excess use of saline enemas
   b. Retention of sodium and water
      1) Steroid therapy
      2) HF
      3) Liver disease (e.g., cirrhosis)
      4) Stress response via ADH secretion, RAA system
      5) Nephrotic syndrome
      6) Acute or chronic renal failure
   c. Interstitial to intravascular shift
      1) Remobilization of fluids after treatment of burns
      2) Administration of hypertonic or hyperosmolar solutions (e.g., 3% saline, albumin)
2. Clinical presentation
   a. Subjective
      1) Dyspnea
      2) Headache
   b. Objective
      1) Tachycardia
      2) Increased BP
      3) JVD
      4) Tachypnea, dyspnea, crackles
      5) Peripheral edema
      6) Ascites
      7) Increased urine output
      8) Muscle weakness
      9) Confusion, apathy, lethargy, coma
      10) Hemodynamic changes: increased CVP and PAOP
      11) Weight gain greater than 5% of body weight
      12) Clinical indications of pulmonary or cerebral edema
   c. Diagnostic studies
      1) Hematocrit and serum osmolality decreased
      2) BUN decreased
      3) Urine specific gravity less than 1.01 if ADH osmoreceptor mechanism is intact.
      4) Chest radiography may show pulmonary vascular congestion.

3. Collaborative management
   a. Monitor urine output, I & O, daily weight, and laboratory studies.
   b. Prevent hypervolemia by closely monitoring intravenous (IV) fluids; volumetric or controller pumps must be used for patients predisposed to hypervolemia.
   c. Decrease excess volume.
      1) Restriction of fluids and/or sodium
      2) Diuretics as prescribed
      3) Hemodialysis or continuous renal replacement therapy (CRRT) may be used, especially if renal insufficiency is present.
   d. Provide frequent oral and skin care.

Water Excess Syndromes
May be referred to as hypo-osmolar (or hypervolemic) hyponatremia
1. Etiology: water gain in excess of sodium gain
   a. Replacement of isotonic body fluids with hypotonic solution (e.g., D_5W)
   b. Excess use of tap water enemas
   c. Psychogenic polydipsia
   d. GI or genitourinary (GU) irrigation with hypotonic fluids (e.g., tap water or distilled water)
   e. Excessive ice chips
   f. Syndrome of inappropriate antidiuretic hormone (SIADH)
   g. Administration of oral hypoglycemic agents and tricyclic antidepressants
2. Clinical presentation
   a. Subjective
      1) Anorexia, nausea, vomiting
      2) Abdominal and muscle cramps
      3) Headache
      4) Weakness
   b. Objective
      1) Edema
      2) Lethargy
      3) Muscle twitching, seizures
      4) Confusion
   c. Diagnostic studies
      1) Serum osmolality less than 280 mOsm/kg
      2) Serum sodium decreased (dilution effect)
      3) Hematocrit decreased
3. Collaborative management
   a. Monitor urine output, I & O, daily weight, and laboratory studies.
   b. Decrease water and normalize osmolality.
      1) Restrict fluids.
      2) Administer diuretics as prescribed.
      3) Administer hypertonic (3%) saline as prescribed for severe hyponatremia.
         a) Usually administered no more rapidly than 100 ml/hr and no more than 400 ml/24 hr
         b) Monitor closely for clinical indications of fluid overload because it pulls fluid into the vascular space.
      4) Initiate CRRT as prescribed.
      5) Administer demeclocycline or lithium as prescribed for nephrogenic SIADH.
   c. Provide frequent oral and skin care.
   d. Monitor for clinical indications of cerebral or pulmonary edema; institute seizure precautions.

Hyponatremia
1. Etiology: both sodium and water decreased
   a. Decreased sodium intake
      1) Sodium-restricted diet
      2) Alcoholism
   b. Increased sodium excretion
      1) Skin losses
         a) Diaphoresis
         b) Burns
      2) GI losses
         a) GI suctioning
         b) Vomiting
         c) Diarrhea
         d) Draining wound or fistula
         e) Laxative abuse
      3) Renal losses
         a) Diuretics: thiazide, loop
         b) Adrenal insufficiency
         c) Cerebral salt-wasting syndrome
      4) Adrenal insufficiency (i.e., Addison disease)
2. Clinical presentation
   a. Subjective
      1) Anorexia, nausea, vomiting, abdominal cramps
      2) Apprehension
      3) Headache
      4) Weakness, fatigue
   b. Objective
      1) Tachycardia
      2) Postural hypotension
      3) Diarrhea
      4) Weight loss
      5) Decreased skin turgor
      6) "Fingerprinting" over sternum
      7) Personality changes
      8) Mental confusion, disorientation
      9) Lethargy progressing to coma
      10) Muscle cramps, muscle twitching, increased deep tendon reflexes (DTRs)
      11) Tremors, seizures
      12) Oliguria
   c. Diagnostic studies
      1) Serum sodium less than 136 mEq/l with normal serum osmolality
3. Collaborative management
   a. Monitor urine output, I & O, daily weight, and laboratory studies.
   b. Restore normal serum electrolyte levels.
      1) Increased dietary sodium for mild deficiency
      2) Parenteral sodium for moderate or severe deficiency
         a) NS as prescribed
         b) Hypertonic (3%) saline as prescribed for severe hyponatremia
            i) Usually administered no more rapidly than 1 to 2 ml/kg/hr and no more than 400 ml/24 hr
            ii) Monitor closely for clinical indications of fluid overload because it pulls fluid into the vascular space.
      3) Potassium replacement may also be needed.
   c. Monitor for neurologic changes; institute seizure precautions.
   d. Provide frequent oral and skin care.

Hypernatremia
1. Etiology: Both sodium and water are increased.
    a. Excess salt (sodium chloride) consumption
    b. Excess or rapid administration of NS or hypertonic saline solution
    c. Administration of sodium bicarbonate, sodium polystyrene sulfonate (Kayexalate)
    d. HF
    e. Renal failure
    f. Cirrhosis
    g. Steroid therapy
    h. Cushing syndrome
    i. Primary hyperaldosteronism
    j. Salt water near-drowning, ingestion of salt water
2. Clinical presentation
    a. Subjective
        1) Thirst
        2) Muscle weakness or cramps
    b. Objective
        1) Tachycardia
        2) Hypertension
        3) Low-grade fever
        4) Edema
        5) Dry, sticky tongue and mucous membranes
        6) Flushed, dry skin
        7) Muscle rigidity, twitching
        8) Increased DTRs
        9) Central nervous system irritability: restlessness, agitation
        10) Mental confusion, disorientation
        11) Tremors, seizures
        12) Oliguria
        13) Weight gain
    c. Diagnostic studies
        1) Serum sodium greater than 145 mEq/l with normal serum osmolality
3. Collaborative management
    a. Monitor urine output, I & O, daily weight, and laboratory studies.
    b. Treat the cause.
    c. Restore normal serum electrolyte levels.
        1) Sodium restriction
            a) Mild restriction: 3 to 4 g/day; commonly referred to as a *"no added salt" diet*
            b) Moderate restriction: 2 g/day; consumption of only foods specifically "low sodium"
            c) Severe restriction: 500 mg/day; only low-sodium foods with avoidance of shellfish and limitation of dairy and meat
        2) Diuretics as prescribed
    d. Provide frequent oral and skin care.
    e. Monitor for change in neurologic status; institute seizure precautions.

Hypokalemia
1. Etiology
    a. Poor potassium intake
        1) Starvation
        2) Alcoholism
        3) Administration of potassium-deficient parenteral fluids or nutrition
        4) Use of low-potassium dialysate
    b. Increased GI losses
        1) GI surgery
        2) Gastric or intestinal suction
        3) Vomiting
        4) Fistula
        5) Diarrhea
        6) Chronic malabsorption syndrome
        7) Laxative abuse
        8) Intestinal bypass surgery
    c. Increased renal losses
        1) Polyuria
        2) Renal tubular acidosis
        3) Sodium restriction
        4) Hypomagnesemia
        5) Hyperaldosteronism
        6) Licorice excess: increases aldosterone effect
        7) HF
        8) Steroid therapy or Cushing syndrome
        9) Cirrhosis
        10) Stress via RAA system and release of corticosteroids
        11) Burns (as fluid shifts back into intravascular space 48 to 72 hours after fluid resuscitation)
        12) Drugs
            a) Diuretics: thiazide; loop
            b) Certain antimicrobials: aminoglycosides, amphotericin B, carbenicillin, penicillin
            c) Corticosteroids
    d. Skin losses
        1) Diaphoresis
    e. Extracellular to intracellular shift
        1) Alkalosis
        2) Insulin
        3) Treatment of DKA
        4) Refeeding syndrome
2. Clinical presentation
    a. Subjective
        1) Anorexia, nausea, vomiting
        2) Malaise, fatigue
        3) Dizziness
        4) Muscle cramps
    b. Objective
        1) Orthostatic hypotension
        2) Decreased GI motility and bowel sounds, paralytic ileus, constipation, abdominal distention
        3) Muscle weakness, possibly flaccid paralysis
        4) Decreased DTR
        5) Irritability, mental confusion, drowsiness to coma
        6) Respiratory muscle weakness causing shallow ventilation, dyspnea progressing to respiratory paralysis and respiratory arrest
        7) Polyuria, polydipsia, inability to concentrate urine
        8) Enhanced digitalis effect
        9) Decreased CO, dysrhythmias, and cardiac arrest may occur.
    c. Diagnostic studies
        1) Serum potassium less than 3.5 mEq/l
        2) Electrocardiogram (ECG) changes
            a) Flat T waves and prominent U waves
            b) Depressed ST segment

c) Prolonged QT and PR intervals
d) Dysrhythmias (e.g., premature ventricular contractions, ventricular tachycardia, ventricular fibrillation, torsades de pointes)
3. Collaborative management
   a. Monitor urine output, I & O, daily weight, and laboratory studies.
   b. Treat the cause.
      1) Correct alkalosis.
      2) Correct hypomagnesemia and/or hypocalcemia; hypokalemia that is refractory to treatment is frequently accompanied by hypomagnesemia and/or hypocalcemia.
      3) Discontinue causative drug if possible.
   c. Restore normal serum electrolyte levels.
      1) Increase dietary potassium for mild hyperkalemia; encourage use of potassium chloride salt substitute.
      2) Administer potassium supplements orally.
      3) Administer potassium parenterally for severe hypokalemia.
         a) Safety
            i) Never administer potassium IV push.
            ii) Always use an infusion pump.
            iii) Do not add to a preexisting infusion; if potassium is to be added to maintenance fluids, a new solution should be mixed to avoid uneven distribution of the potassium.
         b) Potassium "runs" IV as prescribed usually via minibag (usual safe maximum 10 mEq/100 ml over 1 hour but may be administered at 20 mEq/hr if serum potassium is <2.5 mEq/l)
            i) Concentration no greater than 10 mEq/100 ml if given via peripheral catheter or 20 mEq/100 ml if given via a central venous catheter
            ii) Administration in NS unless contraindicated; dextrose may stimulate insulin secretion and intracellular shift of potassium
            iii) NOTE: It takes 100 to 200 mEq of potassium to increase serum potassium by 1 mEq/l.
            iv) Close monitoring of ECG when administering high concentrations of potassium
   d. Monitor for clinical indications of digitalis toxicity if patient receiving digitalis preparation.
   e. Teach patient about adequate potassium replacement if receiving diuretics; potassium-sparing diuretics may be used.

Hyperkalemia

1. Etiology
   a. Increased potassium intake
      1) Excessive administration/ingestion of potassium: oral or parenteral
      2) Excessive or too rapid potassium replacement
      3) Excessive use of KCl salt substitute
      4) Transfusion of banked blood; the longer the blood has been stored, the higher the extracellular potassium content
      5) Cardioplegic solution
      6) Drugs that contain potassium, such as potassium penicillin and potassium phosphate enemas
   b. Decreased potassium excretion
      1) Acute and chronic renal disease
      2) Adrenal insufficiency (i.e., Addison disease)
      3) Drugs
         a) Potassium-sparing diuretics
         b) ACE inhibitors or angiotensin receptor blockers (ARBs)
         c) Nonsteroidal antiinflammatory drugs (NSAIDs)
         d) Cyclosporine
   c. Cellular disruption with leak of intracellular potassium
      1) Crush injuries
      2) Rhabdomyolysis
      3) Hemolysis (e.g., blood transfusion reaction, fresh water near-drowning)
      4) Early burns
      5) Trauma
      6) Catabolism
      7) Lysis of tumor cells from chemotherapy
   d. Intracellular to extracellular shift
      1) Acidosis
      2) Insulin deficiency
      3) Malignant hyperthermia
      4) Drugs
         a) Massive digitalis overdosage
         b) Muscle paralyzing agents (e.g., succinylcholine)
   e. Pseudohyperkalemia
      1) Hemolyzed blood sample
      2) Sample drawn above an IV infusion containing potassium
      3) Traumatic venipuncture
      4) Delay in analysis of sample
2. Clinical presentation
   a. Subjective
      1) Nausea, vomiting, abdominal cramping, diarrhea
      2) Numbness, paresthesia of extremities
      3) Weakness, fatigue
   b. Objective
      1) Initially tachycardia progressing to bradycardia and cardiac arrest
      2) Decreased contractility, decreased CO, hypotension
      3) Abdominal distention
      4) Hyperactive bowel sounds
      5) Muscle weakness progressing to flaccid paralysis
      6) Increased DTRs initially progressing to decreased to absent DTRs
      7) Respiratory muscle weakness may cause hypopnea, respiratory distress
      8) Lethargy, apathy, mental confusion
      9) Oliguria
   c. Diagnostic studies
      1) Serum potassium greater than 5 mEq/l
         a) Mild: 5 to 6 mEq/l
         b) Moderate: 6 to 7 mEq/l
         c) Severe: greater than 7 mEq/l

2) ECG changes
    a) 5.5 to 6 mEq/l: tall, narrow, peaked T waves, shortened QT interval
    b) 6 to 7 mEq/l: wide QRS complexes, prolonged PR intervals
    c) 7 to 7.5: flattened to absent P waves, further widening of QRS complexes
    d) 8 or greater: fusion of QRS complexes and T waves, idioventricular rhythm, asystole
3. Collaborative management
    a. Monitor urine output, I & O, daily weight, and laboratory studies.
        1) Check BUN and creatinine levels for data about renal function.
    b. Treat the cause.
        1) Dialysis for renal failure
        2) Treatment of acidosis
        3) Insulin therapy for hyperglycemia
        4) Discontinuance of any causative drug if possible
            a) Potassium-sparing diuretics
            b) ACE inhibitors or ARBs
            c) NSAIDs
    c. Restore normal serum electrolyte levels
        1) Potassium restriction
            a) Ensure that IV solution or TPN contain no potassium.
            b) Check medications for potassium content.
        2) Diuretics as prescribed: usually 40 to 80 mg furosemide
        3) Emergency treatment if potassium is greater than 6.5 mEq/l or dysrhythmias are present; however, patients with chronic renal failure may tolerate high levels of potassium and not be symptomatic until 7 mEq/l or greater
            a) Dextrose and insulin as prescribed; this moves potassium back into the cell and the effect lasts about 4 to 6 hours; sodium polystyrene sulfonate should be given during this time
                i) Usual dosage is 50 ml of 50% dextrose and 10 units of insulin.
                ii) Monitor for increased or decreased serum glucose.
            b) Sodium polystyrene sulfonate, an exchange resin, as prescribed; exchanges sodium for potassium and moves potassium out of the body via the GI tract
                i) Oral or by retention enema
                    (a) Usual dose is 15 to 50 g in 50 to 100 ml of 20% sorbitol orally
                    (b) 50 g in 200 ml of dextrose as retention enema
                ii) Sorbitol, an osmotic laxative, produces a cathartic effect only when given orally and may contribute to intestinal necrosis when given by enema.
            c) Nebulized albuterol as prescribed
                i) Usual dose is 10 to 20 mg nebulized over 15 minutes
                ii) Adverse effect: tachycardia
            d) Bicarbonate as prescribed to correct acidosis
                i) Usual dose 50 mEq IV over 5 minutes
                ii) This effect lasts 1 to 2 hours.
                iii) Adverse effects: hypernatremia, hyperosmolality
            e) CRRT (e.g., continuous venous-venous hemodialysis) if prescribed
    d. Monitor for or prevent cardiac effects of hyperkalemia.
        1) IV calcium as prescribed
            a) Usual dose 5 to 10 ml of 10% calcium chloride over 2 to 5 minutes
            b) Blocks the neuromuscular and cardiac effects
            c) Contraindicated if patient is receiving digitalis

Hypocalcemia
1. Etiology
    a. Decreased calcium intake or absorption
        1) Chronic insufficient dietary calcium intake
        2) Hypoparathyroidism
            a) Injury to parathyroid gland(s) during thyroidectomy
        3) Hypomagnesemia
        4) Acute and chronic renal failure
        5) Vitamin D deficiency or resistance
        6) Liver disease
        7) Postgastrectomy
        8) Chronic malabsorption syndrome
        9) Alcoholism
        10) Cushing syndrome
        11) Steroid therapy
    b. Increased calcium excretion
        1) Diuretic therapy: loop, osmotic, potassium sparing, carbonic anhydrase inhibitors
        2) Chronic diarrhea
        3) Hyperphosphatemia
        4) Diuretic phase of AKI
    c. Increased calcium binding, decreased ionized calcium
        1) Citrated blood administration
        2) Alkalosis
        3) Acute pancreatitis
        4) Drugs (e.g., aminoglycosides, cimetidine, heparin, theophylline)
2. Clinical presentation
    a. Subjective
        1) Abdominal cramps, biliary colic
        2) Muscle cramps
        3) Paresthesia of fingertips, circumoral area
    b. Objective
        1) Chvostek sign: facial twitching in response to tapping on the facial nerve
        2) Trousseau sign: carpal spasm after 3 minutes of inflation of a BP cuff to a level above systolic pressure
        3) Muscle tremors
        4) Increased DTRs, carpopedal spasm
        5) Irritability, confusion, psychosis
        6) Memory loss
        7) Laryngospasm, stridor
        8) Tetany (characterized by cramps, twitching of the muscles, sharp flexion of the wrist and ankle joints, seizures)
        9) Seizures
        10) Decreased contractility, CO

11) Oliguria, anuria if renal calculi obstructive
12) Bruising, bleeding
c. Diagnostic studies
   1) Serum calcium less than 8.5 mg/dl (<4.5 mEq/l)
      a) If albumin is decreased, corrected total calcium can be calculated: measured total calcium + 0.8 × (4.0 − albumin)
      b) Hypocalcemia is present if serum ionized calcium is less than 4.1 mg/dl.
   2) ECG changes
      a) Prolonged QT interval
      b) Dysrhythmias (e.g., torsades de pointes)
   3) Serum phosphate decreased
3. Collaborative management
   a. Monitor airway patency and ventilation; cricothyroidotomy may be necessary for severe laryngospasm.
   b. Monitor urine output, I & O, daily weight, and laboratory studies.
   c. Treat the cause.
      1) Phosphate-binding antacids as prescribed for hyperphosphatemia
      2) Calcium administration, phosphate restriction, and phosphate-binding agents for renal failure
   d. Restore normal serum electrolyte levels.
      1) High-calcium, low-phosphorus diet
      2) Oral calcium with vitamin D supplements as prescribed for mild hypocalcemia
      3) Calcium gluconate or calcium chloride IV as prescribed
         a) 10 ml of calcium gluconate contains 4.5 mEq of calcium; 10 ml of calcium chloride contains 13.6 mEq of calcium.
            i) Calcium chloride produces higher ionized calcium; however, calcium gluconate is frequently preferred because it is less irritating to tissues.
         b) Administration through central venous catheter if possible; if administered through a peripheral catheter, prevent extravasation, which may cause necrosis and sloughing
         c) Slow administration: Dilute in 100 ml of D_5W and administer over 10 to 30 minutes.
         d) Close monitoring of BP and cardiac rhythm during calcium administration
      4) Magnesium as prescribed (hypocalcemia unresponsive to treatment may indicate concurrent hypomagnesemia)
   e. Monitor for or prevent neurologic complications; institute seizure precautions.

Hypercalcemia
1. Etiology
   a. Increased calcium intake
      1) Excessive intake of calcium supplements or calcium antacids
      2) Milk-alkali syndrome related to milk and antacid intake
   b. Increased calcium absorption: hypophosphatemia
   c. Increased mobilization of calcium from bone
      1) Hyperparathyroidism
      2) Vitamin D excess
      3) Immobility
      4) Osteolytic lesions
      5) Malignancy, especially breast, lung, lymphoma, multiple myeloma
      6) Paget disease
      7) Leukemia
      8) Granulomatous disease (e.g., sarcoidosis, TB, histoplasmosis)
      9) Thyrotoxicosis
   d. Decreased calcium excretion
      1) Thiazide diuretics
      2) Adrenal insufficiency (i.e., Addison disease)
      3) Renal tubular acidosis
      4) Hyperparathyroidism
      5) Oliguric phase of AKI
   e. Increased ionized calcium: acidosis
2. Clinical presentation
   a. Subjective
      1) Thirst
      2) Anorexia, nausea, vomiting, abdominal pain
      3) Malaise, fatigue, weakness
      4) Bone or flank pain; pathologic fractures may occur
      5) Depression
   b. Objective
      1) Decreased bowel sounds, constipation, paralytic ileus
      2) Neuromuscular weakness to flaccidity; decreased DTRs
      3) Agitation, confusion, lethargy, stupor, coma
      4) Subtle personality changes progressing to psychosis
      5) Renal calculi
      6) Polyuria, polydipsia
      7) Azotemia
      8) Enhanced digitalis effect
   c. Diagnostic studies
      1) Serum calcium greater than 10.5 mg/dl (>5.8 mEq/l)
      2) Serum phosphate decreased
      3) ECG changes: shortened QT interval, dysrhythmias and/or blocks
      4) Radiography: osteoporosis
3. Collaborative management
   a. Monitor urine output, I & O, daily weight, and laboratory studies.
   b. Treat the cause.
      1) Discontinuance of causative drugs
      2) Surgery, radiation, antineoplastics for malignancy
      3) Partial parathyroidectomy for hyperparathyroidism
   c. Restore normal serum electrolyte levels.
      1) Decrease calcium absorption.
         a) Low-calcium, high-phosphorus diet
         b) Corticosteroids
      2) Increase calcium excretion.
         a) Oral or parenteral fluids as prescribed; usually isotonic saline at 100 to 200 ml/hr
         b) Any of the following as prescribed:
            i) Loop diuretics (e.g., furosemide)
            ii) Calcitonin
            iii) Phosphorus
            iv) EDTA (disodium salt)

c) Dialysis may be used.
3) Decrease bone resorption of calcium.
   a) Weight-bearing activities
   b) Any of the following as prescribed:
      i) Etidronate
      ii) Pamidronate
      iii) Gallium nitrate
      iv) Corticosteroids
      v) Plicamycin (formerly known as *mithramycin*)
      vi) Inorganic phosphate
d. Monitor for or prevent cardiac effects of hypercalcemia: calcium channel blockers as prescribed.
e. Prevent renal calculi while correcting hypercalcemia: Agents for acidification of urine may be used because acidification of urine increases solubility of calcium.
f. Monitor for clinical indications of digitalis toxicity.

Hypophosphatemia
1. Etiology
   a. Inadequate intake of phosphorus
      1) Malnutrition
      2) Alcoholism
      3) Severe, prolonged vomiting
      4) Prolonged low-phosphorus or phosphate-free IV therapy or TPN therapy
   b. Decreased GI absorption or increased intestinal loss
      1) Excessive use of phosphate-binding gels such as aluminum hydroxide (Amphojel)
      2) Prolonged vomiting, gastric suction, sucralfate (Carafate)
      3) Chronic diarrhea
      4) Chronic malabsorption syndrome
      5) Vitamin D deficiency
   c. Increased renal excretion of phosphorus
      1) Thiazide diuretics
      2) Hypomagnesemia
      3) Hypokalemia
      4) Hyperglycemia
      5) Hyperparathyroidism
      6) Fanconi syndrome
   d. Extracellular to intracellular shifts
      1) Parenteral glucose or insulin administration
      2) Alkalosis
      3) Large amounts of carbohydrate (refeeding syndrome)
      4) Treatment of DKA
      5) Beta-adrenergic drugs (e.g., albuterol)
2. Clinical presentation
   a. Subjective
      1) Anorexia, nausea, vomiting
      2) Malaise, fatigue
      3) Paresthesia
      4) Bone pain
      5) Chest pain
   b. Objective
      1) Tachycardia, hypotension
      2) Tremors
      3) Muscle weakness
      4) Nystagmus, anisocoria
      5) Incoordination, ataxia
      6) Confusion, lethargy, coma
      7) Seizures
      8) Memory loss
      9) Respiratory muscle weakness and decreased respiratory excursion
      10) HF: dyspnea, crackles
      11) Weight loss
      12) Hemolytic anemia
      13) Platelet dysfunction: petechiae, bleeding
      14) Immunosuppression
   c. Diagnostic studies
      1) Serum phosphate less than 3 mg/dl
      2) Increased serum and urine calcium
      3) ECG: dysrhythmias
      4) Radiography: skeletal abnormalities
3. Collaborative management
   a. Monitor urine output, I & O, daily weight, and laboratory studies.
   b. Treat the cause.
      1) Discontinuance of phosphate-binding gels
      2) Correction of hypercalcemia if cause of hypophosphatemia
   c. Restore normal serum electrolyte levels.
      1) High-phosphorus, low-calcium diet
      2) Oral phosphate supplements (e.g., Neutra-Phos [sodium and potassium phosphate], Phospho-Soda [sodium phosphate], K-Phos [potassium phosphate]) as ordered and monitor for signs of hypocalcemia when giving supplements
      3) Parenteral sodium phosphate or potassium phosphate IV as ordered and monitor for signs of hypocalcemia
         a) Usual dose
            i) If phosphate is less than 1 mg/dl without adverse effects, usual dose is 0.6 mg/kg/hr.
            ii) If phosphate is less than 2 mg/dl with adverse effects, usual dose is 0.9 mg/kg/hr.
         b) Utilization of central venous catheter if possible
         c) IV phosphate is contraindicated in hypercalcemia.
   d. Monitor for cardiovascular, pulmonary, and neurologic effects of hypophosphatemia.

Hyperphosphatemia
1. Etiology
   a. Increased phosphorus intake
      1) Cathartic abuse with phosphate-containing laxatives and enemas
      2) Excessive vitamin D
      3) Transfusion of stored blood
      4) Acute elemental phosphorus poisoning
   b. Decreased phosphorus excretion
      1) Acute or chronic renal failure
      2) Hypoparathyroidism
   c. Intracellular to extracellular shifts
      1) Acidosis
      2) Malignant hyperthermia
      3) Severe hypothermia
   d. Cellular destruction
      1) Neoplastic disease treated with chemotherapy

            2) Catabolism
            3) Rhabdomyolysis
    2. Clinical presentation
        a. As for hypocalcemia
        b. Diagnostic studies: serum phosphate greater than 4.5 mg/dl
    3. Collaborative management
        a. Monitor airway patency; cricothyroidotomy may be necessary for severe laryngospasm.
        b. Monitor urine output, I & O, daily weight, and laboratory studies.
        c. Treat the cause.
            1) Correction of hypocalcemia
            2) Dialysis if renal failure is cause
            3) Saline diuresis and urinary alkalization if tumor lysis syndrome or rhabdomyolysis
        d. Restore normal serum electrolyte levels.
            1) Low-phosphorus, high-calcium diet
            2) Sucralfate or aluminum antacids to bind with phosphate in the GI tract as prescribed
            3) Glucose and insulin as prescribed to shift phosphate into the cell (transient effect only)
        e. Monitor for or prevent neurologic complications; institute seizure precautions.

Hypomagnesemia
    1. Etiology
        a. Decreased magnesium intake or absorption
            1) Protein-calorie malnutrition
            2) Starvation
            3) Alcoholism
            4) Prolonged low-magnesium or magnesium-free IV therapy or TPN therapy
        b. Impaired absorption
            1) Alcoholism
            2) Intestinal malabsorption syndrome
            3) Acute pancreatitis
        c. Increased magnesium loss
            1) Drugs
                a) Diuretics
                b) Antimicrobials: aminoglycosides, pentamidine, amphotericin B
                c) Ethanol
                d) Cisplatin
                e) Cyclosporin A
            2) Diuretic phase of AKI
            3) Vomiting, gastric suction, fistula
            4) Chronic diarrhea (e.g., ulcerative colitis; laxative abuse)
            5) Hypoparathyroidism
            6) Hyperaldosteronism
            7) Steroids
            8) DKA
            9) HF
        d. Increased magnesium binding: citrated blood administration
        e. Extracellular to intracellular shift
            1) Refeeding syndrome
            2) Amino acid solutions
            3) Insulin; treatment of DKA
            4) Acute myocardial infarction
    2. Clinical presentation
        a. Subjective
            1) Anorexia, nausea, vomiting, abdominal distention
            2) Paresthesia of fingertips, circumoral area
            3) Muscle cramps
            4) Syncope
        b. Objective
            1) Tachycardia, hypotension
            2) Chvostek and Trousseau signs
            3) Tremors, increased DTRs, carpopedal spasm
            4) Ataxia, nystagmus
            5) Laryngospasm, stridor
            6) Tetany
            7) Seizures
            8) Insomnia
            9) Confusion, psychosis
            10) Memory loss
            11) Decreased contractility, CO
            12) Increased digitalis effect
        c. Diagnostic studies
            1) Serum magnesium less than 1.5 mEq/l
                a) May have concurrent hypocalcemia, hypokalemia, and hypophosphatemia
            2) ECG changes
                a) Prolonged QT interval
                b) Dysrhythmias especially torsades de pointes
    3. Collaborative management
        a. Monitor airway patency; cricothyroidotomy may be necessary for severe laryngospasm.
        b. Monitor urine output, I & O, daily weight, and laboratory studies.
        c. Treat the cause.
            1) Nutritional support for malnutrition
            2) Use of potassium-sparing diuretics if diuretics are needed because they spare magnesium
        d. Restore normal serum electrolyte levels.
            1) High magnesium diet
            2) Oral magnesium supplements in the form of magnesium antacids as prescribed
            3) Magnesium sulfate IV as prescribed
                a) Usually administered slowly so that magnesium will be absorbed
                    i) 1 to 2 g diluted in 100 ml and administered over 1 hour unless critical level, then 4-g dose should be given over 2 hours
                    ii) 1 to 2 g may be diluted in 10 ml and administered over 5 to 20 minutes for when life-threatening dysrhythmias (e.g., torsades de pointes) occur
            4) Calcium replacement as prescribed; most patients with hypomagnesemia also have hypocalcemia
        e. Monitor for or prevent neurologic complications; institute seizure precautions.
        f. Monitor for clinical indications of digitalis toxicity for patients on digitalis preparations.

Hypermagnesemia
1. Etiology
   a. Increased magnesium intake
      1) Magnesium antacids
      2) Magnesium sulfate IV
      3) Magnesium-containing antacids, laxatives, enemas
   b. Decreased magnesium excretion
      1) Acute or chronic renal failure
      2) Hyperparathyroidism
      3) Hypoaldosteronism
      4) Hypothyroidism
   c. Intracellular to extracellular shift
      1) Untreated ketoacidosis
      2) Burns
      3) Rhabdomyolysis
   d. Pseudohypermagnesemia: sample hemolysis
2. Clinical presentation
   a. Subjective
      1) Weakness, fatigue
      2) Nausea, vomiting
      3) Somnolence
      4) Diplopia
   b. Objective
      1) Bradycardia, hypotension
      2) Facial flushing
      3) Muscle weakness progressing to paralysis
      4) Decreased DTRs: Loss of patellar reflex occurs at levels greater than 8 mEq/l.
      5) Respiratory muscle weakness may cause hypoventilation and dyspnea.
      6) Respiratory muscle paralysis and apnea may occur with levels greater than 10 mEq/l.
      7) Confusion, somnolence, lethargy, coma
      8) Cardiopulmonary arrest
   c. Diagnostic studies
      1) Serum magnesium greater than 2.5 mEq/l
      2) ECG: prolonged PR, QRS, QT; bradycardias and blocks
3. Collaborative management
   a. Monitor and maintain airway and ventilation; intubation and mechanical ventilation may be necessary.
   b. Monitor urine output, I & O, daily weight, and laboratory studies.
   c. Treat the cause.
      1) Discontinuance of magnesium-containing antacids or laxatives, IV magnesium
   d. Restore normal serum electrolyte levels.
      1) Low-magnesium diet
      2) Diuresis
         a) NS or ½ NS and furosemide (1 mg/kg) as prescribed if normal renal function
         b) Monitor for hypocalcemia and hypokalemia.
      3) Dialysis if renal failure is cause of hypermagnesemia
      4) Dextrose and insulin may promote movement of magnesium into the cells (transient effect only).
   e. Monitor for or prevent neuromuscular, pulmonary, and cardiovascular complications.
      1) IV calcium as prescribed
         a) Usual dose is 5 to 10 ml of 10% calcium chloride over 2 to 5 minutes.
         b) Blocks the neuromuscular and cardiac effects
         c) Contraindicated if patient is receiving digitalis

Urinary Incontinence

Definition
The involuntary leakage of urine

Etiology
1. Bladder dysfunction
   a. Urge incontinence: related to detrusor over activity, involuntary detrusor contractions, or poor compliance
   b. Overflow incontinence: associated with overdistention of the bladder with resultant overflow or bladder outlet obstruction
2. Urethral dysfunction
   a. Stress incontinence: The involuntary loss of urine with physical activities that increase abdominal pressure in the absence of a detrusor contraction or an overdistended bladder.
3. Other causes (Table 8.5)

Clinical Presentation
1. Subjective
   a. Frequency, dysuria, urgency, or nocturia
   b. Feeling of incomplete emptying, hesitancy, straining, or weak stream
   c. In women: feeling of vaginal fullness or pressure
   d. Constipation
   e. new lower extremity weakness
   f. If UTI: dysuria, pelvic pain
2. Objective
   a. Altered mental status
   b. Weakness or altered gait
   c. If UTI: fever, hematuria
   d. Pelvic organ prolapse

Diagnostic Studies
1. Laboratory testing
   a. Urinalysis and cytology
   b. Prostate specific antigen (PSA)
   c. BUN/creatinine
   d. Serum glucose
2. Imaging studies
   a. Computed tomography (CT) or intravenous pyelography (IVP) to rule out upper tract abnormalities, developmental anomalies, bladder configuration, and fistula
   b. Renal ultrasound if contrast study is contraindicated
   c. Postvoid residual
3. Specialized studies
   a. Simple cystometrogram
   b. Complex urodynamics for leak point pressures and uroflowmetry

TABLE 8.5 Transient Causes of Incontinence

Delirium	Result of underlying illness or medication; incontinence is secondary and abates once the cause of delirium is corrected
Infection	Acute, symptomatic UTI causes incontinence, but the far more common asymptomatic bacteriuria does not
Atrophic urethritis or vaginitis	Characterized by vaginal erosions, telangiectasia, petechiae, and friability; may cause or contribute to incontinence. Although oral estrogen may worsen incontinence, a 3- to 12-mo course of topical estrogen can be useful.
Pharmaceuticals	**Drug Type** / **Potential Effects on Continence**
	Sedative–hypnotics (e.g., long-acting benzodiazepines; alcohol) — Sedation, delirium, decreased mobility
	Anticholinergics (dicyclomine, disopyramide, sedating antihistamines, antipsychotics, TCAs, antiparkinson agents, antidepressants; *not* SSRIs) — Urinary retention, overflow incontinence, delirium, impaction; the antipsychotics also decrease mobility
	Opiates — Urinary retention, stool impaction, sedation, delirium
	α-Adrenergic antagonists — Relax sphincter; may induce stress incontinence in women
	α-Adrenergic agonists — Urinary retention in men (tighten sphincter, prostate)
	Calcium channel blockers, especially the dihydropyridines — Urinary retention; nocturnal diuresis due to fluid retention
	"Loop" diuretics (thiazide-like agents only rarely cause it) — Polyuria, frequency, urgency
	NSAIDs — Nocturnal diuresis caused by fluid retention
	Thiazolidinediones — Nocturnal diuresis caused by fluid retention
	Some nociceptives (gabapentin, pregabalin) — Nocturnal diuresis caused by fluid retention; sedation; delirium
	Dopamine receptor agonists (e.g., ropinirole, pramipexole) — Nocturnal diuresis caused by fluid retention
	ACE inhibitors — Drug-induced cough leads to stress incontinence in women
	Vincristine — Urinary retention caused by neuropathy
Excess urine output	From large intake, diuretic agents (theophylline, caffeinated beverages, alcohol), and metabolic disorders (hyperglycemia, hypercalcemia); nocturnal incontinence may result from mobilization of peripheral edema (HF, venous insufficiency, side effects of medications)
Restricted mobility	Often results from overlooked, correctable conditions such as arthritis, pain, foot problems, postprandial hypotension, or fear of falling
Stool impaction	May cause both fecal and urinary incontinence that remit with disimpaction

ACE, Angiotensin-converting enzyme; *HF,* heart failure; *NSAID,* nonsteroidal antiinflammatory drug; *SSRI,* selective serotonin reuptake inhibitor; *TCA,* tricyclic antidepressant; *UTI,* urinary tract infection.
Adapted from Resnick, N. M., Tadic, S. D., & Yalla, S. V. (2010) Geriatric incontinence and voiding dysfunction. In: Wein AJ, Novick AC, Partin AW, et al, eds. *Campbell-Walsh urology* (10th ed.). St. Louis: Elsevier.

   c. Endoscopic evaluation
   d. Cystogram

Collaborative Management
1. Provide stepped care plan by type beginning with non-invasive behavioral modifications and pharmacologic interventions in nonresponders:
   a. Urge incontinence
      1) Kegel exercises
      2) Anticholinergic and antimuscarinic agents
      3) Surgical removal of obstructing or other pathologic lesions
   b. Overflow incontinence
      1) Surgical removal of any obstructing lesions
      2) Catheterization (clean intermittent or indwelling)
   c. Stress incontinence
      1) Pelvic floor muscle training (PFMT) or Kegel exercises
      2) Midurethral sling surgery
   d. Transient incontinence
      1) Treat underlying medical condition
      2) Behavioral therapy, including habit training and timed voiding

Urinary Tract Infection

Definitions
Pyelonephritis: UTI affecting one or both kidneys
Cystitis: UTI in the bladder that does not involve the kidneys

6) Fatigue, weakness
7) Anxiety
c. Dyspnea if pulmonary edema is present
d. Headache
e. Pruritus
f. Decreased libido
g. Weight loss or weight gain
2. Objective
a. GU
1) Decrease in urine volume
a) Nonoliguria: dilute urine output greater than 400 ml/24 hr
b) Oliguria: urine output less than 400 ml/24 hr
c) Anuria: urine output less than 100 ml/24 hr
i) Rare but may be seen in complete obstruction (postrenal)
2) Altered excretion of drugs; toxic drug levels
3) Bladder distention may be noted with postrenal failure.
b. Neurologic
1) Change in behavior
2) Confusion
3) Change in level of consciousness
4) Focal neurologic deficits
5) Tremors, twitching, increased DTR
6) Asterixis
7) Seizures
c. GI
1) Bleeding gums
2) Uremic breath
3) Abdominal distention
4) Malnutrition
5) GI bleeding, melena
6) Constipation or diarrhea
7) May have paralytic ileus
d. Respiratory
1) Deep, rapid breathing (i.e., Kussmaul respirations)
2) Pulmonary edema
a) Bilateral crackles
3) Hemoptysis may be seen along with AKI in Goodpasture syndrome
e. Cardiovascular
1) Tachycardia
2) Dysrhythmias
3) Uremic pericarditis
a) Pericardial friction rub
4) Hypertension
5) Vascular access
a) Bruit
b) Thrill
c) Neurovascular assessment of limb
f. Musculoskeletal
1) Impaired mobility
2) Muscle weakness
g. Integument
1) Dry skin
2) Pruritus
3) Edema
4) Bruising
5) Pallor
6) Uremic frost (end stage)
h. Hematologic and immunologic
1) Increased susceptibility to infection, sepsis
2) Petechiae, bruising, bleeding
3. Diagnostic studies
a. Blood
1) Elevated BUN, creatinine
2) Hyperkalemia
3) Hyperphosphatemia
4) Hypocalcemia
5) Hypermagnesemia
6) Sodium level is dependent on water balance.
a) Normal or dilutional hyponatremia
7) Hyperuricemia
8) Arterial blood gases: metabolic acidosis with increased anion gap
9) Hematology
a) Hematocrit, hemoglobin usually decreased; may be increased in prerenal failure due to dehydration
b) Platelets: decreased
10) Clotting profile: Bleeding time may be increased.
b. Urine
1) Varies; dependent on type of AKI
2) Decreased creatinine clearance
c. Radiologic
1) Kidneys, ureters, and bladder (KUB) radiography, renal ultrasonography, or CT may indicate cause of postrenal failure.
2) Chest radiography may show:
a) Pericardial effusion
b) Pleural effusion
c) Pulmonary edema
d. Renal biopsy: most definitive diagnostic test, especially for glomerulonephritis
4. Diagnostic studies by type of AKI
a. Prerenal
1) Oliguria
2) Urinary sodium less than 20 mEq/l
3) Increased BUN with BUN:creatinine ratio greater than 10:1 (usually 20:1)
4) Urine specific gravity greater than 1.02
5) Urine osmolality increased except with metabolic acidosis or diuretics
6) Urine pH less than 6
7) No protein in urine or only minimal amount of protein in urine
8) Sediment in urine: hyaline casts, finely granular casts
b. Intrinsic
1) Cortical
a) Urine output may be normal (nonoliguria), oliguria, or polyuria.
b) Urine sodium greater than 20 mEq/l
c) BUN:creatinine increased with 10:1 ratio
d) Urine specific gravity varies
e) Urine pH greater than 6
f) Moderate to heavy proteinuria
g) Sediment in urine: RBCs, WBCs, casts

2) Medullary
    a) Urine output may be normal (nonoliguria), oliguria, or polyuria.
    b) Urine sodium greater than 20 mEq/l
    c) Urine specific gravity 1.010
    d) BUN:creatinine increased with 10:1 ratio
    e) Urine specific gravity 1.01 to 1.015
    f) Urine pH greater than 6
    g) Minimal to moderate proteinuria
    h) Sediment in urine: tubular epithelial cells, tubular casts, rare RBCs
c. Postrenal
    1) Oliguria with partial obstruction; anuria with complete obstruction
    2) Urine sodium, 20 to 40 mEq/l
    3) BUN:creatinine increased with 10:1 ratio
    4) Urine specific gravity, 1.01 to 1.015
    5) Urine pH greater than 6
    6) Sediment in urine: RBCs, WBCs, calculi, uric acid crystals, hyaline casts
    7) KUB radiography, IVP may show obstruction and/or ureteral dilatation
    8) May have positive culture for bacteria
5. RIFLE classification system (Table 8.6): correlates with outcomes
6. Stages of acute renal injury (Table 8.7)
    NOTE: Some patients (especially when acute renal injury is related to nephrotoxins) go through only three phases: onset, nonoliguric, and recovery.

Collaborative Management
1. Prevent or treat the cause.
    a. Administer oral N-acetylcysteine (NAC) as prescribed along with adequate hydration with an intravascular isotonic crystalloid to prevent contrast-induced AKI.
    b. Administer fluids, diuretics (usually mannitol), and sodium bicarbonate as prescribed for rhabdomyolysis with myoglobinuria.
    c. Monitor serum creatinine when using nephrotoxic agents (e.g., aminoglycosides, amphotericin B, vancomycin).

Table 8.6 Rifle Classification System for Degrees of Acute Kidney Injury

Grades of Severity	Serum Creatinine	Glomerular Filtration Rate	Urine Output
Risk	1.5× normal	Decreased by >25%	<0.5 ml/kg/hr for 6 hr
Injury	2× normal	Decreased by >50%	<0.5 ml/kg/hr for 12 hr
Failure	3× normal or ≥3 mg/dl	Decreased by >75%	<0.3 ml/kg/hr for 24 hr or anuria for 12 hr
Loss	Complete loss of renal function for >4 wk		
End-stage kidney disease	Complete loss of renal function with need for renal replacement therapy for >3 mo		

Adapted from Bellomo, R., Ronco, C., Kellum, J. A., Mehta, R. L., & Palevsky, P. (2004). Acute renal failure—definition, outcome measures, animal models, fluid therapy and information technology needs: the Second International Consensus Conference of the Acute Dialysis Quality Initiative (ADQI) Group. *Crit Care, 8*(4), R204–212.

Table 8.7 Stages of Acute Kidney Injury*

	Onset	Oliguric-Anuric	Diuretic	Recovery
Definition	Period of time from the precipitating event to the beginning of oliguria or anuria	Period of time when urine output is less than 400 ml/24 hr	Period of time between urine output of greater than 400 ml/24 hr until when laboratory values stabilize	Period of time between when the laboratory values stabilize until they are normal
Duration	Hours to days	1–2 wk	1–2 wk	3–12 mo
BUN/creatinine	Normal or slight increase	Increased	Begins to decrease	Almost normal
Urine output	Decreased; about 20% of normal	Less than 400 ml/24 hr; about 5% of normal	May exceed 3 l/24 hr; about 150%–200% of normal	Back to 100% of normal
Mortality	5%	50%–60%	25%	10%–15%
Other characteristics		• Metabolic acidosis • Water gain with dilutional hyponatremia • Hyperkalemia • Hypocalcemia • Hyperphosphatemia • Hypermagnesemia • Azotemia	• Metabolic acidosis • Sodium may be normal or decreased • Hyperkalemia continues	• Uremia, acid–base imbalances, and electrolyte imbalances gradually resolve

*Some patients (especially when acute kidney injury is related to nephrotoxins) go through only three phases: onset, nonoliguric, and recovery.
Adapted from Kidney Disease: Improving Global Outcomes (KDIGO) Acute Kidney Injury Work Group. (2012). KDIGO Clinical Practice Guideline for Acute Kidney Injury. *Kidney Int*, Suppl, 2, 1–138.

d. Prevent or treat abdominal hypertension and abdominal compartment syndrome.
e. Support renal perfusion and improve GFR through appropriate treatment.
   1) Volume to improve preload in patients with hypovolemia as evidenced by decreased RAP or PAOP
   2) Inotropes to improve contractility in patients with decreased contractility as evidenced by decreased right ventricular stroke work index (RVSWI) or left ventricular stroke work index (LVSWI).
   3) Vasopressors to increase afterload in patients with massive vasodilation as evidenced by decreased SVR
   4) Low-dose dopamine or fenoldopam should not be used for the treatment or prevention of AKI (Inker et al., 2014).
   5) Diuretic trial as prescribed if patient is not anuric
      a) Controversial because diuretics in acute renal injury may increase mortality (Mehta, Pascual, Soroko, & Chertow, 2002).
      b) Agents
         i) Loop diuretics (e.g., furosemide [Lasix], bumetanide [Bumex])
         ii) Osmotic diuretics (e.g., mannitol)
            (a) Frequently used for rhabdomyolysis
            (b) Contraindicated in HF, pulmonary edema
f. Administer immunosuppressants and initiate plasmapheresis for immune-mediated causes of acute renal injury (e.g., Goodpasture syndrome).
2. Maintain fluid, electrolyte, and acid–base balance.
a. Fluid
   1) Monitor for clinical indications of fluid overload.
   2) Maintain sodium and water restriction and encourage the patient to remain within prescribed restrictions.
      a) Restrict fluid: 24-hour restriction usually determined by adding 500 ml (for insensible loss) to the previous day's urine output
      b) Space fluid allowances over the entire 24-hour period.
      c) Treat thirst by offering ice chips (must be included as intake), wet washcloths, misting the mouth, and providing mouth care.
      d) Restrict sodium (usually 1–2 g/day).
b. Potassium
   1) Monitor for clinical indications of hyperkalemia.
   2) Maintain potassium restriction (usually 40 mEq/day); do not allow salt substitute (KCl) on dietary trays.
c. Phosphorus
   1) Monitor for clinical indications of hyperphosphatemia.
   2) Maintain phosphorus restrictions.
   3) Administer phosphate-binding agents (e.g., Basaljel, Amphojel).
      a) These aluminum-containing phosphate-binding agents may contribute to dialysis encephalopathy due to accumulation of aluminum; calcium carbonate or calcium acetate may be prescribed instead.
   4) Treat hypocalcemia with calcium administration; increasing calcium will decrease phosphorus.
d. Magnesium
   1) Monitor for clinical indications of hypermagnesemia.
   2) Maintain dietary magnesium restrictions.
   3) Do not administer magnesium-containing medications (e.g., magnesium sulfate, magnesium citrate).
e. Monitor arterial blood gases for acid–base imbalance.
   1) Initiate dialysis to eliminate nitrogenous wastes as prescribed for metabolic acidosis.
   2) Administer sodium bicarbonate or Carbicarb as prescribed.
      a) Generally used only for severe metabolic acidosis (pH <7.1)
      b) Monitor for hypernatremia.
      c) Monitor for hypocalcemia caused by increased binding between albumin and calcium and decrease in ionized calcium.
3. Diminish the accumulation of nitrogenous wastes.
a. Maintain protein restriction; usually 0.6 g/kg/day initially but may be as high as 1 to 1.5 g/kg/day if on hemodialysis or CRRT; 1.5 to 2 g/kg/day if on peritoneal dialysis
b. Provide protein foods of high biological value (i.e., contain all essential amino acids).
c. Provide adequate caloric intake to prevent catabolism and utilization of dietary protein for energy needs: usually greater than or equal to 35 to 40 kcal/kg/day.
d. Initiate dialysis as indicated and prescribed.
   1) Indications for dialysis in patients with AKI generally include the following:
      a) Volume overload (especially with pulmonary edema)
      b) Uncontrollable hyperkalemia
      c) Uncontrollable hyperphosphatemia
      d) Uncontrollable acidosis
      e) Symptomatic uremia (e.g., neurologic changes)
      f) Pericarditis
      g) Seizures or coma
      h) BUN 80-100 mg/dl or greater but may be initiated at BUN greater than 50–60 mg/dl
      i) Serum creatinine 10 mg/dl or greater
   2) Contraindications for dialysis
      a) Hemodynamic instability: CRRT may be used in these situations.
      b) Inability to tolerate anticoagulation
      c) Lack of vascular access
   3) Maintenance of patency and prevention of infection of vascular access (if present)
      a) Palpate shunt, fistula, AV graft for thrill; auscultate for bruit; note change in bright red color in tubing in shunt; palpate pulses and check capillary refill distal to access.
      b) Do not allow venipuncture, IV cannulation, injections, BP measurements in limb with shunt, fistula, or AV graft.
      c) Monitor for constrictive clothing or dressing in limb with shunt, fistula, or AV graft.

d) Monitor for bleeding; use pressure dressing to stop bleeding; bulldog clamps (always kept clamped to dressing) are used on shunt tubing to stop bleeding.
e) Note any redness, induration, or purulent drainage around access; culture any purulent drainage; change dressing as for central venous catheter.
f) Instruct patient not to disturb scabs at puncture sites at fistula or AV graft for hemodialysis.
4) Maintenance of patency and prevention of infection of peritoneal access
a) Note any redness, induration, or purulent drainage around access; culture any purulent drainage.
b) Provide aseptic catheter care.
i) Wash with antibacterial soap.
ii) Dress with light gauze dressing.
iii) Aseptic catheter manipulation
c) Culture peritoneal dialysate outflow fluid periodically or as indicated.
4. Prevent further damage to the kidney by nephrotoxic agents.
a. Note that dosages of drugs eliminated by the kidney are decreased and the interval between doses is increased.
b. Monitor peak/trough serum drug levels when appropriate (e.g., aminoglycosides).
c. Monitor urine creatinine clearance when patient is receiving nephrotoxic agents.
d. Prevent contrast dye-related nephrotoxicity.
1) IV volume expansion with either isotonic crystalloid or sodium bicarbonate.
2) Administer N-acetylcysteine (NAC) as prescribed.
a) Acts as an oxygen free radical scavenger
b) Usual dose is 600 mg orally every 12 hours the day before and the day of the radiologic procedure that requires contrast.
e. Monitor for changes in urine color that may indicate the presence of heavy pigments that may cause acute tubular necrosis.
1) Myoglobinuria: tea or cola colored
2) Hemoglobinuria: wine colored
5. Provide adequate nutrition while maintaining dietary restrictions.
a. Provide high biological protein within protein restriction.
b. Provide enough calories to prevent catabolism of somatic protein stores.
c. Increase dietary calcium.
d. Decrease dietary sodium, potassium, and phosphorus.
6. Prevent fluid volume deficit during the diuretic phase.
a. Monitor for clinical indication of fluid volume deficit.
b. Volume may be replaced hourly during this phase by replacing the last hour's urine output during the following hour.
7. Prevent infection: Initiate dialysis as prescribed when BUN level greater than 80–100 mg/dl because BUN values above this level are associated with increased risk of infection.
8. Prevent injury: Initiate dialysis as prescribed when BUN level greater than 80–100 mg/dl because BUN values above this level are associated with neurologic changes.
9. Monitor for and treat anemia and platelet dysfunction.
a. Monitor hemoglobin, hematocrit, and RBCs.
b. Treat anemia as prescribed.
1) Folic acid, iron, vitamin B_{12}
2) Recombinant erythropoietin
a) Cannot be used with CRRT as it is dialyzed
3) Packed RBCs: only prescribed if the patient is symptomatic of anemia (e.g., dyspnea, chest pain, syncope, hypotension)
c. Monitor for clinical indications of platelet dysfunction (e.g., petechiae, ecchymosis, bleeding).
d. Administer desmopressin (DDAVP) as prescribed for platelet dysfunction.
10. Promote comfort.
a. Administer antipyretics as prescribed.
b. Utilize emollient or cornstarch baths.
11. Monitor for complications.
a. Renal: Chronic renal failure will develop in 25%–30% of patients with AKI.
b. Cardiovascular
1) Dysrhythmias
2) Hypertension
3) Pericarditis, cardiac tamponade
4) Pulmonary edema
c. Neurologic
1) Coma
2) Seizures
d. Metabolic
1) Electrolyte imbalances
a) Hyperkalemia
b) Hyperphosphatemia
c) Hypermagnesemia
d) Hypocalcemia
2) Acid–base imbalance: metabolic acidosis
e. GI
1) Peptic ulcer disease
2) GI hemorrhage
f. Hematologic
1) Anemia
2) Uremic coagulopathies
g. Infection
1) Increased susceptibility to pneumonias
2) Septicemias
3) Urinary tract and wound infections
h. Miscellaneous: drug toxicity

Chronic Kidney Disease

Definition
1. "Abnormalities of kidney structure or function, present for >3 months, with implications for health" (Acute Kidney Injury Work Group, 2012)
2. Stages (Table 8.8)

Etiology
1. Diabetes mellitus
2. Hypertension
3. Glomerulonephritis
4. Polycystic kidney disease
5. Irreversible AKI

Table 8.8 Classification of Chronic Kidney Disease

GFR and ACR Categories and Risk Adverse Outcomes			ACR Categories (mg/mmol), Description and Range		
			<3: Normal to Mildly Increased ACR	3–30: Moderately Increased ACR	>30: Severely Increased ACR
			A1	A2	A3
GFR categories (ml/min/1.73m), description and range	≥90: normal and high GFR	G1	No chronic kidney disease in the absence of markers of kidney damage		
	60–89: mild reduction in GFR rationed to normal range for a young adult	G2			
	45–59: mild to moderate reduction in GFR	G3a			
	30–44: moderate to severe reduction in GFR	G3b			
	15–29: severe reduction in GFR	G4			
	<15: kidney failure	G5			

Increasing risk of adverse outcomes →

- ☐ Low risk of adverse outcomes (if no other markers of kidney disease, no chronic kidney disease)
- ☐ Moderately increased risk
- ☐ High risk
- ■ Very high risk

ACR, Albumin:creatinine ratio; *GFR*, glomerular filtration rate
From Carville, S., Wonderling, D., Stevens, P.; Guideline Development Group. (2014). Early identification and management of chronic kidney disease in adults: summary of updated NICE guidance. *BMJ* 349:g4507.

Pathophysiology
Fig. 8.8.

Collaborative Management
1. As for AKI
2. Maintain ventilation, oxygenation, and circulation.
   a. Assessment for clinical indications of pericarditis, HF, hypertension, and assistance with treatment
   b. Assessment for clinical indications of life-threatening fluid, electrolyte, or acid–base imbalance and assistance with treatment
      1) Hypervolemia
      2) Hyperkalemia
      3) Hypermagnesemia
      4) Metabolic acidosis
3. Initiate and maintain renal replacement therapy.
4. Maintain safety.
   a. Adjustment of drug dosages
   b. Monitoring for delirium and uremic encephalopathy
   c. Mobility assistance to prevent fracture
   d. Avoidance of invasive procedures and monitoring for bleeding
5. Provide patient and family education.
   a. Dietary restrictions
   b. Prevention of complications
   c. Participation in care and decision-making

Renal Replacement Therapy

Dialysis
1. Definition: separation of solutes by differential diffusion through a semipermeable membrane that is placed between the two solutions (Fig. 8.9).
2. Purposes
   a. Eliminate excess body fluids.
   b. Maintain or restore electrolyte balance.

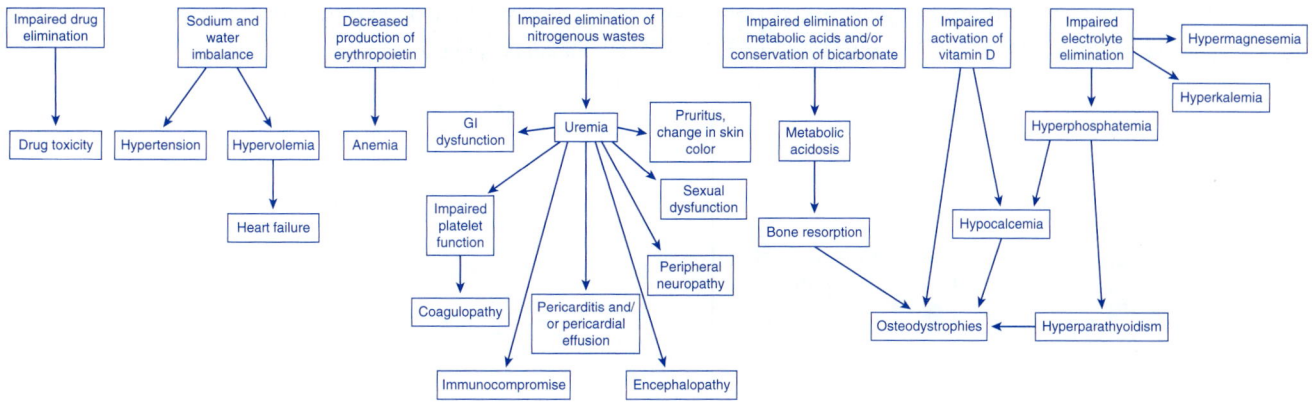

Fig. 8.8 Pathophysiology of chronic kidney disease. *GI,* Gastrointestinal.

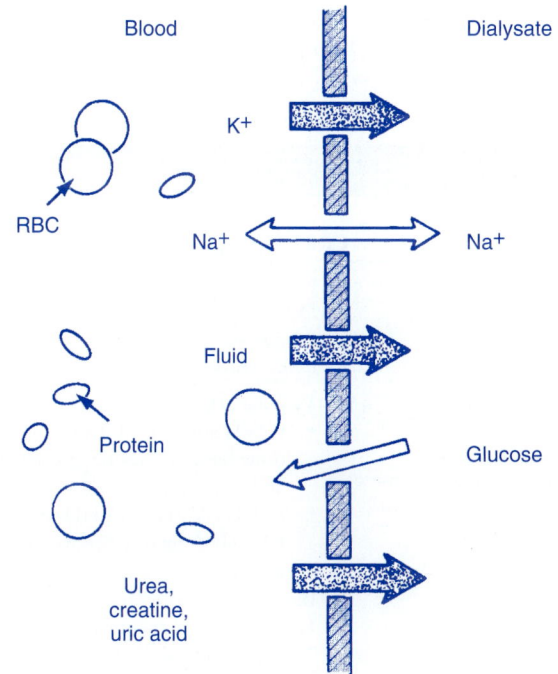

Fig. 8.9 Osmosis and diffusion in dialysis. Net movement of major particles and fluid is illustrated. (From Long, B. C., Phipps, W. J., & Cassmeyer, V. L. [1993]. *Medical-surgical nursing: A nursing process approach* [3rd ed.]. St Louis: Mosby.)

    c. Maintain or restore acid–base balance.
    d. Eliminate nitrogenous wastes and toxins from the blood.
  3. Indications
    a. Acute or chronic renal failure
      1) Symptomatic uremia
      2) Uremic pericarditis
    b. Severe water intoxication
    c. Severe electrolyte imbalance
    d. Drug intoxication (drug must be dialyzable [e.g., alcohol, salicylates, lithium, barbiturates, some poisons])
    e. Hepatic encephalopathy or coma
  4. Components
    a. Dialysate: solution of water, electrolytes (sodium, chloride, magnesium, bicarbonate), nonelectrolytes (glucose), buffer (acetate, lactate, or bicarbonate)
      1) Electrolyte concentration in the dialysate is adjusted to the patient's needs.
    b. Semipermeable membrane: peritoneum, extracorporeal membrane
    c. Patient's blood in contact with the membrane
  5. Principles (Fig. 8.10)
    a. Osmosis: A hypertonic solution is used as the dialysate to move water across the semipermeable membrane.
    b. Diffusion: The dialysate solution contains a concentration of selected solutes lower than the blood so that these solutes will move across the semipermeable membrane and into the dialysate solution.
    c. Filtration: In some forms of dialysis, there is a pressure difference between the sides of the semipermeable membrane with the highest pressure on the forward side of the membrane to act as a hydrostatic force pushing against the membrane to provide a filtration effect.
    d. Convection (in CRRT): the transfer of solutes and solutions simultaneously moving across the semipermeable membrane
  6. Variables affecting efficiency
    a. Size and number of the pores in the semipermeable membrane
    b. Surface area of the semipermeable membrane
    c. Thickness of the semipermeable membrane
    d. Size of the solute molecules
    e. Concentration of solutes in the blood
    f. Osmotic concentration
    g. Pressure gradients
    h. Temperature of the solution
    i. Rate of blood flow
  7. Comparison of various types of dialysis (Table 8.9)
    a. Choice of right dialysis option
      1) Intermittent hemodialysis: therapy of choice for hemodynamically stable patients in hospital setting
      2) Peritoneal dialysis: suited for hemodynamically stable patients with intact peritoneum but has low efficiency
      3) CRRT: suitable for critically ill or hemodynamically unstable patients and has a higher efficiency than peritoneal dialysis
  8. Collaborative management
    a. Peritoneal dialysis
      1) Preparation
        a) Prepare patient for insertion of peritoneal catheter (Fig. 8.11, *A*)
          i) Explain procedure to patient.

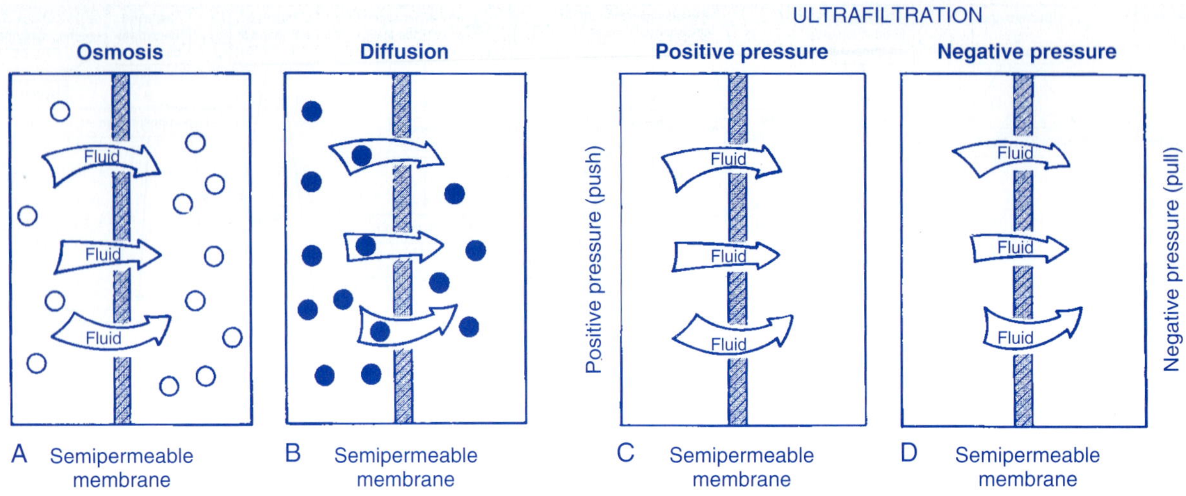

Fig. 8.10 Dialysis is based on the following principles: osmosis (**A**), diffusion (**B**), and ultrafiltration. Ultrafiltration occurs when either positive pressure (**C**) or negative pressure (**D**) is placed on the system. Ultrafiltration is maximized by exerting both positive and negative pressure on the system simultaneously. (From Long, B. C., Phipps, W. J., & Cassmeyer, V. L. [1993]. *Medical-surgical nursing: A nursing process approach* [3rd ed.]. St Louis: Mosby.)

Table 8.9 Types of Dialysis

	Hemodialysis	Intermittent Peritoneal Dialysis	CRRT Therapies
Principles	• Osmosis • Diffusion • Filtration	• Osmosis • Diffusion • Filtration	• Osmosis • Diffusion • Filtration • Convection

Treatment requirements	• Membrane: extracorporeal membrane or high coefficient membrane
	• Blood pump
	• Dialyzer
	• Dialysate
	• Vascular access
	• Anticoagulation
		• Membrane: peritoneum
		• Dialysate: 1.5%, 2.5%, 4.25%
		• Access: peritoneal catheter
			• Vascular access:
			  • CAVH and CAVHD are rarely done because they require arterial and venous access
			  • SCUF, CVVH, CVVHD, and CVVHDF require venovenous access
			• Blood pump
			• High-coefficient membrane hemofilter
			• Therapy fluid: predilution, postdilution, or dialysate

Specific indications	• Need for rapid treatment • Hemodynamically stable patient • Fluid overload unresponsive to diuretics • Electrolyte imbalance • Acute or chronic renal failure • Drug overdose or poison intoxication with dialyzable agent • Pulmonary edema refractory to diuretics	• Fluid overload • Electrolyte imbalance • Acute or chronic renal failure • Drug overdose or poison intoxication with dialyzable agent • Intact peritoneum • Inability to anticoagulate • Hemodynamic instability	• Fluid overload unresponsive to diuretics • Acute or chronic renal failure in hemodynamically unstable patient • Electrolyte imbalance • Drug overdose or poison intoxication with dialyzable agent • Inability to tolerate hemodialysis • May also be used in HF, sepsis, lactic acidosis, rhabdomyolysis, MODS, hepatic failure
Contraindications	• Hemodynamic instability • Hypovolemia • Inadequate vascular access • Coagulopathy	• Rapid treatment required • Acute peritonitis • Recent abdominal surgery • Known abdominal adhesions • Abdominal trauma • Intraperitoneal hematoma • Recent vascular anastomosis of abdominal vessels • Respiratory distress • Sepsis • Extreme obesity • Coagulopathy	• Rapid treatment required • Systolic blood pressure less than 60 mm Hg for CAVH, CAVHD • Lack of venovenous access for SCUF, CVVH, CVVHD • Coagulopathy: relative; may increase risk during vascular access placement

Table 8.9	Types of Dialysis—cont'd		
	Hemodialysis	**Intermittent Peritoneal Dialysis**	**CRRT Therapies**
Advantages	• Rapid and efficient; only 3–4 hr per session (usually 3 times weekly) unless overdose treatment, which may require 8–16 hr • Very efficient for small molecules; corrects biochemical disturbances quickly for time on therapy	• Equipment is easily and readily assembled • Fairly simple; requiring less staff and patient education • Relatively inexpensive • Minimal danger of acute electrolyte imbalance or hemorrhage • Dialysate can be individualized easily • Anticoagulation not required	• Removes solutes gradually • Decreased risk of hemodynamic instability • Provides flexibility in fluid administration • Allows adequate nutritional intake • Requires only minimal anticoagulation • Requires less staff education because it requires only catheter access instead of fistula or autograft • Can be used for physiologically unstable patients
Disadvantages	• Complex procedure requiring extensive staff training • Equipment expensive • Machine availability may be limited • Requires anticoagulation • Vascular access necessary	• Relatively slow to alter biochemical imbalances, usually requiring 36 hours for therapeutic effect • May cause protein loss • May be difficult to gain and maintain peritoneal access	• Patient must be in bed during entire treatment if femoral line in place or if unstable • May require anticoagulation • Vascular access necessary • Increased nursing care requirements • Complicates dosing of certain drugs such as antibiotics and agents which are dialyzable

Complications	• Access complications: bleeding, clotting, infection
	• Acute fluid and electrolyte imbalances
	• Hemorrhage
	• Hypovolemia
	• Air embolus
	• Disequilibrium syndrome caused by too rapid removal of waste products
	• Allergic reaction to membrane
	• Hepatitis
	• Dialysis encephalopathy (related to accumulation of aluminum from water used to prepare dialysate)
	• Infection
	• Dysrhythmias
		• Access complications: infection, dialysate leak, bleeding, and peritonitis
		• Too rapid fluid removal, causing the following:
		  • Hypovolemia
		  • Hypernatremia
		• Hypervolemia caused by dialysate retention
		• Hypokalemia caused by potassium-free dialysate usage
		• Alkalosis caused by alkaline dialysate usage
		• Disequilibrium syndrome caused by too rapid a removal of waste products
		• Hyperglycemia caused by high glucose concentration of dialysate
		• Protein loss
		• Respiratory distress
			• Hypotension
			• Hypothermia
			• Hypovolemia or hypervolemia if too rapid or too slow fluid removal
			• Electrolyte imbalance of potassium, calcium, magnesium, and phosphate, depending on therapy
			• Acid–base imbalances
			• Access complications: bleeding, clotting, infection
			• Depletion syndrome: loss of vitamins and amino acids
			• Hemorrhage related to the following:
			  • Anticoagulation
			  • Disruption of filter or tubing
			• Infection
			• Air embolism

BP, Blood pressure; *CRRT*, continuous renal replacement therapy; *CVVH*, continuous venovenous hemofiltration; *CVVHD*, continuous venovenous hemodialysis; *CVVHDF*, continuous venovenous hemodiafiltration; *HF*, heart failure; *MODS*, multiple organ dysfunction syndrome; *SCUF*, slow continuous ultrafiltration therapy.

      ii) Ask patient to void or insert urinary catheter before abdominal puncture.
   b) Weigh patient before treatment and daily after draining dialysate.
 2) Procedure (Fig. 8.11, *B*)
   a) Warm dialysate to body temperature.
   b) Ensure that prescribed medications have been added to dialysate: heparin; potassium chloride; antibiotics; lidocaine; etc.
   c) Instill 1 to 3 l of dialysate (usually 2 l) (inflow phase); this volume is usually infused at a rate of 2 l in 10 to 20 minutes.
   d) Allow to dwell in intraperitoneal space for 20 to 30 minutes. (NOTE: If first exchange, do not allow dialysate to dwell; drain immediately to ensure catheter patency and placement.)
   e) Drain and measure dialysate (outflow phase).
   f) Assess appearance of dialysate.
      i) Normal: clear, pale yellow or straw-colored
      ii) Cloudy: Suspect infection; culture and sensitivity is indicated.
      iii) Bloody: if occurs after the first four exchanges, suspect intraabdominal bleeding or coagulopathy

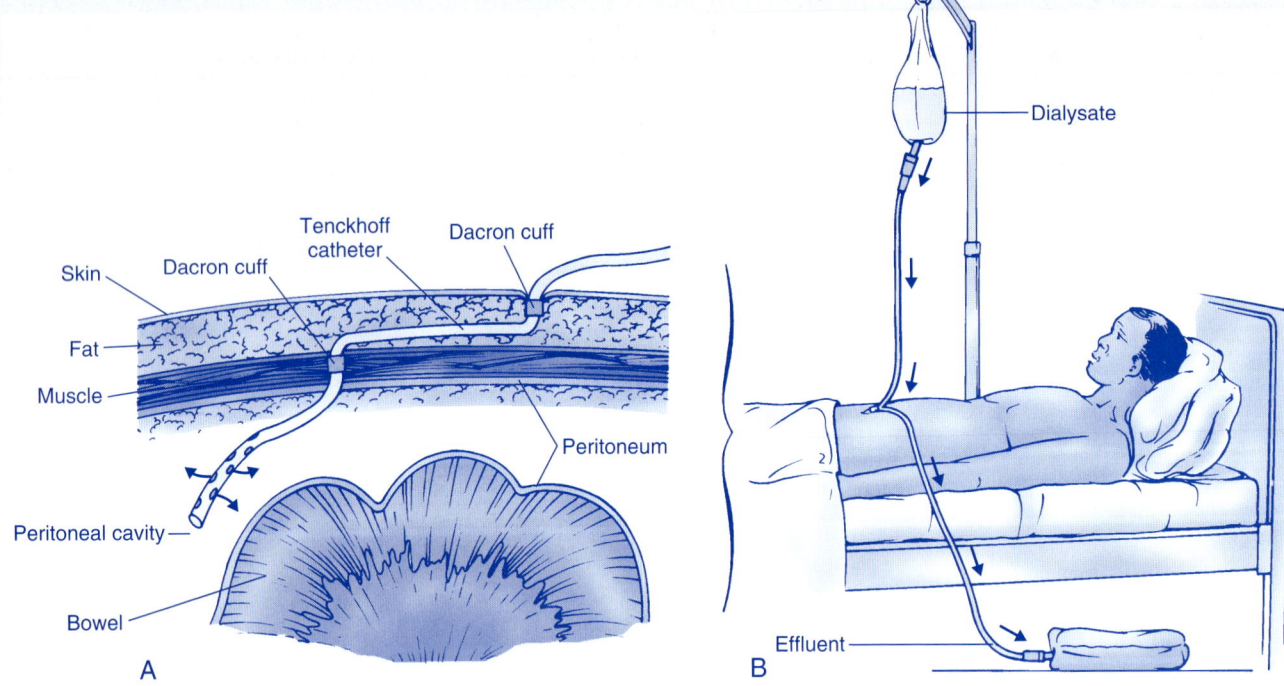

Fig. 8.11 Manual peritoneal dialysis via an implanted Tenckhoff catheter. **A,** Catheter position in peritoneal cavity. **B,** Manual peritoneal dialysis process. (From Ignatavicius, D. D., & Workman, M. L. [2006]. *Medical-surgical nursing: Critical thinking for collaborative care* [5th ed.]. Philadelphia: Saunders.)

        iv) Amber: Suspect bladder perforation.
        v) Brownish: Suspect bowel perforation.
    g) If the amount drained is less than the amount instilled
        i) Turn patient side to side.
        ii) Apply gentle pressure to the abdomen.
  3) Keep meticulous cumulative intake and output records (e.g., if drain is 300 ml less than the amount instilled [+300 ml] during one exchange but the next exchange yields a drain volume of 400 ml more than the amount instilled [−400 ml], the cumulative volume is −100 ml).
  4) Monitor for hypotension and respiratory distress, especially during inflow phase.
  5) Monitor vital signs during outflow phase.
  6) Monitor blood glucose levels in all patients; hyperglycemia is likely to occur in patients with diabetes or when 4.25% dialysate is used.
  7) Provide peritoneal catheter exit site care.
b. Hemodialysis
  1) Preparation
    a) Patient must have vascular access (Table 8.10 and Figs. 8.12 and 8.13).
    b) Weigh patient before hemodialysis.
    c) Do not administer drugs that may cause hypotension before hemodialysis.
        i) Antihypertensives
        ii) Antiemetics
        iii) Narcotics
        iv) Beta-blockers
        v) Calcium channel blockers
    d) Do not administer dialyzable drugs immediately before hemodialysis.

  2) Procedure (usually performed by specially trained hemodialysis nurse rather than critical care staff)
    a) Vascular access is cannulated or connected to the dialyzer.
    b) Anticoagulation is maintained.
    c) Blood chemistries are monitored throughout the treatment.
    d) Vital signs are monitored frequently for evaluation of hemodynamic stability and tolerance.
    e) Hematocrit is monitored for changes that may indicate too rapid removal of fluid.
    f) Monitor the vascular access and the hemofilter for indications of clotting.
c. Selected complications
  1) Disequilibrium syndrome
    a) Caused by toxins (e.g., urea being rapidly removed from the blood but not as rapidly removed from the cerebrospinal fluid)
    b) The higher concentration of toxins in the brain cells may cause a shift of fluid into brain cells and cerebral edema.
    c) Clinical indications may include nausea, vomiting, headache, hallucinations, and seizures.
    d) Collaborative management
        i) Use a smaller dialyzer.
        ii) Reduce blood pump speed.
        iii) Shorten dialysis time and dialyze more frequently.
        iv) Administer diazepam and phenytoin as prescribed for seizures.
  2) Muscle cramps
    a) Caused by rapid water removal and sodium shifts

Table 8.10 Forms of Vascular Accesses for Dialysis

Access	Advantages	Disadvantages	Management
Double-lumen vascular catheter (Fig. 8.12) inserted into the subclavian, jugular, or femoral vein	• Easy insertion • Immediate use • High flow rates are achieved • No venipuncture required for access	• Externally located • Can be easily dislodged • Prone to infection and thrombosis • Femoral catheters are associated with a higher incidence of infection	• Monitor site daily and provide site care • Restrict use of this catheter to dialysis only • Administer heparin into catheter if prescribed • A fibrinolytic may be used to reestablish patency of an occluded catheter
Fistula (Fig. 8.13, *A*)	• Located internally • Greater longevity • Lower clotting and infection rates than external devices • No danger of disconnect	• Requires 4–6 wk to mature before use • Requires venipuncture for access • May result in ischemia to affected limb (referred to as "vascular steal syndrome") • May thrombose	• Do not use limb for BP or venipuncture • Listen for bruit, feel for thrill: indicate patency • Assess neurovascular status of affected limb frequently • Teach patient exercises to increase blood flow in fistula (e.g., squeezing a ball) • Warn patient not to wear constrictive clothing
AV graft (Fig. 8.13, *B*)	• As for fistula • May be used for patients with vessels inadequate for fistula formation • Can be used earlier than traditional fistula	• As for fistula • Infection is more serious than with traditional fistula because of the risk of disintegration and hemorrhage • May cause aneurysm formation	• As for fistula • Rotating puncture sites and applying pressure on needle removal aids in prevention of aneurysm and pseudoaneurysm

AV, Arteriovenous; *BP,* blood pressure.

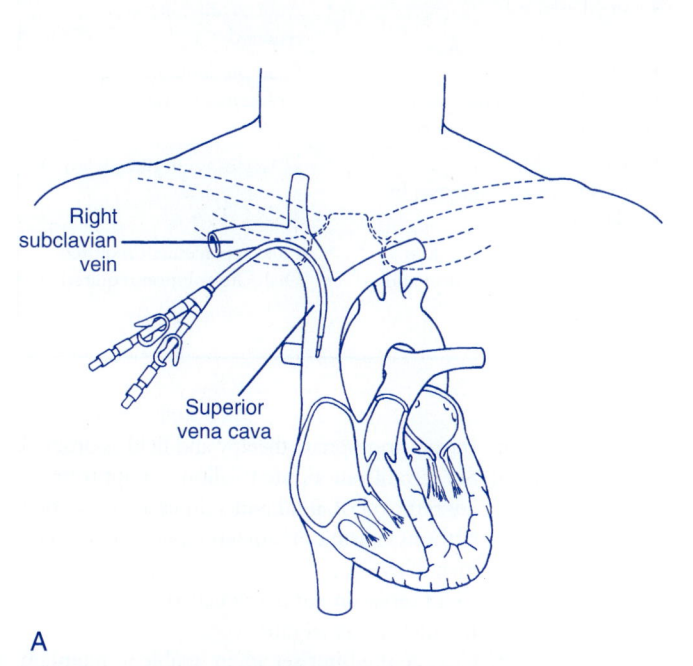 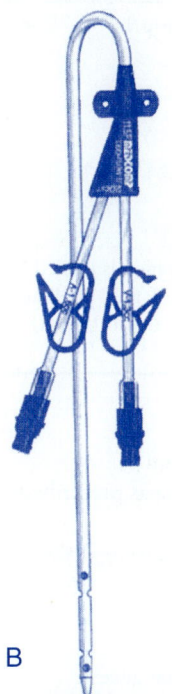

Fig. 8.12 A, Temporary vascular access using subclavian dual-lumen venous catheter. **B,** Dual-lumen temporary catheter. (Courtesy of MEDCOMP Corporation, Harleysville, PA.)

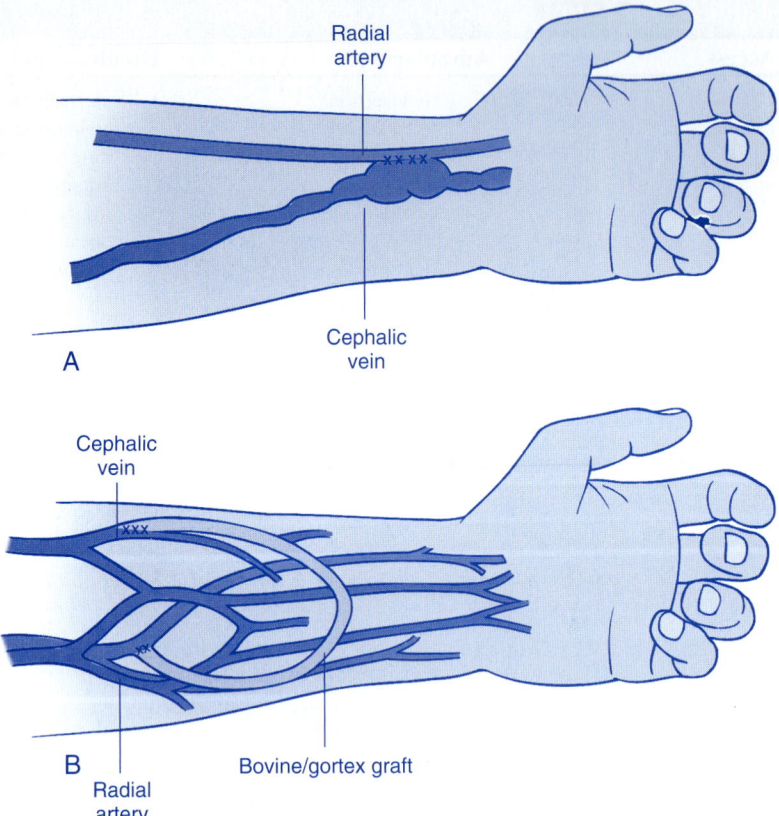

Fig. 8.13 Permanent vascular accesses. **A,** Arteriovenous (AV) fistula. **B,** AV graft. (From Urden, L. D., Stacy, K. M., & Lough, M. E. [2010]. *Critical care nursing: Diagnosis and management* [6th ed.]. St. Louis: Mosby.)

Table 8.11	Continuous Renal Replacement Therapy		
Type	**Ultrafiltration Rate**	**Function**	**Nursing Considerations**
SCUF (slow, continuous ultrafiltration)	100–300 ml/hr	• Fluid removal	• Anticoagulation may be required
CVVH (continuous venovenous hemofiltration)	35 ml/kg/hr	• Fluid removal • Small- to moderate-sized solute removal by convection	• Fluid predilution or replacement required
CVVHD (continuous venovenous hemodialysis)	35 ml/kg/hr	• Fluid removal • Maximal solute removal by diffusion	• Dialysate solution is required
CVVHDF (continuous venovenous hemodiafiltration); not available on all equipment	Ultrafiltration is limited by amount of fluid predilution or postdilution or dialysate fluid infused	• Maximal fluid and solute removal by convection and diffusion	• Fluid replacement required • Dialysate solution required

   b) Collaborative management
      i) Administer quinine as prescribed before dialysis.
      ii) Hypertonic saline during dialysis may also be prescribed.
   d. CRRT (Table 8.11)
      1) Preparation
         a) Patient must have vascular access.
         b) Heparin, citrate, and other combinations are placed in the port and need to be removed before initiation of treatment.
      2) Procedure
         a) Prepare hemofilter with dialysate solution.
         b) Connect vascular access to hemofilter.
         c) Initiate appropriate therapy and fluid as ordered.
         d) Set ultrafiltration rate to allow for appropriate removal of fluid and solutes as prescribed without causing or worsening hemodynamic instability.
         e) Fluid replacement if calculated according to the ultrafiltration rate.
         f) Change the filter set when unable to maintain prescribed rate or if filter clots and flow is stopped.

Renal Transplant

Renal replacement therapy for patients with chronic kidney disease

Learning Activities

CHAPTER 8

1. Complete the following crossword puzzle related to renal anatomy and physiology.

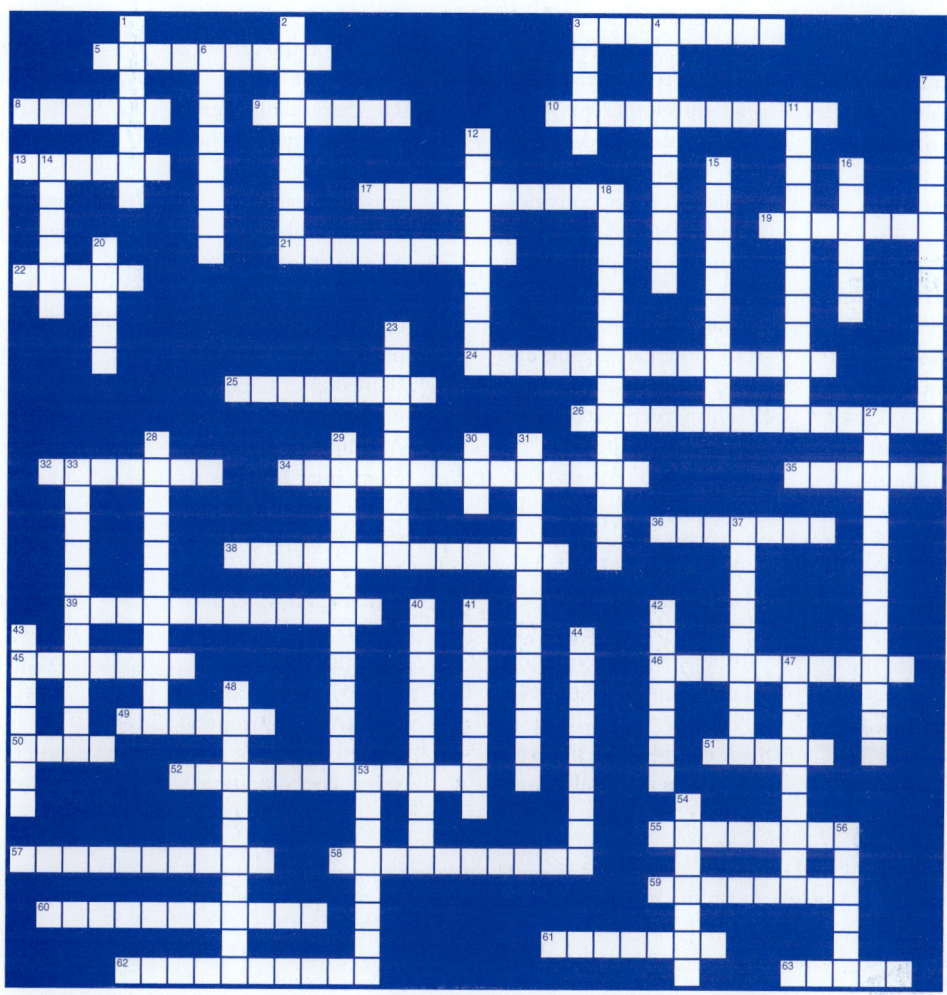

ACROSS

3. This electrolyte works with sodium to maintain body fluid osmolality
5. The passage of a substance from the capillary into the tubule
8. The primary extracellular cation
9. A positively charged ion
10. This pressure is a pushing pressure
13. This structure includes proximal convoluted, loop of Henle, and distal convoluted segments
17. Indicates that the fluid has an osmolality more than body fluids: example 3% saline
19. The passageway for expulsion of urine from the bladder to the urinary meatus
21. This electrolyte is crucial for neuromuscular transmission
22. The substance is secreted by the juxtaglomerular apparatus in response to low perfusion
24. The hormone that stimulates the release of RBCs from the bone marrow
25. The concentration of this ion determines pH
26. The process which maintains constancy in GFR
32. Vitamin D is necessary for the absorption of this mineral
34. This type of nephron is important in the kidney's ability to concentrate urine
35. Site of the glomerulus, proximal, and distal tubules
36. This organ is a collapsible bag of smooth muscle
38. Fluid inside cells
39. The human body is composed mostly of this substance
45. The endocrine gland that is referred to as the suprarenal gland
46. This electrolyte is crucial for cellular energy
49. A small funnel tapering into the ureter
50. The end product of protein metabolism
51. A negatively charged ion

607

52. The movement of substances from the tubule back into the capillaries
55. Indicates that the fluid has approximately the same osmolality as body fluids; example normal saline
57. The movement of solutes and solutions from an area of high pressure to an area of low pressure
58. This area of the kidney includes the renal cortex and medulla
59. This type of nephron has a short loop of Henle
60. The state of internal equilibrium within the body
61. Urea is the result of the breakdown of this macronutrient
62. Cluster of tightly coiled capillaries in the nephron
63. Loop diuretics such as furosemide work at the loop of

DOWN
1. Composed of 6 to 10 pyramids
2. The primary intracellular cation
3. Cup-like structures that drain the papillae
4. Number of osmols per kilogram of solution; expressed as mOsm/kg
6. This arteriole leads out of the glomerulus
7. This substance is made by the kidney and modulates the vasoconstrictive effects of angiotensin and norepinephrine
11. Fluid between cells
12. This structure consists of Bowman capsule and the glomerulus
14. This structure collects urine from the renal pelvis and propels it to the bladder by peristaltic waves
15. Waste product of muscle metabolism
16. This type of transport is against concentration gradients and requires energy
18. A complex physiologic process which allows for concentration of urine
20. Cavity filled with adipose tissue, minor and major calices, the renal pelvis, and origin of the ureter
23. An estimate of a known substance in the plasma compared with the amount in the urine
27. Fluid inside vessels
28. The extracellular anion that is essential in the maintenance of acid-base balance
29. Fluid outside cells
30. This hormone is produced in the hypothalamus and released by the posterior pituitary; it causes water retention in the renal tubule
31. Another term for glomerular filtrate
33. The hormone of the adrenal cortex that causes retention of sodium and water and excretion of potassium
37. The movement of solutes from an area of high solute concentration to an area of low solute concentration
40. The type of fluid loss (or gains) that cannot be measured
41. This arteriole leads into the glomerulus
42. Microscopic functional unit of the kidney
43. The thin layer of fibrous membrane that surrounds each kidney
44. The capillary network that runs parallel to the ascending and descending loop of Henle
47. Indicates that the fluid has an osmolality less than body fluids; example 1/2 normal saline
48. The extracellular anion that is essential in the maintenance of acid-base balance
53. Triangular wedges of medullary tissue; composed of collecting tubules
54. The movement of solution from an area of low solute concentration to an area of high solute concentration
56. The inward extension of cortical tissue between the pyramids

2. Number the structures below according to the order of their involvement in urine formation.
   ___Ureters
   ___Glomerulus
   ___Loop of Henle
   ___Proximal convoluted tubule
   ___Bladder
   ___Bowman capsule
   ___Collecting ducts
   ___Distal convoluted tubule
   ___Urethra

3. Complete the following statements related to the movement of solutes and solutions.
   Water moves by the process of _____.
   Electrolytes move by the process of _____.
   The sodium-potassium pump is an example of _____.
   The use of a pushing pressure, such as hydrostatic pressure, is called _____.

4. A 72-year-old woman is brought to the emergency department from a long-term care facility. She had recently been started on enteral feedings. She has had a change in level of consciousness. Her sodium level is 150 mEq/l, her BUN is 80 mg/dl, and her serum glucose is 1000 mg/dl. Calculate her serum osmolality and identify what this serum osmolality indicates. What is the most likely cause of this abnormal serum osmolality? _____
_____
_____

5. Identify the electrolyte or electrolytes that the statement describes.
   a. Serum levels of this electrolyte go up in acidosis and down in alkalosis _____
   b. These three electrolytes frequently go down together. _____
   c. Serum levels of this electrolyte go down in hypoalbuminemia. _____
   d. These two electrolytes have an inverse relationship: When one goes down, the other goes up. _____
   e. These two electrolytes are frequently deficient in malnourished patients. _____
   f. Loss of either of these electrolytes causes hydrogen ions to move into the cell resulting in metabolic alkalosis. _____

6. Specify whether the following causes of metabolic acidosis would have a normal anion gap or an increased anion gap.

Condition	Normal Anion Gap	Increased Anion Gap
Shock		
Renal failure		
Diarrhea		
Diabetic ketoacidosis		
Salicylate overdose		
Renal tubular acidosis		
Rhabdomyolysis		
Carbonic anhydrase inhibitors		
Ethylene glycol poisoning		

7. Identify three major reasons for the BUN to be elevated in a patient with a normal creatinine.
8. Identify whether these signs and symptoms are indicative of electrolyte deficit or excess.

Sign or Symptom	Excess (Hyper)	Deficit (Hypo)
Sodium		
Weight gain		
Abdominal cramps		
Flushed, dry skin		
Postural hypotension		
Headache		
Hypertension		
Potassium		
Flat T waves, prominent U waves		
Decreased GI motility, paralytic ileus		
Intestinal colic, diarrhea		
Muscle cramps → flaccid paralysis		
Decreased cardiac contractility		
Tall, peaked T waves, widened QRS complex		

Sign or Symptom	Excess (Hyper)	Deficit (Hypo)
Calcium		
Tetany		
Decreased deep tendon reflexes		
Neuromuscular weakness, flaccidity		
Seizures		
Bone or flank pain		
Laryngospasm		
Phosphorus		
Tetany		
Fatigue		
Chest pain		
Dyspnea		
Increased deep tendon reflexes		
Abdominal cramps		
Magnesium		
Decreased deep tendon reflexes		
Anorexia, nausea, vomiting		
Cardiopulmonary arrest		
Lethargy		
Dysrhythmias, especially torsades de pointe		
Facial flushing		

9. Identify three electrolyte imbalances that enhance the digitalis effect and increase the chance of digitalis toxicity.

10. Identify the fluid, electrolyte, or acid–base imbalances to which these patients would be predisposed:
    a. A patient receiving regular doses of furosemide.
    b. A patient with persistent vomiting.
    c. A patient with acute kidney injury (oliguric phase).
    d. A patient with diabetic ketoacidosis (before treatment).
    e. A patient receiving multiple units of banked blood.

11. List seven reasons for transient causes of incontinence:
    D: _____
    I: _____
    A: _____
    P: _____
    E: _____
    R: _____
    S: _____

12. Answer the following questions related to urinary tract infections (UTIs).
    a. What is a common UTI risk factor in adults?
    b. Bacteria from the intestines, most commonly _____, often infect the urinary tract by ascending from the perineal area in the lower urinary tract.
    c. Why are women more susceptible to UTIs than men?
    d. How often should the need for an indwelling catheter be assessed?

13. List three indications for dialysis in a patient with acute kidney injury. _____

14. Categorize the following causes of acute kidney injury as prerenal, intrarenal, or postrenal.

Condition	Prerenal	Intrarenal	Postrenal
Acute pyelonephritis			
Benign prostatic hypertrophy			
Contrast dyes			
Diuretics			
Aminoglycosides			
Glomerulonephritis			
Goodpasture syndrome			
Hemorrhage			
Hepatorenal syndrome			
Hypersensitivity reactions			
Intraabdominal tumor			
Malignant hypertension			
Neurogenic bladder			
Prolonged hypotension			
Renal calculi			
Rhabdomyolysis with myoglobinuria			
Septic shock			

15. Identify the following characteristics as occurring during the oliguric or diuretic phase of acute kidney injury or both.

Characteristic	Oliguric Phase	Diuretic Phase	Both
Elevated BUN			
Hyperkalemia			
Metabolic acidosis			
Volume deficit			
Volume excess			

612 Chapter 8 The Renal System

16. Complete the following crossword puzzle related to renal assessment, conditions, and treatments.

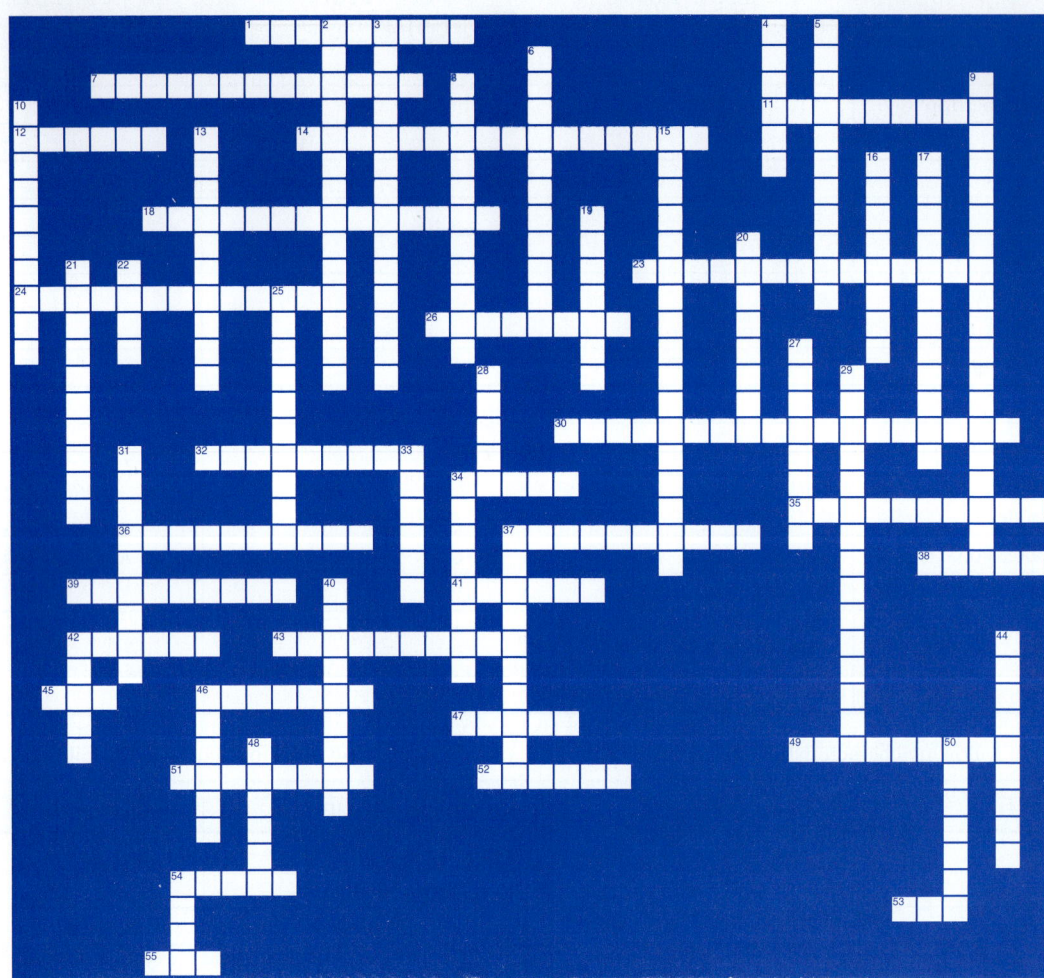

ACROSS

1. Significant changes in serum levels of this electrolyte causes T wave change and dysrhythmias
7. Electrolyte imbalance that occurs with osteolytic lesions
11. This type of intrarenal failure is caused by nephrotoxic agents or prolonged ischemic injury
12. This condition that occurs in renal failure is caused by deficiency of erythropoietin
14. The electrolyte imbalance primarily associated refeeding syndrome
18. The condition characterized by the breakdown of skeletal muscle
23. Tenderness over this "angle" may indicate pyelonephritis
24. A carbonic anhydrase inhibitor; frequently used to treat metabolic alkalosis (abbrev.)
26. The separation of solutes by differential diffusion through a semipermeable membrane that is placed between two solutions
30. An acute inflammation of the kidney associated with beta-hemolytic streptococcal infection
32. The hand-flapping tremor seen in uremia
34. Pain in this area is frequently associated with renal conditions
35. This serum value goes down in overhydration and up in dehydration
36. A potentially permanent renal replacement therapy for patients with chronic renal failure
37. A dopaminergic agent which increases renal flow (generic)
38. The amount of time that the dialysate solution remains in the peritoneal cavity is referred to as the _____ time
39. This categorization of acute renal failure is caused by disrupted renal flow; renal stone is an example of a cause of this type of renal failure
41. This is palpable over a fistula
42. Glomerulonephritis requires renal _____ for definitive diagnosis
43. High levels of this electrolyte occur in renal failure; low levels occur in malnutrition
45. Another term for this x-ray is "flat plate of abdomen" (abbrev.)
46. A long-term vascular access consisting of an internal artery-vein anastomosis
47. Calculation of this gap differentiates metabolic acidosis caused by acid gain from metabolic acidosis caused by bicarbonate loss
49. Solution of glucose and electrolytes used on one side of the semipermeable membrane to pull fluid and electrolytes
51. This phase of acute renal failure is heralded by a dramatic increase in urine output
52. A condition characterized by cramps, convulsions, twitching of the muscles, and sharp flexion of the wrist and ankle joints

53. This lab value is normally 10x the creatinine value (abbrev.)
54. The most common form of CRRT today (abbrev.)
55. The most common type of acute renal failure in critically ill patients (abbrev.)

DOWN

2. An oxygen free scavenger which may be used after contrast dyes especially if the patient has an elevated creatinine
3. An aldosterone antagonist (also referred to as a potassium-spacing diuretic [generic])
4. Increased levels of urea in the blood
5. Syndrome characterized by basement membrane damage and manifested by renal failure and hemoptysis
6. The surgical procedure performed for renal fracture
8. A cause of hypoproteinemia is renal failure
9. A thiazide diuretic (generic)
10. An ion exchange agent used to decrease serum potassium (brand)
13. The breakdown at body protein
15. Drugs used to prevent organ rejection in a post-transplant patient cause _____
16. The categorization of acute renal failure that is caused by disrupted blood flow to the kidney
17. The electrolyte imbalance that occurs with crush injury, renal failure, and hemolysis
19. A deficiency of this electrolyte may cause paresthesia, tetany, seizures
20. Type of intrarenal failure that is caused by infectious processes
21. Presence of this substance in the urine is the result of massive hemolysis; may cause renal failure
22. Precipitation from the kidney that takes the shape of the tubule where it was formed
25. This categorization of acute renal failure that is caused by damage to renal tissue
27. An osmotic diuretic (generic)
28. Renal patients may taste _____
29. Calcium may be administered for hypocalcemia, hyperkalemia, and _____
31. This type of renal injury is caused by compression of the kidney between the lower ribs and the vertebral column
33. Levels of this electrolyte are greatly affected by water balance
34. The renal injury that involves multiple lacerations extending into the renal collection system
37. A loop diuretics (generic)
40. Presence of this substance in the urine is the result of the breakdown of skeletal muscle; may cause renal failure
44. High levels of this electrolyte may cause respiratory paralysis and cardiopulmonary arrest
46. This type of edema is frequently associated with nephrotic syndrome
48. To move the kidney down to palpable range the patient is asked to take a deep _____
50. This plasma protein which has the most significant effect on intravascular oncotic pressure
54. A renal replacement therapy that may be used in patients who can not tolerate hemodialysis (abbrev.)

The Hematologic and Immunologic Systems

CHAPTER 9

Selected Concepts in Anatomy and Physiology

Purposes of the Hematologic and Immunologic Systems
1. Hematologic
   a. Provides the medium for transportation of oxygen, carbon dioxide, and nutrients to the tissues
   b. Facilitates removal of waste products
   c. Maintains hemostasis
   d. Maintains internal environment, including participation in regulation of temperature and acid–base balance
2. Immunologic
   a. Protects the body's internal milieu against invading organisms and the development, growth, and dissemination of abnormal cells
   b. Maintains homeostasis by removing damaged cells from the circulation

Bone Marrow
1. Adults have 30 to 50 ml of bone marrow per kilogram of body weight.
   a. Two types of bone marrow
      1) Red (i.e., active)
      2) Yellow (i.e., inactive)
2. Most functioning bone marrow in adults is located in flat bones (vertebrae, skull, pelvic and shoulder girdles, clavicle, ribs, sternum) and proximal epiphysis of long bones.
3. The functions of the bone marrow include:
   a. Production of the following:
      1) Erythrocytes (red blood cells [RBCs])
      2) Leukocytes (white blood cells [WBCs]), including granulocytes (i.e., neutrophils, eosinophils, basophils), agranulocytes (i.e., monocytes), and lymphocytes
      3) Thrombocytes (platelets)
   b. Recognition and removal of senescent cells
   c. Participation in cellular and humoral immunity

Spleen
1. The largest of the secondary lymphoid organs
2. Stores about 300 ml of blood
3. White pulp: primarily supports humoral immunity; performs the following functions:
   a. Production of lymphocytes
   b. Stimulation of B-cell activity to produce immunoglobulins; therefore, splenectomized patients have an increased risk of leukocytosis and sepsis with encapsulated microorganisms (e.g., *Streptococcus pneumoniae*, *Haemophilus influenzae*, and *Neisseria meningitidis*) (McCance & Huether, 2014)
   c. Storage site for splenic reticuloendothelial tissue and immunoglobulins
4. Red pulp: contains reticuloendothelial tissue; performs the following functions:
   a. Storage and release of RBCs into the circulation
      1) Caused by contraction of smooth muscle in the capsule surrounding the spleen and in invaginations of the capsule, called *trabeculae*
      2) When stimulated by the sympathetic nervous system (SNS), as much as 200 ml of concentrated RBCs can be released into the circulation, raising the hematocrit (Hct) by .3-4%
   b. Filtering and destruction (by the process of phagocytosis) of damaged or old erythrocytes (referred to as *culling*)
      1) Removes particles from intact RBCs without destroying them (referred to as *pitting*)
      2) Catabolizes hemoglobin (Hgb) released from RBCs that have been destroyed by the spleen; iron returned to the bone marrow for reuse
   c. Filtering and trapping foreign material, including bacteria and viruses
   d. Storage and release of platelets; destruction of damaged or senescent platelets

Liver
Performs the following functions:
1. Filtering of blood as it comes from the gastrointestinal (GI) tract
   a. Removal of foreign material, including microorganisms, damaged or old RBCs, and other degradation products by the Kupffer cells lining the sinusoidal beds of the liver
   b. Destruction of RBCs produces bilirubin, which the liver converts to bile, necessary for fat digestion
2. Elimination of immune complexes (e.g., antigen–antibody complexes) from the blood

3. Detoxification of toxic substances that enter the blood
4. Manufacture of some clotting factors (i.e., vitamin K–dependent factors II, VII, IX, X) and antithrombin
5. Storage of blood (e.g., in heart failure, the liver becomes engorged with blood)

Lymphatic System

1. The lymphatic system is part of the circulatory system and essential to the immune system, made up of a complex network of lymphatic vessels that carry lymph fluid.
2. Lymph: pale yellow fluid that transports lymphocytes
   a. Composition
      1) Mostly water
      2) Contains lymphocytes, granulocytes, enzymes, and antibodies
      3) Deficient in platelets and fibrinogen, so it coagulates very slowly
   b. Function: return of proteins and fat from GI tract, excess interstitial fluid, and certain hormones to the blood
   c. Flow is unidirectional.
3. Lymph circulation
   a. Lymphatic capillaries are somewhat larger than blood capillaries and irregular in diameter.
   b. Lymphatic vessels are formed by lymphatic capillaries.
   c. Lymph ducts drain into the subclavian vein.
      1) The right lymphatic duct collects lymph from the right side of the head, neck, and thorax and from the right arm, right lung, right side of heart, and right upper surface of the diaphragm and drains into the right subclavian vein.
      2) The thoracic duct collects lymph from all other parts of the body.
   d. Lymph nodes are small, bean-shaped organs located along lymph vessels.
      1) Spongy and multichanneled on inside
      2) Bone marrow is the site for B- and T-cell lymphocyte production; then T cells mature in the thymus, and B cells go directly into circulation.
      3) Functions
         a) Lymph nodes filter and allow WBCs to phagocytose bacteria and foreign material carried by lymph.
         b) Granulocytes, macrophages, and lymphocytes pass through the lymph node to return to the blood circulation.
      4) Enlargement of lymph nodes
         a) This occurs with inflammation, infection, or malignancy.
         b) Enlargement of superficial nodes can be palpated; enlarged deep nodes can only be visualized on radiography or computed tomography (CT).
   e. Additional lymphoid tissue synthesizes immunoglobulins A (IgA) and E (IgE) and is located in the submucosa of the respiratory, intestinal, or genitourinary (GU) tracts.
      1) Mucosa-associated lymphoid tissues (MALT): clusters of T and B lymphocytes, macrophages, and phagocytes dispersed in the mucosal linings of the respiratory, GI, and GU tracts
      2) Gut-associated lymphoid tissue (GALT): Peyer patches in the intestinal tract
4. Thymus
   a. Location: anterosuperior mediastinum below the thyroid gland; each lobe is packed with lymphocytes
   b. Function
      1) Site of maturation and distribution of T lymphocytes
      2) Secretes a hormone, thymosin, which is thought to stimulate immune function
5. Microglia cells
   a. Location: white matter of the brain
   b. Function: lymphocyte-rich tissue that functions to destroy foreign matter that crosses the blood–brain barrier; also clears debris (phagocytosis)

Blood

1. Plasma is 55% of total blood volume.
   a. Composed of plasma and plasma proteins, including prealbumin, albumin, serum globulins, fibrinogen, prothrombin, and plasminogen
   b. Hct expresses the percentage of RBCs in the total blood volume; affected by the fluid component of the blood
      1) Increased Hct may indicate polycythemia or hemoconcentration.
      2) Decreased Hct may indicate anemia or hemodilution.
2. All blood cells originate from pluripotential stem cells that differentiate into myeloid and lymphoid lineage cells.
   a. Erythroid stem cells (i.e., pronormoblasts) develop into reticulocytes and finally into erythrocytes.
   b. Myeloid stem cells (myeloblasts or monoblasts) develop into granulocytes and monocytes.
   c. Lymphoid stem cells (i.e., lymphoblasts) develop into B and T lymphocytes.
   d. Thrombocytic stem cells (i.e., megakaryoblasts) develop into thrombocytes.
3. Erythrocytes are also referred to as *red blood cells* or *RBCs*.
   a. Structure
      1) Erythrocytes are nonnucleated round biconcave cells; they lack mitochondria.
      2) The inner part of RBCs (referred to as *stoma*) is the location of Hgb attachment and contains the antigens that determine ABO and Rh blood type.
   b. Function of RBCs
      1) Transport oxygen from lungs to tissues
      2) Participate in maintenance of acid–base balance
      3) Provide insulation and weight to the blood
      4) Are highly permeable to hydrogen, chloride, and bicarbonate ions and water
   c. Types of RBCs
      1) Reticulocytes: immature RBCs
         a) Useful in assessing erythrocyte production; elevated reticulocyte count (i.e., greater than 25% of total RBC count) means that production of new RBCs is greater

b) Mature in 1 to 4 days after release and function like normal RBCs but may have a shortened life span
c) May be released after sudden blood loss, such as hemorrhage; repeated challenges to this compensatory mechanism lead to exhaustion of reserve reticulocytes
2) Erythrocytes: mature RBCs
a) Life span is approximately 120 days.
b) The spleen acts as an RBC reservoir; contains 1% to 2% of circulating RBCs.
d. Erythropoiesis
1) Regulation
a) Determined by relationship of cellular oxygen requirement and general metabolic activity
i) Increased muscle mass causes higher RBC levels.
ii) Whereas androgens increase RBC production, estrogens decrease production.
b) Bone marrow is stimulated to make more RBCs by the hormone erythropoietin; erythropoietin is secreted by the kidney in response to hypoxemia.
2) Nutritional requirements for RBC and Hgb production
a) Iron and iron precursors such as ferritin
b) Vitamin B_{12}, B_6, B_2, C, and E
c) Folic acid
d) Essential elements: zinc, selenium, copper, and niacin
3) Process
a) Stem cell
b) Erythroblast (has a nucleus)
c) Expulsion of nucleus
d) Erythrocyte
4) Hgb synthesis
a) Synthesis takes place in bone marrow.
b) Hgb consists of four globin chains and four heme groups per Hgb molecule; each Hgb molecule has two different types of globin (e.g., normal adult Hgb [referred to as HbA]), two alpha chains and two beta chains.
c) The heme portion of Hgb molecules contains iron: more than two thirds of the body's iron is contained in Hgb and myoglobin.
i) Oxygen binds to the heme protein within the erythrocyte.
ii) The binding affinity of oxygen to Hgb is dependent upon acid–base balance, temperature, and levels of 2,3-diphosphoglyceric acid (2,3-DPG).
(a) Alkalosis, hypothermia, and decreased levels of 2,3-DPG cause the oxyhemoglobin dissociation curve to shift to the left, increasing the affinity between oxygen and Hgb; this facilitates the pickup of oxygen at the lung but impairs drop-off of oxygen at the tissues.
(b) Acidosis, hyperthermia, and increased levels of 2,3-DPG cause the oxyhemoglobin dissociation curve to shift to the right, decreasing the affinity between oxygen and Hgb; this impairs the pickup of oxygen at the lung but facilitates drop-off of oxygen at the tissues.
e. Destruction (hemolysis) of erythrocytes
1) Destruction of old and immature RBCs occurs in the liver and spleen.
2) Destruction of immature RBCs occurs primarily because they are misshapen or damaged.
3) Presenescent RBCs are removed from the circulation by the spleen, liver, or bone marrow for any of the following reasons:
a) RBC membrane abnormalities
b) Hgb abnormalities
c) Abnormal metabolic functions
d) Physical trauma to the RBC
e) Antibodies
f) Infectious agents and toxins
4) Hgb and iron are returned to the bone marrow for reuse.
a) Heme is bound to haptoglobin for recirculation.
b) Iron is bound to transferrin for recirculation.
5) Erythrocyte destruction increases bilirubin production; bilirubin is transported to the liver attached to albumin.
a) Indirect bilirubin is unconjugated; this is before the liver has converted it to a water-soluble substance; indirect bilirubin becomes elevated in hemolytic states that overwhelm the liver's ability to conjugate or in liver disease when the liver is unable to adequately conjugate.
b) Direct bilirubin is conjugated; this is after the liver has converted it to a water-soluble substance that will be excreted into the bile; direct bilirubin becomes elevated in biliary obstruction.
c) Bilirubin is excreted via the GI tract or as urobilinogen in the urine.
4. Leukocytes: phagocytic and immunologic systems
a. Cytokines: protein hormones synthesized by the various leukocytes
1) Act as chemical mediators of immunity and inflammation
2) Important in regulation of normal immune and inflammatory responses
3) Are causative factors in systemic inflammatory response syndrome (SIRS) (see Chapter 11)
4) Types of cytokines

Table 9.1	Definitions of Selected Leukocyte Activities
Opsonization	The process by which opsonins render bacteria more susceptible to phagocytosis by leukocytes; an opsonin is an antibody or complement split product that, when attached to foreign material, microorganism, or antigen, enhances phagocytosis of the substances by leukocytes and other macrophages
Chemotaxis (Fig. 9.1)	The movement toward (positive) or away from (negative) a chemical stimulus; movement of neutrophils and monocytes toward an invading microorganism
Margination (Fig. 9.1)	The process of the WBC sticking to the wall of the capillary
Diapedesis (Fig. 9.1)	The passage of WBCs through the walls of the vessels that contain them without damage to the vessels
Phagocytosis	The process by which certain cells engulf and destroy microorganisms and cellular debris; involves invagination, engulfment, internalization and formation of phagocyte vacuole, digestion of phagocytosed material by lysosomes and oxygen-derived radicals, and release of digested microbial products
Lysis	The destruction or dissolution of a cell through the action of a specific agent

WBC, White blood cell.

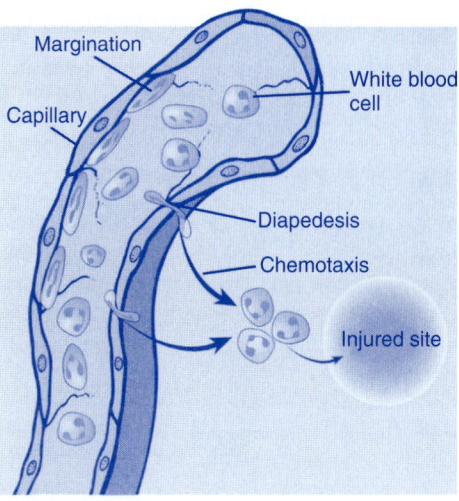

Fig. 9.1 Illustration of margination, diapedesis, and chemotaxis. (From Lewis, S. M., Heitkemper, M. M., Dirksen, S. R., & O'Brien, P. G. [2007]. *Medical-surgical nursing: Assessment and management of clinical problems* [7th ed.]. St. Louis: Mosby.)

  a) Monokines are synthesized by mononuclear phagocytes.
  b) Lymphokines are synthesized by lymphocytes.
  c) Macrophages secrete nonspecific cytokines such as tumor necrosis factor (TNF), interleukins (ILs), and interferons.
 b. Granulocytes: active phagocytes
  1) Neutrophils (also known as *polymorphonuclear leukocytes [PMNs]*); largest component of granulocytes and the circulating WBC mass (40%–80%)
   a) Function
    i) Neutrophils leave the blood vessel, migrate through the tissues, and search for microorganisms or damaged or old body cells; they then engulf, kill, and digest them through the process of phagocytosis. (Table 9.1 and Fig. 9.1 describe some selected cellular processes of leukocytes, including phagocytosis.)
     (a) Neutrophils are the most actively phagocytic of granulocytes.
     (b) Neutrophils are attracted to inflammation and bacterial microorganisms.
     (c) After phagocytosis, the neutrophil dies.
     (d) Pus is the endproduct of neutrophil death.
     (e) Neutrophils exhibit a burst of oxygen consumption during phagocytosis known as a *respiratory burst*; this produces superoxide, hydrogen peroxide, and hydroxyl radicals; these oxygen-derived radicals normally function in destruction of microorganisms but may be injurious to normal body tissue.
    ii) Neutrophils contain cytoplasmic granules that include lysosomal enzymes, which aid in killing the microorganism.
   b) Life span after maturation: half-life, 4 to 10 hours
   c) Maturity
    i) Bands are immature neutrophils.
     (a) Phagocytic
     (b) Increase in bands seen in acute bacterial infection; frequently referred to as a *shift to the left*
    ii) Segmented neutrophils (referred to as *segs*) are mature neutrophils.
     (a) Phagocytic
     (b) Increase in mature segmented neutrophils seen in inflammation, liver disease, and pernicious anemia; frequently referred to as a *shift to the right*
   d) Recruitment
    i) Movement into the tissues is stimulated by microorganisms or antigen–antibody reactions.
    ii) The bone marrow speeds maturation and release when more neutrophils are needed for phagocytosis.
   e) Destruction: lost from the blood via the GI tract, pulmonary or oral secretions, and urine and into the tissues

2) Eosinophils: comprise 0% to 5% of WBC mass
   a) Functions
      i) Ingest immune complexes (antigen–antibody complexes) and inactive mediators of allergic response
      ii) Some phagocytic activity
      iii) Probably most important during parasitic infections and allergic reactions; especially important in helminth infections because these parasitic worms are too large to be phagocytized, and eosinophils secrete chemicals that destroy the surface of the helminth
      iv) Also elevated in pulmonary and dermatologic inflammation and infection
      v) Effect against viruses
   b) Life span after maturation: half-life in circulation is approximately 30 minutes; in tissues, it is 12 days
   c) Tissue eosinophils are present in large numbers on mucosal surfaces of the respiratory and GI systems and the skin because these locations are common entry points for foreign material.
   d) Releases leukotrienes, prostaglandins, platelet-activating factor (PAF), and a variety of cytokines
   e) Pivotal in asthma exacerbation caused by allergic reaction
3) Basophils: comprise 0% to 2% of WBC mass
   a) Function
      i) Similar to mast cells, basophils contain heparin and histamine, which are released as they degranulate during acute local or systemic allergic reactions; mast cells stay in the tissue, and basophils stay in the circulatory system.
      ii) Basophils do not participate in phagocytic activity.
   b) Life span after maturation: unknown
c. Agranulocytes
   1) Mononuclear phagocytes
      a) Monocytes: comprise 3% to 8% of WBC mass
         i) Function
            (a) Some phagocytic activity
            (b) Differentiate into macrophages as they migrate into the tissues
         ii) Life span after maturation: circulating half-life, 8 to 10 hours
      b) Macrophages (not measured in WBC count because of their location)
         i) Function
            (a) Greater phagocytic ability than PMNs or monocytes; especially involved in removal of damaged or senescent cells, cellular debris, and mutant or cancer cells
            (b) Produce the cytokine IL-1, which increases proliferation of T cells, stimulates the growth and development of B lymphocytes, causes fever, and stimulates the release of prostaglandin
            (c) Produce the cytokine alpha interferon, which is important in the body's defense against viruses and tumors
            (d) Also produce IL-6, IL-8, and TNF
         ii) Fixed or mobile
            (a) Fixed (or tissue) macrophages: stay in one organ and phagocytize live and dead debris
               (i) Lung: alveolar macrophages
               (ii) Brain: microglia
               (iii) Liver: Kupffer cells
               (iv) Bone: osteoclast
               (v) Peritoneum: peritoneal macrophages
               (vi) Kidney: mesangial cells
               (vii) Spleen: splenic mononuclear cells
            (b) Mobile macrophages: found primarily at sites of inflammation and in peritoneal, pleural, and synovial spaces; migrate through the circulatory system as monocytes
         iii) Life span: months or years
   2) Lymphocytes: comprise 10% to 40% of WBC mass
      a) Primary cells of the immune response, circulate shortly in the blood before transition into secondary lymph organs.
      b) T cells: comprise approximately 70% to 80% of lymphocytes
         i) Develop in the bone marrow; mature and differentiate in the thymus and the lymph node
         ii) Function: cellular immunity
         iii) Types of T cells
            (a) Helper T cells (also referred to as *CD4 T lymphocytes, T4 lymphocytes, or T$_H$*) detect foreign cells and produce lymphokines to stimulate the production or activation of other cells to fight infection; lymphokines are soluble proteins that function as chemical communicators to transmit instructions to macrophages, lymphocytes, and tissue cells.
            (b) Cytotoxic T cells (also referred to as *killer cells or T$_c$*) emit chemicals that dissolve the foreign cell's membrane to kill the cell before the invader can use it as a base for multiplication.
            (c) Suppressor T cells (also referred to as *CD8 T lymphocytes, T8 lymphocytes, or T$_S$*) modulate the overall immune system by signaling B cells and T cells to slow down or stop their activity.

(d) Memory T cells circulate in blood and lymph after the initial infection to allow ready response to subsequent invasion by the same organism.
(e) Helper T cells typically carry the CD4 surface molecule; suppressor and cytotoxic T cells typically carry the CD8 surface molecule; normally, there are twice as many CD4 cells as CD8 cells.
c) B cells: comprise approximately 10% to 20% of lymphocytes
i) Develop and mature in the bone marrow (bursa); migrate to lymph nodes and lymphoid tissue for differentiation and antibody production or plasma cell differentiation
ii) Function: production of immunoglobulins (humoral immunity)
(a) After being activated, B cells become plasma cells.
(i) Recognize specific foreign material
(ii) Develop specific immunoglobulins to that antigen
(b) Memory B cells circulate in blood and lymph after the initial infection to allow ready response to subsequent invasion by the same organism.
d) Natural killer (NK) cells (also referred to *as null cells*): comprise approximately 10% of lymphocytes
i) Large granular cytotoxic lymphocytes that are neither T cells nor B cells (i.e., no surface marker exists on these lymphocytes)
ii) Functions
(a) Kill nonspecifically and do not need prior exposure for activation
(b) Involved in surveillance against tumors, some parasites, and viruses
(c) Can activate T cells
(d) Have phagocytic properties
(e) Produce cytokines

Inflammation

1. Sequential physiologic response the body makes to injuries, immunologic processes, or foreign substances in the body; may be acute or chronic
    a. Occurs at sites of tissue damage irrespective of etiology
    b. May be local only or can become systemic; systemic response is now referred to as SIRS (discussion of SIRS and multiple organ dysfunction syndrome [MODS] is in Chapter 11)
2. Process
    a. Stage I: vascular stage
       1) Phases
          a) Phase 1: immediate but temporary vasoconstriction caused by trauma to vascular smooth muscle
          b) Phase 2
             i) Warmth, redness, swelling, pain, and loss of function are the five classic symptoms of the inflammatory response.
             ii) Injured tissues and cells secrete chemical mediators (Table 9.2); The predominant effect is vasodilation and increase in capillary permeability, causing warmth, redness, and swelling.
                (a) Healing is enhanced by the increase in mobilization of nutrients to the area.
                (b) Tissue injury is decreased by diluting toxins or microorganisms that enter the area.
                (c) Pain is caused by tissue stretching and release of histamine and prostaglandin.
                (d) Loss of function is caused by tissue swelling and pain.
       2) The major leukocyte in this stage of inflammation is the tissue macrophage.
          a) Response is immediate because the tissue macrophage is already in the tissue.
          b) Granulocyte colony-stimulating factor (G-CSF) is secreted by the macrophage to stimulate the bone marrow to speed up the maturation and release of leukocytes.
          c) Cytokines secreted by the macrophage attract neutrophils to the area of injury or invasion.
    b. Stage II: cellular stage
       1) Major leukocyte in this stage of inflammation is the neutrophil, which attacks and destroys foreign material and removes necrotic tissue.
       2) Thromboxane (procoagulant) and prostacyclins (anticoagulants) act to wall off the site of injury and are part of the inflammatory process.
    c. Stage III: tissue repair and replacement
       1) Initiated at the time of injury
       2) Regeneration: replacement of lost cells with the same type of cells
       3) Repair: replacement of lost cells with connective tissue cells to form scar tissue; some loss of function occurs with the degree of loss dependent on the percentage of previously functional tissue replaced by scar tissue

Immunity

1. Definition: protection of the body against pathogenic organisms or other foreign material; dependent on ability to recognize self from nonself
    a. Self is determined genetically; it is anything synthesized by a person's own particular DNA code.
    b. Nonself describes anything that is different in its chromosome structure and evokes a response from the immune system; antigens are chemical substances (almost always protein) that are viewed by the body as foreign (nonself).

Table 9.2 Chemical Mediators of the Inflammatory Process

Chemical Mediator	Actions
Bradykinin	• Causes vasodilation • Increases capillary permeability • Enhances chemotaxis • Causes pain • Converts plasminogen to plasmin • Produces smooth muscle contraction (e.g., bronchospasm)
Collagenase	• Degrades clots
Complement cascade	• Triggers neutrophil aggregation • Increases capillary permeability • Activates mast cells and basophils
Elastase	• Degrades clots
Endorphin	• Causes vasodilation • Produces analgesia
Fibrinolysin	• Digests fibrin
Histamine	• Causes vasodilation • Increases capillary permeability • Increases heart rate and contractility • Produces bronchospasm • Increases secretion of mucus and gastric acid • Inhibits T cells
Interleukin-1	• Stimulates protein catabolism • Causes fever • Activates lymphocytes • Stimulates fibroblasts
Interleukin-2	• Activates B lymphocytes to make antibodies • Activates macrophages
Leukotriene	• Causes vasoconstriction • Increases capillary permeability • Produces smooth muscle contraction (e.g., bronchospasm)
Lipase	• Degrades fat
Plasminogen	• Degrades clots when activated to plasmin
Prostacyclin	• Causes vasodilation • Inhibits platelet aggregation • Increases capillary permeability
Prostaglandin (PGD_2, PGF_{2a})	• Vasoconstriction • Bronchoconstriction
Prostaglandin (PGE_2, PGI_2)	• Causes vasodilation • Produces smooth muscle relaxation (e.g., bronchodilation) • Promotes platelet aggregation • Increases capillary permeability • Activates lysosomal enzymes • Potentiates leukotrienes • Causes pain
Serotonin	• Causes vasodilation • Increases capillary permeability • Causes pulmonary vasoconstriction • Produces smooth muscle contraction (e.g., bronchospasm)
Thromboxane	• Causes vasoconstriction and endothelial damage • Causes pulmonary vasoconstriction • Acts as a potent platelet aggregator
Tumor necrosis factor	• Causes necrosis of bacteria or tissue • Stimulates muscle catabolism • Induces fever

1) Nonself proteins may be normally pathogenic and warrant an immunologic response (e.g., foreign microbes).
2) Nonself antigens or proteins that are not pathogenic but precipitate an immunologic response include allergens such as animal dander and plant pollens; the response is called a hypersensitivity reaction.
3) When the body perceives an existing body cell as foreign because of surface markers or cellular changes and mounts a response against it, the response is called an autoimmune reaction.
2. Lines of defense are categorized into physical, mechanical, and biochemical barriers.
   a. First: skin and mucous membranes, acid secretions and enzymes, natural immunoglobulins
   b. Second: macrophages and neutrophils (i.e., inflammatory response)
   c. Third: cellular and humoral immunity
3. Innate immunity: body's inherent immune mechanisms; present at birth; does not require prior exposure to antigen for activation
   a. Anatomical: skin and mucous membranes
   b. Chemical
      1) Acid secretions in stomach, vagina, and mouth
      2) Digestive enzymes in the GI tract
      3) Tears and perspiration
      4) Lysosomes
      5) Natural immunoglobulins
      6) Cytokines
      7) Pyrogen (produced by granulocytes to cause an increase in body temperature)
   c. Cellular
      1) Normal bacterial flora: GI tract, vagina, and respiratory tract
      2) Tissue macrophages
      3) Leukocytes and mobile macrophages
      4) Inflammatory process
4. Acquired immunity: immunity developed by the body through the creation of antibodies and formation of T and B memory cells in response to exposure to foreign material (i.e., antigen)
   a. Types
      1) Passive acquired immunity: produced by the injection of antibodies or sensitized lymphocytes
      2) Active acquired immunity: produced by natural exposure to an antigen (e.g., infection) or administration of live attenuated vaccines (e.g., rubella, mumps) that triggers a direct response from the body
   b. Cell-mediated immunity
      1) Particularly effective against viruses, parasites, some fungi, and bacteria harbored inside of cells; responsible for delayed hypersensitivity, transplant rejection, and malignancy surveillance and possibly destruction
      2) Primarily mediated by T cells
      3) Induced and regulated primarily through the production and activity of cytokines
      4) Process

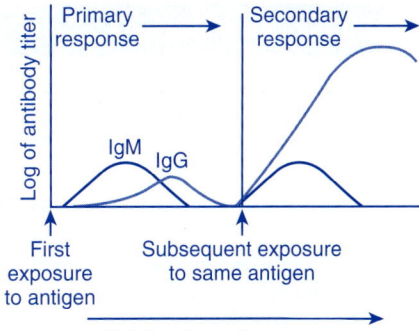

Fig. 9.2 Primary and secondary immune responses. The introduction of antigen induces a response dominated by two classes of immunoglobulins, IgM and IgG. IgM predominates in the primary response, with some IgG appearing later. After the host's immune system is primed, another challenge with the same antigen induces the secondary response, in which some IgM and large amounts of IgG are produced. (From Lewis, S. M., & Dirksen, S. R. [2011]. *Medical-surgical nursing: Assessment and management of clinical problems* [8th ed.]. St. Louis: Mosby.)

   a) The macrophage is the first cell to detect most antigens.
   b) The macrophage processes the antigen and "presents" it to both T and B cells.
   c) T cells recognize the antigen as foreign when it is on the macrophage cell membrane.
   d) The antigen binds with an antigen receptor on the surface of the T cell, sensitizing the T cell.
   e) Sensitized T cells secrete lymphokines, which regulate and coordinate the immune response to combat foreign cells, protect the body against mutant or cancer cells, and destroy foreign tissue; IL-8 is secreted by the macrophage and stimulates T cell division.
   f) T cells are programmed to recognize the body's own tissue (self) from nonself (antigenic); autoimmune diseases are caused when the immune system cannot recognize self, and the body is damaged by the immune system.
   g) NK cells also contribute to cellular immunity, especially in relation to cancer cell surveillance.
   c. Humoral-mediated immunity
      1) Primarily effective against bacteria and viruses
      2) Primarily mediated by B cells
      3) Process (Fig. 9.2)
         a) After being activated, B cells become plasma cells and recognize specific foreign cells or antigens.
         b) Plasma cells make antibodies (also called *immunoglobulins*) (Table 9.3).
            i) Immunoglobulins (antibodies) are plasma proteins that bind to specific antigens; they begin the process that causes lysis or phagocytosis of an offending antigen.

Table 9.3 Immunoglobulins (Igs)

Ig	Actions	Comments
IgG	• Coats microorganisms (primarily bacteria and viruses) to enhance phagocytosis • Activates complement system	• Most abundant Ig (75%–80% of total) • Present in intravascular and extravascular spaces • Crosses the placental barrier and provides natural immunity
IgA	• Protects epithelial surfaces against antigen adhesion and invasion • Protects against entry via the respiratory tract, GU tract, or GI tract • Activates complement system	• Present in many body secretions (e.g., saliva, tears, sweat, mucus, breast milk) • 10%–15% of total
IgM	• Kills bacteria in bloodstream • Activates complement system	• First responder to bacterial or viral invasion • Present mostly in intravascular space • 5%–10% of total Igs
IgD	• Not well understood • May activate B cells	• 1% of total Igs
IgE	• Attaches to mast cells and basophils and causes them to release their contents (e.g., histamine) in response to contact with specific antigens	• Present in serum, interstitial space, and exocrine secretions and on basophils and mast cells • Very small (0.002) percentage of total Igs

GI, Gastrointestinal; *GU,* genitourinary.

   ii) One end of the immunoglobulin (Ig) molecule has a constant fragment with a fixed sequence of amino acids that is constant within the category of the immunoglobulin (e.g., IgG, IgM).
   iii) The other end of the Ig has an antigen-binding fragment with an amino acid sequence specific to the antigen for which it was formed.
  c) The first exposure to an antigen is followed by a latent phase in which no antibody levels are detected.
  d) Primary response follows as serum antibody levels rise rapidly; maximal antibody response takes 3 to 5 days.
  e) Levels plateau and finally decline.
  f) Subsequent exposure to the antigen results in more rapid production of antibodies to that antigen and higher concentrations of the antibody; this is the basis for immunizations and the consequence of increasing severity of allergic reactions.
  g) Inflammation occurs because antigen–antibody complexes (referred to as *immune complexes*) attract WBCs.
 4) Immune complexes activate the complement cascade.
  a) Complement is a group of blood proteins: there are more than 20 of these proteins, but 11 are considered the primary complement elements.
   i) These are labeled C1 to C9, with C1 having three subunits (C1q, C1r, C1s).
   ii) C1 is primarily synthesized by the intestinal epithelium.
   iii) C2 and C4 are produced by macrophages.
   iv) C3, C6, and C9 are synthesized by the liver.
   v) C5 and C8 are synthesized by the spleen.
  b) When activated, they function as mediators to enhance various aspects of inflammatory response; they also do the following:
   i) Attract and stimulate PMNs
   ii) Kill microorganisms by punching holes in their cell membranes, allowing intracellular fluid to leak out; mononuclear phagocytes and monocytes then clear the debris from the bloodstream
   iii) Agglutinate the bacteria
   iv) Activate basophils and mast cells
   v) Complement deficiencies may be congenital or acquired and result in unusual infections and abnormal hypersensitivity reactions.
  c) They may be activated with or without previous exposure to the antigen.
   i) Anaphylactoid reaction: no previous exposure to the antigen; no true antigen–antibody interaction
   ii) Anaphylactic reaction: previous exposure to the antigen; involves antigen–antibody interaction. (A more detailed description of anaphylactoid and anaphylactic reactions is in Chapter 11.)
 d. Hypersensitivity (allergic) reactions
  1) Type I: immediate hypersensitivity reactions ranging from mild reaction with localized response to a severe systemic reaction referred to as *anaphylaxis*
   a) Reaction occurs within minutes (usually 5–20) of exposure to even a miniscule amount of the antigen.
   b) Caused by IgE specific to the antigen; the antigen binds to one end of IgE; IgE is bound to a mast cell or basophil; when the antigen attaches, the mast cell or basophil degranulates and histamine is released; slow-reacting

substance of anaphylaxis (SRS-A) and eosinophil chemotactic factor of anaphylaxis (ECF-A) are also released; eosinophils are recruited to the site
- c) Example: anaphylactic reaction to a penicillin, insect venom, foods, or pollen
2) Type II: cytotoxic hypersensitivity
- a) Reaction is usually within minutes to days.
- b) Caused by the combination of IgG, IgM, or IgA antibody and antigenic receptors on membranes of cells; complement cascade is activated; NK cells are involved in destruction of the immune complex and the cell to which it is attached, and macrophages may phagocytize the immune complexes
- c) Example: mismatched blood transfusion reaction
3) Type III: immune complex–mediated reaction
- a) Reaction is usually within hours.
- b) Caused by large quantities of antigen–antibody (IgG, IgM, or IgA) complexes that cannot be quickly and efficiently cleared by the reticuloendothelial system; complement cascade is activated; neutrophils are activated at the site of deposition; inflammatory process is stimulated, and mediators are released
- c) Example: vasculitis and renal damage caused by immune complexes
- d) The fundamental difference between type II and type III hypersensitivity reactions hinges on where the immune complex occurs. A type II reaction is a tissue-specific reaction, and type III reaction occurs in the vascular system and later migrates into a tissue.
4) Type IV: delayed or cell-mediated hypersensitivity mediated by T lymphocytes without the involvement of antibodies
- a) Reaction is within 1 or more days.
- b) Cause is poorly understood but is presumed to be cells that require time to migrate to the site; probably caused by previously sensitized lymphocytes and lymphokines that activate the inflammatory response at the site
- c) Example: skin testing for tuberculosis (TB), contact dermatitis, and latex allergy

Hemostasis

1. Definition: the termination of bleeding by a complex process that involves integrated interactions among blood vessels, platelets, clotting factors, and the fibrinolytic system
2. Hemostatic mechanisms
   a. Vascular response
      1) Disruption of vascular integrity causes a SNS response, resulting in vasospasm and blood vessel constriction in the injured vessel.
      2) Thromboxane A_2, endothelin, the alpha-adrenergic system, and serotonin are thought to mediate this response.
   b. Platelet aggregation
      1) Thrombocytes (platelets)
         a) Produced in bone marrow
         b) Life span is 9 to 12 days.
         c) Thrombopoiesis
            i) Thrombopoietin (a hormonelike erythropoietin for RBCs) is postulated to stimulate the production and release of thrombocytes.
            ii) Iron is needed for thrombopoiesis.
         d) Thrombocytes are stored in and destroyed by the spleen
      2) Process
         a) Endothelial damage exposes the basement membrane of the subendothelial collagen.
         b) Damaged tissues release chemicals (e.g., thromboplastin) to activate platelets.
         c) Activated platelets swell and develop hairlike projections.
         d) Swelling increases the surface area of the platelets for platelet adhesion and makes platelets more likely to aggregate.
         e) Granules and components necessary for the clotting process are released from the platelets; adenosine diphosphate (ADP) released by degranulation of the platelets enhances adhesiveness and aggregation.
            i) Adhesiveness: stickiness that aids in ability to stick to vessel walls occurs.
               (a) Enhanced by circulating von Willebrand factor (vWF), collagen, and endothelial collagen–specific glycoprotein (GP) Ia/IIb surface receptors.
               (b) Additional GP receptors, such as IIb, IIIa, IV, and V, progress this reaction to aggregation.
            ii) Aggregation: process of platelets adhering or clumping together to form the "platelet plug"
         f) Activated platelets become adhesive and aggregate.
         g) Platelet aggregation becomes large enough to form a platelet plug (sometimes referred to as *a white clot*) that seals the damaged blood vessel.
            i) This platelet plug lasts 2 to 5 hours and dissolves as fibrin clots replace the platelets.
         h) During aggregation of the platelets, platelet factor III (PFIII), an important contributor in the intrinsic pathway, is released.
         i) Platelets contain factor XIII (fibrin-stabilizing factor), essential in the formation of a stable fibrin clot.
      3) Platelet function is affected by qualitative and quantitative factors.
         a) Qualitative changes
            i) Drugs that decrease the ability of the platelets to aggregate
               (a) Alcohol
               (b) Aspirin
               (c) Ticlopidine
               (d) Clopidogrel

(e) GP IIb/IIIa platelet receptor blockers (e.g., abciximab, eptifibatide, tirofiban HCl)
(f) Nonsteroidal antiinflammatory drugs (NSAIDs, e.g., phenylbutazone, ibuprofen)
(g) Quinidine
(h) Dextran 40 (i.e., low-molecular-weight dextran)
(i) Heparin
(j) Aminoglycosides (e.g., gentamicin)
(k) Loop diuretics (e.g., furosemide) and thiazides (e.g., hydrochlorothiazide)
(l) Catecholamines (e.g., epinephrine, norepinephrine, dopamine)
(m) Phenothiazines
(n) Herbs such as ginkgo biloba, Chinese ginseng, chamomile, and ginger
(o) Vitamin E
ii) Disorders that alter platelet quality
(a) Catecholamine release
(b) Diabetes mellitus
(c) Hepatic cirrhosis
(d) Hyperthermia or hypothermia
(e) Malignant lymphomas
(f) Sarcoidosis
(g) Scleroderma
(h) Systemic lupus erythematosus (SLE)
(i) Thyrotoxicosis
b) Quantitative changes
i) Thrombocytopenia: a platelet count of less 150,000 mm^3
(a) Significance
(i) Mild thrombocytopenia: platelet counts greater than 50,000/mm^3 but less than normal; surgery can generally be tolerated
(ii) Moderate thrombocytopenia: platelet counts of 20,000 to 30,000/mm^3; spontaneous bleeding may occur but considered unlikely unless vascular injury occurs
(iii) Severe thrombocytopenia: platelet counts less than 10,000/mm^3; spontaneous intracranial hemorrhages likely; high risk of bleeding without provocation
(b) Causes
(i) Decreased production (e.g., bone marrow depression, vitamin B_{12} or folic acid deficiency, viral illness (e.g., HIV, Epstein-Barr virus [EBV], cytomegalovirus [CMV], rubella), estrogen, metabolic hormones [e.g., thyroxine, cortisol])
(ii) Increased destruction (e.g., idiopathic thrombocytopenic purpura [ITP], disseminated intravascular coagulation [DIC], heat stroke, hypertension, artificial heart valves, large-bore intravenous [IV] catheters [e.g., intraaortic balloon pump], sepsis)
(iii) Hypersplenism (e.g., portal hypertension)
(iv) Heparin-induced thrombocytopenia (HIT)
(v) Dilutional thrombocytopenia: caused by large volumes of fluids that do not contain platelets
ii) Thrombocytosis: a platelet count of greater than 400,000 mm^3
(a) Significance: may cause excessive thrombosis or bleeding, depending on the quality of the platelets
(b) Causes
(i) Malignancy (bone marrow)
(ii) Granulomatous disease
(iii) Polycythemia vera
(iv) Leukemia
(v) Postsplenectomy
(vi) Rheumatoid arthritis (RA)
(vii) Trauma
(viii) Vitamin E deficiency
(ix) Increased production of certain cytokines (IL-6 and IL-11)
c. Coagulation
1) Dependent on presence of clotting factors, active ionized calcium, and functioning of the pathways
2) Blood coagulation factors (Table 9.4)
a) Consist of proteins, lipoproteins, and calcium, which is critical in the intrinsic, extrinsic, and common pathways
b) Circulate as inactive; activated in a cascade fashion
3) Clotting pathways (Fig. 9.3)
a) Pathways are cascades in which one action is dependent upon a preceding action or interaction.
b) A fibrin clot may be produced through activation of either the intrinsic or extrinsic pathway, although the factor VII–initiated extrinsic pathway is a more potent and significant initiator of clotting.
i) Intrinsic pathway
(a) Initiated by damage to RBCs or platelets
(b) Time from activation through intrinsic pathway and common pathway to a clot: 2 to 6 minutes
(c) Tested by activated partial thromboplastin time (aPTT) or factor Xa level

Table 9.4 Blood Coagulation Factors

Factor*	Name(s)	Comments
I	Fibrinogen	• Synthesized in liver • Precursor to fibrin (Ia)
Ia	Fibrin	• Activated fibrinogen (I) becomes fibrin (Ia)
II	Prothrombin	• Synthesized in liver • Vitamin K dependent • Precursor to thrombin (IIa) • Activates fibrinogen, factors V, VII, VIII, XI, XIII, protein C, and platelets
IIa	Thrombin	• Activated prothrombin becomes thrombin
III	Tissue thromboplastin Tissue factor	• First factor of extrinsic pathway
IV	Calcium	• Acts as an enzyme cofactor for most of the activation steps in intrinsic, extrinsic, and common pathways
V	Proaccelerin Labile factor Ac globulin	• Synthesized in liver • Combines with Xa and phospholipid to accelerate conversion of prothrombin (II) to thrombin (IIa)
VI	There is no designated factor VI	
VII	Proconvertin Stable factor	• Synthesized in liver • Vitamin K dependent • Part of extrinsic pathway • Complexes with tissue thromboplastin (III) to activate X
VIII	Antihemophiliac factor A	• Part of intrinsic pathway • Complexes with IXa and platelet phospholipid to activate X
IX	Plasma thromboplastin component Christmas factor Antihemophiliac factor B	• Synthesized in liver • Vitamin K dependent • Associated with factors VIII, XI, and XII in the intrinsic pathway
X	Stuart-Prower factor	• Synthesized in liver • Vitamin K dependent • Part of intrinsic and extrinsic pathways • Complexes with V and phospholipid to accelerate prothrombin (II) conversion
XI	Plasma thromboplastin antecedent	• May be synthesized in liver • May be vitamin K dependent • Part of intrinsic pathway • Associated with factors VIII, IX, and XII in the intrinsic pathway
XII	Hageman factor Contact factor	• First factor in intrinsic factor • Indirectly activates plasmin and complement cascades
XIII	Fibrin-stabilizing factor Fibrinase Laki-Lorand factor	• May be synthesized in liver • Activated by thrombin (IIa) • Produces a stronger, insoluble clot; stabilizes clot formation

*"a" after the factor indicates an activated factor.

    ii) Extrinsic pathway
       (a) Initiated by injured tissue and subsequent release of tissue thromboplastin
       (b) Time from activation through extrinsic pathway and common pathway to a clot: as short as 15 to 20 seconds
       (c) Tested by prothrombin time (PT)
  c) Common pathway
    i) Platelet factor III and tissue thromboplastin combine to become a prothrombin activator.
    ii) Prothrombin is converted to thrombin.
    iii) Fibrinogen is converted to fibrin.
    iv) Fibrin clot is formed.
    v) Pathway is tested by aPTT, factor Xa levels, PT, fibrinogen level, and thrombin time.
  d) Other prothrombotic mechanisms
    i) Inflammation triggers thromboxane.
    ii) Cancer procoagulants, such as cancer procoagulant (CP), or heat shock proteins (HSPs) enhance coagulability.
  d. Anticoagulant mechanisms in normal system
    1) Fibrinolytic system (Fig. 9.4)

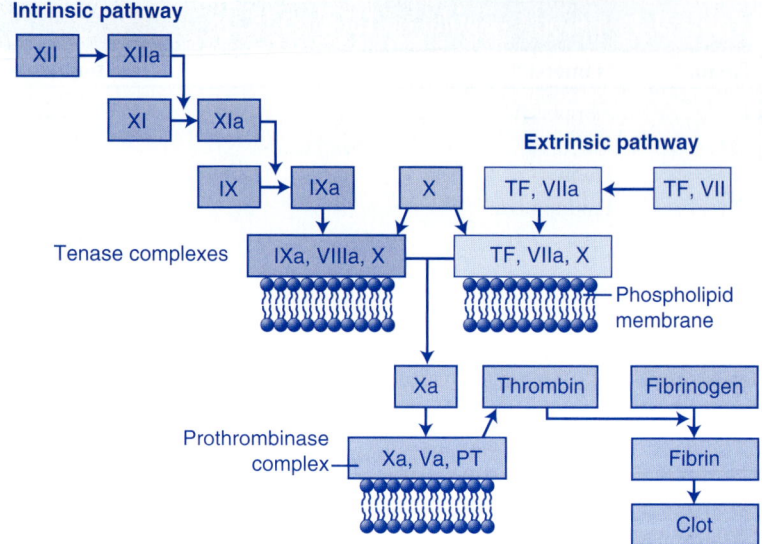

Fig. 9.3 The clotting pathways. (McCance, K. L., & Huether, S. E. [2014] *Pathophysiology. The biologic basis for disease in adults and children* [7th ed.]. St. Louis: Elsevier Mosby.)

a) Activated clotting factors are cleared by the reticuloendothelial system.
b) Clot-lysing activities maintain blood in fluid state.
   i) Process of clot breakdown takes approximately 7 to 10 days.
   ii) Blood (intrinsic pathway) or tissue (extrinsic pathway) plasminogen activators activate plasminogen to plasmin; therefore, after a clot has developed, steps are initiated to eliminate it.
   iii) Plasmin works to lyse fibrin clots producing fibrin degradation products (FDPs) (also referred to as *fibrin split products [FSPs]*) and elevation in D-dimer; FDPs have anticoagulant properties, and increased amounts of FDPs enhance potential for patients to bleed.
   iv) Fibrinolytics speed up this process by either directly providing tissue plasminogen activator (e.g., alteplase, reteplase) or tenecteplase or by triggering the process by adding a complex to cause the activation of the fibrinolytic system (i.e., streptokinase).
c) Controls of fibrinolysis
   i) Plasminogen activator inhibitor type 1 (PAI-1) inactivates tissue plasminogen activator.
   ii) Alpha$_2$-antiplasmin is an inhibitor of plasmin.
   iii) Antithrombin (AT) is a serum protease that degrades specific coagulation factors IXa, Xa, and XIIa.
2) AT system
   a) Defends against excessive clotting
   b) Release of ATIII from mast cells
   c) Neutralizes the clotting capability of thrombin
   d) Extrinsic infusion of ATIII (i.e., ASA, clopidogrel, cilostazol, abciximab)can provide anticoagulant effects.

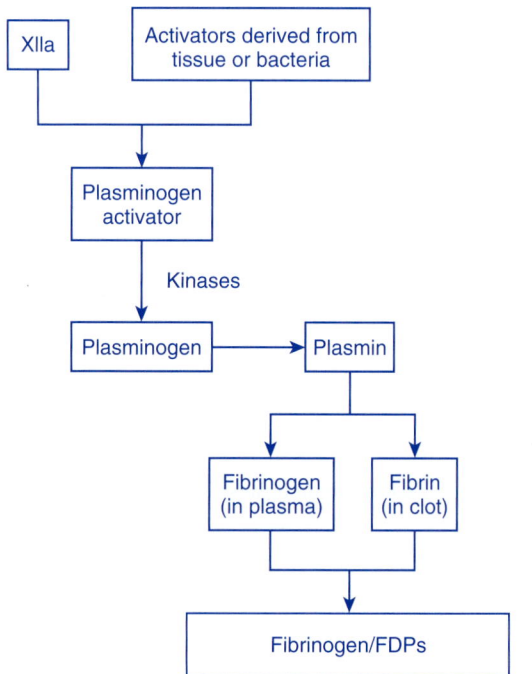

Fig. 9.4 The fibrinolytic process. *FDP*, Fibrin degradation product (From Lewis, S. M. & Dirksen, S. R. [2011]. *Medical-surgical nursing: Assessment and management of clinical problems* [8th ed.]. St. Louis: Mosby.)

e. Regulators of coagulation
   1) Calcium is required for activation of factors.
   2) Tissue factor pathway inhibitor (TFPI) inhibits excessive tissue factor activity.
   3) Protein C and thrombomodulin enhance degradation; absence leads to thrombophilia and excess clotting.
   4) ATIII degradation is affected by intrinsic or extrinsic administration of heparins.
   5) Plasmin cleaved by tissue plasminogen activator (t-Pa)
   6) Prostacyclin (PGI$_2$) released by damaged endothelium or extrinsic administration inhibits platelet aggregation.

Table 9.5 ABO Blood Groups

Patient's ABO Group	Percentage of Population	Antigen on RBC	Antibodies in Plasma	Compatible RBCs	Compatible Plasma
O	47	None	Anti-A, anti-B	O	O, A, B, AB
A	41	A	Anti-B	O, A	A, AB
B	9	B	Anti-A	O, B	B, AB
AB	3	A and B	None	O, A, B, AB	AB

RBC, Red blood cell.

Blood Groups

1. Three systems describe the most important antigens on RBCs, tissues, and other cells.
    a. ABO system (Table 9.5)
        1) This system is concerned with antigens on the RBC that are designated A and B; the presence of these antigens is genetically controlled.
        2) Blood type is named for the antigen that is present on the RBC.
        3) Antibodies are present in the plasma for the antigen or antigens that are not present (e.g., B antibodies are found in group A blood because B antigens are absent).
            a) Blood that contains both A and B antigens is termed *type AB blood*.
            b) Blood that contains neither A nor B antigens is termed *type O blood*.
        4) Agglutination that occurs in mismatched blood is the basis for typing and crossmatching.
            a) Blood typing detects the major antigens: A, B, and Rh.
            b) Crossmatching detects the presence of major or minor RBC antigens in donor blood that can lead to reactions for a specific recipient.
    b. Rh system (Table 9.6)
        1) This system is concerned with a series of six common types of Rh antigens, each called an Rh factor.
        2) Each person has one of each of three pairs, so they have three of these Rh factors designated c, C, d, D, e, and E.
        3) Only C, D, and E are antigenic enough to cause significant development of anti-Rh antibodies (and therefore to potentially cause blood transfusion reaction if nonmatched blood is administered).
        4) If C, D, or E antigens are present, the person is Rh+; if none of these three antigens is present, the person is Rh−; most (85%) of Americans are Rh+.
        5) Rh antibodies do not develop spontaneously; they only occur after exposure to Rh antigen (e.g., second exposure to non–Rh-matched blood or Rh− mothers pregnant with the second Rh+ fetus if anti-Rh globin [Rho-gam] was not given); delayed transfusion reactions can occur even after the first exposure to Rh+ blood and cause a mild transfusion reaction.

Table 9.6 Rh Compatibility

Patient's Rh Type	RBC Rh Type for Transfusion	Plasma Rh Type for Transfusion
Positive	Positive or negative	Positive or negative
Negative	Negative	Positive or negative

   c. Other RBC antigens
        1) Cold agglutinins
            a) These are antibodies that cause erythrocytes to coagulate when blood plasma temperature is below normal body temperature (below 31°C).
            b) Banked blood must be warmed to normal body temperature (37°C) before giving the blood to a patient who has cold agglutinins.
            c) Cold agglutinins more commonly occur in nonwhites, older adults, patients with autoimmune disease, or after viral infection; may be a temporary or permanent condition occurs mostly in the winter.
        2) Coombs test: used to determine presence of hemolyzing antibodies
            a) Direct: detects antibodies attached to RBCs
            b) Indirect: detects antibodies in serum
        3) Other RBC antigens include Kell (third most common), Duffy, and Kidd.
    d. Uncrossmatched type O negative packed RBCs may be used safely in exsanguinating patients.
        1) Whole blood is avoided to decrease the risk of reaction caused by anti-A and anti-B antibodies in type O plasma.
        2) Blood antigen–antibody complexes may complicate later crossmatching and may cause future blood transfusion reaction to own blood type unless it is O negative.
        3) Type-specific blood may be preferable, and type matching takes only 5 to 15 minutes.
    e. Human leukocyte antigen (HLA)
        1) Concerned with a group of antigenic substances found on many cell types (including WBCs and platelets but not on erythrocytes)
        2) Detected serologically by cytotoxicity assays; HLA-A, HLA-B, HLA-C are found on all nucleated cells, but HLA-D and HLA-DR antigens are only located on B lymphocytes, monocytes, epidermal, and endothelial cells.
        3) Very important in organ and tissue transplantation histocompatibility

Assessment of the Hematologic and Immunologic Systems

Interview
1. Chief complaint: why the patient is seeking help and duration of the problem
    a. Symptoms that may be related to hematologic or immunologic conditions
        1) General
            a) Fatigue
            b) Weakness
            c) Chills
            d) Fever
            e) Weight loss
            f) Night sweats
            g) Apathy
            h) Lethargy
            i) Malaise
            j) Abnormal bleeding, bruising, or swelling
            k) Chronic or recurrent infections
            l) Poor wound healing
            m) Enlarged or tender lymph nodes
            n) Blood in urine
            o) Craving for ice (pica)
        2) Specific
            a) Skin
                i) Dry, coarse skin
                ii) Bruising or bleeding
                    (a) Mucosal bleeding: oral, GI, urogenital
                    (b) Prolonged bleeding
                    (c) Petechiae
                    (d) Bruising easily
                iii) Color changes
                    (a) Jaundice
                    (b) Pallor
                    (c) Cyanosis
                iv) Rash
                v) Pruritus
                vi) Lesions
                vii) Wounds: poor healing
                viii) Inflammation
            b) Eyes
                i) Visual disturbances (e.g., blurring, diplopia)
                ii) Blindness related to retinal hemorrhage
                iii) Conjunctival pallor or inflammation
                iv) Scleral hemorrhage
            c) Ears
                i) Vertigo
                ii) Tinnitus
            d) Nasopharynx and mouth
                i) Epistaxis
                ii) Dysphagia
                iii) Gingival bleeding
                iv) Painful lesions on mouth and lips
                v) Sore or red, beefy tongue
                vi) Sore throat
                vii) Persistent hoarseness
                viii) Cracks in corners of mouth (i.e., angular cheilitis)
            e) Neck: nuchal rigidity
            f) Lymph nodes
                i) Swelling greater than 2 cm for longer than 2 weeks
                ii) Tenderness
                iii) Irregular and immovable
            g) Cardiovascular
                i) Chest pain
                ii) Sternal tenderness
                iii) Palpitations
                iv) Known murmurs
            h) Pulmonary
                i) Exertional dyspnea
                ii) Cough
                iii) Sputum
                iv) Orthopnea
                v) Respiratory tract infections
                vi) Hemoptysis
            i) GI
                i) Anorexia
                ii) Abdominal pain and cramping
                iii) Abdominal fullness
                iv) Eructation
                v) Bloody or black stools
                vi) Vomiting of blood or coffee-ground material
                vii) Ulcers: oral, esophageal, gastric
                viii) Change in bowel habits
                    (a) Diarrhea
                    (b) Constipation
                ix) Rectal pain or bleeding
            j) GU
                i) Hematuria
                ii) Pyuria
                iii) Abnormal menstrual flow: menorrhagia, amenorrhea
                iv) Incontinence, dysuria, hesitancy, frequency
                v) Urinary retention
                vi) Pelvic or flank pain
            k) Neurologic
                i) Change in level of consciousness
                ii) Confusion
                iii) Irritability
                iv) Memory loss
                v) Headache
                vi) Ataxia
                vii) Sensory changes: paresthesia, anesthesia
                viii) Syncope, vertigo
            l) Back and extremities
                i) Pain or tenderness in joints, back, shoulder, or bone
                ii) Joint stiffness or swelling
                iii) Muscle weakness
2. Past medical history
    a. Surgical history
        1) Splenectomy
        2) Thymectomy
        3) Tonsillectomy
        4) Tumor removal
        5) Total or partial gastrectomy

6) Surgical excision of duodenum
7) Organ or tissue transplant
8) Prosthetic heart valves
9) Response to dental extractions (e.g., excessive bleeding)
   b. Medical problems
      1) Anemia
      2) Asthma
      3) Autoimmune disease (e.g., lupus erythematosus)
      4) Deep vein thrombosis (DVT) or pulmonary embolus (PE)
      5) Diabetes mellitus
      6) Human immunodeficiency virus (HIV) or acquired immunodeficiency syndrome (AIDS)
      7) Liver disease
      8) Malabsorption syndrome
      9) Malignancy, especially leukemia, lymphoma, multiple myeloma
      10) Mononucleosis
      11) Problems with wound healing
      12) Prolonged or excessive bleeding (e.g., after dental procedures, injury, or surgery)
      13) Radiation therapy
      14) Recent viral illness exposures or symptoms (e.g., exposure to children with Coxsackie virus, EBV)
      15) Recurrent infections
      16) Renal failure
      17) Sexually transmitted disease
      18) Spleen disorders
      19) Vitamin K deficiency
   c. Allergies
      1) Known allergies and type of reaction
         a) Inhalants
         b) Contactants
         c) Injectables
         d) Ingestibles
      2) Transfusion with blood or blood products and reactions
   d. Immunizations: types, dates, any adverse reactions
3. Family history
   a. Congenital immune deficiency
   b. Congenital bleeding disorder (e.g., hemophilia)
   c. Congenital RBC dyscrasias (e.g., sickle cell disease)
   d. Congenital anemia (e.g., thalassemia)
   e. Asthma
   f. Allergies
   g. Anemia
   h. Jaundice
   i. Malignancies
   j. Autoimmune disease (e.g., SLE, RA)
4. Social history
   a. Relationship with spouse or significant other; family structure
   b. Occupation
      1) Occupational exposure to radiation
      2) Occupational exposure to chemicals (e.g., lead, benzene, ethylene oxide, insecticides, vinyl chloride)
      3) Military service; exposure to toxins
   c. Educational level
   d. Stress level and usual coping mechanisms; lifestyle changes
   e. Recreational habits
   f. Exercise habits
   g. Dietary habits; dietary deficiency: iron, folic acid, vitamin B_{12}
   h. Caffeine intake
   i. Tobacco use: record as pack-years (number of packs per day times the number of years the patient has been smoking)
   j. Alcohol use: record as alcoholic beverages consumed per month, week, or day
   k. Recent foreign travel
   l. Sexuality
      1) Safe sex practices
      2) Sexual preference: heterosexual; homosexual; bisexual
      3) Multiple sexual partners
      4) Sexual activity with prostitutes, homosexuals, or bisexuals
5. Medication history
   a. Agents used to treat existing hematologic conditions
      1) Drugs used for erythropoiesis: iron, vitamin B_{12}, pyridoxine, folic acid, recombinant human erythropoietin
      2) Drugs used for bleeding or clotting disorders: ASA, NSAIDs, aminocaproic acid, cryoprecipitate, anticoagulants
      3) Antineoplastic agents for cancer or autoimmune disease
      4) Antiviral agents
      5) Antiretroviral medications
      6) Drugs to augment the immune system (e.g., interferon, IL-2, and colony-stimulating factors)
      7) Antibody preparations targeting autoimmune disorders (e.g., infliximab for Crohn disease, rituximab for RA)
   b. Agents that may exert a negative effect on the hematologic or immunologic system
      1) Allergy medication
      2) Analgesics
         a) Acetaminophen: may decrease platelets; may cause hemolytic anemia
         b) Antiinflammatory agents
            i) Antigout drugs (e.g., colchicine): may cause aplastic anemia
            ii) ASA: inhibits platelet aggregation; decreases macrophage activity
            iii) Corticosteroids (e.g., prednisone): suppresses the immune and inflammatory process
            iv) Nonsteroidal (e.g., phenylbutazone, ibuprofen): inhibits platelet aggregation; depresses bone marrow and may cause aplastic anemia; lyse T, B, and NK cells; inhibits interferon production; inhibits IL-1 and IL-2 production
         c) Opiates
            i) Heroin: may decrease platelets
            ii) Morphine sulfate: may decrease platelets
      3) Antibiotics
         a) Oral antibiotics: may kill vitamin K–producing bacteria in the GI tract

b) All antibiotics may cause opportunistic infections by altering normal flora in GI tract, mouth, vagina, and so on; *Clostridium difficile* is an example frequently seen in critical care units that causes severe diarrhea.
   c) Tetracyclines: inhibit chemotaxis; inhibit activation of the lymphocytes
   d) Sulfonamides (including trimethoprim sulfamethoxazole): inhibit chemotaxis; inhibit activation of the lymphocytes; may cause aplastic anemia; may decrease platelets
   e) Chloramphenicol: depresses WBC production; may cause aplastic anemia
   f) Penicillin: may decrease platelets
   g) Rifampicin: may decrease platelets
 4) Anticonvulsants
   a) Phenytoin: inhibits the effects of corticosteroids; may cause lymph node hyperplasia; may cause anemia or thrombocytopenia
   b) Phenobarbital: may cause aplastic anemia
 5) Antidysrhythmics
   a) Procainamide: may cause hemolytic anemia, thrombocytopenia; decreases production of WBCs
   b) Quinidine: may cause hemolytic anemia, thrombocytopenia
   c) Propranolol: inhibits platelet aggregation
 6) Antifungals
   a) Amphotericin B: may cause anemia or thrombocytopenia
 7) Antihypertensives
   a) Captopril: may cause pancytopenia
   b) Methyldopa: may cause thrombocytopenia, anemia
 8) Antituberculins (e.g., para-aminosalicylic acid, isoniazid [INH])
 9) Diuretics
   a) Chlorothiazide: may cause anemia or thrombocytopenia
   b) Furosemide: may cause anemia or thrombocytopenia
 10) Heparin: may decrease platelets
 11) Histamine receptor antagonists (e.g., ranitidine): may decrease platelets
 12) Immunosuppressives
 13) Oral contraceptives and diethylstilbestrol: Estrogen products cause anemia.
 14) Oral hypoglycemic agents (e.g., chlorpropamide) may cause anemia or thrombocytopenia.
 15) Sympathomimetics (e.g., epinephrine): decrease chemotaxis; decrease WBC production and response to antigens; alter antibody production
 16) Anesthetic agents (e.g., halothane, nitrous oxide, cyclopropane): decrease phagocytosis and inhibit T cell function
c. Nonprescribed drug use
 1) Over-the-counter drugs
 2) Vitamins, minerals, and herbs
 3) Substance abuse: injectable drug use, especially if needles are shared
   a) IV drug use
   b) Intramuscular steroid use
   c) Intradermal "poppers"

Physical Examination
1. Vital signs
   a. Weight: weight loss
   b. Heart rate: tachycardia frequently seen with anemia, blood loss, or infection
   c. Blood pressure: hypotension seen with blood loss
   d. Temperature
     1) Hyperthermia frequently seen with infection but less likely to be seen in older adults
     2) Hypothermia frequently seen with anemia
2. Inspection
   a. Skin and appendages
     1) Color
       a) Pallor or flushing of mucous membranes and palmar creases
       b) Pallor of conjunctivae
       c) Cyanosis
       d) Jaundice
       e) Signs of inflammation
     2) Bleeding
       a) Petechiae
       b) Ecchymosis
       c) Purpura
       d) Mucous membrane bleeding
       e) Gingival bleeding
       f) Retinal hemorrhages
       g) Hemorrhage from orifices
       h) Blood in stool, urine, sputum
       i) Cold or ashen palms
     3) Moisture
       a) Dry, rough skin (i.e., xeroderma)
       b) Moisture-related skin breakdown may occur at skin folds (e.g., axillae, groin, perineal areas); fungal infections are common in these areas.
     4) Lesions and wounds
       a) Rash
       b) Excoriated skin
       c) Leg ulcers
       d) IV catheter insertion site: erythema or inflammation
       e) Chest tube insertion site: erythema or inflammation
       f) Surgical or traumatic wounds: erythema, inflammation, or poor wound healing
       g) Orthopedic devices
       h) Drains
     5) Pitting edema of extremities
     6) Hair: alopecia
     7) Nail and nailbed
       a) Pallor of nailbeds
       b) Spoon nails
       c) Clubbing
       d) Slow capillary refill (longer than 3 seconds)
   b. Mouth
     1) Dryness of the mouth (i.e., xerostomia)
     2) Gingival and mucosal ulceration
     3) Swollen, reddened, bleeding gums
     4) Red, beefy tongue

5) White coating on tongue (e.g., candidiasis, also called *thrush*)
6) White, irregular lesions on lateral surfaces of tongue (oral hairy leukoplakia frequently seen in HIV-positive patients)
7) Purplish lesions on tongue
  c. GI: nasogastric (NG) tube drainage
  d. Neuromuscular
   1) Decreased level of consciousness
   2) Pupil changes
   3) Decreased sensation
   4) Muscle weakness
3. Palpation
  a. Pulse amplitude
  b. Enlargement or tenderness of superficial lymph nodes
   1) Symptoms of benign or inflammatory lymph nodes include association with pain, movability, and regular borders.
   2) Malignant lymph nodes characterized by irregular shape, lack of movability, decreased discomfort
  c. Tenderness during sternal or rib palpation
  d. Tenderness during abdominal palpation
  e. Hepatomegaly
  f. Splenomegaly
4. Percussion
  a. Decreased deep tendon reflexes
  b. Diaphragmatic excursion
  c. Hepatomegaly
  d. Splenomegaly
5. Auscultation
  a. Cardiovascular
   1) Dysrhythmia
   2) S_3
   3) S_4
   4) Murmur
   5) Rub
   6) Bruits over carotids, aorta, and renal artery
  b. Pulmonary
   1) Crackles
   2) Pleural rub
  c. Abdomen
   1) Bowel sounds
   2) Peritoneal friction rub

Diagnostic Studies

1. Blood
  a. Hematology
   1) RBC: normal 4.7 to 6.1 × 10^6/ml for men; 4.2 to 5.4 × 10^6/ml for women
    a) Quantity
     i) Elevated in dehydration, chronic hypoxemia, and high altitudes; may temporarily increase after a cold shower or with intense emotions
     ii) Decreased in bone marrow suppression, hemorrhage, anemias, leukemias, or pregnancy
    b) Quality
     i) Size
      (a) Microcytic: RBCs too small
      (b) Macrocytic: RBCs too large
     ii) Color
      (a) Hypochromic: Hgb concentration too low
      (b) Hyperchromic: Hgb concentration too high
     iii) Types of anemia
      (a) Macrocytic, normochromic: pernicious anemia, folate deficiency
      (b) Microcytic, hypochromic: iron deficiency anemia
      (c) Normocytic, normochromic: aplastic anemia, posthemorrhagic anemia, hemolytic anemia, sickle cell anemia, and anemia of chronic illness; note that the RBCs are normal size and color, but the numbers are insufficient
   2) Reticulocyte count: normal 0.5% to 2% of RBC
    a) Immature RBCs
    b) Assesses the responsiveness and potential of the bone marrow to respond to bleeding or hemolysis
   3) Erythrocyte sedimentation rate (ESR or sed rate): normal 1 to 13 mm/hr for men; 1 to 20 mm/hr for women
    a) Nonspecific test; measures the amount of RBCs that settle in 1 hour
    b) Elevated in inflammatory processes (e.g., RA, malignancy, rheumatic fever, hemolytic anemia, thyroid disorders, autoimmune disorders, nephrotic syndrome)
    c) Decreased in polycythemia vera; hypofibrinogenemia; sickle cell anemia (not crisis); heart failure
    d) May be used to monitor trends in patients with chronic inflammatory diseases undergoing treatment
   4) Hgb: normal 14 to 18 g/dl for men; 12 to 16 g/dl for women
    a) Elevated in polycythemia, which may occur in chronic hypoxia or high altitudes; dehydration
    b) Decreased in anemia, hemorrhage
   5) Hct: normal 42% to 52% for men; 37% to 47% for women
    a) Elevated in dehydration and polycythemia
    b) Decreased with anemia, leukemia, or with normal Hgb and water overload
   6) RBC indices
    a) Mean corpuscular volume (MCV) (an average of size): normal 80 to 96 fl
     i) Decreased in iron deficiency, pernicious anemia
     ii) Increased in folic acid deficiency, high reticulocyte count
    b) Mean corpuscular Hgb (MCH) (an average of weight of Hgb in an RBC): normal 27 to 31 pg
     i) Decreased in iron deficiency, sickle cell anemia

ii) Increased in polycythemia
c) Mean corpuscular Hgb concentration (MCHC): normal 32 to 36 g/dl
7) Peripheral smear: evaluation of blood cell size, shape, and composition to provide insight but not confirmation of medical disorders
   a) Heinz bodies common with hemolytic anemia and portal hypertension
   b) Schistocytes present with DIC
   c) Spherocytes occur after massive transfusion.
   d) Target cells present with iron deficiency or liver disease.
8) WBCs: 4000 to 11,000/mm^3
   a) Elevated in inflammation, infection, trauma, surgery, acute leukemia, and stress
   b) Decreased in bone marrow depression (e.g., aplastic anemia, agranulocytosis, chronic leukemia, sepsis, chronic illness, autoimmune disorders)
9) Differential (segmented)
   a) Neutrophils: normal 55% to 70%
      i) Elevated in infection, inflammatory processes, malignancy, trauma, hemorrhage, burns, tissue necrosis (e.g., myocardial infarction [MI]), and ketoacidosis
      ii) Decreased in overwhelming infection; bone marrow depression; vitamin B_{12} or folic acid deficiency; and hypersplenism
      iii) Presence of excessive bands rather than mature neutrophils signifies bacterial infection (termed a *left shift*).
      iv) Presence of grossly immature or malformed cells, called *blasts*, are indicative of leukemia.
   b) Eosinophils: normal 1% to 4%
      i) Elevated in:
         (a) Allergic conditions
            (i) Asthma
            (ii) Eczema
         (b) Eosinophilic leukemia
         (c) Autoimmune disorders
         (d) Parasitic infection, especially helminthic infections
      ii) Decreased in:
         (a) Adrenocortical stimulation
         (b) Stress
   c) Basophils: 0.5% to 1%
      i) Elevated in myeloproliferative disease (e.g., myelofibrosis, polycythemia rubra vera), leukemia, uremia
      ii) Decreased in acute allergic reactions, hyperthyroidism, and stress reaction
   d) Monocytes: 2% to 8%
      i) Elevated in chronic inflammatory conditions, viral infections, TB, ulcerative colitis, and parasites
      ii) Decreased in aplastic anemia, hairy-cell leukemia, and drug therapy (prednisone)
   e) Lymphocytes: 20% to 40%
      i) Elevated in chronic bacterial infection, viral infection (e.g., mumps, rubella), lymphocytic leukemia, and multiple myeloma
      ii) Decreased in leukemia, sepsis, immunodeficiency diseases, and SLE
      iii) Lymphocyte assays (Table 9.7)
         (a) T cells
         (b) B cells
         (c) NK cells
   f) Changes in differential
      i) Shift to the left: increased percentage of bands (i.e., immature neutrophils); seen in bacterial infection
      ii) Shift to the right: increased percentage of segs (i.e., segmented neutrophils); seen in inflammation, pernicious anemia, viral illness, and hepatic disease
      iii) Regenerative shift (shift to the left): elevated WBC with increased percentage of bands; indicative of stimulation of bone marrow
      iv) Degenerative shift: decreased WBC with increased percentage of bands; indicative of bone marrow depression
10) Platelets: normal 150,000 to 400,000/mm^3; decreased in SLE, HIV infection, ITP, sepsis, and DIC
    a) 50,000 to 100,000/mm^3: prolonged bleeding times, increased risk of bleeding after severe trauma or surgery
    b) Below 50,000/mm^3: increased risk of bleeding after minor trauma
    c) Below 20,000/mm^3: risk of spontaneous bleeding, including intracranial bleeding
11) Special hematology
    a) Erythropoietin level: normal greater than 5 to 35 IU/l
       i) Increased in anemia, chemotherapy, AIDS, and renal cell carcinoma
       ii) Decreased in polycythemia vera or chronic kidney disease
    b) Ferritin level: normal 12 to 300 ng/ml for men; 10 to 150 ng/ml for women
       i) Iron precursor that demonstrates iron stores and ability to make new RBCs

Table 9.7	Lymphocyte Assays
Lymphocyte Type	**Percentage of Lymphocytes**
Total T cells	60–95
CD4 (helper T cells)	60–75
CD8 (suppressor T cells)	25–30
CD4/CD8 (helper/suppressor ratio)	>1
Total B cells	4–25

ii) Increased in hemochromatosis, hemosiderosis, megaloblastic anemia, hemolytic anemia, alcoholic or inflammatory hepatocellular disease, inflammatory disease, advanced cancers, chronic illnesses (e.g., leukemias, cirrhosis, chronic hepatitis), collagen vascular diseases, hemophagocytic syndromes, and congenital and acquired sideroblastic anemias
iii) Decreased in severe protein deficiency, iron deficiency anemia, and hemodialysis
c) Iron level: normal 80 to 180 mcg/dl for men; 60 to 160 mcg/dl for women; reflects total iron but not ability to create new iron, so this test is only used for iron evaluation in conjunction with ferritin level and iron-binding capacity or transferrin saturation
d) Total iron-binding capacity (TIBC): normal 250 to 460 mcg/dl
   i) Reflects iron binding to Hgb
   ii) Decreased with abnormal Hgb or anemia
e) Transferrin saturation: normal greater than 20%; provides an indication of available iron
f) Haptoglobin levels: normal 50 to 220 mg/dl in a fasting state; decreased in hemolytic anemias
g) Hgb variant or fetal Hgb: normal less than 1% of RBCs; used to detect or monitor the level of hemolysis in sickle cell disease

b. Clotting profile
  1) PT: normal 11 to 12.5 seconds; assesses extrinsic coagulation pathway and the common pathway
     a) International normalized ratio (INR): therapeutic INR is usually 2 to 3 but may be higher, depending on indications for anticoagulant therapy
        i) Mathematical calculation that accounts for the differences in sensitivity between reagents; standardizes PT values
  2) aPTT: normal 30 to 40 seconds; assesses intrinsic coagulation pathway and the common pathway
  3) Activated clotting time (ACT): therapeutic ACT during procedures that require anticoagulation (e.g., percutaneous coronary intervention [PCI]) is usually 300 to 350 seconds
     a) Bedside test used to monitor heparin-induced anticoagulation
     b) Sheath removal is generally delayed until ACT is less than 150 seconds.
  4) Thrombin time: normal 10 to 15 seconds; assesses time for thrombin to convert fibrinogen to a fibrin clot
     a) Used for monitoring fibrinolytic therapy (e.g., recombinant plasminogen activator [r-PA], recombinant tissue plasminogen activator [rt-PA])
     b) Highly sensitive to minimal exposure to anticoagulants and thus used for trending value rather than precise medication dose adjustment
  5) Bleeding time: normal 1 to 4 minutes; assesses platelet function
  6) Lee White clotting time: normal 6 to 12 minutes; rarely used nonspecific test for clotting abnormalities
  7) Fibrinogen level: normal 200 to 400 mg/dl
     a) Elevated in hypercoagulable states and inflammatory conditions; commonly increased in lymphoma, acute leukemia, and autoimmune diseases
     b) Decreased in hypocoagulable states with propensity to bleed
     c) Chronic liver disease may cause increased or decreased levels
  8) FDPs (also referred to as *fibrin split products [FSPs]*): normal 0 to 10 mcg/dl
     a) Elevated in excessive fibrinolysis (e.g., DIC)
  9) D-dimer: normal less than 250 ng/ml; elevated in DIC
     a) Differentiates DIC from abnormal fibrinogen produced by a failing liver
     b) Used to detect PE in some patients without factors that falsely increase D-dimer such as recent surgery, solid malignancies, autoimmune disease, and heart failure
 10) Specific factor assays: measure amounts of each factor in the blood
     a) ATIII levels: normal greater than 50% of control; decreased in clotting disorders such as DIC
     b) Protein C levels: normal 70% to 150% of normal activity; decreased by heparin, DIC, liver disease
     c) Protein S levels: normal 60% to 130% of normal activity; decreased by heparin, DIC, liver disease

c. Serum proteins
  1) Total protein: normal 6.4 to 8.3 g/dl
  2) Albumin: normal 3.5 to 5 g/dl
  3) C-reactive protein: normal less than 0.8 mg/dl; nonspecific test for evaluating the severity and course of inflammatory conditions and bacterial disease
  4) Serum protein electrophoresis: immunoglobulin analysis (Table 9.8)
  5) Complement assay
     a) Components
        i) Total complement: normal 35 to 75 units/ml
        ii) C3: normal 75 to 175 mg/dl
        iii) C4: normal 22 to 45 units/ml
     b) Decreased total complement levels occurs in the following:
        i) SLE
        ii) Glomerulonephritis
        iii) Acute serum sickness
        iv) Cirrhosis
        v) Malnutrition
        vi) Severe immunodeficiency
        vii) Acute renal transplant rejection
        viii) *Neisseria* infections

Table 9.8 Immunoglobulin Analysis

Immunoglobulin	Increased	Decreased
IgG	• Infection • Hepatitis A • Glomerulonephritis • RA • SLE • AIDS • IgG myeloma	• Agammaglobulinemia • Chronic lymphocytic leukemia
IgM	• Hepatitis A and B • Chronic infections • SLE • RA • Sjögren syndrome • AIDS	• Hypogammaglobulinemia • Chronic lymphocytic leukemia • IgG myeloma • IgA myeloma • Agammaglobulinemia
IgA	• SLE • RA • IgA myeloma	• IgA deficiency • Acute and chronic lymphocytic leukemia • Agammaglobulinemia • IgG myeloma • Chronic infections
IgE	• Allergic rhinitis • Allergic asthma • Parasitic infection	• IgA deficiency • Intrinsic asthma
IgD	• Eczema • Skin disorders	• Unknown

RA, Rheumatoid arthritis; *SLE*, systemic lupus erythematosus.

   c) Elevated total complement levels occur in the following:
      i) Acute rheumatic fever
      ii) Acute MI
      iii) Ulcerative colitis
      iv) Cancer
      v) *Neisseria* infections
 d. Chemistry
   1) Calcium: normal 8.5 to 10.5 mg/dl
   2) Bilirubin: normal total bilirubin 0.3 to 1 mg/dl
      a) Indirect (before being conjugated by the liver): 0.2 to 0.8 mg/dl
      b) Direct (after being conjugated by the liver): 0.1 to 0.3 mg/dl
 e. Type and crossmatch
   1) Blood typing: determined by agglutination studies
   2) Rh factor determination
   3) Coombs test: detects immune antibodies important in crossmatching
      a) Direct: normal negative; measures antibodies (IgG) attached to RBCs
      b) Indirect: normal negative; measures antibodies (IgG) in the serum
 f. HLA: evaluates tissue compatibility in transplantation
   1) Tissue
      a) Complement-dependent cytotoxic assay
      b) Mixed lymphocyte culture
   2) Crossmatching
 g. Immune profile
   1) CD4 cell count: normal 800 cells/mm^3; varies with age
      a) Measured helper T cells
      b) Decreased in HIV infection and AIDS; assists in staging HIV infection
      c) Decreased with chronic corticosteroid therapy or immunosuppressive treatment
   2) T4/T8 (CD4/CD8) ratio
      a) Helper cells: suppressor/cytotoxic cells ratio: normal greater than 1
      b) Normally more CD4 cells than CD8 cells
      c) Reverse ratio in HIV infection or AIDS
 h. HIV antibody screening: normal negative
   1) Detects antibodies to HIV; present with exposure to HIV, but absence does not mean that the patient has not been exposed because time is required for development of antibodies
   2) Does not indicate immunity
   3) Types of tests
      a) Enzyme-linked immunosorbent assay (ELISA): screening test subject to error; up to 10% false-positive results
      b) Western blot: more specific than ELISA
 i. HIV virus screening (e.g., polymerase chain reaction [PCR]: normal negative)
 j. HIV viral load testing/HIV RNA quantification
   1) May range from imperceptible (less than 25–5000 copies of HIV/ml) to 1 million or more copies/ml; consider that the higher the viral load, the more rapid the damage from HIV
   2) Used to evaluate the effectiveness of antiretroviral therapy
2. Culture and sensitivity: various body secretions (e.g., blood, urine, wound secretions)

a. Gram stain: identification of gram-positive or gram-negative bacteria
b. Culture: identification of microorganism
c. Sensitivity
   1) Minimum inhibitory concentration (MIC): the smallest concentration of antibiotic that effectively inhibits bacterial growth; reported as antibiotic concentration per milliliter of solution necessary for growth inhibition
   2) This is compared with the achievable blood level of the antibiotic.
      a) If this level is less than the MIC, the bacterium is considered resistant to that antibiotic.
      b) If this level is greater than the MIC, the bacterium is considered sensitive to that antibiotic.
      c) Certain antimicrobials are dosed to achieve a specific MIC level (e.g., vancomycin), and other blood levels are used to assess toxicity (e.g., aminoglycosides).
   3) Other factors, such as known adverse effects of the antibiotic, are also considered.
3. Urine
   a. RBCs: normal 0 to 2/low-power field; RBCs in the urine may indicate trauma (e.g., renal calculi), severe thrombocytopenia, or bleeding disorder (e.g., DIC)
   b. WBCs: normal 0 to 4/low-power field; WBCs in the catheterized urine specimen indicate urinary tract infection
   c. Bilirubin: normal none; urobilinogen indicates biliary obstruction or liver disease
4. Stool
   a. Blood: may be grossly bloody or guaiac positive in bleeding disorders
   b. Clostridial toxin assay: normal negative; positive indicates the presence of a toxin that is released by *C. difficile*
5. Radiologic and radioisotope studies
   a. Chest radiography: may show infiltrates indicative of infection or bleeding
   b. Flat plate of abdomen: may show gross bleeding or hematoma
   c. Lymphangiography: visualizes the lymph system after injection of a dye; assists in node assessment
   d. Isotopic lymphangiography: uses technetium 99m and is less invasive than radiographic lymphangiography
   e. CT scans: chest, liver, spleen; detection of enlarged lymph nodes
   f. Positron emission tomography (PET) scans: demonstrate metabolic activity and glucose uptake that can indicate the presence of malignancy, abnormal lymph nodes
6. Biopsy
   a. Bone marrow
      1) Aspirate reveals cell numbers and maturation to diagnose bone marrow suppression.
      2) Biopsy of the bone and bone marrow is necessary for diagnosis of leukemia or stage of cancer.
   b. Lymph node
      1) Open: direct visualization; performed in operating room
      2) Closed or needle: performed at bedside
   c. Synovial
   d. Biopsy of transplanted organs to look for indications of rejection
7. Anergy panel testing
   a. Administration of antigen for observation of a delayed inflammatory skin reaction
      1) TB, mumps, *Candida* spp., and trichophytin are most frequently used.
      2) Mumps antigen is contraindicated for patients allergic to chicken or eggs.
   b. Normal response: a negative response to TB (unless the patient has been previously exposed to TB) and a positive reaction to several of the other antigens within 24 to 72 hours
   c. Abnormal responses
      1) Anergy: failure to respond to any of the injections
      2) Immunodeficiency: induration of less than 5 mm in diameter

Blood and Blood Component Administration

Blood Conservation and Salvaging Techniques
1. Avoiding blood transfusion
   a. Nonblood substitutes should be used if possible because they are safer and easier to use, and some are less costly than blood products.
   b. Substitutes
      1) Crystalloids
      2) Synthetic colloids (e.g., dextran)
      3) Noninfectious plasma derivatives
   c. Intraoperatively
      1) Restrict preoperative diagnostic phlebotomy
      2) Use meticulous intraoperative surgical hemostasis
      3) Use blood or cell salvage
         a) A collection of the siphoned blood that has escaped from the operative site of noncontaminated surgeries is filtered and returned to the patient.
         b) Reduces need for donated blood, safer
         c) Evidence supports use in cardiac and orthopedic surgery
      4) Employ hemodilution
      5) Use pharmaceutical hemostasis agents
      6) Maintain normothermia
      7) Position patients to minimize blood loss and hypertension
   d. Postoperatively
      1) Use blood or cell salvage
      2) Tolerate anemia
      3) Optimize fluid and volume management
      4) Restrict diagnostic phlebotomy
2. Indications for transfusion depend on:
   a. The patient's clinical condition
      1) Critically ill, nonbleeding adult patients younger than 55 years old and without evidence of an acute MI or unstable angina: keep Hgb greater than 7.0 g/dl rather than greater than 10 g/dl.

b. The patient's ability to compensate for reduced tissue oxygenation
1) Patients with severe cardiac or respiratory disease or with preexisting anemia have a limited ability to compensate.

Actions

1. Replacement of circulating volume, blood, or blood component
2. Improvement of oxygen-carrying capacity (RBCs, whole blood)
3. Replenishment of clotting factors (fresh-frozen plasma [FFP], cryoprecipitate) and platelets
4. Replenishment of granulocytes

Blood and Blood Products
Table 9.9.

Collaborative Management

1. Administer blood safely.
    a. Insert or ensure patency of IV catheter; do not use a catheter (or lumen) smaller than 24 gauge; if using central venous access device, verify that lumen is no smaller than 1.9 French.
    b. Ensure that the type and crossmatch has been done and blood or blood component is available.
    c. Assess vital signs; notify physician if temperature is 37.8°C (100°F) or higher.
    d. Request blood or blood component from blood bank when ready to administer it within 20 to 30 minutes; if you cannot begin the transfusion within 30 minutes after receiving it, return it to the blood bank.
    e. Check all of the following before administration of blood or blood component:
        1) Physician prescription for blood or blood product
        2) Consent form signed by the patient (according to hospital policy)
        3) Confirm at the bedside the following with another registered nurse:
            a) Patient's name and date of birth
            b) Type of blood component
            c) Patient's blood group and Rh factor
            d) Donor's blood group and Rh factor
            e) Unit number of blood or blood component
            f) Expiration date of the blood or blood component
        4) Contact the blood bank if there are any discrepancies
    f. Sign the transfusion record, along with the RN who confirmed the above information.
    g. Prime the blood administration set with normal (0.9%) saline, allowing the normal saline to cover the filter; use only normal saline, do not use dextrose-containing solutions or lactated Ringer's solution.
    h. Warm the blood if indicated.
        1) Blood may be warmed to avoid hypothermia in the patient receiving 4 or more units over 6 hours or in a patient who has tested positive for cold agglutinins.
        2) Warm the blood to 32° to 37°C using a blood-warming device in these situations.
    i. Clamp off the saline and start the blood or blood component.
    j. Adjust rate to administer slowly 25 to 50 ml within the first 15 minutes.
    k. Monitor for transfusion reaction (Table 9.10 and Box 9.1).
        1) Ask the patient to notify the nurse if he or she develops chills, low back pain, shortness of breath, nausea, sweating, itching, hives, or anxiety.
        2) Assess for clinical indications of transfusion reaction (Table 9.10).
        3) Take appropriate action for transfusion reactions (Table 9.10 and Box 9.2) if they occur.
    l. Monitor vital signs every 15 minutes for the first hour and then every 30 minutes until transfusion is complete or according to hospital policy.
    m. Adjust rate to infuse blood within 4 hours of initiating the infusion; FFP, platelets, and granulocytes are administered rapidly; if the blood slows, do the following:
        1) Ensure that the roller clamp is open.
        2) Increase the height of the blood bag.
        3) Gently squeeze the bag several times to agitate the blood cells.
        4) Gently squeeze the tubing and flashbulb.
        5) Remove dressing and check site.
        6) Close the blood and open the saline to allow 50 to 100 ml to irrigate the line; then restart the blood.
    n. Flush administration set tubing with saline after transfusion is complete.
    o. Disconnect the empty blood bag from the administration set and dispose of them according to hospital policy.
2. Monitor for adverse effects (Table 9.11) and complications.
    a. Complications
        1) Hepatitis
            a) Hepatitis B transmission has been reduced by mandatory testing of all donor blood for hepatitis B surface antigen.
            b) Non-A, non-B hepatitis (also referred to as type C hepatitis) accounts for 90% of cases of transfusion-related hepatitis.
        2) HIV
            a) HIV transmission through blood transfusion has been greatly reduced by screening for HIV antibody, which started in 1985, and by careful history taking of potential donors for risk factors for HIV.
        3) CMV
            a) CMV usually is not a problem for immunocompetent patients but may be life threatening in immunodeficient patients.
            b) Clinical indications of CMV infection include mild fever, mild splenomegaly, and atypical serum lymphocytes.
            c) CMV-negative blood products are indicated for immunodeficient patients.
        4) Transfusion-related acute lung injury or acute respiratory distress syndrome (ARDS)

Table 9.9 Blood and Blood Products

Product	Contents	Compatibility Required	Uses	Volume/Unit	Comments
Whole blood	RBCs, WBCs, platelets, plasma, and clotting factors	ABO, Rh specific NOTE: In emergency situations, type-specific blood or O− blood may be used.	Restores blood volume and oxygen-carrying capacity	≈500 ml	• Must be fresh (less than 4 hr old) to preserve platelet function • Administer over 2–4 hr • Best for hemorrhagic shock
Packed RBCs	RBCs and 20% plasma	ABO, Rh specific preferred; ABO, Rh compatible required	Restores oxygen-carrying capacity	≈250 ml	• Increases Hgb by 1 g/dl/unit and Hct by 2%–3%/unit; this change takes at least 6–12 hr • Administer over 2–4 hr
Washed RBCs	RBCs and 20% plasma with fewer WBCs and platelets than packed RBCs	ABO, Rh specific preferred; ABO, Rh compatible required	Restores oxygen-carrying capacity in patients previously sensitized by transfusions	≈250 ml	• As for packed RBCs • Must be administered within 24 hr of washing
Leukocyte-poor RBCs	RBCs, plasma but no leukocytes	ABO, Rh specific preferred; ABO, Rh compatible required	Restores oxygen-carrying capacity in patients susceptible to febrile reactions	≈250 ml	• As for packed RBCs
Platelets	Platelets, WBCs, plasma	ABO, Rh specific or compatible	Corrects low platelet levels to aid in clotting	≈50 ml	• Administer 1 unit over 10 min • Will increase platelet count by 5000–10,000/mm^3 • Agitate often as platelets tend to settle
Fresh-frozen plasma (FFP)	Water, plasma proteins, clotting factors	Rh compatibility required; ABO compatibility preferred	Expands blood volume Restores clotting factor deficiencies Contains no platelets	≈250 ml	• Takes 20 min to thaw • Must be given within 6 hr of thawing • Administer 1 unit over 1–2 hr or more rapidly if for hemorrhage
Granulocytes	WBCs, small amount of plasma	ABO, Rh compatible; HLA compatible if possible	Restores granulocytes in life-threatening granulocytopenia	≈300 ml	• Administer rapidly • Chills and fever may occur; steroids and antihistamines may be given; meperidine may be used for shivering • Administer over 2–6 hr
Cryoprecipitate	VIII, XIII, fibrinogen, fibronectin	ABO specific or compatible	Replaces clotting factors	≈10 ml; usually 10 bags pooled	• Administer rapidly immediately after thawing • May administer 30 units at one time
Albumin	Albumin from plasma	No compatibility required	Provides volume expansion (no clotting factors)	5%: 200 or 500 ml 25%: 50 or 100 ml	• Administer 1 ml/min or more rapidly if patient is in shock • Chemically processed so no risk of hepatitis
Plasma protein fraction (PPF)	Albumin and globulin in saline solution	No compatibility required	Provides volume expansion (no clotting factors)	5%: 200–500 ml	• Administer 10 ml/min • Chemically processed so no risk of hepatitis

Hct, Hematocrit; *HLA*, human leukocyte antigen; *RBC*, red blood cell; *WBC*, white blood cell.

Table 9.10 Types of Transfusion Reactions

Type of Reaction	Cause	Clinical Indications	Timing	Treatment
Febrile (nonhemolytic) NOTE: Most common type of transfusion reaction.	Antigen–antibody reaction to WBCs, platelets, or plasma proteins in the blood product	• Fever (rise in temperature greater than 1°C) • Chills • Headache • Nausea, vomiting • Flushing • Anxiety • Muscle pain	Immediately or up to 6 hr after transfusion	• Stop transfusion • Keep vein open with saline • Notify physician and blood bank • Send blood specimens to blood bank • Antipyretics as indicated • Steroids may be prescribed • Washed or leukocyte-poor blood should be considered for future transfusions
Mild allergic (type I hypersensitivity reaction)	Allergic reaction to plasma-soluble antigen in blood product	• Flushing • Itching • Urticaria • Hives	During transfusion or up to 1 hr after transfusion	• If febrile, stop transfusion • If afebrile, slow transfusion to keep-vein-open rate until advised by physician • Notify physician and blood bank • Monitor vital signs • Antihistamines as prescribed
Anaphylaxis (type I hypersensitivity reaction)	Allergic reaction in patients with IgA deficiency sensitized to IgA through previous transfusion or pregnancy	• Anxiety • Urticaria • Facial edema • Dysphagia • Abdominal cramps, diarrhea • Urinary incontinence • Dyspnea • Stridor • Wheezing • Cyanosis • Chest pain or pulmonary edema may occur • Shock may occur • Cardiopulmonary arrest may occur	Immediately; after transfusion of only a few milliliters of blood	• Stop transfusion • Keep vein open with saline • Notify physician and blood bank • Oxygen • Antihistamines, steroids, and/or aqueous epinephrine as prescribed • Emergency airway and/or CPR may be necessary • Washed or leukocyte-poor blood or blood from IgA-deficient donor should be considered for future transfusions

Acute hemolytic (type II hypersensitivity reaction)	ABO group incompatibility; antibodies in recipient's plasma attach to antigens in transfused RBCs, causing RBC destruction	• Burning sensation along vein
		• Lumbar pain
		• Chills
		• Fever
		• Flushing
		• Nausea, vomiting
		• Tachycardia, tachypnea
		• Hypotension (may be the only sign in unconscious patient)
		• May have:
		  • Dyspnea
		  • Chest pain
		  • Hemoglobinemia; hemoglobinuria
		  • Anuria
		  • DIC
		• Shock may occur
		• Cardiopulmonary arrest may occur
			Usually within 15 min after initiation of transfusion, but may occur anytime during transfusion; may be delayed if Rh incompatibility	• Stop transfusion
				• Keep vein open with saline
				• Notify physician and blood bank
				• Send blood unit and blood sample from the patient to the blood bank immediately
				• Monitor vital signs and urine output
				• Fluids for shock as prescribed
				• Diuretics (usually mannitol) may be prescribed, especially if hemoglobinuria occurs
				• Monitor for acute renal failure and shock
				• Request new crossmatch

Delayed hemolytic	Alloimmune response causes slow hemolysis	• Fever • Mild jaundice • Purpura • Anemia	Days to weeks after completion of transfusion	• Monitor urine output and Hgb and Hct levels

Table 9.10 Types of Transfusion Reactions—cont'd

Type of Reaction	Cause	Clinical Indications	Timing	Treatment
TRALI	Donor antibodies react with recipient HLA antigen	• Fever, chills • Dyspnea • Cough • Crackles • Hypoxemia • Shock	During transfusion or shortly after the transfusion	• Stop transfusion • Administer oxygen • Intubation and mechanical ventilation may be necessary • Steroids may be prescribed
TACO	Fluid administered faster that the cardiovascular system can accommodate	• Tachycardia • Hypertension • Headache • Jugular venous distention • Increased RAP, PAP, PAOP • Dyspnea • Cough • Crackles	During transfusion or shortly after the transfusion	• Administer RBCs no more rapidly than 4ml/kg/hr unless severe hemorrhage occurring • Slow or stop transfusion • Continue IV saline slowly if transfusion discontinued • Position patient upright with legs over the side of bed • Oxygen as indicated • Diuretics or venous vasodilators as indicated
Sepsis	Transfusion of contaminated blood components (blood should be infused within 4 hr)	• Chills • Fever • Vomiting • Abdominal pain • Diarrhea (may be bloody) • Hypotension • Shock	During or after transfusion	• Stop the transfusion • Obtain cultures of patient's blood and send with remaining blood to blood bank • Antibiotics as prescribed • Fluids or steroids as prescribed • Vasopressors may be needed
Graft-versus-host disease	Occurs in immunodeficient patients who receive lymphocytes; involves donor's lymphocytes mounting an attack against the recipient's tissues	• Fever • Rash • Stomatitis • Hepatitis • Severe diarrhea • Bone marrow suppression • Infection • Lymphadenopathy • Hepatosplenomegaly	Days to weeks after transfusion	• Steroids as prescribed • Methotrexate or azathioprine (Imuran) may be prescribed

CPR, Cardiopulmonary resuscitation; *DIC,* disseminated intravascular coagulation; *Hct,* hematocrit; *Hgb,* hemoglobin; *HLA,* human leukocyte antigen; *IV,* intravenous; *PAOP,* pulmonary artery occlusion pressure; *PAP,* Pulmonary artery pressure; *RAP,* Right atrial pressure; *RBC,* red blood cell; *TACO,* Transfusion-associated circulatory overload; *TRALI,* transfusion-related acute lung injury; *WBC,* white blood cell.

Box 9.1 Clinical Indications of Blood Transfusion Reaction in an Unconscious or Sedated Patient

Tachycardia or bradycardia
Hypotension
Fever
Visible signs of hemoglobin in urine
Oliguria or anuria
Bleeding
Skin rash
Hives
Respiratory distress

Box 9.2 Nursing Actions for Suspected Transfusion Reaction

1. Stop the transfusion.
2. Maintain intravenous access with normal saline and new administration set.
3. Reassure the patient; stay at the bedside.
4. Notify the physician and blood bank.
5. Recheck blood numbers and type.
6. Treat symptoms appropriately.
7. Return unused portion of blood in blood bag and administration set to the blood bank.
8. Collect and send blood and urine samples to the laboratory; send another urine specimen 24 hours after transfusion reaction.
9. Document the transfusion reaction and treatment administered.

Table 9.11 Potential Adverse Effects of Blood Transfusion

Complications	Clinical Indications	Prevention or Treatment

Citrate intoxication and hypocalcemia caused by binding of citrate with calcium	• Paresthesia of fingertips, circumoral area
	• Chvostek sign
	• Trousseau sign
	• Muscle cramps, tremors
	• Increased DTRs, carpopedal spasm
	• Abdominal cramps, biliary colic
	• Confusion, psychosis
	• Memory loss
	• Laryngospasm, stridor
	• Tetany (characterized by cramps, twitching of the muscles, sharp flexion of the wrist and ankle joints, seizures)
	• ECG changes
	  • Prolonged QT interval
	  • Dysrhythmias
		• Monitor calcium in patients receiving multiple transfusion and patients with hepatic or renal disease
		• Administer 500 mg–1 g of calcium for every 3–5 units of blood as prescribed

Hyperkalemia caused by hemolysis of stored blood and liberation of potassium (NOTE: The older the blood, the higher the potassium in the blood.)	• Tachycardia progressing to bradycardia and cardiac arrest
	• Nausea, vomiting, intestinal colic, diarrhea
	• Muscle weakness progressing to flaccid paralysis
	• Numbness, tingling of extremities
	• Increased deep tendon reflexes
	• Fatigue
	• Lethargy, apathy, mental confusion
	• Respiratory muscle weakness may cause hypopnea, dyspnea
	• Respiratory distress
	• Oliguria
	• Decreased contractility, cardiac output
	• ECG changes
	  • Tall, peaked T waves
	  • Wide QRS complex
	  • Prolonged PR interval
	  • Flattened to absent P wave
	  • Bradycardia
	  • Dysrhythmias
		• Monitor potassium closely in patients receiving stored blood (especially patients with renal insufficiency)
		• Dextrose and insulin may be prescribed acutely for patients with cardiac effects of hyperkalemia

Loss of 2,3-DPG (2,3-DPG is a byproduct of glucose metabolism on the Hgb molecule; banked [refrigerated] blood is low in 2,3-DPG; 2,3-DPG encourages unloading between Hgb and oxygen)	• Clinical indications of hypoxia (e.g., tachycardia, dysrhythmias, cyanosis, restlessness, confusion)	• Especially a problem if massive amounts of banked blood are administered • Give fresh whole blood when possible for patients in need of multiple transfusions
Ammonia intoxication Occurs in older blood; especially a problem for patients with hepatic disease	• Decreased cardiac output: hypotension • Confusion • Altered level of consciousness • Elevated serum ammonia	• Avoid use of older blood, especially for massive transfusion • Monitor for ammonia intoxication in patients with hepatic disease
Dilutional coagulopathy	• Prolonged PT, aPTT • Bleeding from needle site, wound	• Administer 2 units of FFP and/or platelets for every 10 units of packed RBCs as prescribed
Hypothermia	• Decrease in body temperature • Decrease in tissue delivery of oxygen caused by shift of the oxyhemoglobin dissociation curve to the left, resulting in increased affinity between Hgb and oxygen	• Warm blood to 35°–37°C if large quantities of blood are being administered

aPTT, Activated partial thromboplastin time; *DTRs*, deep tendon reflexes; *ECG*, electrocardiogram; *FFP*, fresh-frozen plasma; *Hgb*, hemoglobin; *PT*, prothrombin time; *RBC*, red blood cell; *2,3-DPG*, 2,3-diphosphoglyceric acid.

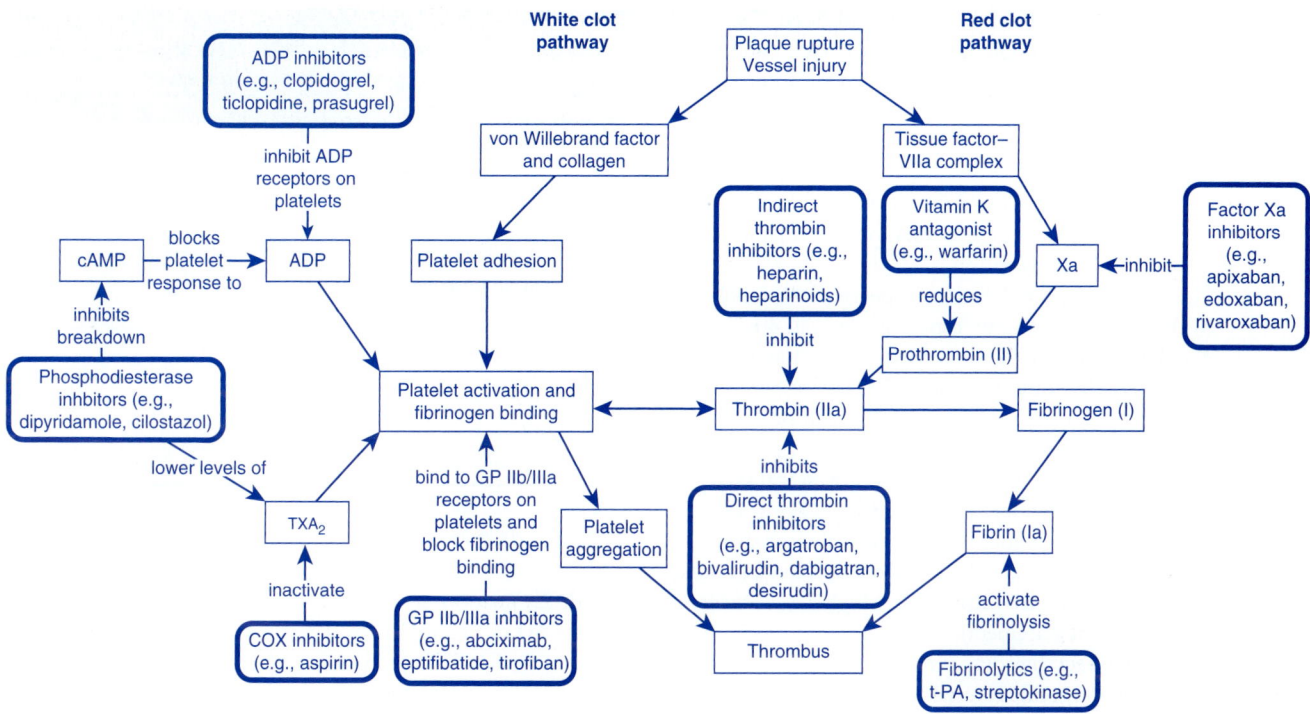

Fig. 9.5 Drugs that inhibit clotting: effects on pathways to thrombus formation. *ADP,* Adenosine diphosphate; *cAMP,* cyclic adenosine monophosphate; *COX,* cyclooxygenase; *GP,* glycoprotein; *t-PA,* tissue plasminogen activator; *TXA₂,* thromboxane A₂.

Drugs Affecting Clotting
Fig. 9.5.

Platelet Aggregation Inhibitors
1. Many drugs inhibit platelet aggregation as an adverse effect (e.g., NSAIDs, quinidine); others (Box 9.3) are prescribed for the specific purpose of impairing platelet aggregation to prevent the development of the platelet plug (i.e., white clot) and the intrinsic pathway.
2. Actions
    a. Inhibits platelet aggregation and platelet-mediated thrombosis
        1) Quality: inhibit platelet aggregation; although this effect has traditionally been thought to last as long as the platelet lives (i.e., 9–12 days), evidence now suggests that the effect decreases after 24 hours
        2) Quantity: may decrease the number of platelets, though this is an undesirable effect
            a) Referred to as *thrombotic thrombocytopenic purpura (TTP)*; treated by discontinuance of the offending drug and may require administration of platelets
            b) Monitor for and report petechiae, ecchymosis, or bleeding.
    b. Cyclooxygenase (COX) inhibitors (e.g., ASA) block synthesis of thromboxane A₂, inhibiting platelet aggregation.
    c. ADP pathway inhibitors (e.g., ticlopidine, clopidogrel, prasugrel) block ADP from binding to its receptor, inhibiting platelet aggregation.
    d. Phosphodiesterase inhibitors (e.g., dipyridamole, cilostazol) increase cyclic adenosine monophosphate (cAMP) and lower levels of thromboxane A₂, inhibiting platelet aggregation.

Box 9.3 Drugs Used to Decrease Platelet Aggregation

Cyclooxygenase inhibitors (e.g., aspirin)
Phosphodiesterase inhibitors (e.g., dipyridamole, cilostazol)
Adenosine diphosphate pathway inhibitors (e.g., ticlopidine, clopidogrel, prasugrel)
Glycoprotein IIb/IIIa platelet receptor blockers (e.g., abciximab, eptifibatide, tirofiban HCl)
Combination agents (e.g., dipyridamole and aspirin combination)
Dextran 40 (LMD)

---

    e. GP IIb/IIIa inhibitors (e.g., abciximab, eptifibatide, tirofiban HCl) block the GP IIb/IIIa platelet receptor; this interrupts the final common pathway for platelet aggregation by interfering with platelet aggregation via fibrinogen, vWF, and fibronectin.
        1) Differences between these agents
            a) Half-life
                i) Abciximab: 10 to 30 minutes
                ii) Tirofiban: 120 minutes
                iii) Eptifibatide: 150 minutes
            b) Duration of platelet inhibition
                i) Abciximab causes the most significant and prolonged (i.e., usually 18–36 hours but may be up to 1 week) reduction in platelet aggregation.
                ii) Tirofiban and eptifibatide: 1 to 2 hours after cessation of infusion
            c) Effect of renal insufficiency on dosing
                i) Abciximab may be used with no adjustment.
                ii) Tirofiban requires dosage adjustment.

iii) Eptifibatide is contraindicated if serum creatinine is 4 mg/dl or higher and requires dosage adjustment if serum creatinine is greater than 2 mg/dl.
3. Indications
   a. Oral agents
      1) Carotid artery disease for stroke prophylaxis (especially clopidogrel, ASA, or dipyridamole and ASA combination)
      2) Peripheral arterial disease (especially cilostazol)
      3) Postvascular surgery (especially dextran 40)
      4) Maintenance of coronary artery stent patency (especially clopidogrel or ASA)
      5) Acute coronary syndrome (ACS) with or without MI (especially ASA)
   b. IV agents: GP IIb/IIIa platelet receptor blockers (e.g., abciximab, eptifibatide, tirofiban HCl)
      1) ACS with or without PCI; note that abciximab is only used for ACS if PCI is planned within 24 hours
      2) PCI when risk for thrombosis is high (i.e., coronary artery stent placement)
4. Evaluation of effect: bleeding time
5. Reversal agent: no specific reversal agent; platelet transfusion may be indicated

Anticoagulants

1. Indirect thrombin inhibitors (e.g., unfractionated heparin [UFH] or low-molecular-weight heparin [LMWH])
   a. Action: accelerates the formation of the ATIII–thrombin complex, which deactivates thrombin and prevents the conversion of fibrinogen to fibrin
      1) Prevents extension of existing clots
      2) Decreases platelet aggregation
      3) Note that there is an unpredictable dose–response relationship with heparin, although prediction of response is improved with weight dosing; there is a more predictable dose–response relationship with heparinoids.
   b. Indications
      1) ACS (UFH or LMWH)
      2) Prevention or treatment of DVT (UFH, LMWH)
      3) PE (UFH or LMWH)
      4) Peripheral arterial emboli (UFH)
      5) Transient ischemic attack or ischemic stroke (UFH)
      6) DIC with clinical evidence of thromboembolism (UFH)
      7) Maintenance of arterial patency after PCI or fibrinolytic therapy (UFH or heparinoid)
      8) Maintenance of arterial line patency (UFH)
      9) Patients with or at risk of HIT having PCI
   c. Differences between unfractionated and LMWH
      1) LMWH is more potent at inactivating factor Xa than inactivating thrombin.
      2) LMWH has a longer half-life (4–6 hours compared with 1–2 hours for UFH).
      3) LMWH has 90% bioavailability, and UFH has only 30% bioavailability, which allows a more predictable anticoagulant response for LMWH.
      4) Less risk of HIT with LMWH than UFH
      5) Cost of LMWH is greater, but there is not a need for ongoing laboratory monitoring.

Table 9.12 Recommended International Normalized Ratio for Selected Indications

Indication	INR
Prophylaxis for venous thrombosis	2–3
Treatment of venous thrombosis	2–3
Treatment of PE	2–3
Prevention of systemic embolism	2–3
Tissue heart valves	
Acute MI	
Valvular heart disease	
Atrial fibrillation	
Mechanical prosthetic valves	2.5–3.5

INR, International normalized ratio; *MI*, myocardial infarction; *PE*, pulmonary embolism.

   d. Evaluation of effect
      1) UFH: aPTT, ACT
      2) LMWH: Monitoring of coagulation parameters is not required but may prolong PT and aPTT.
   e. Reversal agent: protamine
      1) 1 mg of protamine neutralizes approximately 100 units of heparin.
      2) Administer slowly to avoid hypotension.
2. Direct thrombin inhibitors (argatroban [Acova], bivalirudin [Angiomax])
   a. Action: inhibit thrombin activity (note that there is a predictable dose–response relationship)
   b. Indications
      1) HIT and associated thromboembolic complications (specifically argatroban)
      2) ACS undergoing PCI (specifically bivalirudin)
      3) Being evaluated for use in ischemic stroke, DIC, and MI
   c. Evaluation of effect: aPTT or ACT
   d. Reversal agent: none
3. Oral anticoagulants (e.g., warfarin [Coumadin])
   a. Actions: limits the availability of vitamin K, which is necessary for the formation of factors II (prothrombin), VII, IX, and X, along with the anticoagulant proteins C and S
      1) Prevents development of a clot
      2) Prevents extension of an existing clot and secondary thromboembolic complications
   b. Indications
      1) DVT
      2) Valvular heart disease
      3) Arial dysrhythmias
      4) Postvalve replacement
   c. Evaluation of effect: PT, INR (Table 9.12)
   d. Reversal agent: vitamin K

Fibrinolytics

1. Action: activation of plasminogen to accelerate clot lysis
   a. Recombinant plasminogen activators (e.g., alteplase, reteplase, tenecteplase)
      1) Activate plasminogen to plasmin, the active agent, which breaks and degrades the fibrin clot (i.e., speeds up the normal process to allow early reperfusion)

2) Causes clot-specific lysis to reestablish flow; tenecteplase is the most fibrin specific, and reteplase is the least fibrin specific of these agents
3) Do not cause antigenicity because these are recombinant agents
   b. Streptokinase
      1) Activates plasminogen systemically and converts it to plasmin, which then degrades fibrin clots, fibrinogen, and other plasma proteins
      2) Causes systemic lytic state
   c. Comparison of half-life
      1) Tenecteplase: ~20 minutes so dosed as a single bolus over 5 minutes
      2) Reteplase: ~15 minutes so dosed as two boluses 30 minutes apart
      3) Alteplase: ~5 minutes so dosed as a bolus followed by a 90-minute infusion
      4) Streptokinase: ~20 minutes, but effects last 48 to 72 hours because of fibrinogen depletion; dosed as a 30- to 60-minute infusion
2. Indications
   a. MI (within 6 hours or still having ischemic chest pain)
      1) The goal is to have fibrinolytics initiated within 30 minutes of the patient's arrival to the emergency department because time is muscle.
         a) Door
         b) Data
         c) Decision
         d) Drug
      2) Note that primary PCI is preferred if a cardiac catheterization laboratory and an interventional cardiologist is available; the goal is to have the catheter passing the stenosis within 60 to 90 minutes.
   b. Ischemic stroke (within 3 hours): It is necessary to perform CT to rule out hemorrhagic stroke and have that CT interpreted within the 3-hour window before administering the fibrinolytic; note that new evidence suggests that this time window may be extended to 4.5 hours for some subgroups.
   c. Massive PE: as indicated by acute right ventricular failure, refractory hypoxemia, or hemodynamic instability
   d. Acute arterial occlusion: typically administered intraarterially

Selected Drugs That Inhibit Clotting
Table 9.13.

Coagulopathies
Table 9.14.

Disseminated Intravascular Coagulation

Definition
1. A syndrome characterized by thrombus formation and hemorrhage secondary to overstimulation of the normal coagulation process, leading to massive intravascular clotting with resultant depletion in clotting factors and platelets and risk for bleeding
2. DIC may be acute or chronic, but this discussion is limited to acute DIC.

Table 9.13	Selected Drugs that Affect Clotting		
Drug	Administration	Adverse Effects	Nursing Implications
Glycoprotein IIb/IIIa Inhibitors			

Abciximab	• IV injection: 0.25 mg/kg administered 10 min to 1 hour before the start of the PTCA or atherectomy followed by infusion
	• IV infusion: 0.125 mcg/kg/min (10 mcg/min maximum) for 12 hr
		• Bleeding
		  • Intracranial hemorrhage
		  • Hematuria
		  • Hematemesis
		  • Bleeding at sheath site or other puncture point
		• Thrombocytopenia
		• Hypotension
		• Bradycardia
		• Nausea, vomiting, abdominal pain
		• Chest pain
		• Back pain
		• Headache
		• Pain at injection site
		• Allergic reaction, anaphylaxis (especially with repeat administration)
			• Monitor PT, aPTT or ACT, platelet count
			• Administer with aspirin and heparin therapy as prescribed
			• Note contraindications: patients with active internal bleeding, clinically significant bleeding in the GI or GU tract within the past 6 weeks, bleeding diathesis, history of CVA within the past 2 years or CVA with significant residual neurologic deficit, intracranial neoplasm, aneurysm, AVM, severe uncontrolled hypertension, oral anticoagulants within 7 days unless PT is less than 1.2 times control, thrombocytopenia, presumed or documented history of vasculitis, major surgery or trauma within the past 6 weeks, pericarditis, known hypersensitivity to abciximab or murine proteins
			• Use cautiously in patients who weigh less than 75 kg, patients older than 65 years of age, patients with a history of GI disease, and patients receiving thrombolytics
			• Do not administer with dextran
			• Monitor oral secretions, sputum, vomitus, NG aspirate, stool, urine for blood
			• Limit venipuncture and urinary catheterization as much as possible; use IV catheter with saline lock for blood sampling; avoid noncompressible IV sites
			• Avoid nasotracheal and NG tubes if possible
			• Avoid automatic BP cuffs
			• Administer platelets as prescribed for thrombocytopenia
			• Store refrigerated; do not shake (should be clear); administer through filter

Continued

Table 9.13 Selected Drugs that Affect Clotting—cont'd

Drug	Administration	Adverse Effects	Nursing Implications
Glycoprotein IIb/IIIa Inhibitors			

Eptifibatide	For ACS
	• IV injection: 180 mcg/kg over 1–2 min followed by:
	  • IV infusion: 2 mcg/kg/min for up to 72 hr; decreased to 0.5 mcg/kg/min during PCI and continued for 24 hr after PCI
	For PCI without ACS
	• IV injection: 135 mcg/kg over 1–2 min before procedure followed by:
	  • IV infusion: 0.5 mcg/kg/min for 24 hr
		• Bleeding
		  • Intracranial hemorrhage
		  • Hematuria
		  • Hematemesis
		  • Bleeding at sheath site
		• Hypotension
			• Monitor PT, aPTT or ACT, platelet count
			• Note contraindications: active internal bleeding, clinically significant bleeding in the GI or GU tract within the past 6 weeks, bleeding diathesis, history of CVA within the past 2 years or CVA with significant residual neurologic deficit, intracranial neoplasm, aneurysm, AVM, severe uncontrolled hypertension, oral anticoagulants within 7 days unless PT is less than 1.2 times control, thrombocytopenia, presumed or documented history of vasculitis, major surgery or trauma within the past 6 weeks, pericarditis, known hypersensitivity to eptifibatide, renal failure, thrombocytopenia
			• Administer with aspirin and heparin therapy as prescribed
			• Monitor oral secretions, sputum, vomitus, NG aspirate, stool, urine for blood
			• Limit venipuncture and urinary catheterization as much as possible; use IV catheter with saline lock for blood sampling; avoid noncompressible IV sites
			• Avoid nasotracheal and NG tubes if possible
			• Avoid automatic BP cuffs
			• Administer platelets as prescribed for thrombocytopenia
			• Store refrigerated

Tirofiban HCl	• IV infusion: premixed as 25 mg in 500 ml; usual dose is 0.4 mcg/kg/min for 30 min and then continued at 0.1 mcg/kg/min (dosage is decreased in renal failure)	• Bleeding
		  • Intracranial hemorrhage
		  • Hematuria
		  • Hematemesis< • Bleeding at sheath site
		• Hypotension
		• Bradycardia
		• Pelvic pain
			• Monitor PT, aPTT or ACT, platelet count
			• Note contraindications: active internal bleeding, clinically significant bleeding in the GI or GU tract within the past 6 weeks, bleeding diathesis, history of CVA within the past 2 years or CVA with significant residual neurologic deficit, intracranial neoplasm, aneurysm, AVM, severe uncontrolled hypertension, oral anticoagulants within 7 days unless PT is less than 1.2 times control, thrombocytopenia, presumed or documented history of vasculitis, major surgery or trauma within the past month, pericarditis, known hypersensitivity to tirofiban
			• Use cautiously in patients who weigh less than 75 kg, patients older than 65 years of age, patients with a history of GI disease, patients receiving thrombolytics, patients with thrombocytopenia
			• Administer with aspirin and heparin therapy as prescribed
			• Limit venipuncture and urinary catheterization as much as possible; use IV catheter with saline lock for blood sampling; avoid noncompressible IV sites
			• Monitor oral secretions, sputum, vomitus, NG aspirate, stool, urine for blood

Table 9.13   Selected Drugs that Affect Clotting—cont'd

Indirect Thrombin Inhibitors

Unfractionated heparin (UFH)	• SC: usually prophylactic, dose is 5000 units every 12 hr (also called *mini heparin*)
	• IV injection: usually 80 units/kg (maximum, 10,000 units) followed by infusion (only 60 units/kg recommended if patient is receiving fibrinolytics or GP IIb/IIIa inhibitors)
	• IV infusion: mix 25,000 units in 500 ml (50 units/ml) and infuse at 18 units/kg/hr (maximum, 1000 units/hr) (only 12 units/kg recommended if patient is receiving fibrinolytics or GP IIb/IIIa inhibitors); dose is adjusted to achieve aPTT of 1.5–2.5 times the laboratory control
	• NOTE: The trend in IV weight-dosed heparin is to decrease the amount of heparin (60 units/kg for injection followed by 12 units/kg/hr for infusion) and desirable aPTT (45–60 seconds)
	• Maximum: 40,000 units/day
		• Hemorrhage with excessive aPTT
		• Hypertension or hypotension
		• Hypersensitivity reaction, including bronchospasm
		• Fever
		• Hepatitis
		• Hyperkalemia, especially in patients with renal failure
		• Thrombocytopenia (caused by immune response referred to as HIT)
			• Monitor aPTT and platelet count and for signs of hemorrhage
			  Note petechiae and request platelet count if petechiae noted; heparin usually discontinued if platelet count is less than 100,000/mm^3
			  Administer argatroban as prescribed for HIT
			• Note contraindications: known hypersensitivity, active bleeding, blood dyscrasias (except DIC), suspected intracranial hemorrhage, severe hypertension, PUD, open wounds, recent surgery, endocarditis, shock, threatened abortion
			• Use cautiously in alcoholism, liver disease, renal disease, older adults
			• Monitor oral secretions, sputum, vomitus, NG aspirate, stool, urine for blood
			• Ensure that protamine sulfate (antidote) is available
			• Avoid IM, arterial, or venous punctures if at all possible
			• Hold pressure for longer than usual if punctures are necessary
			• Do not discontinue suddenly: warfarin usually will have already been started and the PT within therapeutic range before heparin is discontinued
			• Do not aspirate before SC administration and do not massage after administration
			• Note that NTG interacts with heparin causing more heparin to be required to achieve therapeutic aPTT; monitor aPTT closely with significant NTG dosage changes or discontinuance

Low-molecular-weight heparin (LMWH)	Enoxaparin • SC: 30 mg bid or 40 mg qd Dalteparin sodium (Fragmin) • SC: 2500 units daily starting 1–2 hr before surgery and repeated qd for 5–10 days postoperatively Ardeparin (Normiflo) • SC: 50 antifactor Xa units/kg every 12 hr beginning the evening before surgery and continued until the patient is ambulatory Tinzaparin sodium • SC: 175 antifactor Xa units/kg daily for approximately 6 days or until adequate anticoagulation with warfarin	• Bleeding • Epidural or spinal hematoma (especially when used with patients with epidural or spinal anesthesia) • Fever • Elevation of liver enzymes • Thrombocytopenia • Chest pain	• Note that LMWH does not require routine laboratory monitoring because it does not usually alter PT or aPTT • Note that contraindications and cautions are as for heparin • Obtain baseline platelet count; monitor for petechiae • Monitor oral secretions, sputum, vomitus, NG aspirate, stool, urine for blood • Ensure that protamine sulfate (antidote) is available • Avoid IM, arterial, and venous punctures if at all possible • Hold pressure for longer than usual if punctures are necessary • Administer deep subcutaneously but avoid IM injection

Continued

Table 9.13 Selected Drugs that Affect Clotting—cont'd

Direct Thrombin Inhibitors

Drug	Dosage	Adverse Effects	Nursing Implications
Argatroban	• IV infusion: mix 250 mg in 250 ml of normal saline (1 mg/ml); administer initially at 2 mcg/kg/min; no loading dose is given • Maximum: 10 mcg/kg/min • Reduce dosage in hepatic disease; start at 0.5 mcg/kg/min	• Bleeding: GI, GU, intracranial • Allergic reaction • Dyspnea • Hypotension • Fever • Diarrhea • Sepsis • Cardiac arrest	• Monitor PT, aPTT, CBC, and for signs of bleeding • Note that contraindications and cautions are as for heparin • Obtain baseline platelet count and aPTT; monitor aPTT every 4 hr • Anticoagulant effects are increased in patients receiving platelet aggregation inhibitors, fibrinolytics, or other anticoagulants • Monitor oral secretions, sputum, vomitus, NG aspirate, stool, urine for blood • Avoid IM, arterial, and venous punctures if at all possible • Hold pressure for longer than usual if punctures are necessary • Protect infusion from direct sunlight
Bivalirudin	• IV injection: 0.75–1 mg/kg followed by IV infusion • IV infusion: mix 250 mg in 250 ml of normal saline (1 mg/ml) and infuse at 1.75–2.5 mg/kg/hr for 4 hr then decrease infusion to 0.2 mg/kg/hr for an additional 14–20 hr if needed	• Bleeding • Back pain • Generalized pain • Headache • Nausea • Hypotension	• Monitor PT, aPTT, CBC, and for signs of bleeding • Note that contraindications and cautions are as for heparin • Obtain baseline platelet count and aPTT; ACT may also be used • Anticoagulant effects are increased in patients receiving platelet aggregation inhibitors, fibrinolytics, or other anticoagulants • Monitor oral secretions, sputum, vomitus, NG aspirate, stool, urine for blood • Avoid IM, arterial, and venous punctures if at all possible • Hold pressure for longer than usual if punctures are necessary • Protect infusion from direct sunlight
Dabigatran	Oral: Maximum, 150 mg twice daily	• GI bleed	• Monitor PT, aPTT, CBC, and for signs of bleeding • Note that it is contraindicated in patients with mechanical prosthetic heart valves because of incidence of valvular thrombosis, stroke, TIA, or MI • Instruct the patient that premature discontinuance of dabigatran may increase the risk of thrombotic events. • Note that increased risk of bleeding may occur when drugs such as antiplatelet agents, heparin, fibrinolytic therapy, or NSAIDs are given concomitantly; impaired renal function can also increase the risk of bleeding. • Instruct patient to brush and floss your teeth gently • Note that there is no reversal agent.

Table 9.13 Selected Drugs that Affect Clotting—cont'd

Vitamin K Antagonist

Warfarin	• PO: 2–10 mg daily depending on PT and INR
	• INR 2–3
	  • MI
	  • DVT prophylaxis or treatment
	  • PE
	  • Valvular heart disease
	  • Atrial fibrillation
	  • Tissue heart valve
	• INR 2.5–3.5
	  • Mechanical heart valve
		• Hemorrhage with excessive PT
		• Agranulocytosis, leukopenia
		• Hepatitis
		• Diarrhea
		• Fever
		• Rash
		• Skin necrosis: occurs during the first several days of warfarin therapy; lesions occur on extremities, breasts, trunk, penis
		• Cholesterol microemboli causing purple toe syndrome
			• Monitor PT and for signs of hemorrhage
			• Note contraindications: known hypersensitivity, bleeding disorders, leukemia, PUD, liver disease, severe hypertension, endocarditis, acute nephritis, blood dyscrasias, eclampsia, suspected intracranial hemorrhage, open wounds, recent surgery, threatened abortion
			• Use cautiously in alcoholism, pregnancy, lactation, during menses, during use of any drainage tube, in older adults, and in any patient in whom slight bleeding is dangerous
			• Ensure that vitamin K (Aqua Mephyton) is available
			• Avoid IM, arterial, and venous punctures if at all possible
			• Hold pressure for longer than usual if punctures are necessary
			• Monitor oral secretions, sputum, vomitus, NG aspirate, stool, urine for blood
			• Do not discontinue suddenly
			• Teach patient to avoid trauma and increase amounts of vitamin K (green leafy vegetables) and how to monitor for bleeding
			• Teach the patient to report fever or rash; usually necessitates discontinuance

Factor Xa Inhibitors

Rivaroxaban	PO: 10 mg once daily Feeding tube: 15- or 20-mg tablets by crushing and suspending drug in 50 ml of water	• Bleeding • Risk of thrombosis after premature discontinuance of anticoagulation. • Epidural or spinal hematoma reported with concurrent use of anticoagulants and spinal puncture procedures; neurologic injuries such as temporary or permanent paralysis may occur	• Monitor for bleeding • In patients who have had neuraxial anesthesia or spinal puncture, monitor for manifestations of spinal or epidural hematoma (e.g., back pain; tingling, numbness, or weakness in lower limbs; bowel or bladder incontinence) in patients having neuraxial anesthesia or spinal puncture • Do not remove epidural catheters less than 18 hr after a dose of rivaroxaban; administer next dose 6 hr or more after catheter removal; if traumatic puncture occurred, delay rivaroxaban administration for 24 hr • Emphasize the importance of immediately contacting a health care provider if any neurologic symptoms occur • Teach patients that if they are taking a dosage of 15 mg twice daily and miss a dose, two 15-mg tablets may be taken at the same time to ensure full intake of the 30-mg daily dosage
Edoxaban	PO: 15 mg, 30 mg, 60 mg once daily	• Bleeding • Skin rash	• Monitor for bleeding and for signs of neurologic impairment (e.g., numbness or weakness in lower limbs, bowel or bladder dysfunction, tingling or numbness in lower limbs, muscle weakness, back pain) • Contraindicated in patients with moderate to severe hepatic impairment. • Note risk of thrombosis after premature discontinuance of therapy • Contraindicated in patients with nonvalvular atrial fibrillation patients with Cl_{cr} greater than 95 ml/min because reduced efficacy has been noted in patients • Temporarily interrupt therapy before surgery or other invasive procedure to minimize risk of bleeding
Apixaban	PO: 5 mg twice daily	• Bleeding • Severe hypersensitivity reaction	• Monitor aPTT, PTT, ACT, platelets, INR • Monitor for bleeding • Monitor for fever, skin rash, urticaria, and nuchal rigidity • Note risk of thrombosis with abrupt discontinuance, • May prolong INR • If patient unable to swallow whole tablets, crush

Continued

Table 9.13 Selected Drugs that Affect Clotting—cont'd

Fibrinolytics

Drug	Dose	Adverse Effects	Nursing Implications

Recombinant plasminogen activator (r-PA) reteplase	• IV injection of 10 units over 2 min initially followed by 10 units over 2 min after 30 min
	• Heparin administered concurrently
		• Severe, spontaneous bleeding, including potential cerebral, retroperitoneal, GU, GI bleeding, surface bleeding
		• Reperfusion dysrhythmias
			• Monitor aPTT, PT, thrombin time, neurologic status, and for signs of hemorrhage
			• Note contraindications: active bleeding; history of cerebral hemorrhage, intracranial neoplasm, AVM or aneurysm; recent (within 2 months) intracranial or intraspinal surgery or trauma; known bleeding disorder; severe uncontrolled hypertension; prolonged CPR
			• Use cautiously in recent (within 10 days) major surgery, GI, GU bleeding, or trauma; hypertension with SBP greater than 180 mm Hg or DBP greater than 110 mm Hg; high likelihood of left heart thrombus; acute pericarditis; significant liver dysfunction; pregnancy; retinopathy; septic thrombophlebitis; advanced age (older than 70–75 years); patients receiving oral anticoagulants; any condition in which bleeding constitutes a significant hazard or would be particularly difficult to manage because of its location
			• Identify indications of reperfusion in MI
			  • Cessation of pain
			  • ST segments descending back to baseline
			  • Reperfusion dysrhythmias (ventricular ectopy including PVCs, VT or VF, accelerated idioventricular rhythm, junctional escape rhythms, bradycardia)
			  • Early CK peak
			• Limit venipuncture and urinary catheterization as much as possible; use IV catheter with saline lock for blood sampling; avoid noncompressible IV sites
			• Avoid nasotracheal and NG tubes if possible
			• Avoid automatic BP cuffs
			• Administer all drugs through existing IVs started before initiation of thrombolytic therapy or by mouth
			• Monitor oral secretions, sputum, vomitus, NG aspirate, stool, urine for blood
			• Bleeding precautions are maintained for 12–24 hr

Recombinant tissue plasminogen activator (rt-PA) alteplase	For acute MI • IV injection: 15 mg followed by: • IV infusion: 0.75 mg/kg (not to exceed 50 mg) over next 30 min, followed by 0.5 mg/kg (not to exceed 35 mg) over the next 60 min • Heparin started within 1 hour of initial dose	• Severe, spontaneous bleeding, including potential cerebral, retroperitoneal, GU, GI bleeding, surface bleeding • Reperfusion dysrhythmias	• Monitor aPTT, PT, thrombin time, fibrinogen, neurologic status, and for signs of hemorrhage • Note contraindications: active bleeding; history of cerebral hemorrhage, intracranial neoplasm, AVM or aneurysm; recent (within 2 months) intracranial or intraspinal surgery or trauma; known bleeding disorder; severe uncontrolled hypertension; prolonged CPR • Use cautiously in recent (within 10 days) major surgery, GI, GU bleeding, or trauma; hypertension with SBP greater than 180 mm Hg or DBP greater than 110 mm Hg; high likelihood of left heart thrombus; acute pericarditis; significant liver dysfunction; pregnancy; retinopathy; septic thrombophlebitis; advanced age (older than 70–75 years); patients receiving oral anticoagulants; any condition in which bleeding constitutes a significant hazard or would be particularly difficult to manage because of its location

Table 9.13 Selected Drugs that Affect Clotting—cont'd

Fibrinolytics

	For ischemic stroke
	• Total dose: 0.9 mg/kg with maximum dose of 90 mg or less
	• IV injection: 10% of this total dose over 1 minute followed by:
	  • IV infusion: remaining 90% of this total dose administered over 60 min
	• Anticoagulants and platelet aggregation inhibitors are not used for at least 24 hr
	For acute pulmonary embolism
	• IV infusion: 100 mg at 50 mg/hr for 2 hr
	For acute arterial occlusion
	• 0.05 to 0.1 mg/kg/hr by local intraarterial infusion
	• Reconstitution in sterile water only
			• Monitor for indications of reperfusion in MI
			  • Cessation of pain
			  • ST segments descending back to baseline
			  • Reperfusion dysrhythmias (ventricular ectopy including PVCs, VT or VF, accelerated idioventricular rhythm, junctional escape rhythms, bradycardia)
			  Early CK peak
			• Note that signs of reperfusion are much more subtle in PE and thrombotic stroke
			• Limit venipuncture and urinary catheterization as much as possible; use IV catheter with saline lock for blood sampling; avoid noncompressible IV sites
			• Administer all drugs through existing IVs started before initiation of thrombolytic therapy or by mouth
			• Avoid nasotracheal and NG tubes if possible
			• Avoid automatic BP cuffs
			• Monitor oral secretions, sputum, vomitus, NG aspirate, stool, urine for blood
			• Bleeding precautions are maintained for 12–24 hr

Recombinant tissue plasminogen activator (rt-PA) tenecteplase	• IV injection over 5 seconds
	  • Less than 60 kg: 30 mg
	  • At least 60 but less than 70 kg: 35 mg
	  • At least 70 but less than 80 kg: 40 mg
	  • At least 80 but less than 90 kg: 45 mg
	  • At least 90 kg: 50 mg
	• Heparin administered concurrently
		• Severe, spontaneous bleeding including potential cerebral, retroperitoneal, GU, GI bleeding, surface bleeding
		• Reperfusion dysrhythmias
			• Monitor aPTT, PT, thrombin time, neurologic status, and for signs of hemorrhage
			• Note contraindications: active bleeding; history of cerebral hemorrhage, intracranial neoplasm, AVM or aneurysm; recent (within 2 months) intracranial or intraspinal surgery or trauma; known bleeding disorder; severe uncontrolled hypertension; prolonged CPR
			• Use cautiously in recent (within 10 days) major surgery, GI, GU bleeding, or trauma; hypertension with SBP greater than 180 mm Hg or DBP greater than 110 mm Hg; high likelihood of left heart thrombus; acute pericarditis; significant liver dysfunction; pregnancy; retinopathy; septic thrombophlebitis; advanced age (older than 70–75 years); patients receiving oral anticoagulants; any condition in which bleeding constitutes a significant hazard or would be particularly difficult to manage because of its location
			• Identify indications of reperfusion in MI
			  • Cessation of pain
			  • ST segments descending back to baseline
			  • Reperfusion dysrhythmias (ventricular ectopy including PVCs, VT or VF, accelerated idioventricular rhythm, junctional escape rhythms, bradycardia)
			  • Early CK peak
			• Limit venipuncture and urinary catheterization as much as possible; use IV catheter with saline lock for blood sampling; avoid noncompressible IV sites
			• Avoid nasotracheal and NG tubes if possible
			• Avoid automatic BP cuffs
			• Administer all drugs through existing IVs started before initiation of thrombolytic therapy or by mouth
			• Monitor oral secretions, sputum, vomitus, NG aspirate, stool, urine for blood
			• Bleeding precautions are maintained for 12–24 hr

Continued

Table 9.13	Selected Drugs that Affect Clotting—cont'd		
Fibrinolytics			
Streptokinase	IV: mix 1.5 million units in 250 ml (6000 units/ml) • For acute MI, usual loading dose 750,000 units IV injection followed by 750,000 units IV infusion over next hour • For PE and arterial thromboembolism, usual loading dose 250,000 units over 30 min followed by 100,000 units/hr for up to 72 hr	• Allergic reaction (angioneurotic edema, pruritus, bronchospasm, dyspnea, hypotension, cyanosis, seizures, loss of consciousness) • Severe spontaneous bleeding • Cerebral, retroperitoneal, GU, GI, surface bleeding • Reperfusion dysrhythmias	• Monitor aPTT, PT, thrombin time, neurologic status, and for signs of hemorrhage • Note contraindications: patients who have had recent streptococcal infection or streptokinase within 6 months to 5 years • Note that indications in MI, contraindications, cautions, and signs of reperfusion after use for MI are as for r-PA or rt-PA • Administer diphenhydramine (Benadryl) and hydrocortisone sodium succinate (Solu-Cortef) if chance of allergic reaction • Limit venipuncture and urinary catheterization as much as possible; use IV catheter with saline lock for blood sampling; avoid noncompressible IV sites • Administer all drugs through existing IVs started before initiation of thrombolytic therapy or by mouth • Avoid nasotracheal and NG tubes if possible • Avoid automatic BP cuffs • Monitor oral secretions, sputum, vomitus, NG aspirate, stool, urine for blood • Maintain bleeding precautions for 48–72 hr because of fibrinogen depletion seen with streptokinase

ACS, Acute coronary syndrome; *ACT*, activated clotting time; *aPTT*, activated partial thromboplastin time; *AVM*, arteriovenous malformation; *bid*, twice a day; *BP*, blood pressure; *CBC*, complete blood count; *CK*, creatine kinase; Cl_{cr}, creatine clearance; *CPR*, cardiopulmonary resuscitation; *CVA*, cerebrovascular accident; *DBP*, diastolic blood pressure; *DIC*, disseminated intravascular coagulation; *DVT*, deep vein thrombosis; *GI*, gastrointestinal; *GP*, glycoprotein; *GU*, genitourinary; *HIT*, heparin-induced thrombocytopenia; *IM*, intramuscular; *INR*, international normalized ratio; *IV*, intravenous; *MI*, myocardial infarction; *NG*, nasogastric; *NSAID*, nonsteroidal antiinflammatory drug; *NTG*, nitroglycerin; *PCI*, percutaneous coronary intervention; *PE*, pulmonary embolism; *PO*, oral; *PT*, prothrombin time; *PTCA*, percutaneous transluminal coronary angioplasty; *PUD*, peptic ulcer disease; *PVC*, premature ventricular contraction; *qd*, every day; *SBP*, systolic blood pressure; *SC*, subcutaneous; *TIA*, transient ischemic attack; *VF*, ventricular fibrillation; *VT*, ventricular tachycardia.

Table 9.14	Inherited and Acquired Coagulopathies	
Cause of Coagulopathy	**Pathophysiology**	**Treatment**
Hereditary Coagulopathies		
Hemophilia A	• X-linked recessive disorder; although considered a hereditary disorder, may occur as a new mutation in factor VIII gene • Deficiency of factor VIII • Inadequate factor VIII–vWF complex • Inadequate platelet adhesion	• Either highly purified factor VIII concentrate or recombinant factor VIII administration • DDAVP stimulates the endothelial cells to release vWF and plasminogen activator
Hemophilia B (i.e., Christmas disease)	• X-linked recessive disorder • Deficiency of factor IX	• Highly purified factor IX
von Willebrand disease	• Types 1 and 2 are inherited as autosomal dominant traits and type 3 is inherited as autosomal recessive deficiency of vWF • Decreased platelet adhesion	• Usually mild and does not require treatment, although the risk of bleeding is increased • Either highly purified factor VIII concentrate that contains vWF • DDAVP stimulates the endothelial cells to release vWF and plasminogen activator
Acquired Coagulopathies		
Vitamin K deficiency	• Inadequate synthesis and regulation of prothrombin, procoagulant factors (VII, IX, X), and anticoagulant regulators (proteins C and S)	• Parenteral administration of vitamin K • FFP in life-threatening hemorrhage or in preparation for emergency surgery
Liver disease	• Impaired clotting caused by diminished production of clotting factors, especially factor VII and less so factor IX • Impaired fibrinolysis caused by diminished production of plasminogen and alpha$_2$-antiplasmin • Decreased thrombopoietin results in decreased platelet production	• FFP • Platelets

Chapter 9 The Hematologic and Immunologic Systems

Table 9.14 Inherited and Acquired Coagulopathies—cont'd

	Acquired Coagulopathies	
Immune thrombocytopenic purpura (ITP; formerly known as *idiopathic thrombocytopenia purpura*)	**Acute ITP** • Secondary to infection, particularly viral, or other condition that results in large amounts of antigen in the blood, such as drug allergies or SLE • Antigen and antibodies form immune complexes that bind to receptors on platelets, which causes platelet destruction in the spleen. **Chronic ITP** • Development of autoantibodies against platelet-specific antigens • Removal of the antibody-coated platelets removed by spleen	• Glucocorticoids • IV immunoglobulins • Splenectomy may be considered • Immunosuppressive agents may be used
Thrombotic thrombocytopenic purpura	• Platelets aggregate and cause occlusion of arterioles and capillaries within the microcirculation • Platelet consumption • Organ ischemia	• Plasma exchange with FFP • Glucocorticoids • Splenectomy may be considered • Immunosuppressive agents may be used
Disseminated Intravascular Coagulation (see Hemostasis section)		
Heparin-Induced Thrombocytopenia (see Hemostasis section)		

FFP, Fresh-frozen plasma; *DDAVP*, desmopressin; *IV*, intravenous; *SLE*, systemic lupus erythematosus; *vWF*, von Willebrand factor.

Etiology

Always secondary
1. Vascular injury or inflammation
   a. Shock
   b. Vasculitis
   c. Giant hemangioma
   d. Dissecting aneurysm
   e. Toxemia of pregnancy
2. Infection and sepsis
   a. Bacterial
      1) Gram negative (e.g., *Escherichia coli*, meningococci)
      2) Gram positive (e.g., *Staphylococcus* spp., *Streptococcus* spp.)
   b. Viral (e.g., influenza, herpes, CMV, adenovirus)
   c. Rickettsial (e.g., Rocky Mountain spotted fever)
   d. Protozoal (e.g., malaria)
   e. Fungal (e.g., *Aspergillus, Candida, Histoplasma,* or *Toxoplasma* spp.)
3. Hematologic or immunologic
   a. Hemolytic blood transfusion reaction
   b. Massive blood transfusion
   c. Prolonged cardiopulmonary bypass
   d. Sickle cell crisis
   e. Thalassemia major
   f. Polycythemia vera
   g. Anaphylaxis
   h. SLE
   i. Transplant rejection
4. Trauma
   a. Multiple traumas
   b. Burns
   c. Acute anoxia
   d. Heat stroke
   e. Crush injury
   f. Head injury
   g. Surgery
5. Neoplastic disorders
   a. Adenocarcinoma: produce the procoagulant mucin
      1) Pancreatic cancer
      2) Breast cancer
      3) Prostate cancer
      4) Ovarian cancer
      5) Lung cancer
      6) Colon cancer
      7) Stomach cancer
   b. Cancer of the urinary tract
   c. Sarcoma
   d. Leukemia
   e. Pheochromocytoma
6. Obstetric complications
   a. Abruptio placentae
   b. Retained dead fetus
   c. Retained placenta
   d. Septic abortion
   e. Hydatidiform mole
   f. Amniotic fluid embolism
   g. Acute fatty liver of pregnancy
   h. Toxemia
   i. Placenta previa
   j. Eclampsia
7. Embolism
   a. PE
   b. Fat embolism
   c. Amniotic fluid embolism
8. GI and accessory organs
   a. Necrotizing enterocolitis
   b. Pancreatitis
   c. Obstructive jaundice
   d. Hepatitis
   e. Cirrhosis
   f. Acute hepatic failure

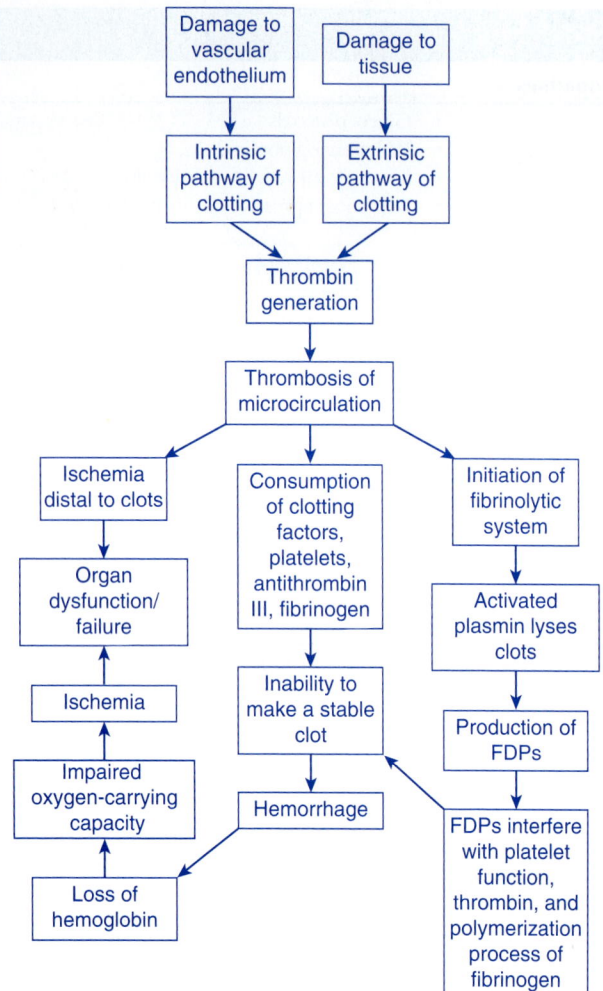

Fig. 9.6 Pathophysiology of disseminated intravascular coagulation (DIC). *FDP*, Fibrin degradation product.

9. Pulmonary
   a. ARDS
   b. PE
10. Toxins
    a. Snake bites
    b. ASA poisoning
    c. Impure IV drugs
11. Prosthetic devices
    a. LeVeen or Denver shunt
    b. Intraaortic balloon pump

Pathophysiology
Fig. 9.6.

Clinical Presentation
1. Subjective
   a. History of predisposing factor
   b. Symptoms related to ischemia
      1) Chest pain
      2) Dyspnea
      3) Abdominal pain
      4) Pain in digits
      5) Visual changes
      6) Headache
2. Objective
   a. Clinical indications of decreased perfusion (subjective included)
      1) Brain: change in level of consciousness, focal neurologic signs, seizures
      2) Heart: chest pain, ST-segment elevation or depression, clinical indications of hypoperfusion
      3) Lung: dyspnea, chest pain, clinical indications of hypoxemia
      4) Kidney: decreased urine output, occult or gross hematuria, proteinuria, electrolyte imbalance
      5) GI tract: abdominal pain, diarrhea, occult or gross blood in stool
      6) Skin: acral cyanosis of toes, fingers, lips, nose, or ears; mottling, coldness, necrosis
   b. Clinical indications of platelet dysfunction
      1) Petechiae: frequently the first indication of DIC
      2) Ecchymoses
      3) Purpura
   c. Clinical indications of hemorrhage
      1) Tachycardia
         a) Initially postural only; then profound tachycardia
      2) Hypotension
         a) Initially narrowed pulse pressure
         b) Then postural hypotension
         c) Then profound hypotension
      3) Tachypnea
      4) Overt bleeding in a patient with no previous bleeding history
         a) Mucosal surfaces: gingival bleeding; epistaxis
         b) GU: hematuria
         c) GI: hematemesis, hematochezia, melena, guaiac-positive stool
         d) Pulmonary: hemoptysis
         e) Gynecologic: vaginal bleeding
         f) Skin: prolonged oozing from puncture points, IV sites, and wounds (referred to as *surface bleeding*), bruising
      5) Occult bleeding
         a) Swollen joints and joint pain may indicate bleeding into the joint.
         b) Abdominal distention and rebound tenderness may indicate intraperitoneal bleeding.
         c) Back pain, leg numbness, and hypotension may indicate retroperitoneal bleeding.
         d) Headache, change in level of consciousness, and pupillary changes may indicate intracerebral hemorrhage.
         e) Visual changes (e.g., blurred vision, loss of visual fields) may indicate retinal hemorrhage.
         f) Alterations in hemodynamic parameters: Right atrial pressure, pulmonary artery wedge pressure, and cardiac output or cardiac index may be decreased.
3. Diagnostic studies: All that bleeds is not DIC; diagnostic studies are definitive.
   a. Serum
      1) Platelet count: decreased (less than 150,000/mm^3); one of the earliest findings
      2) PT: prolonged (usually greater than 40 seconds); less sensitive than other tests

Table 9.15 Disseminated Intravascular Coagulation Scoring System*

Laboratory Test	0	1	2	3
Platelet count/nL	Greater than 100	Greater than 50	Less than 50	
D-Dimer (mcg/ml)	Less than 1		1–5	Greater than 5
Fibrinogen (g/l)	Greater than 1	Less than 1		
Prothrombin index (%)	Greater than 70	40–70	Less than 40	

*The DIC Scoring System requires the presence of a risk factor for disseminated intravascular coagulation (DIC) before the laboratory test results can be evaluated. If greater than or equal to 5, it is compatible with overt DIC. If less than 5, it is suggestive for nonovert DIC in a patient with an underlying disorder known to be associated with DIC.

Adapted from Taylor, F. B., Toh, C. H., Hoots, W. K., Wada, H., & Levi, M. (2001). Towards definition, clinical and laboratory criteria, and a scoring system for disseminated intravascular coagulation. *Thromb Haemost, 86,* 1327–1330.

3) aPTT: prolonged (usually greater than 70 seconds); less sensitive than other tests
4) Thrombin time: prolonged (greater than 15 seconds)
5) Fibrinogen level: decreased by 50% or more or less than 200 mg/dl
   a) Used for patients who have contributing factors that do not permit monitoring platelet count
   b) Because fibrinogen is elevated in pregnancy, sepsis, and neoplastic conditions, a decrease of 50% is a more accurate indicator of DIC than an absolute value in these patients.
6) ATIII complex: decreased (usually less than 70% activity)
   a) Evaluates the activation of the coagulation system that occurs when thrombin is generated
   b) Decreased ATIII indicates accelerated coagulation.
7) FDPs: elevated (usually greater than 40 mcg/ml) but may be reported as positive at a number of dilutions; diagnostic for DIC is positive at greater than 100 dilutions (reported positive at 1:100)
   a) Measures the results of both fibrin and fibrinogen degradation
8) D-dimer (endproduct of fibrin degradation): elevated (greater than 250 ng/ml) or positive at greater than 1:8 dilutions
   a) Specific to the results of fibrin degradation
   b) More specific for DIC than FDPs but less sensitive
   c) May be falsely positive postsurgical in certain malignancies, DVT, and PE
9) Protamine sulfate test: strongly positive
   a) Protamine sulfate is added to plasma to see if fibrin strands are formed.
   b) A positive test reflects the formation of excessive amounts of thrombin.
10) Clotting factor analysis: shows a decrease in factors I, V, VIII, and fibrinogen
11) Peripheral smear: shows presence of schistocytes, helmet cells, and RBC fragments
12) Hgb and Hct: may be decreased if blood loss is significant
13) Arterial blood gases: respiratory alkalosis initially progressing to metabolic acidosis due to lactic acidosis
14) DIC scoring system using diagnostic tests (Table 9.15)
   b. Urine: may be positive for blood
   c. Stool: may be positive for blood
   d. Sputum: may be positive for blood

Collaborative Management
1. Identify and closely assess high-risk groups for clinical indications of DIC.
   a. Monitor closely for thrombosis or bleeding.
      1) Note petechiae, ecchymosis, and acrocyanosis.
      2) Test NG aspirate or vomitus, stools, and urine for blood.
      3) Monitor oral secretions, pulmonary secretions, and gums for bleeding.
      4) Monitor peripheral pulses and capillary refill.
   b. Monitor laboratory studies for diagnostic indications of DIC.
   c. Monitor closely for clinical indications of hypoperfusion or intracranial hemorrhage.
   d. Monitor hemodynamic parameters as indicated; insert indwelling urinary catheter to monitor hourly urine output.
2. Control underlying causative factors.
   a. Surgery
      1) Surgical débridement
      2) Abscess drainage
      3) Evacuation of the uterus
      4) Removal of tumor
   b. Antimicrobials for infection
   c. Antineoplastics for malignancy
3. Maintain airway, ventilation, and oxygenation.
   a. Administer oxygen to maintain PaO_2 of 80 mm Hg and SpO_2 (oxygen saturation in plasma) of 94%.
   b. Assist with intubation and mechanical ventilation as necessary.
   c. Suction only as necessary and with low suction to avoid trauma to the tracheobronchial mucosa.
4. Correct hypovolemia, hypotension, hypoxia, and acidosis.
   a. Insert or ensure patency of peripheral IV catheter.
   b. Administer normal saline to replace volume until type and crossmatch are completed and blood is available.

Table 9.16 Treatments for Disseminated Intravascular Coagulation

Treatment	Rationale	Controversy
Heparin	• Prevents further microclots and prevents platelet aggregation • Works with ATIII to neutralize circulating thrombin	• May perpetuate bleeding
ATIII	• Works with heparin to neutralize circulating thrombin	• May perpetuate bleeding
Clotting factors • FFP • Cryoprecipitate • Platelets	• Reestablishes normal hemostatic potential	• "Fuel to the fire" theory attests that until the clotting process is stopped, clotting factors just increase the thrombosis and microclotting
Epsilon-aminocaproic acid (Amicar)	• Blocks the fibrinolytic system so that stable clots are not degraded • Decreases amount of FDPs that act as anticoagulant	• Clearance of microclots from occluded vessels may be delayed • Indicated only in primary fibrinolysis

ATIII, Antithrombin III; *FDP*, fibrin degradation product; *FFP*, fresh-frozen plasma.

      c. Administer volume replacement, inotropes, or vasopressors as prescribed to maintain mean arterial pressure greater than 60 mm Hg.
5. Stop the microclotting to maintain perfusion and protect vital organ function.
    a. Administer IV low-dose heparin (usually 5–15 units/kg/hr) as prescribed; desirable aPTT is 1.5 to 2 times the control.
      1) Used primarily for patients with thrombosis who continue to bleed despite other rigorous treatment; often effective with underlying malignancy, acute promyelocytic leukemia, and purpura fulminans (may be seen in sepsis)
      2) Prevents further thrombosis in the microvasculature and prevents platelet aggregation; works with ATIII to neutralize circulating thrombin
      3) Continues to be controversial because it may potentiate or prolong bleeding, but it is thrombosis of small vessels, not hemorrhage, that has the greatest impact on morbidity and mortality in DIC
      4) Contraindicated in central nervous system (CNS) or GI hemorrhage, DIC associated with hepatic failure, hemorrhagic obstetric causes (e.g., abruptio placentae), and recent surgical procedures
    b. Administer ATIII as prescribed: ATIII inhibits the action of thrombin; may be administered if AT levels are low
    c. NOTE: Table 9.16 describes rationale and controversies regarding selected treatments.
6. Stop the bleeding by supporting coagulation.
    a. Administer blood products as prescribed to replace missing clotting factors.
      1) Platelets: Maintain platelet count above 50,000/mm^3; platelet replenishment is a priority to assist reinitiation of effective clotting.
        a) Desmopressin acetate may be prescribed to improve platelet function when platelet dysfunction is caused by dextran, NSAIDs, or ASA; monitor for fluid overload, hyponatremia, and tachycardia.
      2) FFP (contains all clotting factors)
        a) Used for bleeding patients with markedly prolonged PT and aPTT
        b) Replenishes fibrinogen levels
      3) Cryoprecipitate (contains factors VIII, XIII, and fibrinogen): maintains fibrinogen levels above 125 mg/dl
      4) Packed RBCs: may be needed if blood loss is significant
      5) May potentiate or prolong the clotting (fuel-to-the-fire theory), so heparin may be given first
    b. Administer hemostatic cofactors as prescribed.
      1) Vitamin K: needed for liver production of several clotting factors
      2) Folic acid: Deficiency may cause thrombocytopenia.
    c. Administer an antifibrinolytic agent (epsilon aminocaproic acid [Amicar], tranexamic acid [Cyklokapron]) as prescribed for primary fibrinolysis.
      1) Should be avoided in all other situations because it may enhance deposition of fibrin in the microcirculation and macrocirculation and lead to fatal DIC
      2) Requires concurrent heparin therapy in DIC
    d. Apply thrombin-soaked gauze, pressure dressings, or ice packs to control bleeding sites; the efficacy of topical hemostatics is unconfirmed.
    e. Maintain normal body temperature because hypothermia contributes to coagulopathy and vasoconstriction, perpetuating tissue ischemia.
    f. Maintain normal vascular volume because low circulating volume exacerbates effects of vascular clotting.
7. Treat ischemic pain.
    a. Administer analgesics as prescribed.
    b. Elevate ecchymotic limbs.
8. Maintain skin integrity and minimize tissue trauma.
    a. Provide meticulous skin care.
      1) Turn gently and frequently and assess skin during care
      2) Keep the skin moist with lubricating lotions.
      3) Use specialized beds as needed.
    b. Provide careful mouth care; use alcohol-free mouthwash and swabs.

Table 9.17 Comparison of Nonimmune and Immune Heparin-Induced Thrombocytopenia

Characteristic	Nonimmune (also referred to as HIT-1)	Immune (also referred to as HIT-2)
Onset	Day 1–4 of heparin administration	Day 5–10 of heparin administration
Route and dose	Primarily with high dose of IV heparin	Any route or dose
Effect on platelets	90,000–150,000/mm^3 for 1–5 days	Greater than 50% drop from baseline on days 7–10
Course	Platelet count may normalize	Thrombosis
	No thrombosis	May be associated with life-threatening complications
Mechanism	Direct toxic effect	Immune mediated
Antibodies	No	Yes
Treatment	Observation	Cessation of heparin and nonheparin anticoagulants

IV, Intravenous.

    c. Provide careful perianal care; avoid rectal thermometers and suppositories.
    d. Alternate activity with rest; mobilize and ambulate patient progressively.
    e. Use an electric, rather than straight-edged, razor.
    f. Avoid tape if possible; use adhesive remover to remove tape.
    g. Apply local pressure to any break in skin integrity.
        1) Avoid intramuscular, subcutaneous infections.
        2) Use an existing vascular access for blood sampling whenever possible.
            a) If venous puncture is necessary, apply pressure for 3 to 5 minutes afterward.
            b) If arterial puncture is necessary, apply pressure for 10 to 15 minutes afterward.
    h. Reduce frequency of taking cuff blood pressure readings: An arterial line is ideal for pressure monitoring and obtaining blood specimens.
    i. Do not give ASA or NSAID because of the effect on platelet aggregation.
    j. Teach patients to avoid the Valsalva maneuver; administer stool softeners to avoid constipation.
    k. Do not disturb any clot.
9. Provide psychological support and reassurance: Tell the patient that treatment is being provided to stop the bleeding (hemorrhage causes extreme anxiety).
10. Monitor for complications.
    a. Intracerebral hemorrhage (a major cause of death)
    b. Hemorrhagic shock
    c. ARDS
    d. GI dysfunction
    e. Renal failure
    f. Infection or sepsis

Heparin-Induced Thrombocytopenia

Definition
A prothrombotic disorder caused by a subset of antibodies against platelet factor 4 (PF4)–heparin complexes with strong platelet-activating properties
1. Differentiation between non–immune-mediated HIT and immune-mediated HIT (Table 9.17)

Etiology
Heparin administration or heparin-coated catheters
1. Risk is greater with UFH (3%–5%) than with LMWH (0.05%).

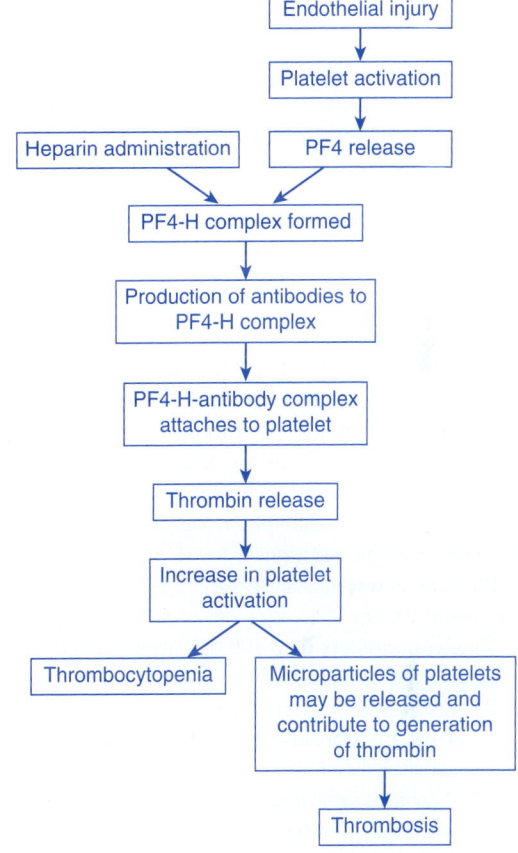

Fig. 9.7 Pathophysiology of heparin-induced thrombocytopenia (HIT). *PF4-H*, Platelet factor 4–heparin.

2. Risk is higher with bovine heparin than with porcine heparin.
3. Risk is higher in postoperative patients.
4. Risk is higher in patients with underlying vascular endothelial cell injury or venous stasis.

Pathophysiology
Fig. 9.7.

Clinical Presentation
1. Subjective: none
2. Objective
    a. Thrombotic events: reason for previous name of heparin-induced thrombosis and thrombocytopenia (HITT)

Table 9.18	4Ts Scoring System for Heparin-Induced Thrombocytopenia		
	2 Points	**1 Point**	**0 Points**
Thrombocytopenia	Platelet count fall greater than 50% from baseline *and* platelet nadir greater than or equal to $20 \times 10^9/l$	Platelet count fall 30%–50% from baseline *and* platelet nadir $10–19 \times 10^9/l$	Platelet count fall less than 30% from baseline *and* platelet nadir less than $10 \times 10^9/l$
Timing of fall in platelet count	Clear onset between days 5 and 10 *or* less than or equal to 1 day if heparin exposure within previous 30 days	Fall in platelet count consistent with onset between days 5 and 10, but timing is not clear because of missing platelet counts *or* onset after day 10 of heparin exposure *or* fall in platelet count less than or equal to 1 day with prior heparin exposure 30–100 days ago	Fall in platelet count less than 4 days after recent heparin exposure
Thrombosis or related occurrence	New thrombosis, skin necrosis, or acute systemic reaction after UFH exposure	Progressive or recurrent thrombosis or unconfirmed but clinically suspected thrombosis	No thrombosis or thrombosis preceding heparin exposure
Thrombocytopenia: possible other causes	None apparent	Possible other causes present	Probable other causes present

*Score less than 4 = low probability of heparin-induced thrombocytopenia (HIT); score of 4–5 = intermediate probability of HIT, score greater than 5 = high probability of HIT.

UFH, Unfractionated heparin;

From Crowther, M. A., Cook, D. J., Albert, M., Williamson, D., Meade, M., Granton, J., et al. (2010). The 4Ts scoring system for heparin-induced thrombocytopenia in medical-surgical intensive care unit patients. *J Crit Care, 25*(2), 287–293.

1) Venous four times more likely than arterial
   a) Venous: DVT, PE, cerebral venous thrombosis, adrenal infarction
   b) Arterial: MI, thrombotic stroke, limb arterial occlusion, renal or mesenteric arterial thrombosis, aortic occlusion
   b. Skin lesions, including petechiae and purpura
   c. Acute systemic reactions
   d. Bleeding is rare.
3. Diagnostic studies
   a. Platelet count less than 100,000/mm³ or a 50% decrease from baseline platelet count
   b. Platelet activation (functional) assays: rely on the ability of the PF4–heparin antibody to activate platelets; less sensitive but more specific
      1) Serotonin release assay: highly sensitive and specific but slow return of results
      2) Platelet aggregation assay such as heparin-induced platelet aggregation
   c. Antigen assays: more sensitive but less specific
      1) ELISA for PF4–heparin antibodies
   d. Platelet serotonin-release assay
4. Scoring system for HIT: 4 Ts score (Table 9.18)

Collaborative Management

1. Correct coagulopathy.
   a. Discontinue the offending agent (i.e., heparin).
   b. Administer an alternative anticoagulant (e.g., argatroban) as prescribed.
      1) Warfarin is contraindicated until platelet counts normalize because it decreases protein C activity and predisposes to microvascular thrombosis and limb gangrene.
   c. Plasmapheresis may be used to remove the pathogenic immunoglobulins.
2. Treat ischemic pain (as for DIC).
3. Maintain skin integrity and minimize tissue trauma (as for DIC).
4. Provide psychological support and reassurance (as for DIC).
5. Monitor for complications.
   a. Arterial or venous thrombosis
   b. Catheter-related thrombosis
   c. PE
   d. Adrenal infarction and acute adrenal crisis
   e. Thrombotic stroke
   f. MI
   g. Mesenteric artery thrombosis

Anemia

Definition

Decrease in the quantity or quality of circulating RBCs caused by:
1. Decrease in RBC or Hgb production
2. Excessive loss of RBCs
3. Excessive lysis of RBCs earlier than the 120-day life expectancy of the RBC

Predisposing Factors

1. Nutritional deficiencies: iron, folic acid
2. Pernicious anemia: deficiency of intrinsic factor necessary for absorption of vitamin B_{12}
   a. Hereditary affecting primarily people of Northern European descent but may also affect people of African and Hispanic descent
   b. Autoimmune disorder
   c. GI disorders (e.g., gastritis, Crohn disease, bowel resection)
   d. Medications such as proton pump inhibitors and antineoplastics
3. Acute blood-loss anemia
   a. GI: esophageal varices, gastric ulcers, lower GI bleed
   b. GU: renal trauma, menorrhagia

c. Trauma: bleeding may be overt or occult
d. Coagulopathies
4. Anemia of chronic illness (e.g., renal failure, cancer)
5. Aplastic anemia: failure of the bone marrow to produce blood cells; some degree of pancytopenia is present
6. Sickle cell anemia: hereditary affecting primarily people of African descent but may also affect people of Hispanic, Mediterranean, or Middle Eastern descent

Pathophysiology
1. General
   a. Reduced oxygen-carrying capacity of the blood
   b. Tissue ischemia
   c. Anaerobic metabolism
   d. Local acidosis
   e. Cellular edema
2. Specific to pernicious anemia
   a. Inherited autoimmune disorder that produces parietal cell antibodies or excessive drinking or smoking or gastric resection
   b. Defective gastric secretion of the GP intrinsic factor
   c. Ineffective erythropoiesis
3. Specific to aplastic anemia: stem cell defect or injury or destruction of hematopoietic cells
4. Specific to sickle cell anemia
   a. Hereditary disorder causing presence of Hgb S, an abnormal form of Hgb A
   b. Crystallization of the abnormal Hgb is promoted by deoxygenation, dehydration, acidosis, or temperature changes
   c. RBCs become crescent or sickle shaped after they release oxygen.
   d. These misshapen RBCs get stuck in the blood vessels, causing occlusion, tissue injury, and pain.
   e. Vascular occlusion may cause MI, ischemic stroke, splenic or hepatic infarction, blindness, or bone necrosis.
   f. Chronic hemolysis occurs because sickled RBCs are destroyed within 15 days.
   g. Immunocompromise occurs because spleen function is compromised.

Clinical Presentation
1. Subjective
   a. Weakness, fatigue
   b. Anorexia, indigestion, epigastric pain, oral pain related to glossitis
   c. Exertional dyspnea
   d. Palpitations
   e. Chest pain
   f. Paresthesia
2. Objective
   a. Pallor
   b. Tachycardia
   c. Tachypnea
   d. Glossitis
   e. Brittle or fine hair
   f. Diarrhea or constipation
   g. Flow murmur (i.e., systolic murmur associated with the turbulence of increased flow of blood through the heart)
   h. Impaired proprioception progressing to ataxia
3. Diagnostic studies
   a. RBC quantity: less than 4.4 to 5.9×10^6/ml for men or 3.8 to 5.2×10^6/ml for women
   b. RBC quality
      1) Microcytic (i.e., smaller), hypochromic (i.e., RBCs pale in color)
      2) Normocytic, normochromic
      3) Macrocytic (i.e., larger), normochromic
   c. Bone marrow biopsy to evaluate RBC production or detect malignancy
   d. Studies for detection of malignancy
4. Specifics depending on type of anemia
   a. Specific to iron-deficiency anemia: microcytic, hypochromic RBCs; iron level, TIBC, ferritin levels
   b. Specific to pernicious anemia
      1) Neurologic changes such as paresthesias and numbness progressing to loss of balance, dementia
      2) Decreased RBC, Hgb, and Hct
      3) Macrocytic, normocytic RBCs
      4) Increased MCV, normal MCH
      5) Increased serum bilirubin
      6) Decreased fasting serum B_{12}
      7) Normal serum folate (to rule out folate deficiency)
      8) Schilling test: abnormal: indicates impaired B_{12} absorption
   c. Specific to folic acid deficiency anemia: macrocytic, normocytic RBCs
   d. Specific to acute blood-loss anemia: normocytic, normochromic
   e. Specific to anemia of chronic illness: normocytic, normochromic or macrocytic, normocytic
   f. Specific to aplastic anemia: normocytic, normochromic
   g. Specific to sickle cell crisis
      1) Chest pain
      2) Fever
      3) Bone or joint pain
      4) Fatigue
      5) Jaundice with chronic hemolysis
      6) Complete blood count (CBC)
         a) Severe reduction in RBC count, Hgb, Hct
         b) Reticulocyte count: decreased
         c) Presence of nucleated RBCs, sickled RBCs
      7) Bilirubin: elevated
      8) Chest radiography: pulmonary infiltrates

Collaborative Management
1. Maintain airway, oxygenation, and ventilation.
   a. Position of comfort
   b. Oxygen by nasal cannula at 2 to 6 l/min if indicated to maintain SpO₂ of 94% unless contraindicated; in patients with chronic obstructive pulmonary disease, use pulse oximetry to guide oxygen administration to SpO₂ of 90%
2. Maintain adequate circulation and perfusion.
   a. Increased oral fluids
   b. IV access for fluid and medication administration as indicated
   c. Blood and blood products as prescribed (Table 9.9)

1) Monitor for transfusion reaction.
    a) Ask the patient to notify the nurse if she or he develops chills, low back pain, shortness of breath, nausea, sweating, itching, hives, or anxiety.
    b) Assess for clinical indications of transfusion reaction (Table 9.10 and Box 9.1).
    c) Take appropriate action for transfusion reactions (Table 9.10 and Box 9.2) if they occur.
    d) Monitor vital signs every 15 minutes for the first hour and then every 30 minutes until transfusion complete or according to hospital policy.
2) Monitor for adverse effects and complications (Table 9.11).
3. Control pain and discomfort.
    a. Analgesics
    b. NSAIDs
    c. Antiemetics
4. Administer drugs and therapies to treat cause.
    a. Iron supplements (iron-deficiency anemia)
    b. Vitamin B_{12} (pernicious anemia)
    c. Folic acid (folic acid deficiency anemia)
    d. Hydroxyurea (sickle cell anemia)
5. Initiate falls precautions caused by weakness, fatigue, altered mental status, or confusion.
6. Monitor for complications.
    a. Shock
    b. Transfusion reactions
    c. Vaso-occlusive crisis in sickle cell anemia

Immunodeficiency

Definition
A state of decreased responsiveness or unresponsiveness of the immune system causing an impaired ability to defend the body against antigens

Etiology
1. Congenital immunodeficiency
2. Acquired immunodeficiency
    a. Acute or overwhelming infections
        1) Bacterial
        2) Viral
    b. Physical agents, chemicals, or drugs
        1) Radiation
        2) Antibiotics
        3) Antineoplastic agents
        4) Steroids
        5) Antacids, histamine$_2$ receptor antagonists
        6) Immunosuppressive agents (e.g., for posttransplant patients)
        7) Anesthetic agents
        8) Alcohol
    c. Surgery
    d. Stress
        1) Physiologic
        2) Psychologic including noise
    e. Bone marrow depression
    f. Post-splenectomy
    g. Cancer, especially leukemia, lymphoma, or multiple myeloma
    h. Chronic diseases (e.g., diabetes mellitus, inflammatory bowel disease, hepatic cirrhosis or failure, chronic renal failure, psychiatric illness)
    i. Malnutrition
        1) Protein-calorie malnutrition
        2) Zinc deficiency
    j. Alcohol or drug abuse
    k. Anaphylaxis
    l. HIV disease or AIDS
    m. Aging (immunosenescence)
    n. CNS depression
    o. Leukopenia

Pathophysiology
1. In addition to the above listed etiological factors, critically ill patients are likely to have:
    a. Invasive catheters, NG tubes, endotracheal tubes, chest tubes, indwelling urinary bladder catheters, trauma, burns, surgery, skin lesions that alters skin barrier or mucous membranes
    b. Stress, which promotes catabolism, impairs healing, and causes immunodeficiency
    c. Sleep deprivation, which alters the immune function by reducing IL-1, reducing cellular immunity
    d. Multiple infections, which may overwhelm the immune system and bone marrow, causing a consumptive leukopenia
    e. Impaired consciousness, artificial airways, or feeding tubes, which cause impaired gag, swallowing, and cough reflexes
    f. Increased gastric pH caused by antacids, histamine$_2$-receptor antagonists, and proton pump inhibitors, which allows proliferation of bacteria in the stomach, which may migrate or be aspirated into the tracheobronchial tree and lungs
    g. Malnutrition caused by preexisting disease or inadequate nutritional replacement
    h. Altered perfusion of the intestinal tract, which results in impaired integrity of the intestinal wall and translocation of microorganisms or their toxins from intestinal lumen into the blood
    i. Prolonged hospitalization, which increases risk of exposure to microorganisms in the hospital environment from contaminated objects, other patients, or transmitted by hospital personnel
2. These factors reduce resistance to infection caused by a decrease in number or effectiveness of leukocytes and lymphocytes and suppression of the immune system.
3. Infection
    a. Chain of infection includes the following components
        1) Source of infection
        2) Mechanism of spread
            a) Understaffing has been linked to increased risk of nosocomial infection because routine nursing interventions, such as turning, suction, and compliance with aseptic standards may decline.
            b) Unit design may also affect risk of nosocomial infection since handwashing needs to be convenient; the use of alcohol-based cleansers at multiple convenient locations is helpful.

c) Avoidance of artificial nails and polish
  d) Avoidance of rings with stores
  e) Careful placement of patients with infections to avoid cross-contamination
 3) Susceptible host
b. Nosocomial infection
 1) 80% of nosocomial infections are within one of the following categories:
  a) Urinary tract infection
  b) Surgical site infection
  c) Pneumonia
  d) Intravascular catheter related bloodstream infection
 2) 70% of nosocomial infections are caused by the following microorganisms
  a) Gram-positive microorganisms
   i) *Staphylococcus aureus*
   ii) Coagulase-negative staphylococci
   iii) Enterococci
  b) Gram-negative microorganisms
   i) *E. coli*
   ii) *Pseudomonas aeruginosa*
   iii) *Enterobacter* spp.
   iv) *Klebsiella pneumoniae*
c. Drug-resistance infections
 1) Underlying principles of antimicrobial resistance
  a) Given sufficient time and antimicrobial use, resistance will occur.
  b) Resistance is progressive, from low to high levels.
  c) Organisms resistant to one antimicrobial are likely to become resistant to others.
  d) Resistance is slow to decline, if it declines at all.
  e) Use of antimicrobials by one person affects others in the immediate and extended environment.
 2) Factors that contribute to microbial resistance include the following:
  a) Increased use and misuse of antimicrobials
  b) Increase in the number of susceptible hosts
  c) Increase in use of invasive procedures and devices
  d) Lack of diligence with infection control practices
 3) Examples
  a) Methicillin-resistant *S. aureus* (MRSA)
  b) Vancomycin-resistant enterococci (VRE)
  c) Vancomycin-resistant intermediate *S. aureus* (VISA)
  d) Vancomycin-resistant *S. aureus* (VRSA)
  e) Penicillin-resistant *Streptococcus pneumoniae*
  f) Extended-spectrum beta-lactamase-producing microorganisms
d. Opportunistic infection
 1) Causes
  a) Immunocompromise
  b) Suppression of normal flora
   i) Candidiasis
    (a) Oral (i.e., thrush)
    (b) Systemic
   ii) *C. difficile*
    (a) Causes diarrhea
    (b) Treated with metronidazole or vancomycin

Clinical Presentation
1. Subjective
   a. History of precipitating condition
   b. Increased susceptibility to infection
      1) Immunodeficiency is suspected when an individual experiences chronic recurrent infections that do not respond to therapy or do respond but recur.
2. Objective
   a. Fever: greater than 101°F or 38.3°C
      1) Fever may be the only sign of infection in patients with leukopenia.
      2) Not all patients can develop a fever because the immune system (cytokines) is responsible for fever, so in immune-deficient patients, temperature may be normal or below normal even in the presence of infection.
   b. Skin rash
   c. Poor wound healing
   d. Redness, swelling, induration at IV site, wounds, incisions
   e. Recurrent abscess
   f. Osteomyelitis
   g. Hepatosplenomegaly
   h. Presence of opportunistic infections (e.g., *Pneumocystis* pneumonia, oral candidiasis)
   i. Presence of opportunistic malignancy (e.g., Kaposi sarcoma)
   j. Chronic diarrhea
   k. Clinical indications of sepsis or septic shock may be seen
3. Diagnostic studies
   a. Serum
      1) WBC: Total WBC may be decreased, or one component of the differential may be decreased.
      2) T-cell count: may be decreased or T-cell count may be normal, but T-cell function may be impaired
      3) Albumin and total proteins: may be decreased if protein malnutrition is a causative factor
   b. Cultures: may show causative organism(s)
   c. Anergy profile: delayed or absent response to skin tests
   d. Antibody titers: may be abnormal

Collaborative Management
1. Prevent or monitor for clinical indications of infection.
   a. Place in private room; limit number of visitors.
   b. Avoid contact with visitors or hospital staff who have any of the following:
      1) Fever
      2) Upper respiratory infection
      3) Diarrhea
      4) Open skin lesions
      5) Exposure to contagious disease

c. Maintain appropriate isolation or precautionary measures.
d. Minimize potential of cross-contamination; do not assign the patient and a patient with an infection to the same nurse.
e. Institute and emphasize good handwashing.
   1) The wearing of gloves does not eliminate the need to wash hands because microorganisms can permeate gloves and applying gloves over dirty hands may transfer microorganisms to the outside of the glove and therefore to the patient.
   2) Hands should be washed at the following times:
      a) Before and after patient contact
      b) Before and after invasive procedures
      c) After contact with soiled items
      d) After toileting
      e) Before and after using gloves
      f) Before handling food
   3) Technique
      a) Alcohol-based cleansers are used when the hands are not obviously soiled.
      b) Handwashing with soap and water is recommended when the hands are soiled and at least every five times of using alcohol-based cleanser.
         i) Wet hands under running water.
         ii) Apply 5 ml of soap and distribute thoroughly over both hands.
         iii) Using friction, wash all surfaces of the hands and fingers for at least 15 seconds, including under nails.
         iv) Rinse and dry thoroughly.
         v) Turn off faucets with a paper towel if there is not an automatic shutoff or fool controls.
f. Ensure proper cleaning, storage, disinfection, and sterilization of medical equipment as appropriate.
g. Provide only food that is cooked, pasteurized, or sterilized; unpeeled fruit should be avoided.
h. Provide sterile water for drinking as indicated.
i. Minimize introduction of organisms.
   1) Avoid cut flowers, potted plants, and standing water.
   2) Damp dust with disinfectant solution at least every 24 hours.
j. Culture common sources of contamination (e.g., ventilator tubing).
k. Avoid intrusive procedures and invasive devices if possible.
l. Teach and encourage necessary personal hygiene techniques.
m. Assess oral mucosa daily and maintain oral hygiene.
n. Decrease stress, noise, bright lights, and so on.
o. Do not administer live vaccines.
p. Encourage high protein and high calories in diet.
q. Administer filgrastim (granulocyte-colony stimulating factor) (Neupogen) and sargramostim (granulocyte macrophage-colony stimulating factor) (Leukine, Prokine) as prescribed.
   1) These drugs stimulate proliferation and differentiation of hematopoietic cells, specifically neutrophils or neutrophils and monocytes.
   2) Indicated to decrease incidence of infection in patients with nonmyeloid malignancy receiving bone marrow suppressive antineoplastic agents and for ganciclovir-induced neutropenia in AIDS patients
2. Provide appropriate nutritional support.
   a. Enteral nutrition is preferred over parenteral nutrition because it helps to prevent translocation of gram-negative bacteria from the GI tract and helps to prevent stress ulcers.
   b. Nutritional support containing glutamine and arginine may also be helpful in prevention of sepsis.
3. Prevent breaks in skin integrity.
4. Maintain activity but provide for adequate rest.
5. Assist in patient and family adjustment: Provide appropriate reassurance that measures are being taken to stop the bleeding.
6. Monitor for complications.
   a. Poor wound healing
   b. Opportunistic infections
   c. Secondary infections
   d. Sepsis
   e. Septic shock

Leukopenia

Definition
A decrease in circulating WBCs (i.e., leukocytes)

Etiology
1. Malignant invasion of the bone marrow is a primary cause of leukopenia, with malnutrition and chemotherapy being contributing factors.
   a. Leukopenia can be drug induced during malignancy treatment.
   b. Hypersplenism and splenomegaly can cause leukopenia.
   c. Stress and exercise, burns, tissue necrosis, chronic inflammatory disorders (e.g., gout, vasculitis)
2. Leukopenia can also occur because of several factors such as:
   a. Decreased production of leukocytes caused by hematopoietic progenitor cell abnormality (i.e., intrinsic factor)
   b. Increased destruction of the precursor cells, resulting from exaggerated apoptosis
   c. Increased removal or utilization of circulating neutrophils
   d. Increased margination of leukocytes (i.e., neutrophils) from circulation into vascular walls
   e. Other disorders in cell production are caused by extrinsic diseases
      1) Tumor infiltration or fibrosis of the bone marrow, HIV, Chédiak-Higashi syndrome
      2) Irradiation or chemotherapy
      3) Vitamin B_{12} deficiency

Pathophysiology
Leukopenia makes the patient vulnerable to opportunistic organisms; infections are difficult to manage because the patient is unable to mount an effective immune response.

Clinical Presentation
1. Subjective
   a. Bone pain
   b. Recurrent infections
   c. Anorexia, weight loss, fatigue, weakness
2. Objective:
   a. Neutropenia with an absolute count of less than 500 cells/microliter, fever
   b. Anemia and thrombocytopenia if associated with bone marrow suppression
   c. CNS dysfunction
   d. Lymphadenopathy, cachexia
   e. Recurrent or serious infections
3. Diagnostic studies
   a. Bone marrow biopsy
   b. CBC
   c. Blood smear

Collaborative Management
1. As for immunodeficiency
2. Administer treatment as prescribed; may be specific to underlying cause
   a. Protective isolation (i.e., neutropenic precautions) to prevent infection
   b. Termination of chemotherapy may stimulate stem cells proliferation of leukocytes
   c. Use of granulocyte-stimulating factors (e.g., Neupogen)
   d. Administration of leukocytes
   e. Splenectomy in severe cases of leukopenia

Learning Activities

CHAPTER 9

1. Complete the following crossword puzzle.

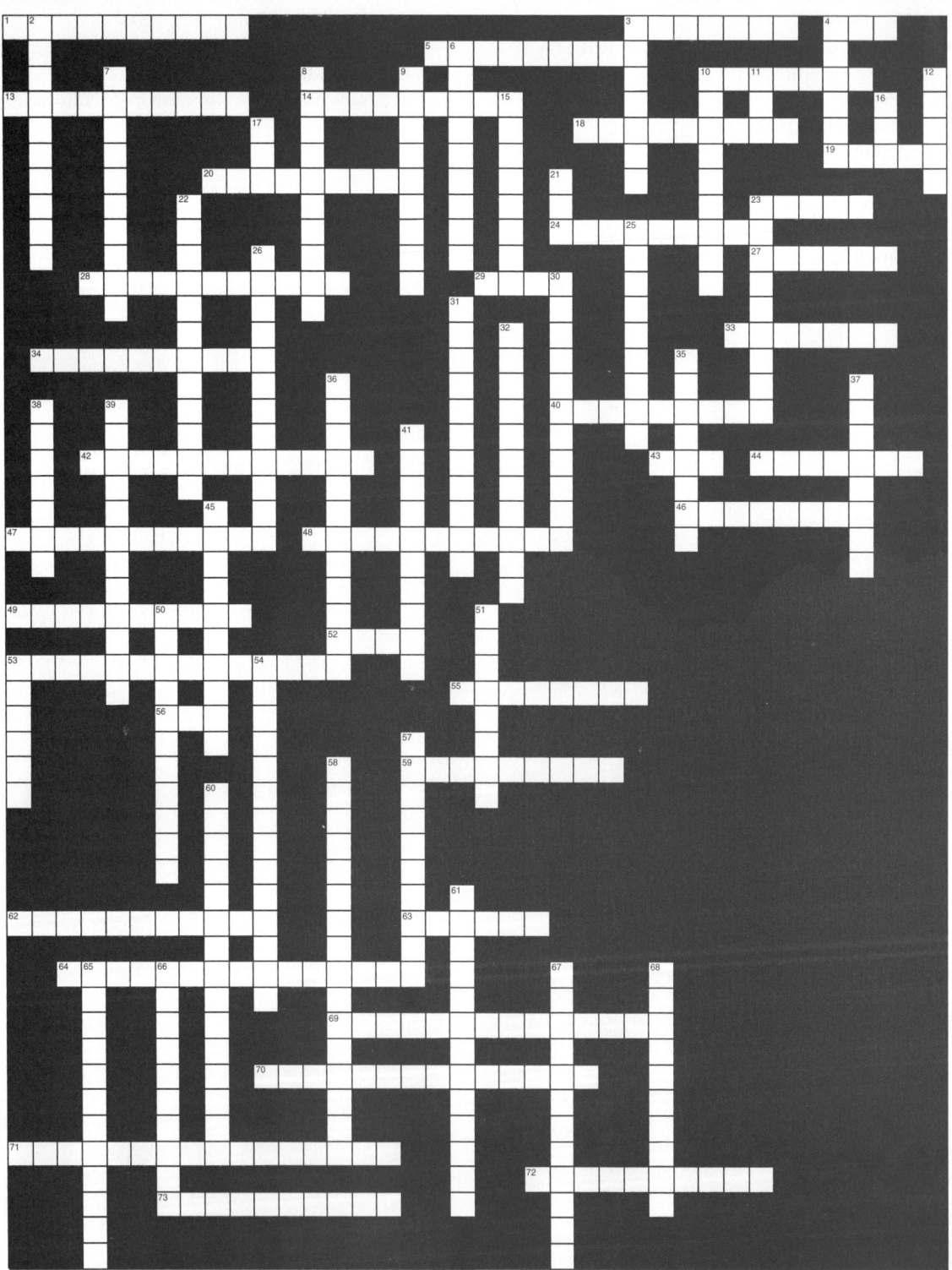

662

Chapter 9 The Hematologic and Immunologic Systems

ACROSS

1. Complex physiologic process for termination of bleeding
3. The major physiologic effect of anemia
4. Characterized by widespread microclots, consumption of clotting factors and platelets, and impaired fibrinolysis (abbrev)
5. This mediator is released by the mast cell in allergic reactions
10. Activated plasminogen; the active agent in the fibrinolytic process
13. Movement of neutrophils and phagocytes through pores of small blood vessels
14. This type of anemia is associated with increased RBC destruction, which causes jaundice
18. Factor X is sometimes referred to as ____ factor; deficient in hemophilia B
19. Increase in segmented neutrophils is referred to as a shift to the ____
20. This type of cell can engulf and digest microorganisms and cellular debris
23. The yellowish fluid that transports lymphocytes
24. The first sign of platelet dysfunction
27. The liquid portion of blood
28. Indirect thrombin inhibitor frequently used post-PCI (generic)
29. Increase in the number of immature neutrophils and other leukocytes in the blood is referred to as a shift to the ____
33. This type of immunity is mediated by B cells; involves the development of antigen-specific antibodies
34. A cascading system that can result in direct killing of invading organisms
40. The product of erythrocyte destruction
42. Leukocyte count that is higher than normal
43. The end result of fibrinolysis (abbrev)
44. These cells are fixed macrophages in the liver
46. This type of immunity is mediated by the T cell
47. This type of platelet analysis determines the ability of platelets to aggregate
48. A mature red blood cell
49. The percentage of RBCs in a given volume of blood
52. Anemia related to a deficiency of ____ causes nail changes and sores at the corners of the mouth
53. The main regulator of the platelet circulating mass
55. The granulocyte that releases heparin and histamine
56. The immunoglobulin most important in allergic reactions
59. Glycoprotein IIb/IIIa inhibitor frequently used before and after PCI (generic)
62. This mediator causes vasoconstriction, pulmonary vasoconstriction and platelet aggregation
63. Reduction in the total number of circulating erythrocytes or a decrease in the quality or quantity of hemoglobin
64. This blood product is administered to replace factor VIII in patients with hemophilia
69. A synonym for antibody; made by B cells
70. The process of erythrocyte production
71. A decrease in the number of platelets
72. A type of agranular leukocyte; B cells and T cells are examples
73. This type of T cell serves to modulate the immune response; increased in AIDS

DOWN

2. This type of granulocyte is most significant in allergic reactions
3. Parenteral anticoagulant that acts as an indirect thrombin inhibitor (generic)
4. The most specific laboratory test for DIC
6. The clotting pathway that is initiated by endothelial injury
7. Leukocyte count that is lower than normal
8. The movement of neutrophils and monocytes toward an antigen
9. These cells are decreased in ITP, DIC, and HIT
10. This electrolyte may increase with administration of banked blood
11. A drug frequently administered to decrease platelet aggregation (abbrev)
12. A platelet plug is sometimes referred to as a ____ clot
15. Chemical mediators of immunity and inflammation
16. The most abundant immunoglobulin
17. Normal adult hemoglobin (abbrev)
21. An autoimmune disorder in which an IgG autoantibody is formed and binds to and destroys the platelets (abbrev)
22. Sequential physiologic response that the body makes to injuries
23. Direct thrombin inhibitor that may be used for HIT (generic)
25. The clotting pathway that is initiated by tissue injury
26. This type of platelet analysis determines the number of platelets
30. A synonym for platelet
31. The adherence of phagocytes to the vessel wall
32. A leukocyte that releases granules when it ruptures
35. This sign may occur with hemolytic anemia
36. Heparin and ____ maintain the fluidity of the blood
37. Vitamin K antagonist; oral anticoagulant (generic)
38. This electrolyte may decrease with administration of banked blood
39. This coagulation study evaluates platelet function (2 words)
41. A cytokine synthesized by lymphocytes
45. This blood protein becomes fibrin when activated
50. Oral platelet aggregation inhibitor prescribed for several months after PCI with stents (generic)
51. This type of anemia is caused by bone marrow suppression
53. The site of T-cell distribution
54. This hormone is released from the kidney in response to low oxygen levels
57. This agranulocyte is the major phagocyte of the leukocytes
58. The first homeostatic mechanism
60. A common presenting symptom of leukemia and lymphoma
61. The process by which stem cells develop and differentiate into different types of blood cells
65. An immature erythrocyte
66. This type of anemia is caused by loss of intrinsic factor and malabsorption of vitamin B12
67. The final stage of the clotting process
68. The reticulocyte count reflects activity of the ____ (2 words)

Chapter 9 The Hematologic and Immunologic Systems

2. List the five major clinical indications of inflammation.
   a. _____
   b. _____
   c. _____
   d. _____
   e. _____

3. Identify which type of hypersensitivity reaction the following situations demonstrate.

Example	Type
Skin testing for tuberculosis	
Poststreptococcal glomerulonephritis	
Anaphylaxis to penicillin	
Hemolytic blood transfusion reaction	

4. Complete the following table.

	Platelet Plug	Intrinsic Pathway	Extrinsic Pathway	Common Pathway	Fibrinolytic System
Activation					
Laboratory test					

5. Match the drug with the laboratory effect.

___ 1.	Aspirin	a.	Prolonged bleeding time
___ 2.	Heparin	b.	Prolonged PT
___ 3.	Warfarin	c.	Prolonged aPTT
___ 4.	rt-PA	d.	Decreased fibrinogen levels
___ 5.	Streptokinase	e.	Increased fibrin degradation products
___ 6.	Clopidogrel	f.	Increased INR

6. Identify the appropriate actions to take for suspected transfusion reaction.

   a.

   b.

   c.

   d.

   e.

   f.

   g.

   h.

   i.

7. Identify the direction of change of the following laboratory values in DIC, ↑ or ↓.

Platelets	
PT	
aPTT	
Fibrin split products	
Factors V, VIII	
Fibrinogen	

8. Match the coagulopathy with the associated pathology.

____ 1. Hemophilia A
____ 2. Hemophilia B
____ 3. von Willebrand disease
____ 4. Heparin-induced thrombocytopenia
____ 5. Disseminated intravascular coagulation
____ 6. Liver disease
____ 7. Immune thrombocytopenic purpura
____ 8. Thrombotic thrombocytopenic purpura

a. Activation of thrombin and consumption of platelets and clotting factors
b. Binding of immune complexes to platelets, which are then destroyed by the spleen
c. Deficiency of von Willebrand factor
d. Deficiency of factor VIII
e. Deficiency of factor IX
f. Development of heparin–platelet factor 4 complex, which increases platelet activation and causes thrombocytopenia
g. Platelet aggregation and consumption
h. Inability to produce clotting factors

9. Discuss the controversy of the following therapies in the treatment of DIC.

a.	Heparin	
b.	Clotting factors	

10.
Match the cause of the anemia to the pathophysiology.

___1.	Esophageal varices	a. Blood loss
___2.	Radiation or drugs	b. Decreased or faulty RBC production
___3.	Hereditary	c. Destruction of RBCs
___4.	Malignancy	
___5.	Lead poisoning	
___6.	Crohn disease	
___7.	Anorexia nervosa	
___8.	Mismatched blood transfusion reaction	
___9.	Trauma	
___10.	Chronic kidney disease	
___11.	Sickle cell anemia	

Integumentary/Musculoskeletal Systems

CHAPTER 10

Integumentary/Musculoskeletal Systems

1. Integumentary/Musculoskeletal Systems are covered in two sections of the CCRN test plan.
   a. Endocrine/hematology/gastrointestinal (GI)/renal/integumentary constitutes 20% of the exam.
   b. Musculoskeletal/neurology/psychosocial constitutes 13% of the exam.

Integumentary System
Selected Concepts in Anatomy and Physiology

Functional Anatomy

1. General characteristics of the skin
   a. Largest and heaviest single organ of the body
   b. Approximately 15% to 20% of body weight
   c. 1 to 2 mm thick
   d. Estimated weight 10 lbs
   e. Covers an area of 1.2 to 2.4 m^2
2. Contains three layers: epidermis, dermis, and hypodermis (Figure 10.1)
   a. Epidermis: outermost and thinnest skin layer
      1) Composed of epithelial tissuxe and devoid of blood vessels; depends on dermis for nutrition
      2) Between 0.3 mm on the eyelids to 1.5 mm on the palms of the hands and soles of the feet
      3) Layers
         a) Stratum corneum: the outermost layer
            i) Made of 25 to 30 layers of dead flat keratinocytes; keratinocytes produce keratin
            ii) Lamellar granules provide water-repellent action and are continuously shed and replaced.
         b) Stratum lucidum: only found in the fingertips, palms of hands, and soles of feet
            i) Made up of three to five layers of flat dead keratinocytes
         c) Stratum granulosum
            i) Made up of three to five layers of keratinocytes
            ii) Site of keratin formation
            iii) Keratohyalin gives the granular appearance.
         d) Stratum spinosum
            i) Appears covered in thornlike spikes
            ii) Provides strength and flexibility to the skin
         e) Stratum basale: deepest layer
            i) Made up of a single layer of cuboidal or columnar cells
            ii) Cells produced here constantly divide and move upward.
      4) Functions
         a) Defensive barrier
         b) Absorption of nutrients
         c) Homeostasis
      5) Major cells: keratinocytes, melanocytes, Langerman cells, and Merkel cells
         a) Keratinocytes
            i) Produce the scleroprotein keratin, which provides protection from mechanical stress and the main constituent of nail, hair, and skin
            ii) Aid in protection
            iii) Serve as a waterproofing protein
         b) Melanocytes
            i) Produce the brown pigment melanin
            ii) Increase in response to exposure to sunlight
            iii) Absorb damaging ultraviolet (UV) light
         c) Langerhans cells
            i) Migrate to the epidermis from the bone marrow
            ii) Participate in the immune response by presenting an antigen to T cells
         d) Merkel cells are associated with the touch receptors and respond when the epidermis is deformed.
      6) Dermis: thicker, middle layer of skin
         a) Composed of dense layers of connective tissue (i.e., collagen and elastin proteins) to provide elasticity. stretching, and flexibility
         b) Between 1 and 4 mm thick
         c) Contains
            i) Collagen and elastic fibers
            ii) Blood and lymph vessels

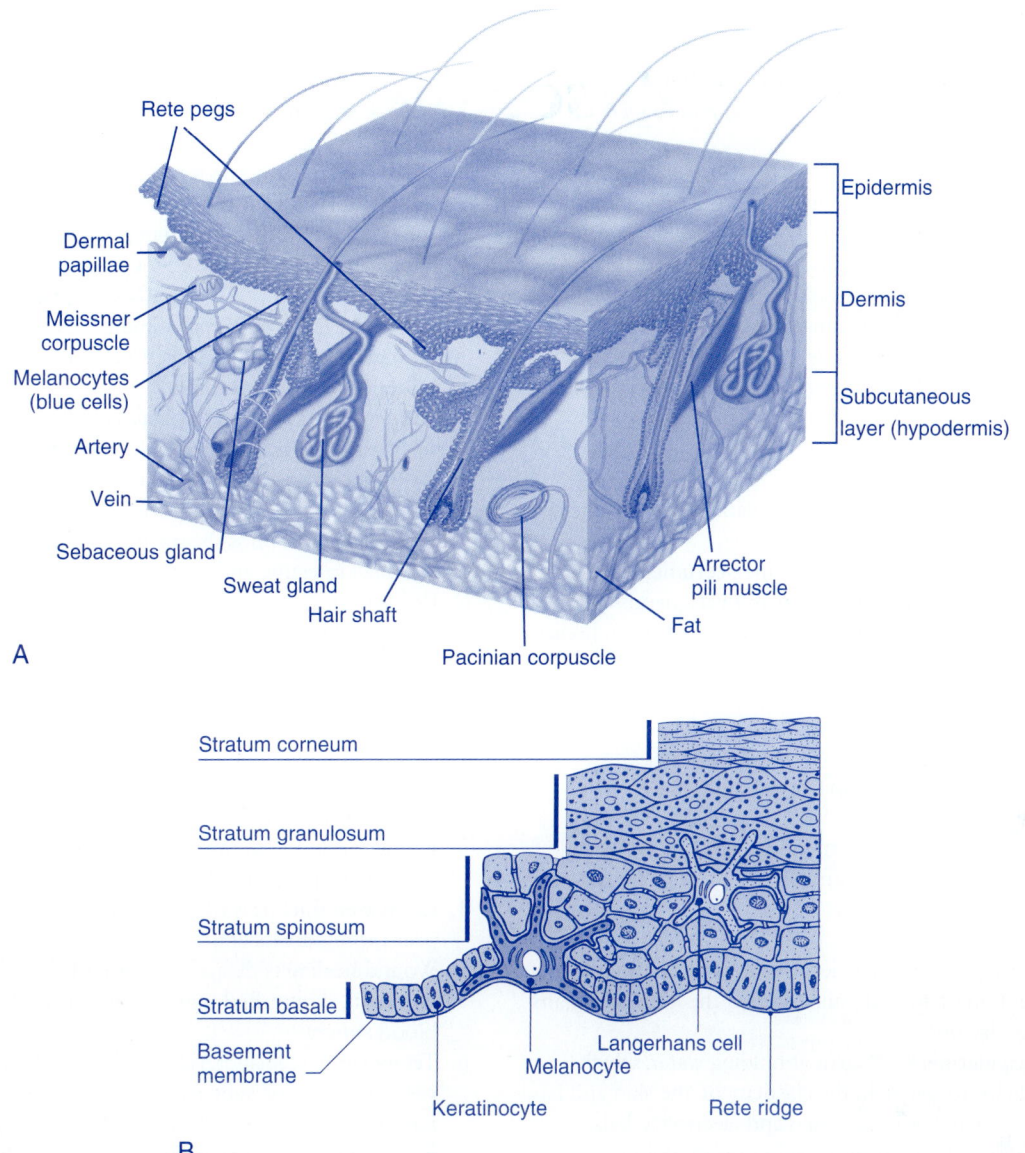

Fig. 10.1 Structure of the Skin. **A,** Cross-section showing major skin structures. **B,** Layers of the epidermis. (From McCance, K. L., & Huether, S. E. (2014). *Pathophysiology. The biologic basis for disease in adults and children* (7th ed.). St. Louis: Elsevier Mosby.)

        iii) Nerves
        iv) Sweat glands
        v) Hair follicles
        vi) Sebaceous glands
        vii) Sensory fibers
    d) Major cells
        i) Fibroblasts, which secrete collagen
        ii) Mast cells, which release histamine, which is important in hypersensitivity reactions in the skin
        iii) Macrophages are phagocytic cells that participate in immunity.
  7) Hypodermis (i.e., subcutaneous layer)
    a) Underlying layer of connective tissues that contains macrophages, fibroblasts, fat cells, nerves, blood vessels, lymphatics, fine muscles, and hair follicle roots
    b) Functions
        i) Acts as an energy reserve
        ii) Supports thermoregulation
        iii) Specializes in accumulating and storing fats
        iv) Area for blood vessel passage
        v) Area for pressure-sensing nerve endings
    c) Major cell: adipocytes
  b. Accessory structures of skin
    1) Hair or pili: present on most skin surfaces except palms, palmar surfaces of digits, soles, and plantar surface
        a) Functions
            i) Prevents heat loss
            ii) Decreases sunburn
            iii) Eyelashes help protect eyes.
            iv) Touch receptor
  c. Nails: tightly packed keratinized cells
    1) Function: protect the distal ends of finder and toes
  d. Sebaceous glands: absent in palms and soles
    1) Usually connected to hair follicles

2) Produce sebum; functions of sebum
   a) Moistens hairs
   b) Waterproofs and softens the skin
   c) Inhibits growth of bacteria and fungi
e. Oil glands
   1) Eccrine sweat glands
      a) Distributed among most areas of skin
      b) Functions
         i) Regulate body temperature through evaporation and perspiration
         ii) Help eliminate wastes (i.e., urea)
   2) Apocrine sweat glands
      a) Limited in distribution to axilla, scalp, face, areolae, abdomen, and genital area
      b) Secretions are more viscous
   3) Ceruminous glands
      a) Modified sudoriferous gland found in external auditory meatus
      b) Produce a waxy substance cerumen that contains secretions of oil and wax glands
      c) Function: barrier for entrance of foreign bodies

Physiology
1. Epidermis growth and keratinization
   a. Stem cells divide to produce keratinocytes
   b. Keratinocytes pushed up toward the surface with keratin
   c. Keratinization is replacement of cell contents with the protein keratin; occurs as cells move to the skin surface over 2 to 4 weeks
2. Function of protection
   a. Physical, protective barrier for the internal organs
   b. Prevention of loss of fluids so that the internal organs do not dry out
      1) Epidermis is efficient at holding water, which helps to maintain the elasticity of the skin and has a role in the body's fluid and electrolyte balance
   c. Acidic secretions from the skin prevent colonization by harmful microorganisms.
3. Function of thermoregulation
   a. Receptors in the skin monitor temperature and transmit impulses to central control mechanisms in the hypothalamus.
   b. The hypothalamus coordinates the autonomic nervous system, including the control of body temperature, thirst, hunger, and other homeostatic systems.
   c. Skin provides insulation, perspiration, and control of blood flow.
      1) The body is insulated by subcutaneous adipose tissue, which is found under the dermis.
      2) Eccrine glands are stimulated to produce sweat when the core temperature rises above 37°C.
      3) Sweat, in turn, cools the body through the process of evaporation.
   d. Skin provides an abundant blood supply, which aids thermoregulation.
      1) When the core temperature is increased, the body cools itself by increasing blood flow to the skin.
         a) Heat is removed from the body by the process of radiation.
         b) Heat is also lost through the skin by conduction and convection.
      2) When the core temperature is decreased, heat loss is reduced by the process of vasoconstriction, which reduces the flow of warm blood to the extremities from the body's core if the body becomes too cold.
      3) As people age, their thermoregulatory mechanisms become less efficient, which makes it more difficult for older people to detect and respond to temperature variations.
4. Function of sensation (i.e., touch, pressure, pain, heat, and cold)
   a. Skin reacts to external stimuli; supplied with approximately one million nerve fibers, most of which end in the face and extremities.
5. Function for vitamin D synthesis
   a. Vitamin D is synthesized by the skin as a consequence of the exposure of the skin to UV light.
   b. Vitamin D is necessary for controlling the amount of calcium and phosphorus that is absorbed through the small intestine and mobilized from the bone.
6. Psychological and body image function: The skin is highly visible and has cosmetic, aesthetic, and cultural significance.

Changes in Older Adults
1. Skin becomes thinner, drier, and less elastic; the appearance of the skin is wrinkled with changes in pigmentation.
2. Reduction in the number of melanocytes reduces protection against UV radiation and graying of the hair.
3. Reduction in the number of Langerhans cells reduces the immune response of the skin.
4. Decreased thickness of the dermis causes the skin to appear more translucent.
5. Wound healing is delayed because of decreased cell proliferation, diminished immune response, and diminished blood supply.
6. Temperature regulation is less effective because of decreased vascularity, loss of subcutaneous fat, loss of cutaneous vasomotor response, and decreased eccrine sweat production.
7. Reduced sensory perception is caused by the decrease in the number of pressure and touch receptors.

Assessment
Interview
1. Chief complaint: why the patient is seeking help and duration of the problem
2. Nonspecific problems or complaints
3. Changes in appetite
4. Environmental exposure
5. Home medication regimen

Vital Signs
Inspection and Palpation of the Skin
1. Color
2. Temperature
3. Moisture
4. Capillary refill
5. Color
6. Moisture
   a. Temperature
   b. Texture
   c. Mobility and turgor
   d. Lesions

Table 10.1	Complex Wounds
Surgical wounds	• Open nonhealing postsurgical wounds • Localized incisions • Infection or draining wounds • Complicated surgical wounds
Pressure injury (i.e., ulcer)	• Multiple stage II injury • Stage III or IV injury
Other wounds	• Infected wounds requiring IV antibiotics • Wounds requiring frequent dressing changes • Amputation • Diabetic ulcers • Necrotizing fasciitis • Osteomyelitis • Ischemic ulcers related to peripheral vascular disease • Venous stasis ulcers • Wounds related to trauma • Burn wounds • Fistula

IV, Intravenous.

7. Diagnostic study
   a. Biopsy

Complex Wounds

Definitions
1. Complex wounds: difficult wounds, either chronic or acute, that defy cure using conventional and simple dressing therapy
   a. Major groups of complex wounds (Table 10.1)
2. Pressure injury

Etiology: One or Several of the Following Factors
1. Trauma
2. Burns
3. Surgery
4. Chronic illnesses that impair wound healing (e.g., diabetes mellitus, peripheral vascular disease)
5. Infection
6. Pressure injury, specifically
   a. Immobility
   b. Friction and shear
   c. Malnutrition
   d. Medical condition
   e. Contracture
   f. Pressure injury in critically ill patients (Cox, 2017b)
      1) Age
      2) Prolonged critical care stay
      3) Diabetes mellitus
      4) Cardiovascular disease
      5) Hypotension
      6) Prolonged mechanical ventilation
      7) Vasopressor administration

Pathophysiology
1. Injury to the epidermis, dermis, or subcutaneous tissue
2. Hemostasis
   a. Immediately after injury to the skin, small vessels within the wound constrict to provide at least a measure of hemostasis for 5 to 10 minutes.
   b. Platelets aggregate in severed vessels and trigger the clotting cascade and release essential growth factors and cytokines that are important for the initiation and progression of wound healing.
   c. The fibrin matrix that results stabilizes the wound and provides a provision scaffold for the wound healing process.
3. Inflammation
   a. This phase is completed within 1 to 4 days, except in the presence of infection or other causes of wound chronicity.
   b. Key components of this phase are increased vascular permeability and cellular recruitment.
   c. The presence of necrotic tissue, foreign material, and bacteria results in the abnormal production of metalloproteases, which alter the balance of inflammation and impair the function of the cytokines.
4. Proliferation
   a. Also called *migration*, it refers to basal cell proliferation and epithelial migration occurring in the fibrin bridgework inside a clot.
   b. It continues until the individual cells are surrounded by cells of similar type.
   c. In a clean surgical wound, the epithelial cells migrate downward to meet deep in the dermis. Migration ceases when the layer is rejuvenated; this is normally completed within 48 hours of surgery.
   d. The superficial layer of epithelium creates a barrier to bacteria and other foreign bodies. However, it is very thin, easily traumatized, and gives little tensile strength.
   e. Fibroblast proliferation occurs and is an accumulation of ground substance and collagen production.
   f. Fibroblasts are transformed from local mesenchymal cells, are usually present in the wound within 24 hours, and predominate by the 10th postoperative day.
   g. They attach to the fibrin matrix of the clot, multiply, and produce glycol protein and mucopolysaccharides, which make up ground substance.
   h. Fibroblasts also synthesize collagen, the primary structural protein of the body.
   i. Collagen production begins on the second postoperative day. Maximum collagen production does not begin until day 5 and continues for at least 6 weeks.
   j. The developing collagen matrix stimulates angiogenesis.
   k. Granulation tissue is the result of the combined production of collagen and growth of capillaries.
5. Remodeling (i.e., maturation)
   a. Key elements of remodeling include collagen cross-linking, collagen remodeling, and wound contraction.
   b. The tensile strength of the wound is directly proportional to the amount of collagen. As disorganized collagen is degraded and reformed, covalent cross-links are formed that enhance tensile strength.
   c. Maximum strength depends on the interconnection of collagen subunits.
   d. Approximately 80% of the original strength of the tissue is obtained by 6 weeks after surgery, but the diameter and morphology of collagen fibers do not have the appearance of normal skin until 180 days.

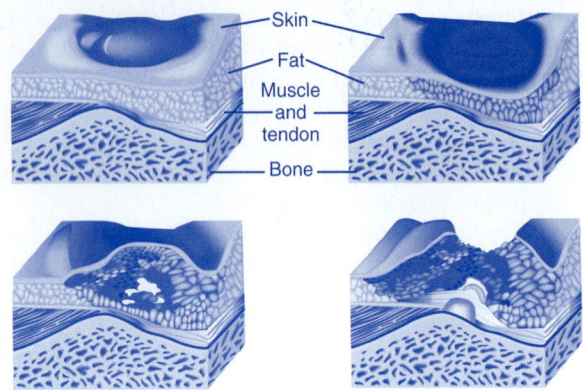

Fig. 10.2 Progression of decubitus ulcer. Sustained pressure over a bony prominence compresses the tissue and reduces blood flow, resulting in progressive ischemia and necrosis of tissue. (From McCance, K. L., & Huether, S. E. (2014). *Pathophysiology. The biologic basis for disease in adults and children* (7th ed.). St. Louis: Elsevier Mosby.)

    e. Remodeling can take up to 2 years after the initial wound injury. This explains why closed wounds can quickly break down if attention is not paid to the initial causative factors.
6. Pressure injury, specifically
    a. Constant pressure sufficient to impair local blood flow to soft tissue (>32 mm Hg) for an extended period
    b. Shear forces and friction accentuate the effects of pressure.
    c. Maceration, such as occurs with incontinence or oozing wounds, also increases the risk of skin injury.

Clinical Presentation

1. Obvious wound or laceration
2. Redness or blanching caused by burn
3. Drainage, possibly purulent
4. Pressure injury staging (Mackintosh, Gwilliam, & Williams, 2014; National Pressure Ulcer Advisory Panel, 2016) (Figure 10.2)
    a. A pressure injury is damage to the skin and underlying soft tissue that is localized and usually over a bony prominence or related to a device.
        1) The sacral area, greater trochanter, ischial tuberosity, heel, and lateral malleolus locations account for 95% of all pressure injury sites.
    b. Stage 1
        1) Intact skin with nonblanchable redness of a localized area usually over a bony prominence; color changes do not include purple or maroon, which may indicate deep injury
        2) Painful, firm, soft, warmer, or cooler area compared with the adjacent area
        3) May be difficult to detect in individuals with dark skin tones
        4) May be compared to a tomato
    c. Stage 2
        1) Partial-thickness loss of dermis presenting as a shallow open ulcer with a red pink wound bed without slough
        2) May also present as an intact or ruptured serum-filled blister
        3) Does not include moisture-associated skin damage (MASD); intertriginous dermatitis (ITD); medical adhesive-related skin injury (MARSI); or traumatic wounds such as skin tears, burns, or abrasions
        4) There is partial loss of the dermis.
        5) May be compared to a potato that has had a potato peeler swiped across the surface
    d. Stage 3
        1) Full-thickness tissue loss; subcutaneous fat may be visible, but bone, tendon, or muscle is not visible or palpable
        2) Slough may be present; there may be undermining, epibole, or tunneling.
        3) Depth varies with local because some areas do not have subcutaneous tissue; in areas such as the nose, ear, occiput, and malleolus, the ulcer may be shallow.
        4) May be compared to an apple with a bite removed
    e. Stage 4
        1) Full-thickness tissue loss with exposed bone, tendon, or muscle; exposed bone or tendon is visible or palpable
        2) Slough or eschar may be present on parts of the wound bed; undermining, epibole, and tunneling are common.
        3) Depth varies with local because some areas do not have subcutaneous tissue; in areas such as the nose, ear, occiput, and malleolus, the ulcer may be shallow.
        4) Because these ulcers extend into muscle and supporting structures, osteomyelitis is possible.
        5) May be compared to a peach with a deep bite removed; the pit is visible
    f. Unstageable pressure injury
        1) Full-thickness skin or tissue loss in which the stage cannot be determined because it is obscured by slough or eschar
    g. Deep tissue pressure injury
        1) Persistent nonblanchable discoloration that is deep red, maroon, or purple; this color varies with dark skin
        2) Pain and temperature changes frequently precede color changes.
        3) May evolve to reveal full-thickness pressure injury

Collaborative Management

1. Identify patients at high risk.
    a. Braden Scale for Predicting Pressure Sore Risk is a commonly used tool.
        1) Consists of six categories
            a) Sensory perception: measures a patient's ability to detect and respond to discomfort or pain that is related to pressure on parts of her or his body
            b) Moisture: assesses the degree of moisture the skin is exposed to
            c) Activity: evaluates a patient's level of physical activity
            d) Mobility: evaluates the capability of a patient to adjust her or his body position independently
            e) Nutrition: assesses a client's nutritional status and looks at her or his normal patterns of daily nutrition

f) Friction and shear: determines the amount of assistance a client needs to move and the degree of sliding on beds or chairs that they experience
2) Scoring
   a) Each category is rated on a scale of 1 to 4, excluding the "friction and shear" category, which is rated on a 1 to 3 scale, for a total of 23 points.
   b) A higher score indicates a lower risk of developing a pressure ulcer and vice versa.
      i) Very high risk: total score of 9 or less
      ii) High risk: total score of 10 to 12
      iii) Moderate risk: total score of 13 to 14
      iv) Mild risk: total score of 15 to 18
      v) No risk: total score of 19 to 23
2. Institute preventive measures for pressure injury.
   a. Reduce pressure and turn on a regular schedule, usually at least every 2 hours.
   b. Encourage patient mobility.
   c. Protect the patient's heels.
   d. Use mattresses that distribute pressure.
   e. Manage any situation that causes moisture (e.g., incontinence).
   f. Ensure adequate nutrition.
   g. Prevent friction and shearing forces.
3. Consider use of the InSPiRE skin integrity care bundle (Coyer et al., 2015).
   a. Assessment of skin integrity on admission and ongoing assessment performed and documented every 12 hours
   b. Strategies to prevent pressure injuries
      1) Skin hygiene: bathing once daily with pH-balanced cleansing agent and use of a topical moisturizer if skin is dry and flaky
      2) Repositioning: Turning at least every 3 hours and more often is indicated.
         a) Use of a "turn team"
         b) Left lateral–supine–right lateral is recommended if possible with lateral turns being a full lateral if tolerated.
         c) Foam wedges to maintain position
      3) Elimination of pressure and friction
         a) Support surface depending on need: nonpowered pressure-redistribution support surface, dynamic powered alternating pressure support surface, or other support surface
         b) Examination of nares, lips, and mouth every 12 hours
         c) Securing of nasogastric and endotracheal tubes
         d) Repositioning of nasogastric and endotracheal tubes at least every 12 hours or more often if necessary
      4) Elimination of heel pressure: elevation of heels using heel protectors and foam pads under calf
   c. Protection from forces of pressure and friction
      1) Maintenance of normal skin temperature
      2) Avoidance of skin contact with plastic surfaces
      3) Interprofessional collaboration
         a) Nutritional assessment by a dietician and early enteral feeding
         b) Assessment and assistance of physical therapy to promote mobility: patient to sit in chair out of bed daily if clinically possible
4. Use appropriate collaborative therapies depending on the type and severity of wound
   a. Nonoperative
      1) Reduction of pressure
      2) Control of infection: cleansing; antimicrobials when appropriate
         a) Cultures: There is confusion regarding the significance of a positive wound swab and the risk of invasive infection.
            i) Wound healing is only significantly retarded when a sufficient bacterial load (>105 bacteria/g of tissue) is present.
            ii) An open draining wound without necrotic tissue will be colonized, but the bacteria present are usually insufficient in number to affect healing.
         b) Wound cleaning: Invasive infection retards healing and leads to wound breakdown, but for most wounds, all that is required to reduce bacterial counts to tolerable levels is to clean away accumulated debris with saline.
         c) Topical antiseptics may be used to irrigate, cleanse, and debride wounds.
            i) Chlorhexidine 0.05% is the most widely used antiseptic; it has a lower incidence of contact dermatitis and less tissue toxicity.
            ii) Cetrimide 1% has a marked detergent action and is often used for soiled traumatic wounds; however, the agent's in vitro cytotoxicity makes it unpopular for routine use.
            iii) Povidone–iodine is particularly useful against staphylococci but is less effective against *Pseudomonas* species; it is also associated with contact hypersensitivity as well as toxicity from systemic absorption, which limits its use as an irrigant in large, deep cavities.
            iv) Hypochlorite solutions (bleach) are rarely used because of concerns about tissue toxicity.
         d) Antimicrobials as prescribed
            i) Systemic antimicrobials do not penetrate necrotic tissue and have little to offer in the management of chronic wounds.
            ii) Topical antimicrobial applications should also be avoided because they are ineffective and foster multiple drug resistant strains of bacteria.
            iii) Antimicrobials are only appropriate when there is invasive infection, such as cellulitis or osteomyelitis.
      3) Negative-pressure device (e.g., vacuum-assisted closure [VAC]): removes drainage and helps wounds close
      4) Dressings to nurture the cellular environment of the wound for healing
         a) The ideal dressing must be easy to apply, painless to remove, and require few changes;

it must maintain the wound temperature and moisture level, permit respiration, and allow epithelial migration.
- i) Wet-to-dry dressings are no longer advocated as a method of debridement; these are painful and remove granulating tissue along with necrotic tissue.
- b) The most favorable environment for the mobility and respiration of cells is a moist wound because a moist wound environment has shown enhanced epithelial migration, fibroblast function, and collagen production. These findings supported the development of occlusive dressings.
- c) Occlusive dressings allow in situ degradation of necrotic material, which is then absorbed into the fluid phase of the dressing.
    - i) Semipermeable adhesive films, such as OpSite and Tegaderm, are permeable to gas and water vapor but are a barrier to bacteria and water.
        - (a) Generally reserved for the definitive closure of superficial, partial-thickness wounds in which comfort and ease of management are important
        - (b) Can be left in place for several days but usually leak if exudate builds up
        - (c) Removal is easier if the film is stretched before being pulled off.
    - ii) Hydrocolloid dressings, such as Comfeel and DuoDERM, are adhesive, water- and gas-impermeable membranes.
        - (a) The inner layer forms a gel when it comes into contact with exudate.
        - (b) Warn patients that the wound may, at first, become smelly and appear to enlarge.
        - (c) Provide an excellent seal around the edges of the wound and can protect pressure areas.
        - (d) Absorb exudate and help to debride the wound.
        - (e) Change when the gel leaks out.
        - (f) To avoid frequent changes, the dressing should have a diameter at least 2 cm bigger than the wound.
        - (g) Can be used in the presence of necrotic material but tend to have problems with overwhelming exudate buildup in large wounds or when there is anaerobic colonization
    - iii) Alginate dressings such as Kaltostat and other alginates are derivatives of seaweed.
        - (a) Activated by wound exudate to produce a hydrophilic gel
        - (b) Absorb the noncellular components of the exudate.
        - (c) Provide a satisfactory dressing for lightly contaminated wounds and cavities.
        - (d) Generally unsatisfactory in the presence of dry, necrotic tissue because there is no exudate to activate them
        - (e) Because they are not adhesive, they are easily removed by lavage, but they must be held in place by another dressing
        - (f) Depending on the amount of exudate, alginates can be changed twice a week.
    - iv) Foam dressings such as Lyofoam and Alleryn are highly absorbent synthetic foams.
        - (a) Absorb large volumes of exudate from discharging wounds, reducing the need for dressing changes.
        - (b) Can be used in combination with a hydrogel for necrotic wounds that require debriding
    - v) Hydrogel dressing, including IntraSite, are based on starch polymers.
        - (a) Provide moisture to the wound and encourage debridement.
        - (b) Best suited to dry necrotic wounds, but they also absorb exudate while maintaining the products of tissue repair and degradation, including growth factors and lysosomes, in contact with the wound
        - (c) If the wound is clean, it only needs to be replaced once or twice a week; daily dressings may be needed if the wound is necrotic or infected.
    - vi) Suitable dressings should be determined by wound assessment.
        - (a) Definitive protocols for these dressings have not yet been developed; choices of dressings increasingly represent a cost–benefit analysis in which the high cost of the latest dressing is balanced against savings in time and labor involved in dressing changes
        - (b) Choice of dress should also consider the following:
            - (i) Depth of wound
            - (ii) Amount of exudate
            - (iii) Degree of contamination
- b. Operative, especially when extent of skin and subcutaneous tissue loss is extensive
    - 1) Debridement: removal of necrotic tissue from wound edges and cavity; may take place at the bedside or in surgery
    - 2) Reconstruction with graphs and flaps
    - 3) Vascular surgery for peripheral vascular disease with nonhealing vascular ulcers

4. Support wound healing
     a. Nutritional support to include adequate protein
     b. Hydration
     c. Glucose control

Intravenous Infiltration

Definitions
1. Infiltration: leakage of intravenous (IV) fluids or medications into the tissue around an IV catheter
2. Extravasation: leakage of a potentially damaging medication into the tissue around an IV catheter

Etiology and Risk Factors (Infusion Nurses Society, 2016)
1. Catheter insertion location susceptible to catheter movement with patient movement (e.g., hand, wrist, antecubital space, ankle, foot)
2. Infusion of antibiotics or corticosteroids
3. Presence of patient infection
4. Multiple attempts at venous cannulation
5. Patient difficulty or inability to communicate pain, discomfort, or swelling, including altered level of consciousness or cognition
6. Medications that alter pain response (e.g., opiates) or suppress inflammation (corticosteroids)
7. Aging or diseases that cause changes in vascular system (e.g., diabetes mellitus, systemic lupus, peripheral vascular disease)
8. Difficulty with peripheral vascular access (e.g., obesity, multiple venipunctures, IV drug abuse)
9. Peripheral catheters indwelling for more than 24 hours
10. Length of time for injection or infusion of vesicant medications
11. Patient movement causing erosion of the vein wall
12. Restriction of the blood flow in the area near the IV site

Pathophysiology
1. Puncture of vein wall
2. Leakage of fluid into the subcutaneous tissue surrounding catheter insertion site causes swelling.
3. Swelling causes discomfort.
4. Extravasation may cause tissue damage.
   a. Extravasation of a vesicant causes tissue damage.
      1) Cytotoxic drugs (e.g., vincristine, vinblastine, cisplatin, doxorubicin)
      2) Noncytotoxic drugs (e.g., alcohol, diazepam, digoxin, phenytoin)
   b. Extravasation of a vasopressor (e.g., epinephrine, norepinephrine, phenylephrine, dopamine) causes vasoconstriction and ischemia, which may cause tissue damage.

Clinical Presentation
1. Subjective
   a. Discomfort, burning, or pain
   b. Tightness
2. Objective
   a. Cool skin around IV catheter insertion site
   b. Blanched skin around IV catheter insertion site
   c. Swelling at or above the IV insertion site
   d. Dressing over IV catheter may be damp
   e. Slowed or stopped IV infusion flow rate
   f. Absence of backflow of blood into the IV tubing if the solution container is lowered
   g. Blistering may occur if vesicant extravasation occurs.
   h. Skin sloughing if vasopressor or vesicant extravasation occurs
3. Grading scale (Infusion Nurses Society, 2000)
   a. 0: no symptoms
   b. 1
      1) Skin blanched, cool to touch, with less than 1 inch of edema in any direction from the IV catheter insertion site
      2) The patient may or may not have pain.
   c. 2
      1) Skin blanched, cool to touch, with between 1 and 6 inches of edema in any direction from the IV catheter insertion site
      2) The patient may or may not have pain.
   d. 3
      1) Skin blanched and translucent, cool to touch, with more than 6 inches of edema in any direction from the IV catheter insertion site
      2) The patient complains of mild to moderate pain.
      3) The patient may complain of numbness.
   e. 4
      1) Skin blanched and translucent and cool to touch; may be discolored or bruised
      2) More than 6 inches of edema in any direction from the IV catheter insertion site with deep pitting possible
      3) The patient complains of moderate to severe pain and possibly numbness.
      4) Pulses and capillary refill may be impaired.
      5) Inflammation at the insertion site may be noted.

Collaborative Management
1. Prevention of infiltration or extravasation
   a. Careful select IV catheter insertion site
      1) Avoid areas of joint flexion, such as the hand, wrist, or antecubital fossa; the preferred site is the forearm.
      2) Avoid small or fragile veins.
      3) Avoid veins in areas with edema or neurologic impairment.
   b. Secure the IV catheter with tape and dressing according to hospital protocol to prevent movement of catheter.
   c. Use central venous access devices for vesicants and vasopressors if possible.
2. Detection of infiltration or extravasation
   a. Frequently monitor the IV site.
   b. Instruct the patient and family to report signs or symptoms of infiltration or extravasation, such as swelling or discomfort.
   c. Aspirate for blood return if infiltration is suspected; aspiration of blood return does not definitely rule out infiltration because there could be a venous puncture even though catheter tip is in the venous lumen.
3. Prevention of complications of infiltration or extravasation when infiltration or extravasation noted
   a. Stop the IV infusion immediately if infiltration occurs.
   b. Do not flush the catheter; aspirate from the catheter with a small syringe.
   c. Remove the catheter if indicated by hospital protocol; note that some protocols recommend that the

catheter not be clamped but not removed because the catheter may be used for insertion of substance-specific medications for extravasation (e.g., phentolamine for vasopressors, dexrazoxane for anthracyclines) or hyaluronidase, which is nonsubstance-specific and aids in fluid reabsorption.
    d. Mark the area of infiltration or extravasation with a skin marker; estimate the volume of solution that has infiltrated.
    e. Perform frequent assessments for changes in perfusion, sensation, or movement.
    f. Elevate the extremity unless it causes patient discomfort.
    g. Apply compresses as indicated.
        1) Dry, cold compresses to localize the medication and reduce inflammation
            a) Indicated for nonirritant and hyperosmolar fluid and medications
            b) Contraindicated with extravasation of vinca alkaloids and vasopressors
        2) Dry, warm compresses to increase blood flow and disperse medications
4. Prepare the patient for surgical procedures if required.
    a. Decompression with fasciotomy
    b. Surgical washout procedure
    c. Debridement with skin grafting

Musculoskeletal System
Selected Concepts in Anatomy and Physiology

General Information About the Musculoskeletal System
1. The human skeleton has 206 bones.
2. Functions
    a. Provide structure and support for soft tissue
    b. Protect vital organs

Functional Anatomy
1. Types of bone
    a. Compact bone
        1) Smooth and dense
        2) Forms shaft of long bones and outside layer of other bones
        3) Spongy bone
            a) Contains spaces
            b) Spongy sections contain bone marrow.
                i) Red bone marrow
                    (a) Found in flat bones of sternum, ribs, and ileum
                    (b) Produces blood cells and hemoglobin
                ii) Yellow bone marrow
                    (a) Found in shaft of long bones
                    (b) Contains fat and connective tissue
2. Joints: area where two or more bones meet
    a. Function: holds skeleton together while allowing the body to move
    b. Types of joints
        1) Synarthrosis: immovable (e.g., skull)
        2) Amphiarthrosis: slightly movable (e.g., vertebral joints)
        3) Synovial: freely movable (e.g., shoulders, hips)
            a) Found at all limb articulations; types include hinge, ball and socket, and pivot
            b) Surface covered with cartilage
            c) Joint cavity covered with tough fibrous capsule
            d) Cavity lined with synovial membrane and filled with synovial fluid
3. Ligaments: bands of connective tissue that connect bone to bone
    a. Functions
        1) Either limit or enhance movement
        2) Provide joint stability
        3) Enhance joint strength
4. Tendons: fibrous connective tissue bands that connect bone to muscles; enable bones to move when muscles contract
5. Muscles
    a. Skeletal (i.e., striated voluntary): allows voluntary movement
        1) 600 skeletal muscles
        2) Made up of thick bundles of parallel fibers
        3) Each muscle fiber is made up of smaller structure myofibrils.
        4) Myofibrils are strands of repeating units called sarcomeres.
        5) Skeletal muscle contracts with the release of acetylcholine.
        6) The more fibers that contract, the stronger the muscle contraction.
    b. Smooth (i.e., nonstriated involuntary): muscle movement controlled by internal mechanism (e.g., muscles in bladder wall and GI system)
    c. Cardiac (i.e., striated involuntary): found in heart

Physiology
1. Bone cells
    a. Osteoblasts: bone-forming cells that become osteocytes after they lay down new bone
    b. Osteocytes: make up 90% to 95% of bone cells; they maintain bone by signaling osteoblasts to form bone or osteoclasts to break down bone
    c. Osteoclasts: bone-resorbing cells
2. Bone healing (McCance & Heuther, 2013)
    a. Hematoma formation: If vessels have been damaged, fibrin and platelets within the hematoma form a meshwork as initial framework for healing.
    b. Procallus formation: Fibroblasts, osteoblasts, and capillary buds migrate into the wound to produce granulation tissue referred to procallus.
    c. Callus formation: Osteoblasts in the procallus form callus.
    d. Callus replacement: Osteoblasts replace callus in lamellar bone and trabecular bone.
    e. Remodeling: The surfaces of the bone are remodeled to the size and shape of the bone before injury.

Changes in Older Adults
1. Musculoskeletal changes can be caused by
    a. Loss of calcium and organic material; bones have reduced strength and are more brittle
    b. Diminished estrogen and testosterone levels cause a decrease in new bone growth and bone mass, contributing to osteoporosis and decreased skeletal muscle atrophy.

c. Tendons and ligaments are less flexible, and joints have decreased range of motion.
   d. Intervertebral discs shrink, compression of the discs, and loss of bone mass contribute to loss of body height and kyphosis (i.e., hunchback).
   e. Decreased activity contributes to decreased muscle strength and reduced joint mobility.
   f. Changes in balance contribute to risk of falls.

Musculoskeletal Assessment

Health history
1. Chief complaint and duration
   a. Examine complaints of pain for location, duration, radiation, character, aggravating, and alleviating factors
2. Effect on activities of daily living (ADLs)
3. Precipitating events (e.g., trauma)
4. Possible related symptoms: fever, fatigue, weight changes, rash, or swelling

Physical Examination
1. Inspection
   a. Posture
   b. Gait: ability to walk with or without assistive devices
   c. ADLs: ability to feed, toilet, and dress self
   d. Visible bone or joint deformity or swelling; compare with corresponding bone or joint
   e. Muscle mass symmetry
2. Palpation
   a. Joint warmth
   b. Range of motion (ROM); note complaints of pain with ROM
      1) Note any crepitus.
      2) Note: Do not attempt to move a joint past normal ROM or past the point where the patient experiences pain.
   c. Muscle strength (Table 10.2)

Diagnostic Studies
1. Serum
   a. Electrolytes: calcium, phosphorus
   b. Rheumatoid factor
   c. Lupus erythematosus (LE) prep/antinuclear antibodies
   d. Erythrocyte sedimentation rate (ESR)
   e. Alkaline phosphatase
   f. Acid phosphatase
   g. Enzymes: creatine kinase
2. Urine: 24-hour creatine-to-creatinine ratio

Table 10.2	Grading Muscle Strength
Grade	Description
0	No contractions; paralysis
1	Contraction felt but no limb movement
2	Passive ROM
3	Full ROM against gravity
4	Full ROM against some resistance
5	Full ROM against full resistance

ROM, Range of motion.

3. Radiography
4. Bone density scan
5. Bone scan
6. Computed tomography (CT)
7. Magnetic resonance imaging (MRI)
8. Ultrasonography
9. Endoscopy: arthrocentesis, arthroscopy
10. Electromyography
11. Myelography

Osteomyelitis

Definition
A condition caused by the invasion of one or more pathogenic microorganisms that stimulates the inflammatory response in bone tissue
1. May be acute or chronic
2. The most common sites in adults are the pelvis and vertebrae.

Etiology
1. Trauma
2. Surgery
3. IV drug use
4. Most common microorganism: *Staphylococcus aureus*; other causative organisms include streptococci, *Haemophilus influenzae, Pseudomonas, Escherichia coli,* and fungi

Pathophysiology
1. Infective organisms gain access to the medullary cavity of the bone.
   a. By direct access such as an open wound (i.e., open fracture) or surgery
   b. Hematogenous spread from acute infection elsewhere in the body
2. Infection begins in the soft, medullary tissue.
   a. May remain localized or spread through the bone to the marrow, cortex, and periosteum
3. Granulocytic leukocytes infiltrate the area.
4. Leukocytes are destroyed by the bacteria, which causes release of proteolytic enzyme.
5. Inflammation causes thrombosis of blood vessels, which cause bone ischemia and eventually necrosis.
6. Necrotic bone separates from the viable bone, forming a fragment called a sequestrum.
7. Sinuses in the involucrum allow pus to escape from the inside.
8. Some pockets of infection are walled off.
9. New granulation may close sinuses, but infection within causes building of pressure that causes reopening and formation of new channels.

Clinical Presentation
1. Subjective
   a. Sudden pain and tenderness in the affected bone
   b. Chronic fatigue is chronic osteomyelitis.
2. Objective
   a. Fever
   b. Redness, warmth, and swelling over the affected area
   c. Movement restriction
   d. Purulent drainage if skin opening

3. Diagnostic studies
   a. White blood cell count: elevated
   b. ESR: elevated
   c. Blood cultures: positive
   d. Radiography: may show periosteal elevation and sequestrum
   e. Bone scan: positive for active infection; shows changes earlier than radiography
   f. CT or MRI: positive for sinus tracts, abscesses

Collaborative Management

1. Treat infection.
   a. IV antibiotics; frequently required for 4 to 6 months
   b. IV fluids
   c. Incision, drainage, and culture of an abscess or sinus tract; wound care may include continuous wound irrigation
   d. Surgical management may be required
      1) *Sequestrectomy:* surgical removal of a sequestrum (i.e., dead bone)
      2) Bone grafts
      3) Bone segment transfers
      4) Muscle flaps
      5) Amputation
2. Manage pain.
   a. Immobilization of affected body part
   b. Nonnarcotic analgesic or opiates (or both)
3. Facilitate healing: Hyperbaric oxygen may be used.
4. Monitor for complications.
   a. Pathologic fracture
   b. Abscess
   c. Extensive bone destruction
   d. Amyloidosis

Immobility in Critical Care

1. Critical illness is associated with immobility and physiological deterioration.
   a. Cardiovascular effects
      1) Orthostatic hypotension
      2) Deep vein thrombosis
   b. Pulmonary
      1) Orthostatic pneumonia
      2) Pulmonary embolism
   c. Musculoskeletal
      1) Decreased muscle mass and strength
      2) Loss of bone density
      3) Contractures
   d. GI
      1) Constipation
      2) Ileus
   e. Genitourinary
      1) Urinary tract infection
      2) Calculus formation
   f. Central nervous system
      1) Emotional and behavioral changes
      2) Anxiety, emotionally labile
      3) Decreased attention span
      4) Depression
   g. Integumentary
      1) Pressure injury
   h. Metabolic
      1) Fluid retention
      2) Increased excretion of calcium nitrogen, phosphorus
   i. Altered sleep pattern (i.e., sleep deprivation)
      1) Perceptual or coordination deficits
      2) Diminished intellectual performance
      3) Learned helplessness syndrome
2. Prevention of complications of immobility
   a. Position change every 2 hours
   b. Active or passive ROM every 4 to 8 hours
   c. Head of the bed elevation to 30 degrees while in bed
   d. Progressive activity as tolerated
      1) Cardiac chair
      2) Dangle legs while sitting on side of the bed.
      3) Stand for any amount of time the patient can toleration; beneficial for expanding lung capacity.
      4) Pivot out of bed to chair; the patient should not be out of bed to chair for more than 1 to 2 hours at a time.
      5) Levels of ADLs: Encourage participation in hygiene and feeding as appropriate.
      6) Progress to steps and ambulation.
      7) Use occupational and physical therapy to reduce risks associated with health comorbidities, provide early intervention for rehabilitation, and contribute to the patient's well-being and quality of life.

LEARNING ACTIVITIES

CHAPTER 10

1. Complete the following crossword puzzle related to the integumentary and musculoskeletal systems.

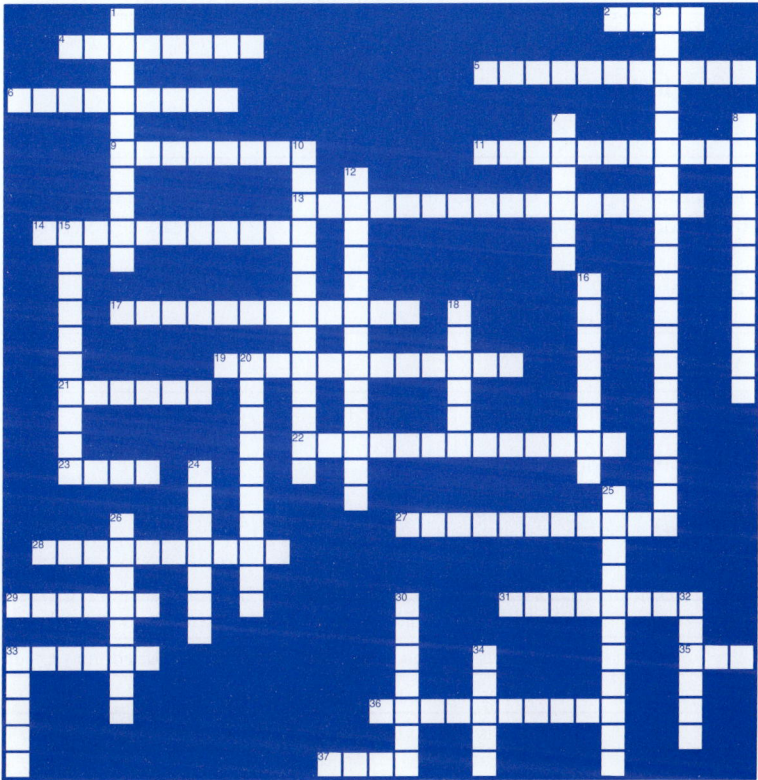

ACROSS

2. Injury to the skin caused by moisture (acronym)
4. A break in the continuity of a bone
5. These cells are phagocytes that participate in immune responses
6. The other layer of the skin
9. These sweat glands are primarily in the axillae, scalp, abdomen, and genital area
11. These cells synthesize and secrete the melanin with exposure to UV light
13. A primary function of the skin that is diminished with aging
14. This type of drug increases the risk of pressure injury in critically ill patients
17. Leakage of IV fluids or medications into the tissue around an IV catheter
19. This type of osteomyelitis has migrated from an infection elsewhere in the body
21. This type of bone marrow contains fat and connective tissue
22. Infection of the bone that potentially leads to localized ischemia and necrosis
23. Largest single organ of the body
27. These cells secrete connective tissue that creates a matrix across wound edges in the healing process
28. Subcutaneous layer of the skin
29. A commonly used scoring system to predict risk for pressure injury
31. Type of fracture that causes a break in the skin
33. These cells function as mechanoreceptors when stimulated by deformation of the epidermis
35. This type of bone marrow produces blood cells and hemoglobin
36. These cells initiate an immune response by presenting processed antigens to T cells
37. These cells release histamine

DOWN

1. A risk to the skin when there is constant moisture, such as incontinence
3. Most likely organism in osteomyelitis (2 words)
7. Immature new bone; bone healing is complete when this has been replaced by mature bone
8. Cells that break down bone
10. Leakage of a potentially damaging medication into the tissue around an IV catheter
12. These cells produce keratin, a protein substance that protects the skin from mechanical stress
15. Connective tissues that help regulate energy balance
16. Outward curvature of the spine that occurs with osteoporosis
18. This type of bone contains red and yellow bone marrow
20. Loss of this skin quality with aging causes wrinkles
24. The greatest number of these sweat glands are on the palms of the hands, soles of the feet, and the forehead; very important for thermoregulation
25. Cells that build bone
26. Patient ____ is a significant risk for infiltration, especially when the IV catheter is in the wrist, hand, or antecubital space
30. Smooth, dense bone; example is shaft of long bone
32. The middle layer of the skin
33. Injury to the skin caused by tape (acronym)
34. This type of force occurs when patients slide down in bed and increases the risk of skin injury

677

2. Match the grade of pressure injury to the fruit descriptive of the injury.

Pressure Injury Grade	Fruit Description
____1. 1	a. peach
____2. 2	b. tomato
____3. 3	c. bitten apple
____4. 4	d. partially peeled potato

3. Describe the difference between infiltration and extravasation.

_____

_____

_____

_____

4. Match the grade of infiltration with the description.

Infusion Nurses Society Infiltration Grade	Description
____1. 1	a. edema extending no more than 6 inches from the catheter insertion site
____2. 2	b. skin is blanched and translucent and the patient may experience pain or numbness
____3. 3	c. pulses may be impaired
____4. 4	d. skin is cool to touch with minimal edema

Multisystem

CHAPTER 11

NOTE: The blueprint includes Cardiogenic and Hypovolemic Shock in Cardiovascular, Anaphylactic Shock in Hematology/Immunology, and Neurogenic Shock in Neurologic, but this text discusses all shock states together and then discusses their differences.

Definitions
1. Shock: inadequate perfusion of cells and vital organs, causing tissue hypoxia that leads to cellular, metabolic, and hemodynamic alterations
   a. Alteration in either of the four main circulatory components can lead to shock:
      1) Cardiac function
      2) Blood volume
      3) Vascular tone
      4) Resistance
   b. NOTE: Shock is not a blood pressure (BP) level, and the patient may not be significantly hypotensive, especially early in shock.
   c. Shock is often associated with systemic inflammatory response syndrome (SIRS) and can lead to multiple organ dysfunction syndrome (MODS)
2. SIRS: the systemic response to a variety of insults that begin as local inflammation; the local vasodilation and increased capillary permeability of local inflammation that is part of the normal healing process becomes systemic, leading to intravascular volume loss, activation of the clotting cascade, and vasodilation
3. MODS: a clinical syndrome in which progressive and potentially irreversible physiologic dysfunction of two or more organ systems is caused by primary or secondary injury

Classification by Etiology
1. Hypovolemic: caused by inadequate intravascular volume
2. Cardiogenic: caused by impaired ability of the heart to pump blood effectively
   a. Obstructive shock is sometimes considered as a separate type of shock but this text will consider it as a subcategory of cardiogenic shock; it is caused by blood flow that is impaired by a blockage or compression such as cardiac tamponade or pulmonary embolism (PE).
3. Distributive: caused by massive vasodilation, resulting in relative hypovolemia
   a. Septic: resulting from massive vasodilation caused by release of mediators of the inflammatory process in response to overwhelming infection
   b. Anaphylactic: resulting from massive vasodilation caused by release of histamine in response to a severe allergic reaction
   c. Neurogenic: resulting from massive vasodilation caused by suppression of the sympathetic nervous system (SNS)

Pathophysiology
1. Stages of shock
   a. Initial stage: subclinical hypoperfusion caused by inadequate oxygen delivery (DO_2), inadequate extraction of oxygen, or both
   b. Compensatory stage: attempts of the neural, endocrine, and chemical compensatory mechanisms activated by the SNS to restore perfusion to vital organs (Fig. 11.1)
   c. Progressive stage: compensatory mechanisms fail to maintain tissue perfusion, leading to anaerobic metabolism, failure of the sodium potassium pump, and cell death (Fig. 11.2)
   d. Refractory stage: tissue hypoxia and ischemia lead to irreversible dysfunctions that are refractory to treatment (Fig. 11.3).

Clinical Presentation (Table 11.1)
1. Initial stage: Cardiac output (CO) and cardiac index (CI) are decreased, but there are no clinical indications of hypoperfusion; this decrease in CO and CI would be detected by invasive hemodynamic monitoring.
2. Compensatory stage
   a. Subjective: nonspecific complaints may include:
      1) Weakness
      2) Feeling cold or hot
      3) Nausea
      4) Confusion
      5) Anxiety
      6) Dyspnea
      7) Thirst

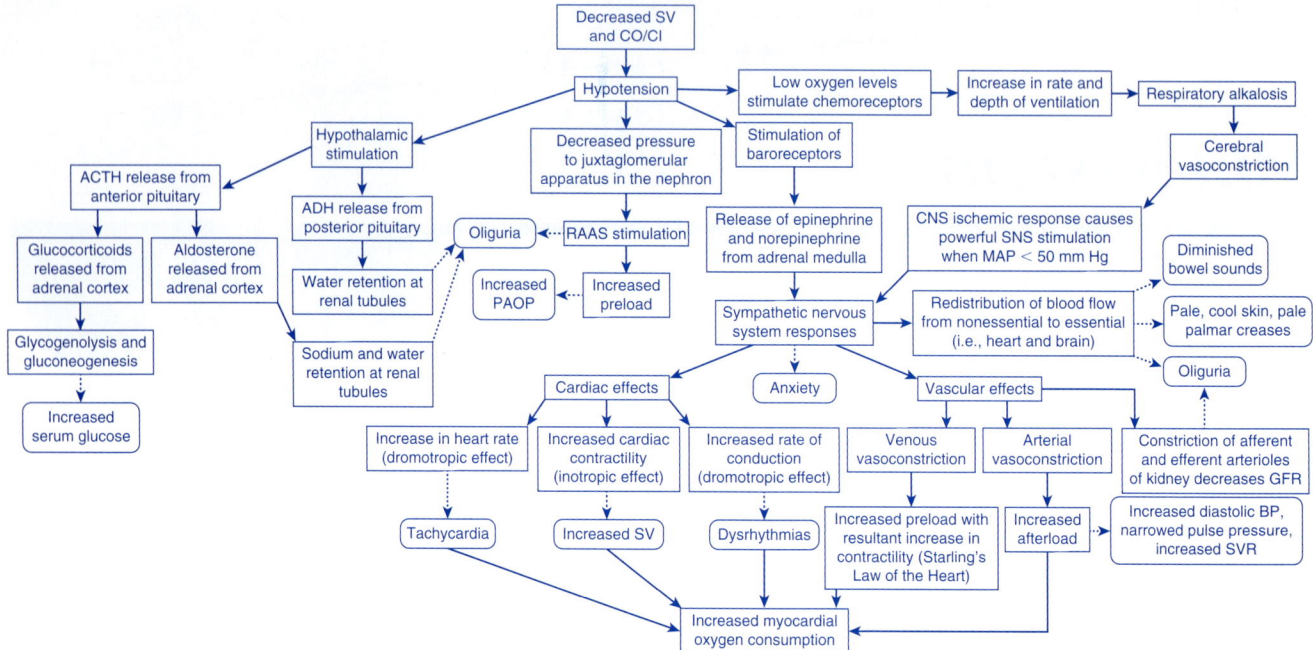

Fig. 11.1 Pathophysiology of shock: compensatory stage. *Dotted lines* connect pathology to clinical presentation. *ACTH*, Adrenocorticotropic hormone; *ADH*, antidiuretic hormone; *BP*, blood pressure; *CI*, cardiac index; *CNS*, central nervous system; *CO*, cardiac output; *GFR*, glomerular filtration rate; *PAOP*, pulmonary artery occlusive pressure; *RAAS*, renin–angiotensin–aldosterone system; *SV*, stroke volume; *SVR*, systemic vascular resistance.

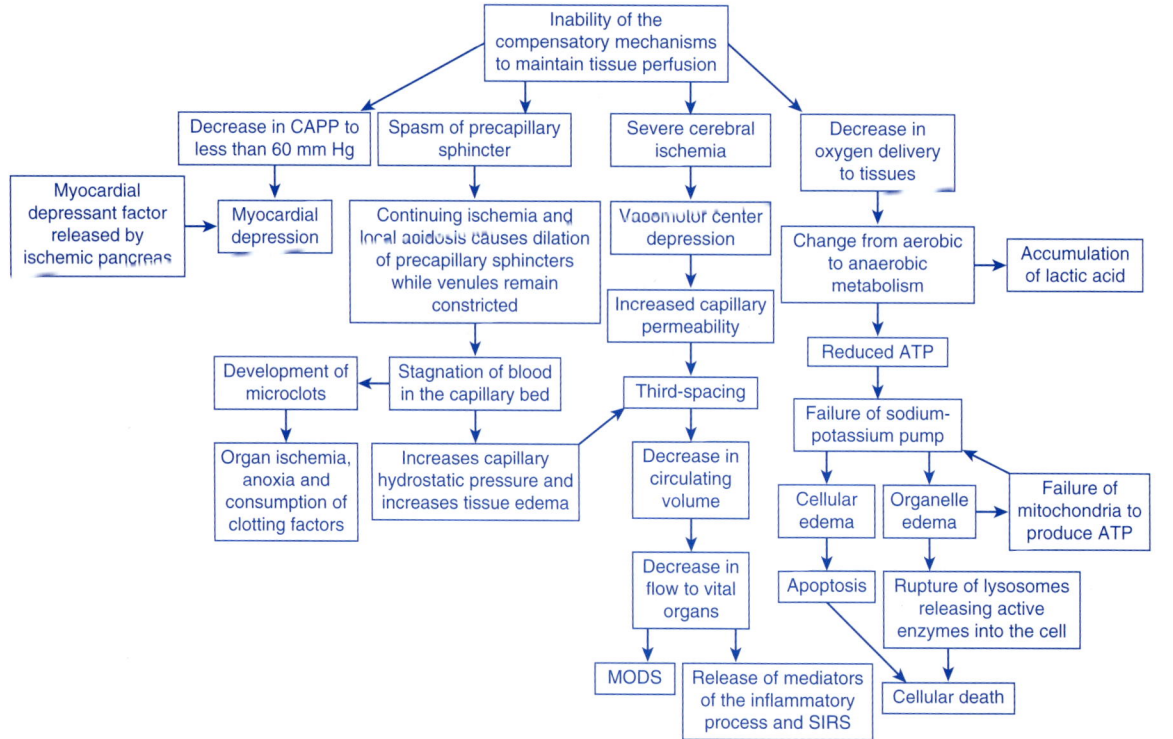

Fig. 11.2 Pathophysiology of shock: progressive stage. *ATP*, Adenosine triphosphate; *CAPP*, coronary artery perfusion pressure; *MODS*, multiple organ dysfunction syndrome.

b. Objective
1) Central nervous system (CNS): Even though the SNS shunts blood to the CNS, neurologic signs occur early because the CNS is very sensitive to changes in oxygen and glucose.
2) Cardiovascular
a) Tachycardia except in the case of neurogenic shock. NOTE: Many patients are prescribed medications to treat hypertension and heart failure (HF) that block the ability of the

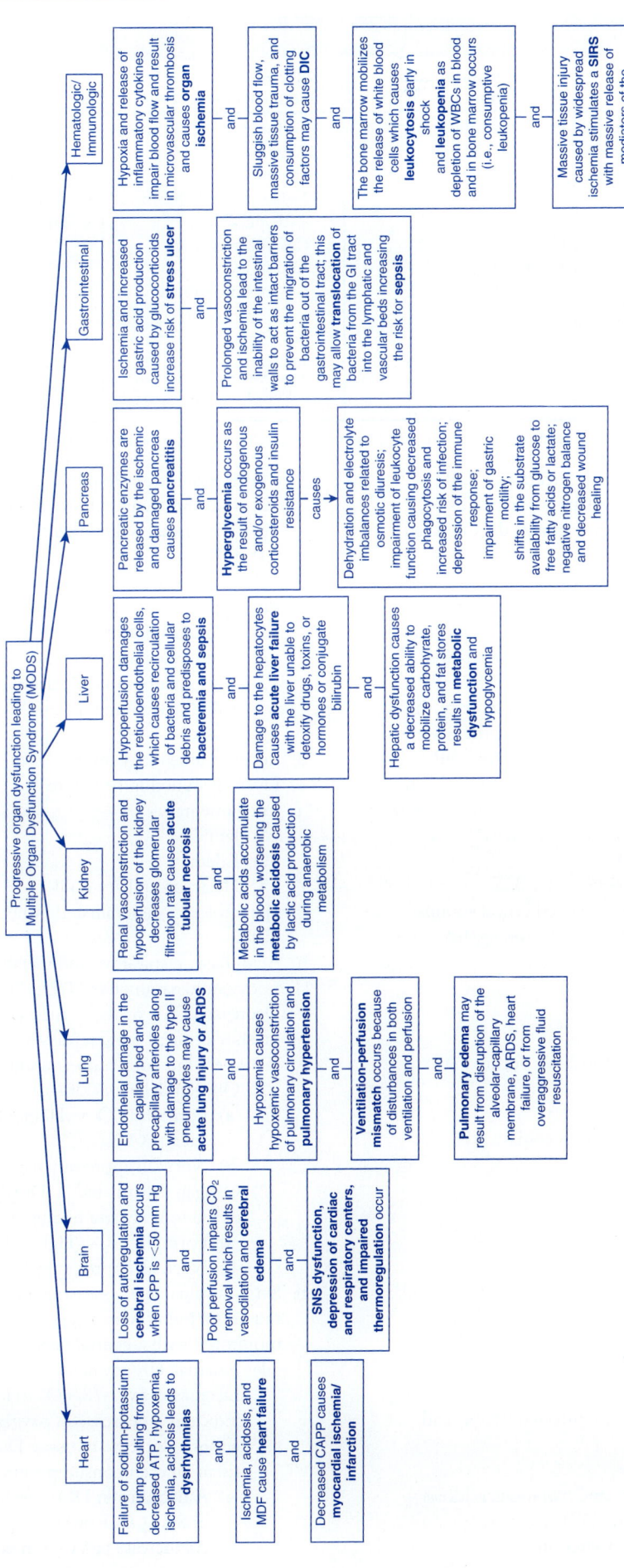

Fig. 11.3 Pathophysiology of shock: refractory stage. *ARDS*, Acute respiratory distress syndrome; *ATP*, adenosine triphosphate; *CAPP*, coronary artery perfusion pressure; *CPP*, cerebral perfusion pressure; *DIC*, disseminated intravascular coagulation; *GI*, gastrointestinal; *MDF*, myocardial depressant factor; *MODS*, multiple organ dysfunction syndrome; *SIRS*, systemic inflammatory response syndrome; *SNS*, sympathetic nervous system; *WBC*, white blood cell.

Table 11.1 Clinical Presentation of the Stages of Shock

	Initial: Subclinical Hypoperfusion	Compensatory: SNS Innervation	Progressive: Hypoperfusion	Refractory: Profound Hypoperfusion
Clinical indications	• No clinical indications of hypoperfusion but "something is different" • Detected by invasive hemodynamic monitoring	• Tachycardia • Narrowed pulse pressure • Tachypnea • Cool, moist skin • Oliguria • Diminished bowel sounds • Restlessness → confusion • Hyperglycemia	• Tachycardia, dysrhythmias • Weak, thready pulse • Hypotension • Narrowed pulse pressure • Tachypnea • Cold, clammy skin • Anuria • Absent bowel sounds • Lethargy → coma • Respiratory and metabolic acidosis	• Life-threatening dysrhythmias • Hypotension despite potent vasopressors • ARDS • DIC • Hepatic dysfunction or failure • ATN • Mesenteric ischemia or infarction • Myocardial ischemia or infarction • Failure • Cerebral ischemia or infarction

ARDS, Acute respiratory distress syndrome; *ATN,* acute tubular necrosis; *DIC,* disseminated intravascular coagulation; *SNS,* sympathetic nervous system.

SNS to raise the BP and heart rate (HR) in response to inadequate tissue perfusion. These patients may not exhibit the expected symptoms.
  b) BP changes
      (i) Systolic BP increases or stays the same while vasoconstriction causes a rise in diastolic BP, resulting in a narrowed pulse pressure. Because diastolic BP is a reflection of arterial elasticity, the vasoconstriction caused by the SNS causes an elevation in diastolic BP and a narrowing of the pulse pressure earlier than a decrease in systolic BP or mean arterial pressure (MAP).
  3) Pulmonary: tachypnea
  4) Integumentary: cool, pale, moist skin
  5) Gastrointestinal (GI): decreased bowel sounds
  6) Renal: oliguria (i.e., less than 0.5 ml/kg/hr)
  7) Endocrine: hyperglycemia
3. Progressive stage: hypoperfusion
  a. Subjective
    1) Anorexia, nausea
    2) Chest pain and palpitations may occur
    3) Dyspnea may occur
  b. Objective
    1) CNS: lethargy progressing to coma
    2) Cardiac
      a) Tachycardia
      b) Dysrhythmias
      c) Weak, thready pulse
      d) Hypotension
    3) Pulmonary: tachypnea
    4) Integumentary: cold, clammy skin
    5) GI: absent bowel sounds
    6) Renal
      a) Anuria (i.e., negligible or less than 100 ml/24 hr)
      b) Increased blood urea nitrogen (BUN) and creatinine
      c) Hyperkalemia
    7) Acid–base: respiratory and metabolic acidosis
4. Refractory stage:
  a. CNS: cerebral ischemia or infarction
  b. Cardiovascular

    1) Hypotension despite vasopressors
    2) Life-threatening dysrhythmias
    3) Myocardial ischemia or infarction
    4) HF
    5) Cardiac arrest
  c. Pulmonary
    1) Acute respiratory failure
    2) Acute respiratory distress syndrome
    3) Note that peripheral vasoconstriction can make SpO_2 measurements unreliable in patients with shock.
  d. Renal: acute kidney injury
  e. Liver: dysfunction or failure
  f. Integumentary
    1) Jaundice
    2) Edema
    3) Delayed capillary refill
  g. Hematologic: disseminated intravascular coagulation (DIC)
  h. Acid–base: respiratory and metabolic acidosis
5. Hemodynamic parameters (Table 11.2)
  a. Decreased DO_2 to the tissues: common to all forms of shock except early septic shock, in which DO_2 is increased, but extraction and utilization are impaired
    1) Oxygen delivery (DO_2)
      a) Formula: CO × (Hemoglobin [Hgb] × 1.34 × SaO_2) × 10
      b) Normal: approximately 1000 ml/min
    2) Oxygen delivery index (DO_2I): oxygen delivery indexed to body size because CI used in calculation
      a) Formula: CI × (Hgb × 1.34 × SaO_2) × 10
      b) Normal: approximately 600 ml/min/m^2
  b. SvO_2 is valuable in assessment of shock states but requires a pulmonary artery catheter; $S_{CV}O_2$ can be monitored with a central venous catheter
    1) Normal: 60% to 80%
    2) Decreased $SvO_2/S_{CV}O_2$ to less than 60% indicates a decrease in oxygen reserve caused by either a decrease in tissue DO_2 or an increase in tissue oxygen consumption (VO_2).
      a) A decrease in DO_2 can be caused by decrease in SaO_2, CO, or Hgb.
      b) An increase in VO_2 can be caused by fever, agitation, seizures, of increased work of breathing.

Table 11.2	Hemodynamic Alterations in Shock				
	Hypovolemic	Cardiogenic	Septic	Anaphylactic	Neurogenic
HR	High	High	High	High	Normal or low
BP	Normal → Low	Normal → Low	Low	Normal → Low	Normal → Low
CO/CI	Low	Low	High → Low	Normal → Low	Normal → Low
RAP/PAOP	Low	High	Low	Low	Low
SVR/SVRI	High	High	Low	Low	Low
SvO_2	Low	Low	High → Low	Low	Low

BP, Blood pressure; *CI*, cardiac index; *CO*, cardiac output; *HR*, heart rate; *PAOP*, pulmonary artery occlusive pressure; *RAP*, right atrial pressure; SvO_2, oxygen saturation of venous blood; *SVR*, systemic vascular resistance; *SVRI*, Systemic vascular resistance index.

    c. Pulse pressure variation (PPV) and stroke volume variance (SVV)
        1) Both measures reflect the change in pressures throughout the respiratory cycle.
        2) Can be used to determine whether or not fluids (i.e., an increase in preload) will increase CO in patients who are mechanically ventilated
        3) Measured via invasive arterial catheter
        4) Increase of 10% to 15% indicates fluid responsiveness
        5) Passive leg raise may provide the same information as PPV and SVV but is noninvasive and reversible. Raise legs 45 degrees with patient in semirecumbant position. Changes can be seen in the first minute (Marik, Monnet, & Teboul, 2011).
    d. Tissue oxygenation (StO_2)
        1) Noninvasive way to measure Hgb concentration in the muscle tissue bed
        2) Measured with infrared spectroscopy
        3) Can be used with hypothermic and pulseless patients
        4) Low values associated with changes in DO_2, base deficit, and lactate levels
        5) Studies have shown correlation between StO_2 an SvO_2 (Mitchell, 2016)
6. Diagnostic studies
    a. Serum
        1) Sodium: decreased after hypotonic fluid replacement; increased because of hemoconcentration after fluid loss
        2) Potassium: increased with renal failure, cell lysis
        3) Chloride: can be increased because of normal saline (NS) infusion
        4) Bicarbonate: normal early; decreased late because of acidosis
        5) CO_2: can be decreased early because of hyperventilation; can be increased as a result of respiratory acidosis caused by respiratory failure
        6) Glucose: can be increased with initial stress response
        7) BUN: increased
        8) Creatinine: increased
        9) Bilirubin: increased late because of liver failure
        10) CK: increased with ischemia to muscle tissues
        11) Liver enzymes (aspartate aminotransferase, alanine aminotransferase, lactate dehydrogenase): increased
        12) Lactate: increased
            a) Correlates with the degree of hypoperfusion but can be elevated for other reasons: liver, local hypoperfusion, prolonged use of tourniquet when obtaining venous sample
            b) Levels above 2 mmol/l are associated with increased mortality
        13) Hgb: decreased if blood loss present
        14) Hematocrit (Hct): increased if patient is not losing blood and is hemoconcentrated because of fluid loss; changes from the usual Hgb:Hct ratio of 3:1 can be used to determine if patient is hemoconcentrated or hemodiluted
        15) White blood cell (WBC) count: can be increased early because of stress response; decreased later because of consumption
        16) Prothrombin time (PT), activated partial thromboplastin time (aPTT): may be prolonged as a result of activation of inflammatory/immune response (IIR)
        17) Platelets: may be decreased
        18) Arterial blood gases (ABGs): respiratory alkalosis progressing to metabolic acidosis; PaO_2 and SaO_2 may be decreased
        19) Blood cultures: may identify organism if shock is due to sepsis
    b. Urine
        1) Urine creatinine clearance: decreased
        2) Urine specific gravity: increased early, decreased late
        3) Urine osmolality: increased early, decreased late
        4) Urine sodium: decreased
        5) Presence of heavy pigments
            a) Myoglobinuria occurs with muscle tissue destruction (e.g., crush injuries, muscle ischemia or necrosis, electrical burns, seizures).
            b) Hemoglobinuria occurs with mismatched blood transfusion reaction and fresh water submersion.
    c. Other diagnostic studies may be done to evaluate the reason for shock.

Collaborative Management

1. Identify and treat cause of shock.
2. Maximize oxygen delivery to the tissues (Hgb, SaO_2, CO/CI).
    a. Maintain optimal Hgb and intravascular volume.

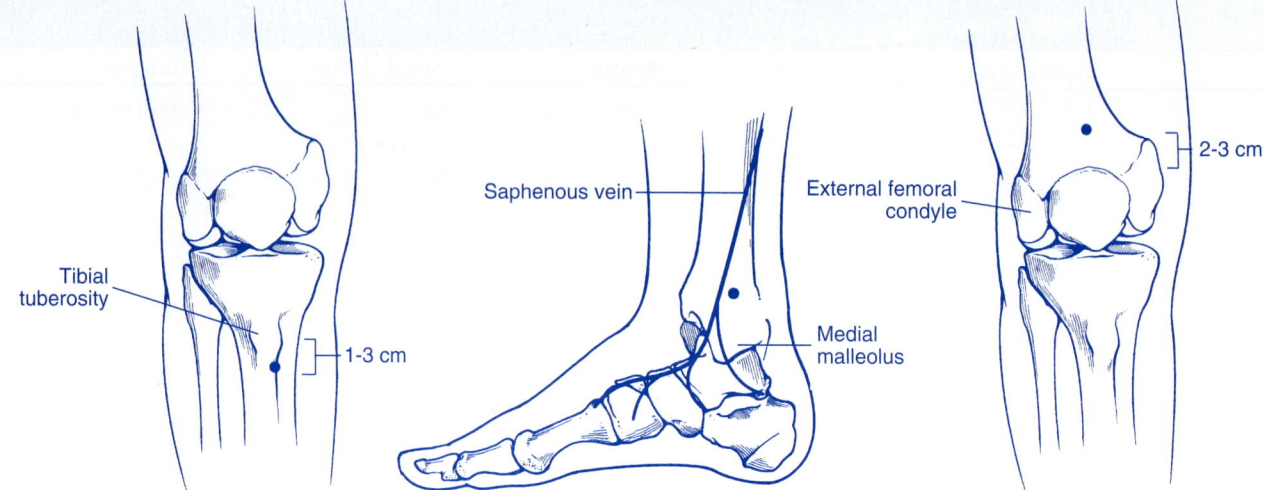

Fig. 11.4 Schematic diagram demonstrating intraosseous (IO) insertion sites. **A,** The proximal tibia. The IO needle is inserted 1 to 2 cm distal to the tibial tuberosity and over the medial aspect of the tibia. The bevel of the needle is directed away from the joint space. **B,** The distal tibia. The IO needle is inserted on the medial surface of the distal tibia at the junction of the medial malleolus and the shaft of the tibia posterior to the greater saphenous vein. The needle is directed cephalad away from the growth plate. **C,** The distal femur. The IO needle is inserted 2 to 3 cm above the external condyles in the midline and directed cephalad, away from the growth plate. (From Howard, P. K., & Steinmann, R. A. [2010]. *Sheehy's emergency nursing principles and practice* [6th ed.]. St. Louis: Elsevier.)

1) Two large-gauge intravenous (IV) catheters, preferably one peripheral and one central, should be inserted immediately.
    a) The intraosseous route may be used to administer fluids and blood products when IV access cannot be obtained (Fig. 11.4)
        i) Placement of rigid needle through the bone cortex into the medullary cavity
        ii) Can be placed in proximal or distal tibia, humerus, or sternum
        iii) Humerus and tibial sites require immobilization of the limb. Sternal site can interfere with cardiopulmonary resuscitation (CPR) but may be helpful with massive extremity trauma.
2) Volume replacement for hypovolemic and vasogenic; may be necessary even in cardiogenic shock to achieve optimal pulmonary artery occlusive pressure (PAOP)
    a) Types of fluids used for fluid resuscitation (Box 11.1)
        i) Crystalloids: solutions with dextrose or electrolytes; safe, effective, inexpensive (Table 11.3)
        ii) Hypertonic crystalloids are not recommended for initial resuscitation of hypovolemic patients and may lead to increased morbidity.
        iii) Colloids: large-molecule (protein or starch) solutions
            (a) Molecules theoretically produce greater expansion of intravascular volume than crystalloids by increasing intravascular oncotic pressure.
            (b) Should not be used over crystalloids routinely
            (c) Hydroxylation of starches results in accumulation in tissues that can lead to increased morbidity as a result of acute kidney injury or liver injury (Lira & Pinksy, 2014).

Box 11.1 Types of Fluids Used for Fluid Resuscitation

Crystalloids*
- Isotonic: NS; LR (D_5NS, D_5LR); Plasmalyte
- Hypotonic: ½NS ($D_5½NS$, D_5W)
- Hypertonic: 3% saline; $D_{10}W$; TPN

Colloids
- Albumin
- Dextran 70/75
- Hetastarch

Blood and Blood Products
- Whole blood
- Packed RBCs
- Fresh-frozen plasma

*Dextrose solutions are in parentheses because even though 5% dextrose adds to osmolality in the bottle or bag, this small amount of dextrose is metabolized so quickly when in the body that it should not be considered in the osmolality of the solution. So consider D_5NS as NS, $D_{5½}NS$ as ½NS, and D_5W as water. This last example is why D_5W is avoided except in extreme hyperosmolar conditions. In significant volumes, D_5W will dilute electrolytes, particularly sodium, and potentially causes neurologic changes, including seizures.

D_5LR, 5% Dextrose in lactated Ringer's solution; D_5NS, 5% dextrose in normal saline; $D_{5½}NS$, 5% dextrose in 0.45% saline; D_5W, 5% dextrose in water; $D_{10}W$, 10% dextrose in water; *NS*, normal (0.9%) saline; *½NS*, 0.45% saline; *LR*, lactated Ringer's solution; *RBC*, red blood cell; *TPN*, total parenteral nutrition (usually 25% dextrose).

Table 11.3 Crystalloids

	Isotonic	Hypotonic	Hypertonic
Osmolality	250–350 mOsm/l (which is similar to blood osmolality of 280–295 mOsm/l)	Less than 250 mOsm/l	Greater than 350 mOsm/l
Uses	• Tend to stay in the vascular space better than other crystalloids • Require replacement with 3 ml for every 1 ml lost because they equilibrate across fluid compartments	• Tend to leave the vascular space and replace the interstitial space better than the vascular space	• Pull fluid from the interstitial space into the intravascular space • Expand intravascular volume over isotonic crystalloid without the adverse effects of colloids • Monitor closely for clinical indications of fluid overload when these solutions are administered

Examples	0.9% saline
	• Composition
	  • 154 mEq of sodium
	  • 154 mEq of chloride
	  • Water
	• Osmolality is 289 mOsm/l
	• pH is 5.7
	• Large volumes may cause metabolic (hyperchloremic) acidosis
	Lactated Ringer's solution
	• Composition
	  • 130 mEq/l
	  • 109 mEq/l of chloride
	  • 4 mEq/l of potassium
	  • 3 mEq/l of calcium
	  • 28 mEq/l of lactate
	  • Water
	• Osmolality is 273 mOsm/l
	• pH 6.7
	• Lactate is added as a buffer to make the solution less acidic (than without the lactate).
	• Lactate is converted to bicarbonate by the liver, so large volumes may cause metabolic alkalosis; this solution should be avoided in patients who have liver disease.
		Half normal (0.45%) saline
		• Composition
		  • 77 mEq of sodium
		  • 77 mEq of chloride
		  • Water
		D_5W
		• Composition
		  • 50 g of dextrose
		  • Water
		• Note that although D_5W is isotonic in the bottle, the body quickly metabolizes the dextrose, and free water is left; avoid this solution except in extremely hyperosmolar patients (e.g., HHS, DI).
			Hypertonic (3% saline)
			• 513 mEq of sodium
			• 513 mEq of chloride
			$D_{10}W$ (10% dextrose in water)
			• Composition
			  • 100 g of dextrose/l
			  • Water
			$D_{50}W$ (50% dextrose in water)
			• Composition
			  • 25 g of dextrose/50 ml ampule
			  • Water
			TPN solution
			• Central
			  • 250 g of dextrose/l
			  • Protein, electrolytes, vitamins vary
			  • Water
			• Peripheral
			  • 100 g of dextrose/l
			  • Protein, electrolytes, vitamins vary
			  • Water

DI, Diabetes insipidus; *HHS*, hyperosmolar hyperglycemic state; *TPN*, total parenteral nutrition.

    (d) Examples
       (i) Albumin: contains plasma protein and available in several concentrations; most costly but least likely to cause complications; however, albumin is associated with increased mortality in patients with traumatic brain injury (TBI) (SAFE Study Investigators, 2007).
      (ii) Dextran: contains polymers of high-molecular-weight polysaccharides
      (iii) Hetastarch: contains polymers of hydroxyethyl starch
  iv) Blood and blood products: used only to achieve a specific physiologic goal, such as to increase oxygen delivery or clotting capability
 (a) Contain plasma proteins that increase the CaO_2 (content of oxygen in arterial blood) because 97% of all oxygen is carried on the Hgb molecule
 (b) Indicated when the patient has lost blood and there are clinical indications of hypoperfusion
 (c) Transfusion should be considered if Hgb is less than 7 g/dl in critically ill patients requiring mechanical ventilation, in resuscitated critically ill trauma patients, and in critically ill patients with stable cardiac disease (Napolitano et al., 2009).
 (d) Major disadvantages of blood and blood products: cost, risk of blood transfusion reaction, blood-

transmitted disease, transfusion-associated lung injury (TRALI), and transfusion-association circulatory overload (TACO)
  b) Volume
     i) Typical fluid challenge is 250 to 500 ml of NS over 5 minutes.
     ii) Monitor BP, central venous pressure (CVP), SVV, PPV, and PAOP for response as available.
     iii) Monitor for clinical indicators of fluid overload (e.g., dyspnea, jugular venous distention, S_3, systolic flow murmur, crackles).
  3) Type and crossmatch immediately if the patient is hemorrhaging; type-specific or O-negative blood may be given in severe hemorrhage but may make future crossmatching more difficult.
  4) Fluid resuscitation can lead to hypothermia; fluids may need to be warmed if the patient's body temperature is low (35°C or less) at the initiation of fluid resuscitation or if multiple units of blood or multiple liters of IV fluids are needed rapid infusers such as the Belmont and Level 1 can warm blood and fluids during administration to assist with maintaining normothermia.
  5) Take care to avoid overresuscitation, which is associated with increased morbidity and mortality.
     a) In trauma patients, increased MAP may cause clot disruption and increased bleeding; permissive hypotension with a MAP of 50 mm Hg may improve outcomes by reducing dilutional coagulopathy and reducing chance of clot dislodgement
  6) Administer venous vasodilators, diuretics, or both as prescribed to decrease the preload (PAOP) in cardiogenic shock.
b. Maintain optimal cardiac contractility and CO and cardiac index (CI)
  1) Monitor the electrocardiogram (ECG), hemodynamic parameters, and neurologic status.
  2) Administer inotropes (e.g., dobutamine) as prescribed.
  3) Administer diuretics (e.g., furosemide) as prescribed.
  4) Administer vasoactive agents.
     a) Administer arterial vasodilators (e.g., nitroprusside [NTP]) to decrease afterload (systemic vascular resistance [SVR]) and/or venous vasodilators (e.g., nitroglycerin [NTG]) to decrease preload (PAOP) as prescribed; these agents may be needed in cardiogenic shock.
     b) Administer vasopressors as prescribed and at the lowest doses necessary to achieve desired effects (Table 11.4).
        i) Vasopressors are sometimes used in an effort to maintain MAP above 65 mm Hg to maintain perfusion pressure, but by constricting the vessels, they may

Table 11.4 Selected Vasopressors

Drug	Administration	Adverse Effects	Nursing Implications
Norepinephrine bitartrate	• IV infusion: Mix 4 mg in 250 ml (16 mcg/ml) and infuse at 0.1–0.5 mcg/kg/min; titrate to BP response. • Administer through CVC if possible; if administered peripherally, use a large vein. • Do not administer with alkaline solutions.	• Bradycardia • Ventricular dysrhythmias • Hypertension • Anxiety • Headache • Tremor • Dizziness • Chest pain • Metabolic (lactic) acidosis • Severe vasoconstriction may cause renal or mesenteric necrosis • Local necrosis with high dosages or if infusion infiltrates	• Monitor HR, BP, ECG, urine output, neurologic status. • Note contraindications: known hypersensitivity, ventricular fibrillation, tachydysrhythmias, pheochromocytoma, narrow-angle glaucoma. • Use cautiously in peripheral vascular disease, mesenteric thrombosis, hyperthyroidism, CAD, hypertension, psychoneurosis, diabetes, patients receiving MAO inhibitors or TCAs, and in older adults. • Taper gradually to wean. • Do not use discolored solution. • Prevent extravasation because necrosis may occur; treat with phentolamine
Dopamine hydrochloride	• IV infusion: Mix 400 mg in 250 ml (1600 mcg/ml) and infuse at 0.5–20 mcg/kg/min, depending on desired effect. • Maximum: 50 mcg/kg/min • Administer through CVC if possible; if administered peripherally, use a large vein.	• Tachycardia • Ventricular ectopy • Hypertension or hypotension • Nausea, vomiting • Dyspnea • Headache • Palpitations • Chest pain • Tissue necrosis with high dosages or extravasation	• Monitor HR, BP, ECG, PAP, PAOP, SVR, CI, and urine output. • Note contraindications: known hypersensitivity, uncorrected tachydysrhythmias, ventricular fibrillation, pheochromocytoma, hypertrophic cardiomyopathy, and in patients receiving MAO inhibitors. • Use cautiously in peripheral vascular disease. • Taper gradually to wean. • Do not administer if discolored. • Prevent extravasation because necrosis may occur; treat extravasation with phentolamine.

Table 11.4 Selected Vasopressors—cont'd

Drug	Administration	Adverse Effects	Nursing Implications
Phenylephrine	• IV infusion: Mix 30 mg in 500 ml (60 mcg/ml); usual dose is 0.5–10 mcg/kg/min. • Rapid onset and short duration • Preferred agent in patients with tachycardia	• Reflex bradycardia • Ventricular dysrhythmias • Hypertension • Nausea, vomiting • Paresthesia • Palpitations • Anxiety • Restlessness • Headache • Tremor • Chest pain	• Monitor BP, HR, and ECG. • Note contraindications: known hypersensitivity, ventricular fibrillation, tachydysrhythmias, pheochromocytoma, and narrow-angle glaucoma. • Use cautiously in older adults and those with hyperthyroidism, CAD, hypertension, psychoneurosis, diabetes mellitus, and peripheral vascular disease. • Prevent extravasation because necrosis may occur; treat with phentolamine. • Treat reflex bradycardia with atropine. • Discard if discolored or precipitate is present.
Epinephrine hydrochloride	• IV infusion: Mix 1 mg in 250 ml (4 mcg/ml) and infuse at 1–10 mcg/min (0.05–1 mcg/kg/min); titrate to desired effect. • Administer through CVC if possible; if administered peripherally, use a large vein. • Do not administer with alkaline solutions.	• Tachycardia • Dysrhythmias • Palpitations • Anxiety • Restlessness • Headache • Dizziness • Tremor • Cerebral hemorrhage • Chest pain • Hyperglycemia	• Monitor BP, HR, and ECG. • Note contraindications: glaucoma, organic brain damage, and cardiomegaly. • Use cautiously in older adults and those with hyperthyroidism, chest pain, hypertension, psychoneurosis, and diabetes mellitus. • Prevent extravasation because necrosis may occur; treat with phentolamine. • Discard if discolored or precipitate is present.
Vasopressin	• IV infusion: 0.01–0.04 units/min	• Bradycardia • Hypertension • Fever • Water intoxication (SIADH), hyponatremia • Nausea, abdominal cramps • Tremor • Headache • Seizures • Coma • Constriction of cardiac arteries, resulting in chest pain and myocardial ischemia	• Monitor HR, BP, daily weight, and serum sodium. • Note contraindications: known hypersensitivity and nephritis. • Use cautiously in CAD.

BP, Blood pressure; *CAD*, coronary artery disease; *CI*, cardiac index; *CVC*, central venous catheter; *ECG*, electrocardiogram; *HR*, heart rate; *IV*, intravenous; *MAO*, monoamine oxidase inhibitor; *PAOP*, pulmonary artery occlusive pressure; *PAP*, pulmonary artery pressure; *SIADH*, syndrome of inappropriate antidiuretic hormone secretion; *SVR*, systemic vascular resistance; *TCA*, tricyclic antidepressant.

actually decrease blood flow to organs even though the MAP is normal.
   ii) Consider the cause of hypotension instead of automatically initiating dopamine to increase the BP; improve perfusion by treating the cause of hypotension (e.g., volume replacement, inotropes, preload or afterload correction).
   iii) Vasopressors are generally contraindicated in patients with cardiogenic shock because they increase afterload (SVR) and myocardial oxygen consumption.
5) Correct metabolic acidosis because it affects cardiac contractility.
   a) Improve oxygenation and perfusion by improving Hgb, SaO_2, and CO/CI.
c. Maintain optimal oxygen saturation and ventilation.
   1) Monitor SpO_2, SvO_2, $S_{CV}O_2$, and ABGs.
   2) Ensure adequate airway.
   3) Administer oxygen to maintain SpO_2 of 94 mm Hg.
      a) Continuous positive airway pressure or positive end-expiratory pressure (PEEP) may be required for refractory hypoxemia.
   4) Initiate mechanical ventilation as prescribed for respiratory muscle fatigue, respiratory acidosis, or refractory hypoxemia.
   5) Monitor closely for changes in SpO_2, ABGs, pulmonary vascular resistance, chest radiographs, and lung compliance indicative of acute respiratory distress syndrome (ARDS).
   6) Assist with extracorporeal membrane oxygenation (ECMO) as required.
      a) ECMO is a form of cardiopulmonary life support in which blood is drained from the vascular system, circulated outside the body by a mechanical pump, and then reinfused

into the circulation. It can be used helpful during cardiogenic shock and ARDS (Makdisi & Wang, 2015)
3. Minimize oxygen consumption of the tissues.
   a. Control body temperature: Hyperthermia may cause vasodilation; hypothermia may cause vasoconstriction and shivering, both of which can negatively affect DO_2 and VO_2
   b. Treat pain and anxiety.
      1) Administer analgesics and anxiolytics as prescribed and indicated.
      2) Provide patient and family support.
         a) Keep the patient and family informed.
         b) Encourage the patient and family to discuss their fear and concerns.
4. Prevent injury caused by decreased perfusion.
   a. Limit sedatives and other CNS depressants.
   b. Administer drugs only IV because peripheral perfusion and drug absorption is impaired.
5. Maintain or improve nutritional status.
   a. Provide enteral feedings unless absolutely contraindicated (e.g., paralytic ileus or structural obstruction).
      1) Use of the GI tract is important to prevent bacterial translocation.
   b. Provide parenteral feeding if enteral feedings are contraindicated or if parenteral supplementation of enteral feedings is needed to meet calorie and protein requirements.
   c. Closely monitor serum potassium, magnesium, and phosphate; replace or restrict as indicated.
   d. Add trace elements and vitamins as prescribed.
6. Maintain renal perfusion and glomerular filtration rate (GFR).
   a. Insert indwelling urinary catheter to monitor hourly urine output.
   b. Monitor BUN and creatinine.
   c. Replace volume as indicated by CVP and PAOP.
   d. Monitor closely for change in color of urine, which may indicate myoglobinuria or hemoglobinuria.
7. Maintain glycemic control.
   a. Recognize that hyperglycemia is related to stress and insulin resistance and occurs in patients without a diagnosis of diabetes mellitus.
   b. Maintain serum glucose at 140 to 180 mg/dl; the previous target of 110 is no longer recommended because of evidence of increased mortality (Clain, Rannar, & Salim, 2015).
      1) Measure glucose every 1 to 2 hours.
      2) Administer continuous infusion of short acting insulin as required.
      3) Titrate insulin according to protocol.
      4) Transition to subcutaneous insulin before discontinuation of insulin infusion.
      5) Treat hypoglycemia as required with dextrose (available in various concentrations).
8. Monitor for complications.
   a. Dysrhythmias: close monitoring and administration of appropriate antidysrhythmic agents depending on rhythm
   b. GI ulceration: stress ulcer prophylaxis with H2 receptor antagonists or proton pump inhibitors
   c. Venous thromboembolism (VTE): prophylaxis with low-molecular-weight heparin subcutaneously
   d. Mesenteric ischemia, infarction: monitoring for abdominal pain, bloody diarrhea
9. Monitor for indications of organ failure and MODS.
   a. Acute lung injury progressing to respiratory distress syndrome (ARDS)
   b. Disseminated intravascular coagulation (DIC)
   c. Liver failure
   d. Acute tubular necrosis (ATN)
   e. Myocardial infarction (MI)
   f. Cerebral infarction
10. Provide emotional support to the patient and family.
    a. Inform the patient regarding what is going to occur and why.
    b. Provide the family with accurate information; maintain hope but do not give false reassurance.

Hypovolemic Shock
Definition
Shock caused by inadequate intravascular volume

Etiology
1. External losses
   a. Blood
      1) GI (e.g., esophageal varices, peptic ulcer, hemorrhoids)
      2) Genitourinary (e.g., antepartal or postpartum bleeding, hematuria)
      3) Trauma
      4) Major blood vessel disruption (aortic dissection)
      5) Coagulopathy
         a) Congenital coagulopathy (e.g., hemophilia)
         b) Acquired coagulopathy (e.g., DIC)
   b. Fluid
      1) GI (e.g., vomiting, diarrhea, nasogastric suction)
      2) Renal
         a) Diabetic ketoacidosis
         b) Hyperosmolar hyperglycemic state
         c) Diabetes insipidus
         d) Hypoaldosteronism (Addison disease)
         e) Diuretics
      3) Integumentary
         a) Burns
         b) Exudative wounds
         c) Excessive perspiration (e.g., heat exhaustion)
2. Internal sequestration
   a. Blood
      1) Hemoperitoneum or retroperitoneal (e.g., hemorrhagic pancreatitis, ruptured spleen, lacerated liver)
      2) Thoracic trauma with hemothorax, hemomediastinum
      3) Dissecting aortic aneurysm
      4) Pelvic or long bone fractures
   b. Fluid
      1) Ascites: peritonitis; pancreatitis; cirrhosis; intraabdominal malignancies (e.g., liver, ovarian)
      2) Pleural effusion
      3) Intestinal obstruction

Pathophysiology
Fig. 11.5.

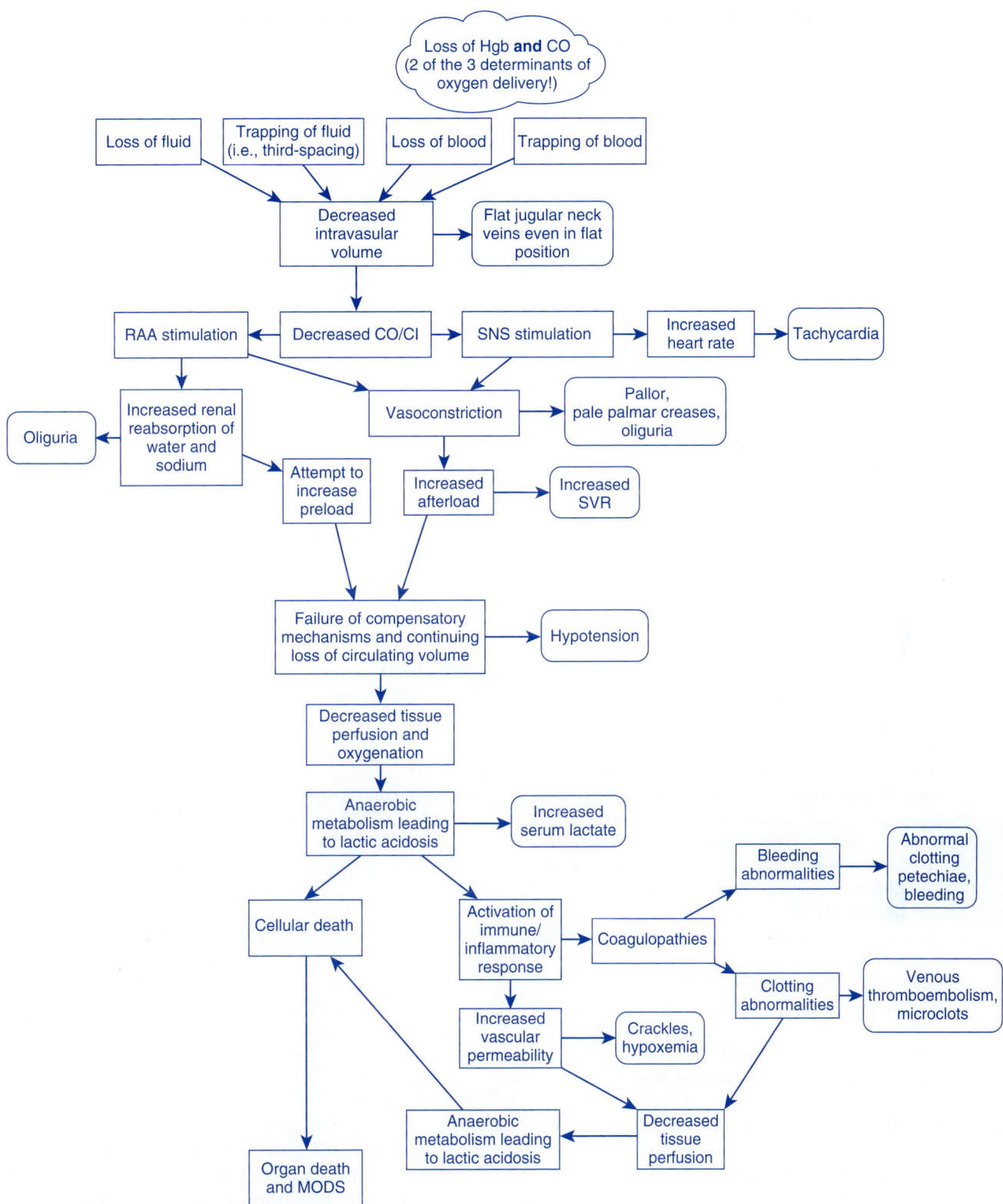

Fig. 11.5 Pathophysiology of hypovolemic shock. *Dotted lines* connect pathology to clinical presentation. *CI*, Cardiac index; *CO*, cardiac output; *Hgb*, hemoglobin; *MODS*, multiple organ dysfunction syndrome; *RAA*, renin-angiotensin-aldosterone; *SNS*, sympathetic nervous system; *SVR*, systemic vascular resistance.

Clinical Presentation
Same as for shock and including the following:
1. Subjective: history of precipitating factor
2. Objective
   a. Flat neck veins
   b. Abdominal girth
      1) Measure at same location on the abdomen and mark with a pen.
      2) A 1-inch increase in abdominal girth is equal to an increase in intraabdominal volume of 500 to 1000 ml.

Table 11.5 Severity of Hemorrhagic Shock

Indicator	Class I	Class II	Class III	Class IV
Blood loss (percent of blood volume)	Less than 15	15–30	30–40	Greater than 40
Blood loss (ml)	Less than 750	750–1500	1500–2000	Greater than 2000
Heart rate (beats/min)	Less than 100	Greater than 100	Greater than 120	140 or greater
Blood pressure	Normal	Normal	Decreased	Decreased
Pulse pressure	Widened or normal	Narrowed	Narrowed	Narrowed
Capillary refill	Normal	Delayed	Delayed	Delayed or absent
Ventilatory rate (breaths/min)	14–20	20–30	30–40	Greater than 35
Urine output (ml/hr)	30 or greater	20–30	Less than 20	Negligible
Skin appearance	Cool, pink	Cool, pale	Cold, moist, pale	Cold, clammy, cyanotic
Neurologic status	Slightly anxious	Mildly anxious	Anxious, confused	Confused, lethargy

Adapted from American College of Surgeons (2008). *ATLS: Advanced trauma life support for doctors* (8th ed.). Chicago: Author.

    c. Daily weight
       1) Use the same scale, same time of day, and same clothing and linens.
       2) 1-kg increase or decrease indicates a gain or loss of 1 liter (1000 ml) respectively
    d. Intake and output
       1) Consider insensible losses.
       2) Weigh dressings and convert to volume, using 1 kg equal to 1000 ml.
       3) Include all drainage tubes.
    e. Parameters used for evaluation of severity of hemorrhagic shock (Table 11.5)
  3. Hemodynamics: Table 11.2
  4. Diagnostic studies
    a. Hct (Note: The Hgb:Hct ratio is normally 3:1; Hct can be erroneously high with dehydration or hemoconcentration and erroneously low with hemodilution because it represents a percentage of red blood cells to total blood volume.)
       1) Elevated if caused by dehydration
       2) Decreased if caused by blood loss
    b. Diagnostic peritoneal lavage to detect intraabdominal bleeding
    c. Computed tomography (CT) of the chest or abdomen to detect source of bleeding
    d. Focused assessment sonography for trauma (FAST)
       1) Can be performed rapidly
       2) Can detect free intraperitoneal bleeding

Collaborative Management

Same as for shock and including the following:
1. Identify high-risk patients and monitor for clinical indications of hypoperfusion.
2. Treat the cause.
    a. Compress any compressible vessels.
    b. Surgery may be necessary to control bleeding.
    c. Antidiarrheals for diarrhea, insulin for hyperglycemia, and so on.
3. Administer appropriate volume replacement.
    a. Two large-caliber IV catheters
    b. NS at rapid rate initially; blood is indicated for class III and class IV when fluid loss is blood. Over-resuscitation with fluids can lead to a number of complications. Goal-directed therapy instead of volume-directed therapy is used.
    c. Monitor for fluid overload; goal-directed therapy instead of volume-directed therapy is recommended.
4. Use autotransfusion if appropriate; used primarily in chest trauma (or chest surgery) to decrease the risk of transfusion-transmitted disease and transfusion reactions

Cardiogenic Shock

Definition

Shock caused by impaired ability of the heart to pump blood effectively

Etiology

1. Decreased contractility
    a. Coronary artery disease
       1) Acute MI
          a) Loss of 40% of left ventricular myocardium is associated with increased risk of cardiogenic shock such as large anterior MI or acute MI in patient with history of previous MI or MIs and preexisting left ventricular dysfunction.
    b. Myocardial contusion
    c. Cardiac surgery
    d. Dilated cardiomyopathy
    e. Myocarditis
    f. Severe HF
    g. Ventricular aneurysm
    h. Overdosage of myocardial depressant drugs (e.g., beta-blockers, calcium channel blockers, barbiturates)
    i. Stunned or hibernating myocardium: transient cardiogenic shock
       1) Cardiac surgery: related to hypothermia, cardioplegic arrest
       2) Reperfusion injury
       3) Post-CPR
       4) Hypoxemia
       5) Acidosis
       6) Hypoglycemia
       7) Electrolyte imbalance
    j. Acute rejection of cardiac transplant

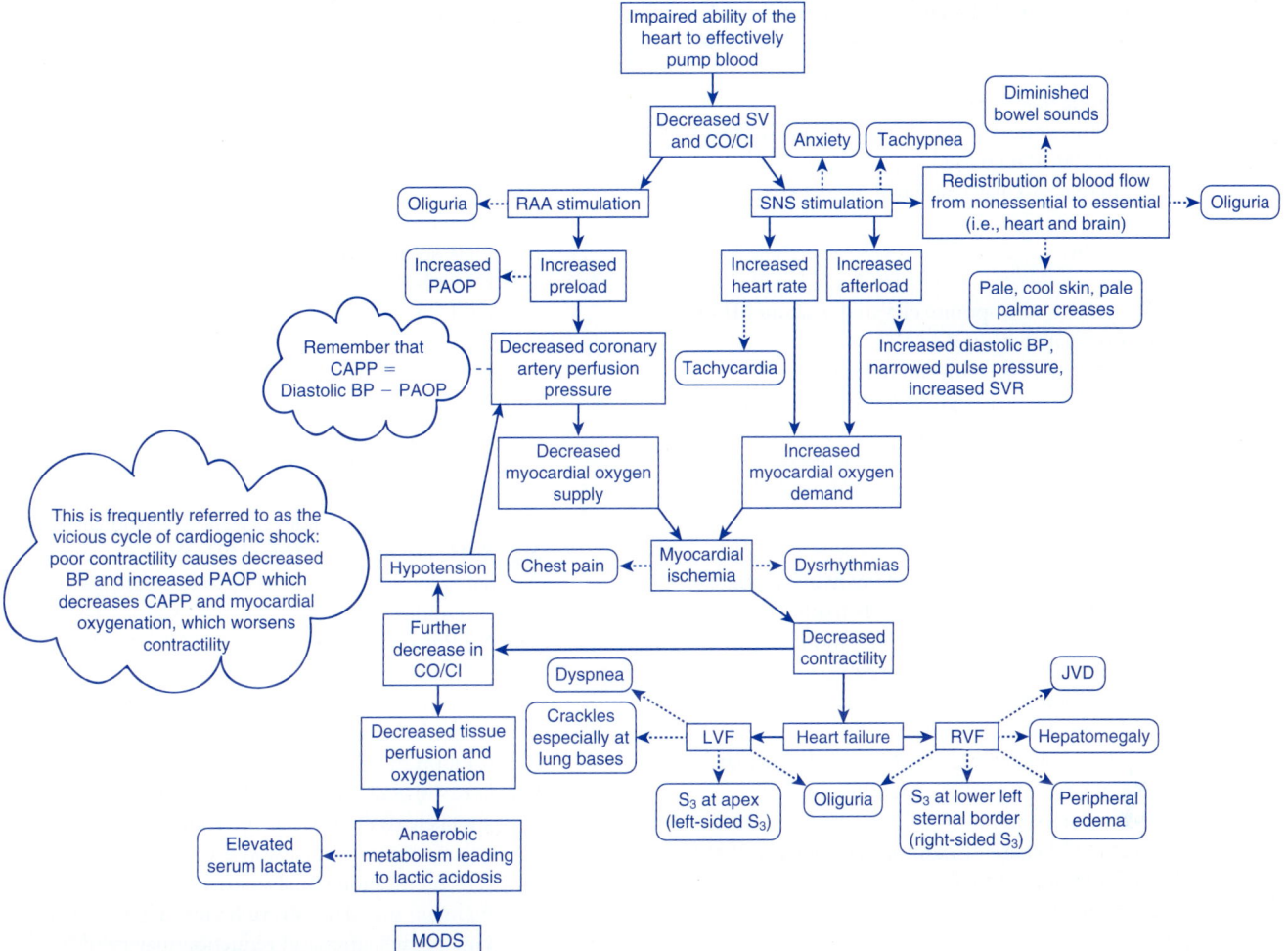

Fig. 11.6 Pathophysiology of cardiogenic shock. *Dotted lines* connect pathology to clinical presentation. *BP,* Blood pressure; *CAPP,* coronary artery perfusion pressure; *CI,* cardiac index; *CO,* cardiac output; *LVF,* left ventricular failure; *MODS,* multiple organ dysfunction syndrome; *PAOP,* pulmonary artery occlusive pressure; *RAA,* renin-angiotensin-aldosterone; *RVF,* right ventricular failure; *SNS,* sympathetic nervous system; *SV,* stroke volume; *SVR,* systemic vascular resistance.

2. Impaired filling
   a. Dysrhythmias
   b. Cardiac tamponade
   c. Noncompliant ventricle (e.g., left ventricular hypertrophy, right ventricular hypertrophy)
3. Impaired emptying (may be referred to as obstructive)
   a. Valvular dysfunction
      1) Chronic: stenosis or regurgitation
      2) Acute: papillary muscle rupture
   b. Ventricular septal rupture or rupture of ventricular free wall
   c. Intracardiac tumor
   d. Massive PE
   e. Tension pneumothorax
   f. Dissecting thoracic aortic aneurysm
   g. Coarctation of the aorta
   h. Restrictive or hypertrophic cardiomyopathy

Pathophysiology

Fig. 11.6.

Clinical Presentation

Same as for shock and including the following:
1. Subjective
   a. History of precipitating factor
   b. Chest pain
   c. Dyspnea
   d. Anxiety, fear, feeling of impending doom
2. Objective
   a. Clinical indicators of left ventricular failure
      1) Tachycardia: This effect may be reduced if patient is receiving beta-blockers.
      2) Dysrhythmias
      3) Pulsus alternans
      4) Tachypnea
      5) Heart sound changes: S_3
      6) Breath sound changes: crackles, wheezes
   b. Clinical indicators of right ventricular failure
      1) Jugular venous distention
      2) Peripheral edema
      3) Hepatosplenomegaly

3. Hemodynamics: Table 11.2; defining characteristics of cardiogenic shock:
   a. CO/CI decreased
   b. Stroke volume decreased
   c. Right atrial pressure, CVP, pulmonary arterial pressure (PAP), and PAOP increased
   d. SVR/Systemic vascular resistance index (SVRI) increased
4. Diagnostic studies
   a. Serum
      1) Enzymes and troponin: elevated if acute MI or myocardial contusion
      2) Electrolytes: Note any abnormality.
      3) ABGs: may reveal significant hypoxemia in pulmonary edema, respiratory acidosis as the patient fatigues and acute respiratory failure occurs, and eventually metabolic acidosis with tissue hypoxia causing lactic acidosis
   b. ECG
      1) May reveal acute (i.e., ST-segment elevation, pathologic Q waves) or old MI (pathologic Q waves without ST-segment elevation)
      2) May reveal ventricular aneurysm (i.e., persistent ST-segment elevation in anterior leads)
      3) May reveal dysrhythmias
   c. Chest radiography: may show pulmonary vascular congestion and enlarged cardiac silhouette
   d. Cardiac catheterization
      1) May reveal cause of cardiogenic shock
      2) May reveal abnormal intracardiac pressures
   e. Echocardiography: may reveal cause of cardiogenic shock
      1) Ventricular wall motion abnormality
         a) Regional wall motional abnormality can identify location of myocardial ischemia or infarction
         b) Global wall motion abnormality in cardiomyopathy or myocarditis
      2) Valvular abnormality (e.g., ruptured ventricular septum, ruptured papillary muscle with acute mitral regurgitation)
      3) Cardiac tamponade

Collaborative Management

Same as for shock and including the following:
1. Identify high-risk patients and monitor for clinical indications of hypoperfusion; use invasive hemodynamic monitoring if appropriate for early detection of changes.
2. Prevent and treat the cause.
   a. Early reperfusion for acute MI with percutaneous coronary intervention or fibrinolytic agents
   b. Control dysrhythmias.
   c. Pericardiocentesis for cardiac tamponade
   d. Fibrinolytics and anticoagulants for pulmonary embolus
   e. Surgery for removal of intracardiac tumors, valve replacement, septal repair, and so on
   f. Emergency decompression followed by chest tube for tension pneumothorax
3. Improve oxygenation.
   a. Oxygen to maintain SpO_2 at least 94%; oxygen delivery methods required to achieve varies from nasal cannula to mechanical ventilation
4. Improve myocardial perfusion.
   a. Nitrates for ischemia while being careful not to decrease BP and coronary artery perfusion pressure
      1) Remember that one NTG sublingually is 400 mcg, so titratable IV NTG is preferred in shock.
      2) Oral phosphodiesterase inhibitors such as sildenafil, tadalafil, vardenafil, udenafil, or avanafil can cause a drastic decrease in BP if treated with NTG.
5. Optimize CO and improve tissue perfusion.
   a. Inotropes (e.g., dobutamine) to increase *contractility*; note that increasing contractility leads to increased myocardial oxygen demand
   b. Diuretics (e.g., furosemide) or venous vasodilators (e.g., NTG) to decrease *preload* (PAOP)
   c. Arterial vasodilators (e.g., NTP) to decrease *afterload* if no contraindications
      1) NTP is contraindicated in acute myocardial ischemia because of the risk of coronary artery steal with shunting of blood from ischemic areas to nonischemic areas
      2) Caution must be exercised with all arterial vasodilators in acute myocardial ischemia because they are likely to decrease aortic root pressure and coronary artery perfusion pressure
      3) Careful titration of all vasodilators is required to maintain the MAP above 65 mm Hg to perfuse vital organs; afterload reduction may need to be achieved nonpharmacologically through the use of an intraaortic balloon pump
   d. Antidysrhythmics as required to control *HR* and *rhythm*.
      1) Anxiolytics (e.g., lorazepam) may be helpful to decrease HR by decreasing anxiety.
      2) Beta-blockers are contraindicated during cardiogenic shock states because they decrease contractility.
   e. Mechanical supports (e.g., IABP) (Chapter 3, Figs. 2-75 through 2-77 and Table 2-27) or ventricular assist devices (Table 2-39)
      1) IABP may be used when pharmacologic treatment is not effective and is especially helpful in patients who have very high afterload that is refractory to arterial vasodilators or who are too hypotensive to use arterial vasodilators to reduce afterload.
      2) IABP or ventricular assist devices may also serve as a bridge to transplant if the patient is a candidate for cardiac transplantation.
      3) A left ventricular assist device or biventricular assist device may be used when desired response is not achieved with IABP and pharmacologic treatment; it may be inserted percutaneously (i.e., Impella).
6. Register the patient for cardiac transplantation if appropriate.
7. Provide pain control and anxiolysis.

Anaphylactic Shock
Definitions
1. Anaphylaxis: a systemic response to a specific antigen, usually occurring within 1 hour of exposure; this immunoglobulin E (IgE)–mediated response is an example of a type I hypersensitivity reaction, and prior exposure to the antigen is required, which allows development of antibodies. Mast cells and basophils release histamine and histamine-like substances that cause vasodilation.
2. Anaphylactoid reaction: an anaphylaxis-type reaction triggered by direct activation of the mast cell; this nonimmune response does not require previous exposure to the antigen; clinically indistinguishable from anaphylaxis, and acute treatment is the same as for anaphylaxis
3. Anaphylactic shock: shock resulting from massive vasodilation caused by release of histamine in response to a severe allergic reaction

Etiology
1. Examples of substances causing anaphylactic (IgE-mediated) reactions
   a. Foods are the most common cause of anaphylaxis (Lieberman et al, 2015); any food can lead to anaphylaxis, but the most common causes are:
      1) Fish
      2) Shellfish
      3) Eggs
      4) Milk and milk products
      5) Soy
      6) Wheat
      7) Strawberries
      8) Legumes (e.g., peanuts, soybeans)
      9) Nuts (e.g., walnuts, pecans, cashews, almonds)
      10) Chocolate
      11) Food additives
         a) Artificial coloring
         b) Preservatives: sulfites and MSG
   b. Drugs
      1) Angiotensin-converting enzyme inhibitors (e.g., captopril, enalapril)
      2) Acetylcysteine
      3) Allergic extracts in hyposensitization therapy
      4) Allopurinol
      5) Anesthetics
         a) Local anesthetics: lidocaine, procaine, cocaine
         b) General anesthetics: thiopental, etomidate, ketamine
      6) Animal serums: antitoxins, antivenoms
      7) Antibiotics
         a) Beta-lactam antibiotics
            i) Penicillin
            ii) Cephalosporins
         b) Tetracycline
         c) Macrolides
      8) Barbiturates
      9) Blood and blood products: blood transfusion incompatibilities, albumin
      10) Enzymes
         a) Pancreatic enzyme
         b) Papaya enzyme
            i) Chymopapain (used in chemical discectomy)
            ii) Meat tenderizer
      11) Iodine-containing contrast media (e.g., Renografin)
      12) Narcotics: morphine, meperidine, codeine
      13) Neuromuscular blockers
      14) Protamine sulfate
      15) Thiazide diuretics (e.g., hydrochlorothiazide)
      16) Vaccines
   c. Venoms
      1) Snake
      2) Hymenoptera (e.g., wasps, hornets, bees, yellow jackets, fire ants)
      3) Spider
      4) Jellyfish
      5) Stingray
      6) Deer fly
      7) Scorpion
   d. Other chemicals or biologicals
      1) Materials (e.g., latex)
      2) Hand lotions
      3) Soap
      4) Perfume
      5) Iodine-containing solutions
      6) Animal dander
2. Examples of substances causing anaphylactoid (non–IgE-mediated) reactions
   a. Drugs
      1) Aspirin
      2) Nonsteroidal antiinflammatory agents: aspirin, ibuprofen, indomethacin
      3) Opiates
      4) Thiamine
      5) Dextran
      6) Gamma globulin
   b. Dyes
      1) Radiopaque contrast media
      2) Fluorescein

Pathophysiology
Fig. 11.7.

Clinical Presentation
Same as for shock and including the following:
1. Subjective
   a. History of precipitating factor
   b. Anxiety, vague uneasiness
   c. Warmth
   d. Nausea, abdominal cramping, abdominal pain, vomiting, diarrhea
   e. Chest tightness, palpitations, substernal pain
   f. Dyspnea
   g. Dizziness, vertigo, syncope
   h. Pruritus
   i. Feeling of a lump in throat
2. Objective
   a. Cutaneous
      1) An identifiable site of allergen exposure, bite, sting, or envenomation may be evident as localized redness, swelling, and pruritus.

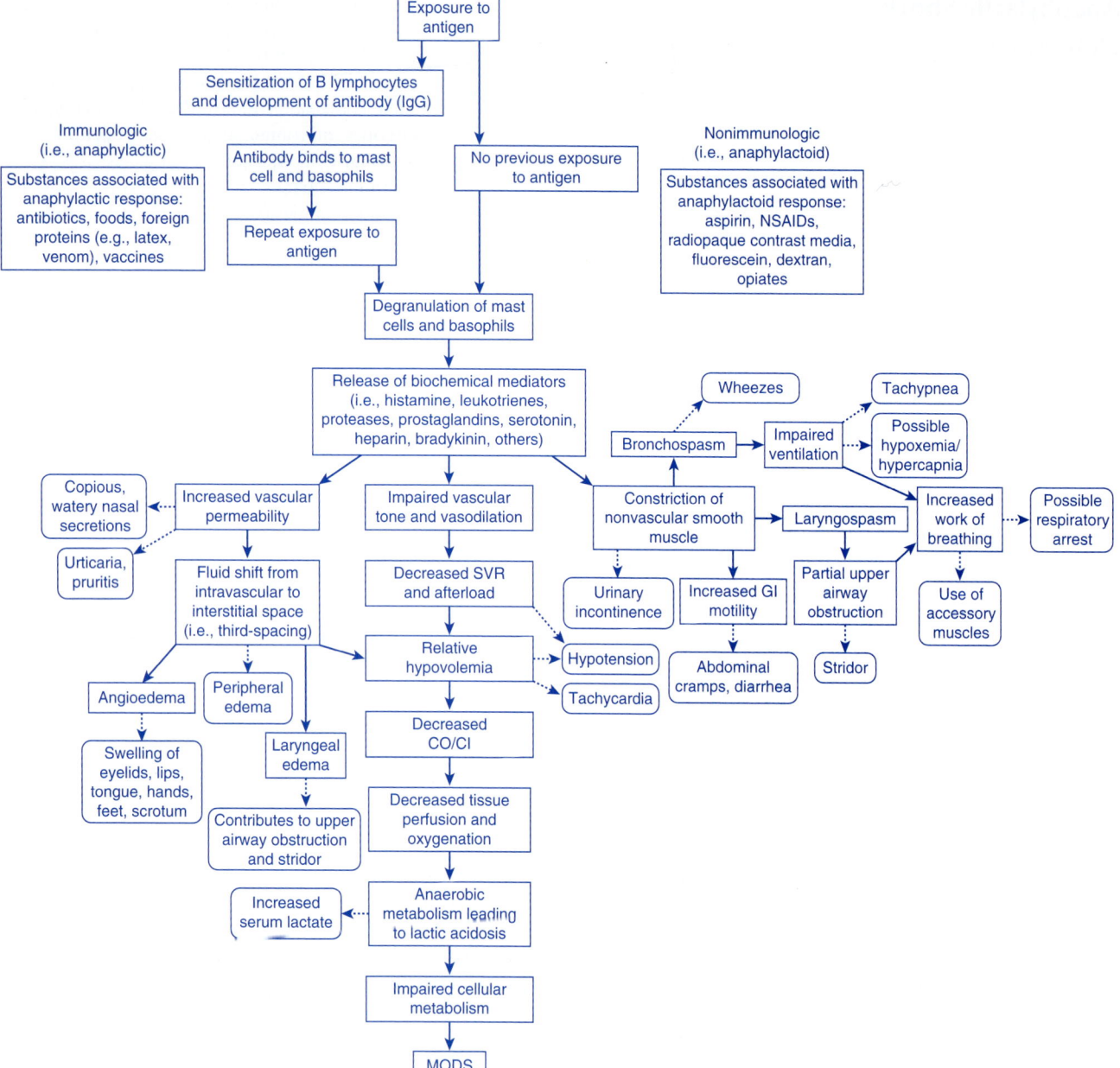

Fig. 11.7 Pathophysiology of anaphylactic shock. *Dotted lines* connect pathology to clinical presentation. *CI,* Cardiac index; *CO,* cardiac output; *GI,* gastrointestinal; *NSAID,* nonsteroidal antiinflammatory drug; *SVR,* systemic vascular resistance.

      2) May be generalized
         a) Angioedema (edema of membranous tissues): swelling of eyes, lips, tongue, hands, feet, and genitalia
         b) Flushing, diaphoresis
         c) Warm to hot skin
         d) Urticaria
         e) Conjunctival injection, tearing
         f) Watery rhinorrhea, sneezing
    b. Cardiovascular
      1) Tachycardia
      2) Hypotension
      3) Dysrhythmias
      4) ST-segment and T-wave changes consistent with ischemia
      5) Shock
      6) Cardiac arrest may occur.
    c. Pulmonary
      1) Hoarseness, dysphonia
      2) Cough
      3) Breath sound changes: stridor, wheezing, crackles, rhonchi
      4) Respiratory arrest may occur.
    d. CNS
      1) Restlessness
      2) Headache
      3) Change in level of consciousness (LOC)
      4) Seizures
    e. Genitourinary
      1) Urinary incontinence
      2) Urine output: may be decreased
      3) Vaginal bleeding

f. GI
      1) Dysphagia
      2) Vomiting
      3) Hyperactive bowel sounds
      4) Diarrhea
3. Hemodynamics: Table 11.2
4. Diagnostic studies
   a. Serum
      1) IgE levels may be used to confirm allergic origin.
      2) Eosinophils elevated
      3) ABGs: initially respiratory alkalosis with hypoxemia and eventually respiratory and metabolic acidosis as hypoventilation and tissue hypoxia occur

Collaborative Management
Same as for shock and including the following:
1. Identify high-risk patients and monitor for clinical indications of allergic reaction and hypoperfusion.
2. Maintain airway, oxygenation, and ventilation.
   a. Airway
      1) Assess airway for clinical indications of angioedema (i.e., edema of uvula, respiratory distress, stridor, hypoxemia).
      2) If angioedema is present, assist with endotracheal tube insertion early to prevent complete airway obstruction; cricothyrotomy may be necessary because of laryngeal edema.
   b. Oxygen to maintain SpO_2 at 94%; the method of oxygen delivery required varies from nasal cannula to mechanical ventilation.
   c. Mechanical ventilation as prescribed
3. Remove or slow absorption of the offending antigen.
   a. Removal of stinger if anaphylaxis is caused by a sting and if the stinger can be removed without squeezing
   b. Apply ice to sting or bite.
   c. Discontinue infusion of dye, drug, or blood.
   d. Dermal decontamination with soap and water if skin exposure to allergen
   e. Gastric lavage is not recommended to remove an ingested antigen.
4. Modify or block the effects of biochemical mediators.
   a. Sympathomimetic agents
      1) Epinephrine is the first-line drug for anaphylaxis; it promotes vasodilation and vasoconstriction; the preferred route is IM but may be given IV.
         a) IM into lateral thigh: 0.2 to 0.5 mg (1:1000 concentration) repeated every 5 to 15 minutes with a maximum of 0.3 mg; higher doses can be given as required.
         b) IV
            i) IV injection: 0.1 to 0.25 mg (1:10,000 concentration); start with a small dose, giving only as much as required to alleviate undesirable symptoms, and repeat as necessary (usually every 20 to 30 minutes), gradually increasing dose depending on need. (Nazareno, Gahart & Adrienne, 2017).
            ii) IV infusion: 1 to 10 mcg/min if inadequate response to IV injection
      2) Glucagon 1 to 5 mg over 5 minutes followed by infusion of 5 to 15 mg/min IV for patients taking beta-blockers with hypotension refractory to epinephrine and fluids; can be repeated if there is no BP response in 10 minutes
         a) Glucagon can stimulate an increase in HR and contractility even with beta blockade.
         b) Monitor for nausea, vomiting, hypokalemia, and hyperglycemia.
   b. Crystalloids: 1 to 2 l of NS
   c. Antihistamines as prescribed to block histamine receptors.
      1) Diphenhydramine 25 to 50 mg IV, IM, or orally (PO)
      2) Ranitidine 50 mg IV or famotidine 20 mg IV
   d. Steroids as prescribed to stabilize mast cells, decrease capillary permeability, and prevent delayed reaction.
      1) Methylprednisolone sodium succinate 100 mg IV or hydrocortisone sodium succinate 100 to 200 to 500 mg IV
      2) Prednisone 40 to 60 mg PO daily
   e. Bronchodilators as prescribed to reverse the bronchoconstriction caused by histamine, Slow reacting substance of anaphylaxis (SRS-A), and bradykinin.
      1) Albuterol, intermittent or continuous nebulizer, for wheezing refractory to epinephrine
      2) Ipratropium bromide or magnesium may also be used.
5. Maintain MAP and tissue perfusion: Fluids, inotropes, and/or vasopressors may be necessary.

Neurogenic Shock
Definition
Shock resulting from massive vasodilation caused by disturbance of the SNS

Etiology
1. Cervical spinal cord injury (most common cause); Note that this is not the same as spinal shock, which is loss of neurologic function below the level of the injury but not necessarily associated with inadequate tissue perfusion.
2. Head injury
3. Hypoglycemia
4. General anesthesia
5. Spinal anesthesia
6. Epidural block
7. Drugs
   a. Barbiturates
   b. Phenothiazines
   c. Sympathetic blocking agents (e.g., antihypertensives)
8. Exposure to unpleasant circumstances (e.g., fright or pain)

Pathophysiology
Fig. 11.8.

Clinical Presentation
1. Subjective: history of precipitating factor
2. Objective
   a. Bradydysrhythmias: may progress to asystole
   b. Hypotension
   c. Hypothermia

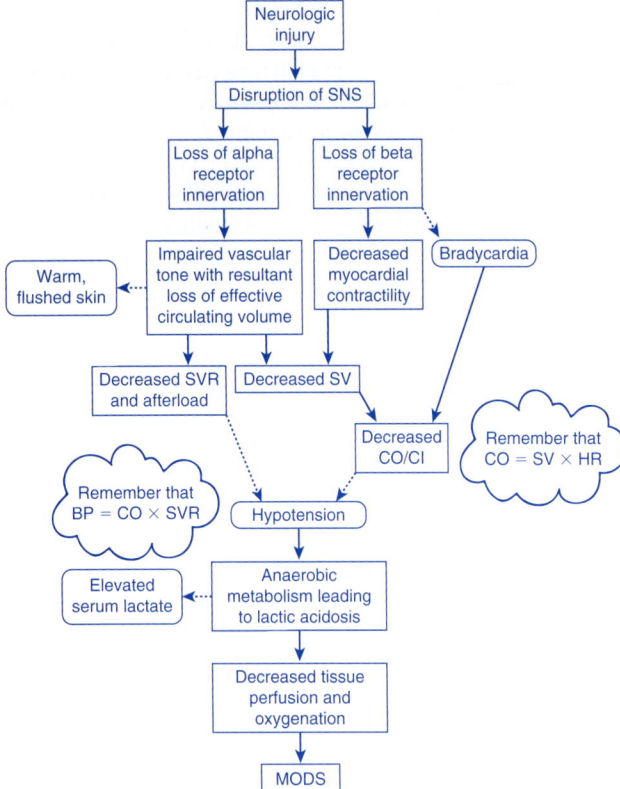

Fig. 11.8 Pathophysiology of neurogenic shock. *Dotted lines* connect pathology to clinical presentation. *BP*, Blood pressure; *CI*, cardiac index; *CO*, cardiac output; *HR*, heart rate; *MODS*, multiple organ dysfunction syndrome; *SNS*, sympathetic nervous system; *SV*, stroke volume; *SVR*, systemic vascular resistance.

   d. Skin warm, dry, flushed
   e. Neurologic deficit (e.g., paralysis below level of spinal cord injury, neurologic changes related to head injury)
3. Hemodynamics: Table 11.2.

Collaborative Management
Same as for shock and including the following:
1. Identify high-risk patients and monitor for clinical indications of hypoperfusion.
2. Prevent and treat the cause.
   a. Spinal cord injury: early immobilization of the spine
   b. Anesthesia: Reverse anesthesia.
   c. Hypoglycemia
      1) Measure serum glucose as required.
      2) Administer 10 to 15 g of carbohydrate if the patient is conscious or 50 ml of $D_{50}W$ if unconscious.
3. Maintain MAP and tissue perfusion.
   a. Maintain MAP greater than 70 mm Hg.
      1) Fluids
         a) Crystalloids
         b) Monitor closely for pulmonary or cerebral edema.
      2) Inotropes, vasopressors, or both may be necessary.
         a) Alpha- and beta-adrenergic medications
         b) Dopamine and norepinephrine are preferred to pure alpha-adrenergic agents.
   b. Maintain a HR of 60 to 100 beats/min: atropine, a pacemaker, or both may be necessary.
4. Treat hypothermia if necessary; rewarm slowly to decrease further vasodilation.
5. Administer VTE prophylaxis.

Septic Shock
Definitions
1. Infection: an inflammatory response to the presence of microorganisms
2. Bacteremia: the presence of viable bacteria in the blood
3. SIRS: an inflammatory response to the invasion of microorganism aimed at restoring homeostasis
   a. Can also occur as a result of trauma and other events that elicit an immune response that are not associated with infection.
   b. SIRS criteria
      1) Temperature greater than 38°C (100.4°F) or less than 36°C (96.8°F)
      2) HR greater than 90 beats/min
      3) Respiratory rate greater than 20 or $PaCO_2$ less than 32 mm Hg
      4) WBC count greater than 12,000/mm³, less than 4000/mm³, or greater than 10% bands
   c. The inflammatory cascade maintains balance, but as a result, capillary permeability is increased, allowing fluid to leave the vascular space, which can cause hypovolemia and pulmonary edema.
   d. SIRS is associated with coagulopathies and vasodilation, which can lead to clotting issues and relative hypovolemia.
   e. SIRS + infection = sepsis
4. Sepsis: life-threatening organ dysfunction caused by a dysregulated host response to infection. Organ dysfunction is represented by an increase in the Sequential Organ Failure Assessment (SOFA) score of 2 points or more (Singer et al, 2016)
5. Septic shock
   a. Subset of sepsis in which particularly profound circulatory, cellular, and metabolic abnormalities are associated with a greater risk of mortality than with sepsis alone
   b. Clinically identified by a vasopressor requirement to maintain a MAP of 65 or greater and serum lactate level of greater than 2 in the absence of hypovolemia
   c. Before 2016, severe sepsis was defined separately from sepsis.
   d. Current clinical practice guidelines still reflect severe sepsis as a subcategory of the infection continuum, although definitions have changed (Singer et al, 2016).

Etiology
1. Factors that cause immunosuppression
   a. Aging
   b. Malnutrition
   c. Alcoholism or drug abuse
   d. Debilitation
   e. Malignancy
   f. Immune deficits and disorders (e.g., AIDS, bone marrow suppression, splenectomy, immunosuppressive drugs)

g. Disease processes: burns, cancer, cardiovascular disease, diabetes, GI disease, liver disease, pulmonary disease, renal disease, traumatic injuries, infections
2. Factors that cause bacteremia and septicemia
   a. Invasive procedures and devices
   b. Pulmonary procedures
   c. Diagnostic procedures
   d. Surgical procedures or wounds
   e. Traumatic wounds or burns
   f. Genitourinary infection
   g. Untreated GI disease (cholelithiasis, intestinal obstruction, appendicitis, diverticulitis)
   h. Peritonitis
   i. Food poisoning
   j. Blood transfusion
   k. Prolonged hospitalization
   l. Translocation of GI bacteria: nothing by mouth (NPO) status, decreased peristalsis, and GI ischemia contribute to proliferation of GI bacteria and translocation of these bacteria into blood or lymph.
3. Microorganisms that are common causes of infections in adults
   a. Gram-negative bacteria
      1) *Escherichia coli*
      2) *Klebsiella* spp.
      3) *Pseudomonas* spp.
      4) Common sites of gram-negative infections: pulmonary system, urinary tract, GI system, wounds
   b. Gram-positive organisms
      1) *Staphylococcus aureus*
      2) *Staphylococcus epidermidis*
      3) *Streptococcus pneumoniae*
      4) *Clostridium* organisms
      5) *Pneumococcus* spp.
      6) Common causes of gram-positive infections: toxic shock syndrome, vaginal and cesarean section delivery, surgical wounds, abscesses, infected burns abrasions, insect bites, herpes zoster, cellulitis, septic abortion, and osteomyelitis

Pathophysiology
Fig. 11.9.

Clinical Presentation
1. Documented or suspected infection
2. General variables
   a. Temperature greater than 38.3°C or less than 36°C
   b. HR greater than 90 beats/min
   c. Tachypnea
   d. Significant edema or positive fluid balance greater than 20 ml/kg over 24 hours
   e. Hyperglycemia
   f. Altered mental status
3. Inflammatory variables
   a. WBC count greater than 12,000/mm^3 or less than 4000/mm^3 or normal WBC count with greater than 10% immature forms
   b. CRP or procalcitonin greater than 2 standard deviations above the normal value
4. Organ dysfunction variables
   a. Cardiovascular: systolic BP 90 mm Hg or less (or decreased by >40 mm Hg from the patient's normal) or MAP of 70 mm Hg or less
   b. Pulmonary: hypoxemia with PaO$_2$/FiO$_2$ less than 250 mm Hg
   c. Renal: urine output less than 0.5 ml/kg/hr for 2 hours despite adequate fluid resuscitation, increased BUN and creatinine
   d. Liver: serum bilirubin greater than 2 mg/dl
   e. GI: decreased bowel sounds
   f. Hematologic: thrombocytopenia; international normalized ratio greater than 1.5
5. Tissue perfusion variables
   a. Lactate greater than 1 mmol/l
   b. Decreased capillary refill or mottling
6. Evidence of infection, sepsis, and hypotension if septic shock
   a. Sepsis with hypotension despite adequate fluid resuscitation along with the presence of perfusion abnormalities
7. Hemodynamics: Table 11.2.

Collaborative Management
Same as for shock and including the following:
1. Identify high-risk patients and monitor for clinical indications of infection and sepsis.
   a. Risk factors for infection in the critically ill patient (Table 11.6)
2. Prevent infection and sepsis.
   a. Use good handwashing techniques and prevent cross-contamination.
   b. Avoid invasive procedures if possible.
   c. Participate in early identification of infection.
      1) Monitor color, characteristics of sputum, urine, stools, wounds, and so on.
      2) Culture secretions and wounds as indicated.
   d. Prepare the patient for surgery as indicated for any of the following:
      1) Removal of all necrotic tissue
      2) Drainage of abscess
      3) Early débridement of burn eschar
      4) Prompt stabilization of fractures to minimize soft tissue damage, inflammation, and infection
   e. Perform meticulous oral and airway care; silent aspiration of oral, nasopharyngeal, and sinus secretions around the endotracheal tube cuff occurs and is a cause of nosocomial pneumonia.
   f. Perform meticulous IV, intraarterial, pulmonary arterial, and urinary catheter care according to Centers for Disease Control and Prevention (CDC) guidelines or hospital policy.
   g. Perform meticulous wound care as indicated by type and appearance of wound.
   h. Avoid NPO status to prevent translocation of enteric bacteria into the lymphatics and vascular bed.
      1) Enteral feedings should be given if at all possible.
      2) Selective gut decontamination (gut sterilization) has been advocated for use with parenteral nutrition for patients who must be NPO; provide parenteral nutrition for nutritional support.

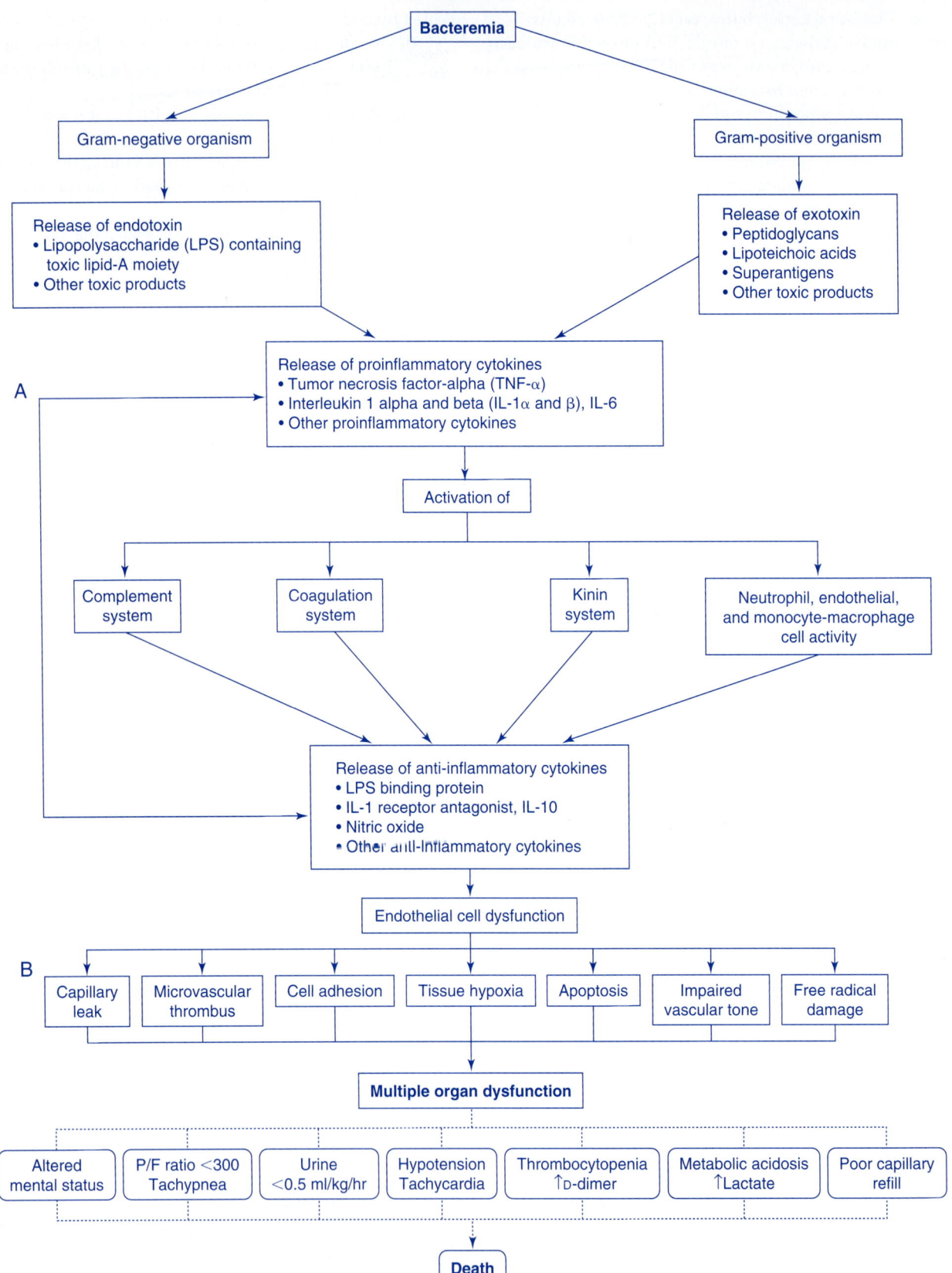

Fig. 11.9 Pathophysiology of sepsis and septic shock. *Dotted lines* connect pathophysiology to clinical presentation. P/F, PaO$_2$/FiO$_2$. (A, From Lazaron, V., & Barke, R.A. [1999]. Gram-negative bacterial sepsis and the sepsis syndrome. *Urol Clin North Am, 26*[4], 687–699. B, Copyright © 2003, Eli Lilly and Company. All rights reserved. Reprinted with permission from Eli Lilly and Company.)

Table 11.6	Risk Factors for Infection in Critically Ill Patients
Risk Factor	**Possible IIR Consequence**
Invasive lines, drains, monitoring devices	Increased risk of infection caused by direct access for microbes
Medications	H_2 blockers alter the normal environment of the GI tract
	Antibiotics alter normal flora, leading to opportunistic infections
IIR activation	Increased capillary permeability increases risk of pulmonary edema, leading to pulmonary complications; increased edema, slowing wound healing
	Activation of the clotting cascade increases risk of VTE
NPO	Bacterial translocation from GI tract
	Inadequate nutrition to produce key components of the IIR
Poor perfusion	Tissue ischemia leading to cell death and further activation of IIR
Complications from bedrest	VTE
	Pressure wounds
	Pulmonary complications caused by reduced tidal volume
Complications from altered LOC	Reduced cough response can lead to respiratory complications; immobility can lead to pressure wounds
Hyperglycemia	Hyperglycemia increases risk of infection
Health care workers	Risk of contamination from clothes, hands, and instruments
Altered sleep	Sleep deprivations alters the immune system

GI, Gastrointestinal; *IIR*, Inflammatory immune response; *LOC*, level of consciousness; *NPO*, nothing by mouth; *VTE*, venous thromboembolism

Box 11.2	Intrinsic and Extrinsic Risk Factors for CLABSI

Intrinsic Risk Factors (nonmodifiable characteristics of the patient)
- Patient's age
- Underlying diseases or conditions
- Patient's gender

Extrinsic Risk Factors (potentially modifiable factors associated with CVC insertion or maintenance)
- Prolonged hospitalization before CVC insertion
- Multiple CVCs
- Parenteral nutrition
- Femoral or internal jugular access site
- Heavy microbial colonization at insertion site
- Multilumen CVCs
- Lack of maximal sterile barriers for CVC insertion
- CVC insertion in an ICU or ED

CVC, Central venous catheter; *ED*, emergency department; *ICU*, intensive care unit.
Adapted from The Joint Commission. (2012). *Preventing central line-associated bloodstream infections*. Oak Brook, IL: Joint Commission Resources. https://www.jointcommission.org/assets/1/18/CLABSI_Monograph.pdfafety Program for Reducing CAUTI in Hospitals.

i. Use appropriate evidence-based bundles to prevent hospital-acquired infections (HAIs) (i.e., infection acquired as a result of hospitalization).
   1) Central line–associated blood stream infection (CLABSI)
      a) Definition: a primary bloodstream infection that develops in a patient with a central line in place within the 48-hour period before onset of the bloodstream infection that is not related to infection at another site
      b) Risk factors for CLABSI (Box 11.2)
      c) CLABSI bundle
         i) Insertion
            (a) Perform hand hygiene.
            (b) Disinfect skin with chlorhexidine (CHG).
            (c) Allow the antiseptic solution to dry before placing the catheter.
            (d) Maximal sterile barrier precautions.
               (i) Person inserting the central venous catheter (CVC) should wear a mask and cap, a sterile gown, and sterile gloves.
               (ii) Use a large (head-to-toe) sterile drape over the patient.
         ii) Catheter selection
            (a) Select a catheter with the minimum number of ports or lumens necessary.
            (b) Avoid the femoral vein.
            (c) Use a subclavian site for a non-tunneled CVC (except in dialysis patients).
            (d) When adherence to aseptic technique cannot be ensured (i.e., catheters inserted during a medical emergency), replace the catheter as soon as possible.
         iii) Maintenance
            (a) Perform hand hygiene immediately before and after each episode of patient contact.
            (b) Apply sterile dressing (gauze, transparent dressing, gauze and transparent dressing, antimicrobial foam disc). Change gauze dressing every 2 days and clear dressings every 7 days (and more frequently if soiled, damp, or loose).
            (c) Use sterile endcaps or needleless connectors on all unused lumens.
            (d) Change caps after administering blood and if there is visual observation of blood in the caps.
            (e) Replace administration sets and add-on devices no more frequently than every 96 hours and at least every 7 days unless contamination occurs.
            (f) Replace sets and add-on devices within 24 hours of start of infu-

sion if fluids that enhance microbial growth are infused (e.g., fat emulsions combined with amino acids and glucose).
- (g) Sanitize access ports with alcohol, CHG, povidone–iodine, and iodophor before and after (each use, a method known as "scrub the hub").
- iv) Removal. Review the necessity every day, with prompt removal of unnecessary CVC

2) Catheter-associated urinary tract infection (CAUTI)
   a) Definition: A urinary tract infection in which an indwelling urinary catheter was in place for more than two calendar days on the date of event and an indwelling urinary catheter was in place on the date of event or the day before
   b) Expected practice
      i) Assess for accepted indications before placement of any indwelling urinary catheter.
      ii) Adhere to aseptic technique for placement, manipulation, and maintenance of indwelling urinary catheters.
      iii) Document all instances of indwelling urinary catheters, including insertion date, indication, and removal date.
      iv) Discontinue indwelling urinary catheters promptly as soon as indications expire
   c) Indications for indwelling urinary catheters
      i) Acute urinary retention or obstruction
      ii) Accurate measurement of urinary output in critically ill patients
      iii) Perioperative use in selected surgeries
      iv) Assistance with healing of stage III or IV perineal and sacral wounds in incontinent patients
      v) Hospice, comfort, and palliative care
      vi) Required immobilization for trauma or surgery (Association of Healthcare Research and Quality [AHRQ], 2015)
   d) Appropriate maintenance (AHRQ, 2015)
      i) If there are breaks in aseptic technique, disconnection of drainage tubing from the catheter, or malfunction of the catheter or drainage system, replace the catheter and the drainage system.
      ii) Make sure urinary flow is not obstructed.
      iii) Drainage bags should always be placed below the level of the patient's bladder to facilitate drainage and to prevent stasis of urine.
      iv) Urine in drainage bags should be emptied at least once each shift and before any transfer off the unit (e.g., going to radiology) using a container designated for that patient only.
      v) Keep the outlet valve from becoming contaminated.
      vi) Follow standard precautions by using gloves and performing proper hand hygiene before and after handling the drainage device.
      vii) Do not change catheters or urinary drainage systems routinely for the purpose of preventing CAUTIs. Consider changing the urinary system in the event of infection, obstruction, or a break or leak of the closed system.
      viii) Do not remove any seals between the catheter and the drainage tubing or disconnect the closed system.
      vix) Avoid irrigation; if catheter obstruction is determined and the catheter remains indicated, replace the catheter and drainage system.
      x) When obtaining a sample of urine from the system, disinfect the sampling port and allow the disinfectant to dry before accessing the port.
      xi) Frequent meatal cleaning may be associated with increased risk of CAUTI. The CDC recommends routine perineal hygiene using soap and water during daily bathing.

3) Ventilator-associated pneumonia (VAP) and ventilator-associated events (VAEs)
   a) Definition: pneumonia in a patient who is intubated and ventilated at the time or within 48 hours before the onset of infection
   b) Expected practice
      i) Elevate the head of the bed (HOB) 30 to 45 degrees.
         (a) Reduces the risk of aspiration
         (b) Improves ventilation
      ii) Daily sedative interruption and daily assessment of readiness to extubate
         (a) Decreases the amount of time spent on mechanical ventilation
      iii) Peptic ulcer disease (PUD) prophylaxis.
      iv) DVT prophylaxis (unless contraindicated).
      v) Daily oral care with chlorhexidine (Institute for Healthcare Improvement, 2010)

4) Surgical site infection (SSI)
   a) Expected practice
      i) Proper use of antibiotics
         (a) Delivery of IV antimicrobial prophylaxis within 1 hour before incision (2 hours is allowed for the administration of vancomycin and fluoroquinolones)
         (b) Use of an antimicrobial prophylactic agent consistent with published guidelines

(c) Discontinuation of the prophylactic antimicrobial agent within 24 hours after surgery (discontinuation within 48 hours is allowable for cardiothoracic procedures in adult patients)
       ii) Proper hair removal
           (a) Do not remove hair at the operative site unless the presence of hair will interfere with the operation.
           (b) If hair removal is necessary, remove hair outside the operating room using clippers or a depilatory agent.
           (c) Use of razors is considered inappropriate with the exception of use on the scrotal area or on the scalp after a traumatic head injury.
       iii) Maintain postoperative blood glucose of 180 mg/dl or lower.
       iv) Maintain perioperative temperature of 35.5°C or more.
       v) Optimize tissue oxygenation by administering supplemental oxygen during and immediately after surgical procedures involving mechanical ventilation (Anderson, 2014).
   5) Multidrug-resistant organisms (MDROs)
       a) Include methicillin-resistant staphylococcus aureus (MRSA), vancomycin-resistant enterococci (VRE), and certain gram-negative bacilli (GNB).
       b) Associated with increased lengths of stay, costs, and mortality
       c) Strategies to control MDROs include infection prevention, accurate and prompt diagnosis and treatment, prudent use of antimicrobials, and prevention of transmission.
3. Restore tissue perfusion and normalize cellular metabolism.
   a. Provide early goal-directed therapy during first 6 hours after severe sepsis or septic shock is recognized.
       1) Initiate surviving sepsis bundle (Dellinger et al, 2013).
           a) To be completed within 3 hours:
               i) Measure lactate level.
               ii) Obtain blood cultures before administration of antibiotics.
               iii) Administer broad-spectrum antibiotics.
               iv) Administer 30 ml/kg of crystalloid for hypotension (MAP <65 mm Hg) or lactate at 4 mmol/l or greater.
           b) To be completed within 6 hours:
               i) Apply vasopressors for hypotension that does not respond to initial fluid resuscitation to maintain MAP greater than 65 mm Hg.
                   (a) Use norepinephrine as the first choice.
                   (b) Add epinephrine when a second pressor is required.
                   (c) Insert the arterial line if vasopressors are required.
                   (d) Add dobutamine in the presence of myocardial dysfunction.
               ii) Reassessment of volume status and tissue perfusion for MAP less than 65 mm Hg or initial lactate greater than 4 mmol/l
                   (a) Repeat focused examination or two of the following:
                       (i) Measure CVP.
                       (ii) Measure $S_{cv}O_2$.
                       (iii) Perform bedside cardiovascular ultrasonography.
                       (iv) Perform dynamic assessment of fluid responsiveness with passive leg raise or fluid challenge.
               iii) Remeasure lactate if initial lactate was elevated.
       2) Goals include the following:
           a) CVP of 8 to 12 mm Hg
           b) MAP of 65 mm Hg or greater
           c) $S_{cv}O_2$ or SvO_2 of 70% or 65% respectively or greater
           d) Urine output greater than 0.5 ml/kg/hr
           e) Normal serum lactate
       3) Resuscitation and management (Dellinger et al, 2004; Marik, 2011; Nguyen et al, 2007; Rivers et al, 2001)
           a) Antimicrobial agents after blood cultures
               i) Cultures
                   (a) One blood draw should be percutaneous.
                   (b) One blood draw should be through each vascular access that has been in place for more than 48 hours.
                   (c) Other cultures from other sites (e.g., cerebrospinal fluid, pulmonary secretions, urine, wound) may be indicated as possible sources of infection.
               ii) Antimicrobials
                   (a) Initiated within 1 hour of recognition of severe sepsis
                   (b) Initial empiric antiinfective therapy of one or more drugs that have activity against all likely pathogens and that penetrate in adequate concentrations into tissues presumed to be the source of sepsis (Dellinger et al, 2013)
                   (c) Reassessed daily
           b) Preload correction
               i) Initial fluid challenge in patients with hypoperfusion or hypovolemia to achieve 30 ml/kg
               ii) Crystalloids are the initial fluid of choice.
               iii) Albumin may be added when patients require substantial amounts of crystalloids.

c) Afterload correction
    i) Norepinephrine (2–20 mcg/min) as the first-choice vasopressor to maintain MAP of 65 mm Hg
    ii) Epinephrine may be added and potentially substituted for norepinephrine.
    iii) Vasopressin may be added to other vasopressors but should not be the only agent used.
    iv) Dopamine may be used as an alternative to norepinephrine in selected patients; low-dose dopamine should not be used for renal protection.
    v) Phenylephrine is not recommended.
    vi) An arterial catheter for continuous monitoring of BP is indicated for patients requiring vasopressors.
    vii) Inotropic therapy: Dobutamine can be used alone or in combination with vasopressor in presence of myocardial dysfunction.
    viii) Corticosteroids should be considered if hemodynamic stability cannot be achieved with fluids and vasopressors.
    viv) The cosyntropin stimulation test is no longer recommended.
    x) Hydrocortisone 200 mg/day, administered continuously; taper when vasopressors are no longer required
    xi) Blood and blood products to maintain Hgb between 7 and 9 g/dl
d) Optimize oxygen delivery
    i) Intubation and mechanical ventilation when required for respiratory distress; use the following settings to avoid ventilator-induced lung injury
        (a) Tidal volume at 6 ml/kg
        (b) Peak inspiratory plateau pressure of no more than 30 cm H_2O
        (c) High levels of PEEP may be required.
        (d) Positioning: HOB elevation to 30 to 45 degrees; prone positioning may be used for a P/F ratio less than 100 mm Hg
e) Maintain glucose control.
    i) Initiate glucose control protocol when two consecutive serum glucose levels are greater than 180 mg/dl.
    ii) Target serum glucose levels between 110 to 150 mg/dl.
4. Control hyperthermia.
    a. Monitor core body temperature.
    b. Administer antipyretics as indicated with recognition that fever is an important defense mechanism (Cunha, 2012).
        1) Indications for treatment of fever
            a) Severe cardiopulmonary disease with body temperatures greater than 38.8°C (102°F)
            b) Brain injury
            c) Extreme hyperpyrexia (i.e., body temperature greater than 41.1°C [106°F])
        2) Treatment guidelines
            a) Reduce temperatures slowly to 38.8°C (102°F) to prevent chills and rebound increase in body temperature.
            b) Use antipyretics (e.g., acetaminophen) and environmental cooling methods such as fans.
    c. Use cooling blankets and tepid soaks.
5. Provide nutritional support as appropriate.
6. Monitor for complications of shock and clinical indications of organ failure.

Multiple Organ Dysfunction Syndrome
Definition
Progressive dysfunction of two or more organ systems as a result of an uncontrolled inflammatory response to severe illness or injury (Sole, Klein, & Moseley, 2017)

Etiology
1. Primary caused by acute direct injury to an organ or organs
2. Secondary caused by SIRS; organs are involved in MODS that were not involved in the initial insult

Pathophysiology
Fig. 11.10

Clinical Presentation
1. MODS: dysfunction of more than one of the following organs:
    a. SOFA score; an increased SOFA score is associated with an increased probability of death in patients with sepsis (Table 11.7).
    b. Quick SOFA (qSOFA) (Singer et al, 2016)
        1) Bedside adaptation of the SOFA. qSOFA uses three criteria.
        2) One point for each of the following
            a) Low BP (i.e., SBP ≤100 mm Hg)
            b) High respiratory rate (i.e., ≥22 breaths/min)
            c) Altered mentation (i.e., Glasgow coma scale score <15)
        3) The presence of 2 or more qSOFA points near the onset of infection is associated with a greater risk of death or prolonged intensive care unit stay

Collaborative Management
1. Prevent and treat infection (see Septic Shock section).
2. Maximize oxygen delivery to the tissues (see Shock section).
3. Monitor for complications.
    a. Shock (if not caused by shock)
    b. Death

Multisystem Trauma
Definitions
1. Trauma: injury to the body caused by acute exposure to mechanical, thermal, electrical, radiation, or chemical energy
    a. Unintentional and deliberate or violence related
    b. Intentional: deliberate acts of violence such as shootings, stabbings, assaults, and child or elder abuse

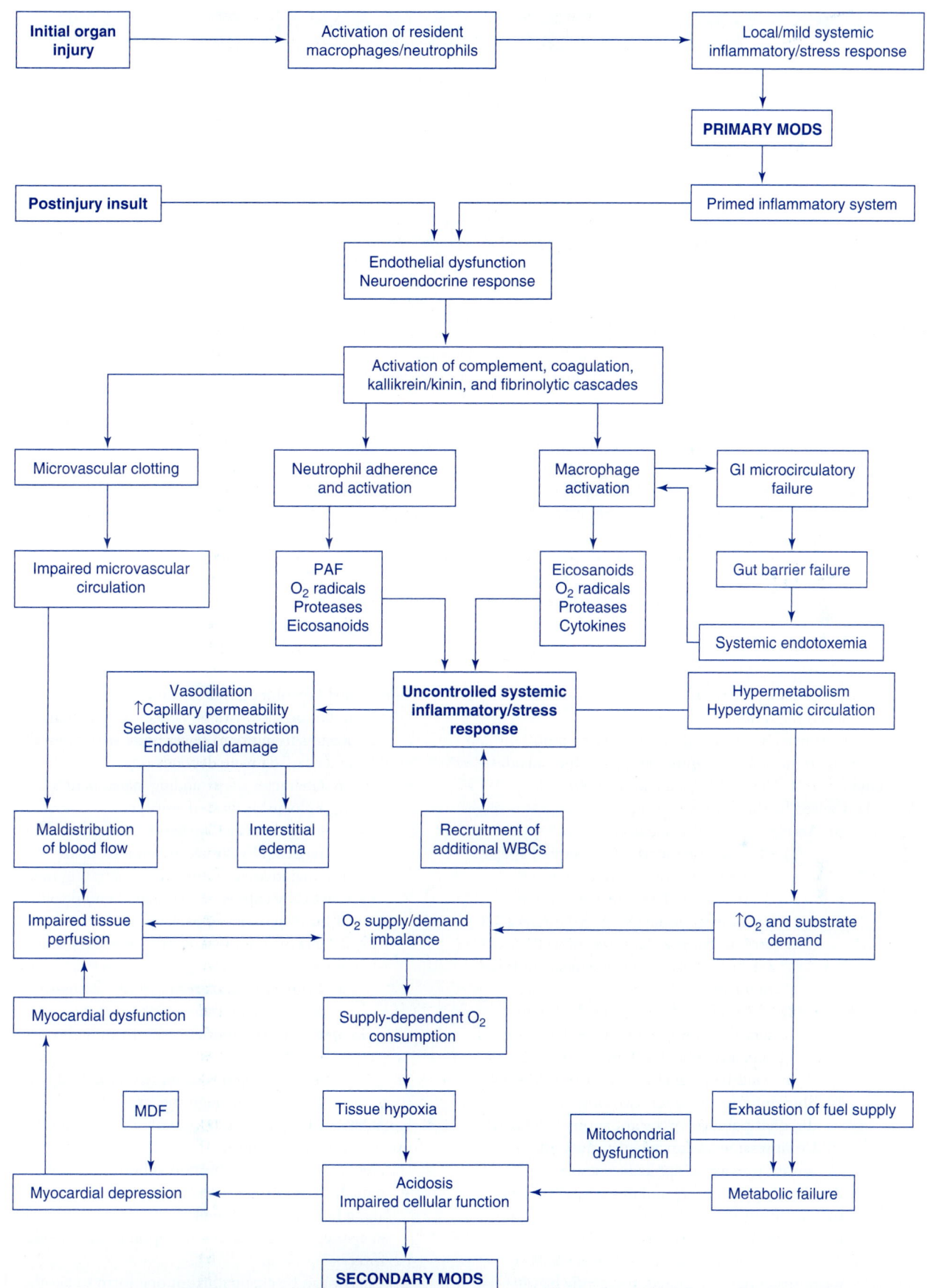

Fig. 11.10 Pathophysiology of multiple organ dysfunction syndrome (MODS). *GI,* Gastrointestinal; *MDF,* myocardial depressant factor; *PAF,* platelet-activating factor; *WBC,* white blood cell. (From McCance, K. L., & Huether, S. E. [2010]. *Pathophysiology. The biologic basis for disease in adults and children* [6th ed.]. St. Louis: Mosby.)

Table 11.7 Sequential [Sepsis-Related] Organ Failure Assessment Score (SOFA)

System	Score 0	1	2	3	4
Respiration					
PaO_2/FiO_2 (mm Hg)	≥400	300–399	200–299	<200 with respiratory support	<100 with respiratory support
Coagulation					
Platelets (×10^3/μl)	≥150	<150	<100	<50	<20
Liver					
Bilirubin (mg/dl [μmol/l])	<1.2 (20)	1.2–1.9 (20–32)	2.0–5.9 (33–101)	6.0–11.9 (102–204)	>12.0 (204)
Cardiovascular					
BP and BP support	MAP ≥70 mm Hg	MAP <70 mm Hg	Dopamine <5 or dobutamine (any dose)	Dopamine 5.1–15, epinephrine ≤0.1, or norepinephrine ≤0.1	Dopamine >15, epinephrine >0.1, or norepinephrine >0.1
Central nervous system					
Glasgow Coma Scale score	15	13–14	10–12	6–9	<6
Renal: creatinine (mg/dl [micromol/l])	<1.2 (110)	1.2–1.9 (110–170)	2.0–3.4 (171–299)	3.5–4.9 (300–440)	>5.0 (440)
Urine output (ml/day)				<500	<200

BP, Blood pressure; *FiO_2*, fraction of inspired oxygen; *MAP*, mean arterial pressure; *PaO_2*, partial pressure of oxygen.

Adapted from Singer, M. et al. (2016). The third international consensus definitions for sepsis and septic shock (sepsis-3). *Journal of the American Medical Association*. 315(8), 801-810. https://doi.org/10.1001/jama.2016.0287.

2. Mechanism of injury: circumstances and energy forces that produced the trauma
    a. Blunt trauma: characterized as an injury with no opening in the skin or communication to the outside environment (Howard & Steinmann, 2010)
        1) Caused by the following forces:
            a) Acceleration or deceleration
                (1) Occurs with increased velocity or speed of a moving object followed by a sudden decrease. The vehicle stops while the body continues to move forward until it strikes a stationary object (e.g., the head strikes the windshield, and the brain strikes the skull).
                (2) The vehicle stops while the body continues to move forward until it strikes a stationary object (e.g., the head strikes the windshield, and the brain strikes the skull).
            b) Shearing: occurs when two oppositely directed parallel forces are applied to tissue
            c) Compression: occurs when a squeezing inward pressure is applied to tissues
        2) Results in more injuries and more types of injury such as contusions, lacerations, fractures, or ruptures of solid tissue masses
        3) Tends to be more difficult to manage because more structures are injured; frequently has an occult presentation, so diagnosis may be delayed, resulting in more significant complications
    b. Penetrating trauma
        1) Caused by direct contact with an instrument that penetrates the body, such as stabbing with a sharp object, bullet wound, high-pressure injections, or foreign object impalement
        2) Results in injury to fewer body structures; the extent of damage depends on:
            a) Character of wounding instrument
            b) Velocity at time of impact
            c) Characteristics of tissue through which it passes (Howard & Steinmann, 2010)
    c. Blast trauma: involves blunt and penetrating trauma
        1) Caused by explosives detonated and displacement of air by gaseous expansion
        2) Results in result in primary, secondary, and tertiary injuries
            a) Primary injuries result from concussive effects of pressure wave.
            b) Secondary injuries result from high velocity projectiles.
            c) Tertiary injuries result from the body being propelled through the air.
3. Kinematics: study of the motion of objects; allows the prediction of likely injuries
    a. Newton's first law of motion: a body at rest will remain at rest unless acted upon by an outside force, and a body in motion will remain in motion traveling in a straight line unless acted upon by an outside force.
    b. Energy can be changed from one form to another, but it can neither be created nor destroyed.
        1) Consider the transformation of the kinetic energy of a moving object (e.g., motor vehicle) that suddenly stops, causing damage to the motor vehicle and occupants.

       a) Four collisions occur in vehicle collisions.
          i) A: auto collision
          ii) B: body collision
          iii) C: cavity contents collision
          iv) D: debris collision
   c. Kinetic energy: the energy of motion
      1) Formula:

$$\frac{Mass \times Velocity^2}{2}$$

      2) Consider that doubling the size of an object results in doubling the kinetic energy, and doubling the velocity quadruples the kinetic energy; this explains why a bullet (small mass with significant velocity) can cause such tissue damage.
      3) Force applied slowly over a large surface area results in less tissue destruction than that same force applied to a small surface area.

Predisposing Factors

1. Blunt trauma
   a. Vehicular collision motor vehicle, motorcycle, bicycle, watercraft, pedestrian struck by motor vehicle
   b. Falls
   c. Assault with a blunt object
   d. Sports-related injuries
2. Penetrating trauma
   a. Gunshot wounds
   b. Stab wounds
   c. Impalement
   d. Projectiles from a blast
3. Blast trauma
   a. Explosions at industrial sites
   b. Terrorist activity
4. Alcohol is a major factor in both intentional and unintentional trauma; in 40% of all traffic-related fatalities, the driver has an elevated blood-alcohol concentration (Schulman, 2009).
5. Another risk to vehicular safety is talking on cellular phones or texting while driving.

Mechanism of Injury

1. Motor vehicle collision
   a. Useful information
      1) Speed of vehicle(s)
      2) Size of vehicle(s)
      3) Location of impact
         a) Head-on
         b) Rear impact
         c) Lateral
         d) Ejection
         e) Rollover
      4) Position of patient in vehicle before and after the impact
         a) If thrown from the vehicle, distance from the vehicle
      5) Use of safety devices
         a) Lap belt
         b) Shoulder belt
         c) Child car seat
         d) Air bags
            i) Did they deploy?
            ii) Location: front or side
      6) Damage to vehicle
         a) Indications of impact
            i) Bent steering wheel
            ii) Broken windshield
            iii) Broken rearview mirror
            iv) Broken gearshift
      7) Smoke or fumes on scene
      8) Condition of other occupants
   b. Anticipated injury
      1) By type of collision (Table 11.8)
      2) By position in vehicle
         a) Driver may strike steering column, instrument panel, gearshift, rearview mirror, windshield, pillar between windshield and door, and door.
            i) Facial laceration, facial bone fractures
            ii) Scalp lacerations, skull fracture, TBI
            iii) Spinal injuries
            iv) Chest wall lacerations, pulmonary contusion, rib, clavicle or sternal fractures, pneumohemothorax
            v) Thoracic aorta tear
            vi) Abdominal wall lacerations; rupture or avulsion of liver, spleen, kidney, pancreas, bowel, and bladder
            vii) Fractured humerus, radius, ulna, wrist, hand
            viii) Fractured pelvis; hip dislocation; fractured femur, tibia, fibula, ankle, or foot; ligamentous injury to the knee
         b) Front seat passenger: higher incidence of head and abdominal injuries and upper torso fractures but fewer thoracic injuries and lower torso fractures
         c) Rear seat passenger: similar to front seat passenger if not restrained
   c. Injury caused by protective devices
      1) Lap belt only worn
         a) Fractured ribs, sternum, clavicle
         b) Myocardial contusion
         c) Aortic tear
         d) Mesenteric tear, bowel perforation
         e) Bladder rupture
         f) Lower thoracic or lumbar vertebral fracture
      2) Shoulder harness only
         a) Cervical spine injuries
         b) Abrasions to neck, chest, abdomen
         c) Carotid artery injuries
         d) Laryngeal injuries
      3) Air bag deployment
         a) Cervical spine injuries
         b) Bag slap injuries to face and neck
         c) Temporary hearing deficit
         d) Corneal abrasion, corneal burns, retinal detachment
         e) Respiratory distress or anaphylaxis from inhaled particles from within the bag and propellant
         f) Upper extremity contusion
         g) Fracture or dislocation of thumb or wrist

Table 11.8	Anticipated Injuries in Motor Vehicle Collisions
Type of Collision	**Anticipated Injuries**
Head-on: up-and-over pathway	• Cervical spine compression injury • Skull fractures, traumatic brain injury • Rib, sternal fractures, flail chest • Pulmonary contusion, pneumothorax, hemothorax • Myocardial contusion • Liver, spleen, duodenum, diaphragmatic lacerations • Great vessel tear
Head-on: down-and-under pathway	• Cervical spine flexion injury • Laryngeal trauma • Carotid shearing • Rib, sternal fractures, flail chest • Pulmonary contusion, pneumothorax, hemothorax • Myocardial contusion • Aortic tears • Pelvic or acetabular fractures • Femur, tibia, fibula fractures
Rear-end	• Whiplash • Rib, sternal fractures, flail chest • Pulmonary contusion, pneumothorax, hemothorax
Lateral	• Cervical ligamentous injuries • Lateral rib fractures, flail chest • Pulmonary contusion, pneumothorax, hemothorax • Spleen or liver lacerations • Pelvic, hip, acetabular fractures • Humerus and clavicle fractures
Ejections	• Skull fractures, traumatic brain injury • Cervical and thoracic spine compression fractures • Rib fracture, pneumothorax, hemothorax • Liver, spleen, pancreas lacerations • Aortic tears • Pelvic fractures, straddle fractures

Adapted from Schulman, C. S. (2009). Trauma. In K. K. Carlson (Ed.), *Advanced critical care nursing*. St. Louis: Saunders.

2. Motorcycle collision
    a. Useful information
        1) Length of skid marks
        2) Deformity of the motorcycle
        3) Stationary objects impacted
        4) Helmet: Cracks in a helmet are likely to result in significant brain injury.
    b. Anticipated injury
        1) TBI is the leading cause of death, especially if the rider is not wearing a helmet.
        2) Tibial and radial injuries are the most common injuries.
        3) Facial fractures
        4) Spinal injuries, especially thoracic
        5) Pulmonary injuries (i.e., pulmonary contusion, pneumothorax, hemothorax)
        6) Pelvic fractures result from straddling position; may have coexisting bladder or urethral injury
        7) Traumatic amputation
        8) Specific to type of impact
            a) Head-on: Bike flips forward, so the rider strikes or travels over the handlebars.
                i) Injury to abdomen and chest as the rider strikes handlebars
                ii) Bilateral femur fractures
                iii) Head and neck injuries
            b) Angular: cycle hit at an angle and collapses on the rider
                i) Tibia and fibula fractures; may be open
                ii) Crushed legs
                iii) Ankle dislocation
            c) Ejection: Rider is thrown off the motorcycle.
                i) Serious injury likely, especially head injury
            d) Laying the bike down
                i) Fractures, abrasions, crush injuries, road burns to lower leg
3. Bicycle collision
    a. Useful information: forward, sideward, or backward unseating
    b. Anticipated injury
        1) If over the handlebars, facial injuries or fractures, head injury
        2) Blunt trauma caused by handlebars
            a) Serious abdominal injury may not be apparent until later in children.
        3) Fractures of the feet from spokes of wheel
        4) Straddle injuries such as vaginal tears, scrotal injuries, perineal contusions, and anal or rectal injuries
        5) Injury to rider from rearview mirror extending from truck or van can cause serious, even fatal, injury to the head, neck, or face
4. Watercraft collision
    a. Useful information
        1) Description of event: collision with another boat or obstruction with an object in the water or on shore
    b. Anticipated injuries
        1) Drowning
        2) Hypothermia
        3) Other injuries as for ejection from a vehicle
5. Pedestrian struck by motor vehicle
    a. Useful information: type of vehicle
    b. Anticipated injury: three points of impact
        1) Bumper: impact to lower leg in adults, causing tibia and fibula fractures
        2) Hood
            i) Thoracic injuries
            ii) Abdominal injuries
            iii) Spinal fractures
            iv) Hip, pelvis, or femur fractures
        3) Ground: head, cervical spine, chest, or abdominal injuries
6. Falls
    a. Useful information
        1) Distance of fall: a fall from more than three times the person's height results in significant injury (McSwain, 2000)
        2) Surface of impact
        3) Area of body that made initial impact
        4) If objects were struck during the fall
        5) Patient's activity before and after fall

b. Anticipated injuries
  1) Compression fractures: os calcis (i.e., heel), femur, tibia, fibula, pelvis, lumbar spine; may be referred to as "Don Juan syndrome"
  2) Bilateral wrist (i.e., Colles) fractures if arms are forward for protection in forward propulsion
  3) Vascular injuries: pelvis and thorax
  4) Renal injury
  5) TBI
  6) Axial loading injury
7. Penetrating injury
  a. Useful information
    1) Wounding agent (e.g., knife, bullet, arrow, ice pick)
    2) Number and location of wounds
    3) Size and length of the agent
    4) If gunshot, caliber and distance of the weapon from the patient
      a) Low-velocity bullets travel at less than 1000 feet per second (fps).
      b) Medium-velocity bullets travel at 1000 to 2000 fps.
      c) High-velocity bullets travel at greater than 2000 fps.
    5) Trajectory
    6) Contaminants
  b. Anticipated injury: dependent on previously indicated factors
8. Blast injuries
  a. Useful information
    1) Proximity to explosion
  b. Anticipated injuries
    1) Primary injuries result from concussive effects of pressure wave and cause injuries to air-filled organs, such as the tympanic membrane, lungs, GI tract, or CNS.
    2) Secondary injuries result from high-velocity projectiles and cause varied injuries depending on the size of the projectiles and tissue impacted.
    3) Tertiary injuries result from the body being propelled through the air and cause injuries similar to ejection from Motor vehicle collision (MVC) or fall.

Pathophysiology

1. Hemorrhage: may be overt or occult
  a. Caused initially by injury but secondarily by coagulopathy
  b. Results in decreased oxygen delivery to tissues (DO_2)
    1) Decrease in CO caused by loss of circulating blood volume
    2) Loss of Hgb to carry oxygen
2. Hypoperfusion
  a. Caused by decrease in Hgb and CO, which results in a decrease in DO_2
  b. Results in the following:
    1) Organ ischemia and possible organ failure
    2) Rhabdomyolysis with muscle ischemia, necrosis, or crush injury
    3) Bowel ischemia with resultant translocation of intestinal bacteria into lymphatics or vascular bed, potentially causing sepsis
    4) Acidosis
3. Hypothermia: Most trauma patients arrive in the emergency department with hypothermia.
  a. Caused by the following:
    1) Exposure: lack of clothing
    2) Open body cavities, especially if long surgery required
    3) Administration of refrigerated blood
    4) Administration of room-temperature IV fluids
    5) Alcohol
  b. Results in the following:
    1) Shift in oxyhemoglobin dissociation curve that impairs oxygen delivery to the tissues
    2) Shivering, which increases oxygen consumption
    3) Impairs platelet function and causes coagulopathy that perpetuates hemorrhage
    4) Increased blood viscosity
    5) Myocardial depression
    6) Acidosis
4. Hypertension (i.e., compartment)
  a. Potential intracranial hypertension and brain herniation (Chapter 5)
  b. Abdominal hypertension and abdominal compartment syndrome (Chapter 7)
  c. Compartment syndrome to the extremities
    1) Clinical indications
      a) Pain: more intense than would be expected by the injury
      b) Pallor
      c) Pulselessness
      d) Polar (i.e., cold); also referred to as poikilothermism
      e) Paresthesia (late)
      f) Paralysis (late)
    2) Collaborative management: fasciotomy with later closure and possible skin graft

Clinical Presentation
This is specific to the injury.

Collaborative Management
1. Initiate primary survey to identify and treat life-threatening conditions
  a. A: airway
  b. B: breathing
  c. C: circulation
  d. D: disability
  e. E: exposure
2. Provide resuscitation measures
  a. A: airway and B: breathing
    1) Maintain airway, oxygenation, and ventilation.
      a) Assess airway patency and restore airway immediately.
        i) Jaw thrust until the cervical spine has been cleared either clinically or radiologically; then may use head tilt–chin lift. Note that any patient with blunt or penetrating trauma above the nipple line must have the cervical spine immobilized with assessment of the airway.
        ii) Oropharyngeal (if no gag reflex) or nasopharyngeal (if basal skull fracture is not suspected) to hold the tongue

away from the hypopharynx in patients with altered levels of consciousness
iii) Intubation may be required; Rapid sequence intubation (RSI) methods should be used
b) Suction oropharynx as needed
c) Oxygen by whatever delivery method necessary to maintain SpO_2 of 94%: nasal cannula, 100% nonrebreathing mask, or intubation with mechanical ventilation with PEEP may be required
d) If no spontaneous breathing, use bag-valve-mask to deliver breaths until mechanical ventilator available.
b. C: circulation
1) Assess for pulse; initiate chest compressions if there is an inadequate pulse.
2) Control of bleeding
a) Pressure on site or artery above site
b) Reinforcement and stabilization of impaled object before surgical procedure for removal
c) Emergent surgery may be required.
3) Maintain adequate circulation and perfusion.
a) IV access with two large-caliber catheters for fluid and medication administration; intraosseous route may be necessary
b) Fluid replacement
i) Crystalloids: usually 0.9% saline or lactated Ringer's solution
ii) Red packed cells or other blood products as prescribed; trauma patients with hemorrhagic shock who require massive transfusion may benefit from 1:1:1 transfusion: 1 unit of packed red blood cells, 1 unit of plasma, and 1 unit of platelets (Holcomb et al, 2015)
iii) Should be given early if significant blood loss is suspected to prevent tissue hypoxia; replacement of platelets, clotting factors, and calcium should be considered, especially if multiple transfusions are given
iv) Colloids generally are not recommended in trauma; albumin is associated with increased mortality in patients with TBI (SAFE Study Investigators, 2004).
v) Avoidance of overresuscitation, which can cause complications of pulmonary edema, cerebral edema, and abdominal compartment syndrome
c. D: disability
1) Neurologic assessment, including Glasgow Coma Scale score or AVPU
a) A: alert; patient is awake, alert, and responsive to voice and is oriented.
b) V: verbal; patient responds to voice but is not fully oriented.
c) P: pain; patient does not respond to voice or pain.
d) U: unresponsive; patient does not respond to voice or pain.
2) Protection of the cervical spine
d. E: environment
1) Expose: Remove all clothing but do not leave the patient uncovered; care must be taken to prevent or treat hypothermia.
2) Evacuate if necessary: Prompt transfer should be achieved if the patient's needs are beyond the resources available at the facility.
3. Conduct secondary survey to identify serious threats that may require emergency surgery or emergency procedures.
a. F
1) Full set of vital signs
2) Focused adjuncts
a) Cardiac monitoring
b) Pulse oximetry to measure SpO_2
c) Nasogastric or orogastric tube to low suction if indicated and not contraindicated
d) Indwelling urinary catheter if indicated and not contraindicated
e) Diagnostic studies
i) Serum
(a) Complete blood count with differential, Hgb, Hct
(b) Chemistry profile, including glucose, BUN, and creatinine
(c) Coagulation profile
(d) Serum lactate
(e) Toxicology, including alcohol
(f) Type and crossmatch
ii) Urine
(a) Pregnancy test if female of childbearing age
(b) Toxicology
iii) X-ray
(a) Spine
(b) Chest
(c) Pelvis
iv) FAST
(a) Can be performed in less than 4 minutes
(b) Can rapidly identify free intraperitoneal fluid in hypotensive patients with blunt abdominal trauma
v) CT scan
(a) Head
(b) Chest
(c) Abdomen
vi) Diagnostic peritoneal lavage
3) Facilitate family presence.
a) Facilitate and support the family's involvement.
b) Provide explanations about procedures.
c) Support the family's emotional and spiritual needs.
b. G: Give comfort measures.
1) Positioning for comfort
2) Anxiolytics
3) Analgesics: nonsteroidal antiinflammatory drugs, narcotics, anesthetics
4) Ice if appropriate
5) Splinting and stabilization of fractures

        6) Cutaneous stimulation (e.g., massage)
        7) Distraction (e.g., music)
    c. H
        1) History
            a) Prehospital: MIVT
                i) Mechanism of injury
                ii) Injuries sustained
                iii) Vital signs
                iv) Treatment initiated and response
            b) Past medical history
        2) Head-to-toe assessment
    d. I: Inspect posterior surfaces while maintaining cervical spine protection.
4. Continue assessment during admission; frequency depends on patient acuity
    a. ABCs
    b. Vital signs: BP, pulse, respiratory rate, and temperature
    c. Oxygen saturation
    d. Respiratory effort
    e. Cardiac rate and rhythm
    f. Pain level
    g. Intake and output
    h. Serum electrolytes
    i. LOC
    j. Close monitoring for progression of symptoms
5. Reverse hypothermia
    a. Passive warming
        1) Removal of wet linens and clothing
        2) Application of warm blankets
        3) Warm room
        4) Head covering
    b. Active external warming: warming blankets, radiant lights
    c. Active internal warming
        1) Warm IV fluid
        2) Warm humidified oxygen
        3) Lavage of stomach, chest, colon, and/or bladder with warm isotonic fluids
        4) Extracorporeal systems such as hemodialysis, cardiopulmonary bypass, or continuous arteriovenous or venovenous warming
    d. Monitoring for hypotension caused by vasodilation with rewarming
6. Reverse acidosis
    a. Measures to treat underlying cause of decrease in tissue delivery (DO_2)
        1) Hgb
            a) Stop the bleeding: apply pressure, prepare the patient for surgery, and so on.
            b) Administer blood and blood products as prescribed.
        2) CO
            a) Administer isotonic fluids and blood and blood products.
            b) Administer vasopressors (e.g., phenylephrine, norepinephrine, dopamine) as prescribed.
                i) Vasopressors should be used only when hypotension persists despite adequate fluid resuscitation.
                ii) Phenylephrine causes the least tachycardia of these vasopressors; norepinephrine causes less tachycardia than does dopamine.
            c) Administer inotropic agents (e.g., dobutamine) to improve contractility as prescribed.
        3) SaO_2
            a) Ensure airway, ventilation, and oxygenation to maintain SaO_2 at least 94%.
    b. Treatment of hypothermia that can impair oxygen delivery to the tissues
    c. Avoidance of the use of sodium bicarbonate unless the pH is less than 7; adverse effects of sodium bicarbonate include the following:
        1) Shifts the oxyhemoglobin dissociation curve to the left, impairing the dissociation of oxygen from the Hgb at the tissue level, which may worsen metabolic acidosis
        2) Increased CO_2 production that may cause or worsen respiratory acidosis
        3) Hypokalemia by shifting potassium from serum to intracellular space
        4) Hypocalcemia by increasing the amount of calcium bound to albumin, thereby reducing ionized calcium
7. Correct coagulopathy
    a. Treat hypothermia that can adversely affect platelet function.
    b. Replace clotting factors as prescribed.
8. Assist with measurement and treatment of compartment hypertension (e.g., intracranial hypertension, abdominal hypertension, compartment syndrome).
9. Treat infection (if present) and prevent sepsis.
    a. Antimicrobials as prescribed
    b. Tetanus prophylaxis if indicated
    c. Cleansing and dressing wounds
    d. Stabilization of fractures
10. Monitor for complications.
    a. Shock
    b. MODS
        1) ARDS
        2) Renal failure
        3) Liver failure
        4) Myocardial failure
        5) Cerebral failure
    c. Infection, sepsis, septic shock
    d. DIC
    e. VTE and PE
    f. Compartment syndrome
    g. Hyperkalemia: potassium levels peak approximately 12 hours after injury and can be worsened by hypoperfusion and acidosis.
    h. Fat embolism syndrome
        1) Associated with long bone and multiple fractures
        2) Develops 24 to 48 hours after injury
        3) Clinical indications include low-grade fever, new-onset tachycardia, dyspnea, hypoxemia, change in LOC, sudden thrombocytopenia, petechiae, ECG changes, and lipuria.
        4) Collaborative management includes oxygen; steroids may be used but have not been shown to be beneficial.

LEARNING ACTIVITIES

CHAPTER 11

1. Complete the following crossword puzzle related to shock, SIRS, and MODS.

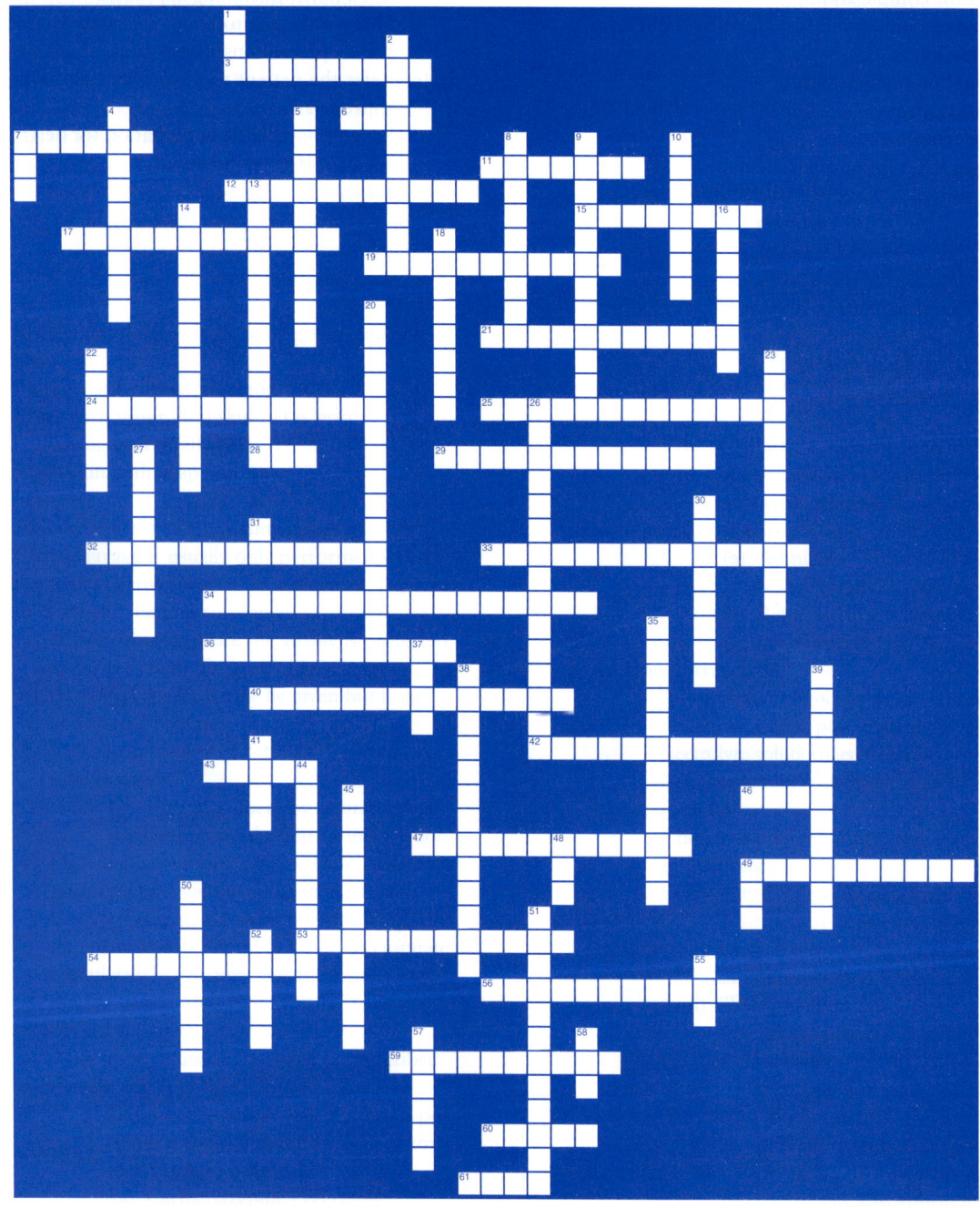

ACROSS

3. An oral antiprostaglandin (generic)
6. A systemic response of the immune system to microorganism, tissue trauma, toxins, burns, and so on (abbrev)
7. Infection with SIRS
11. Elevated serum ____ is an indication of lactic acidosis

714

12. Tension pneumothorax and cardiac tamponade are examples of this subtype of cardiogenic shock
15. Urine output of less than 0.5 ml/kg/hr
17. The stage of shock dominated by neuroendocrine responses to hypoperfusion
19. Type of shock caused by loss of intravascular volume
21. A complication of administering large volumes of IV fluid and blood, which may cause shifting of the oxyhemoglobin dissociation curve to the left
24. The increased or normal systolic BP, along with the increased diastolic BP, causes the decrease in _____ seen in compensatory stage of shock (2 words)
25. The movement of GI bacteria through the bowel wall and into the lymphatics
28. The hemodynamic parameter that is increased in hypovolemic and cardiogenic shock (abbrev)
29. This type of IV fluid contains solutes and may be categorized as hypotonic, isotonic, or hypertonic
32. The consequence of muscle destruction; may cause acute kidney injury
33. A consequence of hemolytic blood transfusion reaction; may cause acute kidney injury
34. Predominant acid–base disorder in shock (2 words)
36. The type of shock caused by the inability of the heart to pump effectively
40. A consequence of hemolytic blood transfusion reaction; may cause renal failure
42. First choice of vasopressor in septic shock (generic)
43. This type of IV infusion is required for hemorrhage, leading to hypoperfusion
46. This hemodynamic parameter differentiates between hypovolemic from cardiogenic shock and cardiac from noncardiac pulmonary edema (abbrev)
47. This type of shock is caused by antigen–antibody response, IgE, and the release of histamine and other mediators
49. Swelling beneath the surface of the skin or mucous membranes associated with anaphylaxis; most often on the face, hands, feet, genitals, and airways
53. Third spacing is the shift of fluid from the intravascular space to the _____ space, pleural space, pericardial space, and peritoneal space
54. The drug most common associated with anaphylactic shock (generic)
56. The stage of shock when compensatory mechanisms are no longer effective in maintaining tissue perfusion
59. The type of shock caused by suppression of the SNS
60. The condition of insufficient perfusion of cells and vital organs
61. The type of acute respiratory failure seen in MODS (abbrev)

DOWN
1. Preferred method of reperfusion for acute MI (abbrev)
2. The stage of shock associated with irreversible organ damage
4. The mediator seen in anaphylactic shock that causes vasodilation and increased capillary permeability
5. The presence of viable bacteria in the blood
7. The branch of the autonomic nervous system responsible for the early compensatory response to hypoperfusion in shock (abbrev)
8. Increased _____ permeability is a systemic effect of SIRS that can lead to decreased preload
9. This type of drugs may be used to decrease preload or afterload in cardiogenic shock (plural)
10. The plasma protein with the greatest effect on plasma oncotic pressure
13. Patients taking this class of medication may not exhibit the expected signs of hypoperfusion
14. Alternative route for fluid administration when IV access cannot be obtained
16. This stage of shock is associated with a decrease in tissue oxygenation but no clinical indications of hypoperfusion
18. Vasopressor that increases risk of tachycardia and dysrhythmia (generic)
20. H1 receptor antagonist (generic)
22. This type of shock is associated with mediator release in response to overwhelming infection
23. VO_2 is oxygen _____
26. A method of returning the patient's hemorrhaged blood to his or her intravascular volume; greatest risks are infection and coagulopathy
27. Type of IV fluids that are used to increase intravascular colloidal oncotic pressure; may worsen outcomes in patients with head injury
30. DO_2 is oxygen _____
31. The most common cause of cardiogenic shock (abbrev)
35. This category of shock includes the three forms of shock that result in massive vasodilation and resultant relative hypovolemia
37. A mechanical therapy used in cardiogenic shock to increase coronary artery perfusion pressure and decrease afterload (abbrev)
38. An anaphylactic-like reaction that does not require previous exposure; not mediated by IgE, probably triggered by the complement system
39. The first-line drug for anaphylactic shock (generic)
41. The frequently fatal result of SIRS; previously referred to as multisystem organ failure (abbrev)
44. The inotropic agent used most often in cardiogenic shock (generic)
45. The decrease in BP when a patient is repositioned from lying to standing is referred to as _____ changes or being tilt positive
48. S_3, crackles, and dyspnea are manifestations of _____ seen in cardiogenic shock (abbrev)
49. The type of acute kidney injury seen in MODS (abbrev)

50. This drug may be used for anaphylaxis in patients who have been receiving beta-blockers (generic)
51. This type of drugs may be used in vasogenic shock to restore normal vascular tone (plural)
52. Pulse pressure variation and stroke volume variation can be used to determine whether or not patients will respond to _____
55. JVD, peripheral edema, and hepatomegaly are manifestations of _____ seen in cardiogenic shock (abbrev)
57. This legume is a common cause of anaphylactic shock
58. The type of coagulopathy seen in MODS (abbrev)

2. Identify which type of shock the following pathologic conditions or procedures may cause.

Condition	Hypovolemic	Cardiogenic	Septic	Anaphylactic	Neurogenic
Myocardial infarction					
Bee sting					
Head injury					
Diarrhea					
Pulmonary embolism					
Ruptured gallbladder					
Esophageal varices					
Ruptured papillary muscle					
Insulin shock					
Ascites					
Intravenous pyelogram (IVP) dye					
Spinal cord injury					
Invasive procedures					
Burns					
Blood transfusion reaction					
Spinal anesthesia					
Trauma					
Malnutrition					
Chemotherapy					

3. Match the pathophysiology with the type of shock.

____ 1. Anaphylactic   a. Massive vasodilation caused by the release of inflammatory mediators in response to overwhelming infection
____ 2. Cardiogenic   b. Inability of the heart to effectively pump
____ 3. Hypovolemic   c. Inadequate intravascular volume
____ 4. Neurogenic   d. Vasodilation caused by the release of histamine from mast cells
____ 5. Septic   e. Vasodilation resulting from suppression or loss of the sympathetic nervous system

4. Identify the following signs and symptoms of shock as occurring during the compensatory, progressive, or refractory stages of shock.

Sign or Symptom	Compensatory	Progressive	Refractory
Acute respiratory distress syndrome			
Anuria			
Cool, pale skin			
Decreased bowel sounds			
Disseminated intravascular coagulation			
Dysrhythmias			
Hypotension			
Mottling of extremities			
Narrow pulse pressure			
Nausea			
Neurologic changes: coma; focal signs			
Neurologic changes: irritability, confusion			
Neurologic changes: lethargy, coma			
Oliguria			
Profound hypotension despite vasopressors			
Tachycardia			
Thirst			

5. Complete this table by putting ↑, ↓, or normal in the empty cells.

Type of Shock	CO/CI	RAP, PAP, and PAOP	SVR	SvO_2
Hypovolemic				
Cardiogenic				
Septic				
Anaphylactic				
Neurologic				

CI, Cardiac index; *CO*, cardiac output; *PAOP*, pulmonary artery occlusive pressure; *PAP*, pulmonary artery pressure; *RAP*, right atrial pressure; SvO_2, oxygen saturation of venous blood; *SVR*, systemic vascular resistance.

6. List two fluids in each category.

Crystalloids		
Isotonic		
Hypotonic		
Hypertonic		
Colloids		
Blood or blood products		

Chapter 11 Multisystem

7. Match these general treatments of shock with the factor of oxygen delivery or consumption that they are intended to affect.

____ 1. Isotonic crystalloids	a. Improved DO_2 by improving SaO_2
____ 2. Red blood cells	b. Improved DO_2 by improving hemoglobin
____ 3. Oxygen	c. Improved DO_2 by improving cardiac output
____ 4. Mechanical ventilation	d. Diminished VO_2
____ 5. Inotropic agents	
____ 6. Sedation	
____ 7. PEEP	
____ 8. Surgical intervention to stop bleeding	
____ 9. Treatment of metabolic acidosis	
____ 10. Hypothermia	

8. Match the following specific therapies with the type of shock for which they may be used. You may list more than one therapy for each form of shock, and the therapies may be used more than once.

____ 1. Anaphylactic	a. IV fluids
____ 2. Cardiogenic	b. Corticosteroids
____ 3. Hypovolemic	c. Blood
____ 4. Neurogenic	d. Vasopressors
____ 5. Septic	e. Inotropes
	f. Intraaortic balloon pump (IABP)
	g. Pacemaker
	h. Epinephrine
	i. Antihistamines
	j. Antimicrobials
	k. Treatment of cause
	l. Oxygen
	m. Vasodilators

9. Match the sign/symptom of dysfunction with the organ that is dysfunctional.

____ 1. Brain	a. Decreased PaO_2/FiO_2 ratio
____ 2. Heart	b. Oliguria
____ 3. Blood	c. Hypoglycemia
____ 4. Kidneys	d. Decrease in Glasgow Coma Scale score
____ 5. Liver	e. Prolonged PT, aPTT, decreased platelets
____ 6. Lungs	f. Increased PAOP

10. Complete the following table that describes the four physiologic alterations that are likely to be seen in SIRS. The criteria for SIRS are two of these four parameters.

Heart rate	Greater than ____			
Respiratory rate	Greater than ____	or	$PaCO_2$	Less than ____
Temperature	Greater than ____	or	Less than ____	
WBC	Greater than ____	or	Less than ____	

11. Identify the three actions which may be used in toxicities or overdosages to decrease absorption of the toxin or drug.

   a. _____
   b. _____
   c. _____

12. Complete the following crossword puzzle related to drug toxic ingestion and trauma.

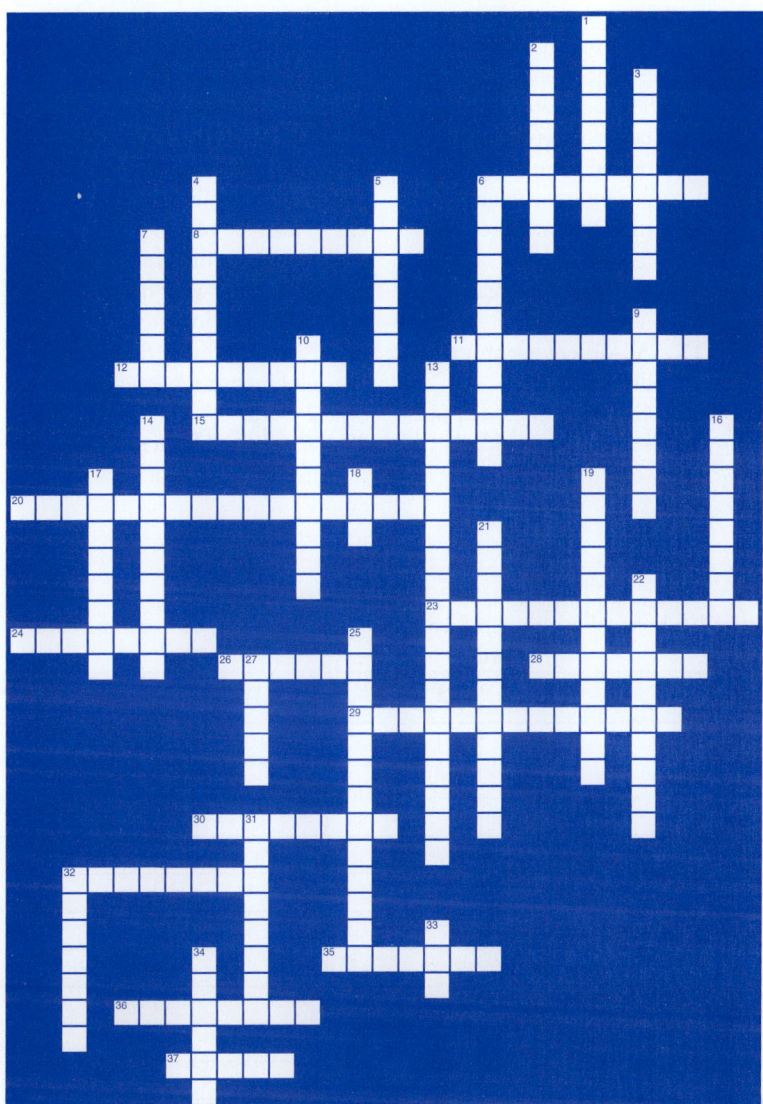

ACROSS
6. Accidental exposure to a toxic substance
8. This device may be required for the bradycardia seen in beta-blocker or calcium channel blocker overdose
11. This drug is used for malignant hyperthermia that occurs in some drug overdosages (generic)
12. Dilated pupils
15. The affinity between hemoglobin and this substance is much greater than the affinity between hemoglobin and oxygen (2 words)
20. This condition causes hypoxia and may be caused by nitrates, sulfa drugs, and local anesthetics
23. The drug most often involved in intentional and unintentional drug overdose in the United States
24. This B vitamin must be given with dextrose to malnourished patients to prevent Wernicke encephalopathy
26. Procedure to flush the drug or toxin from the stomach; may be used if the patient arrives within 1 hour of ingestion for most substances
28. This electrolyte is given for calcium channel blocker overdose
29. This blood cleansing procedure is more effective than hemodialysis for plasma protein-bound drugs
30. This antidote is given if digoxin level is greater than 10 ng/ml (trade)
32. Osmotic laxative added to first dose of activated charcoal if multiple doses are going to be used
35. Drug intoxication in an attempt to get attention is referred to as a suicide ____
36. Antidote for acetaminophen (trade)
37. This organ is most likely to be injured by acetaminophen overdose

DOWN
1. This drug can stimulate the beta-receptors even in the presence of beta-blockade; used for beta-blocker overdose
2. Drug used for the treatment of bradycardia (generic)
3. This type of syndrome may cause generalized seizures
4. High pressure; this type of oxygen therapy is used in carbon monoxide poisoning

5. Usually intentional but may be inadvertent exposure to toxic levels of a substance
6. This type of consult should always be requested for patients with drug overdosage
7. Priority intervention in all cases of toxic ingestion
9. A coma cocktail consists of oxygen, _____, thiamine, and naloxone
10. 20% lipid infusions have been shown to effectively treat overdoses of _____ toxins
13. This procedure is used to assess injury after ingestion of caustic agents
14. This antidote for benzodiazepines should not be given if the patient has coingested tricyclic antidepressants (generic)
16. Antidote for opiates (generic)
17. Adsorbent agent used in drug overdose
18. Carbon monoxide poisoning causes the skin to be very _____
19. Blood cleansing procedure which may be used to remove some drugs or toxins from the blood
21. This complication of drug overdose is the result of excessive muscle rigidity
22. This type of blood screen is done to determine what drugs have been ingested
25. Antidote for methemoglobinemia (generic and 2 words)
27. This "gap" is increased in alcohol intoxication
31. Bowel irrigation with this solution is used for overdose of sustained-release drugs (trade)
32. This complication requires airway maintenance and protection from injury
33. This radiologic procedure may be used to identify the presence of radiopaque agents (abbrev)
34. Pinpoint pupils

13. Match each intervention with a hospital-acquired infection. Interventions can be used more than once.

	CAUTI	CLABSI	VAP	SSI	MDRO
Elevate HOB 30–45 degrees					
Proper hair removal techniques					
Hand hygiene before touching device					
Maintain normothermia					
Administer PUD prophylaxis					
Remove device when no longer required					
Antibiotic stewardship					
Maximum barrier precautions during insertion of device					
Antibiotic stewardship					
Disinfect skin with chlorhexidine					
Use standard precautions					

HOB, head of bed; PUD, peptic ulcer disease.

14. Name three types of traumatic injury.
    a. _____
    b. _____
    c. _____

15. Primary survey of the trauma patient consists of:
    A _____
    B _____
    C _____
    D _____
    E _____

16. Compartment syndrome of an extremity is a complication associated with trauma. List six clinical manifestations of compartment syndrome.
    a. _____
    b. _____
    c. _____
    d. _____
    e. _____
    f. _____

Behavioral/Psychosocial on the Blueprint

CHAPTER 12

Behavioral/Psychosocial Assessment
Interview
Chief Complaint
Identify chief complaint.
History of Present Illness
Identify current symptoms.
Current Medications
Include dose, type, how long the medication has been ordered, time last taken, and any changes related to medication use. Identify current use or abuse of substances, including prescribed, over-the-counter (OTC), alcohol, supplements, or herbal medications and other drugs.
Past Medical History
1. Previous illnesses or injuries
2. Previous hospitalizations
3. Review of body systems
4. Allergies
5. Psychiatric review of systems
    a. Depression
    b. Mania
    c. Anxiety
    d. Psychosis
    e. Attention-deficit/hyperactivity disorder (ADHD) symptoms
    f. Eating disorder symptoms
    g. Trauma-related symptoms
6. Past psychiatric history
    a. History of psychiatric treatment
    b. Psychiatric hospitalizations
    c. Psychiatric medications

Social History
1. Family structure: Identify who makes or influences health care decisions.
2. Substance abuse history
3. Support system: These are the individuals who are in regular contact with the patient and may include immediate or extended family or friends.
4. Educational level
5. Responsibilities: This may include job, financial, spouse, parents, children, and pets.
6. Major family traumas

Family History
1. Family history of psychiatric conditions
2. Family history of medical conditions
3. Family history of substance use disorders

Mental Status Exam
1. Presentation
    a. Dress (e.g., is it clean, age appropriate, fit, and appropriate for the season)
    b. Eye contact (consistent, intermittent, poor)
    c. General appearance (e.g., hygiene and grooming)
    d. Motor activity (purposeful, restless, tremulous, cooperative)
2. Affect: the emotion that the patient expresses outwardly
    a. Anxious, worried
    b. Flat: demonstrates no emotion
    c. Inappropriate: Emotions demonstrated are not consistent with the situation or maturity.
    d. Labile: Emotions demonstrated fluctuate high to low rapidly and inconsistently without respect to the situation.
    e. Guarded: appears wary or overly cautious in conversation
    f. Restricted: reduced in intensity that is less severe than blunted but clearly reduced
    g. Blunted: severe reduction in intensity of externalized feeling tone
    h. Broad: considered "normal" affect; responsive to emotion
3. Mood: the emotion that the patient reports
    a. Hostile
    b. Sad
    c. Elated
    d. Anxious
    e. Agitated
    f. Anger
    g. Fear
    h. Surprise
    i. Disgust
    j. Happy
4. Speech
    a. Pressured: rapid, forced speech
    b. Slurred

c. Loud
d. Soft
e. Patterns
f. Idiosyncrasies
5. Thought processes
   a. Blocking: cessation in the flow of thought or speech
   b. Flight of ideas: leap from one idea to another; distracted from thoughts and speech by things in the environment
   c. Looseness of association: no logical connection between sentences
   d. Circumstantial: thoughts or speech that contains excessive details about the topic but finally reaches the intended point
   e. Tangential: thoughts that are logical and directed that may be related to the topic but take off in a different direction and do not address the question or specific topic
6. Thought content
   a. Suspicious
   b. Hopeless
   c. Guilty
   d. Delusion: persistent belief or perception held by a person despite evidence to the contrary; examples include the following:
      1) Being controlled
      2) Grandeur
      3) Persecution
      4) Nihilistic
      5) Somatic
   e. Ideation (thought): Assess for any distortion of thought in addition to thoughts or plan of suicide or homicide
7. Perceptual disturbances
   a. Pathological hallucinations: false sensory perception occurring in the absence of any relevant external stimulation of the sensory modality involved. Any of the five senses may be affected by hallucinatory experiences (Table 12.1).
   b. Nonpathological hallucinations
      1) Hypnagogic: associated with the semiconsciousness immediately preceding sleep
      2) Hypnopompic: associated with the semiconsciousness preceding waking
   c. Illusion: a false interpretation of an external sensory stimulus (e.g., a coat hanging over a chair is perceived as a person sitting there)
   d. Depersonalization: sensation of unreality concerning oneself, parts of oneself, or one's environment that occurs under extreme stress or fatigue, seen in some psychiatric disorders
   e. Derealization: sensation of changed reality or that one's surrounding have altered, seen in psychiatric disorders such as psychosis and panic attacks.
8. Cognition
   a. Orientation: person, place, time, and situation
   b. Memory
      1) Immediate: minutes
      2) Short term: hours to days
      3) Long term: weeks to years
   c. Intelligence: cognitive ability
   d. Concentration: the ability to focus and pay attention
   e. Judgment: the ability to make sound decisions
   f. Insight: the understanding one has of the current situation
9. Diagnostic studies to rule out medical conditions and/or substance abuse
   a. Complete blood count (CBC)
   b. Hemoglobin
   c. Hematocrit
   d. Thyroid panel
   e. Liver and renal function
   f. Drug toxicology
   g. Pregnancy exam for women 10 to 50 years old
   h. Urinalysis
   i. Vitamin B_{12} and folate
   j. Syphilis serology
   k. Human immunodeficiency virus (HIV)
   l. Substances (medications and drugs of abuse)

Table 12.1 Types of Hallucinations

Type	Perception of:	Description of:
Auditory	Voices or other sounds	Typical in psychosis and schizophrenia. Voices are often threatening, obscene, accusatory, or insulting. Also common in persons with alcoholism, but voices are most commonly unstructured, maligning, reproachful, or threatening. Usually resolve within 1 week of alcohol withdrawal.
Visual	Images	Also common in psychosis and schizophrenia
Gustatory	Taste	Unusual in psychosis; should prompt concern about underlying medical or neurologic disorder rather than psychiatric
Tactile	Touch	Unusual in psychosis; should prompt concern about underlying medical or neurologic disorder rather than psychiatric
Olfactory	Odors	Unusual in psychosis; should prompt concern about underlying medical or neurologic disorder rather than psychiatric
Hypnogogic	Intense dreamlike imagery just before falling asleep	Considered normal hallucinations associated with sleep
Hypnopompic	Intense dreamlike imagery just after awakening	Considered normal hallucinations associated with sleep

Psychosocial Characteristics (Erikson, 1968)

Young Adulthood (18–40 Years of Age)
1. Intimacy versus self-isolation or self-absorption
2. Developmental tasks
   a. Accepts self
   b. Establishes independence
   c. Establishes a vocation to make worthwhile contributions
   d. Learns to appraise and express love responsibly
   e. Establishes intimate bond with another
   f. Establishes and manages residence
   g. Finds congenial social group
   h. Decides on option of a family
   i. Formulates philosophy of life
   j. Establishes role in community

Middle Adulthood (40–60 Years of Age)
1. Generativity versus self-absorption and stagnation
2. Developmental tasks
   a. Develops new satisfaction as a mate
   b. Supportive to mate
   c. Develops sense of unity with mate
   d. Assists offspring to become happy, responsible adults
   e. Takes pride in accomplishments of self and mate
   f. Balances work with other roles; assists aging parents
   g. Achieves social and civic responsibility
   h. Maintains active organizational membership
   i. Accepts physical changes of middle age
   j. Makes an art of friendship
   k. Balances leisure with service pursuits
   l. Develops more depth of personal philosophy by reevaluating values and examining assets

Older Adulthood (60 Years of Age to Death)
1. Integrity versus despair
2. Developmental tasks
   a. Continued self-development
   b. Adapts to family responsibilities
   c. Maintains self-worth, pride, and usefulness
   d. Deals with loss of spouse, friends, upcoming end to life

Basic Human Needs
Basic needs may be the same, but the manner in which they are fulfilled depends on personal abilities, environment, and life experience.

Maslow's Hierarchy of Needs
Progressive; primary needs must be met before dealing with higher level needs (Table 12.2)

Human Needs of Critically Ill Patients
Fig. 12.1.

Responses to Illness and Environment

Stress
1. Definition: mental, emotional, or physical tension or strain
2. Stressors in the critical care setting (Box 12.1)
   a. Distress: stress as a result of noxious stimuli
   b. Eustress: stress as a result of nonthreatening stimuli
3. Admission to a critical care unit is frightening and anxiety producing.
4. Sensory deprivation and sensory overload are stress factors within a critical care unit.
5. Interventions to decrease or eliminate stress
   a. Maintain a calm, restful environment.

Table 12.2	Maslow's Hierarchy of Needs
Physiologic	Oxygen, food, water, and sleep
Safety and security	Protection and freedom from anxiety
Love and belonging	Freedom from loneliness and alienation
Esteem and recognition	Freedom from a sense of worthlessness, inferiority, and helplessness
Self-actualization	Aesthetic needs, self-fulfillment, creativity, and spirituality

From Maslow, A. (1968). *Toward a psychology of being* (2nd ed.). Princeton, MA: Van Nostrand.

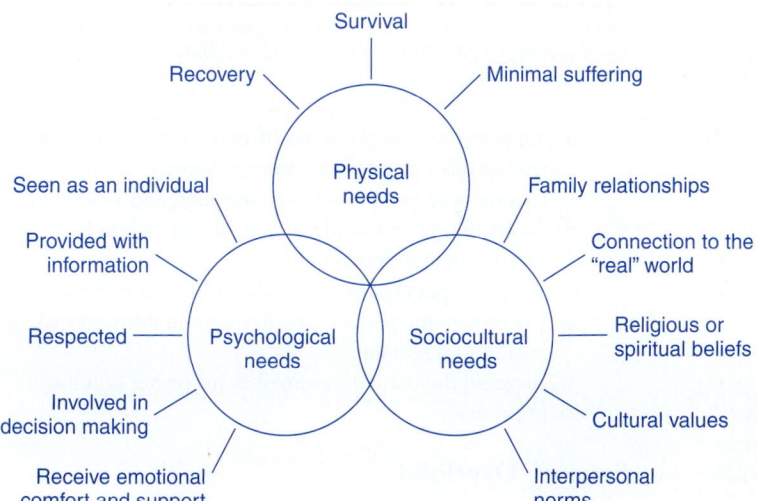

Fig. 12.1 Human needs of critically ill patients.

Box 12.1	Potential Stressors in the Critical Care Setting

Threat of death
Threat of disability
Threat of body image alteration
Pain or discomfort
Separation from family and loved ones
Loss of usual role in family, community, or workplace
Loss of autonomy
Loss of privacy or dignity
Powerlessness and loss of control over environment
Sleep disturbances
Sensory overload
Sensory deprivation
Inability to communicate (if aphasic or intubated)

Adapted from Urden, L., Stacy, K., & Lough, M. (2014). *Critical care nursing: Diagnosis and management* (7th ed.). St. Louis: Elsevier/Mosby.

Table 12.3 Coping Mechanisms for Stress

Type	Example
Action	Taking walks, cleaning house, gardening, singing
Cognitive	Problem solving, reading about issue
Spiritual	Prayer
Interpersonal	Talking with support person
Emotional	Use of psychological defense mechanisms (Table 12.4)

Table 12.4 Psychological Defense Mechanisms

Defense Mechanisms	Level	Description
Anticipation Affiliation Altruism Humor Self-assertion Self-observation Sublimation	Highly adaptive	Optimal in handling stressors; maximize gratification and allow the conscious awareness of feelings, ideas, and their consequences
Displacement Dissociation Intellectualization Isolation of affect Reaction formation Repression Undoing	Compromise formation	Keep potentially threatening ideas, feelings, memories, wishes, or fears out of awareness
Devaluation Idealization Omnipotence	Minor image-distortion	Distortions in self, body, or others that help regulate self-esteem
Denial Projection Rationalization	Disavowal	Keep unpleasant or unacceptable stressors, impulses, ideas, affects, or responsibility out of awareness with or without a misattribution of these to external causes
Acting out Apathetic withdrawal Help-rejecting complaining Passive aggression	Major image distortion	Deal with internal or external stressors by action or withdrawal
Delusional projection Psychotic denial Psychotic distortion	Defensive dysregulation	Failure of defensive regulation to contain reaction to stressors, leading to a pronounced break with objective reality

American Psychiatric Association. (2000). *Diagnostic and statistical manual of mental disorders* (4th ed., text rev.). Washington, DC: Author.

    b. Provide for as much independence of the patient as possible.
    c. Provide contact with reality and outside world.
    d. Encourage use of coping mechanisms (Tables 12.3 and 12.4).

Loneliness

1. Definition: discomfort caused by separation from significant relationships, places, events, and objects
2. Manifestations may include crying and withdrawal.
3. Interventions to decrease loneliness
    a. Encourage participation in decision making and self-care.
    b. Encourage discussion of fears and asking of questions.
    c. Encourage the patient to talk about his or her life, family, work, or pet.
    d. Ask the family to bring in familiar and loved objects.

Powerlessness

1. Definition: a perceived lack of control over the outcome of a specific situation or problem and the patient's perception that any action he or she takes will not affect the outcome
2. May be manifested by apathy, withdrawal, resignation, fatalism, lack of decision making, aggression, or anger
3. Interventions to decrease feelings of powerlessness
    a. Recognize the potential for feelings of powerlessness; particularly at risk are individuals who usually are in a position of power or control in their daily life.
    b. Support the patient's sense of control by offering alternatives related to activity times, treatment times, diet, routine hygiene, diversionary activities, and visitation.
    c. Assist the patient in identifying activities that he or she can perform independently.
    d. Keep the patient informed about his or her treatment.
    e. Encourage the patient's involvement in decision making related to treatment.
    f. Increase the patient's control as his or her condition improves.

Sensory Overload

1. Definition: increased frequency and intensity of stimulation of the senses with nonmeaningful stimuli

2. Contributing factors: constant noise and lights, alarms, chatter of unfamiliar voices
3. Intervention: Eliminate or limit nonmeaningful sensory stimulation.

Sensory Deprivation
1. Definition: decreased frequency, intensity, or variety of stimulation of the senses with meaningful stimuli
2. Contributing factors: absence of windows, clocks, and calendars; constant noise, lights, technical language, and lack of familiar faces; deprivation of familiar touches, sounds, smells, and tastes of their usual environment
3. Interventions
   a. Encourage family visitation.
   b. Encourage the family to bring familiar objects to the hospital.
   c. Place calendar and clock where the patient can see them.

Anger
1. Definition: feeling of great displeasure, hostility, and exasperation
2. May be manifested by clenching of teeth or muscles, avoidance of eye contact, sarcasm, insulting comments, screaming, argumentativeness, and demanding behavior
3. Interventions to decrease feelings of anger
   a. Assist in identifying the cause of anger.
   b. Give the patient permission to be angry.
   c. Assist the patient in identifying appropriate ways to express the anger.

Depression
1. Definition: feeling of sadness and hopelessness
2. May be manifested by loss of interest in people, dissatisfaction, difficulty making decisions, and crying; patient may say that he or she is a failure, being punished, or is considering hurting himself or herself
3. Interventions to decrease feelings of depression
   a. Provide information necessary to identify the patient's needs and to realistically visualize the future.
   b. Inspire hope and facilitate coping.

Denial
1. Definition: refusal to acknowledge the truth; allows the patient to come to grips with reality a little at a time
2. Denial may be manifested by shrugging off symptoms, refusing to discuss the illness, appearing cheerful, and verbalizing the illness while ignoring restrictions.
3. Interventions
   a. Allow the patient to express his or her feelings.
   b. Do not confront the patient with the truth.

Near-Death Experience
1. Definition: a vivid series of events reported by some individuals after periods of clinical death
2. Manifestations may include the following events:
   a. Time interval without feeling
   b. Separation of mind and body
   c. Propulsion through space or a long, dark tunnel
   d. Interaction with a bright light
   e. Meeting an escort (often a decreased family member or friend) who accompanies the patient to a warm, peaceful, bright area
   f. Experiencing a life review
   g. The choice of whether to go back or being told to go back
   h. Return to the body
3. Interventions
   a. Be alert for indications that the patient has had a near-death experience (NDE), especially if the patient has experienced cardiac arrest, electrophysiologic studies, or any life-threatening crisis; the patient may do either of the following:
      1) Say, "I had the strangest dream" or something similar.
      2) Be angry, withdrawn, or unusually calm.
   b. Provide the patient with an opportunity to discuss the experience, such as, "Did anything happen when you were very sick yesterday that you want to talk about?"
   c. Explore your own feelings about NDE.
   d. Listen to the patient and avoid judgment.
   e. Reassure the patient who has a NDE that he or she is not "crazy" and that many persons have had this experience.
   f. Refer the patient to books to read or a support group if available.

Crisis
1. Definition: a state that occurs when one's usual ways of coping are inadequate to deal with the stress (Caplan, 1970)
   a. Involves an attempt to regain equilibrium
   b. Self-limited and allows for growth
2. Types of crises
   a. Situational crises
      1) Occurs suddenly
      2) Can be devastating
      3) Is not part of normal development
         a) Motor vehicle collisions
         b) Acts of nature such as a tornado or flood
         c) Sexual assault
         d) Robbery
         e) Legal difficulties
         f) Separation or divorce
         g) Unemployment
         h) Terminal illness diagnosis
   b. Maturational crises
      1) Occurs over time
      2) Recognized as common and occurs as part of normal development such as:
         a) Pregnancy
         b) Childbirth
         c) Adolescence
         d) Leaving home
         e) Marriage
         f) Midlife events
         g) Aging
         h) Death
3. Stages
   a. Shock and disbelief
   b. Disorganization: may be demanding, irrational, angry

c. Reorganization: difficulty making decisions, forced to confront critical questions
     d. Resolution
  4. Clinical indications of crisis
     a. Crying, screaming
     b. Angry, pacing, hitting out at others
     c. Silent, unresponsive to questions, appears in shock
  5. Crisis intervention
     a. Alleviate crisis state.
        1) Many will abate over time without interventions.
        2) Problem-solving techniques for others
        3) End result is to return person to precrisis functioning.
     b. Use interventions that have been shown to be helpful.
        1) Listen to the patient's story.
        2) Offer empathy.
        3) Ask about attempts to cope.
           a) Identify coping behaviors that have been successful in the past.
           b) Identify current attempts to cope, such as friends, family, prayer, crying, or substance use or abuse.
           c) Suicidal thoughts or plans
        4) Aid the patient in organization of the next few hours or days.
        5) Ensure that basic needs, such as safety, nutrition, and sleep, are being met.
        6) Connect the patient to support services or family support.

General Principles of Care
1. Focus on initial signs and symptoms, methods of assessment for specific disorders, principles of safe care, and pharmacologic agents appropriate to the presentation.
2. Emergency personnel are frequently confronted by individuals or families who appear out of control, in a state of extreme distress, confused, or numb.
3. It is the job of the clinician to assess the reason behind the distress; diagnose any accompanying disorders; treat effectively; and release, refer, or hospitalize the person for additional care.

Therapeutic Milieu
1. An environment where the focus is designed to heal
   a. Healthy social interactions
   b. Respect for all persons
   c. Recognition of patient's rights
   d. Freedom of speech
   e. Sense of support
   f. Honesty in interactions
2. Staff responsibilities
   a. Adhere to schedules.
   b. Maintain safety at all times.
   c. Focus interactions and activities on growth and understanding.
   d. Encourage responsibility; allow the patient to do for self as much as possible.
   e. Inform patient of all changes.
   f. Incorporate patients in the government of environment.

3. Ethical care
   a. Fundamental concept used in making decisions for patient care
      1) Each patient must be treated equal and fair with respect to patient dignity.
      2) Provide no harm (i.e., nonmalfeasance) and do what is in the patient's best interest (i.e., beneficence).
      3) Be honest with the patient and build a trusting relationship.
      4) Impartial treatment of all patients (i.e., justice)
      5) Patients have the independence and freedom to select their treatment (i.e., autonomy).
   b. Patients with a psychiatric emergency have the same rights as other patients to make decisions; it is the health care provider's responsibility to intervene in the freedom of decision making if the patient's safety is at risk (Hamilton, 2007). Short-acting medications can be administered against the patient's will only if the patient is posing an imminent risk to self or others.
   c. Care should be provided in accordance with the provider's standards of care as defined on a state-by-state basis.
4. Confidentiality
   a. Health care agencies and providers must provide confidentiality and privacy of an individual's health care information that is collected and maintained; only those needing the information to provide further care are permitted access.
   b. Health Insurance Portability and Accountability Act (HIPAA) of 1996
      1) Protects the privacy of an individual's identifiable health information and identifiable information
      2) Requirements must be followed by each institution.
5. Civil rights
   a. Civil rights protect an individual from unfair treatment or discrimination because of race, color, national origin, disability, age, gender, or religion.
   b. Civil rights laws ensure that everyone has equal access to and opportunity to participate in certain health care and human services programs without facing unlawful discrimination.
   c. Patients with mental illness have the same patient rights as any other patient.
   d. Hospitalization of the Mentally Ill Act of 1964: All patients in public or private hospitals have a right to treatment (Hamilton, 2007).

Agitation

Definition
Characterized by excess motor activity and driven by internal factors such as disease, pain, anxiety and delirium

Predisposing Factors
1. Potentially life-threatening factors
   a. Impaired gas exchange (e.g., hypoxemia, hypercarbia)
   b. Metabolic factors (e.g., hypoglycemia, acidosis)
   c. Ventilator-related factors (e.g., endotracheal tube malposition, tension pneumothorax)

d. Infection (e.g., central nervous system infection, sepsis)
   e. Drugs and alcohol-related factors (e.g., intoxication, withdrawal)
   f. Ischemia (e.g., myocardial, intestinal, or cerebral ischemia)
2. Miscellaneous factors
   a. Patient–ventilator dyssynchrony (e.g., inadequate flow rates, excessive tidal volumes)
   b. Uncomfortable bed position
   c. Fear
   d. Inability to communicate
   e. Sleep deprivation
   f. Full bladder
   g. Nausea
   h. Need to defecate
   i. Nicotine withdrawal
   j. Drug side effects (anticholinergic, paradoxical response to benzodiazepines)

Pathophysiology
1. Depends on the identification and treatment of underlying cause
2. Not the natural consequence of critical illness, but it occurs frequently in critically ill patients and is associated with adverse clinical outcomes

Clinical Presentation
Ranges from restless to combative
1. Restless: anxious, apprehensive, but movements are not aggressive or vigorous
2. Agitated: fights ventilator, frequent nonpurposeful movement
3. Very agitated: aggressive, pulls or removes tubes
4. Combative: immediate danger to self or staff

Collaborative Management
1. Perform hourly assessment for changes in level of agitation
2. Assess the possible underlying cause of the agitation
   a. Pain or discomfort
      i) Positioning
      ii) Analgesics if required
      iii) Proper temperature
3. Consider use of pharmacologic agents (e.g., sedatives) if agitation continues
   a. Sedating agents
      i) Midazolam, dexmedetomidine, and propofol are most frequently used in the critical care environment with decreasing use of lorazepam.
      ii) Barbiturates, diazepam, and ketamine are occasionally used.
   b. Titrated to maintain light sedation
      i) A light level of sedation is associated with improved clinical outcomes (i.e., shorter duration of mechanical ventilation and critical care unit length of stay).
      ii) Light levels of sedation increase the physiologic stress response and are not associated with myocardial ischemia.

Antisocial Behaviors

Definition and Description
1. Pervasive disregard for and violation of the rights of others
2. Exhibits three or more of the following:
   a. Unlawful behavior resulting in potential for or history of arrests
   b. Deceitfulness or lying
   c. Impulsive or restless
   d. Irritable or aggressive
   e. Irresponsibility/blame
   f. Lack of remorse
   g. Callous, arrogant, disregard for others
3. Not caused by schizophrenia or mania (American Psychological Association [APA], 2013)
4. Consider how individuals will change the way they respond to the environment and relationships after exposure to trauma. Be transparent and trustworthy.
5. Empower the patient; give her or him choices when possible and let her or his voice be heard.
6. Offer peer support if able.

Predisposing Factors
1. Gender: both, although predominately female
2. Familial: biological relatives of females with the disorder
3. Somatization disorders
4. Substance-related disorders
5. Risks
   a. More likely than the general population to die prematurely by violence (suicide, homicide, accidents) (APA, 2013)
   b. Harm to self or others
   c. Unit, staff, or milieu disruption: These individuals may pit staff members against each other or create chaos on the unit.

Collaborative Management
1. Ensure therapeutic milieu.
   a. Use a calm, nonjudgmental approach.
   b. Maintain therapeutic relational boundaries.
   c. Clearly explain and consistently enforce rules and behavioral expectations.
   d. Clearly communicate plan of care with patient.
   e. Establish communication within the health care team so that patient issues, concerns, and progress are clearly communicated with each other and that a consistent approach is used.
2. Maintain a safe environment for patient, other patients, staff, and visitors.
   a. Assessment of psychiatric status, especially suicidal ideation
   b. Removal of any object that can be used for harm

Delirium

Definition and Description
1. An acute change (hours to days) in consciousness and cognition not caused by dementia (Table 12.5)

Table 12.5 Delirium versus Dementia

	Delirium	Dementia
Onset	Rapid: hours to days	Gradual: months to years
Orientation	Impaired	Impaired
Memory	Impaired: short-term and remote	Predominantly short-term memory impaired; remote memory stays intact
Level of consciousness	Disturbed, often fluctuates over 24-hr period	Alert, steady
Sleep–wake cycle	Erratic, disturbed over the course of the day, no patterns	No acute change; however, day–night reversal is common over time
Etiology	Evidence of general medical condition, trauma, substance use or withdrawal, or toxin	No evidence of medical illness, trauma, substance use or withdrawal, or toxin to account for changes
Electroencephalogram	Diffuse slowing	Slowing may occur
Duration	Brief (if effectively treated)	Chronic
Symptoms	Fluctuate over 24 hr	Consistent pattern
Sensory or perception	Hallucinations common	Misidentification, delusions

2. May result from or be related to: a general medical condition (i.e., trauma, infection); use or abuse of or withdrawal from a prescribed, illegal, or OTC substance; exposure to a toxin; or a combination of these.
3. May be accompanied by personality, behavioral, emotional, and functional change
4. Acute and fluctuating in nature

Predisposing and Risk Factors (Box 12.2)
1. Age: Children and older adults are more susceptible to delirium.
2. Gender: males at higher risk
3. History of delirium
4. Existing dementia

Pathophysiology
1. Depends on etiology
2. An acute (hours to days) deterioration of cognition with fluctuating level of awareness
3. Prodromal symptoms
    a. Emotional: anxiety, irritability
    b. Behavioral: restlessness
    c. Cognition: disorientation
    d. Sleep–wake cycle disturbance
4. Cognitive malfunctioning in the following:
    a. Memory
    b. Intellect
    c. Learning
    d. Orientation
    e. Comprehension
    f. Calculation
    g. Language
    h. Judgment

Clinical Presentation
1. Subjective
    a. Memory loss
    b. Confusion
    c. Decline in cognitive functioning, judgment

Box 12.2 Predisposing Risks for Delirium

History or Clinical Course
- History of delirium
- History of dementia
- History of mental illness or psychological problems
- History of alcohol or substance abuse
- History of falls
- Severe illness
- Cardiac surgery
- Cardiopulmonary bypass
- Prolonged surgery
- Electrolyte imbalance: sodium and potassium
- Hypoxia
- Infection
- Severe pain
- Impaired eyesight or hearing
- Malnutrition
- Renal or hepatic disease
- Fracture or trauma

Environmental Factors
- Critical care
- Sleep deprivation
- Sensory overload/sensory deprivation
- Noise
- Hypothermia or hyperthermia
- Physical restraints

Pharmacologic Agents
- Anticholinergics, including antihistamines (e.g., diphenhydramine and disopyramide)
- Opioids
- Benzodiazepines
- Tricyclic antidepressants
- Corticosteroids
- General anesthetics
- H_2 receptor blockers
- Diuretics
- Withdrawal from alcohol, nicotine, or drugs

2. Objective
    a. Lack of orientation to situation, time, place, and person
    b. Behavioral disturbances
    c. Functional decline
    d. Progression if underlying etiology not effectively treated: stupor, coma, seizures, death

3. Diagnostic studies
   a. Mini mental status exam (Folstein, Folstein, & McHugh, 1975)
   b. Diagnostic studies to determine cause of delirium
   c. Confusion Assessment Method (Eli 2001, Inouye et al, 1990)
      1) Commonly used tool to diagnose delirium
      2) Four components
         a) Acute change or fluctuating course of mental status
         b) Inattention
         c) Altered level of consciousness
         d) Disorganized thinking
      3) Interpretation
         a) If features a and b and either c or d are present, delirium is present.

Collaborative Management
1. Maintain airway, breathing, and ventilation.
   a. Oxygen by nasal cannula at 2 to 6 l/min if indicated to maintain SpO$_2$ of 94% unless contraindicated; in patients with chronic obstructive pulmonary disease (COPD), use pulse oximetry to guide oxygen administration to SpO$_2$ of ~90%
   b. Intravenous (IV) access for fluid and medication administration if indicated
2. Provide a safe environment.
   a. Quiet room with minimal stimulation, which allows continuous observation
   b. Use of patient's name during conversation
   c. Conversations should be kept simple and short.
   d. Frequent reorientation to person, place, time, and situation
   e. Determination of additional information to ensure safety
      1) Interview family for additional information.
      2) Presence of familiar persons may be calming and helpful.
      3) Evaluate risk for making unsafe decisions.
      4) Evaluate potential for falling.
   f. Restraints should be avoided if possible but may be required to ensure patient safety.
3. Monitor for complications.
   a. Violence
   b. Falls
   c. Decreased awareness of environment
   d. Decreased self-care (e.g., feeding, toileting, hygiene)

Intensive Care Unit Delirium

Definition
1. Confusion or psychosis associated with the critical care environment
2. Also called intensive care unit psychosis, postcardiotomy delirium, postoperative psychosis, intensive care delirium, acute confusion, and impaired psychological response
3. Usually occurs after 48 hours in the critical care unit; usually clears within 48 hours after transfer from the critical care unit

Contributing Factors
1. Sleep deprivation
2. Sensory deprivation
3. Sensory overload
4. Age
5. Severe illness
6. History of mental illness or psychological problems
7. Noise
8. Isolation
9. Immobilization
10. Cardiopulmonary bypass
11. Prolonged surgery
12. Electrolyte imbalance
13. Hypothermia
14. Endocrine disorders
15. Medications especially corticosteroids

Clinical Presentation
1. Altered consciousness
2. Decreased attention span
3. Disorientation, confusion
4. Memory loss
5. Labile emotions
6. Perceptual distortions such as hallucinations, paranoia
7. Combativeness

Collaborative Management
1. Eliminate possible causes.
   a. Plan uninterrupted sleep time; do not awaken the patient unless truly necessary.
      1) In a study by Tamburri, DiBrienza, Zozula, and Redeker (2004), the mean number of care interactions per night was 42.6, and patients had 2 to 3 hours of uninterrupted sleep on only 6% of the nights observed.
   b. Provide continuity of nursing staff to lessen the number of adjustments required by the patient.
   c. Reorient the patient frequently.
   d. Decrease noise level on alarms, and decrease extraneous conversation and other noise; earplugs may also be used.
      1) The Environmental Protection Agency (1974) recommends that daytime noise levels in a hospital not exceed 45 dB and that nighttime levels not exceed 35 dB.
   e. Adjust lighting to simulate night and day and maintain sleep–wake cycles while allowing for short naps throughout the day.
2. Provide frequent reorientation.
   a. Place a clock and calendar in the room.
   b. Encourage the family to visit and reorient the patient.
   c. Encourage placement of personal belongings at bedside.

Predisposing Factors
1. Genetic
2. Chromosomal abnormality
3. Pregnancy and perinatal problems
4. Environmental: exposure to toxins, deprivation, abuse, neglect

Major or Minor Neurocognitive Disorders (e.g., Dementia)

Definition
1. A chronic global deterioration of cognitive functioning (Table 12.5)
2. Results from a disorder of the brain or an organic disease
3. May be accompanied by personality, behavioral, emotional, and functional change
4. Chronic or progressive in nature

Predisposing Factors
1. Aging
2. Alzheimer disease
3. Frontotemporal lobar degeneration
4. Lewy body disease
5. Vascular disease
6. Traumatic brain injury
7. Substance or medication use
8. HIV infection
9. Prion disease
10. Parkinson disease
11. Huntington disease
12. Other medical conditions such as the following
    a. Neurosyphilis
    b. Subdural hematoma
    c. Brain tumor
    d. Normal-pressure hydrocephalus
    e. Hypothyroidism
13. Deficiencies in the following
    a. Folic acid
    b. Vitamin B_{12}
    c. Niacin
14. Hypercalcemia

Pathophysiology
1. Depends on etiology
2. A chronic global deterioration of cognition
3. Cognitive malfunctioning preceded by deterioration in the following:
    a. Emotional control
    b. Social behavior
    c. Motivation
4. Cognitive malfunctioning in the following six domains:
    a. Complex attention
    b. Executive function
    c. Learning and memory
    d. Language
    e. Perceptual
    f. Social cognition

Clinical Presentation
1. Subjective
    a. Memory loss
    b. Confusion
    c. Decline in cognitive functioning and judgment
2. Objective
    a. Lack of orientation to situation, time, place, and person
    b. Aphasia
    c. Apraxia
    d. Agnosia
    e. Behavioral disturbances
    f. Shallow to flat affect
    g. Focal neurologic signs
        1) Exaggeration of deep tendon reflexes
        2) Extensor plantar response
        3) Pseudobulbar palsy
        4) Gait abnormalities
        5) Weakness of an extremity
3. Diagnostic studies
    a. Mini mental status exam (Folstein, Folstein, & McHugh, 1975)
    b. Mini Cog (Tsoi, Chan et al., 2015)
    c. Other diagnostic testing as appropriate to rule out other causes

Collaborative Management
1. Maintain airway, breathing, and ventilation.
    a. Oxygen by nasal cannula at 2 to 6 l/min if indicated to maintain SpO_2 of 94% unless contraindicated; in patients with COPD, use pulse oximetry to guide oxygen administration to SpO_2 of ~90%
    b. IV access for fluid and medication administration if indicated
2. Provide a safe environment.
    a. Assessment of psychiatric status, especially suicidal ideation and sensory status, such as hearing and visual deficits
    b. Quiet room with minimal stimulation, which allows continuous observation
    c. Use of patient's name during conversation
    d. Conversations should be kept simple and short
    e. Frequent reorientation to person and place
    f. Determination of additional information to ensure safety
        1) Interview family for additional information.
        2) Evaluate risk for making unsafe decisions.
        3) Evaluate potential for wandering and falling.
    g. Restraints should be avoided if possible but may be required to ensure patient safety.
3. Monitor for complications.
    a. Violence
    b. Falls
    c. Decreased awareness of environment
    d. Decreased self-care

Anxiety

Definition and Description
1. Anxiety
    a. Anticipation of future threat, more often associated with muscle tension and vigilance in preparation for future danger and cautious or avoidant behaviors
    b. Subjective experience that differs from one individual to another
    c. Both physiologic and psychological components
    d. Person often does not know cause
    e. Unpleasant emotional state with increased feelings of tension and helplessness

2. Fear: emotional response to real or perceived imminent threat, more often associated with surges of autonomic arousal necessary for fight or flight, thoughts of immediate danger, and escape behaviors.
3. Types of anxiety disorders include the following:
    a. Panic disorder: sudden-onset anxiety in the form of fear and panic (i.e., panic attack)
    b. Phobia: irrational or illogical fear of an object, situation, or event
    c. Generalized anxiety disorder: excessive anxiety and worry, characterized by restlessness, fatigue, poor concentration, irritability, muscle tension, and sleep disturbances
    d. Substance-induced anxiety disorder: anxiety symptoms that develop with substance withdrawal or within a month of substance-abuse cessation

Predisposing Factors
1. Genetic predisposition
2. Preexisting diseases
    a. Physical: hyperthyroidism, hyperparathyroidism, pheochromocytoma, vestibular disorders, seizure disorders, arrhythmias, and other cardiac disorders
    b. Psychological: major depressive disorder
3. Developmental causes
    a. Children: separation from parents, perceived loss of love
    b. Adolescents: peer pressure related to appearance, substance abuse, pressure to achieve, puberty
    c. Adults: life changes such as marriage, divorce, childbirth, menopause, career pressures, loss of parents
    d. Older adult: loss of spouse, significant other, or friends; diminished independence and health
    e. Exposure to high levels of stress over time
    f. Sleep deprivation
    g. Acute changes in health status
    h. Related to substance use: This may include central nervous system (CNS) stimulants (i.e., cocaine, amphetamine, and caffeine) and withdrawal from CNS depressants (i.e., alcohol and barbiturates).
    i. Trauma

Pathophysiology
1. Not well understood
2. Thought to be caused by a disruption of modulator within the CNS
3. Several neurotransmitter systems are thought to be involved.
    a. Serotonin
    b. Norepinephrine
    c. Gamma-aminobutyric acid (GABA)
    d. Peptides
    e. Corticotropin
4. Autonomic nervous system mediates the majority of the symptoms.

Clinical Presentation
1. Subjective
    a. May have history of:
        1) Excessive anxiety or worry for more than 6 months
        2) Inability to control feelings
        3) Three or more of the following symptoms:
            a) Restlessness, keyed up
            b) Fatigue
            c) Difficulty concentrating
            d) Irritability
            e) Muscle tension
            f) Sleep disturbances: difficulty falling or staying asleep, not rested
            g) Sexual problems
        4) Apprehensive, fearfulness, helplessness
        5) Tightness in chest, shortness of breath
        6) Dizziness
        7) Choking feeling
2. Objective
    a. Tachycardia, tachypnea, may have elevated blood pressure
    b. Pallor
    c. Tremors
    d. Dilated pupils, nystagmus
3. Diagnostic studies
    a. Serum blood and urine drug screen as indicated
    b. Electrocardiogram (ECG): may show dysrhythmias, particularly sinus tachycardia, premature atrial contractions (PACs), premature ventricular contractions (PVCs)
    c. Other diagnostic studies to rule out medical conditions

Collaborative Management
1. Maintain airway, breathing, and ventilation.
    a. Oxygen by nasal cannula at 2 to 6 l/min if indicated to maintain SpO$_2$ of 94% unless contraindicated; in patients with COPD, use pulse oximetry to guide oxygen administration to SpO$_2$ of ~90%
    b. IV access for fluid and medication administration if indicated
2. Provide a safe, quiet environment.
    a. Decrease stimulation by providing a quiet, darkened room.
    b. Assess psychiatric status, especially suicidal ideation and agitation level.
    c. Ensure continuous observation.
3. Establish a trusting relationship.
    a. Maintain a calm manner when approaching the patient.
    b. Acknowledge patient's feelings and fears.
    c. Use a calm tone, speak clearly and distinctly.
    d. Maintain eye contact when speaking with the patient.
    e. Communicate honestly.
    f. Assist in problem solving.
4. Reduce anxiety.
    a. Anxiolytics as directed (e.g., diazepam, lorazepam, chlordiazepoxide)
    b. Benzodiazepines are synergistic with alcohol, so assess for recent alcohol usage.
    c. Beta-blockers may also be prescribed.
    d. Antidepressants as prescribed
5. Monitor for complications.
    a. Dysrhythmias
    b. Suicide
    c. Paradoxical reaction to medications, particularly benzodiazepines

Depression

Definition
Disturbance of mood associated with anhedonia (loss of interest or pleasure in usual activities) or an increase in sadness or negative thinking not associated with medication withdrawal, bereavement, or another medical condition

Predisposing Factors
1. Genetic predisposition
2. Severe psychosocial stressors
3. Hormonal imbalance
4. Sudden increase or decrease in substance use
5. Medical conditions such as diabetes, myocardial infarction, carcinomas, or stroke
6. Medication side effects

Pathophysiology
1. Not well defined but thought to be a disturbance in CNS serotonin activity
2. Dysregulation of neurotransmitter system
3. Serotonin deficiency
4. Norepinephrine and dopamine are also thought to be involved.

Clinical Presentation
1. Subjective: symptoms last longer than 2 months
   a. Presence of depressed mood (irritability in a child or adolescent) or anhedonia (loss of interest or pleasure)
   b. Expressions of the following:
      1) Guilt, worthlessness, hopelessness
      2) Feelings of suicide
      3) Recurrent thoughts of death
   c. History of attempted suicide, thoughts or plans of suicide, or recurrent thoughts of death
   d. Sleep disturbance: insomnia, hypersomnia, feeling unrested
   e. Low energy or fatigue
   f. Inability to concentrate
   g. Changes in appetite
   h. Weight loss or gain
   i. Decreased libido
   j. Amenorrhea
   k. Constipation
   l. Psychomotor symptoms
      1) Psychomotor agitation: restless, need to keep moving
      2) Psychomotor retardation: generalized slowing down of movements, physical reactions, and speech.
2. Objective
   a. Appearance indicative of poor hygiene, lack of concern regarding appearance
   b. Flat affect
   c. Tearful
   d. Quiet speech
   e. Little eye contact
   f. Psychomotor retardation
   g. Evidence of psychotic symptoms (i.e., hallucinations, delusions)
3. Diagnostic studies
   a. Serum blood and urine drug screen
   b. Serum alcohol
   c. Thyroid function test to rule out hypothyroidism
   d. CBC with differential to rule out anemia
   e. Computed tomography (CT) scan and possible magnetic resonance imaging of the head to rule out medical cause

Collaborative Management
1. Maintain airway, breathing, and ventilation.
   a. Oxygen by nasal cannula at 2 to 6 l/min if indicated to maintain SpO_2 of 94% unless contraindicated; in patients with COPD, use pulse oximetry to guide oxygen administration to SpO_2 of ~90%
   b. IV access for fluid and medication administration if indicated
2. Provide a safe environment.
   a. Assessment of psychiatric status especially suicidal ideation
   b. Quiet room with minimal stimulation, which allows continuous observation
   c. Nonjudgmental approach
   d. Frequent contacts to assure patient of staff concern
   e. If suicide is a concern, someone to stay with patient at all times
3. Assist with treatment of depression.
   a. Antidepressant therapy
   b. Counseling
   c. Electroconvulsant therapy
   d. Light therapy
   e. Transcranial magnetic stimulation
4. Monitor for complications.
   a. Violent behavior
   b. Suicide

Mania

Definitions
1. Mania: elevated, irritable, or expansive mood
   a. Episode of irritable or elevated mood lasting at least 1 week
   b. Marked impairment in functioning
   c. Symptoms are not due to substance or general medical condition
2. Bipolar: a combination of mood swings from mania to depression

Predisposing Factors
1. Genetic predisposition
2. Severe psychosocial stressors
3. Hormonal imbalance
4. Sudden decrease in substance use

Pathophysiology
Thought to involve the dysregulation of neurotransmitters

Clinical Presentation
1. Subjective
   a. History of manic or hypomanic episodes
   b. Racing thoughts
   c. Little need for sleep
   d. Increase in use of prescribed or illegal drugs to calm down
   e. Risky behaviors
   f. Abuse of credit cards and reckless spending

g. Multiple sex partners
h. Arrests
i. Interference with job performance
j. Unrealistic future plans
k. Previous suicide attempts: past and current plans
2. Objective
   a. Fidgeting, pacing
   b. Difficulty staying on topic; flight of ideas
   c. Elation or euphoria; laughing
   d. Grandiosity
   e. May have injuries
3. Diagnostic studies
   a. Serum blood and urine drug screen
   b. Serum alcohol
   c. ECG: tachycardia, atrial dysrhythmias, PACs, PVCs
   d. Other diagnostic studies to rule out other causes

Collaborative Management
1. Maintain airway, breathing, and ventilation.
   a. Oxygen by nasal cannula at 2 to 6 l/min if indicated to maintain SpO$_2$ of 94% unless contraindicated; in patients with COPD, use pulse oximetry to guide oxygen administration to SpO$_2$ of ~90%
   b. IV access for fluid and medication administration if indicated
2. Provide a safe environment.
   a. Assessment of psychiatric status especially suicidal ideation
   b. Quiet room with minimal stimulation, which allows continuous observation
   c. Nonjudgmental approach
   d. Restraints should be avoided if possible but may be required to ensure patient safety.
3. Control mania.
   a. Antipsychotics for psychosis, if present, until mood stabilizers take effect
   b. Anticonvulsants for regulation of mood (helps stabilize mania and depression in bipolar disorder)
   c. Antidepressants for depression
   d. Beta-blockers to block effects of catecholamines
   e. Counseling to deal with cycling of moods, behavior, and interpersonal relationships
4. Monitor for complications: self-injury or suicide.

Trauma, Violence, and Abuse

Definition
1. Injury caused by violence, accidental injuries, or criminal activity
2. Abuse: mistreatment of another (can be physical, mental, or emotional)
3. Neglect: lack of care for physical, mental, or emotional well-being
4. Sexual assault
5. Posttraumatic stress disorder (PTSD): symptoms after exposure to a traumatic or stressful event (or learning of an event or repeated exposure to details) and show symptoms in four domains: intrusion, avoidance, negative alterations, and hyperarousal.
6. Acute stress disorder: symptoms within 3 days to one month after a traumatic or stressful event with a number of similar symptoms, but not in certain clusters such as PTSD.

Predisposing Factors
1. Substance abuse
2. Stress reactions
3. Inability to cope
4. Direct intent to injure (i.e., assault)
5. History of trauma, violence, or abuse

Clinical Presentation
1. Subjective: Use collaborative information provided by family, friends, and significant others.
   a. Pain related to injury
   b. Extreme emotional distress
      1) May be unable to report symptoms
      2) Injury and history of incident may not seem to match.
      3) Inconsistency with the report of what happened prior to coming into the emergency department or changes in the story
2. Objective
   a. Sudden unexpected physical or emotional injury
      1) Injury can be obvious or not obvious.
   b. Clinical presentation related to location and severity of injury
   c. Bruises in various stages may indicate physical abuse.
   d. Injury with identifiable pattern (e.g., cigarette burn)
3. Diagnostic studies
   a. Serum: tests to rule out medical concerns
   b. Forensic testing as indicated (e.g., DNA)
   c. Evidence collection following chain of evidence if associated with a crime; photos as indicated
   d. Radiographic films of injured areas; radiographic films that show old fractures may indicate abuse
   e. CT scans as indicated; noncontrast head CT if hemorrhage suspected
   f. Other diagnostic studies to rule out other causes

Age-Related Considerations
1. Adults (likely causes): gunshot wounds, lacerations, fractures, rape, penetrating injuries, domestic violence, single car collision
2. Older adults (likely causes): fractures, nutritional deficits, domestic violence, self-injuries, neglect

Collaborative Management
1. Maintain airway, breathing, and ventilation.
   a. Oxygen by nasal cannula at 2 to 6 l/min if indicated to maintain SpO$_2$ of 94% unless contraindicated; in patients with COPD, use pulse oximetry to guide oxygen administration to SpO$_2$ of ~90%
   b. Artificial airway and mechanical ventilation may be necessary, depending on severity of injury.
   c. IV access for fluid and medication administration if indicated
2. Ensure patient safety.
   a. Assessment of psychiatric status, especially suicidal ideation
   b. Clothing and other personal articles must be secured as a protection of chain of evidence if there are potential legal ramifications.
   c. Be aware of duty-to-protect regulations for health care providers.

d. Notification of authorities if abuse or neglect suspected
e. Maintenance of safe environment for patient
f. Protection against unwanted visitors or potential abusers who may attempt to control care
g. Documentation of what patient reports using exact quotes
3. Relieve pain and discomfort.
   a. Position of comfort
   b. Analgesics
   c. Complementary therapies such as heat and cold
4. Prepare patient and assist with procedures as indicated by type, location, and severity of injury. Determination of patient wishes as able
5. Monitor for complications: dependent upon type, location, and severity of injury
   a. Homicide
   b. Suicide

Posttraumatic Stress Disorder

Definition
Exposure to a traumatic event (e.g., directly experiencing, witnessing, learning of the event a close family member involved, repeated exposure to details); does not include electronic media, television, movies, or pictures resulting in a sequela of symptoms

Predisposing Factors
1. Risks include:
   a. Childhood adverse events or emotional problems
   b. Prior behavioral health disorders
   c. Lower socioeconomic status
   d. Lower education
   e. Childhood adversity
   f. Lower intelligence
   g. Female gender
   h. Younger age at time of exposure
   i. Severity of trauma
   j. Dissociation during the trauma
2. Symptoms usually begin within 3 months of the trauma, but delayed expression can occur; can occur at any age after the first year of life

Pathophysiology
1. Fear response may be characterized in part by endocrine effects such as increases in cortisol, because of amygdala activation of the hypothalamic–pituitary–adrenal (HPA) axis.
2. Prolonged HPA activation and cortisol release has other health implications as well such as coronary artery disease, type 2 diabetes, and stroke.

Clinical Presentation
1. Intrusion: one or more of the following
   a. Distressing memories or repetitive play in children
   b. Recurrent distressing dreams; content or affect related to the event
   c. Dissociative reactions
   d. Psychological distress at cues
   e. Physiological reactions to cues
2. Avoidance: one or both of the following
   a. Avoidance of memories, thoughts, feelings
   b. Avoidance of external reminders
3. Negative alterations: two or more of the following
   a. Inability to remember (i.e., dissociative amnesia)
   b. Negative beliefs about oneself, others, the world
   c. Distorted cognitions about cause or consequences leading to blame
   d. Persistent negative emotional state
   e. Diminished interest
   f. Feelings of detachment/estrangement
   g. Persistent inability to experience positive emotions
4. Alterations in arousal: two or more of the following
   a. Irritable behavior or angry outbursts
   b. Reckless or self-destructive behavior
   c. Hypervigilance
   d. Exaggerated startle
   e. Poor concentration
   f. Sleep disturbances
5. Duration is more than 1 month and causes significant distress or impairment and not attributable to a substance.
6. Specify with dissociative symptoms (depersonalization or derealization).
7. Specify if delayed expression (criteria not met until at least 6 months after event).

Collaborative Management
1. Use trauma-focused approach.
   a. Establish trust.
   b. Be transparent.
   c. Do not retraumatize.
   d. Be collaborative.
   e. Give choices when able.
   f. Let the patient's voice be heard.
   g. Be aware of safety and the patient's interpretation of the world or environment.
2. Administer appropriate pharmacologic agents.
   a. Antidepressants
   b. Antianxiety
   c. Sleep aids
   d. Antipsychotics for symptom control
3. Assist with prescribed therapies.
   a. Cognitive behavioral therapy (CBT)
   b. Prolonged exposure (PE)
   c. Eye movement desensitization and reprocessing (EMDR)
   d. Cognitive processing therapy (CPT)
   e. Accelerated resolution therapy (ART)

Risk-Taking Behavior

Definition
Tendency to engage in activities that have the potential to be harmful or dangerous

Predisposing Factors
Impulsivity and aggressive behaviors occur frequently in variety of psychological and neurological disorders including the following
1. Neurocognitive disorders
2. ADHD

3. Autistic spectrum disorders
4. Tourette syndrome and tic disorders
5. Obsessive-compulsive disorder (OCD)
6. Body dysmorphic disorder
7. Hoarding
8. Trichotillomania
9. Skin picking
10. Compulsive shopping
11. Binge eating
12. Hypochondriasis
13. Somatization
14. Intermittent explosive disorder
15. Antisocial personality disorder
16. Conduct disorder
17. Self-harm behaviors
18. Impulsive violence in psychosis, mania, borderline personality disorder
19. Oppositional defiant disorder
20. Substance use disorders

Pathophysiology
1. Impulsivity and compulsivity resulting in risk-taking behaviors suggest that behaviors themselves may be reinforcing and addicting.
2. Rewarding behaviors and addictions share the same brain circuitry.
3. Behaviors are difficult to prevent because the short-term reward is chosen over the long-term gain.
4. Rewarding behavior can become a habit, making it difficult to stop because it reduces tension and there is the potential for withdrawal effects.

Clinical Presentation
1. Depends on the diagnosis
2. During levels of high stress, the patient's perceptual field is very narrow, and he or she is not able to process information.
3. The patient might be a danger to him- or herself or others, be unable to problem solve, and be irrational (flight, fight, freeze).

Collaborative Management
1. Maintain therapeutic approach.
    a. Set limits on behaviors.
        1) Be simple and direct.
        2) Be clear, calm, and nonthreatening.
        3) Be firm yet supportive, and respectful and encouraging.
    b. Use verbal deescalation.
    c. Assess the patient's level of stress.
        1) Avoid the need to be right.
        2) Do not respond to "button pushing."
        3) Do not bring up the past.
        4) Avoid being defensive.
        5) Be flexible and provide specific choices as able.
2. Administer appropriate pharmacologic agents.
    a. Lithium
    b. Anticonvulsants
    c. Beta-blockers
    d. Antidepressants
    e. Atypical antipsychotics
    f. Methylphenidate
    g. Buspirone
    h. Clonidine
    i. Other pharmacologic agents depending on the diagnosis

Substance-Related Disorders
1. Encompasses separate classes of drugs: alcohol, caffeine, cannabis, hallucinogens, inhalants, opioids, sedatives, hypnotics, anxiolytics, stimulants, tobacco, and other substances.

Definitions and Descriptions
1. Substance use disorder: cluster of cognitive, behavioral, and physiological symptoms indicating that the individual continues using the substance despite significant substance-related problems (*Diagnostic and Statistical Manual of Mental Disorders,* 2013) manifested with:
    a. Impaired control
    b. Unsuccessful attempts to cut down or discontinue use
    c. Great deal of time is spent obtaining, using and recovering from its effects.
    d. Craving: intense desire or urge for the substance
    e. Social impairment as evidenced by failing to fulfill major role obligations, using substance despite recurrent problems, or giving up or withdrawal from important activities
    f. Risky use as evidence by using in situations in which it is physically hazardous or use despite knowledge of having problems from the substance physically or psychologically
    g. Tolerance: requiring a markedly increased dose of the substance to achieve the desired effect
    h. Withdrawal: syndrome that occurs when concentrations of a substance declines usually that results in the person using more of the substance to relieve the withdrawal effects
2. Substance-induced disorders
    a. Substance intoxication: development of a reversible substance-specific syndrome caused by the ingestion of the substance. The problematic behavioral or psychological changes associated with intoxication are attributable to the physiological effects of the substance on the CNS and develop during or shortly after use. This includes mood lability, impaired judgment, belligerence, disturbances of perception, thinking, interpersonal behavior, wakefulness, and attention.
    b. Substance withdrawal: development of substance-specific problematic behavioral change, with physiological and cognitive concomitants caused by the cessation of or reduction of the drug

Predisposing Factors
1. Subjective
    a. Family history of substance abuse or dependence
    b. Inability to cope effectively
    c. Group modeling especially in adolescence
    d. Genetic predisposition
    e. Related history of usage
    f. History of request for help with addictions
    g. Report of emotional distress

2. Objective
   a. May be weeping
   b. Drug-seeking behavior: a pattern of seeking a particular medication (e.g., narcotic pain medication or tranquilizers) without an organic basis; may demonstrate abusive or threatening behavior when denied drugs

Clinical Presentation
1. Will depend on the substance involved and on the category of use (withdrawal, intoxication)
2. Subjective
   a. Self-report of use
   b. Family or friends report use.
   c. Request for help with addictions
   d. Emotionally distressed, weeping
3. Objective
   a. Person exhibits intoxication or erratic behavior, including impaired judgment, aggression, mood lability.
   b. Speech can be slurred or rambling.
   c. Unsteady gait
   d. Nystagmus
   e. Impaired memory or attention
   f. Stupor or coma
4. Diagnostic: serum and urine drug screens

Collaborative Management
1. Maintain airway, breathing, and ventilation.
   a. Oxygen by nasal cannula at 2 to 6 l/min if indicated to maintain SpO_2 of 94% unless contraindicated; in patients with COPD, use pulse oximetry to guide oxygen administration to SpO_2 of ~90%
   b. IV access for fluid and medication administration if indicated
2. Provide a safe environment.
   a. Assessment of psychiatric status especially suicidal ideation
   b. Close monitoring for progression of symptoms: The Clinical Institute Withdrawal Assessment of Alcohol Scale (CIWA-Ar) is a widely accepted tool to facilitate assessing and treating alcohol withdrawal (Sullivan et al., 1989).
   c. Quiet room with minimal stimulation, which allows continuous observation
   d. Determination of suicidal ideation or plan for suicide
   e. Restraints should be avoided if possible but may be required to ensure patient safety.
   f. Prevent seizures: benzodiazepines as prescribed
   g. Frequent reorientation
   h. Nonjudgmental attitude
   i. Conversations should be kept simple and short.
3. Monitor for complications.
   a. Cardiac dysrhythmias
   b. Hypertension or hypotension
   c. Respiratory depression
   d. Seizures
   e. Coma
   f. Delirium tremens
   g. Death

Suicidal Ideation and Behaviors

Definition
Thoughts of taking one's own life that may or may not be accompanied by the intent to die

Predisposing factors
1. Family history of suicide
2. Prior attempts
3. Substance abuse
4. Psychiatric illness (e.g., depression, schizophrenia)
5. Physical illness and chronic pain issues
6. Hopelessness
7. Means (e.g., availability of weapon)
8. Recent discharge from inpatient behavioral health hospitalization
9. Situational stressors (e.g., divorce, personal loss, unemployment, financial or legal issues)

Pathophysiology
1. Poor coping skills
2. Most suicidal people do not want to end their biological existence but want to end their psychological pain and suffering.
3. Most suicidal people tell someone that they are thinking about suicide as an option to cope with their pain.

Clinical Presentation
1. No characteristic presentation; risk factors alone are neither sensitive or specific
2. Persons who self-mutilate and injure themselves do not usually wish to die; they frequently use self-harm as a way to respond to anger at themselves or others or the relief of tension.
3. All suicide attempts should be taken seriously even if you believe the actions or thoughts to be manipulative in nature.

Collaborative Management
1. Determine level of risk and mitigate risk factors.
   a. Seek collateral information from family or friends if possible.
   b. Determine the following:
      1) Desire to die
      2) Reasons for living
      3) Frequency of ideation
      4) Intensity of ideation
      5) Intent to die
      6) Lack of deterrents to attempt suicide
      7) Access and means
      8) Plans and preparation
   c. Remove any potential threats from the room.
2. Maintain therapeutic approach.
   a. Be aware of your reactions; clinicians are often angry, anxious, helpless, indifferent, or reject persons who attempt suicide or have suicidal ideation.
   b. Maintain a caring approach.

Medical Nonadherence

Definition
Patient not engaging in treatment as prescribed

Predisposing Factors
1. Lack of trust in provider or effectiveness of treatments
2. Adverse childhood events
3. Lack of readiness for change
4. Education level affects understanding of instructions
5. Financial means for compliance affects ability to purchase drugs and other treatments
6. Other social factors (e.g., transportation, child care)

Pathophysiology
1. Psychological factors play a significant role in health care.
2. Medications and treatments can work better when there is more of an alliance with the provider and can account for 25% to 75% of efficacy for antidepressants and other psychiatric medication (i.e., placebo effect).
3. Managing human feelings
   a. Sense of control or loss of control or helplessness with chronic illness (i.e., self-efficacy versus being told what to do by an authority figure [e.g., provider])
   b. Change on self-concept (i.e., individual with chronic, terminal, or life-threatening condition)

Clinical Presentation
1. Negative consequences for the patient
   a. Worsening illness or illness not improving within expected time period
   b. Nonadherence frequently worse for prevention than for curative treatments
   c. Treatments may worsen relationship with friends or family (e.g., side effects, inability to do things because of financial costs or time of treatments)
2. Negative consequences for the patient–provider relationship
   a. Litigation
   b. Ambivalence toward patient or staff
   c. Negative evaluations
   d. Provider burnout
3. Ambivalence, resistance, and transference can result in:
   a. Misuse of medications
   b. Nonadherence with treatment
   c. Negative attitudes about providers or treatments
   d. Acceptance of the sick role in the patient's life (i.e., may not want to get better)
   e. Help rejecting can have to do with perception of the world as a distrusting place (e.g., patient may say that help is wanted but also insist that nothing you do will help)

Collaborative Management
1. Provide information about recommended treatment(s).
   a. Recommended treatment(s)
   b. Expected effects of treatment(s)
   c. Alternative treatment(s)
   d. Complementary strategies
   e. Instructions for use of treatment(s)
   f. Side effects
   g. What should be reported
2. Develop trust and serve as patient advocate by discussing the following:
   a. Patient's goals of treatment
   b. What the illness means to the patient
   c. What improving their quality of life means to the patient
   d. What the patient is and is not willing to do
   e. The patient's culture and how the patient perceives illness and treatments
   f. Availability of treatment(s)
3. Use talk-back method to evaluate the patient's understanding of their role in the treatment(s).
4. Collaborate and problem solve with the patient, family and friends, and other members of the health care team.

Psychosis

Definition
1. A severe psychiatric disorder characterized by personality disorganization, loss of contact with reality, and deterioration of normal social functioning
2. Acute or chronic: lasting from a few days to several months
3. May be functional or organic

Predisposing Factors
1. Functional type: severe depression, mania, schizophrenic disorder, or brief psychotic episode
2. Organic type
   a. Ingestion of toxic substance
   b. Shock or trauma
   c. Dementia: slow onset
   d. Delirium: rapid onset

Pathophysiology
Poorly understood

Clinical Presentation
1. Subjective: may report any of the following:
   a. Previous history of psychotic episodes
   b. Confusion or amnesia
   c. Paranoid ideation
   d. Fears about safety
   e. Loss of energy
   f. Self-medication
2. Objective
   a. Positive symptoms
      1) Delusions
      2) Hallucinations: usually auditory
   b. Negative symptoms
      1) Avolition: inability to initiate activities (including self-care)
      2) Alogia: absence of speech
      3) Anhedonia: lack of pleasure
      4) Flat affect: absence of emotional responses
   c. Disorganized speech or incoherence

d. Conversation shows confusion, loss of touch with reality, loss of orientation to time, place, and person
   e. Increased agitation or bizarre behavior
   f. Grossly exaggerated behaviors
   g. Psychomotor retardation (i.e., visible generalized slowing down of movements, physical reactions, and speech)
3. Diagnostic studies
   a. Urinalysis, especially if person is an older woman
   b. Urine and serum drug screens
   c. CT scan if changes have been rapid
   d. Other diagnostic studies to rule out other causes

Collaborative Management
1. Maintain airway, breathing, and ventilation.
   a. Oxygen by nasal cannula at 2 to 6 l/min if indicated to maintain SpO_2 of 94% unless contraindicated; in patients with COPD, use pulse oximetry to guide oxygen administration to SpO_2 of ~90%
   b. IV access for fluid and medication administration if indicated
2. Provide a safe environment.
   a. Assessment of psychiatric status, especially suicidal ideation
   b. Quiet room with minimal stimulation, which allows continuous observation.
   c. Nonjudgmental approach
   d. Conversations should be kept simple, short, reality based, and concrete.
   e. Acknowledgement of patient's delusion and/or hallucinations while maintaining reality (e.g., "I believe that you are hearing voices, but I do not hear them.")
   f. Avoidance of arguing with patient about his or her experience; provide support for the feelings that may be generated (e.g., "It must be frightening to hear those voices.")
   g. Frequent reorientation to person, place, time, and situation
   h. Restraints should be avoided if possible but may be required to ensure patient safety.
3. Assist with management of psychosis.
   a. Antipsychotic medications to reduce psychosis
   b. Anxiolytic medications may be used adjunctively with antipsychotic medications to reduce anxiety or induce sleep.
   c. Consult with the patient's current psychiatrist or refer to a psychiatrist if patient has not been previously treated for psychosis.
4. Monitor for complications.
   a. Extrapyramidal symptoms
   b. Neuroleptic malignant syndrome
   c. Incontinence
   d. Coma

Learning Activities

CHAPTER 12

1. Complete the following crossword puzzle related to psychosocial conditions.

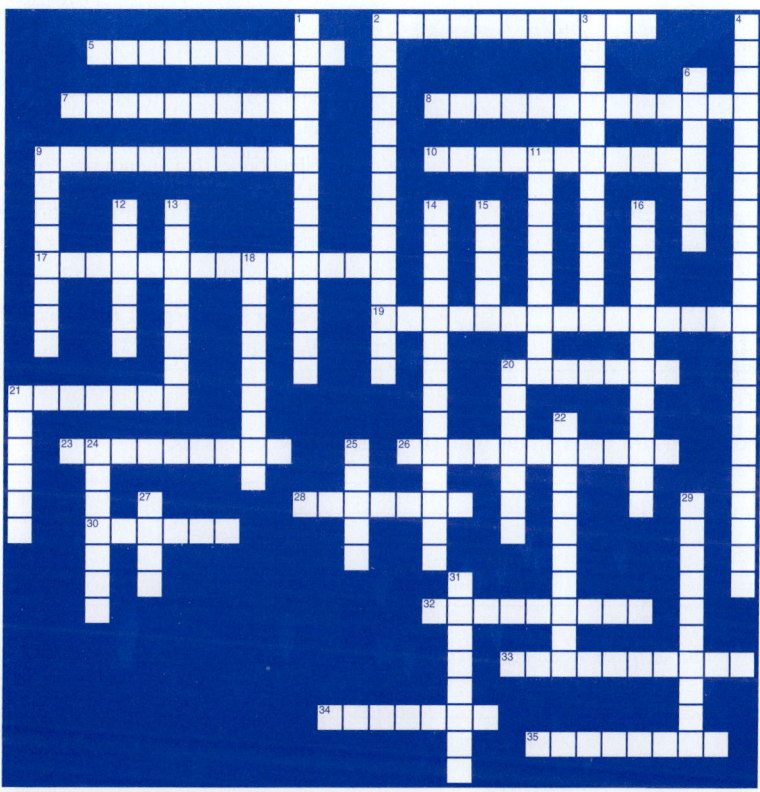

ACROSS
2. Medications that decrease anxiety
5. Logical, directed thought that may "circle the topic" but does not make a point or answer the intended question
7. Physiological and cognitive concomitants caused by the cessation of or reduction in heavy or prolonged substance use
8. Non–goal-directed speech that leaps from one idea to another (3 words)
9. Hallucination that occurs upon awakening
10. This type of crisis occurs suddenly in response to an unexpected stressful event
17. Thoughts or speech that contain excessive details about the topic but finally reach the intended point
19. Altered body image causes aversion to eating in this condition (2 words)
20. This disorder is characterized by feelings of helplessness and tension
21. The inability to perform motor activities despite intact motor function
23. Characterized by hallucinations and delusions and loss of contact with reality
26. A state of sorrow over the loss of a loved one
28. The inability to recognize or identify objects despite intact sensory function
30. State that occurs when one's usual ways of coping are inadequate to deal with the stress
32. Fixed false beliefs
33. Brief test of specific aspects of cognitive function (2 words)
34. Recurrent binge eating and inappropriate compensatory behaviors to prevent weight gain are associated with this condition
35. Involuntary cessation in the flow of thought or speech

DOWN
1. Sensory perceptions when there are no sensory stimuli
2. This class of drugs is also used for mood stabilization
3. Reversible substance-specific syndrome caused by recent ingestion of a substance
4. Thought process in which there is no logical connection between sentences (3 words)
6. Not attending to the emotional, physical, or mental care needs of another who cannot care for him- or herself
9. Willful taking of another person's life
11. The inability to initiate activities that is seen in psychosis
12. Patients with mania have this type of thoughts
13. A chronic global deterioration of cognition
14. This type of drug is administered to decrease the risk of seizures and to decrease anxiety during substance withdrawal
15. Physical, mental, or emotional mistreatment of another

739

16. Stressors expected as part of normal growth and development
18. Lack of pleasure
20. A language disturbance seen in dementia
21. Absence of speech
22. Alteration in mood characterized by sadness and negative self-concept
24. Willful taking of one's own life
25. Elevated or irritable mood of at least 1 week's duration with increased energy or activity and noticeable change from usual behavior
27. This disorder is characterized by eating chalk, paper, or other nonfood objects
29. Hallucinations are this type of disturbance
31. There is an increase in this type of thinking in depression

2. Match the following hallucinations with the correct definition.

____ 1.	Auditory	a. Feeling sensations when not being touched
____ 2.	Visual	b. Seeing images that are not present
____ 3.	Gustatory	c. Smelling odors that are not present
____ 4.	Hypnopompic	d. Perceiving a taste without an identifiable cause
____ 5.	Tactile	e. Hearing voices or sounds that are not there
____ 6.	Olfactory	f. Vivid dreamlike hallucination upon awakening
____ 7.	Kinesthetic	g. Perceiving movement of the body without cause
____ 8.	Somatic	h. Feeling that something is occurring within one's own body

3. List five age-related considerations for older adults with psychological emergencies.
   a. _____
   b. _____
   c. _____
   d. _____
   e. _____

4. Match the level of Maslow's hierarchy of needs to the example.

____ 1.	Physiologic	a. Art and music
____ 2.	Safety and security	b. Water
____ 3.	Love and belonging	c. Promotion at work
____ 4.	Esteem and recognition	d. Marriage
____ 5.	Self-actualization	e. Home security

5. Identify the assessment findings in each of the following conditions that would help you distinguish it from the others.

Condition	Subjective Assessment	Objective Assessment
Anxiety disorder		
Depression		
Mania		
Hallucinations		
Psychosis		
Dementia		
Delirium		

6. Mr. D. is a 67-year-old widower of 2 years who retired 3 months ago from his position as a mechanical engineer. He lives alone in his home of 30 years. His son has accompanied him to the emergency department (ED). He presents to the ED unshaven and disheveled with poor eye contact. He mumbles in response to questions in soft, low tones and is difficult to understand. He keeps stating that he is in awful shape, has no memory, and is of no good use to himself or anyone else, and they should just let him die. When pressed to do so, he reluctantly identifies the correct year, date, and day. He is aware he has been brought to a hospital. His sleep is erratic, his appetite is poor, he has generalized weakness, and his gait is unsteady. His son reports that his father typically is meticulous about his appearance and is very articulate. He states that he last saw his father

2 weeks ago when they had gone out to dinner and had done some grocery shopping. At that time, Mr. D was well groomed, walking steadily and independently, and actively involved in their conversation, his son said. He is concerned that his father has had a stroke or is getting dementia.

a. What additional information might you need about Mr. D?

b. What laboratory tests might be helpful?

c. What would be a preliminary diagnosis for Mr. D and what are the data that support that diagnosis?

d. What would be priority care issues for Mr. D?

7. Ms. B is a 21-year-old college student who is brought to the emergency department by the local police for running naked through her neighborhood. She is cooperative, although she insists that she does not need to be in the hospital. She reports that she feels great, hasn't slept in 2 days, and is not sleepy. She states, "I need to be free, like the birds and the bees." When asked for identification, she responds, "I am a daughter of the world." You notice that she has several bruises and many superficial cuts and scrapes on her body and feet.

a. What additional information might you need about Ms. B?

b. What laboratory tests might be helpful?

c. What are potential diagnoses for Ms. B, and what data support that diagnosis?

d. What would be priority care concerns for Ms. B?

8. Mr. P is a 65-year-old businessman who was admitted in acute respiratory failure. He is intubated and has been on a mechanical ventilator for 2 days. Tonight he is restless and confused. He appears frightened and is pulling at catheters and tubes.

a. What is the most likely cause of Mr. P's symptoms?

b. What are the most likely contributing factors?

c. What are the priorities of care for Mr. P?

Learning Activities Answers

CHAPTER 2

1.

[Crossword puzzle solution]

2.
   a. Autonomy: The right of an individual to make his or her own choice
   b. Beneficence: The principle of acting with the best interest of the other in mind
   c. Nonmaleficence: The principle that "above all, do no harm" as stated in the Hippocratic oath
   d. Justice: A concept that emphasizes fairness and equality

3.
   a. Advance directives are legal documents that express the patient's preferences for end-of-life care. Nurses implement into practice the Patient Self-Determination Act (PSDA), which mandates that providers of health care services under Medicare and Medicaid provide access to information about advance directives and facilitate the ability to create advance directive documents. Nursing is inherently suited to providing the education and support to patients and family members.
   b. Beneficence. The nurse has an obligation to promote good and prevent or remove harm and promote the welfare, health, and safety of society and individuals in accordance with their beliefs, values, preferences, and life goals.
   c. Advocacy refers to respecting and supporting the basic values, rights, and beliefs of the patient. The nurse should be prepared to assist the patient in obtaining information necessary to assist in decision making and monitor and safe guard the quality of care that the patient receives. The nurse in this instance should act as a liaison between the patient, the family, and the health care team.

4. 1. c; 2. e; 3. f; 4. b; 5. d; 6. a

5. Moral distress occurs when one knows the right thing to do but cannot do the right thing either because of internal or external obstacles. Moral distress may occur as a result of end-of-life challenges, nurse–physician conflict, workplace violence, staffing shortages, and so on.
Wavra's "four As" describe a methodology that nurses can use to rise above moral distress or assist others in doing so. Ask: Determine if moral distress is being experienced. Signs and behaviors can be physical, emotional, behavioral, or spiritual. Affirm: Acknowledge the feeling of distress and affirm the professional obligations of the profession. Assess: Identify source and severity of distress and assess readiness to act by analyzing risks and benefits of courses of action. Act: Prepare to take action, implement strategies to initiate the changes you desire, and anticipate and manage setbacks.

6. Any five of the following: aromatherapy, progressive muscle relaxation, biofeedback, meditation, hypnosis, massage, therapeutic touch, purposeful touch, music, pet therapy, humor, acupuncture

7.
   a. Facial expression
   b. Body movements
   c. Compliance with ventilator or vocalization
   d. Muscle tension

8.
   a. Evaluate relationships in the institution and on your unit.
   b. Establish a multidisciplinary critical care committee co-chaired by a physician and a nurse.
   c. Establish multidisciplinary professional activities such as rounding, education, research, and quality and safety programs.
   d. Establish a professional nursing environment.
   e. Implement principles of TeamSTEPPS, shifting the focus to the team rather than the individual.

9.
   a. Identify and eliminate or minimize stress.
   b. Correct misconceptions.
   c. Personalize the message.
   d. Relate information to past experiences and actively involve the patient and family.
   e. Apply appropriate teaching strategies such as explaining the meaning of unfamiliar words, use common words and examples, review content frequently, check back on learning, and use short sentences.

10.
   a. Collect information and identify the problem.
   b. Identify possible solutions or actions.
   c. Analyze the possible consequences of each solution or action.
   d. Select the best possible solution or action.
   e. Implement the solution or action.
   f. Evaluate the results.

11. American Indian, Appalachians, Chinese Americans, Vietnamese Americans

12. 1. f; 2. g; 3. e; 4. d; 5. b; 6. a; 7. c

13. Integration of the best practice, clinician expertise, patient values, and circumstances.

CHAPTER 3

1.

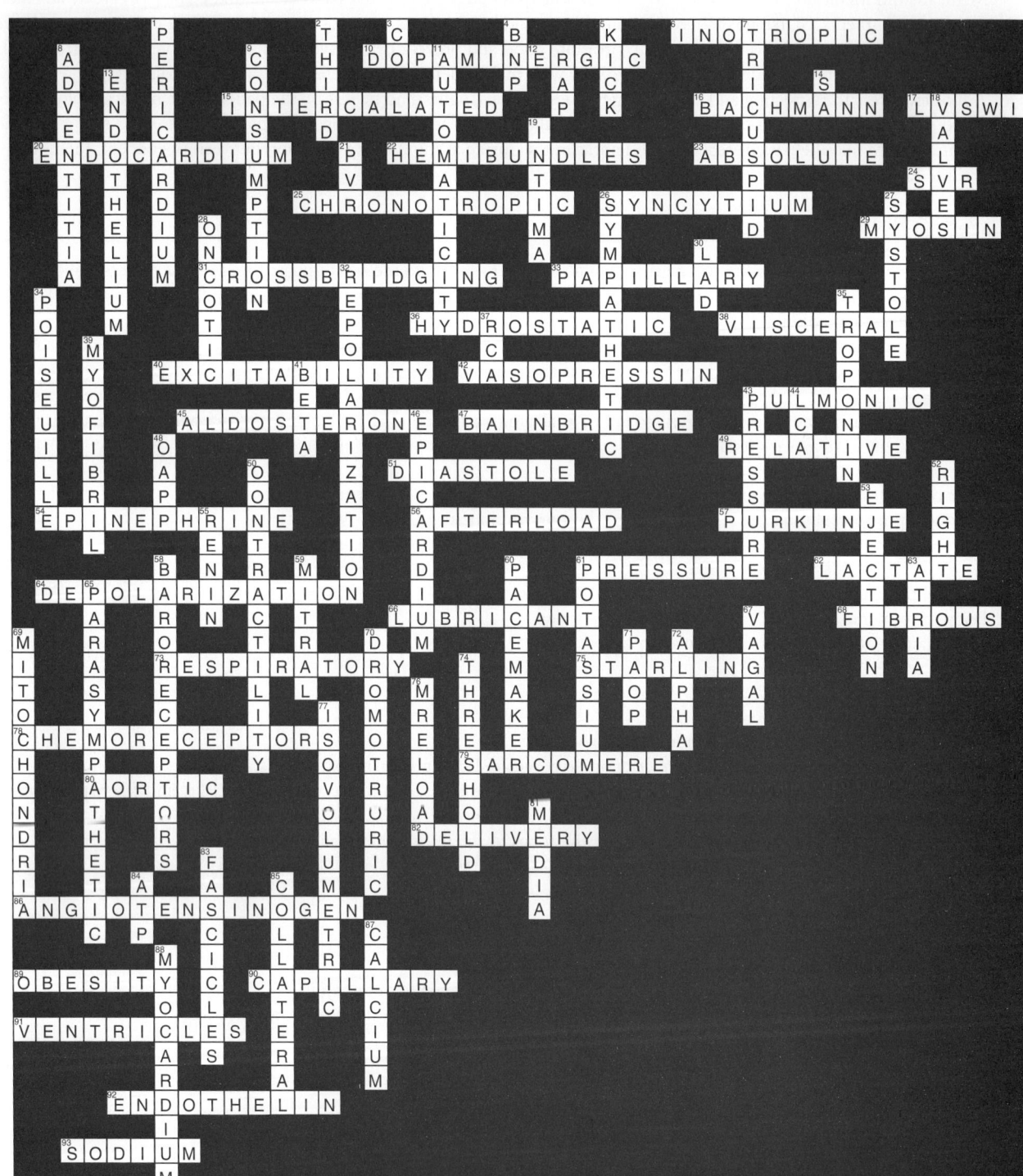

2.

Structure	Coronary Artery
Anterior left ventricle	LAD
AV node	Most commonly RCA; less commonly LCA
Bundle branches	LAD
Inferior left ventricle	RCA
Lateral left ventricle	LCA
Left atrium	LCA
Posterior left ventricle	Most commonly RCA; less commonly LCA
Right atrium	RCA
Right ventricle	RCA
SA node	Most commonly RCA; less commonly LCA
Septum	LAD

3.

Myocardial Oxygen Supply	Myocardial Oxygen Demand
Coronary artery patency	Heart rate
Diastolic pressure	Preload
Diastolic time	Afterload
Oxygen extraction: hemoglobin; SaO_2	Contractility

4. Remember that you were asked to identify primary effects. If you gave answers other than these, perhaps you were thinking of the secondary effects, especially those mediated by the SNS or the resultant effect of a decrease in preload on contractility.

Conditions				
Aortic stenosis	– Heart rate	– Preload	↑ LV afterload	– Contractility
Bradydysrhythmias	↓ Heart rate	↑ Preload	– Afterload	– Contractility
Cardiac tamponade	– Heart rate	↓ Preload	– Afterload	– Contractility
Cardiogenic shock	– Heart rate	↑ Preload	↑ Afterload	↓ Contractility
Cardiomyopathy	– Heart rate	– Preload	– Afterload	↓ Contractility
Heart failure	– Heart rate	↑ Preload	↑ Afterload	↓ Contractility
Hypertension	– Heart rate	– Preload	↑ LV afterload	– Contractility
Hypovolemia	– Heart rate	↓ Preload	– Afterload	– Contractility
Left ventricular myocardial infarction	– Heart rate	– Preload	– Afterload	↓ Contractility
Neurogenic shock	↓ Heart rate	↓ Preload	↓ Afterload	– Contractility
Pulmonary hypertension	– Heart rate	– Preload	↑ RV afterload	– Contractility
Right ventricular myocardial infarction	– Heart rate	↑ RV preload ↓ LV preload	– Afterload	↓ Contractility
Septic shock—early	– Heart rate	↓ Preload	↓ Afterload	↑ Contractility
Septic shock—late	– Heart rate	↓ Preload	↓ Afterload	↓ Contractility
Tachydysrhythmias	↑ Heart rate	↓ Preload	– Afterload	– Contractility
Treatments				
Aminophylline	– Heart rate	– Preload	↓ RV afterload	– Contractility
Digoxin	↓ Heart rate	– Preload	– Afterload	↑ Contractility
Dobutamine	– Heart rate	↓ Preload	↓ Afterload	↑ Contractility
Dopamine (3–5 mcg/kg/min)	↑ Heart rate	– Preload	– Afterload	↑ Contractility

Treatments—cont'd				
Dopamine (5–10 mcg/kg/min)	↑ Heart rate	– Preload	↑ Afterload	↑ Contractility
Dopamine (>10 mcg/kg/min)	↑ Heart rate	– Preload	↑ Afterload	– Contractility
Fluid challenge	– Heart rate	↑ Preload	– Afterload	– Contractility
Furosemide	– Heart rate	↓ Preload	↓ RV afterload	– Contractility
Intraaortic balloon pump	– Heart rate	– Preload	↓ Afterload	– Contractility
Isoproterenol	↑ Heart rate	↓ Preload	↓ Afterload	↑ Contractility
Milrinone	– Heart rate	↓ Preload	↓ Afterload	↑ Contractility
Nesiritide	– Heart rate	↓ Preload	↓ Afterload	– Contractility
Nitroglycerin	– Heart rate	↓ Preload	Afterload*	– Contractility
Nitroprusside	– Heart rate	↓ Preload	↓ Afterload	– Contractility
Phenylephrine	– Heart rate	– Preload	↑ Afterload	– Contractility
Propranolol	↓ Heart rate	– Preload	– Afterload	↓ Contractility
Vasopressin	– Heart rate	– Preload	↑ Afterload	– Contractility

*Nitroglycerin will decrease afterload if dosage is greater than 1 mcg/kg/min or approximately 70 mcg/min in a 70-kg patient.

5.
   1. b; 2. d; 3. a, e; 4. c

6.
   1. c; 2. d; 3. a; 4. b

7.

Parameter	Formula
a. Cardiac output (CO)	Heart rate (HR) × stroke volume (SV)
b. Stroke index (SI)	Cardiac index (CI) ÷ heart rate (HR)
c. Blood pressure (BP)	Cardiac output (CO) × systemic vascular resistance (SVR)
d. Coronary artery perfusion pressure (CAPP)	Diastolic BP − pulmonary artery occlusive pressure (PAOP)
e. Mean arterial pressure (MAP)	[BP systolic + (BP diastolic × 2)] ÷ 3
f. Systemic vascular resistance (SVR)	[(MAP − RAP) × 80] ÷ CO
g. Delivery of oxygen to the tissues (DO_2)	Hgb × SaO_2 × CO × 13.4

8.
   1. k; 2. i; 3. a; 4. f; 5. b; 6. h; 7. m; 8. c; 9. j; 10. g; 11. d; 12. l; 13. e.

9.

Condition	Timing	Location	Pitch
Mitral regurgitation	Systolic	Mitral (apex)	High
Mitral stenosis	Diastolic	Mitral (apex)	Low
Aortic regurgitation	Diastolic	Aortic (base)	High
Aortic stenosis	Systolic	Aortic (base)	High
Mitral valve prolapse	Systolic	Mitral (apex)	High
Papillary muscle dysfunction or rupture	Systolic	Mitral (apex)	High
Ventricular septal defect or rupture	Systolic	LLSB	High

NOTES:
1 To figure out timing, consider when the valve would have been open or closed. For example, in mitral regurgitation, the mitral valve would not be closed when it should be closed, which is during systole, so this is a systolic murmur. Another example is that the aortic valve would not be open when it should be open in aortic stenosis, so this is also a systolic murmur.
2 To figure out location, consider the auscultatory areas; a mitral valve problem would cause a murmur in the mitral auscultatory area which is at the apex.
3 To figure out pitch, remember that all murmurs are high-pitched except murmurs of AV valve stenosis (i.e., mitral or tricuspid stenosis).

10.

1. k; 2. e; 3. j; 4. b; 5. f; 6. c; 7. p; 8. g; 9. h; 10. m; 11. o; 12. d; 13. n; 14. t; 15. s; 16. i; 17. a; 18. l; 19. q, 20. r

11.

a. Ventricular fibrillation
b. Sinus bradycardia with wide QRS (BBB should be assessed for on 12-lead ECG)
c. Supraventricular tachycardia; this is a regular narrow QRS tachycardia with no discernible P waves; the P waves could be hidden in the QRS or T wave, so there is no way to identify where above the ventricle the rhythm originates, but the rate of 180 beats/min
suggests an atrial origin.
d. Idioventricular (escape) rhythm
e. Underlying sinus rhythm (atrial rate is 90 beats/min); there is a third-degree AV block with a ventricular escape rhythm (ventricular rate is 35 beats/min)
f. Underlying rhythm is sinus rhythm (atrial rate is 80 beats/min); there is a second-degree type I (Wenckebach) AV block present; conduction ratio is 3:2 and ventricular rate is 40 to 50 beats/min
g. Ventricular tachycardia (monomorphic)
h. Underlying rhythm is sinus tachycardia (atrial rate is 145 beats/min); there is a second-degree type II block present; conduction ratio is variable but the PR interval of the conducted P wave is consistent
i. Sinus rhythm with two unifocal PVCs

12.

1. g; 2. k; 3. n; 4. b; 5. l; 6. e; 7. f; 8. h; 9. d; 10. m; 11. j; 12. i; 13. c; 14. a

13.

1. g; 2. e; 3. b; 4. f; 5. a; 6. c; 7. d

14.

a. RBBB: Note indicative changes of BBB in V_1 (RV lead) and the wide QRS is totally above the isoelectric line in V_1.
b. LBBB: Note indicative changes of BBB in V_6 (LV lead) and the wide QRS is totally below the isoelectric line in V_1.

15.

a. Right axis deviation: Note negative QRS in I and positive QRS in aVF. Right atrial enlargement: Note tall, peaked P wave in lead II and dominant initial component of the P wave in V_1. Right ventricular hypertrophy: Note dominant R in V_1 along with RAD, RAE, and strain pattern (i.e., asymmetric T wave inversion in V_1 and V_2).
b. Normal axis: Note positive QRS in I and isoelectric QRS in aVF. Left atrial enlargement: Note wide, notched P wave in lead II. Left ventricular hypertrophy: Note deep S wave (must be doubled since voltage was halved when the ECG was recorded) in V_1 and tall R wave in V_5. To check for voltage criteria, add the S in V_1 or V_2 and the R in V_5 or V_6. Because the sum is greater than 35 mm (40 in this case), voltage criteria for LVH are met.

16.

a. Normal axis: Note positive QRS in I and positive QRS in aVF. ST segment elevation is noted from V_1 - V_6. Pathologic Q waves are noted in V_2 and V_3. There is a small R wave in V_1 so the negative wave in that lead is an S wave. This ECG shows evidence of hyperacute anterior MI with injury extending to the septal and lateral walls.
b. Left axis deviation: Note positive QRS in I and negative QRS in aVF. ST segment elevation and pathologic Q waves are noted in II, III, and aVF indicative of acute inferior MI. Reciprocal changes in the V leads (ST-segment depression from V_1–V_5) suggests posterior wall involvement also. Posterior wall leads are indicated.

17.

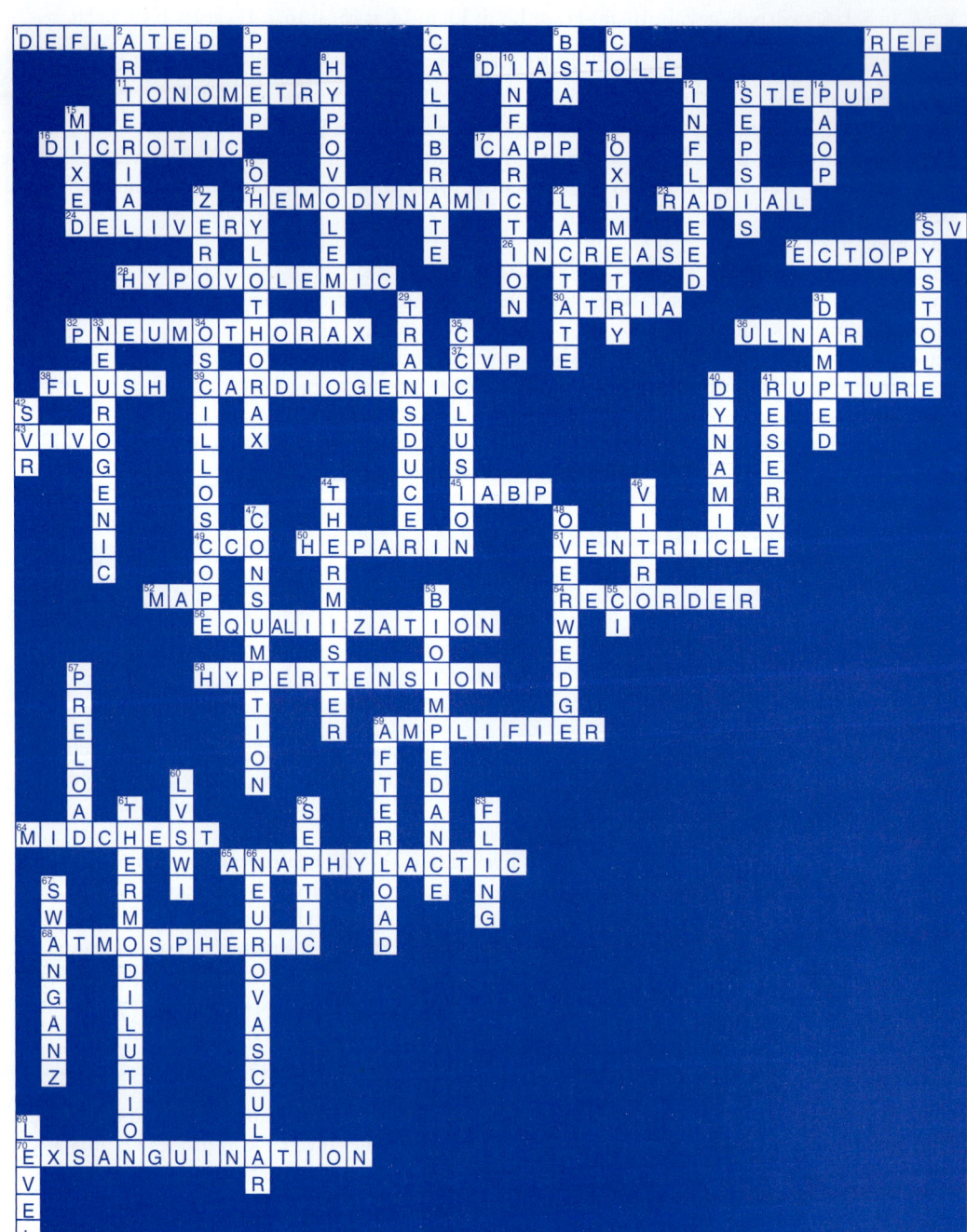

18.

1. i; 2. h; 3. g; 4. b; 5. d; 6. c; 7. a; 8. f; 9. e

Learning Activities Answers

19.

a.

Parameter	↑, ↓, or Normal	Parameter	↑, ↓, or Normal
BP: 88/70 mm Hg	↓	SV: 23 ml/beat	↓
MAP: 76 mm Hg	Normal	SI: 14 ml/m^2/beat	↓
HR: 128 beats/min	↑	SVR: 1813 dynes/sec/cm^{-5}	↑
RAP: 8 mm Hg	↑	SVRI: 3022 dynes/sec/cm^{-5}	↑
PAP: 42/26 mm Hg	↑	PVR: 240 dynes/sec/cm^{-5}	Normal
PAm: 31 mm Hg	↑	PVRI: 400 dynes/sec/cm^{-5}	Normal
PAOP: 22 mm Hg	↑	LVSWI: 10.3 g m/m^2	↓
CO: 3.0 l/min	↓	RVSWI: 2.7 g m/m^2	↓
CI: 1.8 l/min/m^2	↓	SvO$_2$: 51%	↓
SaO$_2$: 88% on 5 l/min via nasal cannula	↓	DO$_2$I: 318 ml/min/m^2	↓

Implications and treatment goals: Patient A is in cardiogenic shock as evidenced by the low cardiac index and increased PAOP and RAP along with the increase in SVR and SVRI. Myocardial oxygen demand is being increased by the increased heart rate, increased preload (note PAOP and RAP), and increased afterload (note SVR). Treatment priorities at this time are to increase contractility (dobutamine), decrease preload (dobutamine will affect preload to some degree but careful IV titration of nitroglycerin or the administration of furosemide may be required), and decrease afterload (IABP may be used since even careful titration of an arterial vasodilator such as nitroprusside may drop the MAP to below 60 mm Hg, which is required to perfuse vital organs).

b.

Parameter	↑, ↓, or Normal	Parameter	↑, ↓, or Normal
BP: 92/70 mm Hg	↓	SV: 24 ml/beat	↓
MAP: 77 mm Hg	Normal	SI: 13 ml/m^2/beat	↓
HR: 122 beats/min	↑	SVR: 2097 dynes/sec/cm^{-5}	↑
RAP: 1 mm Hg	↓	SVRI: 4053 dynes/sec/cm^{-5}	↑
PAP: 20/6 mm Hg	↓	PVR: 221 dynes/sec/cm^{-5}	Normal
PAm: 11 mm Hg	↓	PVRI: 427 dynes/sec/cm^{-5}	Normal
PAOP: 3 mm Hg	↓	LVSWI: 13.1 g m/m^2	↓
CO: 2.9 l/min	↓	RVSWI: 1.8 g m/m^2	↓
CI: 1.5 l/min/m^2	↓	SvO$_2$: 50%	↓
SaO$_2$: 95% on 5 l/min via nasal cannula	Normal with supplemental O$_2$	DO$_2$I: 134 ml/min/m^2	↓
Hgb: 7 g/dl	↓		

Implications and treatment goals: Patient B is in hypovolemic shock evidenced by the low cardiac index with low PAOP and RAP. Heart rate and SVR and SVRI are elevated because of sympathetic nervous system stimulation. The current treatment priority is to replace blood volume because surgery has been accomplished to stop the blood loss. Considering that the primary fluid loss was blood, blood replacement in the form of either whole blood or packed cells is required along with the normal saline as a primary crystalloid. Hemoglobin is critical for oxygen delivery to the tissues, and his history of coronary artery disease accentuates this need. Notice how profound the DO$_2$ is reduced since the hemoglobin and the cardiac output are insufficient to adequately deliver oxygen to the tissues.

20.

1. f; 2. g; 3. a; 4. h; 5. i; 6. d; 7. c; 8. f; 9. j; 10. h; 11. b; 12. e

21.

Drugs	Classification
Adenosine	Unclassified
Amiodarone	III
Atropine	Unclassified
Digoxin	Unclassified
Diltiazem	IV
Dofetilide	III
Esmolol	II

750 Learning Activities Answers

Drugs	Classification
Flecainide	IC
Ibutilide	III
Lidocaine	IB
Metoprolol	II
Procainamide	IA
Propranolol	II
Quinidine	IA
Sotalol	II and III
Verapamil	IV

22.
  a. 24 ml/hr
  b. 2 mcg/kg/min
  c. 5 mcg/kg/min
  d. 10 ml/hr
  e. 30 ml/hr
  f. 45 ml/hr

23.

AOO	VVI		a. DVI
VVI	VAT		b. VDD
AAI	VAT	VVI	c. DDD

24.

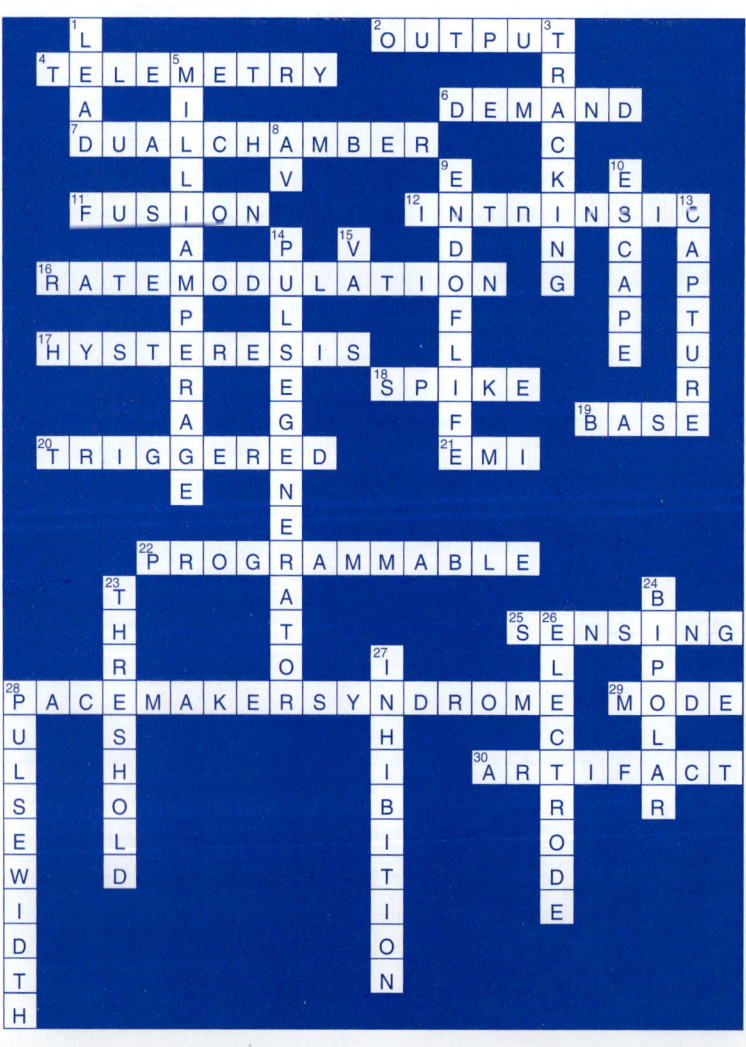

25.
   a. Interpretation: VVI with normal function; complex #4 is a PVC and it is sensed appropriately
   b. Interpretation: DVI function with failure to sense; complex #5 shows atrial pacing with an intrinsic ventricular complex that is not sensed
   c. Interpretation: VVI with intermittent failure to capture; after the third paced complex, there is a nonconducted pacing spike; after the fourth paced complex, there is a nonconducted pacing spike

26.

Nonmodifiable	Modifiable
Heredity	Hypertension
Advancing age	Diabetes mellitus or glucose intolerance
Male gender	Hyperlipidemia
	Hyperhomocysteinemia
	Sedentary lifestyle
	Stress
	Obesity
	Cigarette smoking
	Oral contraceptives (especially in smokers)

27.
   1. a; 2. a; 3. g; 4. d, c; 5. c; 6. b, h; 7. e, h; 8. e, f; 9. e; 10. i, j

28.

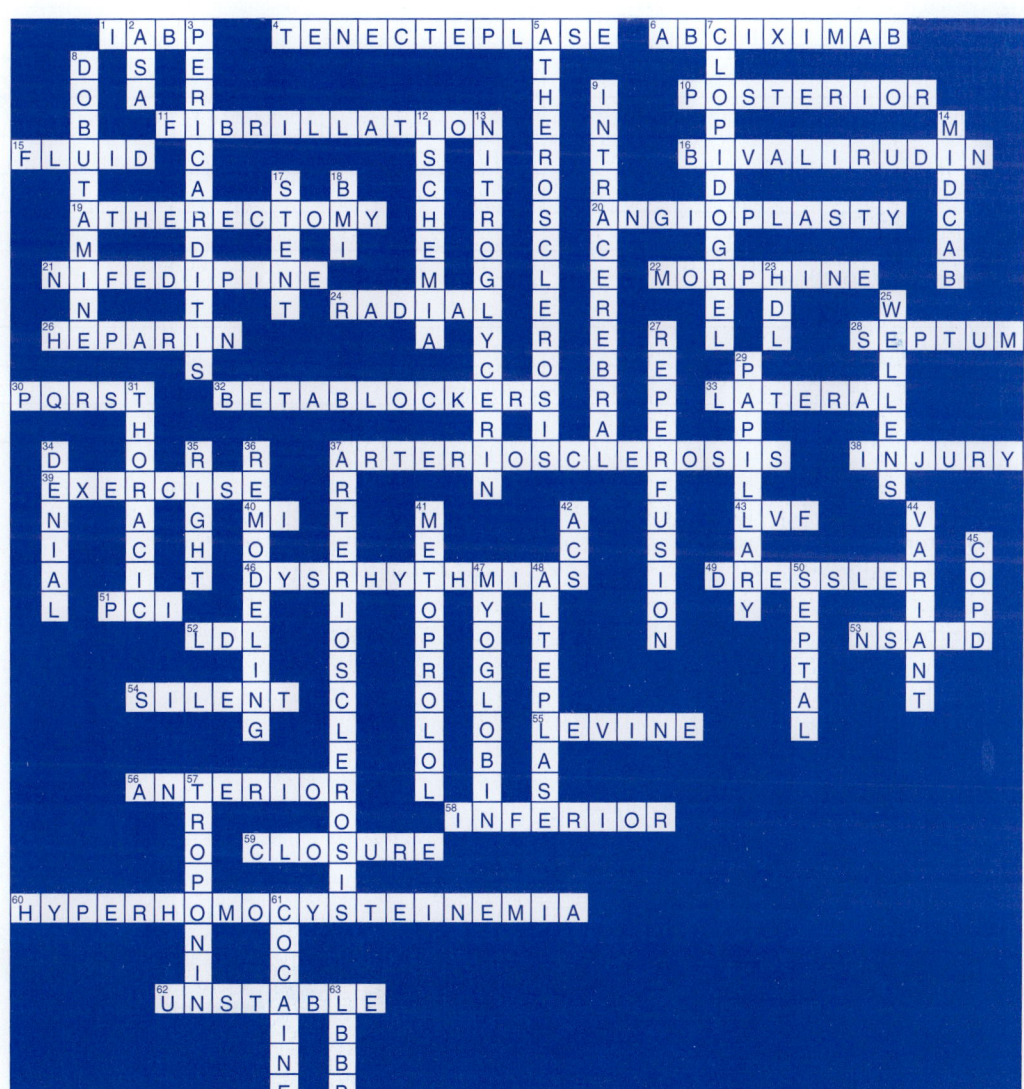

29.
   1. a, b, d, g, j, m; 2. b, c, g, l; 3. e; 4. a, f; 5. a, e, h, n; 6. g; 7. i, k

30.

Causes	Left	Right
Aortic stenosis	✓	
Cardiac tamponade	✓	✓
Cardiomyopathy	✓	✓
Mitral stenosis	✓ (Forward failure)	✓ (Backward failure)
Myocardial infarction (left)	✓	
Myocardial infarction (right)		✓
Pulmonary embolism	✓ (Forward failure)	✓ (Backward failure)
Pulmonary hypertension		✓
Systemic hypertension	✓	
Sign/Symptom	**Left**	**Right**
Abnormal liver function studies		✓
Ascites		✓
Atrial dysrhythmias	✓	✓
Crackles audible over lungs	✓	
Dyspnea	✓	
Elevated PAOP	✓	
Elevated RAP		✓
Hepatomegaly		✓
Jugular venous distention		✓
Mental confusion	✓	
Murmur of mitral regurgitation	✓	
Murmur of tricuspid regurgitation		✓
Orthopnea	✓	
Peripheral edema		✓
S_3, S_4 at apex	✓	
S_3, S_4 at sternum		✓
Weight gain	✓	✓

31.
   a. 1) Increases coronary artery perfusion pressure
      2) Decreases afterload
   b. 1) Aortic regurgitation
      2) Aortic aneurysm
   c. Diastole
   d. Systole
   e. 1) Ischemia of left arm
      2) Renal ischemia

32.
   a. Assisted aortic end-diastolic pressure
   b. Unassisted aortic end-diastolic pressure
   c. Assisted systole
   d. Unassisted systole
   e. Diastolic augmentation

33.
   a. Yes. EF less than 40%
   b. Systolic. This is pump failure as evidenced by S_3.

c. Because she has acute decompensated heart failure, IV diuretics would be warranted. Aldactone, an aldosterone antagonist, would likely be helpful. She is already receiving an ACE inhibitor. Inotropic agents may be used.
   d. Continuous renal replacement therapy, such as continuous venous-venous hemofiltration, might be used. Cardiac resynchronization therapy with a biventricular pacemaker may be indicated. Also, a frank discussion of end-of-life care with the patient and family is indicated.
   e. D
34.

Drug	Arterial Dilator	Venous Dilator
Clevidipine	✓	
Dobutamine	✓	✓
Fenoldopam	✓	
Hydralazine	✓	
Milrinone	✓	✓
Minoxidil	✓	
Morphine sulfate		✓
Nifedipine	✓	✓
Nitroglycerin (less than 1 mcg/kg/min)		✓
Nitroglycerin (>1 mcg/kg/min)	✓	✓
Nitroprusside	✓	✓
Phentolamine	✓	✓
Prazosin	✓	✓

35.
   a.
      - BP 220/140 mm Hg
      - Left ventricular failure (dyspnea, tachypnea, S_3, crackles, hypoxemia, pulmonary edema on chest x-ray)
        - (NOTE: You would expect tachycardia, but remember that the beta-blocker has prevented this sympathetic nervous system compensatory mechanism.)
      - Left ventricular hypertrophy (displaced PMI, cardiomegaly on chest radiography, ventricular strain and large R waves in left ventricular leads)
      - Renal insufficiency (decreased urine output, elevated BUN and creatinine maintaining the normal 10:1 ratio)
      - Occipital headache
   b. Indomethacin (Indocin) and other nonsteroidal antiinflammatory agents inhibit the synthesis of prostaglandins (which are vasodilators) so they increase BP and cause sodium and fluid retention
   c. Heart, brain, kidney, retina
   d. Yes. Hypertensive emergency warrants an admission to a critical care unit.
   e. Reduction of MAP by 25%
   f.

Vasodilator	Nitroprusside, nitroglycerin, hydralazine, nicardipine
ACE inhibitor	Enalapril
Alpha-blocker	Phentolamine
Beta-blocker	Esmolol
Alpha- and beta-blocker	Labetalol

   g. 24 ml/min; because this would result in a significant fluid gain, a more concentrated infusion would be recommended
   h.
      - Nausea, vomiting, abdominal pain: patient report
      - Headache, tinnitus: patient report
      - Coronary artery steal: evidence of myocardial ischemia such as chest pain, ST-segment elevation
      - Nitroprusside-induced intrapulmonary shunt: decrease in SpO_2, decrease in SaO_2 and PaO_2 on ABGs
      - Methemoglobinemia: decrease in SpO_2, decrease in SaO_2 on ABGs, increase in methemoglobin levels
      - Thiocyanate toxicity: metabolic acidosis, confusion, hyperreflexia, seizures, elevated thiocyanate levels
   i. No. Nifedipine has never been approved by the Food and Drug Administration for sublingual (or bite and swallow) use and is no longer recommended because of the precipitous drops in BP that may occur.

j. Labetalol would have been preferable because nitroprusside's effect of causing direct vasodilation may increase intracranial pressure.

k.
- Murmur of aortic regurgitation (high-pitched diastolic murmur) heard best in aortic (second right intercostal space at the right sternal border) area
- BP differences from left arm to right arm or left leg to right leg
- "Ripping" or "tearing" chest pain
- Chest pain that radiates to the back
- Hypotension or shock
- Widening of mediastinum on chest x-ray

36.

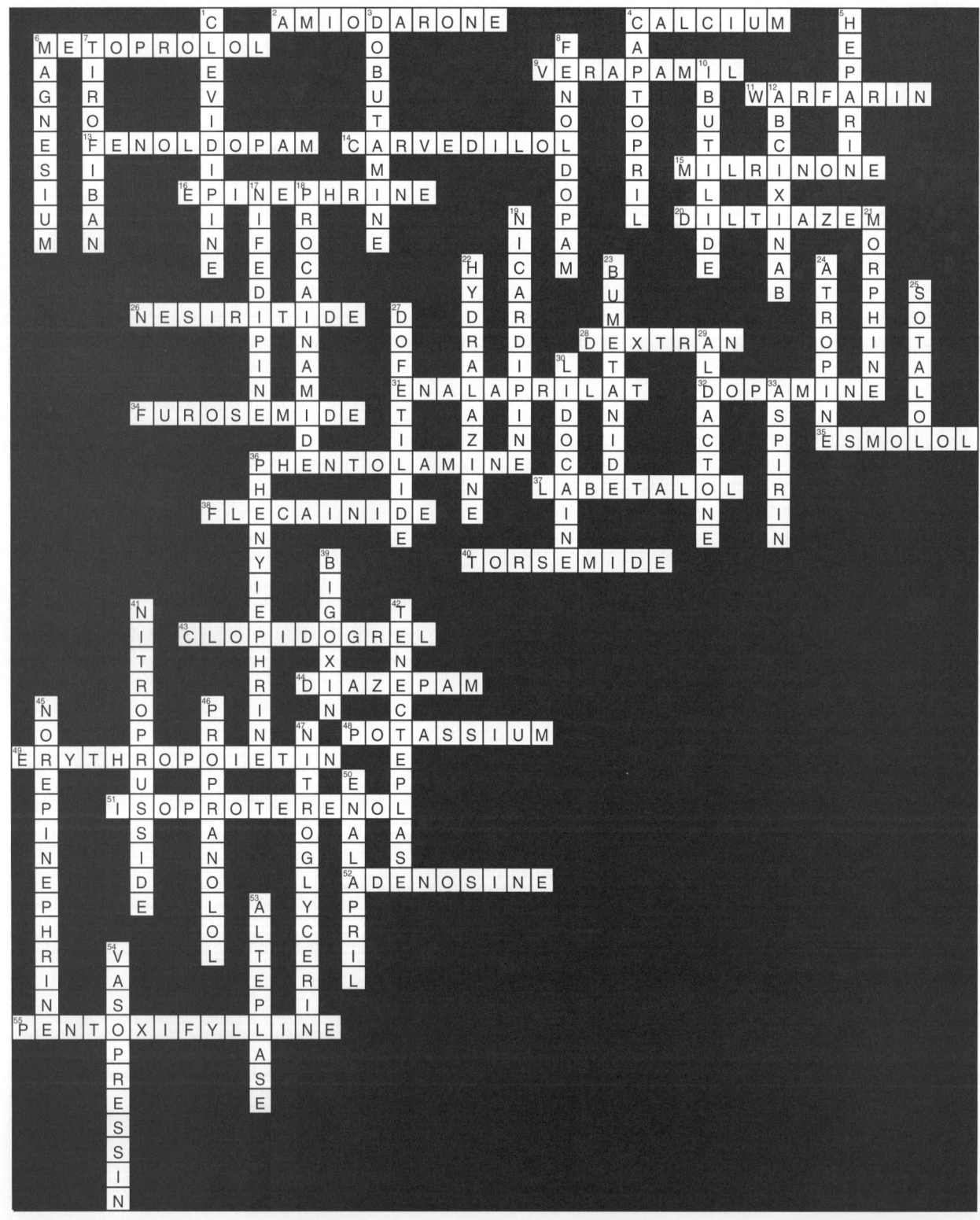

CHAPTER 4

1.

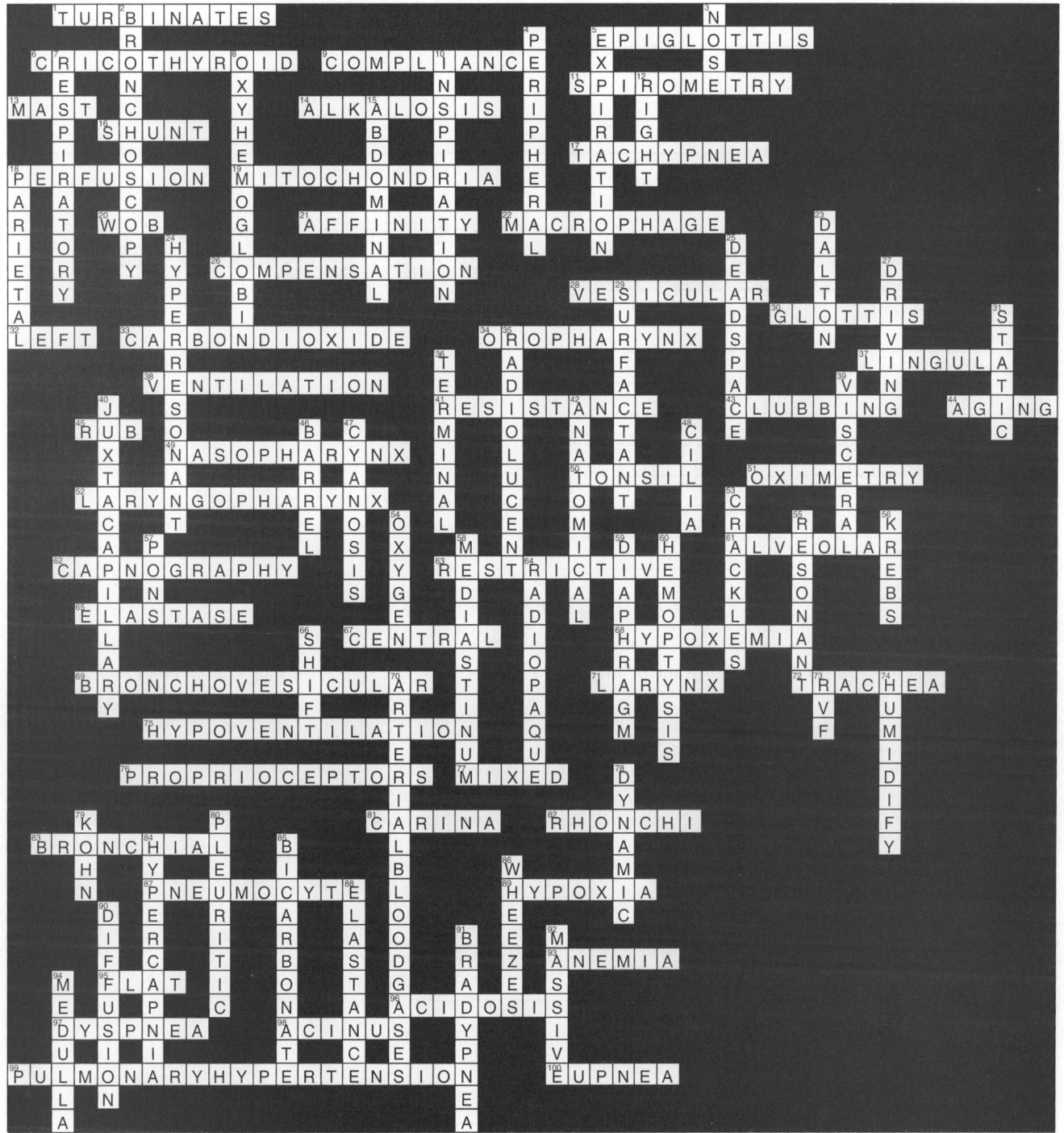

2.

	Primary	**Accessory**
Inspiration	Diaphragm External intercostals	Scalene Sternocleidomastoid
Expiration	None; expiration is normally passive	Internal oblique External oblique Rectus abdominis Internal intercostals Transverse abdominis

3.

	Left	**Right**
Increased 2,3-DPG		X
Hypothermia	X	
Hypercapnia		X
Hyperthermia		X
Acidosis		X
Decreased 2,3-DPG	X	
Hypocapnia	X	
Alkalosis	X	
Hypophosphatemia	X	
Massive blood transfusion	X	

4.

Driving pressure of oxygen = FiO_2 × barometric pressure so FiO_2 of 1.0 × barometric pressure at sea level of 760 mm Hg so driving pressure of oxygen = 760 mm Hg

$PAO_2 = FiO_2 (P_b - 47) - (PaCO_2/ 0.8)$ so 1.0 (760 − 47) − 37/0.8 so PAO_2 = 1.0 × (760−47) − 50/0.8 so 713 − 50 so PAO_2 = 663 mm Hg

A:a gradient = $PAO_2 - PaO_2$ so 663 − 60 so A:a gradient = 603 mm Hg

Estimated shunt = A:a gradient × 0.05 so estimated shunt ≅ 30% (remember that normal is ≈ 5%)

P/F ratio = PaO_2/FiO_2 so 60/1.0 so P/F ratio = 60 mm Hg (remember that P/F ratio of less than 200 is characteristic of ARDS)

5.

	Restrictive	**Obstructive**
Obesity hypoventilation syndrome	X	
Asthma		X
Pneumothorax	X	
Atelectasis	X	
Pneumonia	X	
Kyphoscoliosis	X	
Pulmonary edema	X	
Mucus plugs		X
Lung cancer (bronchial)		X
Lung cancer (parenchymal)	X	
Chronic bronchitis		X
Artificial airway		X
Bronchospasm		X

6.

Condition	Breath Sound Change or Changes
Emphysema	Diminished breath sounds
Atelectasis	Diminished breath sounds Bronchial or bronchovesicular breath sounds Crackles
Pneumonia	Diminished breath sounds Bronchial or bronchovesicular breath sounds Rhonchi may be present
Chronic bronchitis	Rhonchi Wheezes may also be present
Pneumothorax	Diminished or absent breath sounds
Pulmonary fibrosis	Diminished breath sounds Crackles
Asthma	Wheezes Rhonchi
Pulmonary edema	Crackles Wheezes (referred to as *cardiac asthma*) may be present
Pleurisy	Pleural friction rub
Hemothorax	Diminished or absent breath sounds
Pleural effusion	Diminished breath sounds
Pulmonary embolism	Crackles Pleural friction rub if pulmonary infarction develops

7.
   1. b; 2. c; 3. h; 4. a, i; 5. e; 6. i; 7. g; 8. d; 9. e; 10. f

8.
   1. b; 2. d; 3. e; 4. f; 5. a; 6. c; 7. h; 8. g

9.

Tidal volume	~7 ml/kg
Vital capacity	>15 ml/kg
Maximal inspiratory pressure	<(more negative than) −60 cm H_2O
PaO_2	80–100 mm Hg
SaO_2	>95%
SvO_2	60%–80%

10.

a.	Respiratory acidosis
b.	Metabolic alkalosis
c.	Respiratory acidosis (but with elevated bicarbonate; chronic compensated respiratory acidosis with decompensation)
d.	Metabolic alkalosis
e.	Respiratory alkalosis
f.	Metabolic acidosis

11.

	pH	PaCO$_2$	HCO$_3^-$	PaO$_2$	Answer
1.	7.30	54	26	64	Respiratory acidosis with hypoxemia
2.	7.48	30	24	96	Respiratory alkalosis
3.	7.30	40	18	85	Metabolic acidosis
4.	7.50	40	33	92	Metabolic alkalosis
5.	7.35	54	30	55	Compensated respiratory acidosis with significant hypoxemia
6.	7.21	60	20	48	Mixed disorder: respiratory and metabolic acidosis with significant hypoxemia
7.	7.54	25	30	95	Mixed disorder: respiratory alkalosis and metabolic alkalosis
8.	7.40	58	33	72	Mixed disorder: respiratory acidosis and metabolic alkalosis* with mild hypoxemia
9.	7.40	30	18	89	Mixed disorder: respiratory alkalosis and metabolic acidosis*
10.	7.40	40	24	98	Normal
11.	7.33	40	21	62	Metabolic acidosis with hypoxemia
12.	7.34	60	34	70	Respiratory acidosis with partial compensation and hypoxemia
13.	7.29	32	15	98	Metabolic acidosis with partial compensation
14.	7.52	28	22	95	Respiratory alkalosis with partial compensation
15.	7.49	48	38	72	Metabolic alkalosis with partial compensation and hypoxemia

*Without history and previous gases, what looks like a mixed disorder could be compensation and vice versa. Remember that whereas a midline pH makes a mixed disorder with both an acidosis and an alkalosis more likely, a leaning pH makes compensation more likely.

12.

a. The term *hypoxemia* indicates that there is decreased oxygen in the blood; *hypoxia* indicates that there is decreased oxygen in the tissue.

b. Because hypoxemia indicates a decrease in blood oxygen, blood parameters are used, such as PaO$_2$ (<80 mm Hg) or SaO$_2$ or SpO$_2$ (<95%).

c. Clinical indications of oxygen deficit are not evident until the tissues are deficient. The brain is a very sensitive indicator of low oxygen, so restlessness and confusion are indications that brain oxygen levels are low. The adrenal glands are also sensitive to low oxygen levels and they release catecholamines to cause tachycardia and tachypnea. Central cyanosis may also occur. Serum arterial lactate levels would increase because of the shift to anaerobic from aerobic metabolism.

d. Absolutely. Because hypoxemia is present when PaO$_2$ is less than 80 mm Hg and SaO$_2$ is less than 95%, the tissues are still able to maintain normal oxygen levels by increasing the amount of oxygen that they extract. This would be reflected by a decrease in SvO$_2$. Generally, consider a PaO$_2$ of less than 60 mm Hg and SaO$_2$ of less than 90% as consistent with both hypoxemia *and* hypoxia. You can also relate this to the oxyhemoglobin dissociation curve because PaO$_2$ of 60 mm Hg and SaO$_2$ of 90% is when the curve changes from horizontal to vertical, so any decrease in PaO$_2$ results in a more significant decrease in SaO$_2$.

e. Absolutely. Even with a normal PaO$_2$ and SaO$_2$, if the hemoglobin or cardiac output or cardiac index is reduced, oxygen delivery to the tissues is deficient and hypoxia occurs. Some other factors to be considered are shift of the oxyhemoglobin dissociation curve to the left, decreased extraction by the tissues such as occurs in sepsis, and then local perfusion issues such as peripheral vascular disease.

13.

Problem	Preferred Artificial Airway
Tongue against hypopharynx	Oropharyngeal or nasopharyngeal
Need for frequent nasotracheal suctioning	Nasopharyngeal
Inability to open mouth (e.g., seizure)	Nasopharyngeal
Facial or jaw fracture	Nasopharyngeal or nasotracheal tube
Complete upper airway obstruction when endotracheal intubation is impossible (e.g., laryngeal edema or spasm, tracheal fracture)	Cricothyrotomy or tracheostomy
Need for sealed airway (e.g., mechanical ventilation or potential for aspiration)	Endotracheal tube or tracheostomy LMA but less protection from aspiration
Need for long-term lower airway access and sealed airway	Tracheostomy

NOTE: Nasal cannula should be for short-term use only because of the risk of sinus infection.

14.

1. d; 2. e; 3. a; 4. b; 5. c

15.

1. i; 2. q; 3. e; 4. a; 5. j; 6. d; 7. h; 8. f; 9. c; 10. g; 11. m; 12. o; 13. k; 14. p; 15. n; 16. b; 17. l

16.

a. Increase the driving pressure of oxygen
b. Decrease surface tension
c. Decrease intrapulmonary shunt (alveolar recruitment)
d. Aid in prevention of ventilator-induced lung injury

17.

	High Pressure	Low Exhaled Volume
Cuff leak		✗
Bronchospasm	✗	
Need for suctioning	✗	
Disconnect		✗
Water condensation in tubing	✗	
Pneumothorax	✗	
ARDS	✗	

18.

a. Spontaneous tidal volume: at least 5 ml/kg
b. Spontaneous vital capacity: at least 10 ml/kg
c. Maximal inspiratory pressure: greater than (more negative than) −25 cm H_2O
d. PaO_2 of at least 60 mm Hg on a FiO_2 of no greater than 0.5 with no more than 5 cm H_2O PEEP.
e. Rapid shallow breathing index: less than or equal to 105 breaths/min/l

19.

	Patient A	**Patient B**
Age	38	64
Gender	F	M
Diagnosis	Asthma	ARDS
IBW	60 kg	75 kg
ABGs	FiO_2 of 0.28 pH 7.42 $PaCO_2$ 39 mm Hg HCO_3 25 mEq/l PaO_2 88 mm Hg SaO_2 98%	FiO_2 of 0.6 with 10 cm H_2O PEEP pH 7.32 $PaCO_2$ 50 mm Hg HCO_3 23 mEq/l PaO_2 55 mm Hg SaO_2 88%
Spontaneous V_T	350 ml	300 ml
Spontaneous vital capacity	650 ml	600 ml
Spontaneous minute ventilation	7 l	10.8 l
NIF	−40 cm H_2O	−20 cm H_2O
Spontaneous respiratory rate (f)	20/min	36/min
Rapid shallow breathing index (RSBI)	57 breaths/min/l	120 breaths/min/l
Ready for weaning?	Yes	No

Calculations: To calculate the minute ventilation, you would multiply the tidal volume by the respiratory rate. To calculate the RSBI, you would divide the respiratory rate (frequency) by the spontaneous tidal volume (V_T) in liters, so in patient A, f of 20 is divided by 0.35.

Decision making: Patient A is ready for liberation and extubation. Patient B is not ready for liberation and extubation. Note that Patient B's V_T is less than 5 ml/kg of IBW, his vital capacity is less than 10 ml/kg, and his minute ventilation is more than 10 l. His RSBI is greater than 105 breaths/min/l (should be <105 breaths/min/l). His ABGs show mild respiratory acidosis, which is likely to worsen if mechanical ventilation is not continued. His oxygenation status is still impaired despite an FiO_2 of 0.6 and 10 cm H_2O of PEEP. Also, his VC and NIF both indicate that his coughing ability is impaired, and he will likely not be able to clear his airways if extubated.

Learning Activities Answers

20.

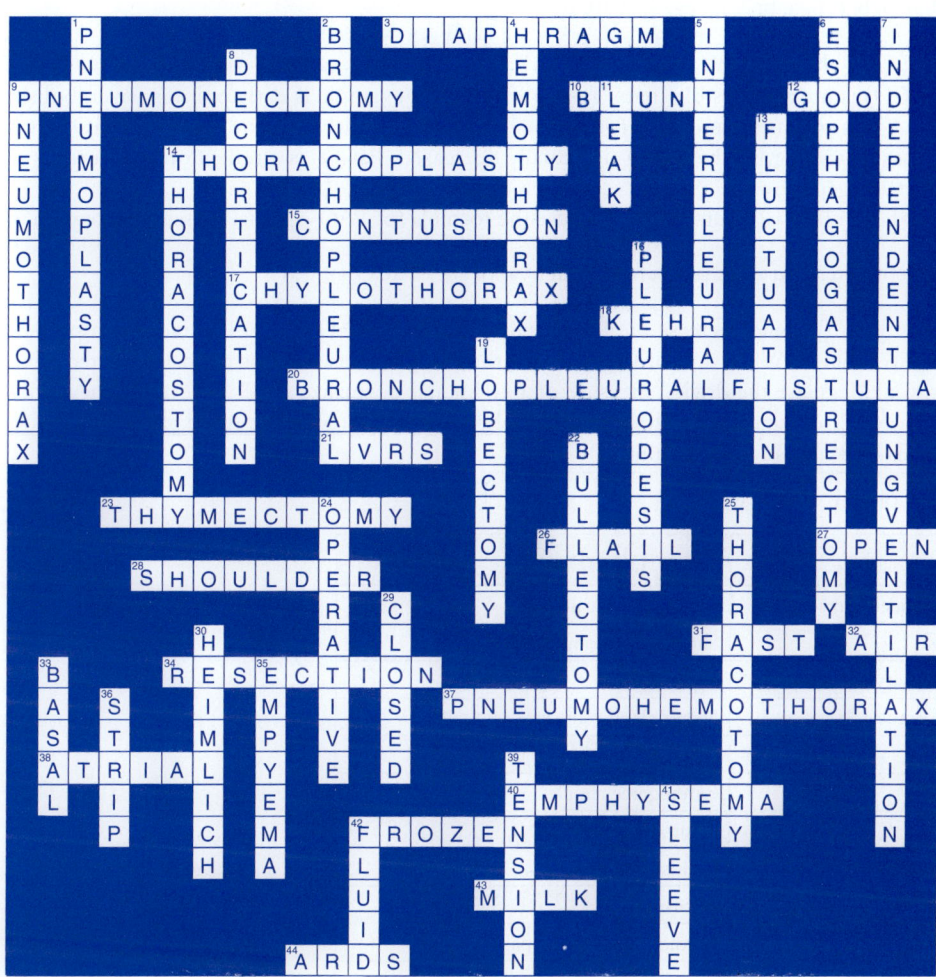

21. Any 10 of the following:

Acute respiratory distress syndrome
Amyotrophic lateral sclerosis
Anesthesia
Aspiration pneumonitis
Asthma
Atelectasis
Chest trauma
CNS depressant drugs
COPD with acute exacerbation
Cystic fibrosis
Epiglottis
Fat embolism
Guillain-Barré syndrome
Head trauma
Kyphoscoliosis
Morbid obesity
Multiple sclerosis
Muscle paralytics

Muscular dystrophy
Myasthenia gravis
Submersion injury
Neuromuscular blocking drugs
Organophosphate poisoning
Pleural effusion
Pneumonia
Pneumothorax
Poliomyelitis
Pulmonary edema
Pulmonary embolism
Pulmonary fibrosis
Sleep apnea
Smoke inhalation
Spinal cord injury
Status asthmaticus
Surgery: especially thoracic, abdominal, flank incision
Tracheal obstruction

22.

1. d; 2. f; 3. i; 4. h; 5. b, c; 6. a, b; 7. j; 8. g; 9. e; 10. b

23.

a. No, because CO_2 is more diffusible than O_2. A great clinical example is early pulmonary embolism, which causes hypoxemia due to a perfusion and therefore diffusion defect. In early PE, the PaO_2 and SaO_2 are decreased, but the patient is hyperventilating, so the $PaCO_2$ is actually decreased. $PaCO_2$ is a reflection of ventilation, and the PaO_2 is a reflection of oxygenation.

b. Yes, because of the effect of Dalton's law. Because the formula for PAO_2 (partial pressure of oxygen in the alveolus) is:

$$(FiO_2 [\text{barometric pressure} - \text{the pressure of water vapor}]) - (PaCO_2 \div 0.8)$$

any increase in $PaCO_2$ would decrease the PAO_2 and therefore the PaO_2. A great clinical example is COPD or any other cause of hypoventilation. When the $PaCO_2$ increases, the PaO_2 decreases unless the patient is receiving supplemental oxygen, which would increase the driving pressure of oxygen and normalize the PaO_2 even if the $PaCO_2$ is increased. This is why the two types of acute respiratory failure are hypoxemic normocapnic (as explained in a. above) and hypoxemic hypercapnic (as explained in b. above).

24. Any five in each column.

Pulmonary	Nonpulmonary
Chest trauma: pulmonary contusion	Sepsis (No. 1 cause)
Near-drowning	Shock or prolonged hypotension
Hypervolemia, pulmonary edema	Septic shock
Inhalation of toxic gases and vapors	Hypovolemic shock
Smoke	Anaphylactic shock
Chemicals	Cardiogenic shock
Oxygen toxicity	Neurogenic shock
Pneumonia	Multisystem trauma
Aspiration pneumonitis	Burns
Radiation pneumonitis	Cardiopulmonary bypass
Pulmonary embolism	Disseminated intravascular coagulation
Radiation	Toxemia of pregnancy
Drugs: bleomycin	Acute pancreatitis
	Diabetic coma
	Head injury
	Drug overdosage
	Multiple blood transfusions

25.

1. b, d; 2. a; 3. b, e; 4. a, d; 5. a, c

26.

Staphylococcus aureus	CAP, HCAP
Serratia marcescens	HCAP
Escherichia coli	HCAP
Legionella pneumophila	CAP, HCAP
Proteus mirabilis	HCAP
Bacteroides fragilis	CAP
Hantavirus	CAP

27.
   a. Elevate the head of the bed 45 degrees.
   b. Ensure appropriate positioning of feeding tube.
   c. Keep cuff of endotracheal tube inflated to 20 to 30 cm H_2O pressure.

28.

Stage	PaO_2	$PaCO_2$	pH	Acid–Base Imbalance
I	↔	↓	↑	Respiratory alkalosis
II	↓	↓	↑	Respiratory alkalosis and mild to moderate hypoxemia
III	↓	↔	↔	Moderate hypoxemia
IV	↓	↑	↓	Respiratory acidosis and critical hypoxemia

29.

Classification	Example
1. Beta$_2$ adrenergic agonists	Salmeterol (Serevent) Metaproterenol (Alupent, Metaprel) Albuterol (Proventil, Ventolin) Pirbuterol (Maxair) Bitolterol (Tornalate) Terbutaline (Brethine, Brethaire)
2. Anticholinergic agents	Ipratropium bromide (Atrovent)
3. Methylxanthines	Aminophylline Theophylline (Theobid, Quibron) Oxtriphylline (Choledyl SA)
4. Electrolyte	Magnesium

30. Any three in each column.

Hypercoagulability	Alteration in Blood Vessel	Venous Stasis
Malignancy	Trauma	Prolonged bed rest or immobilization
Oral contraceptives high in estrogen: especially in smokers	IV drug use	Obesity
Dehydration and hemoconcentration	Aging	Advanced age
Fever	Vasculitis	Burns
Sickle-cell anemia	Varicose veins	Pregnancy
Pregnancy	Diabetes mellitus	Postpartum period
Polycythemia vera	Atherosclerosis	Congestive heart failure
Thrombocytopenia	Inflammatory process	Myocardial infarction
Abrupt discontinuance of anticoagulants		Bacterial endocarditis
Sepsis		Recent surgery especially legs, pelvis, or abdomen
		Thrombus formation in heart (AF)
		Cardioversion

31.

1. e; 2. a, d, f; 3. a, d; 4. b; 5. c; 6. f

32.

Parameter	↑, ↓, or Normal	Parameter	↑, ↓, or Normal
BP: 112/84 mm Hg	Normal	SV: 40 ml/beat	↓
MAP: 93 mm Hg	Normal	SI: 25 ml/m²/beat	↓
HR: 110 beats/min	↑	SVR: 1364 dynes/sec/cm^{-5}	Normal
RAP: 18 mm Hg	↑	SVRI: 2182 dynes/sec/cm^{-5}	Normal
PAP: 55/32 mm Hg	↑	PVR: 618 dynes/sec/cm^{-5}	↑
PAm: 40 mm Hg	↑	PVRI: 989 dynes/sec/cm^{-5}	↑
PAOP: 6 mm Hg	Normal	LVSWI: 30 g m/m²	↓
CO: 4.4 l/min	Normal	RVSWI: 7 g m/m²	Normal
CI: 2.75 l/min/m²	Normal	SvO$_2$: 58%	↓
SaO$_2$: 85% on 5 l/min by nasal cannula	↓	DO$_2$I: 470 ml/min/m²	↓

Implications and treatment goals: The hemodynamic parameters confirm pulmonary hypertension. Note the increase in PAd with a normal PAOP. Remember that if the PAd is more than 5 mm Hg above the PAOP, pulmonary hypertension exists. The increased PVR is further evidence of pulmonary hypertension. Sympathetic nervous system stimulation has caused the tachycardia and the high SVR. Considering her history, you would suspect pulmonary embolism as the cause. V/Q scan or spiral CT would be indicated to aid in the diagnosis of a pulmonary embolism. Arterial blood gases should be analyzed for degree of hypoxemia. Treatment goals for this patient include improving oxygenation (100% by nonrebreathing mask would probably be required and the patient may need to be intubated if fatigue and PaCO$_2$ increases), reestablishing pulmonary perfusion (fibrinolytics are indicated in this patient because she does have acute right ventricular failure and refractory hypoxemia), and prevent extension of the clot and reocclusion (heparin). Note that it has been 2 weeks since her surgery, which is long enough for the surgical clot to have been lysed by the natural fibrinolytic process, so fibrinolytics are not contraindicated on that basis. If fibrinolytics are contraindicated for other reasons, pulmonary artery catheter aspiration or fragmentation of the clot may be attempted. Surgical pulmonary embolectomy is associated with a relatively high mortality rate and should be avoided if possible.

33.

1. c; 2. f; 3. b; 4. e; 5. a; 6. d

34.

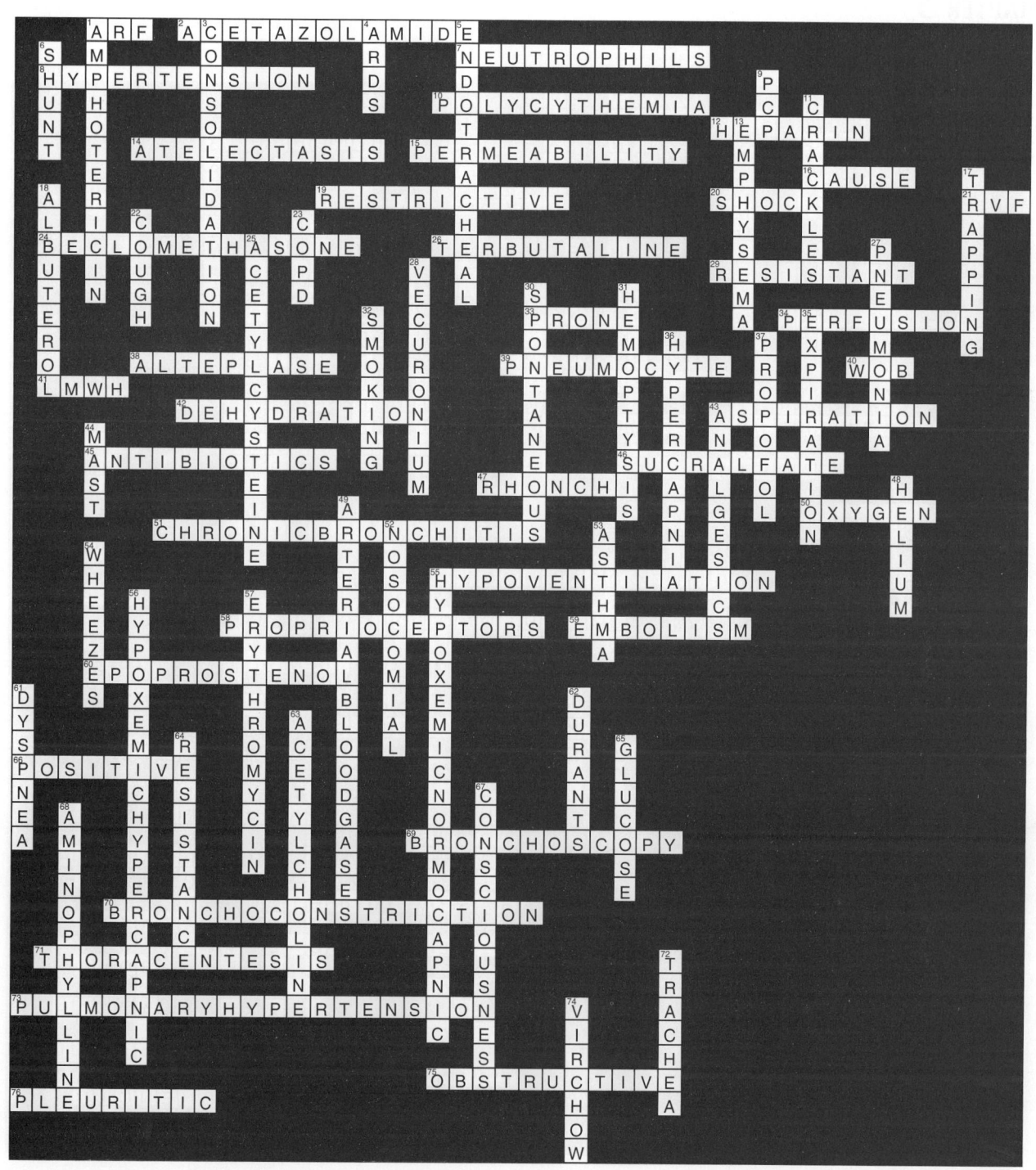

CHAPTER 5

1.

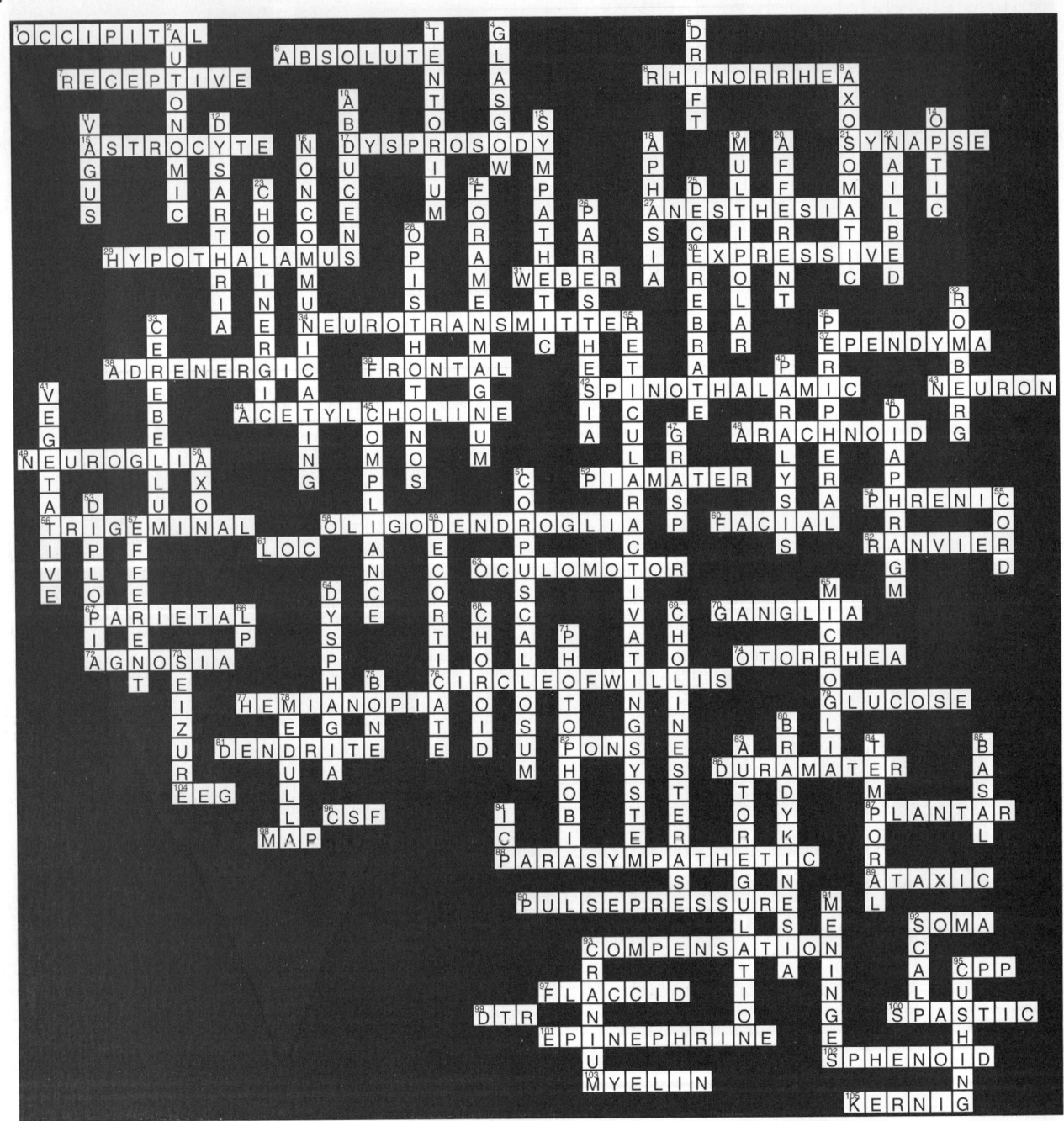

2.
1. k; 2. j; 3. g; 4. c; 5. f; 6. d; 7. b; 8. e; 9. i; 10. l; 11. h; 12. a

3.

To calculate mean arterial pressure:

(SBP + [DBP × 2]) ÷ 3: 80 + (2 × 50) = 180; then divide by 3 = 60

To calculate cerebral perfusion pressure:

MAP − ICP: 60 − 20 = 40 mm Hg

Should you be concerned? YES! CPP less than 50 is associated with loss of autoregulation, hypoperfusion of the brain, and anoxic encephalopathy.

4.

	Sympathetic	Parasympathetic
Bronchodilation	✗	
Coronary artery dilation	✗	
Hypersalivation		✗
Increased blood glucose	✗	
Increased perspiration	✗	
Increased intestinal motility		✗
Pupil constriction		✗
Tachycardia	✗	

5.

Pattern	Site of Lesion
CNS hyperventilation	Lower midbrain or upper pons
Cheyne-Stokes	Cerebral hemispheres, basal ganglia, cerebellar lesion, or upper brainstem
Cluster (or Biot)	Lower pons or upper medulla
Ataxic	Medulla
Apneustic	Mid to lower pons

6.

Cranial Nerve	Name	Method of Assessment
I	Olfactory	• Evaluate the patient's ability to identify familiar odors.
II	Optic	• Evaluate visual acuity using Snellen chart or newsprint. • Evaluate the optic disk during funduscopic examination.
III	Oculomotor	• Evaluate the ability to open eyes widely. • Check the size, shape, position, and reactivity of the pupils. • Have the patient follow your finger with his or her eyes through the six cardinal positions of gaze. • Look for abnormal eye movement (i.e., nystagmus).
IV	Trochlear	• Have the patient follow your finger with his or her eyes through the six cardinal positions of gaze.
V	Trigeminal	• Evaluate the ability of the patient to detect light touch, superficial pain, and temperature on forehead, cheeks, and jaw. • Touch the cornea with a wisp of cotton and check for bilateral blink. • Palpate the strength of the masseter muscles with the patient clinching his or her teeth and the strength of the temporal muscles with the patient squeezing his or her eyes shut.
VI	Abducens	• Have the patient follow your finger with his or her eyes through the six cardinal positions of gaze.
VII	Facial	• Ask the patient to smile and assess symmetry. • Test the patient's ability to taste salt and sugar on the anterior tongue.
VIII	Acoustic	• Evaluate the ability of the patient to hear when speaking at normal voice tones. • Note any vertigo, nystagmus, nausea, vomiting, pallor, sweating, or hypotension.
IX	Glossopharyngeal	• Evaluate the patient's ability to speak; note any hoarseness. • Look for bilateral elevation of the palate with phonation. • Test the patient's ability to taste sour and bitter on the posterior tongue. • Evaluate the patient's ability to swallow. • Test the gag reflex by stroking the palate with a tongue blade and looking for reflex gag. • Evaluate the cough reflex by touching the hypopharynx with a suction catheter.
X	Vagus	• Tested with glossopharyngeal
XI	Spinal accessory	• Ask the patient to shrug his or her shoulders as you push down on them with your hands. • Palpate the sternocleidomastoid and trapezius muscles for size and symmetry.
XII	Hypoglossal	• Look for midline alignment when the patient protrudes his or her tongue. • Look for fasciculations of the tongue.

7.
- a. Neck twisting or flexion
- b. Valsalva maneuver
- c. Airway obstruction
- d. Pain or noxious stimuli
- e. Disturbing conversation
- f. Noise
- g. Bright lights
- h. Tight tracheostomy ties or cervical collar
- i. Seizure activity
- j. Hyperthermia

8.

Intervention	What Is Decreased?
1. Manage blood pressure and brain edema	Blood
2. Maintenance of euvolemia	Brain edema
3. Mannitol	Brain edema
4. Furosemide	Brain edema, CSF
5. Ventriculostomy and CSF drainage	CSF
6. Barbiturate coma	Blood

9.
1. k; 2. h; 3. i; 4. j; 5. g; 6. e; 7. l; 8. a; 9. d; 10. m; 11. c; 12. b; 13. f

10.
GCS: 4
Hunt and Hess aneurysm grade: V

11.

	Vasospasm	Rebleed
Occurs either immediately after the bleed or between 7 and 10 days after the bleed		X
Caused by calcium influx into the vessel	X	
Occurs any time after 3 days	X	
Treated by calcium channel blockers	X	
Caused by lysis of the protective clot		X
Prevented by early clipping if the patient is stable enough		X

12.
- a. Dose: 0.9 mg/kg with maximum dose of less than or equal to 90 mg with the initial bolus being 10% of this total dose over 1 minute and the remaining 90% of this total dose infused over 60 minutes
- b. Time frame: within 4.5 hours of the initial symptoms
- c. Adjuvant therapy: no anticoagulants or platelet aggregation agents for the first 24 hours
- d. Additional contraindications: awakening with symptoms (eliminates ability to determine time of onset of symptoms) and seizure at onset of symptoms (increases risk that the stroke is hemorrhagic rather than ischemic)
- e. Additional contraindications including seizure at symptom onset and awakening with symptoms

13.

Bacterial meningitis	Elevated pressure Increased WBC Normal or elevated protein Decreased glucose Cloudy appearance
Viral meningitis	Elevated pressure Normal or increased WBC Normal or elevated protein Clear appearance
Subarachnoid hemorrhage	Elevated protein Bloody appearance if acute Dark amber (xanthochromic) if more than 5 days old

14.

Observations to Make
Any five of the following:
- Preceding events: Was there an aura?
- Onset:
  - Body movements
  - Deviation of head and eyes
  - Chewing and salivation
  - Posture of body
  - Sensory changes
- Tonic and clonic phases:
  - Progression of movements of the body
  - Skin color and airway
  - Pupillary changes
  - Incontinence
  - Duration of each phase
- Level of consciousness during seizure
  - Postictal phase:
  - Duration
  - General behavior
  - Memory of events
  - Orientation
  - Pupillary changes
  - Headache
  - Aphasia
  - Injuries
- Duration of entire seizure
- Medications given and response

Interventions
Any five of the following:
- Do not leave patient; provide privacy.
- Loosen clothing.
- Open airway but do not try to pry mouth open; nasopharyngeal or nasotracheal airways may be used if necessary.
- Turn patient to side.
- Administer oxygen.
- Do not restrain; gentle guiding of extremities is acceptable.
- Pad side rails with blankets or pillows.
- Administer anticonvulsants (e.g., diazepam, phenytoin).
- Reorient patient after seizure.
- Clean patient if incontinence has occurred.
- Allow patient to sleep.

15.

1. e; 2. b; 3. a; 4. c; 5. d

16.

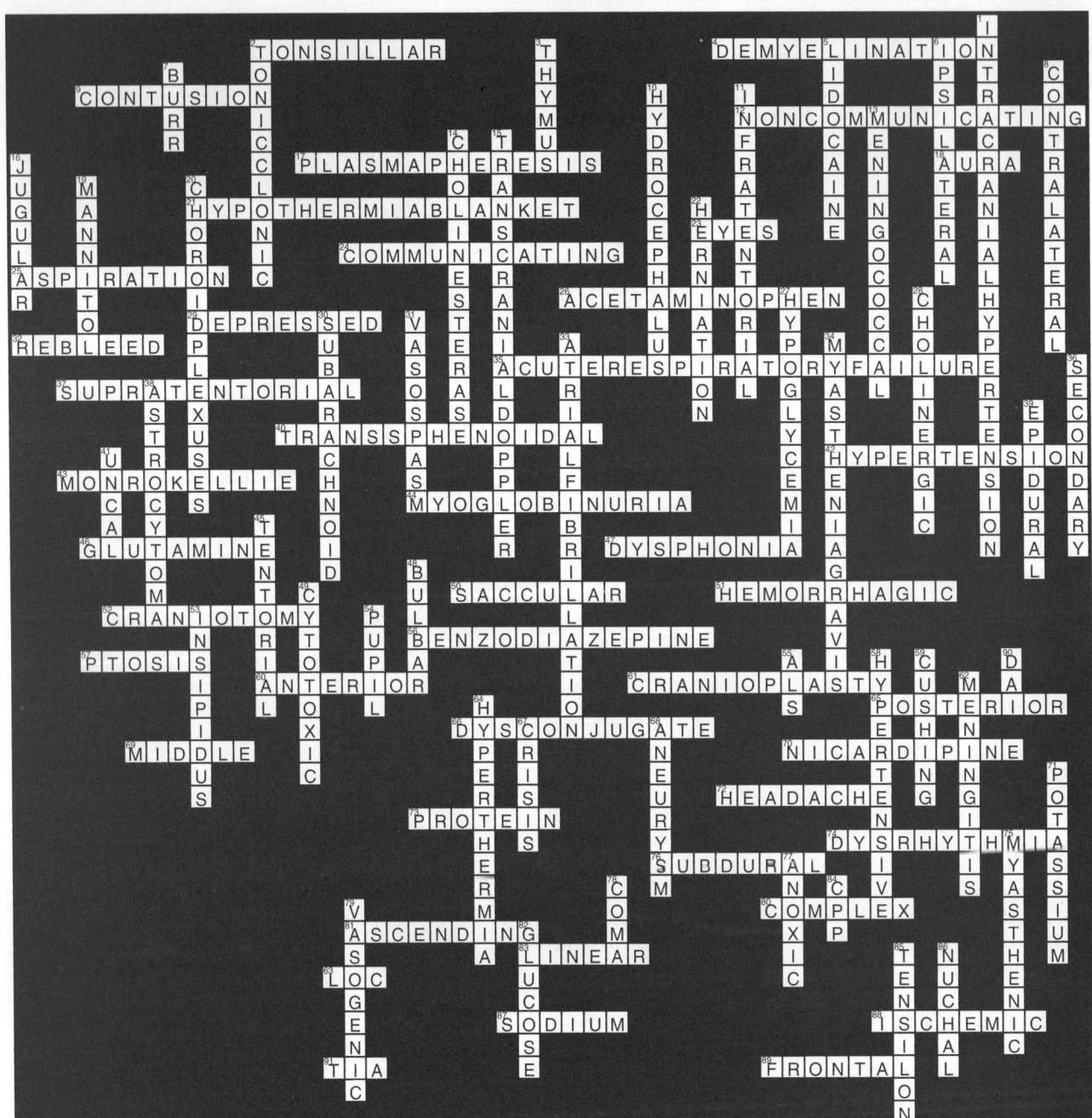

CHAPTER 6

1.

(Crossword puzzle with answers filled in)

2.

Lithium	Decrease
Alcohol	Decrease
Positive pressure ventilation	Increase
Chlorpromazine	Decrease
Phenytoin	Decrease
Hydrochlorothiazide	Increase
Anesthetic agents	Increase
Demeclocycline	Decrease
Beta stimulants	Increase
Morphine sulfate	Increase

3.

	DI	SIADH
Serum ADH	Decreased (if neurogenic DI)	Increased (if neurogenic SIADH)
Urine output	>200 ml/hr	<0.5 ml/kg/hr
Urine specific gravity	<1.005	>1.03
Urine osmolality	Low	High
Serum osmolality	>295 mOsm/l	<280 mOsm/l
Serum sodium	>145 mEq/l	<135 mEq/l
Right atrial/pulmonary artery occlusive pressures	RAP <2 mm Hg; PAOP <4 mm Hg	RAP >6 mm Hg; PAOP >12 mm Hg

4. To calculate the serum osmolality: (serum sodium [158]) × 2 + (BUN [32] ÷ 2.6) + (serum glucose [110] ÷18) = serum osmolality of 334.4 mOsm/kg. The most likely cause of the increase in urine output and the laboratory findings is diabetes insipidus.

5.

	DKA	HHS
Type of diabetes mellitus	1	2 or nondiabetic with intolerance to glucose load (e.g., enteral feeding)
Onset	Gradual or sudden	Gradual
Typical serum glucose range	600 mg/dl	1100 mg/dl
Presence of ketosis	Positive	Negative or minimal
pH	Acidosis	Normal or minimally acidotic
Anion gap	Increased	Normal
Respiratory pattern	Kussmaul (rapid and deep)	Normal or tachypneic (rapid and shallow)
Breath odor	Acetone (fruity)	Normal
Serum osmolality	295–330 mOsm/kg	330–450 mOsm/kg
Serum sodium	Decreased, normal, or increased	Normal or increased
Serum potassium	Increased initially; drops with rehydration and correction of acidosis	Decreased
BUN	Mildly increased	Severely increased
Average fluid deficit	6–9 l	8–15 l

6.

Serum glucose >300 mg/dl	Both
Kussmaul respirations	DKA
pH <7.3	DKA
Positive serum and urine ketones	DKA
Abdominal pain	DKA
Dehydration	Both
Lethargy → coma	Both
Serum glucose >600 mg/dl	HHS

7.

Headache	Hypoglycemia
Serum glucose >300 mg/dl	DKA
Abdominal pain	DKA
Cold, clammy skin	Hypoglycemia
Nervousness, tremors	Hypoglycemia
Polyuria	DKA
Lethargy → coma	DKA
Seizures → coma	Hypoglycemia
Glycosuria	DKA
Tachycardia	Both
Agitation, difficulty with concentration	Hypoglycemia
Weakness, fatigue	DKA
Fruity breath	DKA
Serum glucose <50 mg/dl	Hypoglycemia

8.
   1. b, e; 2. d; 3. b, c, g; 4. b, c, g; 5. a; 6. f, h

CHAPTER 7

1.

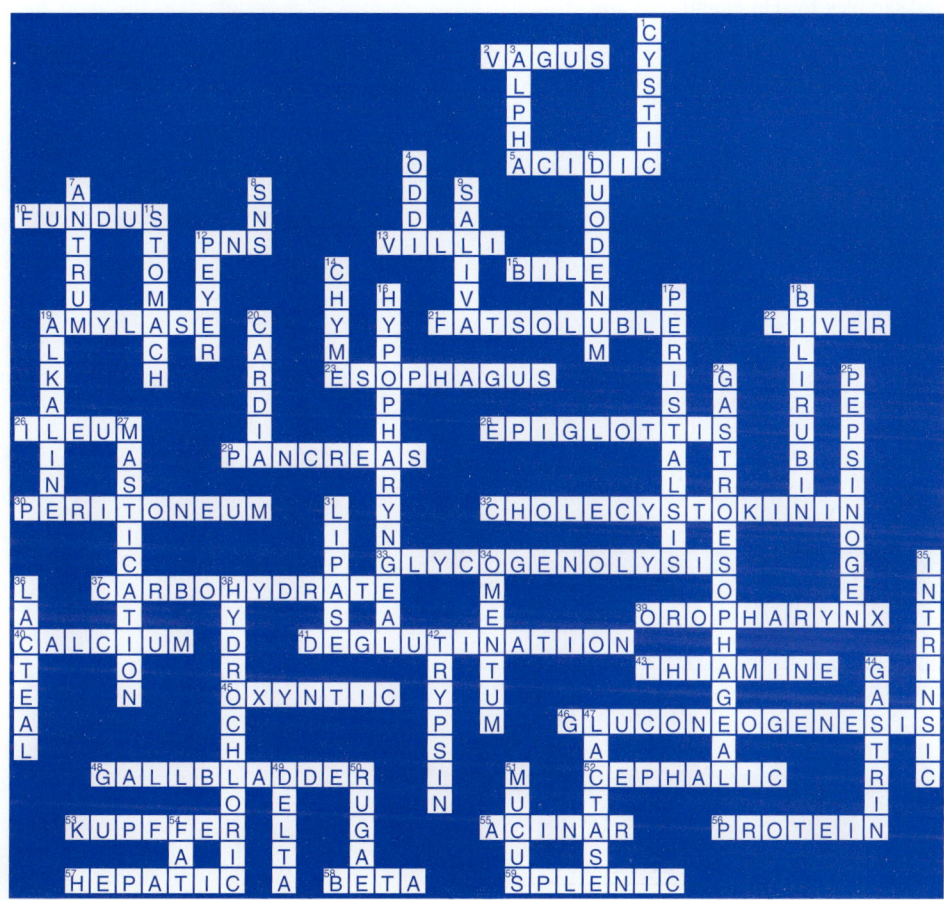

2.

Sign	Description	Indicates
Ballance	Dullness over right flank with patient on left side	Ruptured spleen
Grey Turner	Ecchymosis to flank	Retroperitoneal bleeding
Cullen	Ecchymosis around umbilicus	Intraperitoneal bleeding
Coopernail	Ecchymosis of scrotum or labia	Pelvic fracture
Kehr	Left shoulder pain	Splenic rupture
Chvostek	Spasm of the facial muscles elicited by tapping on the facial nerve	Hypocalcemia
Trousseau	Carpal spasm induced by inflating a BP cuff on the upper arm to a pressure exceeding systolic BP	Hypocalcemia

3.
    a. Liver disease (e.g., cirrhosis, hepatitis)
    b. Biliary obstruction (e.g., cholelithiasis)
    c. Excessive hemolysis (e.g., hemolytic blood transfusion reaction)

4. The half-life of serum prealbumin is 2 to 3 days versus albumin with a half-life of 10 to 20 days. Therefore, serum transferrin will show improvement or decline more quickly.

5. 2428 calories

6.
   a. Administer oxygen (maintain SaO$_2$ of ≥95%).
   b. Insert at least two large-gauge (16 or 18) intravenous catheters.
   c. Obtain blood samples for H&H and type and crossmatch.
   d. Initiate normal saline infusion initially and then blood when prescribed and available.

7.
   a. Peptic ulcer
   b. Esophageal varices
   c. Mallory-Weiss tear
   d. Gastritis
   e. Vascular tumor

8.
   a. Sclerotherapy of varices
   b. Ligation of varices
   c. Intrahepatic (e.g., TIPS) or portosystemic shunt
   d. Balloon tamponade
   e. Octreotide or vasopressin

9.

Type	Example
Antacids	Maalox Mylanta
Histamine (H$_2$) receptor antagonists	Cimetidine Ranitidine Famotidine Nizatidine
Proton pump inhibitors	Omeprazole Lansoprazole Esomeprazole
Mucosal barrier	Sucralfate

10. 1. a, f. Remember that splenic engorgement causes thrombocytopenia and therefore clotting abnormalities; 2. g; 3. d; 4. c; 5. a, c. Remember that many plasma proteins are actually clotting factors; 6. e ;7. a; 8. b

11.

Indicated	Contraindicated
Aldosterone antagonist (potassium-sparing)	Thiazide

12. Any five of the following:
   Abdominal surgery
   Acute cholecystitis
   Hypokalemia
   Intestinal distention
   Intestinal ischemia
   Narcotics (e.g., morphine)
   Pancreatitis
   Pelvic abscess
   Peritonitis
   Pleuritis
   Pneumonia
   Sepsis
   Severe trauma
   Spinal cord injury
   Subphrenic abscess
   Ureteral distention

13. Any five of the following:
    Abdominal pain
    Rebound tenderness
    Abdominal distention
    Rigid "boardlike" abdomen
    Diminished bowel sounds
    Fever
    Leukocytosis
    Nausea, vomiting

14.

Sign or Symptom	Condition
Elevated lipase, amylase	Acute pancreatitis
Sudden, painless hematemesis	Esophageal varices
Decreased protein	Acute pancreatitis, liver disease, malnutrition
Rebound tenderness	Peritonitis
Jaundice	Liver disease, biliary obstruction, hemolysis
Hypocalcemia	Acute pancreatitis
Bleeding tendencies	Liver disease
Elevated ammonia	Hepatic failure, hepatic encephalopathy
Bloody diarrhea	Intestinal infarction
Hyperbilirubinemia	Liver disease, biliary obstruction, hemolysis
Fetor hepaticus	Hepatic failure
High-pitched rushing bowel sounds	Small bowel obstruction
Succussion splash	Pyloric obstruction
Asthma, chronic cough, laryngitis	GERD
Management	**Condition**
Irrigate NG tube until clear	Upper GI bleed
Neomycin and lactulose	Hepatic failure; hepatic encephalopathy
Sclerosis during endoscopy	Esophageal varices
Aldosterone antagonist diuretics	Hepatic failure; hepatic encephalopathy
NPO status	Pancreatitis
Sengstaken-Blakemore tube	Esophageal varices
Volume and blood replacement	GI bleed
Billroth I or II	Gastric ulcer
Proton pump inhibitors	GERD

15.

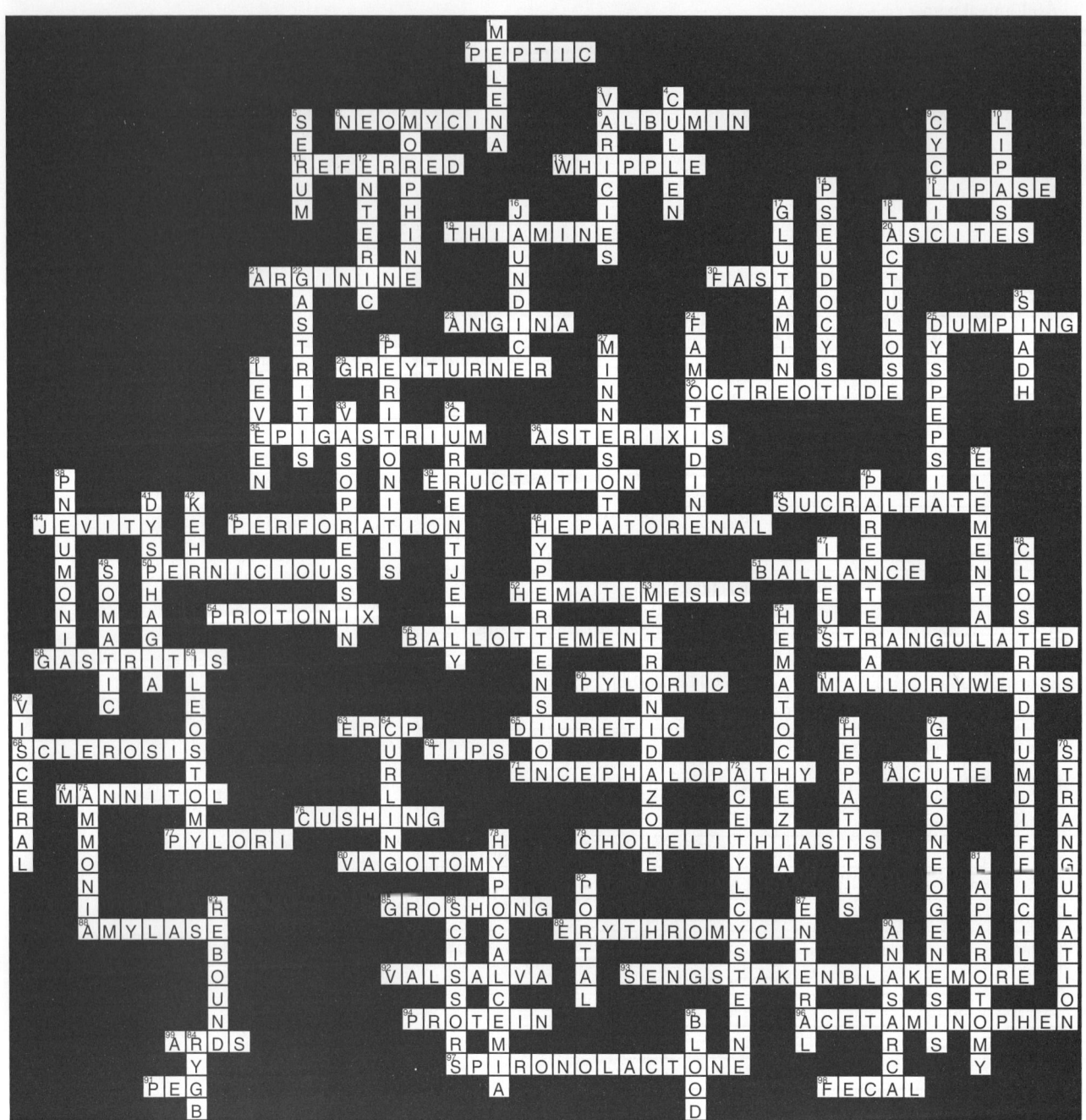

16. Dumping syndrome

17. Pulmonary embolism

18. Serial blood coagulation panels, complete blood count, type and crossmatch; large-bore IV or central line insertion; KUB; Monitor intake and output hourly

19.
  a. Metabolic acidosis with possible respiratory compensation
  b. Bradycardia, hypertension, hyponatremia, seizures, chest pain
  c. Aspiration pneumonia, recurrent bleeding or hemorrhage, gastric outlet syndrome related to ulcer inflammation, sepsis, shock related to hypovolemia or sepsis

20. 1. a; 2. a; 3. a; 4. b; 5. b

CHAPTER 8

1. *[Crossword puzzle with answers filled in]*

2.
   - 7 Ureters
   - 1 Glomerulus
   - 4 Loop of Henle
   - 3 Proximal convoluted tubule
   - 8 Bladder
   - 2 Bowman capsule
   - 6 Collecting ducts
   - 5 Distal convoluted tubule
   - 9 Urethra

3. Water moves by the process of osmosis.
   Electrolytes move by the process of diffusion.
   The sodium-potassium pump is an example of active transport.
   The use of a pushing pressure, such as hydrostatic pressure, is called filtration.

4. Serum osmolality is 433 mOsm/kg, which indicates severe dehydration. This is an example of a hyperglycemic hyperosmolar state caused by glucose intolerance associated with recent initiation of high-glucose enteral feedings.

5.
   a. Potassium
   b. Potassium, calcium, magnesium
   c. Calcium

d. Calcium, phosphorus
e. Magnesium, phosphorus
f. Potassium, chloride

6.

Condition	Normal Anion Gap	Increased Anion Gap
Shock		X
Renal failure		X
Diarrhea	X	
Diabetic ketoacidosis		X
Salicylate overdose		X
Renal tubular acidosis	X	
Rhabdomyolysis		X
Carbonic anhydrase inhibitors	X	
Ethylene glycol poisoning		X

7.
a. Volume depletion (i.e., prerenal)
b. Catabolism
c. GI hemorrhage

8.

Sign/Symptom	Excess (Hyper)	Deficit (Hypo)
Sodium		
Weight gain	X	
Abdominal cramps		X
Flushed, dry skin	X	
Postural hypotension		X
Headache		X
Hypertension	X	
Potassium		
Flat T waves, prominent U waves		X
Decreased GI motility, paralytic ileus		X
Intestinal colic, diarrhea	X	
Muscle cramps → flaccid paralysis		X
Decreased cardiac contractility	X	
Tall, peaked T waves; widened QRS complex	X	
Calcium		
Tetany		X
Decreased deep tendon reflexes	X	
Neuromuscular weakness, flaccidity	X	
Seizures		X
Bone or flank pain	X	
Laryngospasm		X
Phosphorus		
Tetany	X	
Fatigue		X
Chest pain		X
Dyspnea		X

Sign/Symptom	Excess (Hyper)	Deficit (Hypo)
Increased deep tendon reflexes	✗	
Abdominal cramps	✗	
Magnesium		
Decreased deep tendon reflexes	✗	
Anorexia, nausea, vomiting		✗
Cardiopulmonary arrest	✗	
Lethargy	✗	
Dysrhythmias, especially torsades de pointe		✗
Facial flushing	✗	

9.
- a. Hypercalcemia
- b. Hypokalemia
- c. Hypomagnesemia

10.
- a. A patient receiving regular doses of furosemide
    1. Hypovolemia
    2. Hyponatremia
    3. Hypokalemia
    4. Hypocalcemia
    5. Hypomagnesemia
    6. Metabolic alkalosis (caused by hypochloremia and hypokalemia)
- b. A patient with persistent vomiting
    1. Hypovolemia
    2. Hyponatremia
    3. Hypokalemia
    4. Metabolic alkalosis (caused by hypochloremia and hypokalemia)
- c. A patient with acute kidney injury (oliguric phase)
    1. Hypervolemia
    2. Hyponatremia
    3. Hyperkalemia
    4. Hypocalcemia
    5. Hyperphosphatemia
    6. Hypermagnesemia
    7. Metabolic acidosis
- d. A patient with diabetic ketoacidosis (before treatment)
    1. Hyperkalemia
    2. Hypophosphatemia
    3. Hypermagnesemia
    4. Metabolic acidosis
- e. A patient receiving multiple units of banked blood
    1. Hyperkalemia
    2. Hypocalcemia
    3. Hypomagnesemia

11.
D: Delirium
I: Infection
A: Atrophic urethritis or vaginitis
P: Pharmaceuticals
E: Excess urine
R: Restricted mobility
S: Stool impaction

12. a. Catheter usage, diabetes, enlarged prostate
    b. *Escherichia coli*
    c. The female urethra is shorter than the male urethra, and the location of the female urethra provides a convenient entry for bacteria
    d. daily

13. Any three of the following:
    BUN >100 mg/dl
    Volume overload, especially with pulmonary edema
    Uncontrollable hyperkalemia
    Uncontrollable hyperphosphatemia
    Uncontrollable acidosis
    Pericarditis
    Seizures or coma
    Symptomatic uremia

14.

Condition	Prerenal	Intrarenal	Postrenal
Acute pyelonephritis		X	
Benign prostatic hypertrophy			X
Contrast dyes		X	
Diuretics	X	X	
Aminoglycosides		X	
Glomerulonephritis		X	
Goodpasture syndrome		X	
Hemorrhage	X		
Hepatorenal syndrome	X		
Hypersensitivity reactions	X	X	
Intraabdominal tumor			X
Malignant hypertension		X	
Neurogenic bladder			X
Prolonged hypotension		X	
Renal calculi			X
Rhabdomyolysis with myoglobinuria		X	
Septic shock	X		

15.

Characteristic	Oliguric Phase	Diuretic Phase	Both
Elevated BUN			X
Hyperkalemia			X
Metabolic acidosis			X
Volume deficit		X	
Volume excess	X		

16.

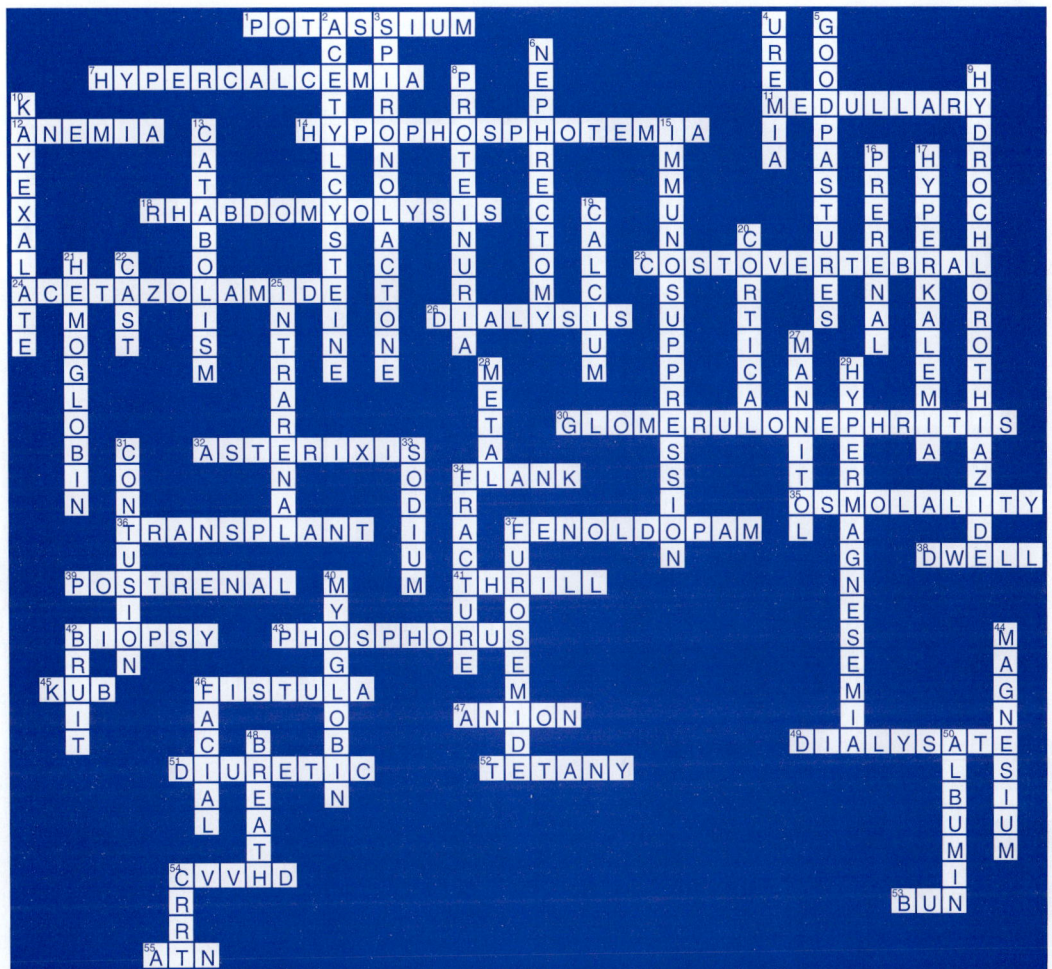

CHAPTER 9

1.

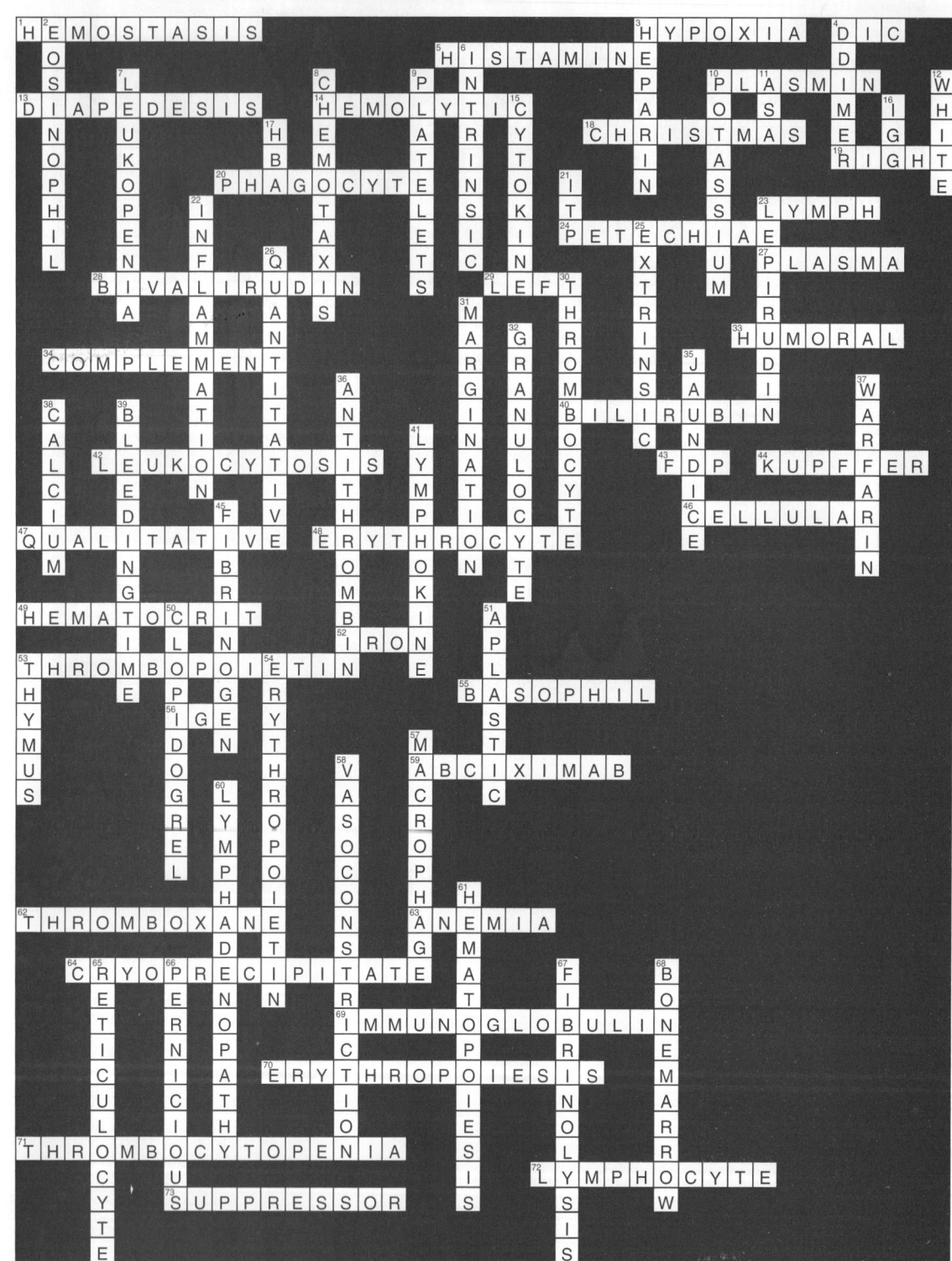

2.
   a. Warmth
   b. Redness
   c. Swelling
   d. Pain
   e. Loss of function

3.

Example	Type
Skin testing for tuberculosis	IV
Poststreptococcal glomerulonephritis	III
Anaphylaxis to penicillin	I
Hemolytic blood transfusion reaction	II

4.

	Platelet Plug	Intrinsic Pathway	Extrinsic Pathway	Common Pathway	Fibrinolytic System
Activation	Intimal defect	Hageman factor (XII)	Tissue thromboplastin (III)	Stuart-Prower factor (X)	Tissue plasminogen activator
Laboratory test	Bleeding time	aPTT	PT	aPTT, TT	Fibrin split products

5. Match the drug with the laboratory effect.
   1. a; 2. c; 3. b, f; 4. e; 5. d, e; 6. a

6.
   a. Stop the transfusion.
   b. Maintain IV access with normal saline and new administration set.
   c. Reassure the patient; stay at the bedside.
   d. Notify the physician and blood bank.
   e. Recheck the blood numbers and type.
   f. Treat the symptoms appropriately.
   g. Return the unused portion of blood in the blood bag and administration set to the blood bank.
   h. Collect and send the blood and urine samples to the laboratory; send another urine specimen 24 hours after the transfusion reaction.
   i. Document the transfusion reaction and treatment administered.

7.

Platelets	↓
PT	↑
aPTT	↑
Fibrin split products	↑
Factors V, VIII	↓
Fibrinogen	↓

8. Match the coagulopathy with the associated pathology.
   1. d; 2. e; 3. c; 4. f; 5. a; 6. h; 7. b; 8. g

9.

a. Heparin	May perpetuate bleeding
b. Clotting factors	May perpetuate clotting

10. 1. a; 2. c; 3. b; 4. b; 5. c; 6. b, 7. b, 8. c; 9. a; 10. b; 11. b, c

CHAPTER 10

1. *[Crossword puzzle with the following answers filled in:]*

Across and down entries include: MACERATION, FRACTURE, MASD, STAPH, EPIDERMIS, APOCRINE, MACROPHAGES, MELANOCYTES, OSTEOCLASTS, THERMOREGULATION, VASOPRESSOR, KERATIN, EXUDATE, DIPOCYTE, INFILTRATION, KYPHOSIS, STAPHYLOCOCCUS AUREUS, HEMATOGENOUS, YELLOW, ELASTICITY, OSTEOMYELITIS, SKIN, ECCRINE, FIBROBLASTS, HYPODERMIS, OSTEOBLASTS, BRADEN, COMPOUND, COMPRESSION, MERKEL, RED, LANGERHANS, MAST, SHARP, SCAR, TARSI

2. 1. b; 2. d; 3. c; 4. a

3. Infiltration is leakage of intravenous fluids or medications into the tissue around an intravenous catheter, but extravasation is the leakage of a potentially damaging medication into the tissue around an intravenous catheter. The difference is the potential for significant tissue injury with extravasation.

4. 1. d; 2. a; 3. b; 4. c

CHAPTER 11

1.

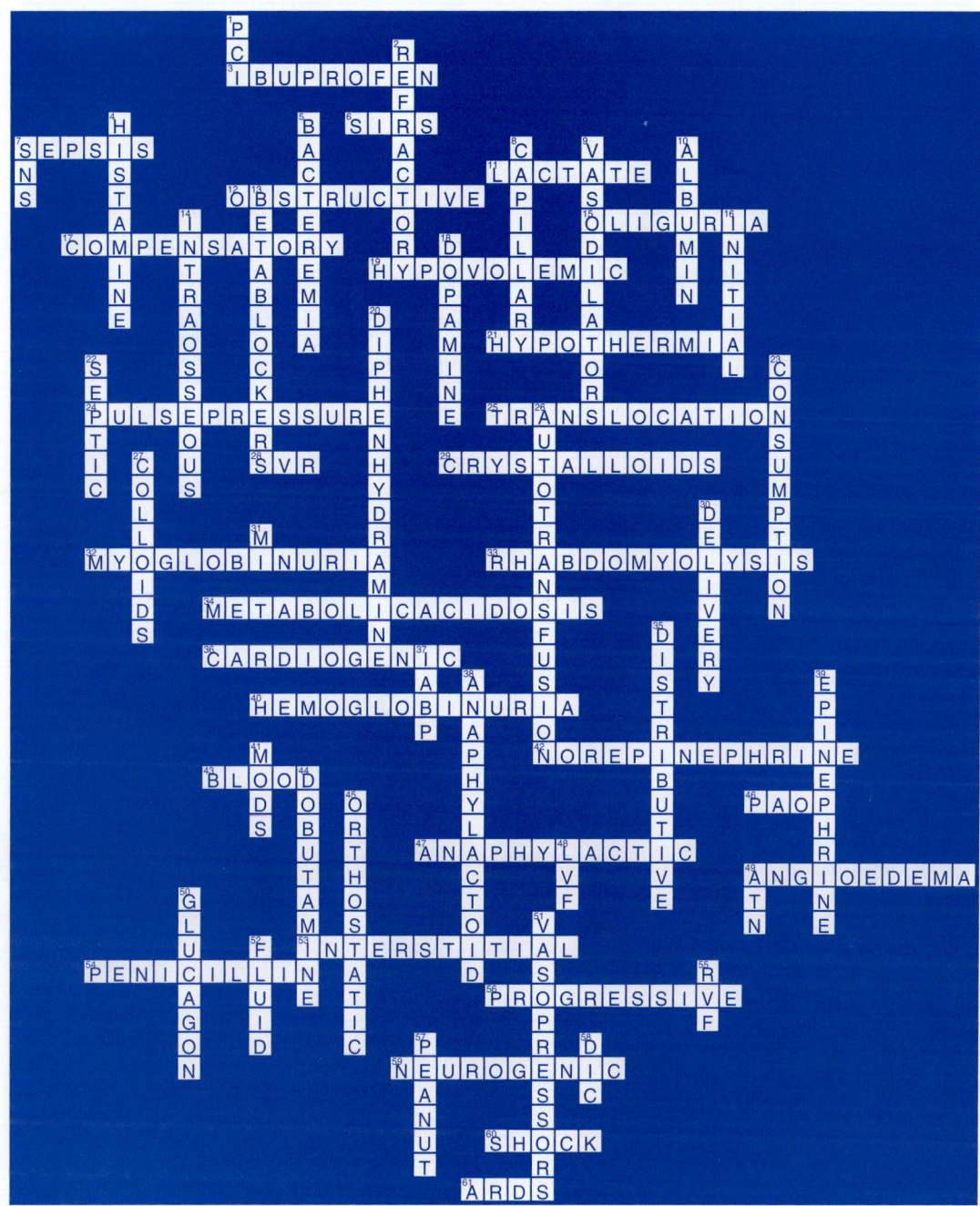

2.

Condition	Hypovolemic	Cardiogenic	Septic	Anaphylactic	Neurogenic
Myocardial infarction		✓			
Bee sting				✓	
Head injury					✓
Diarrhea	✓				
Pulmonary embolism		✓			
Ruptured gallbladder			✓		
Esophageal varices	✓				
Ruptured papillary muscle		✓			
Insulin shock					✓
Ascites	✓				
IVP dye				✓	
Spinal cord injury					✓
Invasive procedures	✓		✓		
Burns	✓		✓		
Blood transfusion reaction				✓	
Spinal anesthesia					✓
Trauma	✓		✓		
Malnutrition			✓		
Chemotherapy			✓		

3.

1. d; 2. b; 3. c; 4. e; 5. a

4.

Sign or Symptom	Compensatory	Progressive	Refractory
Acute respiratory distress syndrome			✓
Anuria		✓	✓
Cool, pale skin	✓		
Decreased bowel sounds	✓	✓	
Disseminated intravascular coagulation			✓
Dysrhythmias		✓	✓
Hypotension		✓	✓
Mottling of extremities		✓	✓
Narrow pulse pressure	✓		
Nausea		✓	
Neurologic changes: coma, focal signs			✓
Neurologic changes: irritability, confusion	✓		
Neurologic changes: lethargy, coma		✓	✓
Oliguria	✓		
Profound hypotension despite vasopressors			✓
Tachycardia	✓	✓	
Thirst	✓	✓	

5.

Type of Shock	CO/CI	RAP/PAP/PAOP	SVR	SvO$_2$
Hypovolemic	↓	↓	↑	↓
Cardiogenic	↓	↑	↑	↓
Septic	↑	↓	↓	↑
Anaphylactic	↓	↓	↓	↓
Neurologic	↓	↓	↓	↓

CI, Cardiac index; *CO*, cardiac output; *PAOP*, pulmonary artery occlusive pressure; *PAP*, pulmonary artery pressure; *RAP*, right atrial pressure; *SVR*, systemic vascular resistance; *SvO$_2$*, oxygen saturation of venous blood.

6.

Crystalloids		
Isotonic	Normal (0.9%) saline	Lactated Ringer solution
Hypotonic	Half-normal (0.45%) saline	5% dextrose in water
Hypertonic	3% saline	10% dextrose in water
Colloids	Albumin	Dextran 70
Blood or Blood Products	Whole blood	Red blood cells

7.
1. c; 2. b, c; 3. a; 4. a; 5. c; 6. d; 7. a; 8. b; 9. c; 10. d

8.
1. a, b, d, h, i, k, l; 2. e, f, k, l, m, and possibly g; 3. a, k, l, and possibly c; 4. a, d, k, l and possibly g; 5. a, d, j, k, l, and possibly b and e

9.
1. d; 2. f; 3. e; 4. b; 5. c; 6. a

10.

Heart rate	>90 beats/min			
Respiratory rate	>20 beats/min	or	PaCO$_2$	<32 mm Hg
Temperature	>38°C (100.4°F)	or	<36°C (96.8°F)	
WBC count	>12,000 cells/mm^3	or	<4000 cells/mm^3	

11.
   a. Gastric lavage
   b. Activated charcoal
   c. Cathartic

12.

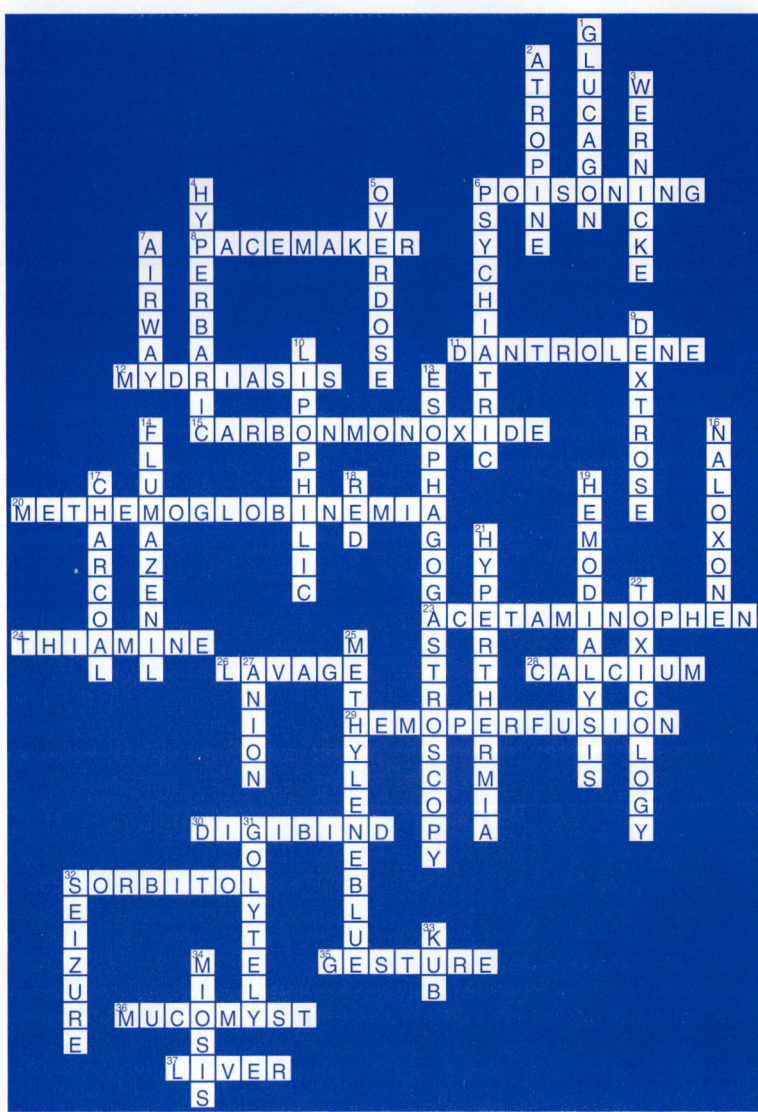

13.

	CAUTI	CLABSI	VAP	SSI	MDRO
Elevate HOB 30–45 degrees			✗		
Proper hair removal techniques				✗	
Hand hygiene prior to touching device	✗	✗	✗		
Maintain normothermia				✗	
Administer PUD prophylaxis			✗		
Remove device when no longer required	✗	✗	✗		
Antibiotic stewardship					✗
Maximum barrier precautions during insertion of device		✗			
Antibiotic stewardship				✗	✗
Disinfect skin with chlorhexidine	✗	✗		✗	
Employ standard precautions	✗	✗	✗	✗	✗

14. a. Blunt; b. Penetrating; c. Blast

15.
A: airway
B: breathing
C: circulation
D: disability
E: exposure

16. a. Pain; b. Pallor; c. Pulselessness; d. Polar; e. Paresthesia; f. Paralysis

CHAPTER 12

1.

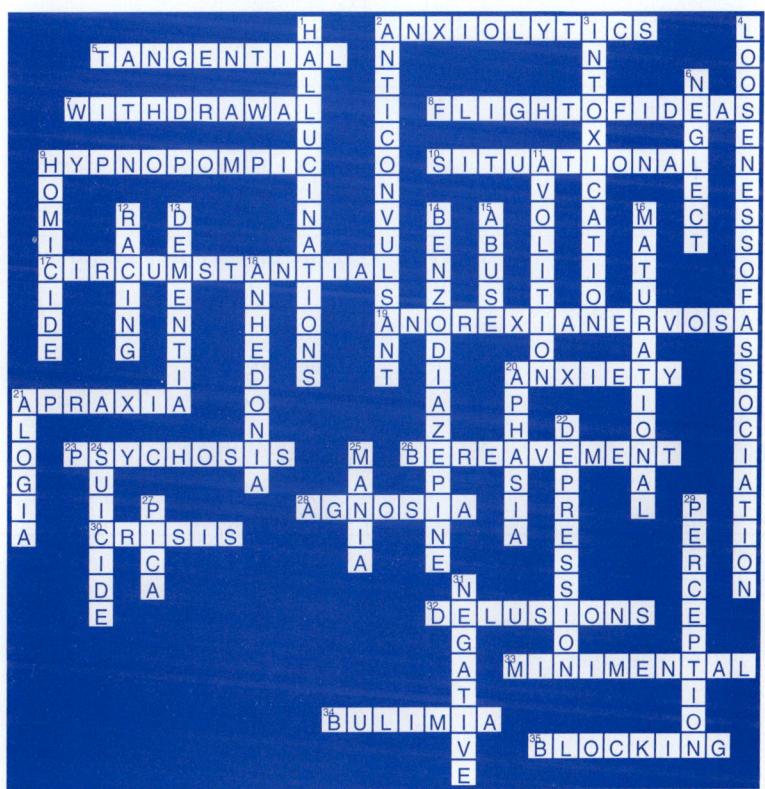

2.
1. e; 2. b; 3. d; 4. f; 5. a; 6. c; 7. g; 8. h

3.
a. Possibility of neglect or abuse
b. Accidental substance abuse related to poor eyesight or decreasing cognitive function
c. Medications take longer to clear because of aging renal function and may cause older adult patients to appear depressed or have flat affect.
d. Intentional substance abuse related to loneliness
e. Depression common in older adult patients with personal loss or faced with losing independence.

4.
1. b; 2. e; 3. d; 4. c; 5. a

5.

Condition	Subjective Assessment	Objective Assessment
Anxiety disorder	Apprehension, nervousness Tremors Tightness in chest Dizziness	Tachycardia, elevated BP, tachypnea Dilated pupils
Depression	Hopeless feeling Inability to concentrate Low energy, fatigue, loss of appetite Depressed mood Decreased libido Recurrent thought of death	Appearance sloppy Flat affect Tearful Little eye contact Slowness of movement Quiet
Mania	Racing thoughts Risky or reckless behaviors Little need for sleep	Increased activity Flight of ideas Distractibility Elation Grandiosity
Hallucinations	Patient reports having visions or hearing voices	Patient is talking or responding to voices or other perceptual disturbances
Psychosis	Paranoid ideas Confusion or amnesia Fears about safety	Delusions, hallucinations Agitation or bizarre behavior Appears out of touch with reality Inability to initiate activities Lack of pleasure
Dementia	Memory loss Speech impairment Decline in cognitive function	Decrease in orientation and judgment Aphasia Apraxia Agnosia Shallow affect Gradual onset Chronic
Delirium	Disorientation Hallucinations Acute onset	Etiology identified; may include medical condition, trauma, substance use/withdrawal, toxins Fluctuating level of consciousness

6.

    a. Does he have a history of medical or emotional issues?
       Is he currently taking any medication?
       Completion of neurologic exam
    b. CBC/electrolyte panel
       Toxicology screen
       Urinalysis
    c. Delirium as evidenced by acute mental status change
       Rule out depression: No reported medical cause for the change. He is oriented to person, place, and time.
       Rule out sepsis, stroke, and substance use: There is no evidence for this, but, given the rapid change, these and other causes of delirium should be ruled out.
       Most likely not dementia due to acute onset
    d. Safety
       Physical stabilization: Assess vital signs and laboratory test results and intervene as indicated. If no abnormality is identified, consider a mental health issue such as depression.
       Emotional stabilization: Consider initiating treatment for depression if no physical problems are identified.

7.
- a. How long has she been exhibiting these behaviors?
  Has she had episodes of this nature previously?
  Is she eating on a regular basis?
  Is she sleeping on a regular basis?
  Has she been harmed by someone else?
  Has she had thoughts of hurting herself or anyone else?
  Is she having any hallucinations?
  Has she had any prescribed medication?
  Has she used any over-the-counter substance?
  Has she used any alcohol or other drugs?
  Has she been physically ill?
- b. CBC and electrolyte panel
  Thyroid level
  Drug screen for alcohol, marijuana, and other hallucinogens
- c. Delirium: need to rule out medical cause of change of behavior
  Mood disorder, such as mania, based on current symptoms and no physical cause identified
- d. Safety
  Physical stabilization: Treat any medical issues identified; normalize sleeping and eating schedule.
  Emotional stabilization

8.
- a. ICU delirium
- b. The most likely cause is sleep deprivation, but other causes should be investigated, including looking at what drugs the patient is receiving or withdrawing from that may be factors.
- c. Safety: prevention of self-extubation and self-harm
  Elimination of causes: uninterrupted sleep to allow REM sleep, extubation and transfer as soon as possible, reduction of noise, and maintenance of normal light–dark cycles

References and Suggested Readings

Aehlert, B. (2009). *ECGs made easy* (4th ed.). St. Louis: Mosby.

Agency for Healthcare Research and Quality. (2016). TeamSTEPPS. Retrieved from https://www.ahrq.gov/teamstepps/index.html.

Alfaro-LeFevre, R. (2013). *Critical thinking, clinical reasoning, and clinical judgment: a practical approach* (5th ed.). St. Louis: Elsevier.

Altman, M. (2011). Let's get certified: best practices for nurse leaders to create a culture of certification. *AACN Adv Crit Care*, 22(1), 68–75.

America Nurses Association. (2017). What is nursing? Retrieved from http://www.nursingworld.org/EspeciallyForYou/What-is-Nursing.

American Association of Critical-Care Nurses. (2013). Assessing pain in the critically ill adult. Retrieved from https://www.aacn.org/clinical-resources/practice-alerts/assessing-pain-in-the-critically-ill-adult.

American Association of Critical-Care Nurses. (2015a). 2013 national practice analysis of critical care nurses. Retrieved from https://www.aacn.org/certification/get-certified/2013-national-practice-analysis-of-critical-care-nurses.

American Association of Critical-Care Nurses. (2015b). Scope and standards of acute and critical care nursing. Retrieved from https://www.aacn.org/~/media/aacn-website/nursing-excellence/standards/scopeandstandardsacutecriticalcare2015.pdf.

American Association of Critical-Care Nurses. (2016a). AACN standards for establishing and sustaining healthy work environments: a journey to excellence (2nd ed.). Retrieved from https://www.aacn.org/~/media/aacn-website/nursing-excellence/standards/hwestandards.pdf.

American Association of Critical-Care Nurses. (2016b). AACN Practice Alert. Family presence during resuscitation and invasive procedures. Retrieved from https://www.aacn.org/~/media/aacn-website/clincial-resources/practice-alerts/fampresresuscpafeb2016ccnpages.pdf.

American Association of Critical-Care Nurses. (2016c). AACN Practice Alert. Family visitation in the adult intensive care unit. Retrieved from https://www.aacn.org/~/media/aacn-website/clincial-resources/practice-alerts/famvisitpafeb2016ccnpages.pdf.

American Association of Critical-Care Nurses. (2016d). CCRN exam handbook. Retrieved from https://www.aacn.org/certification/get-certified/ccrn-adult.

American Association of Critical-Care Nurses. (2016e). Preparation tools and handbooks. Retrieved from https://www.aacn.org/certification/preparation-tools-and-handbooks.

American Association of Critical-Care Nurses. (2016f). Synergy model. Retrieved from https://www.aacn.org/nursing-excellence/aacn-standards/synergy-model.

American Association of Neurological Surgeons. (2017). Patient information: concussion. Retrieved from http://www.aans.org/patient%20information/conditions%20and%20treatments/concussion.aspx.

American Hospital Association. (2003). *The patient care partnership. understanding expectations, rights, and responsibilities*. Chicago: American Hospital Association.

American Nurses Association & National Council of State Boards of Nursing. (2006). Joint statement on delegation. Retrieved from https://www.ncsbn.org/joint_statement.pdf.

American Nurses Association. (2012). Principles for delegation by registered nurses to unlicensed assistive personnel (UAP). Retrieved from http://www.nursingworld.org/principles.

American Nurses Association. (2015a). Code of ethics for nurses with interpretative statements. Retrieved from http://nursingworld.org/MainMenuCategories/EthicsStandards/CodeofEthicsforNurses/Code-of-Ethics-For-Nurses.html.

American Nurses Association. (2015b). *Nursing scope and standards of practice* (3rd ed.). Silver Spring, MD: ANA.

American Nurses Association. (2017). The nursing process. Retrieved from http://www.nursingworld.org/EspeciallyForYou/What-is-Nursing/Tools-You-Need/Thenursingprocess.html.

American Psychiatric Association. (2013). *Diagnostic and statistical manual of mental disorders* (5th ed.). Arlington, VA: American Psychiatric Publishing.

Amidei, C. (2017). Nervous system alterations. In M. L. Sole, D. Klein, & M. Moseley (Eds.), *Introduction to critical care nursing* (7th ed.). (pp. 342–389). St. Louis: Elsevier.

Anderson, D. J. (2014). Strategies to prevent surgical site infections in acute care hospitals: 2014 update. *Infect Control Hosp Epidemiol*, 35(6), 605–627.

Arbour, R. (2004). Intracranial hypertension: monitoring and nursing assessment. *Crit Care Nurse*, 24(5), 19–32.

Arbour, R. (2013). Brain death: assessment, controversy, and confounding factors. *Crit Care Nurse*, 33(6), 27–46.

Armola, R. R., Bourgault, A. M., Halm, M. A., Board, R. M., Bucher, L., Harrington, L., & Medina, J. (2009). AACN levels of evidence: what's new? *Crit Care Nurse*, 29(4), 70–73.

Arnold, E. C., & Boggs, K. U. (2016). *Interpersonal relationships: professional communication skills for nurses* (7th ed.). St. Louis: Elsevier.

Association of Healthcare Research and Quality. (2015). Toolkit for reducing catheter-associated urinary tract infections in hospital units: Implementation guide. HRQ Pub No. 15-0073-2-EF. Retrieved from https://www.ahrq.gov/sites/default/files/wysiwyg/professionals/quality-patient-safety/hais/cauti-tools/impl-guide/implementation-guide.pdf.

Aster, J. C., & Bunn, H. F. (2017). *Pathophysiology of blood disorders*. New York: McGraw Hill Education.

Baggott, C., & Aagaard-Kienitz, B. (2014). Cerebral vasospasm. *Neurosurg Clin North Am*, 25(3), 497–528.

Barill, T. P. (2003). An ECG primer. Retrieved from http://www.nursecom.com/ECGprimer.pdf.

Bartlett, D. (2014). Intravenous lipids: antidotal therapy for drug overdose and toxic effects of local anesthetics. *Crit Care Nurse*, 34(5), 62–66.

Barton, A., Ventura, R., & Vavrik, B. Peripheral intravenous cannulation: protecting patients and nurses. *Br J Nurs*, 26(8), S28–S33.

Beauchamp, T. L., & Childress, J. F. (2013). *Principles of biomedical ethics* (7th ed.). New York: Oxford University Press.

Benner, P. (2001). *From novice to expert: excellence and power in clinical nursing practice*. Upper Saddle River, NJ: Prentice Hall Health.

Benner, P. (2003). Beware of technologic imperatives and commercial interests that prevent best practices! *Am J Crit Care*, 12(5), 469–471.

Berlin, T. (2017). Cerebral blood flow monitoring. In D. Wiegand (Ed.), *Procedure manual for high acuity, progressive, and critical care* (7th ed.). (pp. 811–822). St. Louis: Elsevier.

Berwick, D. M. (2003). Disseminating innovations in health care. *JAMA*, 289(15), 1969–1975.

Boev, C., Xue, Y., & Ingersoll, G. L. (2015). Nursing job satisfaction, certification and healthcare-associated infections in critical care. *Intensive Crit Care Nurs*, 31(5), 276–284.

Boss, B., & Huether, S. (2014). Disorders of the central and peripheral nervous systems and the neuromuscular junction. In K. McCance, & S. Huether (Eds.), *Pathophysiology: the biologic basis for disease in adults and children* (7th ed.). (pp. 527–580). St. Louis: Elsevier.

Bowman, A., Greiner, J. E., Doerschug, K. C., Little, S. B., Bombei, C. L., & Comried, L. M. (2005). Implementation of an evidence-based feeding protocol and aspiration risk reduction algorithm. *Crit Care Nurs Q*, 28(4), 324–333; quiz 334–325.

Bridges, E. (2009). AACN practice alert. Pulmonary artery/central venous pressure measurement. Retrieved from http://www.aacn.org/WD/Practice/Docs/PracticeAlerts/PAP_Measurement_05-2004.pdf.

Caceres, J. A., & Goldstein, J. (2012). Intracranial hemorrhage. *Emerg Med Clin North Am, 30*(3), 771–794.

Callaway, C. W., Donnino, M. W., Fink, E. L., Geocadin, R. G., Golan, E., Kern, K. B., et al. Part 8: Post-cardiac arrest care: 2015 American Heart Association guidelines update for cardiopulmonary resuscitation and emergency cardiovascular care. *Circulation, 132*(18 Suppl. 2), S465–S482.

Campaign for Action. (2016). Retrieved from http://campaignforaction.org.

Cary, A. H. (2001). Certified registered nurses: results of the study of the certified workforce. *Am J Nurs, 101*(1), 44–52.

Cates, M. (2016). Evaluation of peripheral intravenous practices. *Vascular Access, 10*(1), 8–13.

Centers for Disease Control and Prevention. (2018) Healthcare-associated infections. Retrieved from https://www.cdc.gov/hai/surveillance/index.html.

Chapman, S. (2017). Preventing and treating pressure ulcers: evidence review. *Br J Community Nurs, 22*(Suppl. 3), S37–S40.

Choiniere, D. B. (2010). The effects of hospital noise. *Nurs Adm Q, 34*(4), 327–333.

Ciliska, D. K., Pinelli, J., DiCenso, A., & Cullum, N. (2001). Resources to enhance evidence-based nursing practice. *AACN Clin Issues, 12*(4), 520–528.

Clain, J., Rannar, K., & Salim, R. S. (2015). Glucose control in critical care. *World J Diabetes, 6*(9), 1082–1091.

Clark, K., Milner, K. A., Beck, M., & Mason, V. (2016). Measuring family satisfaction with care delivered in the intensive care unit. *Crit Care Nurse, 36*(6), e8–e14.

Connors, A. F., Speroff, T., Dawson, N. V., Thomas, C., Harrell, F. E., Wagner, D., & Knaus, W. A. (1996). The effectiveness of right heart catheterization in the initial care of critically ill patients. *JAMA, 276*(11), 889–897.

Cooper, K. L. (2013). Evidence-based prevention of pressure ulcers in the intensive care unit. *Crit Care Nurse, 33*(6), 57–66.

Copstead-Kirkhorn, L., & Banasik, J. L. (2014). *Pathophysiology* (5th ed.). St. Louis: Elsevier, Saunders.

Cox, J. (2017a). Pressure injuries in critical care: a survey of critical care nurses. *Crit Care Nurse, 37*(5), 46–56.

Cox, J. (2017b). Pressure injury risk factors in adult critical care patients: a review of the literature. *Ostomy Wound Manage, 63*(11), 30–43.

Cox, J., & Rasmussen, L. (2014). Enteral nutrition in the prevention and treatment of pressure ulcers in adult critical care patients. *Crit Care Nurse, 34*(6), 15–27; quiz 28.

Coyer, F., Gardner, A., Doubrovsky, A., Cole, R., Ryan, F. M., Allen, C., & McNamara, G. (2015). Reducing pressure injuries in critically ill patients by using a patient skin integrity care bundle (InSPiRE). *Am J Crit Care, 24*(3), 199–209.

Curley, M. A. Q. (2007). *Synergy: the unique relationship between nurses and patients*. Indianapolis: Sigma Theta Tau Publishing.

Davidson, J. E., Aslakson, R. A., Long, A. C., Puntillo, K. A., Kross, E. K., Hart, J., & Curtis, J. R. (2017). Guidelines for family-centered care in the neonatal, pediatric, and adult ICU. *Crit Care Med, 45*(1), 103–128.

Dellinger, R. P., Levy, M. M., Rhodes, A., Annane, D., Gerlach, H., Opal, S. M., et al. (2013). Surviving sepsis campaign: international guidelines for management of severe sepsis and septic shock: 2012. *Crit Care Med, 41*(2), 580–620.

Dennison, R. (2013). The neurologic system. In R. Dennison (Ed.), *Pass CCRN!* (4th ed.). (pp. 385–475). Maryland Heights. MO: Elsevier.

Dennison, R. D. (2005). Creating an organizational culture for medication safety. *Nurs Clin North Am, 40*(1), 1–23.

Dossey, B. M., & Keegan, L. (2016). *Holistic nursing* (7th ed.). Burlington, MA: Jones & Bartlett Learning.

Dracup, K., & Bryan-Brown, C. W. (1999). Empathy: a challenge for critical care. *Am J Crit Care, 8*(4), 204–205.

Elinson, J. (1987). Advances in health assessment discussion panel. *J Chronic Dis, 40*(Suppl. 1), 83S–91S.

Elliott, R., & McKinley, S. (2014). The development of a clinical practice guideline to improve sleep in intensive care patients: a solution focused approach. *J Int Crit Care Nursing, 30*(4), 246–256.

Ellis, M. (2016). Understanding the latest guidance on pressure ulcer prevention. *J Community Nursing, 30*(4), 29–36.

Elpern, E., Kelleher, A. D., & Oman, K. S. (2016). AACN practice alert: prevention of catheter-associated urinary tract infections in adults. *Crit Care Nurse, 36*(4), e9–e11.

Evidence Summary. (2017). Wound management—chlorhexidine. *Wound Pract Res, 25*(1), 49–51.

Farwell, A. L. (2010). Saving muscle: evidence-based strategies for reducing door-to-balloon times for ST-segment elevation myocardial infarction patients. *J Emerg Nurs, 36*(3), 231–237.

Feldman, V., & Sobrino-Bonilla, Y. (2014). Dim down the lights: implementing quiet time in the coronary care unit. *Crit Care Nurse, 34*(6), 74–75.

Ferri, F. F. (2017). *Ferri's clinical advisor*. St. Louis: Elsevier.

Fitzpatrick, J. C., Campo, T. M., Graham, G., & Lavandero, R. (2010). Certification, empowerment, and intent to leave current position and the profession among critical care nurses. *Am J Crit Care, 19*(3), 218–229.

Folstein, M. F., Folstein, S. E., & McHugh, P. R. (1975). Mini-mental state: a practical method for grading the cognitive state of patients for the clinician. *J Psychiatr Res, 12*, 189–198.

Fowler, M. D. M. (2015). *Guide to the Code of Ethics for Nurses with interpretive statements: development, interpretation, and application.* (2nd ed.). Silver Spring, MD: American Nurses Association.

Frazier, S. (2008). Hemodynamic monitoring. In D. K. Moser, & B. Riegel (Eds.), *Cardiac nursing*. (pp. 705–736). Philadelphia: Saunders.

Freedman, N. S., Gazendam, J., Levan, L., Pack, A. I., & Schwab, R. J. (2001). Abnormal sleep/wake cycles and the effect of environmental noise on sleep disruption in the intensive care unit. *Am J Respir Crit Care Med, 163*(2), 451–457.

Fritter, E., & Shimp, K. (2016). What does certification in professional nursing practice mean? *Med Surg Nursing, 2*, 8.

Garcia-Fernandez, F. P., Agreda, J. J., Verdu, J., & Pancorbo-Hidalgo, P. L. (2014). A new theoretical model for the development of pressure ulcers and other dependence-related lesions. *J Nurs Scholarsh, 46*(1), 28–38.

Gelinas, C. (2016). Pain assessment in the critically ill adult: recent evidence and new trends. *Intensive Crit Care Nurs, 34*(6), 1–11.

Gelinas, C., Arbour, C., Michaud, C., Vaillant, F., & Desjardins, S. (2011). Implementation of the critical-care pain observation tool on pain assessment/management nursing practices in an intensive care unit with nonverbal critically ill adults: a before and after study. *Int J Nurs Stud, 48*(12), 1495–1504.

Gheorghiade, M., Zannad, F., Sopko, G., Klein, L., Pina, I. L., Konstam, M. A., & International Working Group on Acute Heart Failure Syndromes. (2005). Acute heart failure syndromes: current state and framework for future research. *Circulation, 112*(25), 3958–3968.

Giger, J. N. (2013). *Transcultural nursing: assessment and intervention* (6th ed.). St. Louis: Mosby.

Goldman, L., & Schafer, A. I. (2016). *Goldman-Cecil medicine* (25th ed.). St. Louis: Elsevier.

Gosmanov, A. R., Gosmanova, E. O., & Dillard-Cannon, E. (2014). Management of adult diabetic ketoacidosis. *Diabetes Metab Syndr Obes, 7*, 255–264.

Gray, J. A. M. (1997). *Evidence-based healthcare: how to make health policy and management decisions*. London: Churchill Livingstone.

Hall, J. B., Schmidt, G. A., & Kress, J. P. (2015). *Principles of critical care*. New York: McGraw-Hill Education.

Hamilton, P. M. (2007). Psychiatric emergencies: caring for people in crisis. Nursing. Retrieved from CEU.com. http://www.nursingceu.com/courses/358/index_nceu.html.

Hammond, B. B. (2010). Four steps to reducing door-to-balloon time. *J Emerg Nurs, 36*(3), 217–220.

Hardin, S. R., & Kaplow, R. (2017). *Synergy for clinical excellence: the AACN Synergy Model for patient care* (2nd ed.). Burlington, MA: Jones & Bartlett Learning.

Harrington, M., & DeLeskey, K. (2015). Shh! Quiet time in the ICU. *Nurs Manage*, *46*(5), 21–23.

Harris, C. (2014). Neuromonitoring indications and utility in the intensive care unit. *Crit Care Nurse*, *34*(3), 30–40.

Havelock, R. (1973). *The change agent's guide to innovation in education*. Englewood Cliffs, NJ: Educational Technology Publications.

Hayes, C. (2000). The Synergy Model in practice: strengthening nurses' moral agency. *Crit Care Nurse*, *20*(5), 90–94.

Hazinski, M. F., Nolan, J. P., Billi, J. E., Bottiger, B. W., Bossaert, L., de Caen, A. R., et al. (2010). Part 1: Executive summary: 2010 International consensus on cardiopulmonary resuscitation and emergency cardiovascular care science with treatment recommendations. *Circulation*, *122*(16 Suppl. 2), S250–S275.

Hazinski, M. F., Nolan, J. P., Aickin, R., Bhanji, F., Billi, J. E., Callaway, C. W., et al. (2015). Part 1: Executive summary: 2015 International consensus on cardiopulmonary resuscitation and emergency cardiovascular care science with treatment recommendations. *Circulation*, *132*(16 Suppl. 1), S2–S39.

Health Resources and Services Administration. (2016). Cultural, language and health literacy. Retrieved from https://www.hrsa.gov/culturalcompetence/index.html.

Hendricks, J. M., & Cope, V. C. Generational diversity: what nurse managers need to know. *J Adv Nurs*, *69*(3), 717–725.

Holcomb, J. B., Tilley, B. C., Baraniuk, S., Fox, E. E., Wade, C. E., Podbielski, J. M., et al. (2015). Transfusion of plasma, platelets, and red blood cells in a 1:1:1 vs a 1:1:2 ratio and mortality in patients with severe trauma: the PROPPR randomized clinical trial. *JAMA*, *313*(5), 471–482.

Holley, A. B. (2010). Sleep in the ICU. Retrieved from http://www.medscape.com/viewarticle/723907.

Howard, P. K., & Steinmann, R. A. (2010). Epidemiology and mechanisms of injury. In *Sheehy's Emergency Nursing: Principles and Practices* (6th ed.). (pp. 223–253). St. Louis: Elsevier.

How-to guide. (2012). *Prevent ventilator-associated pneumonia*. Cambridge, MA: Institute for Healthcare Improvement.

Hunt, S. A., Baker, D. W., Chin, M. H., Cinquegrani, M. P., Feldman, A. M., Francis, G. S., & International Society for Heart and Lung Transplantation; Heart Failure Society of America. (2001). ACC/AHA guidelines for the evaluation and management of chronic heart failure in the adult: Executive summary, a report of the American College of Cardiology/American Heart Association Task Force on Practice Guidelines (Committee to Revise the 1995 Guidelines for the Evaluation and Management of Heart Failure): Developed in collaboration with the International Society for Heart and Lung Transplantation; endorsed by the Heart Failure Society of America. *Circulation*, *104*(24), 2996–3007.

Infusion Nurses Society. (2016). Infusion nursing standards of practice. *J Infusion Nursing*, *34*(1S), S1–S110.

Inker, L. A., Astor, B. C., Fox, C. H., Isakova, T., Lash, J. P., Peralta, C. A., et al. (2014). KDOQI US Commentary on the 2012 KDIGO Clinical Practice Guideline for the Evaluation and Management of CKD. *Am J Kidney Dis*, *63*(5), 713–735.

Institute for Healthcare Improvement. (2005). Implement the ventilator bundle. Retrieved from http://www.ihi.org/IHI/Topics/CriticalCare/IntensiveCare/Changes/ImplementtheVentilatorBundle.htm.

Institute for Healthcare Improvement. (2011). Science of improvement: how to improve. Retrieved from http://www.ihi.org/resources/pages/howtoimprove/scienceofimprovementhowtoimprove.aspx.

Institute for Safe Medication Practices. (2016). ISMP list of high-alert medications in acute care settings. Retrieved from http://ismp.org/Tools/institutionalhighAlert.asp.

Institute of Healthcare Improvement. (2010). *How-to guide: prevent ventilator-associated by implementing the five components of care called the ventilator bundle*. Cambridge, MA: Institute for Healthcare Improvement.

Institute of Medicine. (2010). The future of nursing: leading change, advancing health. Retrieved from https://www.nap.edu/download/12956.

Institute of Medicine. (2015). Assessing progress on the Institute of Medicine report: the future of nursing. Retrieved from https://www.nap.edu/21838.

Jackson, M., Ignatavicius, D. D., & Case, B. (2004). *Conversations in critical thinking and clinical judgment*. Boston: Jones and Bartlett.

Jauch, E. C., Saver, J. L., Adams, H. P., Bruno, A., Connors, J. J. B., Demaerschalk, B. M., & Yonas, H. (2013). Guidelines for the early management of patients with acute ischemic stroke. *Stroke*, *44*(3), 870–947.

John, C. A., & Day, M. W. (2012). Central neurogenic diabetes insipidus, syndrome of inappropriate secretion of antidiuretic hormone, and cerebral salt-wasting syndrome in traumatic brain injury. *Crit Care Nurse*, *32*(2), e1–e7.

Johnson, S. A., & Romanello, M. L. (2005). Generational diversity. Teaching and learning approaches. *Nurse Educator*, *30*(5), 212–216.

The Joint Commission. (2012). *Preventing central line-associated bloodstream infections*. Oak Brook, IL: Joint Commission Resources. https://www.jointcommission.org/assets/1/18/CLABSI_Monograph.pdfafety Program for Reducing CAUTI in Hospitals.

Kaplow, R. (2011). The value of certification. *AACN Adv Crit Care*, *22*(1), 25–32.

Kasper, D. L., Fauci, A. S., Hauser, S. L., Longo, D. L., Jameson, L., & Loscalzo, J. (2016). *Harrison's Manual of Medicine* (19th ed.). New York: McGraw-Hill Education.

Kendall-Gallagher, D., & Blegen, M. A. (2009). Competency and certification of registered nurses and safety of patients in intensive care units. *Am J Criti Care*, *18*(2), 106–116.

Kidney Disease: Improving Global Outcomes (KDIGO) Acute Kidney Injury Work Group. KDIGO clinical practice guideline for acute kidney injury. *Kidney Int*, *2*(Suppl), 1–138.

Kierszenbaum, A. L., & Tres, L. L. (2016). Nervous tissue. In A. L. Kierszenbaum, & L. L. Tres (Eds.), *Histology and cell biology: an introduction to pathology* (4th ed.). (pp. 239–272). Philadelphia: Elsevier.

Kohn, L. T., Corrigan, J. M., & Donaldson, M. S. (2000). *To err is human. Building a safer health system*. Washington, DC: National Academies Press.

Kollef, M. H. (2004). Prevention of hospital-associated pneumonia and ventilator-associated pneumonia. *Crit Care Med*, *32*(6), 1396–1405.

Kotter, J. P. (1995). Leading change: why transformation efforts fail. *Harv Bus Rev*, *73*(1), 59–68.

Kramlich, D. (2016). Strategies for acute and critical care nurses implementing complementary therapies requested by patients and their families. *Crit Care Nurse*, *36*(6), 52–58.

Kubler-Ross, E. (1969). *On death and dying*. New York: Macmillan.

Langley, G. L., Nolan, K. M., Nolan, T. W., Norman, C. L., & Provost, L. P. (1996). *The improvement guide: a practical approach to enhancing organizational performance*. San Francisco: Jossey-Bass Publishers.

Leske, J. (1991). Overview of family needs after critical illness: from assessment to intervention. *AACN Clin Issues Crit Care Nurs*, *2*(2), 220–229.

Lewin, K. (1951). *Field theory in social sciences*. New York: Harper.

Lieberman, P., Nicklas, R. A., Randolph, C., Oppenheimer, J., Bernstein, D., Bernstein, J., et al. (2015). Anaphylaxis—a practice parameter update 2015. *Ann Allergy Asthma Immunol*, *115*, 341–384.

Link, M. S., Atkins, D. L., Passman, R. S., Halperin, H. R., Samson, R. A., White, R. D., et al. (2010). Part 6: Electrical therapies: automated external defibrillators, defibrillation, cardioversion, and pacing: 2010 American Heart Association guidelines for cardiopulmonary resuscitation and emergency cardiovascular care. *Circulation*, *122*(18 Suppl. 3), S706–S719.

Link, M. S., Berkow, L. C., Kudenchuk, P. J., Halperin, H. R., Hess, E. P., Moitra, V. K., et al. (2015). Part 7: Adult advanced cardiovascular life support. *Circulation*, *132*(Suppl), S444–S464.

Lippett, R., Watson, J., & Westley, B. (1958). *The dynamics of planned change*. New York: Harcourt, Brace, and Company.

Lira, A., & Pinsky, M. R. (2014). Choices in fluid type and volume during resuscitation: impact on patient outcomes. *Ann Intensive Care, 4*, 38.

Liu, J. L., Xu, F., Zhou, H., Wu, X. J., Shi, L. X., Lu, R. Q., et al. (2016). Expanded CURB-65: a new score system predicts severity of community-acquired pneumonia with superior efficiency. *Sci Rep, 6*, 22911. https://doi.org/10.1038/srep22911.

Lundgren, J. (2016). Understanding NPUAP's updates to pressure ulcer terminology and staging. *Wound Care Advisor, 4*, 14.

Mackintosh, R., Gwilliam, A., & Williams, M. (2014). Teaching the fruits of pressure ulcer staging. *J Wound Ostomy Continence Nurs, 41*(4), 381–387.

Maida, V., & Cheung, J. W. (2017). Looking beyond the cell in cellulitis. *Adv Skin Wound Care, 30*(5), 209–212.

Makdisi, G., & Wang, I. (2015). Extra corporeal membrane oxygenation (ECMO): review of a lifesaving technology. *J Thoracic Dis, 7*(7), E166–E176.

Mangurten, J. A., Scott, S. H., Guzzetta, C. E., Sperry, J. S., Vinson, L. A., Hicks, B. A., et al. (2005). Family presence: making room. *Am J Nurs, 105*(5), 40–49.

Marik, P., Monnet, X., & Teboul, J. L. (2011). Hemodynamic parameters to guide fluid therapy. *Ann Intensive Care, 1*, 1.

Marquis, B. L., & Huston, C. J. (2011). *Leadership roles and management functions in nursing. Theory and application* (7th ed.). Philadelphia: Lippincott Williams & Wilkins.

Martin, G. S. (2006). Pulmonary artery catheterization. Retrieved from http://www.medscape.org/viewarticle/521197.

Matthews, E. E. (2011). Sleep disturbances and fatigue in critically ill patients. *AACN Adv Crit Care, 22*(3), 204–224.

Mattox, E. A. (2017). Complications of peripheral venous access devices: Prevention, detection, and recovery strategies. *Crit Care Nurse, 37*(2), e1–e14.

McCaffery, M. (1968). *Nursing practice theories related to cognition, bodily pain and main environment interactions*. Los Angeles: University of California, Los Angeles.

McCaffery, M. (2002). Teaching your patient to use a pain rating scale. *Nursing, 32*(8), 17.

McCance, K. L., & Huether, S. E. (2014). *Pathophysiology. The biologic basis for disease in adults and children* (7 ed.). St. Louis: Elsevier Mosby.

Melnyk, B. M., & Fineout-Overholt, E. (2011). *Evidence-based practice in nursing and healthcare: a guide to best practice* (2nd ed.). Philadelphia: Lippincott Williams & Wilkins.

Mitchell, C. (2016). Tissue oxygenation monitoring as a guide for trauma resuscitation. *Crit Care Nurse, 36*(3), 12–20.

Montalvo, I. (2007). The National Database of Nursing Quality Indicators (NDNQI®). Retrieved from http://www.nursingworld.org/MainMenuCategories/ANAMarketplace/ANAPeriodicals/OJIN/TableofContents/Volume122007/No3Sept07/NursingQualityIndicators.html.

Morton, P. G., & Fontaine, D. K. (2009). *Critical care nursing. A holistic approach* (9th ed.). Philadelphia: Lippincott Williams & Wilkins.

Mtui, E., Gruener, G., & Dockery, P. (2016). Spinal cord: ascending pathways. In E. Mtui, G. Gruener & M. J. T. FitzGerald (Eds.), *Fitzgerald's clinical neuroanatomy and neuroscience* (7th ed.). Philadelphia: Elsevier.

Mudge, E. J. (2015). Recent accomplishments in wound healing. *Int Wound J, 12*(1), 4–9.

Naftel, J. P., Ard, M. D., & Fratkin, J. D. (2013). The cell biology of neurons and glia. In D. E. Haines (Ed.), *Fundamental neuroscience for basic and clinical applications* (4th ed.). Philadelphia: Saunders.

Napolitano, L. M., Kurek, S., Luchette, F. A., Corwin, H. L., Barie, P. S., Tisherman, S. A., & Eastern Association for the Surgery of Trauma Practice Management Workgroup. (2009). Clinical practice guideline: red blood cell transfusion in adult trauma and critical care. *Crit Care Med, 37*(12), 3124–3157.

National Pressure Ulcer Advisory Panel. (2016). NPUAP pressure injury stages. Retrieved from http://www.npuap.org/resources/educational-and-clinical-resources/npuap-pressure-injury-stages/.

Neumar, R. W., Otto, C. W., Link, M. S., Kronick, S. L., Shuster, M., Callaway, C. W., et al. (2010). Part 8: adult advanced cardiovascular life support: 2010 American Heart Association guidelines for cardiopulmonary resuscitation and emergency cardiovascular care. *Circulation, 122*(18 Suppl. 3), S729–S767.

Neville, T. H., Wiley, J. F., Yamamoto, M. C., Flitcraft, M., Anderson, B., Curtis, J. R., et al. (2015). Concordance of nurses and physicians on whether critical care patients are receiving futile treatment. *Am J Crit Care, 24*(5), 403–410.

Nolan, T. W. (1998). Understanding medical systems. *Ann Intern Med, 128*(4), 293–298.

O'Connor, R. E., Brady, W., Brooks, S. C., Diercks, D., Egan, J., Ghaemmaghami, C., et al. (2010). Part 10: acute coronary syndromes: 2010 American Heart Association guidelines for cardiopulmonary resuscitation and emergency cardiovascular care. *Circulation, 122*(18 Suppl. 3), S787–S817.

Ohmart, G. (2013). Nursing peer review. Retrieved from http://nursing.advanceweb.com/Features/Articles/Nursing-Peer-Review.aspx.

Opoku, F. (2015). Ten top tips: improving the diagnosis of cellulitis in the lower limb. *Wounds Int, 6*(1), 4–8.

Pagana, K. D., Pagana, T. J., & Pagana, T. N. (2016). *Mosby's diagnostic and laboratory test reference* (13th ed.). St. Louis: Elsevier.

Page, A. (2004). *Keeping patients safe. Transforming the work environment for nurses*. Washington, DC: National Academies Press.

Palevsky, P. M., Liu, K. D., Brophy, P. D., Chawla, L. S., Parikh, C. R., Thakar, C. V., et al. (2013). KDOQI US commentary on the 2012 KDIGO clinical practice guideline for acute kidney injury. *Am J Kidney Dis, 61*(5), 649–672.

Patel, J., Baldwin, J., Bunting, P., & Laha, S. (2014). The effect of a multicomponent multidisciplinary bundle of interventions on sleep and delirium in medical and surgical intensive care patients. *Anaesthesia, 69*(6), 540–549.

Payen, J. F., Bru, O., Bosson, J. L., Lagrasta, A., Novel, E., Deschaus, I., et al. (2001). Assessing pain in critically ill sedated patients by using a behavioral pain scale. *Crit Care Med, 29*(12), 2258–2263.

Prochaska, J. M. (2000). A transtheoretical model for assessing organizational change: a study of family service agencies' movement to time-limited therapy. *Family Soc, 81*(1), 76–85.

Prochaska, J. M., Prochaska, J. O., & Levesque, D. A. (2001). A transtheoretical approach to changing organizations. *Adm Policy Ment Health, 28*(4), 247–261.

Purnell, L. D. (2014). *Guide to culturally competent health care* (3rd ed.). Philadelphia: F.A. Davis.

Quality and Safety Education for Nurses. (2016). QSEN competencies. Retrieved from http://qsen.org/competencies/pre-licensure-ksas.

Rogers, E. M. (1995). *Diffusion of innovations* (4th ed.). New York: Free Press.

Rushton, C. H. (2016). Moral resilience: a capacity for navigating moral distress in critical care. *AACN Adv Crit Care, 27*(1), 111–119.

SAFE Study Investigators. (2007). Saline or albumin for fluid resuscitation in patients with traumatic brain injury. *N Engl J Med, 357*(9), 874–885.

Savel, R. H., & Munro, C. L. (2013). How much care is too much care? *Am J Crit Care, 22*(2), 86–88.

Savel, R. H., & Munro, C. L. (2015). Moral distress, moral courage. *Am J Crit Care, 24*(4), 276–278.

Shackell, E., & Gillespie, M. (2009). The oxygen supply and demand framework: a tool to support integrative learning. *Dynamics, 20*(4), 15–19.

Siegel, J. D., Rhinehart, E., Jackson, M., & Chiarello, L. (2006). Management of multidrug-resistant organisms in healthcare settings. Retrieved from https://www.cdc.gov/hicpac/pdf/MDRO/MDROGuideline2006.pdf.

Siela, D. (2008). Chest radiograph evaluation and interpretation. *AACN Adv Crit Care, 19*(4), 444–473; quiz 474–475.

Simonneau, G., Robbins, I. M., Beghetti, M., Channick, R. N., Delcroix, M., Denton, C. P., et al. (2009). Updated clinical classification of pulmonary hypertension. *J Am Coll Cardiol, 54*(1 Suppl), S43–S54.

Singer, M., Deutschman, C. S., Seymour, C. W., Shankar-Hari, M., Annane, D., Bauer, M., et al. (2016). The third international consensus definitions for sepsis and septic shock (sepsis-3). *JAMA, 315*(8), 801–810.

Skidmore-Roth, L. A. (2016). *Mosby's 2016 nursing drug reference* (29th ed.). St. Louis: Elsevier.

Sole, M. L., Penoyer, D. A., Su, X., Jimenez, E., Kalita, S. J., Poalillo, E., & Ludy, J. E. (2009). Assessment of endotracheal cuff pressure by continuous monitoring: a pilot study. *Am J Crit Care, 18*(2), 133–143.

Sole, M. L., Klein, D. G., & Moseley, M. J. (2017a). *Introduction to critical care nursing* (7th ed.). St. Louis: Elsevier.

Sole, M. L., Klein, D. G., & Moseley, M. J. (2017b). Shock, sepsis, and multiple organ dysfunction syndrome. In *Introduction to critical care nursing* (7th ed.). (pp. 253–288). St. Louis: Elsevier.

Spasovski, G., Vanholder, R., Allolio, B., Annane, D., Ball, S., Bichet, D., et al. (2014). Clinical practice guideline on diagnosis and treatment of hyponatraemia. *Eur J Endocrinol, 170*(3), G1–G47.

Speroni, K. G., Lucas, J., Dugan, L., O'Meara-Lett, M., Putman, M., Daniel, M., & Atherton, M. (2011). Comparative effectiveness of standard endotracheal tubes vs. endotracheal tubes with continuous subglottic suctioning on ventilator-associated pneumonia rates. *Nurs Econ, 29*(1), 15–20, 37.

Stevens, K. R. (2001). Systematic reviews: the heart of evidence-based practice. *AACN Clin Issues, 12*(4), 529–538.

Stevens, K. R. (2012). Star Model of EBP: knowledge transformation. The University of Texas Health Science Center at San Antonio: Academic Center for Evidence-based Practice. Retrieved from http://nursing.uthscsa.edu/onrs/starmodel/star-model.asp.

Straus, S. E., Glasziou, P., Richardson, W. S., & Haynes, R. B. (2011). *Evidence-based medicine: how to practice and teach it* (4th ed.). Edinburgh: Churchill Livingstone.

Sugarman, R. (2014). Structure and function of the neurologic system. In K. McCance, & S. Huether (Eds.), *Pathophysiology: the biologic basis for disease in adults and children* (7th ed.). (pp. 447–483). St. Louis: Elsevier.

Tachjian, A., Maria, V., & Jahangir, A. (2010). Use of herbal products and potential interactions in patients with cardiovascular disease. *J Am Coll Cardiol, 55*(6), 515–525.

Tainter, C. R., Levine, A. R., Quraishi, S. A., Butterly, A. D., Stahl, D. L., & Lee, J. (2016). Noise levels in surgical ICUs are consistently above recommended standards. *Crit Care Med, 44*(1), 147–152.

Tamburri, L. M., DiBrienza, R., Zozula, R., & Redeker, N. (2004). Nocturnal care interactions with patients in critical care units. *Am J Crit Care, 13*(2), 102–115.

Teal, J. (2011). Certifiably excellent. *AACN Adv Crit Care, 22*(1), 83–88.

Tomte, O., Draegni, T., Mangschau, A., Jacobsen, D., Auestad, B., & Sunde, K. (2011). A comparison of intravascular and surface cooling techniques in comatose cardiac arrest survivors. *Crit Care Med, 39*(3), 443–449.

Urden, L. D., Stacy, K. M., & Lough, M. E. (2018). *Critical care nursing: diagnosis and management*. Maryland Heights, MO: Elsevier.

U.S. Census Bureau. (2014). Projections of the size and composition of the U.S. population: 2014 to 2060. Retrieved from http://www.census.gov/library/publications/2015/demo/p25-1143.html.

Vanderah, T. W., & Gould, D. J. (2016). Introduction to the nervous system. In T. W. Vanderah, & D. J. Gould (Eds.), *Nolte's the human brain: an introduction to its functional anatomy* (7th ed.). (pp. 1–38). Philadelphia: Elsevier.

Vincent, J. L., Pinsky, M. R., Sprung, C. L., Levy, M., Marini, J. J., Payen, D., et al. (2008). The pulmonary artery catheter: in medio virtus. *Crit Care Med, 36*(11), 3093–3096.

Wavra, T. (2006). *The 4 As to rise above moral distress handbook*. Aliso Viejo, CA: AACN.

Wein, A. J., Kavoussi, L. R., Partin, A. W., & Peters, A. W. (2016). *Campbell-Walsh urology* (11th ed.). St. Louis: Elsevier.

Wiener, R. S., & Welch, H. G. (2007). Trends in the use of the pulmonary artery catheter in the United States: 1993–2004. *JAMA, 298*, 423–429.

Xiaohong, D. (2017). Predicting the risk for hospital-acquired pressure ulcers in critical care patients. *Crit Care Nurse, 37*(4), e1–e11.

Yancy, C. W., Jessup, M., Bozkurt, B., Butler, J., Casey, D. E., Jr., Colvin, M. M., et al. (2016). 2016 ACC/AHA/HFSA focused update on new pharmacological therapy for heart failure: an update of the 2013 ACCF/AHA guideline for the management of heart failure. *J Am Coll Cardiol, 134*(13), e282–e293.

Yoder-Wise, P. (2011). *Leading and managing in nursing* (5th ed.). St. Louis: Mosby.

Common Abbreviations and Acronyms Used in Critical Care Nursing

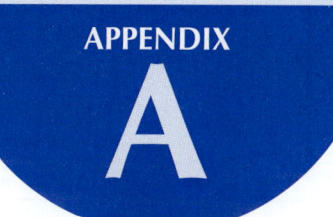

APPENDIX A

2,3-DPG	2,3-diphosphoglyceric acid
A	alveolar
a	arterial
a/A	arterial/alveolar (as in a/A gradient)
A_2	aortic (first) component of S_2
AAA	abdominal aortic aneurysm
AACN	American Association of Critical-Care Nurses
AAL	anterior axillary line
ABG	arterial blood gas
ABI	ankle-brachial index
AC	assist-control
ACC	American College of Cardiology
ACE	Academic Center for Evidence-Based Practice
ACE	angiotensin converting enzyme
ACLS	advanced cardiac life support
ACS	abdominal compartment syndrome
ACS	acute coronary syndrome
ACT	activated clotting time
ACTH	adrenocorticotropic hormone
ADA	American Diabetic Association
ADH	antidiuretic hormone
ADL	activity of daily living
ADP	adenosine diphosphate
AED	automated external defibrillator
AF	atrial fibrillation
AGREE	Appraisal of Guidelines for Research and Evaluation
AHA	American Heart Association
AHA	American Hospital Association
AHRQ	Agency for Healthcare Research and Quality
AIDS	acquired immune deficiency syndrome
AIVR	accelerated idioventricular rhythm
AKI	acute kidney injury
ALF	acute liver failure
ALI	acute lung injury
ALS	amyotrophic lateralizing sclerosis

Appendix A Common Abbreviations and Acronyms Used in Critical Care Nursing

ALT	alanine aminotransferase
AMP	Applied Measurement Professionals
ANA	American Nurses Association
ANCC	American Nurses Certification Corporation
ANP	atrial natriuretic peptide
ANS	autonomic nervous system
AP	anteroposterior
APA	American Psychiatric Association
APRV	airway pressure release ventilation
aPTT	activated partial thromboplastin time
AR	aortic regurgitation
ARB	angiotensin receptor blocker
ARDS	acute respiratory distress syndrome
ARF	acute respiratory failure
AS	aortic stenosis
ASA	acetylsalicylic acid (aspirin)
AST	aspartate aminotransferase
ATN	acute tubular necrosis
ATP	adenosine triphosphate
AV	arteriovenous
AV	atrioventricular
AVM	arteriovenous malformation
BAL	bronchoalveolar lavage
BBB	bundle branch block
BE	base excess
Bi-PAP	positive airway pressure on both inspiration and expiration
BIS	bispectral index
Bi-VAD	biventricular assist device
BLS	basic life support
BM	bowel movement
BMI	body mass index
BNP	brain-type natriuretic peptide
BP	blood pressure
BPOC	barcode point of care
BSA	body surface area
BSN	Bachelor of Science in Nursing
BUN	blood urea nitrogen
C	Celsius (also referred to as centigrade)
CABG	coronary artery bypass graft
CAD	coronary artery disease
CaO_2	oxygen content in arterial blood
CAP	community-acquired pneumonia
CAPM	continuous airway pressure monitoring
CAPP	coronary artery perfusion pressure
CASS	continuous aspiration of subglottic secretions
CAVH	continuous arteriovenous hemofiltration
CAVHD	continuous arteriovenous hemodialysis
CBC	complete blood count
CBF	cerebral blood flow

Appendix A Common Abbreviations and Acronyms Used in Critical Care Nursing

CCO	continuous cardiac output
CCU	critical care unit or cardiac care unit
CDC	Centers for Disease Control and Prevention
CEA	carcinoembryonic antigen
CHB	complete heart block
CHO	carbohydrate
CHP	capillary hydrostatic pressure
CI	cardiac index
CINAHL	Cumulative Index of Nursing and Allied Health Literature
CK	creatine kinase
CKD	chronic kidney disease
CK-MB	creatine kinase–muscle/brain
CLRT	continuous lateral rotation therapy
cm	centimeter
CMV	cytomegalovirus
CNS	central nervous system
CO	cardiac output
CO_2	carbon dioxide
COLD	chronic obstructive lung disease
COP	colloidal oncotic pressure
COPD	chronic obstructive pulmonary disease
CPAP	continuous positive airway pressure
CPB	cardiopulmonary bypass
CPG	clinical practice guideline
CPOE	computerized provider order entry
CPP	cerebral perfusion pressure
CPR	cardiopulmonary resuscitation
CRH	corticotropin-releasing hormone
CRRT	continuous renal replacement therapy
CRT	cardiac resynchronization therapy
CSF	cerebrospinal fluid
CSF	colony-stimulating factor
CSW	cerebral salt wasting
CT	computed tomography
cTnI	cardiac troponin I
cTnT	cardiac troponin T
CVA	cerebrovascular accident
CVA	costovertebral angle
CvO_2	oxygen content in venous blood
CVP	central venous pressure
CVVH	continuous venovenous hemofiltration
CVVHD	continuous venovenous hemodialysis
CVVHDF	continuous venovenous hemodiafiltration
D_5LR	5% dextrose in lactated Ringer solution
D_5NS	5% dextrose in normal saline
D_5W	5% dextrose in water
$D_{10}W$	10% dextrose in water
$D_{50}W$	50% dextrose in water
DAI	diffuse axonal injury

dB	decibel
DBP	diastolic blood pressure
DCA	directional coronary atherectomy
DES	drug-eluting stent
DHA	docosahexaenoic acid
DI	diabetes insipidus
DIC	disseminated intravascular coagulation
DKA	diabetes ketoacidosis
dl	deciliter
DM	diabetes mellitus
DNA	deoxyribonucleic acid
DNR	do not resuscitate
DO_2	oxygen delivery to the tissues
DO_2I	delivery of oxygen to the tissue index
DPL	diagnostic peritoneal lavage
dPP	pulse pressure variation
DT	delirium tremens
DTBT	door-to-balloon time
DTR	deep tendon reflex
DVT	deep vein thrombosis
EAB	extraanatomical bypass
EBCT	electron-beam computed tomography
EBP	evidence-based practice
$ECCO_2OR$	extracorporeal carbon dioxide removal
ECF	extracellular fluid
ECF-A	eosinophil chemotactic factor of anaphylaxis
ECG	electrocardiogram (may also be abbreviated EKG)
ECMO	extracorporeal membrane oxygenator
ED	emergency department
EDH	epidural hematoma
EEG	electroencephalogram
EF	ejection fraction
ELCA	excimer laser coronary atherectomy
ELISA	enzyme linked immunosorbent assay
EMG	electromyogram
EMI	electromagnetic interference
EMS	emergency management system
ENG	electronystagmography
EOM	extraocular movement
EPA	eicosapentaenoic acid
EPA	Environmental Protection Agency
EPS	electrophysiology studies
EPS	extrapyramidal symptoms
ERCP	endoscopic retrograde cholangiopancreatography
ERV	expiratory reserve volume
ESR	erythrocyte sedimentation rate
ET	endotracheal
ETC	Esophageal tracheal Combitube
ETT	exercise tolerance test

EVG	endovascular graft
F	fahrenheit
f	frequency of ventilation
FAST	focused abdominal sonography for trauma
FDA	Food and Drug Administration
FEV	forced expiratory capacity
FFP	fresh frozen plasma
FiO_2	fraction of inspired oxygen
FRC	functional residual capacity
FSP	fibrin split products (also referred to as *fibrin degradation products*)
FT_c	flow time corrected
FTT	failure to thrive
FVC	forced vital capacity
g	gram
GABA	gamma-aminobutyric acid
GALT	gut-associated lymphoid tissue
GCS	Glasgow Coma Scale
GERD	gastroesophageal reflux disease
GFR	glomerular filtration rate
GGT	gamma-glutamyl transferase
GI	gastrointestinal
GP	glycoprotein
GU	genitourinary
H^+	gydrogen ion
H_2O	water
HAP	hospital-acquired pneumonia
HAT	heparin-associated thrombocytopenia
HBV	hepatitis B virus
HCAP	health care–associated pneumonia
HCl	hydrochloric
HCO_3	bicarbonate
Hct	hematocrit
HDL	high-density lipoproteins
HELLP	hemolysis, elevated liver enzyme levels, and low platelet count (as in HELLP syndrome)
HF	heart failure
HFJV	high-frequency jet ventilation
HFO	high-frequency oscillation
HFPPV	high-frequency positive-pressure ventilation
HFV	high-frequency ventilation
Hg	mercury
Hgb	hemoglobin
HHS	hyperglycemic hyperosmolar state
HIPAA	Health Insurance Portability and Accountability Act
HIT	heparin-induced thrombocytopenia
HIV	human immunodeficiency virus
HLA	human leukocyte antigen
HME	heat and moisture exchanger
HOB	head of bed
HR	heart rate

HRSA	Health Resources and Services Administration
HRT	hormone replacement therapy
IABP	intraaortic balloon pump
IAH	intraabdominal hypertension
IAP	intraabdominal pressure
IBW	ideal body weight
IC	inspiratory capacity
ICD	implantable cardiac defibrillator
ICH	intracranial hematoma
ICOP	interstitial colloidal oncotic pressure
ICP	intracranial pressure
ICS	intercostal space
ICU	intensive care unit
I:E	inspiration:expiration
IFD	intermittent flush device
Ig	immunoglobulin
IHP	interstitial hydrostatic pressure
IHSS	idiopathic hypertrophic subaortic stenosis
IL	interleukin
ILV	independent lung ventilation
IM	intramuscular
IMV	intermittent mandatory ventilation
INH	isoniazid
INR	international normalized ratio
INVOS	in vivo optical spectroscopy
IOM	Institute of Medicine (now Academy of Medicine)
IPBH	intraparenchymal brain hemorrhage
IPPB	intermittent positive-pressure breathing
IRA	infarct-related artery
IRV	inspiratory reserve volume
IRV	inverse ratio ventilation
ISMP	Institute for Safe Medication Practices
ITP	idiopathic thrombocytopenia purpura
IU	international units
IV	intravenous
IVP	intravenous pyelogram
IVUS	intravascular ultrasound
JCAHO	Joint Commission on Accreditation of Healthcare Organizations
JVD	jugular venous distention
kg	kilogram
KUB	kidneys, ureters, bladder (same as flat plate of abdomen)
KVO	keep vein open
L	liter
LA	left atrium
LAAL	left anterior axillary line
LAD	left anterior descending (artery)
LAD	left axis deviation
LAH	left anterior hemibundle
LAP	left atrial pressure

Appendix A Common Abbreviations and Acronyms Used in Critical Care Nursing

LBB	left bundle branch
LBBB	left bundle branch block
LCA	left circumflex artery
LDH	lactic dehydrogenase
LDL	low-density lipoproteins
LES	lower esophageal sphincter
LGL	Lown-Ganong-Levine syndrome
LICS	left intercostal space
LLQ	left lower quadrant
LMA	laryngeal mask airway
LMAL	left midaxillary line
LMCL	left midclavicular line
LMN	lower motor neuron
LMWH	low-molecular-weight heparin
LOC	level of consciousness
LP	lumbar puncture
LPAL	left posterior axillary line
LPH	left posterior hemibundle
LPN	licensed practical nurse (aka, licensed vocational nurse)
LR	lactated Ringer solution
LSB	left sternal border
LUQ	left upper quadrant
LV	left ventricle
LVAD	left ventricular assist device
LVEDP	left ventricular end-diastolic pressure
LVEDV	left ventricular end-diastolic volume
LVF	left ventricular failure
LVH	left ventricular hypertrophy
LVMI	left ventricular myocardial infarction
LVSWI	left ventricular stroke work index
M_1	mitral (first) component of S_1
mA	milliampere (unit of measurement for electrical current)
MAL	midaxillary line
MALT	mucosa-associated lymphoid tissues
MAO	monoamine oxidase (as in MAO inhibitors)
MAP	mean arterial pressure
MAP	multidisciplinary action plan
mcg	microgram (unit of measurement for weight)
MCH	mean corpuscular hemoglobin
MCHC	mean corpuscular hemoglobin concentration
MCL	midclavicular line
MCL	modified chest lead
MCT	medium chain triglycerides
MCV	mean corpuscular volume
MDF	myocardial depressant factor
MDMA	methylenedioxymethamphetamine (i.e., ecstasy)
M_E	minute ventilation exhaled
mEq	milliequivalent (unit of measurement for solutes in solution)
mg	milligram (unit of measurement for weight)

MI	myocardial infarction
MIC	minimum inhibitory concentration
MIDCABG	minimally invasive coronary artery bypass graft
MIP	maximal inspiratory pressure (or force) (also referred to as *negative inspiratory pressure* [or *force*])
ml	milliliter (unit of measurement for volume)
mm	millimeter (unit of measurement for length)
mm Hg	millimeters of mercury
MODS	multiple organ dysfunction syndrome
mOsm/kg	milliosmoles per kilogram
mOsm/l	milliosmoles per liter
MR	mitral regurgitation
MRA	magnetic resonance angiography
MRI	magnetic resonance imaging
MRS	magnetic resonance spectroscopy
MS	mitral stenosis
MSG	monosodium glutamate
MSL	midsternal line
MUGA	multiple-gated acquisition scan
MV	mechanical ventilation
MVC	motor vehicle collision
MVO_2	myocardial oxygen consumption
MVP	mitral valve prolapse
MVV	maximal voluntary ventilation
NAC	*N*-acetylcysteine
NASPE	North American Society of Pacing and Electrophysiology
NCLEX	National Council Licensure Examination
NCSBN	National Council of State Boards of Nursing
NDE	near-death experience
NDNQI	National Database of Nursing Quality Indicators
NG	nasogastric
NIF	negative inspiratory force
NIH	National Institutes of Health
NIHSS	National Institutes of Health Stroke Scale
NK	natural killer
NPO	nothing by mouth
NPPV	noninvasive positive-pressure ventilation
NRTI	nucleoside analog reverse transcriptase inhibitor
NS	normal saline
NSAID	nonsteroidal antiinflammatory drug
NSR	normal sinus rhythm
NtRTI	nucleotide reverse transcriptase inhibitor
NYHA	New York Heart Association
O_2	oxygen
O_2EI	oxygen extraction index
O_2ER	oxygen extraction ratio
OCD	obsessive compulsive disorder
OPB	ova, parasites, blood
OPCABG	off-pump coronary artery bypass graft
OPG	oculoplethysmography

Appendix A Common Abbreviations and Acronyms Used in Critical Care Nursing

P_2	pulmonic (second) component of S_2
PA	posterior anterior
PA	pulmonary artery
PAC	premature atrial contraction
PAC	pulmonary artery catheter
$PaCO_2$	partial pressure of carbon dioxide in arterial blood
PAd	pulmonary artery diastolic pressure
PAL	posterior axillary line
PAm	pulmonary artery pressure mean
PaO_2	pressure of oxygen in arterial blood
PAO_2	pressure of oxygen in alveolar blood
PAOP	pulmonary artery occlusive pressure (previously referred to as *pulmonary capillary wedge pressure* or *pulmonary artery wedge pressure*)
PAP	pulmonary artery pressure
PAs	pulmonary artery systolic pressure
PAT	paroxysmal atrial tachycardia
Pb	barometric pressure
PC/IRV	pressure-controlled/inverse-ratio ventilation
PCA	patient-controlled analgesia
PCI	percutaneous coronary intervention
PCP	phencyclidine
PCP	*Pneumocystis carinii* pneumonia
PCR	polymerase chain reaction
PCV	pressure-controlled ventilation
PD	postural drainage
PDA	patent ductus arteriosus
PDE	phosphodiesterase
PDF	probability density function
PDSA	plan–do–study–act
PE	pulmonary embolism
PEA	pulseless electrical activity
P_ECO_2	partial pressure of carbon dioxide in exhaled air
PEEP	positive end-expiratory pressure
PEFR	peak expiratory flow rate
PEG	percutaneous endoscopic gastrostomy
PEJ	percutaneous endoscopic jejunostomy
PET	positron emission tomography
$P_{et}CO_2$	partial pressure of carbon dioxide in end-tidal air
P/F	PaO_2/FiO_2 (as in P/F ratio)
PFT	pulmonary function tests
pH	hydrogen ion concentration
pHi	intramucosal pH
PICC	percutaneously inserted central catheter
PICOT	problem, intervention, comparison, outcome, timing (i.e., format for a clinical question)
PIP	peak inspiratory pressure
PJC	premature junctional contraction
PMI	point of maximal impulse
PML	progressive multifocal leukoencephalopathy
PMN	polymorphonuclear leukocytes

PMR	papillary muscle rupture
PMR	progressive muscle relaxation
PND	paroxysmal nocturnal dyspnea
PNS	parasympathetic nervous system
PO	oral
PPD	purified protein derivative
PPF	plasma protein fraction
PPI	proton pump inhibitor
PPN	peripheral parenteral nutrition
PQRST	provocation, palliation, quality, quantity, region, radiation, severity, timing (i.e., pain description)
PRVC	pressure-regulated volume-controlled
PSB	protected specimen brush
PSV	pressure support ventilation
PSVT	paroxysmal supraventricular tachycardia
PT	physical therapy
PT	prothrombin time
PTCA	percutaneous transluminal coronary angioplasty
$P_{tc}O_2$	transcutaneous partial pressure of oxygen
PTFE	polytetrafluoroethylene
PTMR	percutaneous transmyocardial revascularization
PTSD	posttraumatic stress disorder
PTSMA	percutaneous transluminal septal myocardial ablation
PTT	partial prothrombin time
PTU	propylthiouracil
PV	peak velocity
PVC	polyvinyl chloride
PVC	premature ventricular contraction
PVR	pulmonary vascular resistance
PVRI	pulmonary vascular resistance index
Q	perfusion
QI	quality improvement
QM	quality management
QT_c	QT interval corrected for rate
RA	right atrium
RAA	renin-angiotensin-aldosterone
RAAL	right anterior axillary line
RAD	right axis deviation
RAP	right atrial pressure
RAS	reticular activating system
RBB	right bundle branch
RBBB	right bundle branch block
RBC	red blood cell
RCA	right coronary artery
REF	right (ventricular) ejection fraction
REM	rapid eye movement
RHD	rheumatic heart disease
RICS	right intercostal space
RIND	reversible ischemic neurologic deficit
RLQ	right lower quadrant

Appendix A Common Abbreviations and Acronyms Used in Critical Care Nursing

RMAL	right midaxillary line
RMCL	right midclavicular line
RN	registered nurse
RNA	ribonucleic acid
ROM	range of motion
ROSC	return of spontaneous circulation
r-PA	recombinant plasminogen activator
RPAL	right posterior axillary line
RQ	respiratory quotient
RR	respiratory rate
RSB	right sternal border
RSBI	rapid shallow breathing index
rSO_2	regional oxygen saturation index
RSV	respiratory syncytium virus
rt-PA	recombinant tissue plasminogen activator
RUQ	right upper quadrant
RV	residual volume
RV	right ventricle
RVAD	right ventricular assist device
RVEDP	right ventricular end-diastolic pressure
RVEDV	right ventricular end-diastolic volume
RVESV	right ventricular end-systolic volume
RVF	right ventricular failure
RVH	right ventricular hypertrophy
RVMI	right ventricular myocardial infarction
RVSWI	right ventricular stroke work index
RYGB	roux-Y gastric bypass
SA	sinoatrial
SAED	semiautomatic external defibrillator
SAH	subarachnoid hemorrhage
SaO_2	oxygen saturation of arterial blood
SARS	severe acute respiratory syndrome
SC	subcutaneous
SCI	spinal cord injury
SCUF	slow continuous ultrafiltration
$S_{cv}O_2$	oxygen saturation of central venous blood
SDH	subdural hematoma
SIADH	syndrome of inappropriate antidiuretic hormone
SILV	synchronized independent lung ventilation
SIMV	synchronized intermittent mandatory ventilation
SIRS	systemic inflammatory response syndrome
SjO_2	oxygen saturation of jugular venous blood
SK	streptokinase
SLE	systemic lupus erythematosus
SNS	sympathetic nervous system
SPECT	single-photon emission computed tomography
SpO_2	oxygen saturation in plasma (e.g., pulse oximetry)
SRS-A	slow-reacting substance of anaphylaxis
STEMI	ST-segment elevation myocardial infarction

STTI	Sigma Theta Tau International
SV	stroke volume
SVI	stroke index
SvO_2	oxygen saturation of mixed venous blood
SVR	systemic vascular resistance
SVRI	systemic vascular resistance index
SVT	supraventricular tachycardia
SVV	stroke volume variability
T	temperature
T_1	tricuspid (second) component of S_1
TAA	thoracic aortic aneurysm
TB	tuberculosis
TBI	toe-brachial index
TCA	tricyclic antidepressant
$TcPO_2$	transcutaneous carbon dioxide
TEC	transluminal extraction catheter
TEE	transesophageal echocardiography
TENS	transcutaneous electrical nerve stimulation
TIA	transient ischemic attack
TIBC	total iron-binding capacity
TIPS	transjugular intrahepatic portosystemic shunt
TLC	total lung capacity
TLC	total lymphocyte count
TNA	total nutrient admixture
TNF	tumor necrosis factor
TPN	total parenteral nutrition
TR	tricuspid regurgitation
TRH	thyrotropin-releasing hormone
TSH	thyroid-stimulating hormone
TTP	thrombotic thrombocytopenia purpura
UAP	unlicensed assistive personnel
UES	upper esophageal sphincter
UFH	unfractionated heparin
UMN	upper motor neuron
UTI	urinary tract infection
V	ventilation
V_A	alveolar minute ventilation
VAC	vacuum-assisted closure
VAD	ventricular assist device
VALI	ventilator-associated lung injury
VAP	ventilator-associated pneumonia
VAPSV	volume-assured pressure support ventilation
VBG	vertical banded gastroplasty
VC	vital capacity
V_D	anatomical dead space
V_E	minute ventilation
VF	ventricular fibrillation
VILI	ventilator-induced lung injury
VIP	volume infusion port

Appendix A Common Abbreviations and Acronyms Used in Critical Care Nursing

VO_2	oxygen consumption by the tissues
VO_2I	consumption of oxygen by the tissues index
VPR	volume pressure response
V/Q	ventilation/perfusion ratio
VSD	ventricular septal defect
VT	ventricular tachycardia
V_T	tidal volume
WBC	white blood cell
WPW	Wolff-Parkinson-White syndrome

Normal Laboratory Values

APPENDIX B

I. Blood
   A. Chemistries
      1. Sodium: 136–145 mEq/l
      2. Potassium: 3.5–5.0 mEq/l
      3. Chloride: 96–106 mEq/l
      4. Calcium: 9.0–10.5 mg/dl in adults and 8.8–10.8 mg/dl in children
      5. Ionized calcium: 4.5–5.6 mg/dl in adults and 4.8–5.52 mg/dl in children
      6. Phosphorus: 3.0–4.5 mg/dl
      7. Magnesium: 1.3–2.1 mEq/l in adults, 1.4–1.7 mEq/l in children, and 1.4–2 mEq/l in infants
      8. Glucose: 70–110 mEq/l
      9. Blood urea nitrogen (BUN): 5–20 mg/dl
     10. Creatine: 0.6–1.1 mg/dl in females and 0.8–1.3 mg/dl in males
     11. Uric acid: 3–7 mg/dl
     12. Osmolality: 280–295 mOsm/kg
     13. Lactate: <1 mmol/l
     14. Ammonia: 15–110 mOsm/dl
     15. Iron: 50–150 mcg/dl
     16. Iron-binding capacity: 250–410 mcg/dl
     17. Carcinoembryonic antigen (CEA): <2 ng/ml
     18. Homocysteine: <15 μmol/l
     19. C-reactive protein: <1 mg/dl
     20. Brain-type natriuretic peptide (BNP): <100 pg/ml
     21. Bilirubin
        a. Total: 0.3–1.3 mg/dl
        b. Direct: 0.1–0.3 mg/dl
        c. Indirect: 0.1–1.0 mg/dl
     22. Proteins
        a. Total protein: 6–8 g/dl
        b. C-reactive protein: <0.8 mg/dl
        c. Albumin: 3.5–4.5 g/dl
        d. Prealbumin: 15–35 mg/dl
        e. Transferrin: 250–300 mg/dl
        f. Globulin: 2.3–3.5 g/dl
        g. Albumin/globulin ratio (A/G): 1.5/1–2.5/1
        h. Fibrinogen: 200–400 mg/dl or 2–4 g/l
     23. Lipids
        a. Cholesterol: 150–200 mg/dl
        b. Triglycerides: 40–150 mg/dl
        c. Lipoprotein-cholesterol fractionation
           1) HDL: 29–77 mg/dl
           2) LDL: 62–130 mg/dl
     24. Enzymes
        a. Total CK: 55–170 U/l for males and 30–135 U/l for females
        b. CK-MB: 0% of total CK
        c. LDH: 90–200 IU/l
        d. LDH-1: 17%–25% of total LDH
        e. Alanine aminotransferase (ALT): 5–36 U/ml (formerly called SGPT)
        f. Aspartate aminotransferase (AST): 15–45 U/ml (formerly called SGOT)
        g. Gammaglutamyl transferase (GGT): 5–38 IU/l
        h. Alkaline phosphatase: 30–85 IU/l
        i. Amylase: 56–190 IU/l
        j. Lipase: 0–1.5 IU/ml
     25. Muscle proteins
        a. Myoglobin: <110 ng/ml
        b. Troponin I: <1.5 ng/ml
        c. Troponin T: <0.1 ng/ml
   B. Arterial blood gases
      1. pH: 7.35–7.45
      2. $PaCO_2$: 35–45 mm Hg
      3. HCO_3: 22–26 mM
      4. Base excess: –2 to +2
      5. PaO_2: 80–100 mm Hg
      6. SaO_2: >95% (in elderly >92%)
      7. Arterial lactate: <1 mmol/l
   C. Hematology
      1. Red blood cells (RBC): $4.4–5.9 \times 10^6$/ml for males and $3.8–5.2 \times 10^6$/ml for females; red cell indices include the following:
        a. Mean corpuscular volume (MCV): 80–100 μm^3
        b. Mean corpuscular hemoglobin (MCH): 27–31 pg
        c. Mean corpuscular hemoglobin concentration (MCHC): 32–36 g/dl
      2. Reticulocyte count: 0.5%–1.5% of RBC
      3. Erythrocyte sedimentation rate: ≤15 mm/hr for males and ≤20 mm/hr for females
      4. Hematocrit: 42%–52% for males and 37%–47% for females
      5. Hemoglobin: 14–18 g/dl for males and 12–16 g/dl for females

6. White blood cells (WBC): 4000–11,000 mm³
   a. Differential
      1) Neutrophils: 40%–80%
      2) Eosinophils: 0%–5%
      3) Basophils: 0%–2%
      4) Monocytes: 3%–8%
      5) Lymphocytes: 10%–40%
7. Immune profile
   a. CD4 cell count: 800 cells/mm³; varies with age
   b. T-helper lymphocytes (CD4)/T-suppressor and cytotoxic lymphocytes (CD8) ratio: 1.8
8. HIV antibody screening: negative

D. Clotting profile
1. Prothrombin time (PT): 12–15 sec; therapeutic is 1.5–2.5 times normal
2. Partial thromboplastin time (PTT): 60–90 sec; therapeutic is 1.5–2.5 times normal
3. Activated partial thromboplastin time (aPTT): 25–38 sec; therapeutic is 1.5–2.5 times normal
4. Activated clotting time (ACT): 70–120 sec; therapeutic, 150–190 sec
5. Thrombin time: 10–15 sec
6. Bleeding time: 1–9.5 min
7. Lee White clotting time: 6–12 min
8. International normalized ratio (INR): <2.0
9. Platelets: normal 150,000–400,000/mm³
10. Fibrinogen: 200–400 mg/dl or 2–4 g/l
11. Fibrin split products (FSPs) (also referred to as fibrin degradation products [FDPs]: 0–10 mcg/dl
12. D-dimer: <250 ng/ml

E. Hormones
1. Thyroid-stimulating hormone (TSH): 2–10 mU/ml
2. Triiodothyronine (T3): 0.2–0.3 mcg/dl
3. Thyroxine (T4): 6–12 mcg/dl
4. ACTH: 15–100 pg/ml in AM, 10–50 pg/ml in PM
5. Cortisol: 6–28 mcg/dl at 8 AM, 4–12 mcg/dl at 4 PM, 2–12 mcg/dl at 8 PM
6. ADH: 1–5 pg/ml

F. Toxicology
1. Alcohol: 0 mg/dl
2. Dilantin: therapeutic 10–20 mcg/ml
3. Digoxin: therapeutic 0.5–2.0 ng/ml
4. Lidocaine: therapeutic 1.5–5.0 mcg/ml
5. Phenobarbital: therapeutic 10–40 mcg/ml
6. Theophylline: therapeutic 10–20 ng/dl

II. Urine
A. Glucose: negative
B. Ketones: negative
C. Protein: 0–8 mg/dl; <150 mg/24-hr urine output
D. Amylase: 3–21 IU/hr
E. Bilirubin: negative
F. Bilinogen: 0.3–3.5 mg/dl
G. RBCs: 0–2/low-power field
H. WBCs: 0–4/low-power field
I. Hemoglobin/myoglobin: negative
J. Specific gravity: 1.005–1.030
K. Osmolality: 50–1200 mOsm/l
L. Culture and sensitivity: no bacteria present; if bacteria are present, appropriate antibiotic therapy is identified
M. pH: 4.0–8.0 with average of 6.0
N. Spot urine electrolytes
   1. Sodium: 40–220 mEq/l/day
   2. Potassium: 25–120 mEq/l/day
   3. Chloride: 110–250 mEq/l/day

III. Stool
A. Fecal occult blood test: negative
B. Ova, parasites, blood (OPB): negative
C. Fecal fat: 5 g/24 hr
D. Urobilinogen: 0–4 mg/day
E. Culture: intestinal flora
F. Assay for *Clostridium difficile* toxin A or B: negative; positive if diarrhea is caused by *C. difficile*

Note: Values may vary depending on the laboratory.

Formulae Significant to Critical Care Nursing

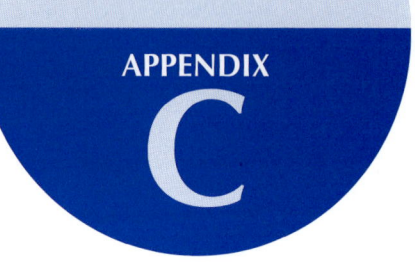

APPENDIX C

General

Conversion

To convert pounds to kilograms	1 lb = 0.45 kg
To convert inches to centimeters	1 in = 2.54 cm
To convert mm Hg to cm H_2O	1 mm Hg = 1.36 cm H_2O
To convert Fahrenheit to Celsius	(°F − 32) ÷ 1.8

Drug Administration

To calculate mcg/kg/min if you know the rate of the infusion	$\dfrac{(mcg/ml) \times (ml/hr)}{(60\ min/hr) \times (kg\ of\ body\ weight)}$
To calculate rate in ml/hr if you know the dose in mcg/kg/min	$\dfrac{(dose\ in\ mcg/kg/min) \times (60\ min/hr) \times (wt\ in\ kg)}{(mcg/ml\ of\ the\ solution)}$
To calculate mg/min if you know the rate of the infusion	$\dfrac{(mg/ml) \times (ml/hr)}{(60\ min/hr)}$
To calculate rate in ml/hr if you know the dose in mg/min	$\dfrac{(dose\ in\ mg/min) \times (60\ min/hr)}{(mcg/ml\ of\ the\ solution)}$
To calculate mcg/min if you know the rate of the infusion	$\dfrac{(mcg/ml) \times (ml/hr)}{(60\ min/hr)}$
To calculate rate in ml/hr if you know the dose in mcg/min	$\dfrac{(dose\ in\ mcg/min) \times (60\ min/hr)}{(mcg/ml\ of\ the\ solution)}$

Cardiovascular

Parameter	Method of Calculation	Normal
Mean arterial pressure (MAP)	[BP systolic + (BP diastolic × 2)] ÷ 3	70–105 mm Hg (normal systolic BP 90–140 mm Hg; normal diastolic BP 60–90 mm Hg)
Cardiac index (CI)	CO ÷ by body surface area (BSA)	2.5–4.0 l/min/m^2
Stroke volume (SV)	CO ÷ HR	60–120 ml/beat
Stroke index (SI)	SV ÷ BSA	30–65 ml/m^2/beat
Systemic vascular resistance (SVR)	[(MAP − RAP) × 80] ÷ CO	900–1400 dynes/sec/cm^{-5}
Systemic vascular resistance index (SVRI)	[(MAP − RAP) × 80] ÷ CI	1700–2600 dynes/sec/cm^{-5}/m^2

Appendix C   Formulae Significant to Critical Care Nursing

Parameter	Method of Calculation	Normal
Pulmonary vascular resistance (PVR)	$[(PAm - PAOP) \times 80] \div CO$	100–250 dynes/sec/cm^{-5}
Pulmonary vascular resistance index (PVRI)	$[(PAm - PAOP) \times 80] \div CI$	225–315 dynes/sec/cm^{-5}/m^2
Left ventricular stroke work index (LVSWI)	$[SI \times (MAP - PAOP)] \times 0.0136$	45–65 g • m/m^2
Right ventricular stroke work index (RVSWI)	$[SI \times (PAm - RAP)] \times 0.0136$	5–12 g • m/m^2
Coronary artery perfusion pressure (CAPP)	Diastolic BP − PAOP	60–80 mm Hg
Right ventricular end-diastolic volume index (RVEDVI)	$RVEDV \div BSA$	60–100 ml/m^2
Right ventricular end-systolic volume index (RVESVI)	$RVESV \div BSA$	30–60 ml/m^2
Arterial oxygen content (CaO$_2$)	$1.34 \times Hgb \times SaO_2$	18–20 ml/dl
Venous oxygen content (CvO$_2$)	$1.34 \times Hgb \times SvO_2$	12–16 ml/dl
Oxygen delivery (DO$_2$)	$CO \times CaO_2 \times 10$	900–1100 ml/min
Oxygen delivery index (DO$_2$I)	$CI \times CaO_2 \times 10$	550–650 ml/min/m^2
Oxygen consumption (VO$_2$)	$CO \times Hgb \times 13.4 \times (SaO_2 - SvO_2)$	200–300 ml/min
Oxygen consumption index (VO$_2$I)	$CI \times Hgb \times 13.4 \times (SaO_2 - SvO_2)$	110–160 ml/min/m^2
Oxygen extraction ratio (O$_2$ER)	$(CaO_2 - CvO_2)/CaO_2$	22%–30%
Oxygen extraction index (O$_2$EI)	$(SaO_2 - SvO_2)/SaO_2$	20%–27%
Corrected QT (QT$_c$)	$QT \div \sqrt{RR}$	0.35–0.43 sec

Pulmonary

Parameter	Method of Calculation	Normal
Static compliance	$\dfrac{\text{Tidal volume}}{\text{Plateau pressure} - \text{PEEP}}$	50–100 ml/cm H$_2$O
Dynamic compliance	$\dfrac{\text{Tidal volume}}{\text{Peak pressure} - \text{PEEP}}$	35–55 ml/cm H$_2$O
a/A ratio	(PaO_2/PAO_2) NOTE: PAO$_2$ is calculated as: $FiO_2 (760 - 47) - (PaCO_2/0.8)$ NOTES: FiO$_2$: fraction of inspired oxygen (written as a decimal) Pb: barometric pressure (760 mm Hg at sea level, adjust for higher altitudes) PaCO$_2$: arterial carbon dioxide tension 47 is the pressure of water vapor at sea level and is subtracted from barometric pressure 0.8 is the usual respiratory quotient	Normal >0.8 Moderately abnormal 0.5–0.8 Significantly abnormal 0.25–0.5 Critically abnormal <0.25
A:a gradient	$PAO_2 - PaO_2$	<10 mm Hg NOTE: A:a gradient × 0.05 ≅ % shunt.
PaO$_2$/FiO$_2$ ratio	$\dfrac{PaO_2}{FiO_2 \text{ (decimal)}}$	>300 300 ≅ 15% shunt 200 ≅ 20% shunt
Respiratory index	$\dfrac{PAO_2 - PaO_2}{PaO_2}$	<1
Rapid shallow breathing index	f/V_T (in liters) using frequency and average tidal volume for 1 minute	No more than 105 breaths/min/l indicates readiness for weaning

Neurologic

Parameter	Method of Calculation	Normal
Cerebral perfusion pressure (CPP)	MAP − ICP	60–100 mm Hg

Nutrition

Parameter	Method of Calculation	Normal
Body mass index (BMI)	Weight (kg)/ht(m) × ht(m)	Optimal: 20–25 Obesity: >25 Underweight: <20

Fluid, Electrolyte, and Acid–Base

Parameter	Method of Calculation	Normal
Serum osmolality	$(2 \times Na) + \dfrac{BUN}{2.6} + \dfrac{glucose}{18}$	280–295 mOsm/l
Anion gap	$(Na + K) - (Cl + HCO_3)$	5–15 NOTE: Some formulae omit potassium; if potassium is omitted, normal is 8–12.
Corrected serum calcium in hypoalbuminemia	$0.8 \times (4 - \text{serum albumin}) + \text{serum calcium}$	8.5–10.5 mg/dl
Corrected serum potassium in acid–base imbalances	0.1 change in pH (from midline normal of 7.4) causes a change in the potassium level by ~0.5 mEq/l in the opposite direction	3.5–5.0 mEq/l NOTE: This formula is especially helpful to estimate the drop in serum potassium expected with pH correction in diabetic ketoacidosis.
Ideal body weight (IBW) using Devine formula	IBW (men) = 50 kg + 2.3 kg × (height [in] − 60) IBW (women) = 45.5 kg + 2.3 kg × (height [in] − 60)	Varies

Dysrhythmias: Etiology, Criteria, Significance, and Management

APPENDIX D

Normal Sinus Rhythm

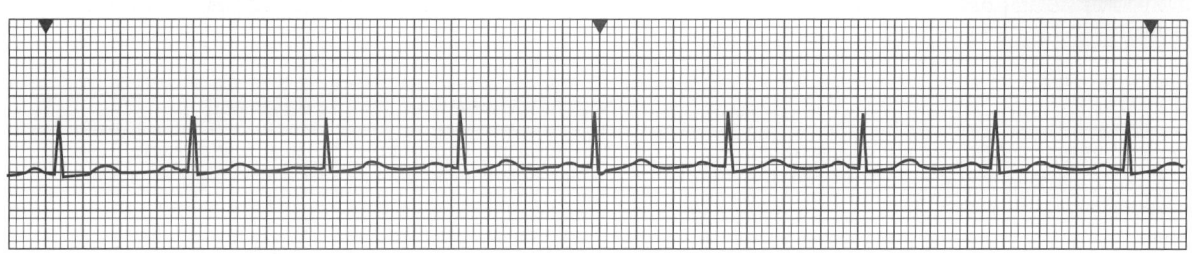

(From Wesley K: *Huszar's basic dysrhythmia and acute coronary syndromes*, ed 4, St. Louis, 2011, Mosby/JEMS.)

Rate	Regularity	P Waves	PR Interval	QRS Duration
60–100 beats/min	Atrial and ventricular rhythms regular	Normal	0.12–0.20 and constant	<0.12

Etiology	Significance	Treatment
Normal	Normal	None

Sinus Bradycardia

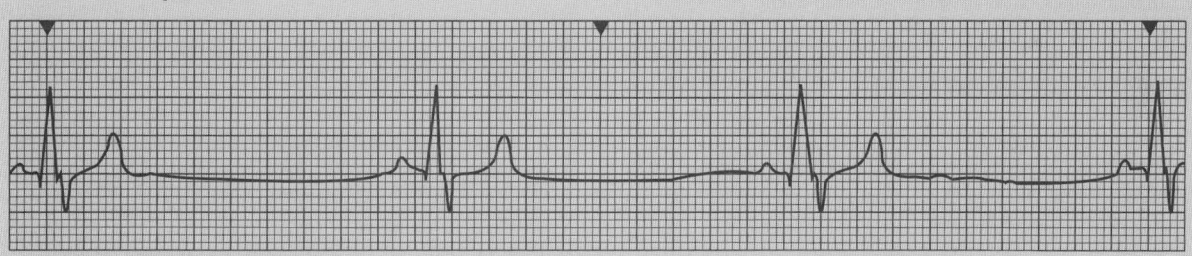

(From Wesley K: *Huszar's basic dysrhythmia and acute coronary syndromes*, ed 4, St. Louis, 2011, Mosby/JEMS.)

Rate	Regularity	P Waves	PR Interval	QRS Duration
<60 beats/min	Atrial and ventricular rhythms regular	Normal	0.12–0.20 and constant	<0.12

Etiology	Significance	Treatment

• Athletic heart
• Sleep
• Vagal stimulation
• Myocardial ischemia or infarction
  • Inferior or posterior MI
• Fibrodegenerative changes of the SA node (e.g., sick sinus syndrome)
• Increased ICP
• Hypothermia
• Hypothyroidism
• Neurogenic shock
• Cervical or mediastinal tumor
• Drug effect: digitalis, β-blockers, calcium channel blockers, opioids
	• Depends on rate
	• If too slow, cardiac output decreases
	  • Clinical manifestations of hypoperfusion may include hypotension, syncope, dyspnea, change in level of consciousness, chest pain, HF, anxiety
	  • Escape beats (e.g., atrial, junctional, ventricular) may occur
		• None if asymptomatic
		• If clinical manifestations of hypoperfusion occur:
		  • Atropine may be used as a temporary treatment in patients who do not have myocardial ischemia
		  • Pacemaker may be necessary if clinical manifestations of hypoperfusion

Sinus Tachycardia

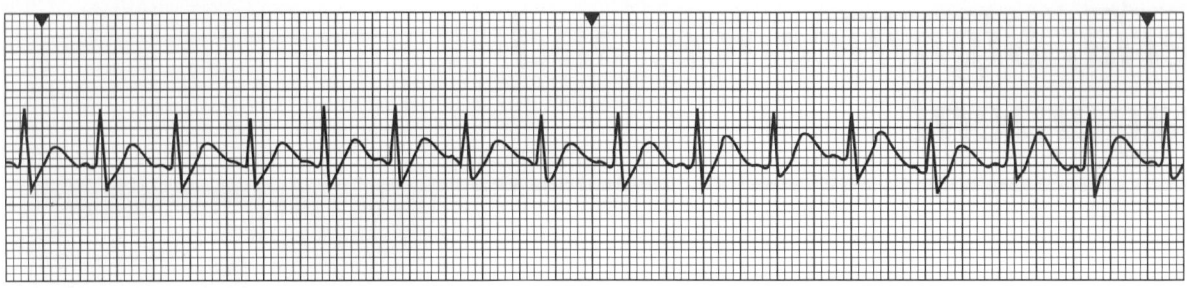

(From Wesley K: *Huszar's basic dysrhythmia and acute coronary syndromes,* ed 4, St. Louis, 2011, Mosby/JEMS.)

Rate	Regularity	P Waves	PR Interval	QRS Duration
>100 beats/min (usually 100–160 beats/min)	Atrial and ventricular rhythms regular	Normal	0.12–0.20 and constant	<0.12

Etiology	Significance	Treatment

• Sympathetic nervous system (SNS) stimulation caused by psychological or physiologic stressors (e.g., stress, fear, anxiety, pain, anger, infection, exercise, dehydration)
• Hypoxia
• Anemia
• Myocardial ischemia or infarction
• Anterior MI
• Hypovolemia or hypervolemia
• Shock
• Hyperthyroidism
• Heart failure (HF)
• Inflammatory heart disease
• Pulmonary embolism
• Fibrodegenerative changes (e.g., sick sinus syndrome with tachy-brady manifestation)
• Drug effect: epinephrine, isoproterenol, dopamine, atropine, caffeine, nicotine, amphetamines, cocaine, alcohol, aminophylline
	• Usually not significant except in patients with heart disease—then may cause angina, MI, HF, or shock	• Treatment of cause
		  • Anxiolytics for anxiety
		  • Analgesics for pain
		  • Antipyretics for fever
		  • Fluids for hypovolemia
		  • Treatment of HF
		  • Avoidance of stimulants
		  • β-Blockers for hyperthyroidism
		• Usually does not require other treatment but the following may also be used:
		  • Oxygen
		  • Sedation and/or β-blocker may be used to decrease or block the effects of catecholamines

Sinus Dysrhythmia (also referred to as sinus arrhythmia)

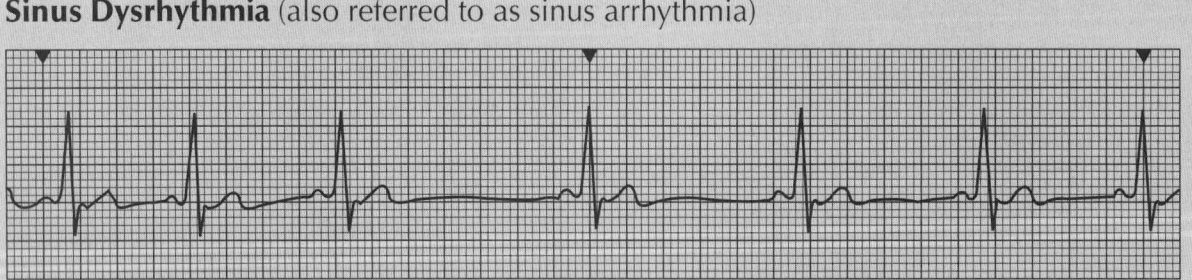

(From Wesley K: *Huszar's basic dysrhythmia and acute coronary syndromes,* ed 4, St. Louis, 2011, Mosby/JEMS.)

Rate	Regularity	P Waves	PR Interval	QRS Duration
Usually 60–100 beats/min but may be slower or faster	Atrial and ventricular rhythms regularly irregular; rate increases with inspiration (so R-R interval shortens) and decreases with expiration (so R-R interval lengthens); difference between shortest and longest R-R intervals <0.12	Normal	0.12–0.20 and usually constant; may vary slightly with rate variation	<0.12

Etiology	Significance	Treatment
• Normal; variation in sympathetic and parasympathetic stimulation during ventilation • In older patients, may indicate sick sinus syndrome • Digitalis toxicity	• Normal variation • May be seen in digitalis toxicity	• None • Discontinuance of digitalis if digitalis toxicity is the cause

Sinus Block (i.e., sinus exit block)

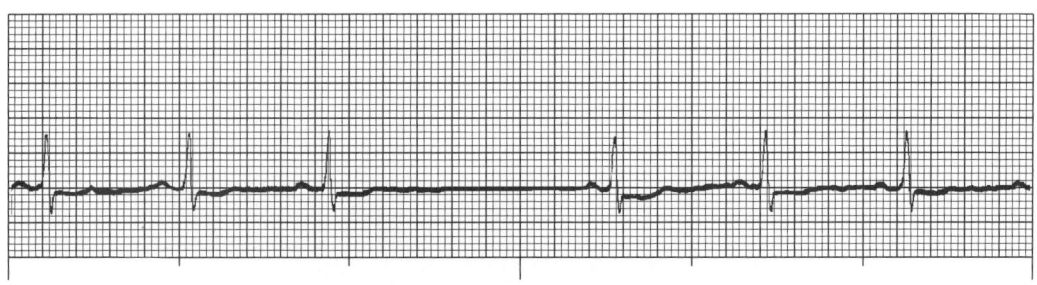

(From Aehlert B: *ECGs made easy*, ed 5, St. Louis, 2013, Elsevier Mosby.)

Rate	Regularity	P Waves	PR Interval	QRS Duration
Dependent on underlying rhythm	Atrial and ventricular rhythms regular with an irregularity; R-R interval at block measures an exact multiple of the normal R-R interval	One or more entire cardiac cycle is absent; P wave absent during block	None during block	QRS absent during block

Etiology	Significance	Treatment
• Fibrodegenerative changes of the sinus node (e.g., sick sinus syndrome) • Ischemia of SA node (e.g., MI) • Vagal stimulation • Carotid sinus hypersensitivity • Inflammatory heart disease (e.g., myocarditis) • Drug toxicity: digitalis, quinidine, procainamide	• Depends on frequency and duration of pauses • If patient loses consciousness (Stokes-Adams attacks), very significant and requires treatment	• Discontinuance of digitalis if digitalis toxicity is cause • Atropine may be used if pauses are frequent or prolonged • Pacemaker may be necessary if pauses are frequent or prolonged or if patient having syncope (i.e., Stokes-Adams attacks) • Transcutaneously initially but permanent pacemaker may be required

Sinus Arrest

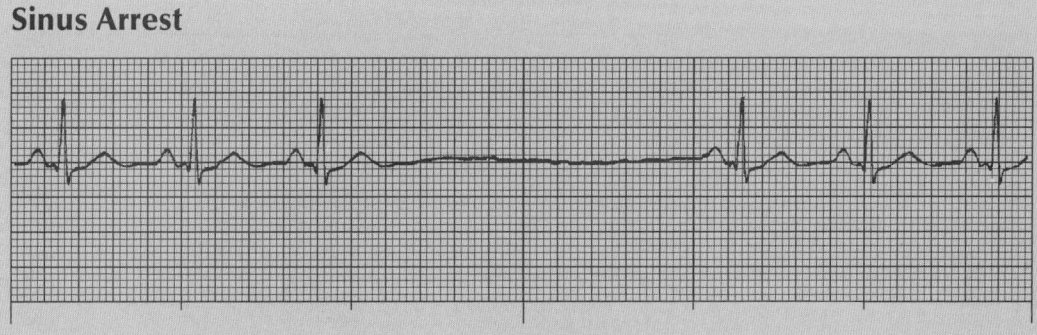

(From Aehlert B: *ECGs made easy*, ed 5, St. Louis, 2013, Elsevier Mosby.)

Rate	Regularity	P Waves	PR Interval	QRS Duration
Dependent on underlying rhythm	Atrial and ventricular rhythms regular with an irregularity (a pause); R-R interval at pause measures more or less than an exact multiple of the normal R-R interval	Indefinite period of time without an entire cardiac cycle; P wave absent during arrest	None during arrest	QRS absent during arrest

Etiology	Significance	Treatment
• Fibrodegenerative changes (e.g., sick sinus syndrome) • Ischemia of SA node (e.g., MI) • Vagal stimulation • Carotid sinus hypersensitivity • Electrolyte imbalance • Drug toxicity: digitalis, β-blockers	• Depends on frequency and duration of pauses • If patient loses consciousness (Stokes-Adams attacks), considered significant and requires treatment	• Discontinuance of digitalis if digitalis toxicity is cause • Atropine may be used if pauses are frequent or prolonged • Pacemaker may be necessary if pauses are frequent or prolonged or if patient having syncope (i.e., Stokes-Adams attacks) • Transcutaneously initially but permanent pacemaker may be required

Premature Atrial Contraction (PAC)

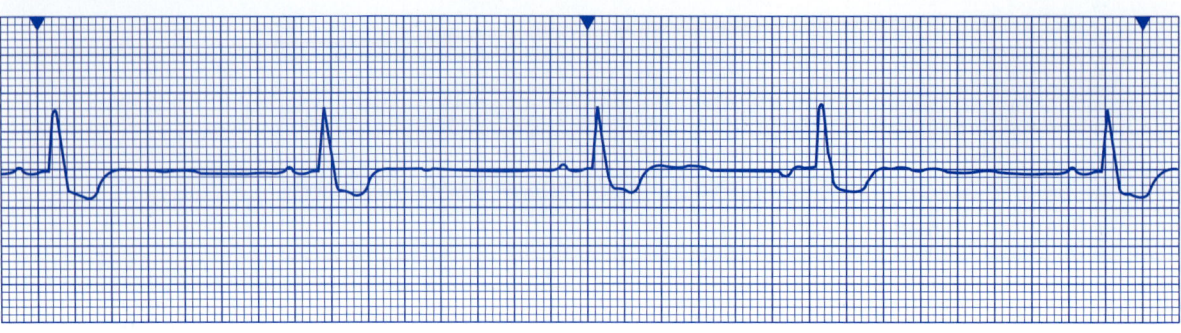

(From Wesley K: *Huszar's basic dysrhythmia and acute coronary syndromes,* ed 4, St. Louis, 2011, Mosby/JEMS.)

Rate	Regularity	P Waves	PR Interval	QRS Duration
Dependent on underlying rhythm	Dependent on underlying rhythm; PAC interrupts underlying rhythm	P wave of this early beat differs from sinus P; the ectopic P wave is early and may be flattened, notched, or lost in preceding T wave	Usually 0.12–0.20 but may be >0.20	<0.12

Etiology	Significance	Treatment
• SNS stimulation caused by psychological or physiologic stressors (e.g., stress, fear, anxiety, pain, anger, infection, exercise, dehydration) • Hypoxia • Myocardial ischemia or infarction • Valvular heart disease (e.g., mitral stenosis, mitral valve prolapse) • Heart failure • Inflammatory heart disease (e.g., myocarditis) • Electrolyte imbalance • Drug effect: caffeine, nicotine, alcohol	• Usually benign but may precede atrial tachycardia, flutter, or fibrillation • Considered significant if >6/min	• Treatment of cause • Usually no treatment necessary; but if frequent, treatment may include digitalis, β-blockers, calcium channel blockers, or anxiolytics

Wandering Atrial Pacemaker

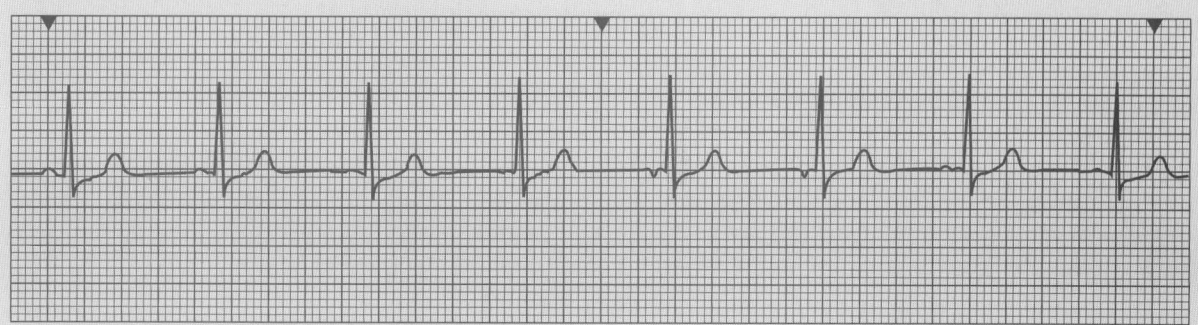

(From Wesley K: *Huszar's basic dysrhythmia and acute coronary syndromes*, ed 4, St. Louis, 2011, Mosby/JEMS.)

Rate	Regularity	P Waves	PR Interval	QRS Duration
Usually 60–100 beats/min	Atrial and ventricular rhythms usually slightly irregular	P waves look different beat to beat; at least 3 different-looking P waves	0.12–0.20 and may vary	<0.12

Etiology	Significance	Treatment
• Vagal stimulation • Sinus bradycardia • Digitalis toxicity	• May represent multiple atrial escape beats	• Usually none needed • Discontinuance of digitalis if digitalis toxicity is suspected • Atropine may be used to increase slow sinus rate

Supraventricular Tachycardia (supraventricular tachycardia refers to any narrow QRS tachycardia whose focus cannot be definitely identified; the term should be used only when a more definitive diagnosis cannot be made)

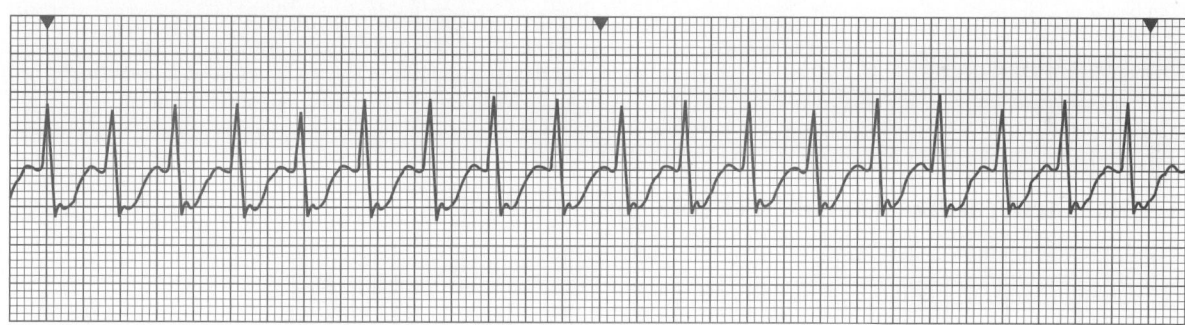

(From Wesley K: *Huszar's basic dysrhythmia and acute coronary syndromes*, ed 4, St. Louis, 2011, Mosby/JEMS.)

Rate	Regularity	P Waves	PR Interval	QRS Duration
>100 beats/min; usually 150–250 beats/min	Atrial and ventricular rhythms regular	P waves are impossible to distinguish; may be lost in QRS or preceding T wave	Cannot measure	<0.12

Etiology	Significance	Treatment
• Depends on whether sinus, atrial, or junctional	• Depends on whether sinus, atrial, or junctional	• Depends on whether sinus, atrial, or junctional; see sinus tachycardia, atrial tachycardia, and junctional tachycardia

Atrial Tachycardia (paroxysmal atrial tachycardia [PAT] refers to the sudden interruption of sinus rhythm by a rapid ectopic focus—starts and ends abruptly)

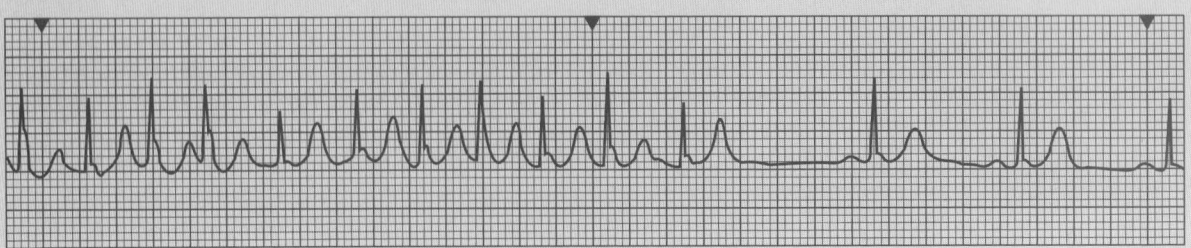

(From Wesley K: *Huszar's basic dysrhythmia and acute coronary syndromes,* ed 4, St. Louis, 2011, Mosby/JEMS.)

Rate	Regularity	P Waves	PR Interval	QRS Duration
150–250 beats/min	Atrial and ventricular rhythms regular	P wave differs from sinus P; may merge with preceding T wave	0.12–0.20	<0.12

Etiology	Significance	Treatment
• SNS stimulation caused by psychological or physiologic stressors (e.g., stress, fear, anxiety, pain, anger, infection, exercise, dehydration) • Hypoxia • Myocardial ischemia or infarction • Valvular heart disease (e.g., mitral valve prolapse) • Chronic obstructive pulmonary disease • Hyperthyroidism • Inflammatory heart disease (e.g., myocarditis) • Wolff-Parkinson-White (WPW) syndrome • Drug effect: caffeine, nicotine, alcohol • Drug toxicity: digitalis (frequently PAT with block)	• Patient may experience palpitations and clinical manifestations of hypoperfusion (e.g., hypotension, syncope, chest pain, HF) because diastolic filling time and preload is greatly reduced • Myocardial oxygen consumption is increased and myocardial oxygen supply is decreased, so myocardial ischemia may occur or worsen	• Depends on patient's tolerance, cause, and history of previous attacks • Discontinuance of digitalis if digitalis toxicity is suspected • Initial treatment: vagal stimulation, adenosine; if the rhythm persists, continue with the following: • Calcium channel blockers (e.g., diltiazem, verapamil) • β-Blockers • Digoxin if not the cause • Synchronized cardioversion • Other considerations • Right atrial pacing • Ablation may be indicated for recurrent AV nodal reentrant tachycardia • NOTE: If QRS is wide (e.g., associated with WPW): do NOT use adenosine, β-blockers, calcium channel blockers, or digoxin; preferred agent in this situation is amiodarone; if WPW, ablation is preferred long-term treatment

Multifocal Atrial Tachycardia (also called chaotic atrial rhythm)

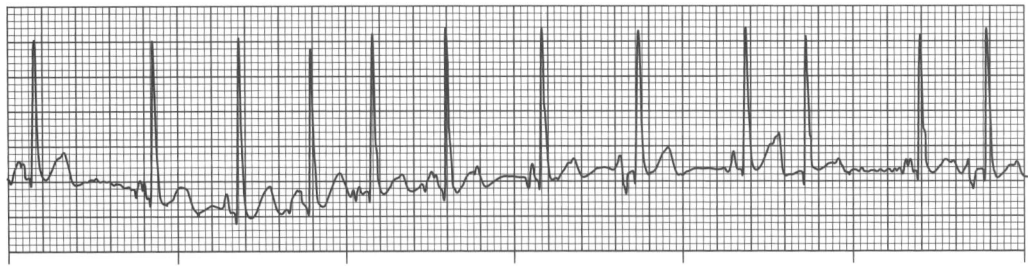

(From Aehlert B: *ECGs made easy,* ed 5, St. Louis, 2013, Elsevier Mosby.)

Rate	Regularity	P Waves	PR Interval	QRS Duration
Usually 100–150 beats/min	Atrial and ventricular rhythms usually slightly irregular	P waves look different beat to beat; at least 3 different-looking P waves	0.12–0.20 and may vary	<0.12

Etiology	Significance	Treatment
• Pulmonary hypertension (e.g., COPD, pulmonary embolism) • Valvular heart disease • Heart failure • Electrolyte imbalance • Drug toxicity: digitalis	• Demonstrates atrial irritability, which may lead to atrial tachycardia, flutter, fibrillation	• Treatment of cause: electrolyte replacement, treatment of heart failure, etc. • Discontinuance of digitalis if digitalis toxicity is suspected • If normal LV function: verapamil, β-blocker, amiodarone, digoxin, flecainide, propafenone • If abnormal LV function: amiodarone, diltiazem, digoxin

Atrial Fibrillation (AF)

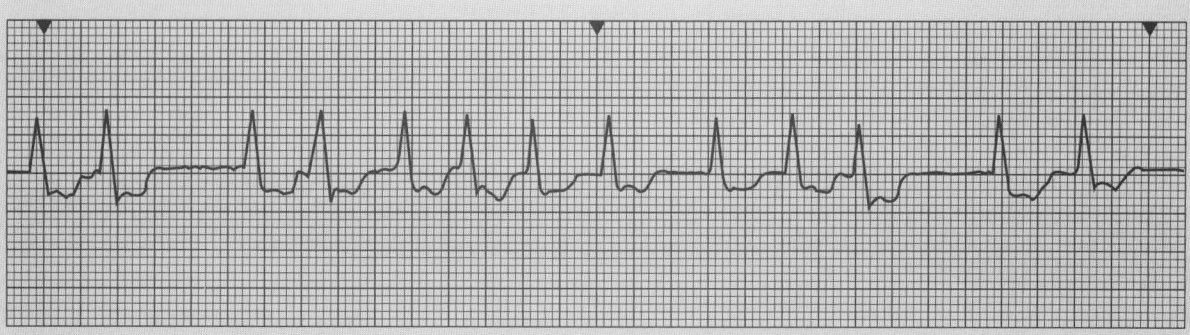

(From Wesley K: *Huszar's basic dysrhythmia and acute coronary syndromes,* ed 4, St. Louis, 2011, Mosby/JEMS.)

Rate	Regularity	P Waves	PR Interval	QRS Duration
Atrial rate >350 beats/min; ventricular rate varies greatly depending on conduction through AV node	Atrial fibrillatory waves irregular; ventricular rhythm irregularly irregular	No true P waves; fibrillatory waves manifested by quivering baseline	No true P waves	<0.12

Etiology	Significance	Treatment
• Myocardial ischemia or infarction • Especially anterior MI • Valvular heart disease (e.g., mitral or tricuspid stenosis or regurgitation) • Heart failure • Cardiomyopathy • Hyperthyroidism • Inflammatory heart disease (e.g., pericarditis) • Hypertension • Post-cardiotomy • Pulmonary hypertension (e.g., COPD, pulmonary embolism) • Wolff-Parkinson-White syndrome • Drug effect: alcohol	• No effective atrial contraction, so loss of atrial kick • Mural thrombi formation predisposes to emboli • Significance varies greatly on rate: may cause clinical manifestations of hypoperfusion (e.g., hypotension, syncope, chest pain, HF)	• Normal LV function: β-blocker or calcium channel blocker for rate control at rest and during exercise; digoxin as a second-line drug (only controls rate at rest) • Abnormal LV function: digoxin, diltiazem, or amiodarone • Although no additional treatment is required acutely if rate is controlled (i.e., between 60 and 100 beats/min), it is desirable to actually convert the AF to normal sinus rhythm if possible to reduce the risk of stroke and increase ventricular diastolic filling volume and cardiac output (considered rhythm control and maintenance) • Normal LV function with duration <48 hours: cardioversion or amiodarone, ibutilide, dofetilide, procainamide, disopyramide, flecainide, propafenone, sotalol • Abnormal LV function of <48 hours, duration: cardioversion or amiodarone • Duration >48 hours or unknown duration: anticoagulation with INR between 2 and 3 for 3 weeks followed by cardioversion • If slow ventricular response rate: atropine or pacemaker may be needed • Digitalis should be considered as cause of slow ventricular response rate; withhold digitalis if it's digitalis toxicity is the cause • NOTE: If associated with WPW: do NOT use adenosine, β-blockers, calcium channel blockers, or digoxin; preferred agent is amiodarone • Other nonacute considerations • Overdrive pacing • Implantable atrial defibrillator • Ablation or Maze procedure may be performed • Long-term anticoagulation is needed for chronic AF to prevent mural thrombi and risk for embolic stroke; desirable INR 2–3

Atrial Flutter

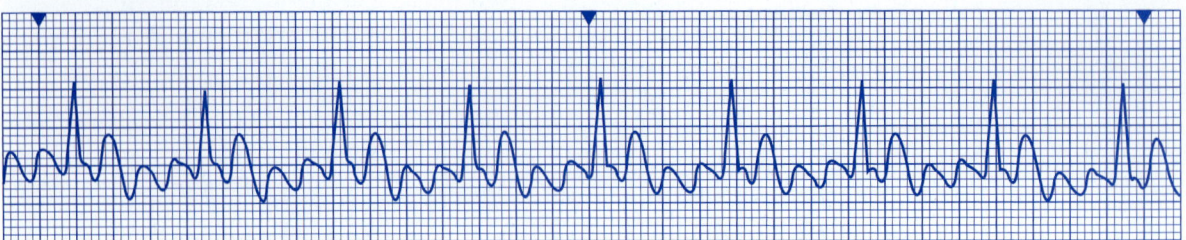

(From Wesley K: *Huszar's basic dysrhythmia and acute coronary syndromes,* ed 4, St. Louis, 2011, Mosby/JEMS.)

Rate	Regularity	P Waves	PR Interval	QRS Duration
Atrial rate approximately 300 beats/min; ventricular rate varies with conduction through the AV node; 2:1 atrial flutter has a ventricular rate of approximately 150 beats/min, 4:1 atrial flutter has a ventricular rate of approximately 75 beats/min	Atrial flutter waves regular; ventricular rhythm (response) usually regular	No true P waves; flutter waves have characteristic sawtooth appearance	No true P waves	<0.12

Etiology	Significance	Treatment
• Myocardial ischemia or infarction • Valvular heart disease • Heart failure • Cardiomyopathy • Hyperthyroidism • Inflammatory heart disease (e.g., pericarditis) • Hypertension • Post-cardiotomy • Pulmonary hypertension (e.g., COPD, pulmonary embolus) • Drug effect: alcohol • Drug toxicity: digitalis	• No effectiveness of atrial contraction • Significance varies greatly depending on rate • If rate is very rapid, may cause clinical manifestations of hypoperfusion (e.g., hypotension, syncope, chest pain, HF) because diastolic filling time and preload is greatly reduced	• As for atrial fibrillation • Although adenosine is not indicated for treatment of atrial flutter, it may slow the rhythm enough to recognize the flutter waves • Anticoagulation may be prescribed for atrial flutter, but the risk of mural thrombi and stroke is considered lower than for atrial fibrillation

Premature Junctional Contraction (PJC)

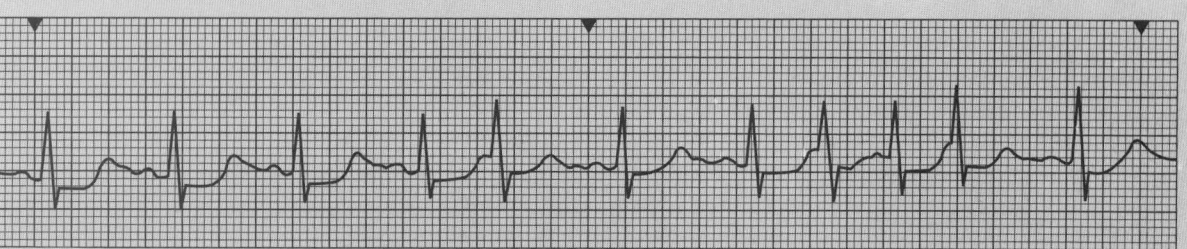

(From Wesley K: *Huszar's basic dysrhythmia and acute coronary syndromes,* ed 4, St. Louis, 2011, Mosby/JEMS.)

Rate	Regularity	P Waves	PR Interval	QRS Duration
Dependent on underlying rhythm	Dependent on underlying rhythm; PJC interrupts underlying rhythm	P wave if visible will be inverted; may be in front of, in, or after the QRS complex	Can be measured only if P wave is in front of QRS; PR will be <0.12 if measurable	<0.12

Etiology	Significance	Treatment
• SNS stimulation caused by psychological or physiologic stressors (e.g., stress, fear, anxiety, pain, anger, infection, exercise, dehydration) • Hypoxia • Myocardial ischemia or infarction • Especially inferior MI • Valvular heart disease • Heart failure • Electrolyte imbalance • Drug effect: nicotine, caffeine, alcohol • Drug toxicity: digitalis • Also etiology as for PACs	• Usually benign but may predispose to junctional tachycardia if frequent	• Usually none necessary but sedation or β-blockers may be used • Discontinuance of digitalis if digitalis toxicity is cause

Junctional ESCAPE Rhythm

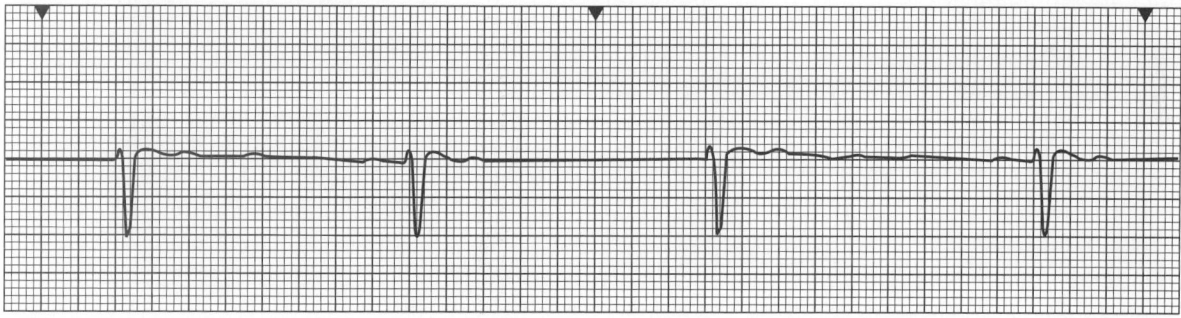

(From Wesley K: *Huszar's basic dysrhythmia and acute coronary syndromes,* ed 4, St. Louis, 2011, Mosby/JEMS.)

Rate	Regularity	P Waves	PR Interval	QRS Duration
40–60 beats/min	Atrial and ventricular rhythms regular	If visible, P wave inverted; may be in front of, in, or after the QRS complex	Can be measured only if P wave is in front of QRS; PR will be <0.12 if measurable	<0.12

Etiology	Significance	Treatment
• Vagal stimulation • SA block • Complete AV block • Myocardial ischemia or infarction • Valvular heart disease • Hypoxia • Post-cardiotomy • Drug toxicity: digitalis	• Protects patient from asystole • Do not suppress	• Note that this is *not* irritability; it is escape, so it is treated by accelerating the sinus node • Atropine • Pacemaker may be needed • Discontinuance of digitalis if digitalis toxicity is cause; it is a frequent cause of this rhythm

Acclerated Junctional Rhythm

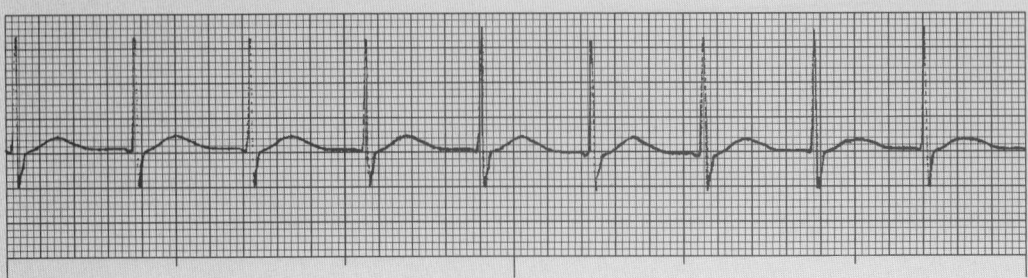

(From Aehlert B: *ECGs made easy*, ed 5, St. Louis, 2013, Elsevier Mosby.)

Rate	Regularity	P Waves	PR Interval	QRS Duration
60–100 beats/min	Atrial and ventricular rhythms regular	If visible, P wave inverted; may be in front of, in, or after the QRS complex	Can be measured only if P wave is in front of QRS; PR will be <0.12 if measurable	<0.12

Etiology	Significance	Treatment
• Vagal stimulation • SA block • Complete AV block • Myocardial ischemia or infarction • Reperfusion of myocardium • Hypoxia • Inflammatory heart disease (e.g., myocarditis) • Post-cardiotomy • Drug toxicity: digitalis	• Protects patient from asystole • Do not suppress	• Treatment of failure of sinus node • Discontinuance of digitalis if digitalis toxicity is cause; it is a frequent cause of this rhythm

Junctional Tachycardia

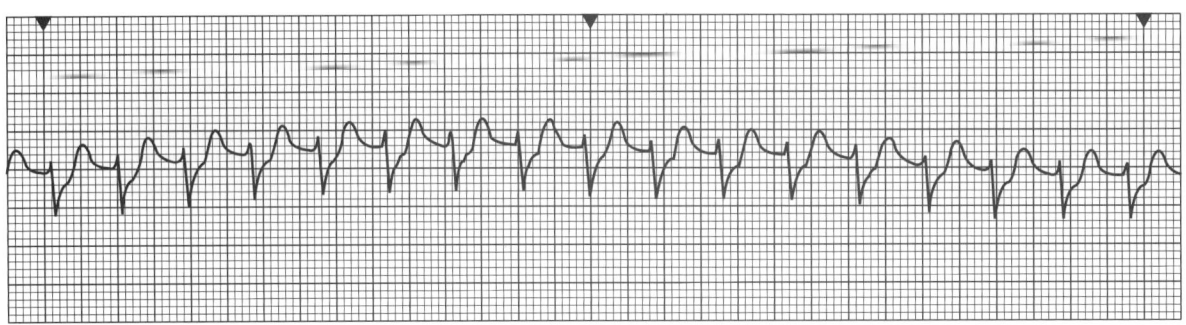

(From Wesley K: *Huszar's basic dysrhythmia and acute coronary syndromes*, ed 4, St. Louis, 2011, Mosby/JEMS.)

Rate	Regularity	P Waves	PR Interval	QRS Duration
>100 beats/min; usually 100–180 beats/min	Atrial and ventricular rhythms regular	If visible, P wave inverted; may be in front of, in, or after the QRS complex	Can be measured only if P wave is in front of QRS; PR will be <0.12 if measurable	<0.12

Etiology	Significance	Treatment
• Myocardial ischemia or infarction • Reperfusion of myocardium • Inflammatory heart disease • Post-cardiotomy • Drug toxicity: digitalis, theophylline	• Usually stops spontaneously and is usually tolerated well	• Treatment of cause • Discontinuance of digitalis if digitalis toxicity is cause • Vagal stimulation • Adenosine • Amiodarone • β-Blockers or calcium channel blockers if normal LV function

First-Degree AV Block

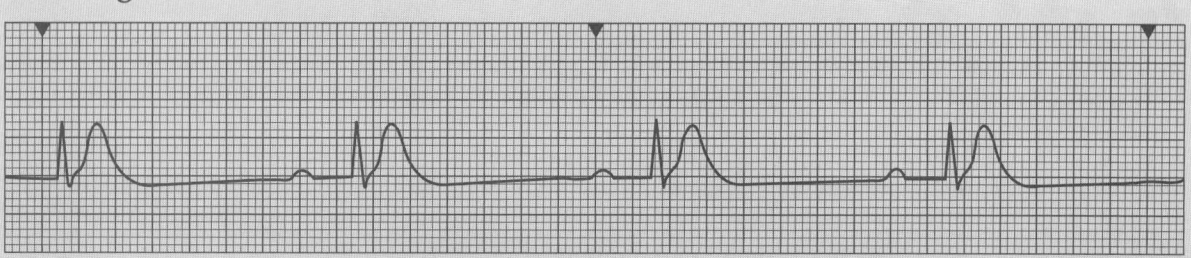

(From Wesley K: *Huszar's basic dysrhythmia and acute coronary syndromes,* ed 4, St. Louis, 2011, Mosby/JEMS.)

Rate	Regularity	P Waves	PR Interval	QRS Duration
Dependent on underlying rhythm	Dependent on underlying rhythm	Normal	>0.20	<0.12

Etiology	Significance	Treatment
• Normal variation • Congenital • Fibrodegenerative changes of the conduction system • Vagal stimulation • Myocardial ischemia or infarction • Myocardial contusion • Cardiomyopathy • Post-cardiotomy • Inflammatory heart disease (e.g., myocarditis) • Electrolyte imbalance • Drug toxicity: digitalis, β-blockers, calcium channel blockers	• Relatively benign but may progress to second- or third-degree block	• Close observation for progression of block • Discontinuance of digitalis if digitalis toxicity is cause • Drugs or pacemaker not needed unless there is also a sinus bradycardia with hypoperfusion

Second Degree AV Block Type I (previously referred to as Mobitz I; also known as Wenckebach)

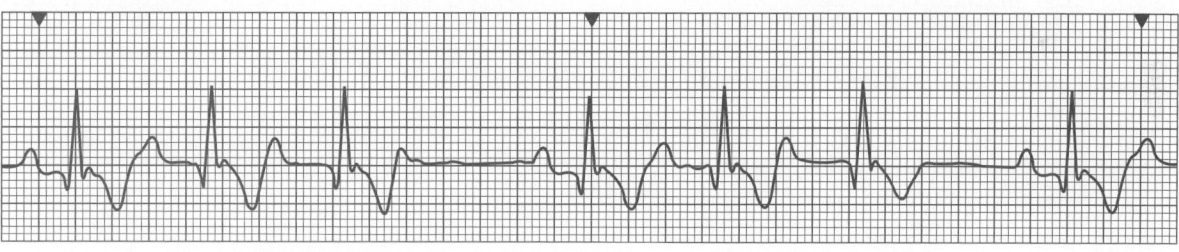

(From Wesley K: *Huszar's basic dysrhythmia and acute coronary syndromes,* ed 4, St. Louis, 2011, Mosby/JEMS.)

Rate	Regularity	P Waves	PR Interval	QRS Duration
Atrial rate dependent on underlying rhythm; ventricular rate dependent on conduction ratio; atrial rate > ventricular rate	Atrial rhythm regular, ventricular rhythm irregular (P-P interval is regular but R-R interval is irregular); groupings identifiable between P waves that were not conducted	Normal, but some P waves not followed by a QRS	Normal PR interval progressively lengthens until a P wave is not followed by a QRS; entire cycle begins again with normal PR interval	<0.12

Etiology	Significance	Treatment
• Fibrodegenerative changes of the conduction system • Myocardial ischemia or infarction • Inferior or posterior MI • Post-cardiotomy • Inflammatory heart disease • Myocardial contusion • Drug toxicity: digitalis, β-blockers, calcium channel blockers	• Block is at AV node • Occurs more often in inferior MIs (RCA lesion) • Relatively benign: usually transient, and does not usually progress to complete heart block	• Does not usually require treatment • Close monitoring for progression of block • Discontinuance of digitalis if digitalis toxicity is cause • Transvenous pacemaker or atropine may be used if rate slow and patient symptomatic

Second-Degree AV Block Type II (previously referred to as Mobitz II) (2:1 block is a second-degree block but may be either type I or type II; the QRS width may be helpful in differentiating between the two: if the QRS is of normal width, it is probably type I; if the QRS is ≥0.12, it is probably type II)

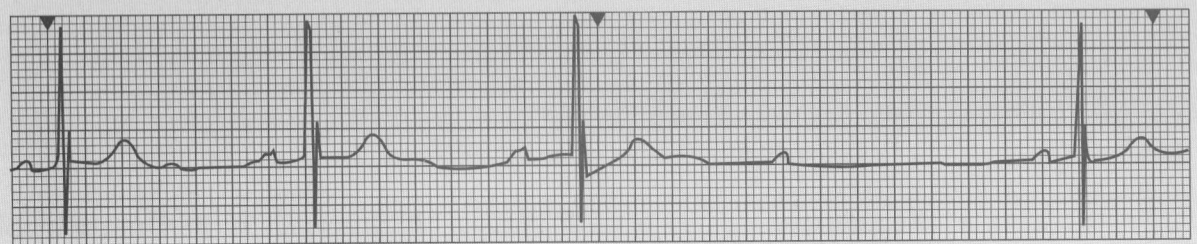

(From Wesley K: *Huszar's basic dysrhythmia and acute coronary syndromes,* ed 4, St. Louis, 2011, Mosby/JEMS.)

Rate	Regularity	P Waves	PR Interval	QRS Duration
Atrial rate dependent on underlying rhythm; ventricular rate dependent on conduction ratio but usually <60 beats/min; atrial rate > ventricular rate	Atrial rhythm regular, ventricular rhythm regular or irregular depending on whether conduction ratio varies or is constant; P-P interval regular, but some R-R intervals may be twice normal	P waves normal, but there are P waves not followed by a QRS without preceding progressive lengthening	Usually 0.12–0.20 of conducted P waves but may be longer; constant for each conducted QRS	≥0.12

Etiology	Significance	Treatment
• Myocardial ischemia or infarction • Anterior MI • Hypertension • Valvular heart disease • Conduction system fibrosis • Inflammatory heart disease (e.g., myocarditis) • Post-cardiotomy • Myocardial contusion	• Block is at bundle of His, which accounts for the slight widening of the QRS complex • Occurs more often in anterior MIs (LAD lesion) • Ominous as it often progresses to third-degree heart block	• Atropine may be used but is not usually helpful • Transcutaneous or transvenous pacemaker

Third-Degree (Or Complete) AV Block

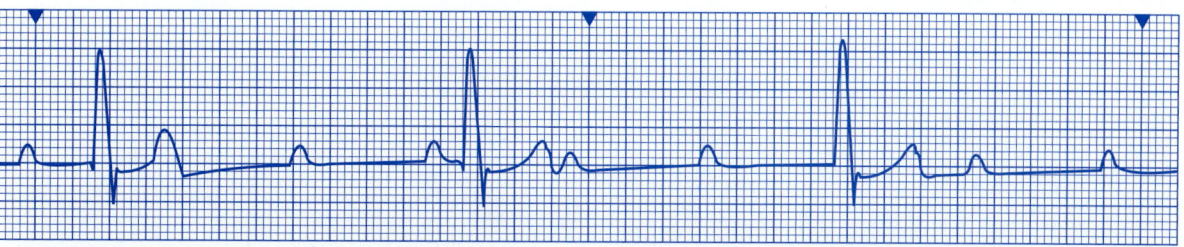

(From Wesley K: *Huszar's basic dysrhythmia and acute coronary syndromes,* ed 4, St. Louis, 2011, Mosby/JEMS.)

Rate	Regularity	P Waves	PR Interval	QRS Duration
Atrial rate dependent on underlying rhythm. Ventricular rate dependent on focus of escape rhythm (40–60 beats/min if escape focus is junctional; 20–40 beats/min if escape focus is ventricular)	Atrial rhythm regular, ventricular rhythm usually regular; P-P interval regular; R-R interval usually regular	Normal but P waves not followed by (associated with) QRS	No consistent PR interval; no relationship between the P waves and the QRS complexes	<0.12 if escape focus is junctional; >0.12 if escape focus is ventricular

Etiology	Significance	Treatment
• Myocardial ischemia or infarction • Conduction system fibrosis • Inflammatory heart disease • Post-cardiotomy • Myocardial contusion • Hypoxia • Electrolyte imbalance • Drug toxicity: digitalis	• If no escape rhythm is established, the patient has ventricular asystole	• Close observation for clinical manifestations of hypoperfusion if inferior MI with junctional escape rhythm • Atropine may be used but is not usually helpful • Pacemaker: transcutaneous initially and permanent if does not resolve

Premature Ventricular Contraction (PVC)

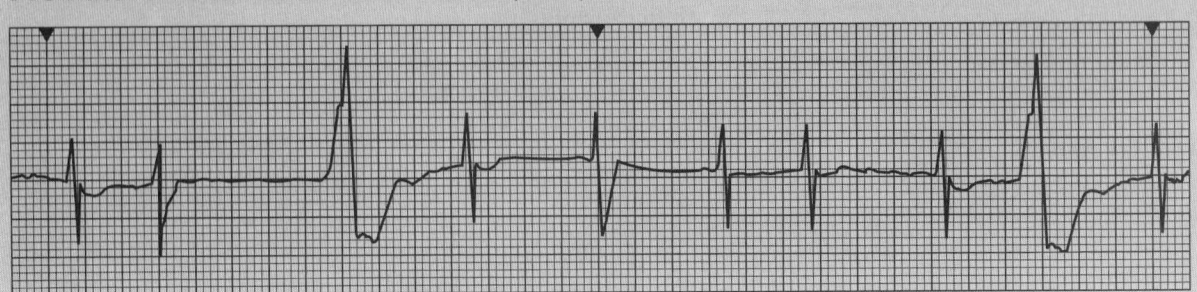

(From Wesley K: *Huszar's basic dysrhythmia and acute coronary syndromes,* ed 4, St. Louis, 2011, Mosby/JEMS.)

Rate	Regularity	P Waves	PR Interval	QRS Duration
Dependent on underlying rhythm	Dependent on underlying rhythm; PVC interrupts underlying rhythm	No associated P wave	No associated P wave; cannot measure PR	≥0.12; QRS of PVC looks different than normal QRS

Etiology	Significance	Treatment

• SNS stimulation caused by psychological or physiologic stressors (e.g., stress, fear, anxiety, pain, anger, infection, exercise, dehydration) or adrenergic drugs (e.g., epinephrine, isoproterenol, dopamine)
• Hypoxia
• Acidosis
• Myocardial ischemia or infarction
• Reperfusion of myocardium
• Heart failure
• Cardiomyopathy
• Myocardial contusion
• Ventricular aneurysm
• Valvular heart disease
• Electrolyte imbalance
• Drugs: caffeine, nicotine, alcohol, cocaine
• Drug toxicity: digitalis; aminophylline
	• PVCs of most significance: may predispose to VT or VF
	  • Frequent (>6/min)
	  • Bigeminal
	  • Multifocal
	  • R on T phenomenon
	  • Couplets
	  • Runs of ventricular tachycardia (3 or more PVCs in a row)
	• Pulse amplitude of PVC is reduced due to decreased filling time
		• Treatment of cause (e.g., oxygen, electrolyte replacement, discontinue digitalis)
		• No treatment required if only occasional, unifocal, and does not occur on previous T wave (R on T)
		• If frequent, multifocal, R on T, couplets, or runs of VT or symptomatic: amiodarone, lidocaine, β-blockers

Monomorphic Ventricular Tachycardia

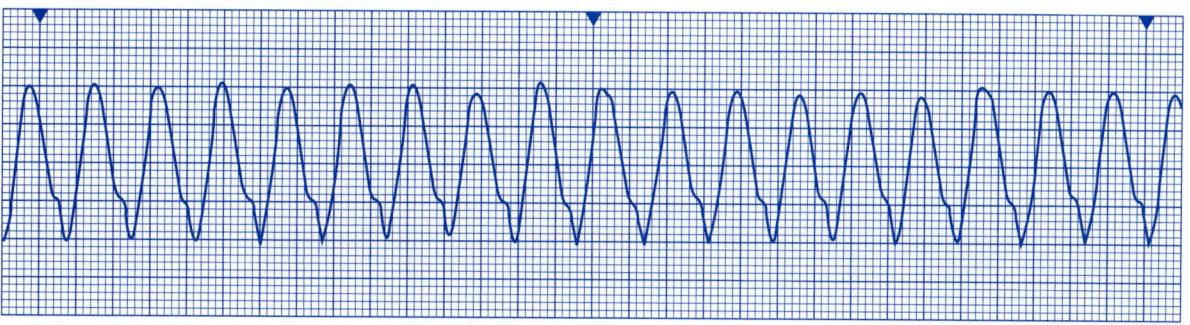

(From Wesley K: *Huszar's basic dysrhythmia and acute coronary syndromes,* ed 4, St. Louis, 2011, Mosby/JEMS.)

Rate	Regularity	P Waves	PR Interval	QRS Duration
100–250 beats/min; VT is usually 150 beats/min; VT at 200–250 beats/min may be called ventricular flutter	Ventricular rhythm usually regular; if dissociated P waves are identifiable, atrial rhythm regular	No associated P waves but may have dissociated P waves scattered through the rhythm	No associated P waves; cannot measure PR	≥0.12; QRS of VT looks different than normal QRSs

Etiology	Significance	Treatment
• SNS stimulation caused by psychological or physiologic stressors (e.g., stress, fear, anxiety, pain, anger, infection, exercise, dehydration) or adrenergic drugs (e.g., epinephrine, isoproterenol, dopamine) • Hypoxia • Acidosis • Myocardial ischemia or infarction • Reperfusion of myocardium • Cardiomyopathy • Myocardial contusion • Ventricular aneurysm • Valvular heart disease • Post-cardiotomy • R on T PVC • Electrolyte imbalance • Drugs: caffeine, nicotine, alcohol, cocaine • Drug toxicity: digitalis	• Ominous as it may progress to ventricular fibrillation • Symptoms depend on underlying heart disease, rate, and duration of VT • May cause angina, HF, and shock	• Treatment of cause • If normal LV function: procainamide, amiodarone, lidocaine, sotalol • If impaired LV function: amiodarone, lidocaine, cardioversion • If having hypotension, chest pain, or pulmonary edema: immediate sedation and cardioversion • If pulseless: treat as VF (e.g., CPR, defibrillation, vasopressin or epinephrine, amiodarone)

Polymorphic Ventricular Tachycardia (torsades de pointes if preceded by prolonged QT)

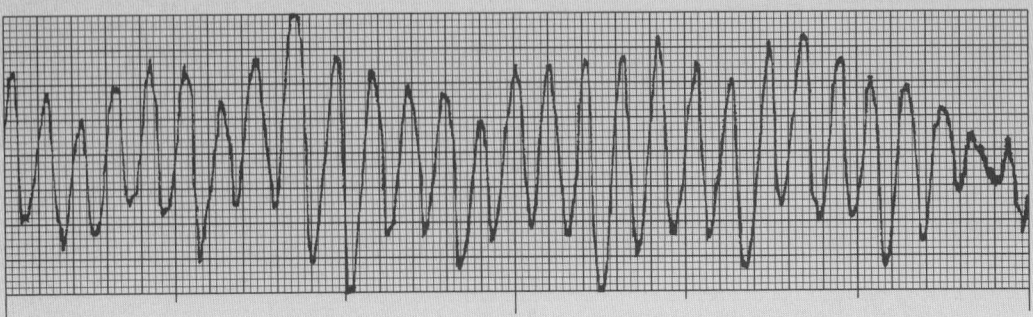

(From Aehlert B: *ECGs made easy*, ed 5, St. Louis, 2013, Elsevier Mosby.)

Rate	Regularity	P Waves	PR Interval	QRS Duration
150–250 beats/min	Ventricular rhythm may be regular	None	None	≥0.12 with QRS that seems to twist around a center line; gradual alteration in the amplitude and direction of the QRS

Etiology	Significance	Treatment

• Class IA antidysrhythmics (e.g., procainamide, quinidine, disopyramide) or class IC antidysrhythmics (e.g., flecainide, propafenone)
• Class III antidysrhythmics (e.g., sotalol, amiodarone)
• Tricyclic antidepressants (e.g., amitriptyline [Elavil])
• Phenothiazines (e.g., chlorpromazine [Thorazine])
• Organic insecticides
• Electrolyte imbalance (especially hypomagnesemia, hypocalcemia, hypokalemia)
• Congenital long QT syndrome or Brugada syndrome
• Marked bradycardia
• Hypothermia
• Subarachnoid hemorrhage
	• No effective perfusion
	• May go into and out of this rhythm
		• Prevention of torsades de pointes: close monitoring of QT interval and discontinuance of any offending drug when QT prolongs to greater than half of the R-R interval
		  • Discontinuance of any offending drug if characteristic torsades pattern seen
		  • Monitor electrolytes and replace as prescribed
		• If QT was previously normal:
		  • Electrolyte replacement
		  • Amiodarone, β-blocker, lidocaine, procainamide, sotalol
		• If QT was previous prolonged (suggests torsades)
		  • Electrolyte replacement especially magnesium
		  • Overdrive pacing
		  • Isoproterenol
		  • Phenytoin
		  • Lidocaine
		• If impaired LV function: amiodarone, lidocaine, cardioversion

Ventricular Fibrillation

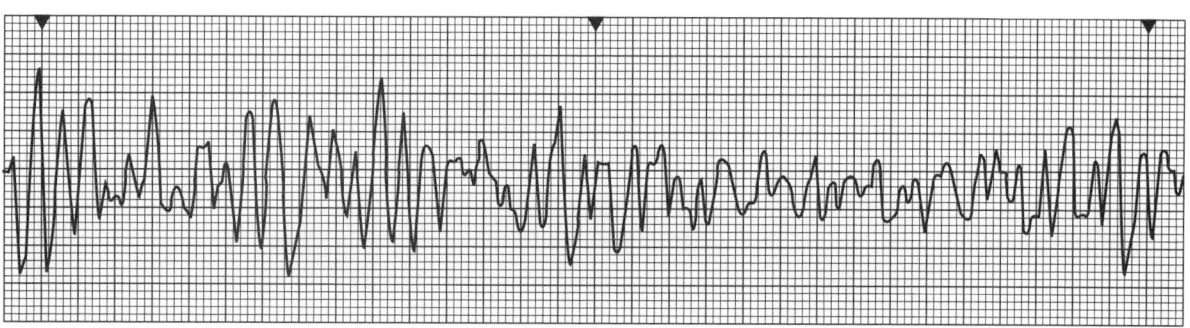

(From Wesley K: *Huszar's basic dysrhythmia and acute coronary syndromes,* ed 4, St. Louis, 2011, Mosby/JEMS.)

Rate	Regularity	P Waves	PR Interval	QRS Duration
None	Irregular; chaotic baseline	None	None	None

Etiology	Significance	Treatment
• SNS stimulation caused by psychological or physiologic stressors (e.g., stress, fear, anxiety, pain, anger, infection, exercise, dehydration) or adrenergic drugs (e.g., epinephrine, isoproterenol, dopamine) • Hypoxia • Myocardial ischemia or infarction • R on T PVC • Electrical shock including microshock • Brugada syndrome (familial) • Drowning • Hypothermia • Drug toxicity: digitalis • Dying heart	• Lethal within 4–6 minutes • No cardiac output • Symptoms include: loss of consciousness, pulse, blood pressure, and ventilation; anoxic seizures	• CPR until defibrillator available and ready then after defibrillation and between successive defibrillation attempts • Immediate defibrillation (150–200 joules [biphasic energy], 360 joules [monophasic energy]) • Vasopressin or epinephrine • Intubation • Antidysrhythmics: amiodarone or lidocaine • Post-resuscitation care

Idioventricular Rhythm

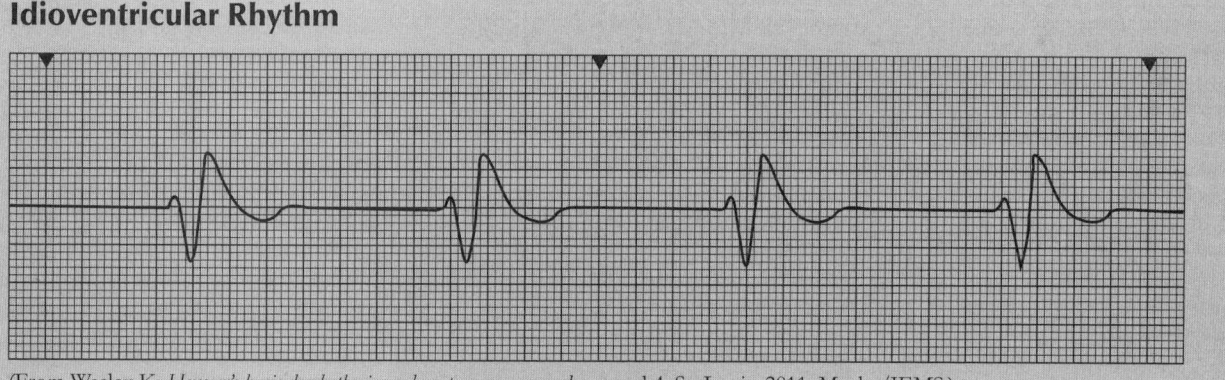

(From Wesley K: *Huszar's basic dysrhythmia and acute coronary syndromes,* ed 4, St. Louis, 2011, Mosby/JEMS.)

Rate	Regularity	P Waves	PR Interval	QRS Duration
20–40 beats/min	Ventricular rhythm usually regular; no atrial activity	None	None	≥0.12

Etiology	Significance	Treatment

• Vagal stimulation
• Failure of higher pacemakers (e.g., ischemia or fibrosis of conduction system)
• Myocardial ischemia or infarction
• Third-degree AV block
• Drug toxicity: digitalis
	• Protects the patient from asystole but very unreliable
	• Do not suppress
		• Acceleration of higher pacemakers with atropine
		• Pacemaker
		• If pulseless:
		  • CPR
		  • Epinephrine
		  • Pacemaker
		  • Consideration and treatment of causes

Accelerated Idioventricular Rhythm

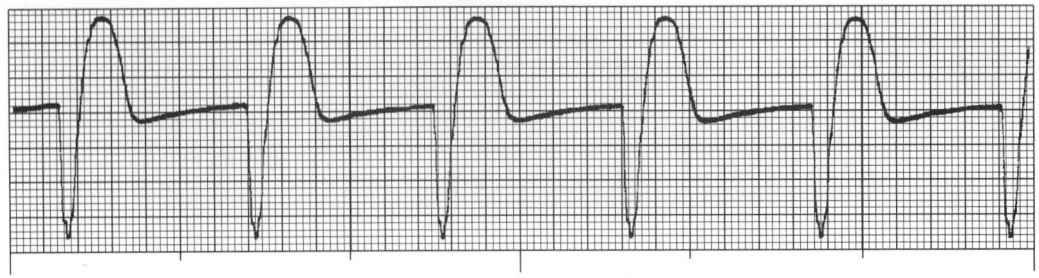

(From Aehlert B: *ECGs made easy,* ed 5, St. Louis, 2013, Elsevier Mosby.)

Rate	Regularity	P Waves	PR Interval	QRS Duration
40–100 beats/min	Ventricular rhythm usually regular; no atrial activity	None	None	≥0.12

Etiology	Significance	Treatment
• Failure of higher pacemakers (e.g., ischemia or fibrosis of conduction system) • Myocardial ischemia or infarction • Reperfusion of myocardium • Drug toxicity: digitalis	• Protects the patient from asystole but very unreliable • Do not suppress	• Acceleration of higher pacemakers with atropine • Pacemaker

Asystole

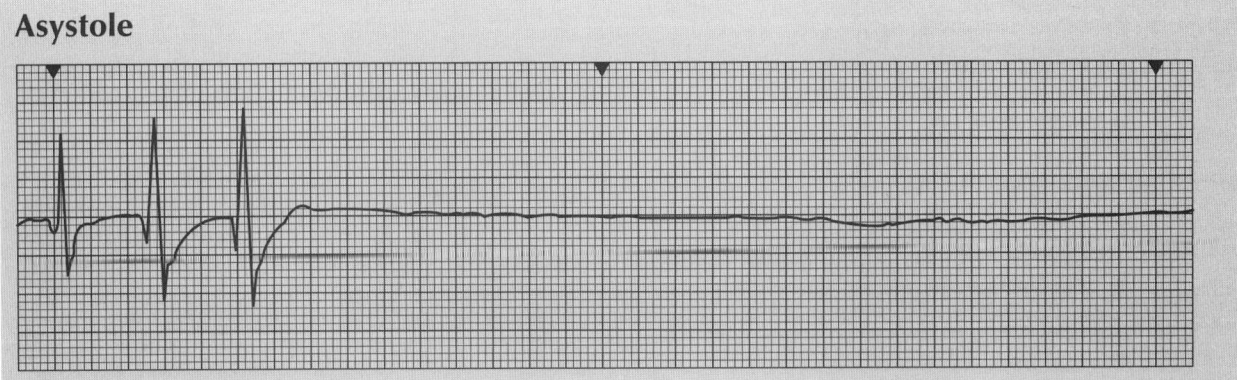

(From Wesley K: *Huszar's basic dysrhythmia and acute coronary syndromes,* ed 4, St. Louis, 2011, Mosby/JEMS.)

Rate	Regularity	P Waves	PR Interval	QRS Duration
None	No atrial or ventricular activity	None	None	None

Etiology	Significance	Treatment

• Vagal stimulation
• Hypoxia
• Acidosis
• Shock
• Myocardial ischemia or infarction
• Third-degree AV block
• Anaphylaxis
• Hypothermia
• Drug overdose
• Dying heart
	• Lethal within 4–6 minutes
	• No cardiac output
	• Symptoms include: loss of consciousness, pulse, blood pressure, and ventilation; anoxic seizures
		• CPR
		• Epinephrine
		• Pacemaker
		• Confirmation of rhythm in second lead to rule out ventricular fibrillation
		• Consideration of causes and treatment accordingly
		  • 5 Hs: hypovolemia, hypoxia, hydrogen ion (acidosis), hyper/hypokalemia, and hypothermia
		  • 5 Ts: tension pneumothorax, tamponade (cardiac), toxins, thrombosis (coronary), and thrombosis (pulmonary)

INDEX

A

A waves, 409, 410t, 411f
AACN Certification Corporation, 5
Abciximab, 641, 643t–644t
   in myocardial infarction, 171t–179t
Abdomen
   acute, 528b
   auscultation of, 506
   in cardiovascular assessment, 79
   computed tomography of, 511t–514t, 580t–581t
   contour of, 504f, 506
   distention of, 501
   flat plate of, 511t–514t
   girth of, 506
   mass in, 507
   movement of, 506
   palpation of, 507
   percussion of, 276–277, 506, 577
   quadrants of, 503, 504f
   regions of, 503, 505f
   in renal assessment, 576–577
   trauma to, 501, 549–552, 549t–550t
   ultrasonography of, 511t–514t
Abdominal aortic aneurysm, 502t
Abdominal compartment syndrome (ACS), 508
Abdominal muscles, in pulmonary assessment, 276
Abdominal pain, 501, 502t
   in acute pancreatitis, 541
   in cardiovascular assessment, 75
   in gastrointestinal assessment, 501
Abdominal perfusion pressure, 508
Abdominal reflex, 404
Abdominal thrusts, 288
Abdominal vessels, injury to, 549t–550t
Abdominal wall, weakness of, 506
Abdominoperineal resection, 552t–553t
Abducens nerve (CN VI), 391t–392t, 401–402
Aberrant conduction, dysrhythmias/blocks from, 133–134, 134t
Ablation, surgical, of dysrhythmias, 570
ABO system, 627, 627t
Abscess
   brain, 447, 451f
   pancreatic, 544
Absence seizure, 445t
Absolute refractory period, 55, 55f
Absorption, 500–501
Abuse, behavioral/psychosocial considerations in, 733–734
Ac globulin, 625t
Accelerated idioventricular rhythm, 94t–96t
Accelerated junctional rhythm, 94t–96t
Acceptability, in culturally competent healthcare, 35

Accessibility, in culturally competent healthcare, 35
Accessory organs of digestion, 496–498, 496f–497f
Accessory pathways, 132–133, 133f
Accommodation, in neurologic assessment, 401
Accountability, 15
Acculturation, 28
ACE inhibitors. *See* Angiotensin-converting enzyme (ACE) inhibitors.
Acetylcholine, 380t
N-Acetylcysteine (NAC)
   for contrast-induced AKI, 597
   for dye-related nephrotoxicity, 599
Acid(s), 283
Acid–base balance, 283–286
   physiology of, 283, 283f
   regulation of, 283–284
   renal system in, 569
Acid–base imbalance, 284–285, 284f, 287t
Acidemia, 283–284
Acidosis, 283–284
   lactic, 70
   metabolic, 285, 287t
   respiratory, 287t
Acinar cells, 498
Acinus, 255
Acoustic nerve (CN VIII), 391t–392t, 402–403, 403f
Acoustic neuroma, 444t
Acova (argatroban), 642, 643t–644t
Acquired immunity, 621–623
Action potential
   of myocardial cells, 54–55, 54f
   of pacemaker cell, 55, 55f
Activated charcoal, for drug intoxication and poisoning, 712
Activated clotting time (ACT), 633
Activated partial thromboplastin time (aPTT), 633
Active transport, 568, 571
Acupuncture, 21
Acute abdomen, 528b
Acute arterial occlusion, 81b, 216–217, 216f
Acute coronary syndromes, 154–185, 155f. *See also* Angina; Myocardial infarction.
   etiology of, 154–158
   stable angina *versus*, 156f
Acute liver failure (ALF), 535, 536t, 537f, 538b
Acute lung injury (ALI), 328
Acute myocardial infarction, chest pain in, 72t–74t
Acute respiratory distress syndrome (ARDS), 328–335. *See also* Respiratory distress; Respiratory failure.

Adaptability, in culturally competent healthcare, 35
Adenohypophysis, hormones of, 466t–469t
Adenoids, 252, 253f
Adenosine, for dysrhythmias/blocks, 137t–146t
ADP pathway inhibitors, 641
Adrenal gland, 564
   hormones of, 466t–469t
β_2-Adrenergic agonists, 324
   short-acting, 327t
Adrenergic blocking agents, for hypertensive crises, 209t–212t
Adrenergic branch, of autonomic nervous system, 390, 392t
Adrenocorticotropic hormone, 466t–469t
Adsorbent therapy, for drug poisoning and intoxication, 712
Adult education, principles of, 42
Advance directive, 18
Advanced cardiac life support, 125, 126f
Adventitia, 64, 65f
Adventitious sounds, 278t
Advocacy, 14–18
   nurses and, 2
Affect, in mental status examination, 721
Afferent sensory neurons, 379
Affordability, in culturally competent healthcare, 35
African Americans, cultural behaviors relevant to nursing care in, 31t
Afterdepolarization, 132
Afterload, 58
   cardiac output and, 60t, 61–62
   for heart failure, 191–192
   preload and, 61
   stroke volume and, 62
Agitation, 726–727
Agnosia, 400
Agranulocytes, 618–619
Air embolism, 353
   during hemodynamic monitoring, 121t–123t
Air-fluid interface, 115
Air leak, with chest tubes, 320–321
Air reference port, 115
Airway(s). *See also* Pulmonary system.
   artificial, 272, 292t–295t
   conducting, 252–255
   lower
      defense mechanisms of, 256
      functional anatomy of, 253–255, 254f
   obstruction of
      clinical presentation of, 286–288
      collaborative management of, 288–297
      etiology of, 286
   resistance in, 263

Note: Page numbers followed by "f" indicate figures, "t" indicates tables, and "b" indicates boxes.

Airway(s) *(Continued)*
  upper
    defense mechanisms of, 256
    functional anatomy of, 252–253, 253f
Airway intubation, 296–297
Airway pressure release ventilation (APRV), 264f, 304t–305t
Albumin, 685
Albuterol, for acute respiratory failure, 327t
Alcohol withdrawal syndrome, 534–535, 535b, 540
Aldosterone antagonists, 582
  for ascites, 538
  for heart failure, 190
Alginate dressings, for complex wounds, 672
Alimentary canal, 489–496, 490f. *See also* Gastrointestinal system.
Alkalemia, 283–284
Alkalosis, 283–284
  metabolic, 285, 287t
  respiratory, 284–285, 287t
Allergic reactions, 622–623
Alpha-blockers, for hypertensive crises, 208
Alpha interferon, 618
Alteplase, 643, 643t–644t
Alternative practices, in culturally competent healthcare, 35
Alveolar-capillary membrane, 256
Alveolar ducts, 255–256, 255f
Alveolar pressure, 265f, 266
Alveolar sacs, 255–256
Alveolar ventilation (V_A), 262t–263t
Alveoli, 255
  defense mechanisms of, 256
  stretch receptors in, 260
Ambrisentan, for acute respiratory distress syndrome, 331t
American College of Cardiology (ACC)/AHA staging system, for heart failure, 585
American Eskimos, cultural behaviors relevant to nursing care in, 31t
American Indians, cultural behaviors relevant to nursing care in, 31t
American Nurses Association Code of Ethics for nurses, 14
Amicar (epsilon-aminocaproic acid), for disseminated intravascular coagulation, 654, 654t
Amino acids, branched-chain, 518
Aminophylline
  for acute respiratory distress syndrome, 331t
  for acute respiratory failure, 327t, 331t
Amiodarone hydrochloride, for dysrhythmias/blocks, 137t–146t
Ammonia intoxication, 640t
Ammonia toxicity, 539–540
Amphiarthrosis joints, 674
Ampulla of Vater, 496f, 497
Amputation, for peripheral arterial disease, 215
Amylase (ptyalin), 489
Amyotrophic lateral sclerosis, 3865, 454
Analgesics
  for acute pancreatitis, 4950
  for chest surgery, 322

Analgesics *(Continued)*
  drug delivery methods for, 19
  in intracranial hypertension, 423
Anaphylactic shock, 119t–120t, 693
  clinical presentation of, 693–695
  collaborative management of, 695
  definition of, 679, 693
  etiology of, 693
  pathophysiology of, 693, 694f
Anaphylactoid reaction, 693
Anaphylaxis, 622–623, 693
Anemia, 656–658
  in acute kidney injury, 599
  clinical presentation of, 657
  collaborative management of, 657–658
  definition of, 656
  in heart failure, 190
  in intraaortic balloon pump, 165t–167t
  pathophysiology of, 657
  pernicious, 532
  predisposing factors of, 656–657
Anergy panel testing, 635
Anesthesia, regional, drug delivery methods for, 19
Aneurysm
  aortic. *See* Aortic aneurysm.
  cerebral, 3840, 434f
    Hunt and Hess grading system for, 435t
  ventricular, in myocardial infarction, 183t–185t
Anger
  in myocardial infarction, 183t
  in responses to illness and environment, 725
Angina
  chest pain in, 72t–74t
  ECG changes in, 102–103
  preinfarction, 159
  stable, acute coronary syndrome *versus*, 156f
  unstable, 570
Angiography
  celiac, 511t–514t
  coronary, 87t–89t
  digital subtraction, 87t–89t
  mesenteric, 511t–514t
  neurologic, 414t–416t
  peripheral, 87t–89t
  pulmonary, 282t–283t
  radionuclide, 87t–89t
  renal, 580t–581t
  spinal cord, 414t–416t
Angiomax (bivalirudin), 642, 643t–644t
Angioplasty
  carotid artery, for ischemic stroke, 442
  percutaneous transluminal coronary, 167t–168t
  transluminal cerebral balloon, for hemorrhagic stroke, 437
Angiotensin-converting enzyme (ACE) inhibitors
  for heart failure, 191
  for hypertensive crises, 208
  for myocardial infarction, 181–182
Angiotensin I, 66
Angiotensin II, 66

Angiotensin II receptor blockers (ARBs), for heart failure, 191
Angle of Louis, 77f–78f
Anion gap, 284, 578, 578t
Anisocoria, 401
Ankle-brachial index (ABI), 85
Anosmia, 400
Antacids, 511–515
Anterior axillary line, 77f
Anterior cerebral arteries, 384t, 385, 385f
  occlusion of, 439b
Antibiotics, for pneumonia, 2615
Antibodies, 621, 622t
Anticholinergics
  for acute respiratory failure, 326, 327t
  for status asthmaticus, 343
Anticoagulant mechanisms, 625–626, 626f
Anticoagulants, 642, 642t–644t
  for ischemic stroke, 3840, 439
  for myocardial infarction, 169, 171t–179t
  for pulmonary embolism, 2685
Anticonvulsants, for status epilepticus, 448t–449t
Antidiuretic hormone, 466t–469t, 572, 572t–574t
  deficiency of, diabetes insipidus from, 474b
  inappropriate, syndrome of, 476–477, 477f
  pharmacology of, 472, 472t
  replacement of, 472t
  syndrome of inappropriate, 426
Antidysrhythmics, 565
  ECG changes from, 97
  Vaughan-Williams classification system of, 135t
Antigens, red cell, 627, 627t
Antihemophiliac factor A, 625t
Antihemophiliac factor B, 625t
Antihistamines, for anaphylactic shock, 695
Antihypertensives
  for hypertensive crises, 208–213
  in ischemic stroke, 440
Antimicrobials, for complex wounds, 671
Antioxidants, for acute respiratory distress syndrome, 335
Antiseptics, for complex wounds, 671
Antisocial behaviors, 727
Antithrombin III (ATIII), for disseminated intravascular coagulation, 654, 654t
Antithrombin (AT) system, 626
Antivirals, for pneumonia, 342
Antrectomy, 530, 534f
Anxiety, 730–731
  during CCRN® examination, 6–7
  complicating mechanical ventilation, 313t–315t
  in myocardial infarction, 183t
Anxiety disorders, 731
Anxiolytics, in myocardial infarction, 182
Aortic aneurysm, 217–221, 218f
  abdominal, 502t
Aortic arch, arterial chemoreceptors in, 260
Aortic auscultatory area, 81, 81f
Aortic ejection click, 83
Aortic pressure, coronary artery perfusion and, 52

Index

Aortic pulsation, 79, 507
Aortic reflex, 63
Aortic regurgitation, 86f, 203–204, 204f
Aortic root pressure, 52
Aortic stenosis, 86f, 204–205, 205f
Aortic valve, 51f, 52
Aortography, coronary, 87t–89t
AP diameter, increased, 274
Apical impulse, 79
Apical-radial pulse deficit, 79
Apixaban, 643t–644t
Apnea, 275t
Apneustic breathing, 275t, 394, 394f
Apocrine sweat glands, 668
Appalachians, cultural behaviors relevant to nursing care in, 31t
Appendages
　in cardiovascular assessment, 77–78
　in pulmonary assessment, 273
Appendicitis, 502t
Approachability, in culturally competent healthcare, 35
Appropriateness, in culturally competent healthcare, 35
Arachnoid mater, 382, 383f
Arcuate vein, 566
Argatroban (Acova), 642, 643t–644t
Arginine, requirements for, 518
Arm strength, in neurologic assessment, 396–398, 398t
Aromatherapy, 19
Arrector pili muscle, 667f
Arterial blood gases (ABGs), 285b, 579
　analysis of, 285–286
　in asthma, 332t
　in cardiovascular assessment, 85
　mechanical ventilation and, 308t
　in neurologic assessment, 413
　in pulmonary assessment, 285–286
Arterial blood pressure, 66, 68f
　systemic, 105–110, 107t–108t
Arterial catheter, 103
Arterial chemoreceptors, in aortic arch, 260
Arterial embolectomy, 215
Arterial occlusion, acute, 81b
Arterial oxygen content, 107t–108t
Arterial oxygen saturation, 107t–108t, 279
Arterial puncture, during hemodynamic monitoring, 121t–123t
Arterial system
　of brain, 384–385, 384t, 385f
　gastrointestinal, 498–500, 499f
Arterial thrombosis, complicating aortic aneurysm, 220
Arterial venous disease, 79, 79t
Arterial wall, 64, 65f
Arteries, 64, 64f–65f
Arterioles, 64
Arteriosclerosis, 154. *See also* Atherosclerosis.
Arteriovenous malformations, 433, 434f
Artificial airways, 272, 292f–295f
Ascending contrast phlebography, 87t–89t
Ascites
　in cardiovascular assessment, 75
　in hepatic failure/encephalopathy, 538–539
　tests for, 506–507

Ashman phenomenon, 565
Aspiration, complicating mechanical ventilation, 313t–315t
Aspiration lung disease, 343–346
Aspiration pneumonia, 343
Assist/control mode ventilation, 304t–305t
Assisted mandatory ventilation, 304t–305t
Asterixis, 577
Asthma, 332t
　cardiac, 71
　pathophysiology of, 347f
Astrocytes, 378
Astrocytomas, 444t
Asystole, 94t–96t
Ataxic breathing, 275t, 394f, 395
Atelectasis, 280
　absorptive, 300
　complicating mechanical ventilation, 313t–315t
Atherectomy, coronary, 167t–168t
Atherosclerosis, 154–158, 155f
Atmospheric pressure, 267
Atonic seizure, 445t
Atria, 50, 50f
　enlargement of, 99–100, 100f
Atrial contraction, 58
Atrial dysrhythmias, in neurologic assessment, 394
Atrial fibrillation, 94t–96t
　maze procedure for, 575
Atrial flutter, 94t–96t
Atrial gallop, 82, 83t
Atrial natriuretic peptide (ANP), 64, 572
Atrial pacemaker, wandering, 94t–96t
Atrial pacing, 148
Atrial septostomy, balloon dilation, for pulmonary hypertension, 337
Atrial tachycardia, 94t–96t
　multifocal, 94t–96t
Atrioventricular (AV) junction, 56, 56f
Atrioventricular (AV) node, 56, 56f
Atrioventricular pacing, 148–150, 149t, 150f
Atrioventricular valves, 51, 51f
Atropine, for dysrhythmias/blocks, 137t–146t
Attitudes, in culturally competent healthcare, 35
Auscultation
　in cardiovascular assessment, 81–85, 81f
　in endocrine assessment, 471
　in gastrointestinal assessment, 506
　in hematologic and immunologic assessment, 631
　in pulmonary assessment, 277
　in renal assessment, 577
Auscultatory areas, cardiac, 81, 81f
Auto-PEEP, 303, 306f
Automatic external defibrillator, 555
Automaticity, altered, dysrhythmias/blocks from, 565
Autonomic nervous system (ANS), 62–63, 63t, 390–392, 392t
　peripheral blood flow and, 66
Autonomy, 14
Autoregulation, cerebral, 386, 418
Availability, in culturally competent healthcare, 35

Avoiding, conflict, 25
Awareness, in culturally competent healthcare, 35
Axons, 378, 379f

B

B cells, 619
B-type natriuretic peptide (BNP), in heart failure, 188, 191
B waves, 409, 410t, 411f
Babinski reflex, 405f
Baby Boomers, 34t
Bachmann bundle, 55, 56f
Bacteremia, definition of, 696
Bad news, guidelines for giving, 23
Bainbridge reflex, 63
Ballance sign, in abdominal trauma, 4955
Balloon rupture, during hemodynamic monitoring, 121t–123t
Balloon tamponade, for esophageal varices, 529, 531f, 532t
Ballottement, 507
Barbiturate-induced coma, for intracranial hypertension, 421–422
Barium enema, 511t–514t
Barium swallow, 511t–514t
Barlow syndrome, 201
Barometric pressure, 267
Baroreceptor reflex, 63
Baroreceptors, 260
　peripheral blood flow and, 66
Barrel chest, 274
Basal ganglia, 382–383
Base, 283
Base excess (BE), 284
Basement membrane, in skin, 667f
Basic life support (BLS), for cardiopulmonary arrest, 123–124
Basilar arteries, 384t, 385, 385f
　occlusion of, 439b
Basophils, 618, 632
Battle sign, 405, 405f
Beck triad, 226
Bedside pulmonary function, 278–280
Behavioral pain scale, 19t
Behavioral/psychosocial considerations, 721–741
　agitation in, 726–727
　antisocial behaviors in, 727
　anxiety in, 730–731
　assessment of, 721–722
　chief complaint in, 721
　current medications in, 721
　delirium in, 727–729, 728t, 728b
　dementia in, 727, 728t
　depression in, 732
　family history in, 721
　history of present illness in, 721
　human needs in, 723, 723f, 723t
　interview in, 721–722
　major or minor neurocognitive disorders in, 730
　mania in, 732–733
　medical nonadherence in, 737
　mental status examination in, 721–722
　past medical history in, 721
　posttraumatic stress disorder in, 734

Behavioral/psychosocial considerations *(Continued)*
  psychosis in, 737–738
  psychosocial characteristics in, 723
  responses to illness and environment in, 723–726, 723t–724t, 724b
  risk-taking behavior in, 734–735
  social history in, 721
  substance-related disorders in, 735–736
  suicidal ideation and behaviors in, 736
  trauma/violence/abuse in, 733–734
Beneficence, 15
Benzodiazepines, 308
  as sedative agents, 309t–310t
  for status epilepticus, 447, 448t–449t
Beta-blockers
  for heart failure, 190
  for hypertensive crises, 208
  in myocardial infarction, 181
Beta-endorphins, 380t
Bi-level ventilation, 304t–305t
Bi-positive pressure ventilation (Bi-PAP), 317
Bicarbonate, 588
Bicuspid valve, 51f
Bicycle collision, 706
Bile, 491t, 497–498, 497f
Bile canaliculi, 497
Bile ducts, 496f, 497
Bilirubin, 498, 498f, 511, 579, 616, 634
Billroth I and II, 530, 534f, 552t–553t
Bilobectomy, 321
Bioartificial liver support, 540
Bioethical principles, 14–15
Biofeedback, 20
Bioimpedance, 114
Biomarkers, cardiac, for myocardial infarction, 159, 160t
Bioprosthetic valves, 206
Biopsy
  cardiac, 87t–89t
  in hematologic and immunologic assessment, 635
  liver, 511t–514t
  lung, 282t–283t
  renal, 580t–581t
Biot's breathing, 275t
Bipolar disorder, 733
Bipolar neurons, 379
Bisoprolol, in heart failure, 190
Bispectral index (BIS) monitoring, 310–311, 412
Bivalirudin (Angiomax), 642, 643t–644t
  for myocardial infarction, 169, 171t–179t
Biventricular failure, 189t
Bladder, 564
  palpation of, 577
  percussion of, 507, 577
Bladder volume, in renal assessment, 577
Blanket consent, 18
Blast trauma, 707
  mechanism of injury in, 704
  predisposing factors in, 705
Bleeding. *See also* Hemorrhage.
  occult, 652
Bleeding time, 633
Blindness, 401

Blood, 615–619
  for shock, 684b, 685–686
Blood-brain barrier, 381
Blood coagulation factors, 624, 625t
Blood gases, arterial. *See* Arterial blood.
Blood groups, 627, 627t
Blood pressure, 66
  arterial, 66, 68f
    systemic, 105–110, 107t–108t
  in cardiovascular assessment, 76–77
  high. *See* Hypertension.
  low. *See* Hypotension.
  in neurologic assessment, 394
  in renal assessment, 576
  renal regulation of, 572
Blood samples, for hemodynamic monitoring, 104
Blood studies, in hematologic and immunologic assessment, 631–634, 632t, 634t
Blood transfusion, 635–636, 637t
  adverse effects of, 636, 640t
  for disseminated intravascular coagulation, 624, 625t
  reactions to, 636, 638t–639t, 639b
  for upper gastrointestinal hemorrhage, 530
Blood urea nitrogen (BUN), 569
Blood vessels, 65f
Blown pupil, 401
Blumberg sign, 507
Blunt cardiac injury, 222–223, 223f–224f
Blunt trauma
  to chest, 356
  mechanism of injury in, 704
  predisposing factors in, 705
"Body packers/stuffers", 712
Bone, 381f
  mineralization of, renal role in, 574
  types of, 674
Bone cells, 674
Bone healing, 674
Bone marrow, functions of, 614
Bosentan, for acute respiratory distress syndrome, 331t
Bowel elimination, changes in, 501
Bowel irrigation, for drug poisoning and intoxication, 712
Bowel sounds, 506, 577
Bowman capsule, 566
Brachytherapy, 167t–168t
Braden Scale for Predicting Pressure Sore Risk, 670–671
Bradycardia
  in cardiac arrest, 127f
  sinus, 94t–96t
Bradykinin, 620t
Bradypnea, 275t, 394, 394f
Brain
  abscess of, 447, 451f
  anatomy and physiology of, 382–384, 384f, 384t
  circulation in, 384–386, 384t, 385f
  coverings of, 382, 383f
  edema of, in intracranial hypertension, 413
  injuries, traumatic, 426–429, 427f

Brain *(Continued)*
  mass of, in intracranial hypertension, 422–423
  metabolism in, 380–381
  tumor, 443–445, 443f, 444t
Brain-blood barrier, 381
Brain death, 395, 406–407
Brain natriuretic peptide (BNP), 64
Brain tissue oxygenation ($PbtO_2$)
  monitoring of, 412
  in traumatic brain injuries, 428–429
Brainstem, 384
  in neurologic assessment, 406
  tumors of, 444t
Brainstem syndrome, 453
Branched-chain amino acids, 518
Breath odor, 505
Breath sounds, 277, 277t–278t, 277f, 577
Breathing
  apneustic, 275t, 394, 394f
  ataxic, 394f, 395
  Biot's, 275t
  Cheyne-Stokes, 275t, 394, 394f
  cluster, 394, 394f
  mindful, 20
  pursed-lip, 272
  work of, 261–263, 264f
Brevibloc. *See* Esmolol.
Bronchi, 254
Bronchial breath sounds, 277f, 277t
Bronchial circulation, 257–258
Bronchioles
  respiratory, 255, 255f
  terminal, 255, 255f
Bronchitis, chronic, 323
Bronchodilators
  for acute respiratory failure, 324–326, 327t
  for anaphylactic shock, 695
  for status asthmaticus, 2630
Bronchography, 282t–283t
Bronchophony, 277
Bronchoplastic reconstruction, 321
Bronchopleural fistula, complicating chest surgery, 323
Bronchoscopy, 2590, 282t–283t
Bronchospasm, beta-blockers and, 181
Bronchovesicular breath sounds, 277f, 277t
Brudzinski sign, 405–406, 406f
Brugada syndrome, 550
Bruits, 85, 506
Brunner glands, 495
Buffer systems, 283–284
Bullectomy, 2595
BUN: creatinine ratio, 578
Bundle branch blocks, 130
  ECG changes in, 99, 99f
Bundle branches, 56, 56f
Bundle of His, 56, 56f
Burr holes, 424
Bypass
  gastric, 552t–553t, 555f
  intestinal, 552t–553t
Bypass graft, for peripheral vascular disease, 214f

C

C-type natriuretic peptide, 64
C waves, 409, 410t, 411f
Calcitonin, 466t–469t
Calcium, 625t, 634
    absorption in, 501
    functions, regulation, and sources of, 572t–574t
Calcium (slow) channel, 54
Calcium channel blockers
    for acute respiratory distress syndrome, 337
    for angina, 163
    for cerebral vasospasm, 437
    for hemorrhagic stroke, 3845
Calf tenderness, in cardiovascular assessment, 75
Callus, formation of, 674
Caloric testing, 403, 403f
Calories, requirements for, 518
Calyces, 565, 565f
Capillaries, 65, 66f
Capillary refill rate, 79
Capnography, 278–279, 279f
    sublingual, 115
Captopril challenge test, 625
Carbohydrates
    absorption of, 500
    digestion of, 500
    for hypoglycemia, 483, 483b
Carbon dioxide
    arterial, partial pressure of ($PaCO_2$), 267f
    diffusion coefficient of, 268
    end-tidal monitoring of, 278–279, 279f
    transport of, 270
Carbonic anhydrase inhibitors, 582
Carboxyhemoglobin, 279
Cardiac arrest. See Cardiopulmonary arrest.
Cardiac asthma, 71
Cardiac auscultation, 81
Cardiac biomarkers, for myocardial infarction, 159
Cardiac biopsy, 87t–89t
Cardiac catheterization, 87t–89t
Cardiac cells, 54
Cardiac chambers, 50–51, 50f
Cardiac conduction system, 55–56, 56f
Cardiac cycle, 52–53, 58, 58f
    components of, 92–93, 92f
Cardiac glands, 494
Cardiac index (CI), 58, 107t–108t
Cardiac muscles, 56–57, 57f, 674
Cardiac output (CO), 58
    abnormal, 108t–109t
    continuous, 113
    decreased, complicating mechanical ventilation, 313t–315t
    determinants of, 59–62, 59f, 60t
    measurement of, 107t–108t
        invasive, 113
        minimally invasive, 113–114
        noninvasive, 114
    therapeutic manipulations to, 121f
Cardiac pulmonary edema, 185
Cardiac resynchronization therapy, 148–150
    in heart failure, 196
Cardiac skeleton, 49–50

Cardiac tamponade, 119t–120t, 225–227
    clinical presentation of, 225–226
    collaborative management for, 226–227
    definition of, 225
    etiology of, 225
    pathophysiology of, 225, 226f
Cardiac transplantation
    in heart failure, 192
    indications for, 201
Cardiac valves, 51–52, 51f
Cardiac wall
    layers of, 49, 50f
    rupture, in myocardial infarction, 183t–185t
Cardiogenic pulmonary edema, clinical presentation, and hemodynamic presentation of, 119t–120t
Cardiogenic shock, 119t–120t, 227, 690
    clinical presentation of, 691–692
    collaborative management of, 692
    definition of, 679, 690
    etiology of, 690–691
    in myocardial infarction, 183t–185t
    pathophysiology of, 691, 691f
Cardiomegaly, 280
Cardiomyopathy, 197–199, 197f
    definition of, 197
    dilated, 197–199, 198f
    hypertrophic, 199–201, 199f
    restrictive, 200–201, 201f
Cardiopulmonary arrest, 120–130
    clinical presentation of, 120
    collaborative management of, 123–129, 126f–127f
    definition of, 120
    etiology of, 120
    evaluation in, 130
    pathophysiology of, 120
    psychosocial considerations and, 129–130
Cardiopulmonary resuscitation, 123
Cardiovascular assessment, 70–87
    auscultation in, 81–85
    diagnostic studies for, 85–87, 87t–89t
    electrocardiography in. See Electrocardiography (ECG).
    hemodynamic monitoring in, 103–120. See also Hemodynamic monitoring.
    inspection and palpation in, 76–81
    interview in, 70–76
    landmarks in, 76, 77f
Cardiovascular system, 49–251
    assessment of, 70–87, 72t–74t. See also Cardiovascular assessment.
    electrocardiography of, 90–103
    in endocrine assessment, 471
    general information about, 49–70
    heart in, 49–64. See also Heart.
    oxygen delivery to tissue (DO_2)/ oxygen consumption by tissues (VO_2) in, 67–70, 69f
    in renal assessment, 575–576
Cardiovascular trauma, 222–225
Cardioversion
    for cardiopulmonary arrest, 128
    for dysrhythmias/blocks, 136
Cardioverter-defibrillator, implantable, 153–154

Care, general principles of, 726
Carina, 254, 254f
Caring practices, 18–24
Carotid arterial stenosis, 221–222
Carotid artery angioplasty, for ischemic stroke, 442
Carotid artery stenting, 221
Carotid bodies, chemoreceptors in, 260
Carotid endarterectomy, 221
Carotid sinus syncope, hypersensitive, 75
Carvedilol, in heart failure, 190
Catecholamines, 466t–469t
Catheter ablation, radiofrequency, 154
Catheter-associated urinary tract infection (CAUTI), 700
Catheter, occlusion of, during hemodynamic monitoring, 121t–123t
Catheterization, cardiac, 87t–89t
Catholicism, religious beliefs in, nursing interventions, 32t–33t
Cavernous sinus, 386
CCRN® certification
    benefits of achieving, 1–2
    maintaining, 9
    synergy model of, 2–3, 2f
CCRN examination, 3–4
    basic information about, 3, 3t
    passing score in, 4
    plans for passing, 4–9, 4f, 5b
    questions in, 3–4
CD4 cell count, 634
Cecum, 495, 495f
Celiac angiography, 511t–514t
Celiac artery, 498, 499f
Cell body, 378, 379f
Cell-mediated hypersensitivity, 623
Cell-mediated immunity, 621
Cellular respiration, 270
Central canal, 387
Central fever, in intracranial hypertension, 423
Central gray horns, 387
Central herniation, 418f, 419t
Central line-associated blood stream infection (CLABSI), 699–700, 699b
Central nervous system
    hyperventilation, 394
    infections, 447–453, 451f
Central neurogenic hyperventilation, 394, 394f
Central sulcus, 382, 384f
Central venous access, 104
Central venous oxygen saturation, 107t–108t, 115
Central venous pressure (CVP), 107t–108t
    in cardiovascular assessment, 78
Cerebellar herniation, 419t
Cerebellar syndrome, 453
Cerebellum, 384
    tumors of, 444t
Cerebral aneurysm, 3840, 434f
Cerebral arteries, 384t, 385, 385f
    occlusion of, 439b
Cerebral balloon angioplasty, for hemorrhagic stroke, 437

Cerebral blood flow (CBF), 385–386
  in intracranial hypertension, 418
  monitoring, 411–412
  regional, 414t–416t
  values, 412
Cerebral circulation, 384–386, 384t, 385f
Cerebral cortical areas, 382–383, 384f, 384t
Cerebral hemispheres, 382–383
Cerebral ischemia and infarction, 645
Cerebral metabolism, 380–381
Cerebral neurotransmitters, 380, 380t
Cerebral perfusion pressure (CPP), 386
  in encephalopathy, 423, 424f
  in intracranial hypertension, 418
  in traumatic brain injury, 428
Cerebral salt wasting syndrome (CSW), complicating craniotomy, 426
Cerebral syndrome, 3860
Cerebral vasospasm, 437
Cerebrospinal fluid (CSF), 386, 387f–388f
  analysis of, in neurologic assessment, 413
  circulation of, 386, 388f
  drainage of, for intracranial hypertension, 421
  excessive accumulation of, 432, 433f
  increased volume of, in intracranial hypertension, 413
  leak, 405, 405f
Cerebrovascular disease, extracranial, 221
Cerebrum, 382–383, 384f, 384t
Certification
  CCRN®
    benefits of achieving, 1–2
    maintaining, 9
    synergy model of, 2–3, 2f
  definition of, 1
  purposes of, 1
Ceruminous glands, 668
Cervical spinal nerves, 388
Cetrimide, for complex wounds, 671
Chain of survival, 540
Chamber enlargement, ECG changes in, 99–100, 100f
Change process, 26–27, 28t
Chaotic atrial rhythm, 94t–96t
Charcoal, activated, for drug intoxication and poisoning, 712
Chemical inflammatory mediators, 619, 620t
Chemoreceptors
  arterial, 260
  cardiac, 63
Chemotaxis, 617f, 617t
Chemotherapy, for brain tumor, 445
Chest
  barrel, 274
  flail, 359f, 361–362
  funnel, 274
  pigeon, 274
  trauma to, 356–363
    general information about, 356
    surgery for, 321
Chest compressions, for cardiopulmonary arrest, 123
Chest pain
  differentiation of, 70–71, 72t–74t
  gastrointestinal, 72t–74t
Chest physiotherapy, 290–291

Chest radiography, 87t–89t, 282t–283t
  in hemodynamic monitoring, 118
  interpretation of, 280–281
Chest tubes, 317–321
  assessment parameters for, 320t
  collaborative management of, 322–323
  drainage systems for, 318, 319f
  purposes of, 317–318
  removal of, 321
Chest wall, 258f
  pain receptors in, 260
  in pulmonary assessment, 274–276
Cheyne-Stokes breathing, 275t, 394, 394f
Chief complaint
  in behavioral/psychosocial considerations, 721
  in cardiovascular assessment, 70
  in endocrine assessment, 466–470
  in gastrointestinal assessment, 501
  in hematologic and immunologic assessment, 628
  in neurologic assessment, 392–393
  in renal assessment, 574–575
Chinese Americans, cultural behaviors relevant to nursing care in, 31t
Chlorhexidine, for complex wounds, 671
Chlorhexidine gluconate, after airway intubation, 297
Chloride, functions, regulation, and sources, 572t–574t
Cholangiography, percutaneous transhepatic, 511t–514t
Cholangiopancreatography, endoscopic retrograde, 511t–514t
Cholecystitis, 502t
Cholecystography, 511t–514t
Cholecystokinin, 499t
Cholinergic branch, of autonomic nervous system, 392, 392t
Cholinergic crisis, 456
Christian Scientist, religious beliefs in, nursing interventions, 32t–33t
Christmas factor, 625t
Chronic obstructive pulmonary disease (COPD), with acute exacerbation, 323
Chvostek sign, 541, 588
Chylothorax, during hemodynamic monitoring, 121t–123t
Chyme, 494
  movement of, 495
Ciliospinal reflex, 402
Cingulate herniation, 418f, 419t
Circle of Willis, 385
Circulation
  bronchial, 257–258
  cerebral, 384–386, 384t, 385f
  of cerebrospinal fluid (CSF), 386, 388f
  pulmonary, 256–257
Cirrhosis, 527, 535
Cisternal puncture, 414t–416t
Cisternography, 414t–416t
Citrate intoxication, 640t
Claudication, intermittent, in cardiovascular assessment, 75
Clearance, glomerular filtration rate and, 568
Clevidipine, 191t
  for hypertensive crises, 208, 209t–212t

Clinical inquiry, 35–41
  nurses and, 3
Clinical judgment, 13–14, 13f
  nurses and, 2
Clinical practice guidelines (CPGs), 37–38
Clinical reasoning, 13–14, 13f
Clonic seizure, 445t
Closing snap, 620, 83
Clot, formation of. *See* Coagulation.
Clotting, drugs affecting, 641–643, 641f, 641b, 643t–644t
Clotting factors, for disseminated intravascular coagulation, 624, 625t, 654, 654t
Clotting pathways, 624–625, 626f
Clotting profile, 579, 633
  in cardiovascular assessment, 85–87
  in gastrointestinal assessment, 510–511
  in neurologic assessment, 413
Clubbing, 273
  in cardiovascular assessment, 78
Cluster breathing, 394, 394f
Coagulation, 624–625
  disseminated intravascular, 643–655, 652f, 653t–654t
Coagulation factors, 624, 625t
Coagulopathy, 643, 650t
  dilutional, 640t
Cocaine, myocardial infarction from, 181
Coccygeal spinal nerves, 388
Cochlear branch, in neurologic assessment, 402
Coercing, conflict, 25
Cognition
  in mental status examination, 722
  in neurologic assessment, 395–396, 396t–398t
Cognitive levels, of questions, in CCRN® examination, 3–4
Cold agglutinins, 627
Colectomy, 548, 552t–553t
Collaboration, 24–26
  nurses and, 3
Collagenase, 620t
Collateral circulation, coronary, 54
Collecting duct, 566
Colloidal oncotic pressures, 65, 66f, 571
Colloids, 684–685, 684b
Colon, 495, 495f
  resection of, 552t–553t
Colon cancer, adjuvant therapy for, 548
Colonic motility, 496
Colonoscopy, 511t–514t
Colostomy, 555–556
Coma
  barbiturate-induced, for intracranial hypertension, 421–422
  cause of, 406
  Glasgow Coma Scale for, 396, 396t
Combitube, 293t–295t
Commissure, 51
Commissurotomy, 205
Common bile duct, 496f, 497
Communication, 25
Community-acquired pneumonia (CAP), 338
Compact bone, 674
Compartment syndrome, abdominal, 508

Compensation, correction *versus*, 285
Competence, cultural, 27
Competing, conflict, 25
Complement assay, 633–634
Complement cascade, 620t
Complementary therapies, 19–21
Complex partial seizure, 445t
Complex wounds
    clinical presentation of, 670, 670f
    collaborative management of, 670–673
    definitions of, 669, 669t
    etiology of, 669
    pathophysiology of, 669–670
Complexity, in patients, 2
Compliance, brain, 418
Compresses, for intravenous infiltration, 674
Compression, for cardiopulmonary arrest, 124
Compromising, conflict, 25
Computed axial tomography (CAT), in neurologic assessment, 414t–416t
Computed tomography (CT), 87t–89t
    abdominal, 511t–514t
    in acute pancreatitis, 543
    for heart failure, 188
    in neurologic assessment, 414t–416t
    thoracic, 282t–283t
Concentration, during CCRN® examination, 8
Concussion, 426
Conduction, aberrant, dysrhythmias/blocks from, 133–134
Conduction system, 55–56, 56f
Confidentiality, 15, 726
Conflict resolution, 25
Conjugate eye movement, 402
Consciousness, level of, in neurologic assessment, 395–396, 397t–398t
Consent, 18
Contact factor, 625t
Continuous airway pressure monitoring (CAPM), 280
Continuous aspiration of subglottic secretions (CASS), 289, 295f
Continuous cardiac output, 113
Continuous drainage system, 409, 409f
Continuous positive airway pressure (CPAP), 316
    for acute respiratory distress syndrome, 333
    for heart failure, 189
Continuous renal replacement therapy (CRRT), 539, 606, 606t
Continuous venovenous hemodiafiltration (CVVHDF), 606t
Continuous venovenous hemodialysis (CVVHD), 606t
Continuous venovenous hemofiltration (CVVH), 606t
Contractility, 58, 60t, 62
    cardiac output and, 62
    stroke volume and, 62, 62f
Contrast dye-related nephrotoxicity, 599
Contusions
    brain, 426
    pulmonary, 356–357
Cooling, initiation of, for hypothermia, 128

Coombs test, 627, 634
Cooperating, conflict, 25
Coopernail sign, in abdominal trauma, 549
Coordination, in neurologic assessment, 398
Coping mechanisms, for stress, 724, 724t
Corneal arcus, in cardiovascular assessment, 78
Corneal blink reflex, 402
Coronary angiography, 87t–89t
Coronary arteries, 52–54, 53f
    left, 53, 53f
    right, 53, 53f
Coronary artery disease, 154
Coronary artery perfusion, 52–53
Coronary artery perfusion pressure (CAPP), 52, 107t–108t
Coronary artery stent, 167t–168t
Coronary atherectomy, 167t–168t
Coronary bypass grafting, for myocardial infarction, 169, 180t–181t
Coronary vasculature, 52–54, 53f
Coronary veins, 54
Corpus callosum, 383
Corrigan pulse, 80f, 81
Cortical nephrons, 565, 565f
Corticospinal syndrome, 453
Corticosteroids
    for acute respiratory distress syndrome, 2590, 335
    for status asthmaticus, 349
Costophrenic angle, 258f
Costovertebral angle, 574
Costovertebral angle pain, in renal assessment, 574
Cough, 270, 288
    in cardiovascular assessment, 71–75
    in neurologic assessment, 403
Coumadin. *See* Warfarin.
Countercurrent mechanism, of kidney, 569
Court cases, types of, 17
Crackles, 278t
Cranial nerves, 388, 391t–392t
    function assessment, 400–404, 402f–404f
    in intracranial hypertension, 418
Craniectomy, 424
Cranioplasty, 424
Craniotomy, 424–426
    for brain tumor, 444
Cranium, 381, 381f–382f
Creatine kinase MB isoenzyme (CK-MB), in myocardial infarction, 159, 160t
Creatinine, 578
    excretion of, 569
Creatinine clearance, 568
Cremasteric reflex, 404
Crescendo angina, 154
Cricothyroid membrane, 253, 253f
Cricothyrotomy, 293t–295t
Crisis, in responses to illness and environment, 725–726
Critical care areas, high-alert medications frequently administered in, 41b
Critical care certification examination, 1–11
Critical care nursing, 12–13. *See also* Professional caring and ethical practice.
Critical-care pain observation tool, 20t
Critical DO_2 point, 70, 70f

Critical thinking, 13–14, 13f
Critically ill adult, family of, 22–24
Crypts of Lieberkühn, 495
Crystalloids, 684, 684b, 685t
    for anaphylactic shock, 695
    for upper gastrointestinal hemorrhage, 529
Cullen sign, 505
Cultural competence, 27
Cultural diversity, 27–31, 29f, 30t
Cultural imposition, 28
Cultural pain, 28
Cultural paradigms, 28
Cultural relativism, 28
Cultural sensitivity, 27
Culturally competent healthcare, barriers to, 35
Culturally congruent nursing care, 27
Culture, 27
    in hematologic and immunologic assessment, 634–635
CURB-65 scoring, for community acquired pneumonia, 341
Cushing triad, 394, 419
Cushing ulcer, 426
Customs, 27
Cyanosis
    in cardiovascular assessment, 77
    in pulmonary assessment, 273
Cyclooxygenase (COX) inhibitors, 641
Cyklokapron (tranexamic acid), for disseminated intravascular coagulation, 654
Cystic duct, 496f, 497
Cystitis, 593
Cystometrography, 580t–581t
Cystoscopy, 580t–581t
Cystourethrography, voiding, 580t–581t
Cytokines, 616–617
Cytomegalovirus (CMV), complicating blood transfusion, 636
Cytotoxic hypersensitivity, 623
Cytotoxic T cells, 618

D

D-dimer, 633
    in pulmonary embolism, 352
Dabigatran, 643t–644t
Dalteparin sodium, in myocardial infarction, 171t–179t
Dalton law of partial pressure, 267–268, 267f
Damped pulmonary artery pressure, 111, 112t, 113f
DDAVP (desmopressin), 472t
De Musset sign, in cardiovascular assessment, 78
Dead space ventilation, 261, 263f
Death and dying, 18
DeBakey classification system, 217
Decision making
    clinical, 13
    ethical, 14–16, 16f
Decompensation, in intracranial hypertension, 418
Deep breathing, during CCRN® examination, 6

Index

Deep tendon reflexes, 404, 404t
Deep vein thrombosis (DVT), complicating craniotomy, 426
Defecation reflex, 496
Defense mechanisms
　immune, 621
　psychological, 724t
Defibrillation, for cardiopulmonary arrest, 124–125
Dehydration, in diabetes insipidus, 474
Delayed hypersensitivity, 623
Delegation, 26
Delirium, 727–729, 728t, 728b
　clinical presentation of, 728–729
　collaborative management of, 729
　definition and description of, 727–729
　ICU, 729
　pathophysiology of, 728
　predisposing and risk factors for, 728
Delivery systems, patient care, 26, 27t
Delta wave, 133f
Delusion, in mental status examination, 722
Dementia, 727, 728t
Dendrites, 378, 379f
Denial
　as defense mechanism, 724t
　in myocardial infarction, 183t
　in responses to illness and environment, 725
Denver shunt, 539
Depression, 732
　in myocardial infarction, 183t
　in responses to illness and environment, 725
Dermal papillae, 667f
Dermatomal levels, for bedside assessment, 400, 400t
Dermatomes, 388, 390f, 391t
Dermis, 666–667, 667f
Desmopressin (DDAVP), 472t
Developmental tasks, 723
Dexmedetomidine, 308t
　as sedative agents, 309t–310t
Dextran, 685
Diabetes insipidus, 473–476, 475f
　clinical presentation of, 474
　collaborative management of, 474–476
　complicating craniotomy, 426
　definition of, 473
　drugs affecting, 474b
　etiology of, 473–474
　pathophysiology of, 474
Diabetes mellitus, 477
　acute coronary syndrome and, 155
Diabetic ketoacidosis (DKA), 477–480, 478f
　clinical presentation of, 478–479
　collaborative management of, 479–480
　definitions of, 477–478
　etiology of, 478
　pathophysiology of, 478
Diagnostic peritoneal lavage (DPL), 4950
Dialysis, 600–606, 601f
　collaborative management of, 601–606, 604f–606f, 605t–606t
　components of, 601
　definition of, 569–5700, 601f
　indication for, 601

Dialysis (Continued)
　principles of, 601, 602f
　purposes of, 569–5705
　types of, 601, 602t–603t
　variables affecting, 601
Diapedesis, 617f, 617t
Diaphoresis, in cardiovascular assessment, 75
Diaphragm, 258f
　rupture of, 362–363
Diaphragma sellae, 382, 383f
Diaphragmatic excursion, 276
Diaphragmatic hernia repair, 321
Diastasis, 58
Diastole, 58, 58f
Diastolic arterial pressure, 105, 108t–109t
Diastolic dysfunction, 59
　heart failure and, 585
Diastolic murmurs, 84, 86f
Diazepam, 308t
　as sedative agents, 309t–310t
　for status epilepticus, 448t–449t
Diencephalon, 383–384
Differential, 632
Diffuse axonal injury, 382–3830
Diffusing capacity, 282t–283t
Diffusion, 569–570
　abnormalities of, in acute respiratory failure, 325t–326t
　gas, 267f
Diffusion pathway, lung, 256, 256f
Digestion, 500
　accessory organs of, 496–498, 496f–497f
Digestive enzymes, 491t
Digital subtraction angiography (DSA), 87t–89t, 414t–416t
Digitalis
　for dysrhythmias/blocks, 137t–146t
　ECG changes in, 97
Dilantin. See Phenytoin.
Dilated cardiomyopathy, 197–199, 198f
Diltiazem, for dysrhythmias/blocks, 137t–146t
Dilutional coagulopathy, 640t
2,3-Diphosphoglycerate (DPG)
　loss of, 640t
　oxyhemoglobin dissociation curve and, 269, 269b
Diprivan. See Propofol.
Disequilibrium syndrome, 604
Dissecting aortic aneurysm, 217
　chest pain in, 72t–74t
Disseminated intravascular coagulation, 643–655
　clinical presentation of, 652–653, 653t
　collaborative management of, 653–655, 654t
　etiology of, 651–652
　pathophysiology of, 652, 652f
Distractions, CCRN® examination and, 6
Distributive shock, 679
Diuretics, 580–582, 583t
　for ascites, 538
　for brain mass, 422–423
　for diabetes insipidus, 475
　for heart failure, 190–191
　for hepatorenal syndrome, 539
　for hypertensive crises, 208–213

Diversity, 27
　cultural, 27–31, 29f, 30t
　generational, 34–35
　religious, 32–34, 32t–33t
　response to, 27–35
　nurses and, 3
Diverticulitis, 502t
Dobutamine, 63t, 192, 192t
Dobutamine hydrochloride, 193t–194t
Dofetilide, for dysrhythmias/blocks, 137t–146t
Doll eyes reflex, 402–403, 404f
Dopamine, 63t, 380t, 582
Dopamine hydrochloride, 193t–194t, 686t–687t
Dopaminergic stimulators, 582–583
Doppler pressure, 85
Doppler pulse, 85
Doppler ultrasonography, 87t–89t
　for CBF measurement, 411–412
　transcranial, in neurologic assessment, 414t–416t
Downward cerebellar herniation, 419t
Dressings, for complex wounds, 671–672
Dressler syndrome, in myocardial infarction, 183t–185t
Droplet precautions, in CNS infection, 452
Drug(s)
　for dysrhythmias/blocks, 136
　effects on ECG, 97
　intoxication and poisoning of, 710
Drug polymorphism, 29–31
Duct of Wirsung, 498
Dumping syndrome, 531
Duodenum, 494
Duplex ultrasonography, 87t–89t
Dura mater, 382, 383f
Durable power of attorney, 18
Dysautonomia, complicating traumatic brain injuries, 429
Dysconjugate eye movement, 402
Dyspepsia, 501
Dyspnea
　in cardiovascular assessment, 71
　in pulmonary assessment, 270
Dysrhythmias/blocks
　clinical presentation of, 134
　collaborative management of, 134–154, 135t
　complicating chest surgery, 2590
　definitions of, 130, 131f
　electrical therapies for, 136
　electrocardiographic changes in, 93–96, 94t–96t
　etiology of, 131
　during hemodynamic monitoring, 121t–123t
　in hypertrophic cardiomyopathy, 200
　with hypothermia, 129
　in myocardial infarction, 183t–185t
　pacemaker for, 565. See also Pacemaker.
　pacemaker-mediated, 153
　pathophysiology of, 131–134
　surgical ablation for, 570

Index 841

E

Ears
  in cardiovascular assessment, 78
  in renal assessment, 576
  trauma to, 405
East Indian Hindu Americans, cultural behaviors relevant to nursing care in, 31t
Eccrine sweat glands, 668
Echocardiography, 87t–89t
  for heart failure, 188
Ectopic SIADH, 476, 477f
Ectopy, ventricular, 134t
Edema
  brain, in intracranial hypertension, 413
  capillary dynamics and, 65
  in cardiovascular assessment, 75, 78
  in endocrine assessment, 471
  pulmonary. See Pulmonary edema.
  in pulmonary assessment, 273
  in renal assessment, 576
Edoxaban, 643t–644t
Education
  adult, principles of, 42
  for low-literacy individuals, 44, 44t
  patient, reasons for, 41
Effective refractory period, 55, 55f
Effort syncope, 75
Egoism, 15
Egophony, 277
Ejection click, 83t
Ejection fraction (EF), 58
Elastase, 620t
Elastic stockings, 2670
Electrical therapies
  for cardiopulmonary arrest, 550
  for dysrhythmias/blocks, 136
Electrocardiography (ECG), 87t–89t, 90–103, 94t–96t
  for cardiac arrest, 120
  components of cardiac cycle in, 92–93, 92f
  continuous derived 12-lead, 91
  drug effects on, 97
  dysrhythmias/blocks in, 93–96
  electrolyte imbalance in, 93, 96–97
  general information on, 90
  for heart failure, 580
  lead selection in, 91–92
  modified chest leads in, 91
  monitoring leads
    five-lead system of, 90, 91f
    three-lead system for, 90–91, 91f
  multiple-lead analysis of, 97–98
    leads for, 97–98, 97f
    mean QRS axis in, 98
  pacing evidence with, 56–570, 150f–151f
  paper for, 90, 90f
  rhythm strip analysis in, 90–97, 93t
  signal averaged, 87t–89t
  ST-segment monitoring in, 103
  stress, 87t–89t
  thallium stress, 87t–89t
Electroencephalography (EEG)
  continuous, 412
  in neurologic assessment, 414t–416t

Electrolytes, 578
  absorption of, 500
  for acute respiratory failure, 327t
  balance of, 572
  imbalance. See Fluid and electrolyte imbalance(s).
  renal regulation, 572
  summary of, 572, 572t–574t
Electromyography (EMG), in neurologic assessment, 414t–416t
Electron-beam computed tomography, 87t–89t
Electronystagmography (ENG), in neurologic assessment, 414t–416t
Electrophysiologic studies (EPS), 87t–89t
Embolectomy
  for ischemic stroke, 3840
  pulmonary, 355
Emboli
  complicating hypertrophic cardiomyopathy, 200
  during hemodynamic monitoring, 121t–123t
  in intraaortic balloon pump, 165t–167t
Embolic stroke, 3845
Emotional responses, in myocardial infarction, 183t
Emphysema, 280, 323
  subcutaneous, 275
Empyema, complicating chest surgery, 323
Enalaprilat, for hypertensive crises, 209t–212t
Encephalitis, 3855, 451f
Encephalopathy, 423–424, 424f
  hepatic, 535–541, 536t, 537f, 538b
  prevention of, 533–534
  stages of, 538b
Enculturation, 28
End-of-life care, 18
Endarterectomy
  carotid, 221
  for ischemic stroke, 442
Endobronchial ultrasound (EBUS), 321
Endocardium, 49, 50f
Endocrine glands, 465, 466f, 466t–469t
Endocrine hormones, 465, 466f, 466t–469t
  pharmacology of, 472–473, 472t–473t
  process of synthesis, secretion, effect, and suppression, 465, 469f
  regulation of, 465
Endocrine system, 465–488
  assessment of, 466–472
  components of, 465, 466f, 466t–469t
  dysfunction, 465–466
  functions of, 465
Endoleak, 220
Endorphin, 620t
Endoscopic retrograde cholangiopancreatography (ERCP), 511t–514t
Endoscopic ultrasound (EUS), 321
Endoscopy
  gastrointestinal, 511t–514t
  for upper gastrointestinal hemorrhage, 530
Endothelin, 64
Endothelin receptor antagonists, for acute respiratory distress syndrome, 336

Endothelium, 65
Endotracheal intubation, 292
  in cardiopulmonary arrest, 125
  complications of, 296–297
  extubation in, 296
  indications for, 292
  insertion of, 292–296
Endotracheal tube, 293t–295t
  for continuous aspiration of subglottic secretions, 289, 295f
  cuffed, 295
Endovascular grafts, for aneurysm repair, 219
Enema, barium, 511t–514t
Enoxaparin, in myocardial infarction, 171t–179t
Enteral nutrition, 518, 519t–523t
Enterogastrone, 499t
Enzymes, in gastrointestinal assessment, 510
Eosinophils, 618, 632
Ependyma, 378
Ependymomas, 444t
Epicardial fat, 49, 50f
Epicardium, 49, 50f
Epidermis, 666–667, 667f
Epidural hematoma, 429, 431, 431f
Epidural sensor or transducer, for ICP measurement, 408f, 408t
Epidural space, 382
Epiglottis, 253
Epinephrine, 63t
  for anaphylactic shock, 695
Epinephrine hydrochloride, 686t–687t
Epoprostenol, for acute respiratory distress syndrome, 331t, 335
Epsilon-aminocaproic acid (Amicar), for disseminated intravascular coagulation, 654, 654t
Eptifibatide, 642, 643t–644t
  in myocardial infarction, 171t–179t
Erb's point, 81, 81f
Erythrocyte sedimentation rate (ESR), 631
Erythrocytes, 615–616
  in hematologic and immunologic assessment, 631
  synthesis and maturation of, 572
Erythroid stem cells, 615
Erythropoiesis, 616
Erythropoietin, 632
  secretion of, 572
Esmolol, for dysrhythmias/blocks, 137t–146t
Esophageal-tracheal airway, 293t–295t
Esophageal varices
  balloon tamponade for, 529, 531f, 532t
  definition of, 527
  nutritional support for, 535
  pathophysiology of, 528f
  sclerotherapy for, 530
  surgery for, 532–533
Esophagitis, 526–527
Esophagoenterostomy, 552t–553t, 554f
Esophagogastrectomy, 321, 4965, 552t–553t, 554f
Esophagogastroduodenoscopy, 511t–514t
Esophagus, 490–493, 492f
  functions of, 491t–492t
  sphincters of, 493

Ethical approaches, 16
Ethical care, 726
Ethical decision making, 14–16, 16f. *See also* Professional caring and ethical practice.
Ethical dilemmas, 16
Ethical issues, 16, 16f
Ethmoid bone, 381f
Ethnic group, 27
Ethnocentrism, 28
Eupnea, 275t
Eustachian tubes, 252–253
Evidence-based practice, 35–36, 36t
Evoked potential studies, in neurologic assessment, 414t–416t
Examination, CCRN®, 3–4
  basic information about, 3, 3t
  passing score in, 4
  plans for passing, 4–9, 4f, 5b
  questions in, 3–4
Excitation-contraction process, 57–58
Excretion, of metabolic waste products, 569
Exercise, acute coronary syndrome and, 158
Exercise testing, 282t–283t
Exercise tolerance test, 87t–89t
Exophthalmos, in cardiovascular assessment, 78
Expectorants
  for acute respiratory failure, 2595
  for status asthmaticus, 265–2665
Expiration (exhalation), 261, 261f
Expiratory maneuvers, with mechanical ventilation, 303
Expiratory reserve volume (ERV), 262f, 262t–263t
Exsanguination, during hemodynamic monitoring, 121t–123t
Extension, abnormal, 399, 399f
External carotid system, 385
External intercostals, 259
External oblique, 259
Extraanatomical bypass (EAB), 215
Extracorporeal carbon dioxide removal (ECCO$_2$R), for acute respiratory distress syndrome, 333
Extracorporeal liver perfusion, 540
Extracorporeal membrane oxygenation (ECMO), 304t–305t
  for acute respiratory distress syndrome, 333
Extraocular movements (EOMs), 402, 402f
Extrapyramidal tracts, 389t
Extremities
  in cardiovascular assessment, 79–81, 79t, 80f
  in renal assessment, 577
Extubation, endotracheal, 296
Eye movements, abnormal, 402
Eyelids, in neurologic assessment, 401
Eyes
  in cardiovascular assessment, 78
  in endocrine assessment, 471
  raccoon, 405, 405f
  in renal assessment, 576
  trauma to, 405, 405f

F

Face
  in cardiovascular assessment, 78
  in endocrine assessment, 471
  trauma to, 404–405
Face mask, 301t–302t
Facial nerve (CN VII), 391t–392t, 402
Facilitator, nurses as, 3
Factor Xa inhibitors, 643t–644t
Factors, coagulation, 624, 625t
Faith, 32
Falls, 706–707
Falx cerebelli, 382, 383f
Falx cerebri, 382, 383f
Family
  of cardiopulmonary arrest patient, 130
  of critically ill adult, 22–24
Family education, 600
Family history
  in cardiovascular assessment, 75
  in gastrointestinal assessment, 503
  in hematologic and immunologic assessment, 629
  in neurologic assessment, 393
  in pulmonary assessment, 272
  in renal assessment, 575
Fascicles, 56, 56f
Fat embolism, 353
Fatigue, in cardiovascular assessment, 75
Fats
  absorption of, 500
  digestion of, 500
  in skin, 667f
Fatty acids, polyunsaturated, 518
Feculent breath, 505
Femoral artery, occlusive disease of, 214
Fenoldopam mesylate, 191t, 582–583
  for hypertensive crises, 635, 209t–212t
Ferritin, 632–633
Fetor hepaticus, 505
Fever, in cardiovascular assessment, 77
Fibrin, 625t
Fibrin clot, 624–625
Fibrin degradation products (FDPs), 626, 633
Fibrin split products (FSPs), 626, 633
Fibrin-stabilizing factor, 625t
Fibrinase, 625t
Fibrinogen, 625t, 633
Fibrinolysin, 620t
Fibrinolytic system, 625–626, 626f
Fibrinolytics, 642–643, 643t–644t
  in ischemic stroke, 440–442, 441b
  for myocardial infarction, 580, 169t–179t
Fibroblasts, 667
Fibrous pericardium, 49, 50f
Fick law of diffusion, 268
Fidelity, 15
Fight or flight response, 62
Filipino Americans, cultural behaviors relevant to nursing care in, 31t
Filtration, 571
Fingertips, in cardiovascular assessment, 78
First-degree AV nodal block, 94t–96t
First rib, 77f
Fissure of Rolando, 382, 384f
Fissure of Sylvius, 382, 384f
Fissures, 382
Fistula, pancreatic, 544
Fixed macrophages, 618
Flaccid posture, 399
Flail chest, 359f, 361–362
Flecainide, for dysrhythmias/blocks, 137t–146t
Flexion, abnormal, 399, 399f
Fling, 111, 112t, 113f
Flow-volume loop studies, 282t–283t
Fluid(s)
  body, regulation of, 571–572
  requirements for, 518
  for shock, 684–686, 684b, 685t
Fluid and electrolyte imbalance(s), 583–592
  electrocardiography and, 93, 96–97
  gastrointestinal losses and, 501
  hypercalcemia as, 589–590
  hyperkalemia as, 587–588
  hypermagnesemia as, 592
  hypernatremia as, 586
  hyperphosphatemia as, 590–591
  hypervolemia as, 584–585
  hypocalcemia as, 588–589
  hypokalemia as, 586–587
  hypomagnesemia as, 591
  hyponatremia as, 585
  hypophosphatemia as, 590
  hypovolemia as, 583–584
  water excess syndrome as, 585
  water loss syndromes as, 584
Fluid balance, 569–572, 570f
Fluid-filled system, 407–409
Fluid overload, during hemodynamic monitoring, 121t–123t
Fluid retention, complicating mechanical ventilation, 313t–315t
Fluid therapy
  for diabetes insipidus, 477
  for diabetic ketoacidosis, 479
Flutter valve, for tracheobronchial secretions removal, 288
Foam dressings, for complex wounds, 672
Focused abdominal sonography for trauma (FAST), 551
Folds of dura mater, 382, 383f
Fondaparinux, for pulmonary embolism, 354
Foramen magnum, 382, 382f
Forced expiratory volume (FEV), 262t–263t
Forced vital capacity (FVC), 262t–263t
Fosphenytoin, for status epilepticus, 448t–449t
Fossae, 382, 382f
Fourth ventricles, 386, 387f
Fraction of inspired oxygen (FiO$_2$), 299
Fractures
  rib, 361–362
  skull, 429–431, 429f
Fragmin. *See* Dalteparin sodium.
Frank-Starling mechanism, 61
Frankincense, 19
Fremitus, 274–275
Frontal bone, 381f
Frontal lobe, 382, 384f, 384t
  tumors of, 444t

Frozen shoulder, complicating chest surgery, 323
Functional residual capacity (FRC), 262t–263t
Functional syncytium, 56
Funnel chest, 274
Furosemide, 583t
Fusiform aortic aneurysm, 217

G

Gag, in neurologic assessment, 403
Gait, in neurologic assessment, 398–399
Gallbladder, 497–498, 497f
   functions of, 491t–492t
   palpation of, 507
Gamma-aminobutyric acid (GABA), 380t
Gas(es)
   diffusion of, 267f
   transport of, 268–270
Gas exchange units, 255–256
Gastrectomy, 531–532, 534f, 552t–553t
Gastric acidity, drugs affecting, 511–515, 514t–515t, 526, 534
Gastric banding, 552t–553t, 555f
Gastric bypass, 552t–553t, 555f
Gastric contents, in gastrointestinal assessment, 511
Gastric dilation, complicating mechanical ventilation, 313t–315t
Gastric emptying, 494
Gastric glands, 494
Gastric inhibitory peptide, 499t
Gastric juice, 491t
Gastric lavage, 529
Gastric motility, 494
Gastric mucosa, drugs affecting, 511–515, 514t–515t, 526
Gastric secretions, 491t, 494
Gastric tonometry, 115
Gastrin, 499t
Gastritis, 502t
   clinical presentation in, 529
   definition of, 527
   etiology of, 527
   pathophysiology of, 528f
Gastroesophageal reflux disease (GERD), 526–527
Gastroesophageal sphincter, 493
Gastrointestinal assessment, 501–511
   auscultation in, 506
   diagnostic studies in, 510–511, 511t–514t
   inspection in, 503–506, 504f–505f
   interview in, 501–503
   intraabdominal pressure in, 508–509, 508f
   landmarks in, 503, 504f
   palpation in, 507
   percussion in, 506–507
   vital signs in, 503
Gastrointestinal chest pain, 72t–74t
Gastrointestinal hemorrhage
   pharmacology for, 514t–515t, 515–516
   upper, 527–535, 528f
Gastrointestinal hormones, 498, 499t
Gastrointestinal surgery
   postoperative management for, 552–556
   procedures in, 552, 552t–553t

Gastrointestinal system
   accessory organs of digestion in, 496–498, 496f–497f
   alimentary canal of, 489–496, 490f
   assessment of, 501–511. *See also* Gastrointestinal assessment.
   blood supply of, 498–500, 499f
   drugs affecting, 511–516, 514t–515t
   esophagus of, 490–493, 492f
   functions of, 491t, 500–501
   gallbladder of, 497–498, 497f
   general information about, 489, 490f, 491t–492t
   innervation of, 500
   large intestine of, 495–496, 495f
   liver of, 496–497, 496f
   oropharynx of, 489–490
   pancreas of, 498
   in renal system, 575
   small intestine of, 494–495
Gastroplasty, vertical banded, 552t–553t
Gaze, cardinal positions of, 402, 402f
General appearance, in neurologic assessment, 395
General survey
   in cardiovascular assessment, 77
   in endocrine assessment, 470
   in gastrointestinal assessment, 503–505
   in pulmonary assessment, 272
Generation X, 34t
Generation Y, 34t
Generational diversity, 34–35
Glabellar reflex, 404
Glasgow Coma Scale (GCS), 396, 396t
Glial cells, 378
Glioblastoma multiforme, 444t
Gliomas, 444t
Glisson capsule, 496
Glomerular filtrate, 568
Glomerular filtration, 567–568
Glomerular filtration rate (GFR), 567–568
Glomerulonephritis, 594
Glomerulus, 566
Glossopharyngeal nerve (CN IX), 391t–392t, 403
Glucagon, 466t–469t, 472–473
Glucocorticoids, 466t–469t
Gluconeogenesis, 380
Glucose, 578
   in cerebral metabolism, 380–381
   for hypoglycemia, 483
Glucose intolerance, acute coronary syndrome and, 155
Glucose oxidase reagent strips, 263–2660
Glutamine, supplementation of, 518
Glycine, 380t
Glycoprotein IIb/IIIa inhibitors, 641–642, 643t–644t
Goblet cells, 495
Granulocytes, 617–618, 617f, 617t
Grasp reflex, 404
Gray matter, 387, 388f
Great vessel injury, 224–225
Grey Turner sign, 505
Growth hormone, 466t–469t

Guessing, during CCRN® examination, 7–8
Guided imagery, 20
Guillain-Barré syndrome, 454–455
Gyri, 382, 384f

H

Haemophilus influenzae, 452
Hageman factor, 625t
Hair, 667
   in endocrine assessment, 471
Hair shaft, 667f
Haitian Americans, cultural behaviors relevant to nursing care in, 31t
Halitosis, 505
Hallucinations
   nonpathological, 722
   pathological, 722, 722t
Halo sign, 405, 405f
Haptoglobin, 633
Haustral shuttling, 495
HCl, as sedative agents, 309t–310t
HCO_3^-, 285
Head
   in cardiovascular assessment, 78–79
   in endocrine assessment, 471
   trauma to, 404–405
Headache
   in cardiovascular assessment, 75
   craniotomy and, 425
   in hemorrhagic stroke, 434
   in neurologic assessment, 392
Healing touch, 21
Health care-associated pneumonia (HCAP), 338
Health history, in musculoskeletal assessment, 675
Health literacy, in culturally competent healthcare, 35
Heart, 49–64. *See also cardiac entries; cardiovascular entries; coronary entries; myocardial entries.*
   biopsy of, 87t–89t
   cardiac cycle and, 52–53, 58, 58f
   cardiac skeleton and, 49–50
   chambers of, 50–51, 50f
   conduction system of, 55–56, 56f
   coronary vasculature, 52–54, 53f
   electrophysiology of, 54–56
   endocrine function of, 64
   excitation-contraction process and, 57–58
   extrinsic control of, 62–64
   intrinsic control of, 59f, 60t
   location of, 50f, 76, 77f
   muscle mechanics of, 56–58, 57f
   neurologic control of, 62–63, 63t
   pathway of blood through, 52, 52f
   valves of, 51–52, 51f
   walls of, 49, 50f
Heart block. *See* Dysrhythmias/blocks.
Heart failure, 185–197
   classifications of, 186–187
   clinical presentation of, 187–188, 189f, 189t
   collaborative management for, 188–197
   complications of, 197
   decompensated, 185
      acute, 185

Heart failure (Continued)
    definitions of, 185
    etiology of, 185, 186t
    hemodynamic parameters for, 188, 189f
    mechanical cardiac support devices for, 192, 195t–196t
    in myocardial infarction, 183t–185t
    pathophysiology of, 186, 187f–188f
Heart-lung transplantation, for pulmonary hypertension, 261§
Heart rate, 59, 60t, 107t–108t
    in cardiovascular assessment, 76
Heart rhythm abnormalities. See Dysrhythmias/blocks.
Heart sounds, 81–84, 83t, 577
Heave, 79, 274
Heimlich maneuver, 288
Heimlich valve, 318, 320f
Helicobacter pylori infection, drug therapy for, 534
Heliox, for status asthmaticus, 349
Helper T cells, 618
Hematocrit, 579, 615, 631
Hematologic and immunologic systems, 614–665
    anticoagulants and, 642, 642t–644t
    assessment of, 628–635
    blood and, 615–619
    blood groups and, 627, 627t
    blood transfusion and, 635–636, 637t–640t, 639b
    bone marrow in, 614
    coagulopathies and, 643, 650t
    drugs affecting clotting and, 641–643, 641f, 641b, 643t–644t
    fibrinolytics and, 642–643, 643t–644t
    hemostasis and, 623–626, 625t, 626f
    immunity and, 619–623, 621f, 622t
    inflammation and, 619, 620t
    liver in, 614
    lymphatic system in, 615
    purposes of, 614
    spleen in, 614
Hematology
    in cardiovascular assessment, 85
    in gastrointestinal assessment, 510
    in hematologic and immunologic assessment, 631–633, 632t, 634t
    in neurologic assessment, 413
    in pulmonary assessment, 281
Hematoma
    formation of, 674
    during hemodynamic monitoring, 121t–123t
    intracerebral, 431, 431f
    intracranial, 431–432, 431f
    subdural, 431, 431f
Hemianopsia, 401
Hemiblocks, 56, 130
Hemicolectomy, 4950
Hemicraniectomy, for ischemic stroke, 442
Hemodialysis, 539
Hemodilution, in triple H therapy for hemorrhagic stroke, 437
Hemodynamic monitoring, 103–120
    abnormal pressure, 106–110, 108t–109t
    clinical decision making, 115–120, 119t–120t

Hemodynamic monitoring (Continued)
    contraindications of, 105
    controversies regarding, 105
    definition of, 103
    general information regarding, 103–105
    indications for, 104–105
    in myocardial infarction, 160
    parameters of, 105–115, 107t–108t
    pressure monitoring system, components of, 105, 106f
    profiles, for selected critical care conditions, 119t–120t
    in renal assessment, 577
    uses of, 103–104, 104f
Hemodynamic pressure, at end-expiration, 116–117, 117f
Hemoglobin, 579, 631
    fetal, 633
    oxygen transport by, 269t
    synthesis of, 616
Hemolysis, 616
Hemoperfusion, 540
Hemophilia, 650t
Hemoptysis, in cardiovascular assessment, 75
Hemorrhage
    complicating chest surgery, 323
    in fibrinolytic therapy and, 169t–170t
    gastrointestinal
        pharmacotherapy for, 514t–515t, 515–516
        upper, 527–535, 528f
    intracranial, 394, 431–432
    intraparenchymal brain, 433
    intraventricular, 433
    splinter, 78
    subarachnoid, 433, 434f
        vasospasm after, 436–437
    in trauma, 707
Hemorrhagic shock, 690, 690t
Hemorrhagic stroke, 433–437, 434f, 435t
Hemostasis, 623–626, 625t, 626f
    in complex wounds, 669
Hemothorax, 360
    during hemodynamic monitoring, 121t–123t
Henderson-Hasselbalch equation, 283
Heparin
    for disseminated intravascular coagulation, 654, 654t
    low-molecular-weight, 642, 643t–644t
    in myocardial infarction, 580, 171t–179t
    for pulmonary embolism, 354–355
    in saline flush system, 118
    unfractionated, 169, 642, 643t–644t
    for pulmonary embolism, 354
Heparin-induced thrombocytopenia, 655–656
    clinical presentation of, 655–656, 656t
    collaborative management of, 656
    definition of, 655, 655t
    etiology of, 655
    pathophysiology of, 655, 655f
Heparin sodium, in myocardial infarction, 171t–179t
Hepatic artery and vein, 499f, 500

Hepatic cells (hepatocytes), 497
Hepatic ducts, 496f, 497
Hepatic failure/encephalopathy, 535–541, 536t, 537f, 538b
Hepatitis
    complicating blood transfusion, 636
    fulminant, 535
    viral, 536t
Hepatobiliary scintigraphy, 511t–514t
Hepatojugular reflux, 78–79
Hepatomegaly, 277
Hepatorenal syndrome, 539
Hepatotoxic drugs, 504b
Herbal supplements, cardiovascular assessment, 76
Hering-Breuer reflex, 260
Hernia
    diaphragmatic, repair of, 321
    strangulated, 502t
Herniation syndromes, brain, 417, 418f, 419t
Hetastarch, 685
Hgb A1C (HbA1C), 85
HIDA scan, 511t–514t
High-frequency ventilation (HFV), 304t–305t
Hill sign, 203
Hilum, 564
Hinduism, religious beliefs in, nursing interventions, 32t–33t
His bundle, 56, 56f
Histamine, 620t
Histamine H_2 receptor antagonists, 514t–515t, 515
History of present illness
    in gastrointestinal assessment, 502
    in neurologic assessment, 393
    in pulmonary assessment, 271
    in renal assessment, 575
"Holiday heart" syndrome, 131–133
Holter monitor, 87t–89t
Homan sign, 81
Homeostasis, 570–571
Homocysteine, 85
Hope, 32
Hormones
    antidiuretic, 466t–469t, 572, 572t–574t
    endocrine, 465, 466f, 466t–469t. See also Endocrine hormones.
Hostile abdomen, 635
Human immunodeficiency virus (HIV)
    antibody screening for, 634
    complicating blood transfusion, 636
Human leukocyte antigen (HLA), 627, 634
Human needs, 723, 723t
    of critically ill patients, 723, 723f
Humor, 21
Humoral-mediated immunity, 621–622, 621f, 622t
Hunchback, 274
Hunt and Hess grading system, for aneurysm, 435t
Hutchinsonian pupil, 401
Hydralazine, 191t
    for hypertensive crises, 630, 209t–212t
Hydrocephalus, 432–433, 433f
    complicating craniotomy, 426
    complicating hemorrhagic stroke, 3840
    in intracranial hypertension, 413–417

Index

Hydrochloric acid, 494
Hydrochloride, as sedative agents, 309t–310t
Hydrocolloid dressings, for complex wounds, 672
Hydrogel dressing, for complex wounds, 672
Hydrostatic pressures, 65, 66f, 571
Hydrothorax, 280
Hyperbaric oxygenation, 300
Hypercalcemia, 589–590
   ECG changes in, 96
Hypercapnia
   clinical indications of, 276, 276b
   complicating mechanical ventilation, 313t–315t
   permissive, for acute respiratory distress syndrome, 333
Hyperglycemia, 381
   Somogyi phenomenon as, 484, 484f
Hyperglycemic crises, 477–478
Hyperglycemic hyperosmolar state (HHS), 480–482, 481f
   clinical presentation of, 481–482
   collaborative management of, 482
   definitions of, 480
   etiology of, 480–481
   pathophysiology of, 481
Hyperhomocysteinemia, acute coronary syndrome and, 570
Hyperkalemia, 587–588
   ECG changes in, 96
   transfusion-related, 640t
Hyperlipidemia, acute coronary syndrome and, 575
Hypermagnesemia, 592
   ECG changes in, 97
Hypernatremia, 586
Hyperphosphatemia, 590–591
Hyperpnea, 275t
Hyperreflexia, 404
Hypersensitive carotid sinus syncope, 75
Hypersensitivity (allergic) reactions, 622–623
Hypertension
   coronary artery disease and, 570
   intraabdominal, 508
   intracranial. See Intracranial hypertension.
   in neurologic assessment, 394
   portal, 527, 540
   pulmonary, 257, 335–337
   in trauma, 707
   in triple H therapy for hemorrhagic stroke, 437
Hypertensive crises, 206–213
   clinical presentation of, 207–208, 207t
   collaborative management for, 208–213
   definitions of, 206
   etiology of, 206–207
   pathophysiology of, 207, 207f
Hypertensive emergencies, 62–630
Hypertensive urgencies, 206
Hyperthermia, in intracranial hypertension, 423
Hypertonic crystalloids, 684
Hypertrophic cardiomyopathy, 199–201, 199f
Hypertrophy, ECG changes in, 99–100
Hyperventilation
   central neurogenic, 394, 394f
   for intracranial hypertension, 421

Hypervolemia, 584–585
   in triple H therapy for hemorrhagic stroke, 437
Hypnosis, 20
Hypocalcemia, 588–589
   ECG changes in, 96
   transfusion-related, 640t
Hypocapnia, complicating mechanical ventilation, 313t–315t
Hypochlorite solutions, for complex wounds, 671
Hypodermis, 667, 667f
Hypoglossal nerve (CN XII), 391t–392t, 403–404
Hypoglycemia, 381, 482–484, 483f–484f, 483b
   clinical presentation of, 482–483
   collaborative management of, 483–484
   definition of, 482
   etiology of, 482
   pathophysiology of, 482
Hypokalemia, 586–587
   ECG changes in, 96
Hypomagnesemia, 591
   ECG changes in, 96
Hyponatremia, 585
Hypoperfusion
   clinical indications of, 61, 61t, 81
   in trauma, 707
Hypopharyngeal sphincter, 493
Hypopharynx, 253
Hypophosphatemia, 590
Hypophysectomy, 474
Hypopnea, 275t
Hyporeflexia, 404
Hypotension
   after cardiopulmonary arrest, 128
   in neurologic assessment, 394
Hypothalamus, 384
   hormones regulated by, 466t–469t
   tumors of, 444t
Hypothermia
   after cardiopulmonary arrest, 129
   cardiac arrest with, 129
   cardiopulmonary arrest with, 129
   ECG changes in, 103
   during hemodynamic monitoring, 121t–123t
   transfusion-related, 640t
   in trauma, 707
Hypothyroidism, ECG changes in, 103
Hypoventilation
   in acute respiratory failure, 325t–326t
   oxygen-induced, 300
Hypovolemia, 541
Hypovolemic shock, 119t–120t, 227, 688
   clinical presentation of, 689–690
   collaborative management of, 690
   complicating pancreatitis, 545
   definition of, 679, 688
   etiology of, 688
   pathophysiology of, 688, 689f
Hypoxemia
   clinical indications for, 276, 276b
   definition of, 297
   etiology of, 298, 298f
   as indication for oxygen therapy, 299

Hypoxemic pulmonary vasoconstriction, 263–265
Hypoxia
   clinical indications for, 276, 276b
   definition of, 297
   etiology of, 298

I

Ibutilide, for dysrhythmias/blocks, 137t–146t
ICP monitoring, 407
ICU delirium, 729
Idioventricular rhythm, 94t–96t
Ileocecal sphincter, 495
Ileostomy, 552t–553t, 555–556
Ileum, 494
Ileus, complicating mechanical ventilation, 313t–315t
Illness and environment
   behavioral/psychosocial responses to, 723–726, 723t–724t, 724b
   human needs related to, 723, 723f
Illusion, 722
Iloprost, for acute respiratory distress syndrome, 331t
Immediate hypersensitivity reactions, 622–623
Immune complex-mediated reaction, 623
Immune complexes, 622
Immune profile, 634
Immune thrombocytopenic purpura (ITP), 650t
Immunity, 619–623, 621f, 622t
Immunocompromised patient, pneumonia in, 338–339
Immunodeficiency, 658–660
   clinical presentation of, 659
   collaborative management of, 659–660
   definition of, 658
   etiology of, 658
   pathophysiology of, 658–659
Immunoglobulin analysis, 634t
Immunoglobulins (Igs), 621, 622t
Immunologic system. See Hematologic and immunologic systems.
Implantable cardioverter-defibrillator, 153–154
Implied consent, 17
Impulse conduction, problems with, 132–134, 132f
Impulse formation, problems with, 560
Impulse transmission, 380
IN-Vivo Optical Spectroscopy (INVOS), 412
Inamrinone, 193t–194t
Incident reports, 18
Incompetent flow, 51
Independent lung ventilation (ILV), 304t–305t
Inderal. See Propranolol.
Indeterminate axis, 98
Infarction, 350–356
Infection
   central nervous system, 447–453, 451f
   complicating chest surgery, 2590
   complicating ICP monitoring, 409–411

Mallory-Weiss tear
    clinical presentation in, 529
    definition of, 527
    endoscopy for, 530
    etiology of, 527
    pathophysiology of, 528f
Malnutrition, 516–526
    clinical presentation in, 516–517
    collaborative management of, 517–526, 519f, 519t–525t
    definitions in, 516
    etiology of, 516
    pathophysiology of, 516
Malpractice, 17–18
Mandible, 381f
Mania, 732–733
Mannitol, 583t
Marasmus, 516
Margination, 617f, 617t
Maslow's hierarchy of needs, 723, 723t
Massage, 21
Mast cells, 667
Maxilla, 381f
Maximal inspiratory pressure (MIP), 278
Maximal voluntary ventilation (MVV), 278
Maze procedure, for atrial fibrillation, 575
McCarty sign, 78
Mean arterial pressure (MAP), 66, 68f, 106, 107t–108t
    in intracranial hypertension, 423
    in traumatic brain injuries, 428
Mean corpuscular hemoglobin (MCH), 631–632
Mean corpuscular hemoglobin concentration (MCHC), 632
Mean corpuscular volume (MCV), 631
Mechanical valves, 62–640
Mechanical ventilation, 300–317
    for acute respiratory distress syndrome, 332–333
    arterial blood gases and, 308t
    assessment of, 307–308
    collaborative management of, 308–312
    complications of, 313t–315t
    expiratory maneuvers with, 303
    for heart failure, 190
    indications for, 300–302
    inspiratory modes of, 303, 304t–305t
    modes of, 304t–305t
    neuromuscular blockade and, 311–312
    noninvasive positive pressure ventilation, 317
    parameters, 306–307
    sedation and, 308t
    for status asthmaticus, 349
    summary of, 301t–302t
    ventilators for, 302–303
    weaning from, inability of, 313t–315t
Media, 64, 65f
Medial lemniscal system, 389t
Mediastinal crunch, 83t, 84
Mediastinal tubes, 318
Mediastinoscopy, 282t–283t
Mediastinum, 258f, 259
Medical nonadherence, 737
Medication errors, 40–41

Medication history
    in cardiovascular assessment, 76
    in gastrointestinal assessment, 503, 504b
    in hematologic and immunologic assessment, 629–630
    in neurologic assessment, 393–394
    in pulmonary assessment, 270
    in renal assessment, 575–576
Meditation, 20, 32
    during CCRN® examination, 7
Medium-chain triglycerides (MCT), 518
Medulla, 260
    vasomotor center in, 67
Medulla oblongata, 384
Medulloblastomas, 444t
Meissner corpuscle, 667f
Melanocytes, 666, 667f
Memory joggers, CCRN® examination and, 6
Memory T cells, 619
Meninges, 382, 383f, 387
    irritation of, 405–406, 406f
Meningioma, 444t
Meningitis, 3850, 451f
Meningococcus, 452
Mental status
    in behavioral/psychosocial assessment, 721–722
    in neurologic assessment, 395–396, 396t–398t
Merkel cells, 666
Mesencephalon, 384
Mesenteric angiography, 511t–514t
Mesenteric ischemia, 502t
Mesentery, 489
Metabolic acidosis, 287t
Metabolic alkalosis, 285, 287t
Metaproterenol, for acute respiratory failure, 327t
Metastatic tumor, brain, 444t
Methemoglobin, 279
Methylxanthines
    for acute respiratory distress syndrome, 331t
    for acute respiratory failure, 326, 327t
Metoprolol, for dysrhythmias/blocks, 137t–146t
Mexican Americans, cultural behaviors relevant to nursing care in, 31t
Mexiletine, for dysrhythmias/blocks, 137t–146t
Microglia, 378, 615
Microshock, during hemodynamic monitoring, 121t–123t
Midaxillary line, 77f
Midazolam, 308t
    as sedative agents, 309t–310t
Midbrain, 384
Middle cerebral arteries, 384t, 385, 385f
    occlusion of, 439b
Midsternal line, 77f
Midsystolic click, 83t, 84
Millennials, 34t
Milrinone, 191t
Mineralocorticoids, 466t–469t
Minimum inhibitory concentration (MIC), 635
Minnesota tube, 531f

Minoxidil, 191t
Minute ventilation (M_E), 262t–263t, 278
Mitral auscultatory area, 81, 81f
Mitral regurgitation, 86f, 201–202, 202f
    pulmonary artery occlusive pressure in, 111, 114f
Mitral stenosis, 86f, 202–203, 203f
Mitral valve, 51, 51f
Mixed disorders, of acid-base imbalances, 285, 285f
Mixed venous oxygen saturation (SvO_2), 280
Mobile macrophages, 618
Model for Improvement, 39, 40f
Monocytes, 618, 632
Monokines, 617
Monomorphic ventricular tachycardia (VT), 94t–96t
Mononuclear phagocytes, 618
Monro-Kellie hypothesis, 417–418
Mood, in mental status examination, 721
Moral agency, 14–18
Moral courage, 16
Moral distress, 15–16
Moral residue, 16
Morphine sulfate, 191t
    for angina, 163
Motor activity assessment scale, 310t
Motor function, in neurologic assessment, 393, 396–400, 398t–399t, 399f
Motor vehicle collision, 705, 706t
Motorcycle collision, 706
Mouth, 252
    in gastrointestinal assessment, 505
    in hematologic and immunologic assessment, 630–631
    in renal assessment, 576
Movement
    involuntary, 399–400, 399f
    symmetrical, 396–398
Mucolytics
    for acute respiratory failure, 326
    for status asthmaticus, 349
Mucosa-associated lymphoid tissues (MALT), 615
Mucous membranes
    in cardiovascular assessment, 77
    in pulmonary assessment, 273
Mucus, 494
Multidrug-resistant organisms (MDROs), 701
Multiple-gated acquisition (MUGA) scan, 87t–89t
Multiple organ dysfunction syndrome (MODS), 702
    clinical presentation of, 702, 704t
    collaborative management of, 702
    definition of, 679, 702
    etiology of, 702
    pathophysiology of, 681f, 703f
Multiple sclerosis, 453, 455
Multipolar neurons, 379–380
Multisystem condition(s), 679–720
    drug intoxication and poisoning as, 710
    multiple organ dysfunction syndrome as, 702, 703f, 704t
    shock as, 679. *See also* Shock.

Multisystem condition(s) *(Continued)*
  systemic inflammatory response syndrome as, 619
  trauma as, 702–705
Murmurs, 84–85, 84f, 86f
Muscle paralysis, in intracranial hypertension, 423
Muscle relaxation, progressive, during CCRN® examination, 6–7
Muscle strength, in neurologic assessment, 396–398, 398t
Muscle-stretch reflexes, 404, 404t
Muscle tone, in neurologic assessment, 398, 399t
Muscular dystrophy, 453
Musculoskeletal chest pain, 72t–74t
Musculoskeletal system, 674
  assessment of, 675, 675t
  changes in older adults, 674–675
  functional anatomy of, 674
  general information about, 674
  physiology of, 674
Music therapy, 21
Muslim, religious beliefs in, nursing interventions, 32t–33t
Myasthenia gravis, 454–456
Myasthenic crisis, 456
Myectomy, ventricular septal, 200
Myelin sheath, 379, 379f
Myelography, in neurologic assessment, 414t–416t
Myeloid stem cells, 615
Myocardial cells, action potential of, 54–55, 54f
Myocardial infarction, 154
  clinical presentation in, 158–160, 160t
  cocaine-induced, 181
  collaborative management of, 160–185, 162f
  complications of, 580, 183t–185t
  ECG changes in, 159–160
  emotional responses in, 183t
  etiology of, 158, 160t
  fibrinolytics, 580, 169t–179t
  hemodynamic monitoring in, 104
  intraaortic balloon pump in, 163, 163f–164f, 165t–167t
  left ventricular, 57–585, 119t–120t
  location of, 57–580, 156t–157t
  pathophysiology of, 160, 161f
  percutaneous coronary intervention for, 580, 167t–168t
  percutaneous coronary intervention in, 580, 167t–168t
  right ventricular, 119t–120t, 154, 161f, 182
  silent, 159
  ST elevation in, 154
Myocardial injury, ECG changes in, 100–102
Myocardial ischemia, ECG changes in, 100–102, 101f, 102t
Myocardial oxygen consumption, 52–53, 53f
  contractility and, 62
  heart rate and, 59
  preload and, 61
Myocardial salvaging techniques, 163–185
Myocardial trauma, ECG changes in, 103

Myocardium, 49, 50f, 52
Myoclonic seizure, 445t
Myoglobin, 579
  in myocardial infarction, 159, 160t
Myosin, 57, 57f

N

Nailbeds
  in cardiovascular assessment, 78
  in pulmonary assessment, 273
Nails, 667
  in endocrine assessment, 471
Naloxone, for opiate intoxication, 711
Nasal bone, 381f
Nasal cannula, 301t–302t
Nasal endotracheal tube, 293t–295t
Nasopharyngeal airway, 293t–295t
Nasopharynx, 252–253, 253f
Nasotracheal suctioning, 289
NASPE/BPEG generic (NBG) pacemaker code, 148t
National Database of Nursing Quality Indicators (NDNQI), 39
National Institutes of Health Stroke Scale (NIHSS), 396, 397t–398t
Nationality, 27
Natural killer (NK) cells, 619
Natural law, 15
Nausea, 501
Navigational bronchoscopy, 322
Near-death experience (NDE), 725
Nebulized albuterol, 588
Neck
  in cardiovascular assessment, 78–79, 78f
  in endocrine assessment, 471
  in pulmonary assessment, 274
Negative-pressure device, for complex wounds, 671
Negative pressure ventilators, 302
Neglect, 733
Negotiating, conflict, 25
Neisseria meningitidis, 452
Nephritis, interstitial, 594
Nephrogenic diabetes insipidus, 473, 474b, 475, 475f
Nephrogenic SIADH, 476, 477f
Nephron, 565–566, 566f
  functions of, 567–569, 568f
Nephrotomography, 580t–581t
Nephrotoxic agents, 575, 594–595
Nerve cells, 378–380
Nerve conduction velocity (NCV) studies, in neurologic assessment, 414t–416t
Nerve palsy, during hemodynamic monitoring, 121t–123t
Nervous system
  autonomic, 62–63, 63t
  parasympathetic, 63
  sympathetic, 62–63, 63t
Nesiritide, 191t
  for heart failure, 191, 191t
Neurilemma, 379, 379f
Neurocognitive disorders, major/minor, 730
Neurofibrils, 378, 379f
Neurogenic diabetes insipidus, 473, 474b, 475f

Neurogenic shock, 119t–120t, 679, 695, 696f
Neurogenic SIADH, 476, 477f
Neuroglia, 378
Neurohypophysis, hormones of, 466t–469t
Neurologic assessment, 392–413
  cranial nerve function in, 400–404, 402f–404f
  diagnostic studies in, 412–413, 414t–416t
  general appearance in, 395
  interview in, 392–394
  meningeal irritation in, 405–406, 406f
  mental status and cognition in, 395–396, 396t–398t
  miscellaneous, 404–407
  monitoring in, 407–412
  motor function in, 396–400, 398t–399t, 399f
  reflexes in, 404, 404t, 405f
  sensory function in, 400
  vital signs in, 394–395, 394f
Neurologic involvement, of hypertensive crises, 208
Neurologic status, in renal assessment, 576
Neurologic system, 378–464
  anatomy and physiology of, 378–392
    macroscopic, 381–392
    microscopic, 378–381, 379f, 380t
  assessment of, 392–413. *See also* Neurologic assessment.
  autonomic, 390–392, 392t
  brain in, 382–384, 384f, 384t. *See also* Brain.
  cerebral circulation in, 384–386, 384t, 385f
  cerebral metabolism in, 380–381
  cerebrospinal fluid in, 386, 387f–388f
  in endocrine assessment, 471
  general information in, 378
  neurophysiology of, 380
  neurotransmitters, 380, 380t
  peripheral nervous system in, 388, 390f, 391t–392t
  in renal assessment, 576
  scalp in, 381
  skull in, 381–382, 381f–382f
  spine and spinal cord in, 386–388, 388f–389f, 389t. *See also* Spinal cord.
  trauma in, 404–405, 405f
Neuroma, acoustic, 444t
Neuromuscular disease
  amyotrophic lateral sclerosis as, 454
  collaborative management of, 455–456
  Guillain-Barré syndrome as, 454
  multiple sclerosis as, 453, 455
  muscular dystrophy as, 453
  myasthenia gravis as, 454–455
Neurons, 378–380, 379f
Neurophysiology, 380
Neurotransmitters
  of autonomic nervous system, 390
  cerebral, 380, 380t
Neurovascular status, in cardiovascular assessment, 81
Neutrophils, 617, 617f, 617t, 632
New York Heart Association (NYHA), classifications of heart failure and, 186

Nexters, 34t
Niacin, 381
Nicardipine, 191t
　for cerebral vasospasm, 437
　for hypertensive crises, 208, 209t–212t
Nicotinic acid, 381
Nimodipine, for cerebral vasospasm, 437
Nissl bodies, 379, 379f
Nitric oxide (NO), for acute respiratory distress syndrome, 331t, 335
Nitrogen, urea, 569
Nitroglycerin, 191t
　for angina, 163
　for hypertensive crises, 208, 209t–212t
Nitroprusside, 191t
　for hypertensive crises, 208, 209t–212t
"No added salt" diet, 586
Nocturia, in cardiovascular assessment, 75
Nodes of Ranvier, 379, 379f
Noise control, 21–22
Non-rebreathing mask, 301t–302t
Noncardiogenic pulmonary edema, clinical presentation, and hemodynamic presentation of, 119t–120t
Noninvasive positive pressure ventilation (NPPV), 317
Nonmaleficence, 15
Nonpathological hallucinations, 722
Norepinephrine, 63t, 380t
Norepinephrine bitartrate, 686t–687t
Norms, 28
Nose
　functions of, 252
　structure of, 252
　trauma to, 405, 405f
Nosocomial malnutrition, 516
Nosocomial pneumonia, 338
Nuchal rigidity, 405
Nucleotides, supplementation of, 518
Null cells, 619
Nursing, 12. *See also* Professional caring and ethical practice.
Nursing Minimum Data Set, 39
Nutrient requirements, of brain, 380
Nutrition
　enteral, 518, 519t–523t
　parenteral, 518, 523t–525t
Nutritional support
　for acute pancreatitis, 543
　for acute respiratory distress syndrome, 335
　for hepatic failure/encephalopathy, 540
　for malnutrition, 517, 519f
Nystagmus, 402

O

Obesity
　acute coronary syndrome and, 158
　gastrointestinal surgery for, 552t–553t, 556
Obstructive breathing, 275t
Obstructive shock, 679
Occipital bone, 381f
Occipital lobe, 384f, 384t
　tumors of, 444t
Occlusive dressings, for complex wounds, 672

Occult bleeding, 652
Octreotide acetate (Sandostatin), 514t–515t, 515–516
Oculocephalic reflex, 402–403, 404f
Oculomotor nerve (CN III), 391t–392t
　functional assessment of, 401–402, 402f
　in intracranial hypertension, 418
Oculoplethysmography (OPG), in neurologic assessment, 414t–416t
Oculovestibular reflex, 403, 403f
Oil glands, 668
Older adults, changes in
　in integumentary system, 668
　in musculoskeletal system, 674–675
Olfactory nerve (CN I), 391t–392t, 400
Oligodendroglia, 378
Oligodendrogliomas, 444t
Omentum, 489
Oncotic pressures, colloidal, 65, 66f
Opening snap, 83, 83t
Opisthotonos, 399
Opsonization, 617t
Optic nerve (CN II), 391t–392t
　functional assessment of, 400–401
　in intracranial hypertension, 418
Oral care, after airway intubation, 297
Oral contraceptives, acute coronary syndrome and, 158
Oral endotracheal tube, 293t–295t
Organ dysfunction, multiple. *See* Multiple organ dysfunction syndrome.
Organizational accountability, in culturally competent healthcare, 35
Organizational structure, 26
Orientation, assessment of, 396
Oropharyngeal airway, 293t–295t
Oropharynx, 253, 253f, 489–490
　functions of, 491t–492t
　suctioning of, 288–289
Orthopnea, 71
Osborne wave, 103
Osler nodes, in cardiovascular assessment, 78
Osmitrol. *See* Mannitol.
Osmolality, 569–570, 579
Osmolarity, 569–570
Osmosis, 569–570
Osmotic diuretics, 582
Osteoblasts, 674
Osteoclasts, 674
Osteocytes, 674
Osteomyelitis, 675–676
　clinical presentation of, 675–676
　collaborative management of, 676
　definition of, 675
　etiology of, 675
　immobility in critical care for, 676
　pathophysiology of, 675
Otorrhea, 405
Overflow incontinence, 592
Oxygen
　arterial, partial pressure of, 269
　deficiency of
　　assessment of, 298–299
　　etiologies of, 298
　　pathophysiology of, 298
　requirements, of brain, 380

Oxygen (Continued)
　supply and demand framework, 70, 71f
　toxicity, 300, 313t–315t
　transport of, 268–270
Oxygen capacity, 269
Oxygen consumption (VO_2), 107t–108t, 270
Oxygen consumption by tissues (VO_2/VO_2I), 68
Oxygen consumption index (VO_2I), 107t–108t
Oxygen content
　arterial (CaO_2), 269
　　noninvasive monitoring of, 279
　venous (CVO_2), 280
Oxygen delivery (DO_2), 107t–108t
　cerebral, 412
Oxygen delivery index (DO_2I), 107t–108t
Oxygen delivery to tissues (DO_2/DO_2I), 67–68, 69f
Oxygen extraction index (O_2EI), 69, 107t–108t
Oxygen extraction ratio (O_2ER), 68–69, 107t–108t
Oxygen saturation
　jugular venous, 412
　mixed venous, 107t–109t, 114–115
Oxygen therapy, 297–300
　for acute respiratory failure, 337
　for cardiopulmonary arrest, 555
　definitions in, 297
　delivery systems for, 300, 301t–302t
　hazards of, 300
　indications for, 299
　principles of, 299
　for status asthmaticus, 346
Oxygenation
　extracorporeal membrane, 304t–305t
　hyperbaric, 300
Oxyhemoglobin dissociation curve, 268–269, 268f, 616
　shifting of, 269
Oxyntic glands, 494

P

P-mitrale, 203
P wave, 92, 92f, 94t–96t
　atrial enlargement and, 99–100, 100f
Pacemaker cell, action potential of, 55, 55f
Pacemaker rule, 96
Pacemaker syncope, 75
Pacemakers, 565
　asynchronous, 148
　collaborative management of, 150–153, 152t
　components of, 565
　definition of, 136, 147t–148t
　electrical malfunctions with, 152t
　indications for, 136
　modes for, 148–150, 149t
　NASPE/BPEG generic (NBG) pacemaker code, 148t
　permanent, 56–575
　synchronous, 560
　temporary, 136–148, 150–151
　　for cardiopulmonary arrest, 128
　types of, 136–148
Pacing, ECG evidence of, 150, 150f–151f
Pacinian corpuscle, 667f

Pain
  abdominal, 501, 502t
    in acute pancreatitis, 541
  chest
    differentiation of, 70–71, 72t–74t
    in gastrointestinal system, 72t–74t
  cultural aspects of, 29, 31t
  management of, 18–19, 19t
Pain response, techniques to elicit, 395
Pain scale, behavioral, 19t
Pallor, in cardiovascular assessment, 77
Palpation
  in cardiovascular assessment, 76–81
  in endocrine assessment, 470–471
  in gastrointestinal assessment, 507
  in hematologic and immunologic assessment, 631
  in musculoskeletal assessment, 675, 675t
  in pulmonary assessment, 272–276
  in renal assessment, 576–577
  of skin, 668
Palpitations, in cardiovascular assessment, 75
Pancreas, 498
  functions of, 491t–492t
  hormones of, 466t–469t
  injury to, 549t–550t
Pancreatectomy, 544
Pancreatic duct, 498
Pancreatic juice, 491t
Pancreaticoduodenectomy, 552t–553t, 553f
Pancreatitis, 502t
  acute, 541–545, 542f
Pancreozymin, 499t
Pancuronium, 311t
Paneth cells, 495
Pantoprazole sodium (Protonix), 514t–515t
Papillary muscle dysfunction, in myocardial infarction, 183t–185t
Papillary muscle rupture, 119t–120t
Papilledema, 401
Paracentesis, 511t–514t
Parasympathetic branch, of autonomic nervous system, 392, 392t
Parasympathetic (vagal) nervous system (PNS), 63
Parasympatholytic drugs, 63
Parathormone, 466t–469t
Parathyroid hormone (parathormone), 466t–469t
Parenteral nutrition, 518, 523t–525t
Parietal bone, 381f
Parietal lobe, 382, 384f, 384t
  tumors of, 444t
Parietal pleura, 258f
Paroxysmal nocturnal dyspnea, 71
Partial pressure, Dalton law of, 267–268, 267f
Partial rebreathing mask, 301t–302t
Passing score, in CCRN® examination, 4
Passive transport, 569
Past medical history
  in cardiovascular assessment, 75
  in gastrointestinal assessment, 502–503
  in hematologic and immunologic assessment, 628–629
  in neurologic assessment, 393
  in pulmonary assessment, 271
  in renal assessment, 575

Paternalism, 15
Pathological hallucinations, 722, 722t
Patient care delivery systems, 26, 27t
Patient education, reasons for, 41
Patient safety, 40–41
Patient-ventilator asynchrony, 311, 313t–315t
Pectoriloquy, whispered, 277
Pectus carinatum, 274
Pectus excavatum, 274
Pedestrian struck, by motor vehicle, 706
Peer review, 41
Penetrating trauma, 707
  chest, 356
  mechanism of injury in, 704
  predisposing factors in, 705
Pentobarbital
  for intracranial hypertension, 421
  as sedative agents, 309t–310t
Peppermint, 19
Pepsinogen, 494
Peptic ulcer, 502t, 527–535
  clinical presentation in, 527–529, 528b
  definition of, 527
  endoscopy for, 530
  etiology of, 527
  nutritional support for, 535
  pathophysiology of, 528f
  pharmacotherapy for, 511, 514t–515t
  surgery for, 527–532, 534f
Perceptual disturbances, in mental status examination, 722, 722t
Percussion
  in endocrine assessment, 471
  in gastrointestinal assessment, 506–507
  in hematologic and immunologic assessment, 631
  in pulmonary assessment, 276–277, 276t
  in renal assessment, 577
Percutaneous coronary intervention (PCI), 200
  in myocardial infarction, 580, 167t–168t
Percutaneous transhepatic cholangiography, 511t–514t
Percutaneous transhepatic portography, 511t–514t
Percutaneous transluminal coronary angioplasty, 167t–168t
Percutaneous transluminal septal myocardial ablation (PTSMA), 200
Perfluorochemical (PFC), for acute respiratory distress syndrome, 2600
Performance, during CCRN® examination, 6–8
Perfusion, in pulmonary system, 265–266, 265f, 266t
Pericardial fluid analysis, 87t–89t
Pericardial friction rub, 82–83, 83t
Pericardial knock, 83, 83t
Pericardial space, 49
Pericardial window, 322
Pericardiocentesis, 87t–89t
Pericarditis
  chest pain in, 72t–74t
  ECG changes in, 103
  in myocardial infarction, 183t–185t
Pericardium, 49, 50f

Periorbital edema, in endocrine assessment, 471
Peripheral angiography, 87t–89t
Peripheral arterial disease, 213–216, 213f–214f
Peripheral blood flow, 66–67
Peripheral fever, in intracranial hypertension, 423
Peripheral nerve stimulation device, 311–312, 311f
Peripheral nervous system, 388, 390f, 391t–392t
Peripheral pulses, 79–81, 79t, 80f
Peripheral smear, 632
Peripheral vascular disease, 79t, 80f
Perirenal fat, 564
Peritoneal dialysis, 601
Peritoneal friction rub, 506
Peritoneal lavage, diagnostic, 4950
Peritoneum, 489
  folds of, 489
Peritubular capillary network, 566
Permission, to take CCRN® examination, 4–5
Pernicious anemia, 532
Personality type, in cardiovascular assessment, 75
Pet therapy, 21
Petechiae, in pulmonary assessment, 273
Peyer patches, 495
PFC (perfluorochemical), for acute respiratory distress syndrome, 2600
pH, 283
Phagocytosis, 617, 617f, 617t
Pharyngeal tonsils, 252
Pharynx
  functions of, 253
  structure of, 252–253
Phenobarbital, for status epilepticus, 448t–449t
Phentolamine, 191t
  for hypertensive crises, 209t–212t
Phenylephrine, 63t, 686t–687t
Phenytoin, for status epilepticus, 448t–449t
Phlebography, ascending contrast, 87t–89t
Phlebostatic axis, 115, 116f
Phonation, in neurologic assessment, 403
Phosphodiesterase inhibitors, 641
Phosphodiesterase type 5 inhibitors, for acute respiratory distress syndrome, 331t
Phosphorus
  functions, regulation, and sources of, 572t–574t
  replacement of, in diabetic ketoacidosis, 480
Physical examination
  in hematologic and immunologic assessment, 630–631
  in musculoskeletal assessment, 675
Physiologic buffers, 283–284
Physiologic dead space, 263f
Pia mater, 382, 383f
Pigeon chest, 274
Pili, 667
Pitressin (vasopressin), 472t, 514t–515t, 516
Pituitary gland
  adenoma, 444t
  tumor of, 444t

Plantar reflex, 404, 405f
Plasma, 615
Plasma exchange, 540
Plasma thromboplastin antecedent, 625t
Plasma thromboplastin component, 625t
Plasminogen, 620t
Platelet aggregation inhibitors, 641–642, 641b
  for ischemic stroke, 384b
  for myocardial infarction, 169, 171t–179t
Platelet plug, 623
Platelets, 632
  aggregation of, 623–624
Plethysmography, 87t–89t
Pleural cavities, 258–259, 258f
Pleural fluid analysis, 281
Pleural friction, 275
Pleural friction rub, 278t
Pleural space, 258f, 259
Pleural tubes, 317–318
Pleurodesis, 322
Pleuropulmonary, chest pain in, 72t–74t
Pneumocytes
  type I, 256
  type II, 255–256
Pneumoencephalography, in neurologic assessment, 414t–416t
Pneumonectomy, 322
Pneumonia, 338–343
  on chest radiography, 280
  clinical presentation of, 340–341
  collaborative management of, 341–343
  definitions in, 338
  etiology of, 338–339
  pathophysiology of, 339, 340f
Pneumoplasty, reduction, 322
Pneumothorax, 280
  chest pain in, 72t–74t
  closed (noncommunicating), 357–358, 358f
  during hemodynamic monitoring, 121t–123t
  open, 359
  recurrent, 358
  tension, 358–359, 359f
    complicating chest surgery, 323
Point of maximal impulse (PMI), 79, 274
Poisoning, of drug, 710
Polymorphic ventricular tachycardia, 94t–96t
Polymorphonuclear leukocytes (PMNs), 617, 617f, 617t
Pons, 384
Pontine, 260
Popliteal artery, occlusive disease of, 214
Portal hypertension, 527, 540
Portal-systemic shunt, 533
Portal triad, 497
Portal vein, 500
Portography, percutaneous transhepatic, 511t–514t
Positive end-expiratory pressure (PEEP), 303
  for acute respiratory distress syndrome, 333
  auto, 303, 306f
Positive-pressure ventilation, 2570
  noninvasive, 580, 317

Positive self-talk, for CCRN® examination, 5, 5b
Positron emission tomography (PET), 87t–89t
  in neurologic assessment, 414t–416t
Postconcussion syndrome, 429
Posterior axillary line, 77f
Posterior cerebral arteries, 384t, 385, 385f
  occlusion of, 439b
Posterior descending artery, 53, 53f
Postganglionic neuron, 390
Postmyocardial infarction syndrome, in myocardial infarction, 183t–185t
Posttraumatic stress disorder, 734
Postural drainage (PD), 290
Posturing, 399, 399f
Potassium
  functions, regulation, and sources of, 572t–574t
  imbalance. See Hyperkalemia.
  replacement of, in diabetic ketoacidosis, 479–480
Povidone-iodine, for complex wounds, 671
Powerlessness, in responses to illness and environment, 724
PPIDA scan, 511t–514t
PQRST format
  for chest pain, 71
  for history of present illness, 75
PR interval, 92, 92f, 94t–96t
  short, in Wolff-Parkinson-White syndrome, 133, 133f
PR segment, 92, 92f
Prayer, 32
  during CCRN® examination, 7
Prazosin, 191t
Precordium, in cardiovascular assessment, 79
Predictability, in patients, 2
Preganglionic neuron, 390
Preload, 58–61, 60t
  cardiac output and, 61, 61f
  for heart failure, 190–191
Premature atrial contractions, 94t–96t
Premature junctional contraction (PJC), 94t–96t
Premature ventricular contraction, 94t–96t
Preparation, for CCRN® examination, 5–6, 5b
Presentation, in mental status examination, 721
Pressure-controlled/inverse ratio ventilation (PC/IRV), 304t–305t
Pressure-controlled ventilation (PCV), 304t–305t
Pressure injury
  etiology of, 669
  preventive measures for, 671
  staging of, 670, 670f
Pressure-regulated volume-controlled ventilation (PRVC), 304t–305t
Pressure support ventilation (PSV), 2580, 304t–305t
Prinzmetal angina, 154
Prinzmetal syndrome, 102
Proaccelerin, 625t
Procainamide hydrochloride, for dysrhythmias/blocks, 137t–146t

Procallus, formation of, 674
Proconvertin, 625t
Proctosigmoidoscopy, 511t–514t
Professional caring and ethical practice, 12–48
  advocacy and moral agency in, 14–18
  caring practices in, 18–24
  clinical inquiry in, 35–41
  clinical judgment in, 13–14, 13f
  collaboration in, 24–26
  critical care nursing, concepts of, 12–13
  ethical decision making in, 14–16, 16f
  legal issues in, 17–18
  response to diversity in, 27–35, 29f, 30t–34t
  systems thinking in, 26–27
Progressive muscle relaxation, 19
Projection, as defense mechanism, 724t
Proliferation, in complex wounds, 669
Prone position, in airway management, 291–292
Propafenone, for dysrhythmias/blocks, 137t–146t
Propofol, as sedative agents, 309t–310t
Propranolol, for dysrhythmias/blocks, 137t–146t
Proprioceptors, 260
Prostacyclin, 620t
  for acute respiratory distress syndrome, 335
Prostaglandin E_1 analog, 515
Prostaglandins, 620t
  synthesis of, 572
Prosthetic valve click, 84
Protamine, 642
Protection, as skin function, 668
Protein
  absorption of, 500
  digestion of, 500
  excretion of, 569
  requirements for, 517–518
  serum, 510, 633–634
Proteinuria, 579
Prothrombin, 625t
Prothrombin time (PT), 633
Protodiastole, 58
Proton pump inhibitors, 514t–515t, 515
Protonix (pantoprazole sodium), 514t–515t
Pseudocysts, pancreatic, 544
Pseudounipolar, 379–380
Psychosis, 737–738
Psychosocial characteristics, 723. See also Behavioral/psychosocial considerations.
Psychosomatic chest pain, 72t–74t
Ptyalin (amylase), 489
Pulmonary angiography, 282t–283t
Pulmonary arterial hypertension, 335–337
Pulmonary artery occlusive pressure (PAOP), 107t–109t, 111, 112t, 113f
  in mitral regurgitation, 111, 114f
Pulmonary artery pressure (PAP), 107t–109t, 110–111, 111b, 112f
  abnormal, 108t–109t, 110
  mean, 257
Pulmonary artery rupture, during hemodynamic monitoring, 121t–123t

Pulmonary assessment, 270–281
    of acid-base balance, 283–286
    of arterial blood gases, 285–286, 285b
    auscultation in, 277
    bedside, 278–280
    chest radiography interpretation in, 280–281, 281f
    diagnostic studies in, 281, 282t–283t
    inspection and palpation in, 272–276
    landmarks in, 272, 281f
    percussion in, 276–277, 276t
Pulmonary autograft, 206
Pulmonary capillaries, blood flow through, 263–266
Pulmonary circulation, 256–257
Pulmonary contusion, 356–357
Pulmonary disorders. *See also specific disease.*
    aspiration, 343–346
        pathophysiology of, 344f
    chronic obstructive, acute exacerbation of, 323
Pulmonary edema, 580
    complicating chest surgery, 323
    neurogenic, complicating traumatic brain injuries, 429
Pulmonary embolectomy, 355
Pulmonary embolism, 350–356
    chest pain in, 72t–74t
    clinical presentation in, 352–353
    complicating chest surgery, 350–356
    definition of, 350
    etiology of, 350
    massive, 354
    pathophysiology of, 350–352, 351f
Pulmonary function studies, 282t–283t
Pulmonary hypertension, 119t–120t, 257
    in acute respiratory distress syndrome, 335–337
    classification and etiology of, 336
    clinical presentation of, 336
    collaborative management of, 336–337
    definition of, 335
    pathophysiology of, 337f
Pulmonary infarction
    during hemodynamic monitoring, 121t–123t
    in pulmonary embolism, 355
Pulmonary stenosis, 86f
Pulmonary system, 252–377. *See also* Airway(s); Lung.
    airway management for, 286–297
    chest tubes in, 317–321, 319f, 320t
    circulation in, 256–258, 257f
    defense mechanisms of, 256
    diffusion in, 268
    in endocrine assessment, 471
    functional anatomy of, 252–260
    general information about, 252
    lymphatics of, 256
    mechanical ventilation for, 300–317. *See also* Mechanical ventilation.
    mediastinum in, 258f, 259
    muscles of ventilation in, 259f
    neuroanatomy of, 260
    oxygen therapy for, 297–300
    physiology of, 260–270, 260f
    pleural cavities in, 258–259, 258f

Pulmonary system *(Continued)*
    in renal assessment, 575
    thoracic cage in, 258, 258f
    ventilation of, 260f
Pulmonary vascular resistance, 107t–108t
Pulmonary vascular resistance index (PVRI), 107t–108t
Pulmonary vasodilators
    for acute respiratory distress syndrome, 331t
    for pulmonary hypertension, 331t
Pulmonic auscultatory area, 81, 81f
Pulmonic ejection click, 83–84
Pulmonic regurgitation, 86f
Pulmonic valve, 51f, 52
Pulse
    in neurologic assessment, 394
    in renal assessment, 576
Pulse contour, 80–81, 80f
Pulse contour waveform analysis method, 113–114
Pulse pressure, 66, 68f
    in neurologic assessment, 394
Pulseless electrical activity, 120
Pulsus alternans, 80, 80f
Pulsus bisferiens, 80f, 81
Pulsus magnus, 80, 80f
Pulsus paradoxus, 80, 80f
Pulsus parvus, 80, 80f
Pupils, in neurologic assessment, 401–402
Purkinje fiber system, 56, 56f
Purposeful touch, 21
Pyelography, retrograde, 580t–581t
Pyelonephritis, 593
Pyloric glands, 494
Pyloroplasty, 530
Pylorus, 495
Pyramidal tracts, 389t
Pyridoxine (B_6), 381

Q

Q wave, 92, 92f
    in myocardial infarction, 102
QRS axis, 98
    ventricular hypertrophy and, 100
QRS complex, 92, 92f
    in Wolff-Parkinson-White syndrome, 565
QT interval, 92f, 93, 94t–96t
    indications for monitoring of, 93
Quadrant method, of axis determination, 98, 99f
Quadruple rhythm, 82, 83t
Quality improvement (QI), 38–39
Quality management (QM), 38–39
Questions, in CCRN® examination, 3–4
Quincke sign, 620

R

R wave, 92, 92f
Raccoon eyes, 405, 405f
Race, 27
Radial artery, for pressure monitoring, 105
Radiation, for brain tumor, 444
Radiofrequency catheter ablation, 154

Radiography
    chest, 87t–89t
        in hemodynamic monitoring, 118
        interpretation in, 280–281, 281f
    skull, 414t–416t
    spine, 414t–416t
Radioisotope brain scan, in neurologic assessment, 414t–416t
Radionuclide angiography, 87t–89t
Radionuclide imaging, gastrointestinal, 511t–514t
Radiosurgery, for brain tumor, 444–445
Ramsay sedation scale, 310t
Ranitidine (Zantac), 514t–515t
Ranson's prognostic criteria for pancreatitis, 543
Ranvier, nodes of, 379, 379f
Rapid shallow breathing index (RSBI), 278
Rationalization, as defense mechanism, 724t
Reasoning, clinical, 13–14, 13f
Recertification, 9
Recombinant tissue plasminogen activator, in myocardial infarction, 171t–179t
Rectum, 495, 495f
Rectus abdominis, 259, 259f
Red blood cell (RBC) indices, 631–632
Red blood cells (RBCs). *See* Erythrocytes.
Red bone marrow, 674
Red pulp, 614
Reduction pneumoplasty, 322
Reentry, 132, 132f
Refeeding syndrome, 523t–525t
Referred pain, 501
Reflex arc, 387–388, 389f
Reflexes, in neurologic assessment, 404, 404t, 405f
Refractoriness, 55, 55f
Refractory periods, 380
Regional anesthesia, drug delivery methods for, 19
Regitine. *See* Phentolamine.
Regurgitant flow, 51
Relative refractory period, 55, 55f
Religion, 32
Religious diversity, 32–34, 32t–33t
Religious symbols, 32
Remodeling
    in complex wounds, 669–670
    in musculoskeletal system, 674
Renal angiography, 580t–581t
Renal assessment, 574–580
Renal biopsy, 580t–581t
Renal blood flow, 566–567
Renal capsule, 564
Renal corpuscle, 566
Renal cortex, 565, 565f
Renal disease, hypertensive crises and, 206
Renal fascia, 564
Renal involvement, of hypertensive crises, 207
Renal ischemia and infarction, 645
Renal medulla, 565, 565f
Renal pelvis, 565, 565f
Renal plexus, 567
Renal radionuclide scan (renogram), 580t–581t

Renal replacement therapy, 600–606
  dialysis as, 600–606, 601f–602f, 602t–603t
Renal sinus, 565
Renal system, 564–613
  in acid-base regulation, 284, 569
  assessment of, 574–580. *See also* Renal assessment.
  auscultation in, 577
  diagnostic studies, 580t–581t
  drugs affecting, 580–583, 580t–581t
  fluid and electrolyte imbalances in. *See* Fluid and electrolyte imbalance(s).
  functional anatomy of, 564–567, 565f–566f
  general information about, 564, 565f
  inspection and palpation in, 576–577
  interview in, 574–576
  percussion in, 577
  physiology of, 567–574
  vital signs in, 576
Renal transplant, 606
Renal tubules, 566
Renin-angiotensin-aldosterone (RAA) system, 66, 67f, 571–572
Reocclusion, in fibrinolytic therapy and, 169t–170t
Reperfusion dysrhythmias, in fibrinolytic therapy and, 169t–170t
Reperfusion therapies, for angina, 163
Repression, as defense mechanism, 724t
Research studies, 37
Residual volume (RV), 262t–263t
Resiliency, in patients, 2
Resistance, airway, 263
Resource availability, patients and, 2
Respiration, cellular, 270
Respiratory acidosis, 284–285, 287t
Respiratory alkalosis, 284–285
Respiratory bronchioles, 255, 255f
Respiratory burst, 617
Respiratory distress
  acute, 323, 328–335
    clinical presentation in, 324, 329
    collaborative management of, 324–335, 331t
    complicating chest surgery, 323
    criteria for, 260b
    definitions in, 323, 328
    etiology of, 323–324, 328
    pathophysiology of, 324, 325t–326t, 329, 330f
    phases, 331t
  clinical indications for, 276b
  collaborative management of, 288–297
Respiratory failure, acute, 323
  clinical presentation in, 324, 329
  collaborative management of, 324–335, 331t
  complicating chest surgery, 323
  definitions in, 323
  etiology of, 323–324
  pathophysiology of, 324, 325t–326t, 329, 330f
Respiratory patterns, in neurologic assessment, 394, 394f
Respiratory process, 260f
Respiratory quotient (RQ), 270

Respiratory rate
  in pulmonary assessment, 262t–263t, 274, 275t
  in renal assessment, 576
Respiratory (ventilatory) rate, in cardiovascular assessment, 76
Respiratory reflex, 63–64
Respiratory system. *See* Pulmonary system.
Rest requirement, 21–22
Resting membrane potential, 54, 54f
Restrictive cardiomyopathy, 200–201, 201f
Resuscitation
  cardiopulmonary, 555, 123
  fluid, 684–686, 684b, 685t
Rete pegs, 667f
Rete ridge, 667f
Reteplase, 643, 643t–644t
Reticular activating system, 384
Reticulocyte count, 631
Reticulocytes, 615–616
Retinal involvement, of hypertensive crises, 207
Retrograde pyelography, 580t–581t
Return of spontaneous circulation (ROSC), care after, 128
Rh system, 627, 627t
Rhinorrhea, 405, 405f
Rhonchal fremitus, 275
Rhonchi, 278t
Rhythm, in renal assessment, 576
Rib fracture, 361–362
Ribs, 77f
RIFLE classification system, 597, 597t
Right anterior axillary line, 77f
Right atria (RA), 50, 50f
  enlargement of, 99, 100f
Right atrial pressure, 107t–108t, 110, 110f
Right-axis deviation (RAD), 98
Right bundle branch (RBB), 56, 56f
Right bundle branch block (RBBB), 550, 94t–96t, 99, 99f
Right cerebral hemisphere, 383
Right coronary artery (RCA), 53, 53f
Right midclavicular line, 77f
Right ventricle, 50f, 51
  failure of, 189t
  hypertrophy of, 100, 100f
  infarction, 154
Right ventricular ejection fraction, 107t–108t
Right ventricular end-diastolic volume (RVEDV), 107t–108t
Right ventricular end-diastolic volume index (RVEDVI), 107t–108t
Right ventricular end-systolic volume (RVESV), 107t–108t
Right ventricular end-systolic volume index (RVESVI), 107t–108t
Right ventricular pressure, 108t–109t, 110, 111f
Right ventricular stroke work index (RVSWI), 107t–108t
Rights, 16–17
Rinne test, 402
Risk-taking behavior, 734–735
Rituals, 27
Rivaroxaban, 643t–644t
Rolando fissure, 382, 384f

Romano-Ward syndrome, 131
Romberg test, 399
Ross procedure, 206
Rotational therapy bed, in airway management, 291
Roux-Y gastric bypass, 552t–553t, 555f
Rovsing sign, in abdominal trauma, 4955
Ruddiness, in cardiovascular assessment, 77

S

S wave, 92, 92f
S_1, 82
  split, 82
S_2, 82
  split, 82
S_3, 82, 83t
S_4, 82, 83t
Saccular aortic aneurysm, 217
Sacral spinal nerves, 388
Safety, patient, 40–41
Saliva, 489, 491t
Salt wasting syndrome, cerebral, complicating craniotomy, 426
Sandostatin (octreotide acetate), 514t–515t, 515–516
Sarcomere, 57, 57f
Sarcoplasmic reticulum, 57, 57f
Saturation of venous blood (SvO_2), 68
Scalene muscles, 259
Scalp, 381
Scapula, 77f
Schilling test, 511t–514t
Scoliosis, 274
Seat belt sign, in abdominal trauma, 549
Sebaceous glands, 667–668, 667f
Sebum, 668
Second-degree AV nodal block type I$^+$ (Wenckebach), 94t–96t
Second-degree AV nodal block type II$^+$, 94t–96t
Second intercostal space, 77f
Second rib, 77f
Secretin, 499t
Sedation-agitation scale, 310t
Sedation, in mechanical ventilation, 308t
Sedative-hypnotics, 2580
Sedatives, 308–311, 309t–310t
  for intracranial hypertension, 423
Segmented neutrophils, 617
Segs, 617
Seizures
  complicating hemorrhagic stroke, 437
  definition of, 445
  in neurologic assessment, 392
  status epilepticus and, 445–446, 446f
  types of, 445t
Self-governance, 26
Semilunar valves, 51f, 52
Sengstaken-Blakemore tube, 531f
Sensation, as skin function, 668
Sensitivity, in hematologic and immunologic assessment, 634–635
Sensory deprivation, in responses to illness and environment, 725
Sensory function, in neurologic assessment, 393, 400

Sensory overload, in responses to illness and environment, 724–725
Sepsis, definition of, 696
Septal rupture, ventricular, 183t–185t
Septic shock, 119t–120t, 696
    clinical presentation of, 697
    collaborative management of, 697–702, 699t, 699b
    definition of, 679, 696
    etiology of, 696–697
    pathophysiology of, 697, 698f
Sequential [sepsis-related] organ failure assessment score (SOFA), 702, 704t
Serotonin, 380t, 620t
Serous pericardium, 49, 50f
Serum chemistries
    in cardiovascular assessment, 85
    in disseminated intravascular coagulation, 652–653
    in endocrine assessment, 471–472
    in gastrointestinal assessment, 510
    in heart failure, 58–645
    myocardial infarction and, 159, 160t
    in neurologic assessment, 412–413
    in pulmonary assessment, 281
    in renal assessment, 577–579
Serum lipids, 579
Serum proteins, 579
Sestamibi-dipyridamole stress test, 87t–89t
Sestamibi exercise testing, 87t–89t
Seventh-Day Adventist, religious beliefs in, nursing interventions, 32t–33t
Sexual assault, 733
Sexual behavior, aggressive, in myocardial infarction, 183t
Shared-governance, 26
Shock
    anaphylactic, 679, 693, 694f
    cardiogenic, 679, 690, 691f
        in myocardial infarction, 183t–185t
    clinical presentation of, 679–683, 682t
    collaborative management of, 683–688, 684f, 684b, 685t
    complicating chest surgery, 323
    definition of, 679
    distributive, 679
    etiology of, classification by, 679
    hemodynamic alterations in, 682–683, 683t
    hemorrhagic, 690t
    hypovolemic, 227, 679, 688, 689f
        complicating pancreatitis, 545
    neurogenic, 679, 695, 696f
    obstructive, 679
    pathophysiology of, 679, 680f–681f
    septic, 679, 696, 698f
    stages of, 679
    vasopressors for, 686–687, 686t–687t
Shortness of breath, in pulmonary assessment, 270
Shoulder, frozen, complicating chest surgery, 323
Shunts, 265–266
    in acute respiratory failure, 325t–326t
    portal-systemic, 533
Sick sinus syndrome, with syncope, 136

Sildenafil, for acute respiratory distress syndrome, 331t
Silent Generation, 34t
Silent ischemia, 103
Simple partial seizure, 445t
Single-photon emission-computed tomography (SPECT), in neurologic assessment, 414t–416t
Sinoatrial (SA) node, 55, 56f
Sinus arrest, 94t–96t
Sinus block, 94t–96t
Sinus bradycardia, 94t–96t
    in neurologic assessment, 394
Sinus dysrhythmia, 94t–96t
Sinus exit block, 94t–96t
Sinus rhythm, 94t–96t
Sinus tachycardia, 94t–96t
    in neurologic assessment, 394
Sinusoids, 497
Skeletal muscles, 674
Skeleton
    cardiac, 49–50
    facial, 381–382, 381f–382f
Skin
    accessory structures of, 667
    in cardiovascular assessment, 77–78
    characteristics of, 666
    in endocrine assessment, 471
    in gastrointestinal assessment, 505
    in hematologic and immunologic assessment, 630–631
    inspection and palpation of, 668
    layers of, 666–668, 667f
    peripheral changes of, in cardiovascular assessment, 75
    in pulmonary assessment, 273
    in renal assessment, 576
Skin tests, in pulmonary assessment, 281
Skull, 381–382, 381f–382f
    fractures, 429–431, 429f
    radiography of, in neurologic assessment, 414t–416t
Sleep quality, 21
Sleep studies, 282t–283t
Slow continuous ultrafiltration (SCUF), 606t
Small intestine, 494–495
    absorption in, 500–501
    enzymes of, 491t
    functions of, 491t–492t
    infarction/obstruction/perforation of, 545–549, 546f
Smoking, coronary artery disease and, 155
Smooth muscles, 674
Smoothing, conflict, 25
Snaps, 83
Snellen chart, 400
Social contract theory, 15
Social history
    in cardiovascular assessment, 75–76
    in gastrointestinal assessment, 503
    in hematologic and immunologic assessment, 629
    in neurologic assessment, 393
    in pulmonary assessment, 272
Sodium (fast) channel, 54
Sodium, functions, regulation, and sources of, 572t–574t

Sodium polystyrene sulfonate, 588
Sodium-potassium pump, 54
Soma, 378, 379f
Somatic pain, 501
Somatosensory evoked potentials (SSEP), in neurologic assessment, 414t–416t
Somatotropin, 466t–469t
Somnography, in neurologic assessment, 414t–416t
Somogyi phenomenon, 484, 484f
Sotalol, for dysrhythmias/blocks, 137t–146t
Speech
    in mental status examination, 721
    in neurologic assessment, 396, 403
Sphenoid bone, 381f, 382
Sphincter of Oddi, 497
Spinal accessory nerve (CN XI), 391t–392t, 403
Spinal cord, 386–388, 388f–389f, 389t
    function of, 387–388, 389f
    structure of, 386–387, 388f, 389t
Spinal cord angiography, in neurologic assessment, 414t–416t
Spinal nerves, 388, 390f, 391t–392t
Spinal processes, 77f
Spinal shock, 695
Spinal tracts, 387, 389t
Spine, 386–388
Spine radiography, in neurologic assessment, 414t–416t
Spinocerebellar tracts, 389t
Spinothalamic tracts, 389t
Spiritual distress, 32
Spirituality, 32
Spirometry, 278, 282t–283t
Spleen
    functions of, 614
    injury to, 549t–550t
    palpation of, 507
    percussion of, 507
Splinter hemorrhage, 78
Splits, 82
Spongy bone, 674
Spontaneous breathing trial (SBT), 316
Spontaneous wedge, 118
Sputum analysis, in pulmonary assessment, 281
Sputum production, in pulmonary assessment, 270–271
Square wave test, 117–118, 117f
ST segment, 92, 92f
    elevation of, 154
    in myocardial infarction, 102
Stability, in patients, 2
Stable factor, 625t
Stanford classification systems, 217
Starling's law, 61, 571
Station, in neurologic assessment, 399
Status asthmaticus, 346–350. *See also* Asthma.
    collaborative management of, 348–350
    definitions of, 346
    etiology of, 346
    pathophysiology of, 346
Status epilepticus, 445–447, 445t, 446f, 448t–449t
Stem cells, 615

Stenosis, 51
  aortic, 204–205, 205f
Stent, coronary artery, 167t–168t
Sternal angle, 77f–78f
Sternocleidomastoid, 259
Sternum, 77f
  fracture of, 361–362
Steroids, for anaphylactic shock, 695
Stevens Star Model, of Knowledge Transformation, 36–38, 36f
Stockings, elastic, 2670
Stokes-Adam attack, 75
Stomach, 492f–493f, 493–494. *See also gastric entries.*
  functions of, 491t–492t
  injury to, 549t–550t
  percussion of, 507
Stool
  in gastrointestinal assessment, 511
  in hematologic and immunologic assessment, 635
Strangulated hernia, 502t
Stratum basale, 666, 667f
Stratum corneum, 666, 667f
Stratum granulosum, 666, 667f
Stratum lucidum, 666
Stratum spinosum, 666, 667f
Streptokinase, 643, 643t–644t
  for pulmonary embolism, 354
Stress
  acute coronary syndrome and, 158
  in responses to illness and environment, 723–724, 724t, 724b
Stress electrocardiography, 87t–89t
Stress incontinence, 592
Stress ulcer
  complicating craniotomy, 426
  complicating mechanical ventilation, 313t–315t
Stretch receptors, alveolar, 260
Stridor, 278t
Stroke
  algorithm for, 440f
  hemorrhagic, 433–437, 434f, 435t
  ischemic, 437–443, 438f, 438b–439b, 440f, 441b
  National Institutes of Health Stroke Scale (NIHSS) for, 396, 397t–398t
Stroke index (SI), 58, 107t–108t
Stroke volume (SV), 58, 107t–108t
  afterload and, 62, 62f
  contractility and, 62, 62f
  preload and, 61
Strokes-Adams attack, 75
Stuart-Prower factor, 625t
Study groups, CCRN® examination and, 6
Subarachnoid bolt or screw, for ICP measurement, 408f, 408t
Subarachnoid hemorrhage, 433, 434f
  vasospasm after, 436–437
Subarachnoid space, 382, 383f
Subdural hematoma, 431, 431f
Subdural space, 382, 383f
Subglottic secretions, continuous aspiration of, 289, 295f
Sublimation, as defense mechanism, 724t
Sublingual capnography, 115

Suboccipital puncture, in neurologic assessment, 414t–416t
Substance-induced disorders, 735
Substance P, 380t
Substance-related disorders, 735–736
Substance use disorders, 735
Succussion splash, 506
Sucking chest wound, 359–360, 359f
Sucking reflex, 404
Sudden cardiac death, in myocardial infarction, 183t–185t
Suicidal ideation and behaviors, 736
Sulci, 382, 384f
Summation gallop, 82, 83t
Superficial reflexes, 404, 405f
Superior mesenteric artery, 499f, 500
Superior sagittal sinus, 386
Suppressor T cells, 618
Suprasternal notch, 77f
Supraventricular tachycardia, 94t–96t
Surfactant, 255
  aerosolized, for acute respiratory distress syndrome, 333
Surgical ablation, of dysrhythmias, 570
Surgical site infection (SSI), 700–701
Swallowing, 490
  in neurologic assessment, 403
Sweat glands, 667f
  apocrine, 668
  eccrine, 668
Sylvian fissure, 382, 384f
Sympathectomy, 215
Sympathetic branch, of autonomic nervous system, 390, 392t
Sympathetic nervous system (SNS), 62–63, 63t
Sympathetic storm, complicating traumatic brain injuries, 429
Sympathomimetic agents, for anaphylactic shock, 695
Sympathomimetic drugs, 63, 63t
Synaptic knobs, 379, 379f
Synaptic transmission, 380
Synarthrosis joints, 674
Synchronized intermittent mandatory ventilation (SIMV), 304t–305t
Syncope, in cardiovascular assessment, 75
Syncytium, functional, 56
Syndrome of inappropriate antidiuretic hormone (SIADH), 426, 476–477, 477f
Synergy
  assumptions of, 2–3
  core concept of, 2
  definition of, 2
Synergy model, 2–3, 2f
Synergy model nurse competencies, 13, 13b
Synovial joints, 674
System, 26
Systemic inflammatory response syndrome (SIRS), 619
  definition of, 679, 696
Systemic vascular resistance, 107t–108t
Systemic vascular resistance index, 107t–108t
Systems thinking, 26–27
  nurses and, 3

Systole, 58, 58f
Systolic arterial pressure, 105, 108t–109t
Systolic dysfunction, heart failure and, 186
Systolic murmurs, 84, 86f

T
T cells, 618–619
T-piece or tube, 301t–302t
T wave, 92f, 93
  myocardial ischemia and, 100–102
T4/T8 (CD4/CD8) ratio, 634
Tachycardia
  atrial, 94t–96t
  junctional, 94t–96t
  pacemaker-mediated, 153
  sinus, 94t–96t
  supraventricular, 94t–96t
  ventricular
    monomorphic, 94t–96t
    polymorphic, 94t–96t
    pulseless, defibrillator for, 124–125
Tachycardia overdrive, 136
Tachypnea, 275t
Tadalafil, for acute respiratory distress syndrome, 331t
Tamponade, balloon, for esophageal varices, 529, 531f, 532t
Taste, in neurologic assessment, 403
Teaching
  barriers to, 42
  process, 42–44
Technetium-99 pyrophosphate scan, 87t–89t
Teleology, 16
Temperature
  in neurologic assessment, 395
  in renal assessment, 576
Temporal bone, 381f
Temporal lobe, 384f, 384t
  tumors of, 444t
Tendons, 674
Tenecteplase, 643, 643t–644t
Tension pneumothorax, 358–359, 359f
  complicating chest surgery, 323
Tentorium cerebelli, 382, 383f
Terminal bronchioles, 255, 255f
Tetany, 588
Tezosentan, 590
Thalamus, 383
Thallium-201 scan, 87t–89t
Thallium stress electrocardiography, 87t–89t
Thebesian veins, 54
Therapeutic touch, 21
Thermal diffusion flowmetry, for CBF measurement, 411
Thermoregulation, as skin function, 668
Thiamine (B_1), 381
Thiazide diuretics, 582
  for diabetes insipidus, 475
Third-degree block, 94t–96t
Third spacing, 65, 571
Third ventricles, 386, 387f
Thirst, 571
Thoracentesis, 282t–283t
Thoracic cage, 258, 258f
Thoracic catheters. *See* Chest tubes.
Thoracic computed tomography, 282t–283t
Thoracic spinal nerves, 388

Index

Thoracoplasty, 322
Thoracostomy
  closed, 321
  exploratory, 321
  open, 322
Thoracostomy tubes. *See* Chest tubes.
Thoracotomy, 322
Thorax
  internal structures of, 258f
  landmarks of, 76, 77f
  in pulmonary assessment, 274–276
Thought processes and content, in mental status examination, 722
Threshold potential, 54, 54f
Thrill, 79
Thrombin, 625t
Thrombin inhibitors
  direct, 642, 643t–644t
  indirect, 642, 643t–644t
Thrombin time, 633
Thrombocytes, 623
Thrombocytic stem cells, 615
Thrombocytopenia, 624
  heparin-induced, 655–656
    clinical presentation of, 655–656, 656t
    collaborative management of, 656
    definition of, 655, 655t
    etiology of, 655
    pathophysiology of, 655, 655f
Thrombocytopenic purpura
  immune, 650t
  thrombotic, 641, 650t
Thrombocytosis, 624
Thromboendarterectomy, 215
Thrombopoiesis, 623
Thrombosis
  during hemodynamic monitoring, 121t–123t
  in intraaortic balloon pump, 165t–167t
Thrombotic stroke, 3840
Thrombotic thrombocytopenic purpura (TTP), 641, 650t
Thromboxane, 620t
Thrombus, pulmonary embolism from, 2665
Thymectomy, 322
Thymus, 615
Thyrocalcitonin, 466t–469t
Thyroid cartilage, 253
Thyroid gland
  in endocrine assessment, 471
  hormones of, 466t–469t
Thyroid-stimulating hormone (thyrotropin), 466t–469t
Thyroxine (T_4), 466t–469t
Tidal volume (V_T), 262t–263t
Time management, during CCRN® examination, 8
Tirofiban (Aggrastat), 641, 643t–644t
Tirofiban HCl, in myocardial infarction, 171t–179t
Tissue factor, 625t
Tissue plasminogen activator
  for pulmonary embolism, 354
  recombinant, 441b
Tissue thromboplastin, 625t
Toe/brachial index (TBI), 85

Tongue
  in endocrine assessment, 471
  in neurologic assessment, 403
Tonic-clonic seizure, 445t
Tonic seizure, 445t
Tonometry, gastric, 115
Tonsils, pharyngeal, 252
Torsades de pointes, 94t–96t
Total iron-binding capacity (TIBC), 633
Total lung capacity (TLC), 262f, 262t–263t
Touch, 21
Toxicology, 710
Trach collar, 301t–302t
Trachea, 77f, 253–254, 254f
  deviation, 274
  resection of, 322
Tracheobronchial injury, 363
Tracheobronchial tree, suctioning of, 289–290
Tracheostomy, 293t–295t
  weaning from, 296
Tranexamic acid (Cyklokapron), for disseminated intravascular coagulation, 654
Transcalvarial herniation, 418f, 419t
Transcatheter aortic valve replacement (TAVR), 206
Transcranial Doppler, 414t–416t
Transesophageal Doppler, 114
Transferrin saturation, 633
Transfusion, blood. *See* Blood transfusion.
Transient ischemic attack, 437, 438b
Transjugular intrahepatic portosystemic shunt (TIPS), 533, 533f
Transluminal cerebral balloon angioplasty, for hemorrhagic stroke, 437
Transplantation
  cardiac, indications for, 201
  heart-lung, for pulmonary hypertension, 337
Transtentorial herniation, 418f, 419t
Transthoracic needle lung biopsy, 282t–283t
Transvenous sinus, 386
Transverse abdominis, 259
Trauma
  to abdomen, 501, 549–552, 549t–550t
  behavioral/psychosocial considerations in, 733–734
  to brain, 426–429, 427f
  to chest, 356–363
    general information about, 356
    surgery for, 321
  clinical presentation of, 707
  collaborative management of, 707–710
  definitions of, 702–705
  kinematics of, 704–705
  mechanism of injury in, 705–707
  multisystem, 702–705
  to neurologic system, 404–405, 405f
  pathophysiology of, 707
  predisposing factors in, 705
Tremor, 399
Treprostinil, for acute respiratory distress syndrome, 331t
Tricuspid auscultatory area, 81, 81f
Tricuspid regurgitation, 86f
Tricuspid stenosis, 86f

Tricuspid valve, 51, 51f
Trigeminal nerve (CN V), 391t–392t, 402
Triggered activity, dysrhythmias/blocks, 132
Triglycerides, medium-chain, 518
Triiodothyronine (T_3), 466t–469t
Triple H therapy, for hemorrhagic stroke, 437
Trochlear nerve (CN IV), 391t–392t, 401–402
Tropomyosin, 57, 57f
Troponin, 57, 57f
  in myocardial infarction, 159, 160t
  in pulmonary embolism, 2665
Trousseau sign, 541, 588
Trumpet airway, 293t–295t
Tubular reabsorption, 567f, 568–569
Tubular secretion, 567f, 569
Tumor, brain, 443–445, 443f, 444t
Tumor necrosis factor, 620t
Turbulence, causes of, 84, 84f
Turgor, in cardiovascular assessment, 77

U

U wave, 92f, 93
Ulcers
  peptic, 502t, 527–535. *See also* Peptic ulcer.
  stress
    complicating craniotomy, 426
    complicating mechanical ventilation, 313t–315t
Ultrasonography, 282t–283t, 580t–581t
  of abdomen, 511t–514t
  Doppler, 87t–89t
    for CBF measurement, 411–412
    transcranial, in neurologic assessment, 414t–416t
Umbilicus, in gastrointestinal assessment, 506
Uncal herniation, 418f, 419t
Unexplained joint pain, in cardiovascular assessment, 75
Unipolar neurons, 379–380
Unstable angina, 570
Upper esophageal sphincter (UES), 493
Upper gastrointestinal hemorrhage, 527–535, 528f
Upper motor neurons (UMNs), 380, 387, 399t
Upward transtentorial herniation, 418f, 419t
Urea, excretion of, 569
Urea nitrogen, 569
Uremia, 578
Ureters, 564
Urethra, 564–565
Urge incontinence, 592
Urinary incontinence, 592–593, 593t
  clinical presentation, 592
  collaborative management of, 593
  definition of, 592
  diagnostic studies, 592–593
  etiology of, 592
Urinary tract infection, 593–594
  clinical presentation of, 594
  collaborative management of, 594
  definition of, 593
  etiology of, 594

Index

...ation, changes in, in renal assessment, 574
...ine
  appearance of, 574
  in cardiovascular assessment, 87
  composition of, 569
  formation of, 567–569, 567f–568f
  in gastrointestinal assessment, 511
  in hematologic and immunologic assessment, 635
  in neurologic assessment, 413
  in renal assessment, 579–580
Urine output, 569, 577
Urokinase, for pulmonary embolism, 354
Utilitarianism, 16

V

Vaccination, in CNS infection, 452–453
Vagolytic drugs, 63
Vagotomy, 530, 534f
Vagus nerve (CN X), 391t–392t, 403
Values, 14, 28
Valve replacement, 625
Valves
  bioprosthetic, 206
  cardiac, 51–52, 51f
  mechanical, 62–640
Valvular heart disease, 201–206
  collaborative management for, 205–206
  complications of, 205
Valvuloplasty, 205
Variant angina, 154
Varices, esophageal. See Esophageal varices.
Varicose veins, in cardiovascular assessment, 75
Vasa recta, 566
Vascular access, in cardiogenic arrest, 125
Vascular disease, 213–222
  peripheral, 79t, 80f
Vascular sounds, 85, 506, 577
Vascular system, 64–67, 64f
  blood pressure and, 66, 68f
  pathway of blood through, 52, 52f
Vasoactive intestinal peptide, 499t
Vasodilator testing, for pulmonary arterial hypertension, 336
Vasodilators, for myocardial infarction, 182
Vasomotor center, 67
Vasopressin, 472t, 514t–515t, 516, 686t–687t
Vasopressin test, in diabetes insipidus, 474
Vasopressors, for shock, 686t–687t, 686t–687t
Vasospasm, cerebral, 437
Vasospastic angina, 102
Vaughan-Williams antidysrhythmic classification system, 135t
Vectorcardiography, 87t–89t
Veins, 66
Venography, 87t–89t
Venous humidification, 506
Venous oxygen content (CvO_2), 68, 107t–108t
Venous oxygen saturation
  jugular, 412
  mixed, 107t–109t, 114–115, 280
Venous system
  of brain, 386
  gastrointestinal, 500

Ventilation
  alveolar (V_A), 262t–263t
  for cardiopulmonary arrest, 124
  dead space, 262t–263t, 263f
  liquid, 304t–305t
    for acute respiratory distress syndrome, 260D
  mechanical, 300–317. See also Mechanical ventilation.
  minute, 278
  muscles of, 259, 259f
  positional changes in, 266f
  process of, 261f
  pulmonary, 260f
Ventilation/perfusion (V/Q) mismatching, in acute respiratory failure, 325t–326t
Ventilation/perfusion (V/Q) ratio, 265–266, 266f, 266t
Ventilation/perfusion (V/Q) scan, 282t–283t
Ventilation scan, 282t–283t
Ventilator-associated events (VAEs), 700
Ventilator-associated lung injury (VALI), 313t–315t
Ventilator-associated pneumonia (VAP), 338, 700
Ventilators, types of, 302–303
Ventilatory arrest, 120. See also Cardiopulmonary arrest.
Ventilatory failure, acute, 324
Ventilatory mechanics, 278, 282t–283t
Ventilatory rate, in neurologic assessment, 394–395, 394f
Ventilatory rhythm, in neurologic assessment, 394–395, 394f
Ventilatory support, in pulmonary assessment, 276
Ventricles, 50–51, 50f
  fourth, 386, 387f
  lateral, 386, 387f
  left. See also Left ventricle.
    infarction, 57–585
  right. See also Right ventricle.
    infarction, 154
  third, 386, 387f
Ventricular aneurysm, in myocardial infarction, 183t–185t
Ventricular assisted device (VAD), 192, 195t–196t
Ventricular contraction, premature, 94t–96t
Ventricular ectopy, 134t
Ventricular fibrillation, 94t–96t
  defibrillation for, 550
Ventricular gallop, 82, 83t
Ventricular hypertrophy, 100, 100f
Ventricular pacing, 148, 149t, 150f
Ventricular septal defect or rupture, 86f
Ventricular septal myectomy, 200
Ventricular septum, rupture of, 119t–120t
  in myocardial infarction, 183t–185t
Ventricular system, cerebral, 386, 387f
Ventricular tachycardia (VT)
  monomorphic, 94t–96t
  polymorphic, 94t–96t
  pulseless, defibrillator for, 124–125
Ventriculography, 87t–89t
  in neurologic assessment, 414t–416t

Venturi mask, 301t–302t
Veracity, 15
Verapamil, for dysrhythmias/blocks, 137t–146t
Versed. See Midazolam.
Vertebral artery, occlusion of, 439b
Vertebral line, 77f
Vertebrobasilar system, 384t
Vertical banded gastroplasty (VBG), 552t–553t
Vesicular breath sounds, 277f, 277t
Vestibular branch, in neurologic assessment, 402–403, 403f–404f
Veteran Generation, 34t
Video-assisted thoracoscopic surgery (VATS), 322
Vietnamese Americans, cultural behaviors relevant to nursing care in, 31t
Villi, 495
Villikinin, 499t
Violence, behavioral/psychosocial considerations in, 733–734
Virchow triad, 2665
Visceral pain, 501
Visceral pleura, 258f
Vision
  in endocrine assessment, 471
  in neurologic assessment, 392
Visual acuity, 400
Visual fields, 400–401
Vital capacity (VC), 262f, 262t–263t, 278
Vital signs
  in cardiovascular assessment, 76–77
  in endocrine assessment, 470
  in gastrointestinal assessment, 503
  in hematologic and immunologic assessment, 630
  in intracranial hypertension, 419
  in neurologic assessment, 394–395, 394f
  in pulmonary assessment, 272
Vitamin B_1, 381
Vitamin B_6, 381
Vitamin B_{12}, 381
Vitamin D synthesis, as skin function, 668
Vitamin K antagonist, 643t–644t
Vitamin K deficiency, 650t
Vitamins
  absorption in, 500
  in cerebral metabolism, 381
Vocal folds, 253, 253f
Vocal fremitus, 274–275
Voice sounds, 277
Voiding cystourethrography, 580t–581t
Volume-assured pressure support ventilation (VAPSV), 304t–305t
Volume replacement, for upper gastrointestinal hemorrhage, 529–530
Vomiting, 501
  in intracranial hypertension, 418
Von Willebrand disease, 650t
Vulnerability, in patients, 2

W

Wandering atrial pacemaker, 94t–96t
Warfarin, 642, 643t–644t
  in myocardial infarction, 169, 171t–179t
  in pulmonary embolism, 355

Water, absorption of, 500
Water deprivation test, in diabetes insipidus, 477f
Water excess syndrome, 585
Water exchanges, 571
Water-hammer pulse, 81
Water load test, in SIADH, 476
Water loss syndromes, 584
Watercraft collision, 706
Waterhouse-Friderichsen syndrome, 453
Weaning
　from mechanical ventilation, inability of, 313t–315t
　from tracheostomy, 296
　from ventilatory support, 312–317
Weber test, 402
Weight
　changes in renal assessment, 576
　gain, in cardiovascular assessment, 75

Wellens syndrome, 102, 103f, 154
Wells criteria, 266–2685
Wenckebach block, 94t–96t
Wheezing, 271, 278t
Whipple procedure, 4965, 552t–553t, 553f
Whisper test, 402
Whispered pectoriloquy, 277
White blood cells (WBCs), 632
White clot, 623
White matter, 387, 388f
White pulp, 614
Will, living, 18
Wirsung duct, 498
Withdrawal, as defense mechanism, 724t
Wolff-Parkinson-White syndrome, 133f
Work of breathing, 261–263, 264f

X
X-rays. *See* Radiography.
Xanthelasma, in cardiovascular assessment, 78
Xanthines, for status asthmaticus, 348
Xanthoma palpebrarum, in cardiovascular assessment, 78
Xenon (^{133}Xe) inhalation, 414t–416t

Y
Yellow bone marrow, 674

Z
Zantac (ranitidine), 514t–515t
Zygomatic bone, 381f